CARE OF THE ADULT
WITH A CHRONIC ILLNESS OR DISABILITY

A Team Approach

CARE OF THE ADULT
WITH A CHRONIC ILLNESS
OR DISABILITY

A Team Approach

LESLIE JEAN NEAL, PhD, RN, FNP-C
Associate Professor of Nursing
Marymount University
Arlington, Virginia

SHARRON E. GUILLETT, PhD, RN
Assistant Professor and Chair
AAS Nursing Program
Marymount University
Arlington, Virginia

ELSEVIER
MOSBY

ELSEVIER
MOSBY

11830 Westline Industrial Drive
St. Louis, Missouri 63146

Notice

Pharmacology is an ever-changing field. Standard safety precautions must be followed, but as new research and clinical experience broaden our knowledge, changes in treatment and drug therapy may become necessary or appropriate. Readers are advised to check the most current product information provided by the manufacturer of each drug to be administered to verify the recommended dose, the method and duration of administration, and contraindications. It is the responsibility of the licensed health care provider, relying on experience and knowledge of the patient, to determine dosages and the best treatment for each individual patient. Neither the publisher nor the author assumes any liability for any injury and/or damage to persons or property arising from this publication.

The Publisher

International Standard Book Number 0-323-02330-4

Executive Publisher: Darlene Como
Executive Editor: Loren Wilson
Senior Developmental Editor: Nancy L. O'Brien
Publication Services Manager: Deborah L. Vogel
Project Manager: Deon Lee
Design Manager: Gail Morey Hudson

Printed in the United States of America

Last digit is the print number: 9   8   7   6   5   4   3   2   1

Contributors

LEE A. BAZZARONE, DC, CCSP
Vienna, Virginia

BETH CAMERON, ND, FNP
Professor and Director of Nursing Department
Trinity College of Nursing & Health Sciences
Rock Island, Illinois

THERESA PERFETTA CAPPELLO, PhD, RN
Dean and Professor
School of Health Professions
Marymount University
Arlington, Virginia

ROSALYN COUSAR, MSN, RN, AACRN
Inova Juniper Program
Fairfax, Virginia

DEYANN D. DAVIS, MSN, RN
Advanced Clinical Nurse, Pain Management and Palliative Care
Board of Directors, Northwestern Community Services
Front Royal, Virginia

MARY C. EWALD, MS, RN
Assistant Professor
Trinity College of Nursing & Health Sciences
Rock Island, Illinois

DOT GOODMAN, BS, RN, WOCN
Inova VNA
Fairfax, Virginia

KIMBERLY HAYNES, MS, RN, CS, ONC, ARNP
Clinical Nurse Specialist
Mid America Sarcoma Institute
Overland Park, Kansas

DIANA JORDAN, MS, RN, ACRN
Nurse Educator
Pennsylvania Mid-Atlantic AIDS Education and Training Center
Inova Juniper Program
Fairfax, Virginia

MARCIA H. KRUGLER, MSN, APRN, BC
Clinical Specialist Psychiatry/Mental Health
Lecturer, Department of Nursing
University of Vermont
Burlington, Vermont

JUNA MACKEY-PADILLA, PhD, MSN, RN
Site Director
Pennsylvania/MidAtlantic AIDS Education and Training Center
Inova Juniper Program
Fairfax, Virginia

SHARON MAILEY, PhD, RN
Professor of Nursing
Division of Nursing and Respiratory Care
Shenandoah University
Winchester, Virginia

JENNIFER H. MATTHEWS, PhD, APRN,BC
Associate Professor of Nursing
Division of Nursing and Respiratory Care
Shenandoah University
Winchester, Virginia

HELEN MAUTNER, MS, RN
Assistant Professor of Nursing
Marymount University
Arlington, Virginia

LORETTA NORMILE, PhD, RN
Assistant Professor
College of Nursing and Health Science
George Mason University
Fairfax, Virginia

LIN E. NOYES, PhD, RN
Clinical Director
Alzheimer's Family Day Center
Falls Church, Virginia

TRACY L. POELVOORDE, MSN, BSN, BA
Assistant Professor
Trinity College of Nursing & Health Sciences
Rock Island, Illinois

KAREN REA, MSN, RN, BC
REAsource for Health Education
Arlington, Virginia

JULIE RIES, MA, PT, GCS
Assistant Professor
Program in Physical Therapy
Marymount University
Arlington, Virginia

DOTTIE ROBERTS, MSN, MACI, CMSRN, RN, BC, ONC
Clinical Nurse Specialist
Rehabilitative & Medical Services
Palmetto Health Baptist
Columbia, South Carolina

JUDITH ROGERS, RNC, MSN, PhD(c)
Marymount University
Arlington, Virginia

DAWN RUDE, MS, BSN
Associate Professor
Trinity College of Nursing & Health Sciences
Rock Island, Illinois

MARYELLEN ZARNIK SILVA, MS, RN, CRNP
Adjunct Faculty
Marymount University
Arlington, Virginia

SHEILA SPARKS, DNSc, RN
Professor and Director
Division of Nursing and Respiratory Care
Shenandoah University
Winchester, Virginia

KAREN S. WILSON, MSN, RN
Assistant Professor
Trinity College of Nursing & Health Sciences
Rock Island, Illinois

FATMA YOUSSEF, DNSc, RN
Professor of Nursing
Marymount University
Arlington, Virginia

Reviewers

CAROL BOSWELL, EdD, RN
Associate Professor, School of Nursing
Texas Tech University Health Sciences Center
Odessa, Texas

PAULA DiBENEDETTO, RN, MSN
Assistant Professor, School of Nursing
Texas Tech University Health Sciences Center
Lubbock, Texas

MITZI FORBES, PhD, RN, CHTP
Assistant Professor
University of Wisconsin–Milwaukee
Milwaukee, Wisconsin

CHERYL GRAHAM-EASON, MEd, MS, RN
Professor, Community College of Allegheny County
Pittsburgh, Pennsylvania

MARY HANSON-ZALOT, MSN, RN, AOCN
Nursing Faculty
Methodist Hospital School of Nursing
Philadelphia, Pennsylvania

DALICE L. HERTZBERG, MSN, RN, FNP-C, CRRN
Instructor, JFK Partners and the School of Nursing
University of Colorado Health Sciences Center
Denver, Colorado

PHYLLIS G. PETERSON, MN, RN, AOCN
Assistant Professor, Division of Nursing
Our Lady of Holy Cross College
New Orleans, Louisiana

JANET JOHNSON PRINCE, BSN, RN, CWOCN, CGRN
Cardiovascular Nurse Clinician
St. Joseph Hospital
Nashua, New Hampshire

TERRY SAVAN, BSN, RN, MA, PA, CRNP
Certified Registered Nurse Practitioner
Lehigh University Health Center
Bethlehem, Pennsylvania

KAREN TOMAJAN, MS, RNC, CRRN
Director, Clinical Education, Integris Health
Oklahoma City, Oklahoma

Clinical Consultants

CATHY S. ELROD, MS, PT
Assistant Professor
Physical Therapy Program
Marymount University
Arlington, Virginia

ELAINE LEONARD PUPPA, MEd, MSN, CRNP
Research Consultant
Center for Health Policy Development and Management
University of Maryland, Baltimore County
Baltimore, Maryland

Preface

We are pleased to present *Care of the Adult with a Chronic Illness or Disability: A Team Approach.* As instructors in medical-surgical nursing with more than 50 years of combined nursing experience, we realized that the usual texts lacked depth and breadth regarding chronic care. Additionally, although health care is provided in primarily non–acute care settings, most medical-surgical texts continue to focus on acute care with only brief references to home and community care. This book addresses the "chronic care gap" found in other texts. We believe it is a book whose time has come.

Increasingly, persons with chronic illnesses or disabilities are being discharged from hospitals to community settings. Therefore, nursing students, nurses, and other health care professionals need a solid resource to enable them to provide the best possible care to their patients. Many medical-surgical texts lack an interdisciplinary perspective. However, we contend that quality chronic care cannot be provided without using a team approach, so this text was written to include other health care disciplines, with professionals from fields other than nursing providing review and input.

CLINICAL ACCURACY

Dr. Neal's home health care and rehabilitation nursing background and Dr. Guillett's experience working with persons with disabilities and persons with sensory impairments have prepared us well to write and co-edit this book. Our 20 contributing authors are experts in their fields and have brought vast practical experience to the book's content.

All are active in clinical practice or education, and most participate in both areas of nursing. All of the authors used the most current research and knowledge of clinical and evidenced-based practice to write the chapters and consulted with professionals outside of nursing to broaden their perspectives. Authors injected their chapters with down-to-earth practical instructions and tips as well as the latest information from the published literature. The chapters are intentionally written in a style that is not overloaded with references or research to enhance readability and the likelihood that the reader will apply the information to practice. However, all of the information contained herein is based on the most current practice in the field of chronic care.

ORGANIZATION

The book is organized into three major units:
- Unit I: General Concepts of Chronic Care Nursing
- Unit II: Care of the Adult with a Chronic Illness or Disability
- Unit III: Care of the Adult Living with Cancer or HIV/AIDS

Unit I provides the principles and theories on which the remaining chapters are grounded. It also sets the tone of the book, emphasizing the importance of the person with the chronic illness or disability as a decision maker and interpreter of his or her own quality of life. In addition, because research shows that more than 80% of people with chronic illnesses use some form of alternative or complementary therapy, an entire chapter is dedicated to a discussion of these modalities.

Unit II focuses on the chronic illnesses and disabilities that occur most often among adults, subdivided into body systems: the senses, integumentary, respiratory, hematology, cardiovascular, gastrointestinal, genitourinary, endocrine, neurologic, and musculoskeletal. A particularly notable feature is Chapter 22, which is devoted exclusively to a discussion of dementias.

Cancer, HIV infection, and AIDS are now recognized as chronic illnesses. We believe that there are unique issues with regard to the care of persons with these diseases and have therefore devoted a complete unit to the discussion of that care. Unit III is subdivided into cancers of the upper body, cancers of the lower body, and HIV and AIDS.

Most chapters within the sections begin with specific learning objectives and an introduction to the system or disease set covered within. Most chapters discuss the assessment, pathophysiology, diagnosis, clinical manifestations, and interdisciplinary care (including drug therapy) of a particular chronic disease or of a set of chronic diseases or disabilities. There may be slight variation among or between chapters based on the material that is most appropriate to each.

To facilitate ease of use and to clearly illustrate the interdisciplinary nature of chronic care, we included specific features in each chapter. A complete functional health assessment using Gordon's Functional Health Patterns

(1994) appears in most chapters to assist readers to identify the lifestyle changes that can occur with each disease or disability. Students will find the Think S for Success feature, which summarizes the important components of chronic care, particularly useful for organizing their plans of care. Each chapter is rich with discussions of the interdisciplinary team members involved and their specific roles in patient care. Most chapters have a case study followed by a case conference to clarify how the team members might collaborate regarding a particular patient. Additionally, ethnic variations, alternative therapies, family/caregiver issues, and ethical considerations are other components of each chapter that support the premise that chronic illness engenders lifestyle changes to which the patient and family may need to adapt.

AUDIENCE

This book is appropriate for both nursing students and nursing and other health care professionals. When used as a supplement to a standard medical-surgical nursing textbook, the book will assist nursing students to understand and differentiate the special needs of the patient with a chronic illness or disability as opposed to the needs of a patient with acute illness. The professional nurse and other health care providers (such as therapists, medical social workers, dietitians, and physicians) will find this book an excellent resource because the information contained herein is not otherwise easily located in one reference book. Typically, health care professionals must search a variety of sources to find this material.

There are no true prerequisites to using this book. However, a basic knowledge of anatomy and physiology is helpful because each chapter was written with the assumption that the reader either has this knowledge or will use a good reference to review anatomy and physiology while reading the book.

As medical-surgical nursing instructors, we understand that nursing students are often required to purchase a standard, often huge, medical-surgical nursing text. If the primary focus of the course is acute care, such a text is an important purchase. However, many medical-surgical courses today incorporate the care of the person with a chronic illness or disability. Several schools devote an entire course to chronic care. Courses that cover chronic care will significantly benefit from this book because it will provide students with a comprehensive perspective of persons with a chronic illness or disability and the specifics of the care of these persons. Students and professionals of health care disciplines other than nursing might use this book as a resource when counseling a patient about lifestyle changes and tips to maximize quality of life. Nursing home, home health care, and community health professionals may find this book invaluable in its applicability to their clientele.

We are confident that the reader will find this book to be an indispensable tool unlike any other resource currently available. We hope that it will contribute to the body of knowledge about persons with chronic illness or disability and thereby assist health care professionals to approach the care of these persons differently than they would the care of persons with acute illnesses. We hope that others will see that the person with a chronic illness or disability is a *person first*, who happens to have an illness or disability and who needs the health care professional to assist her or him to adapt to the subsequent changes in lifestyle. We believe that the traditional approach of *doing to* or *doing for* a patient should be changed to the approach of *doing with* a patient who leads a team of interdisciplinary professionals in her or his own care.

ACKNOWLEDGMENTS

To the editors, contributing authors, and reviewers who assisted in the creation of this book.

Leslie Jean Neal
Sharron E. Guillett

Contents

UNIT I
GENERAL CONCEPTS OF CHRONIC CARE NURSING

1 Understanding Chronic Illness and Disability, 1

2 Settings of Chronic Care, 11

3 Alternative Approaches and Therapies for Chronic Care, 21

UNIT II
CARE OF THE ADULT WITH A CHRONIC ILLNESS OR DISABILITY

Section 1 ■ *THE SENSES*

4 Disorders of the Eyes, 35

5 Disorders of the Ears, 50

Section 2 ■ *INTEGUMENTARY*

6 Disorders of the Skin, 63

7 Wounds, 83

Section 3 ■ *RESPIRATORY*

8 Obstructive Airway Disease, 107

9 Tuberculosis, 126

Section 4 ■ *HEMATOLOGY*

10 Disorders of the Blood, 135

11 Malignancies of the Blood, 149

Section 5 ■ *CARDIOVASCULAR*

12 Disorders of the Heart, 161

13 Disorders of the Vasculature, 181

Section 6 ■ *GASTROINTESTINAL*

14 Nutritional and Eating Disorders, 197

15 Disorders of the Esophagus, Diaphragm, and Stomach, 213

16 Disorders of the Intestines and Rectum, 228

17 Disorders of the Liver, Pancreas, and Gallbladder, 241

Section 7 ■ *GENITOURINARY*

18 Chronic Kidney Disease, 261

19 Disorders of the Urinary Bladder, 271

Section 8 ■ *ENDOCRINE*

20 Disorders of Hormone Regulation, 284

Section 9 ■ *NEUROLOGIC*

21 Disorders of the Brain, 314

22 Dementias, 348

23 Disorders of the Spinal Cord, 362

24 Neuromuscular Disorders, 378

Section 10 ■ *MUSCULOSKELETAL*

25 Disorders of the Joints and Connective Tissues, 393

26 Musculoskeletal Disorders, 412

UNIT III
CARE OF THE ADULT LIVING WITH CANCER OR HIV/AIDS

Section 11 ■ *CANCERS OF THE UPPER BODY*

27 Living with Cancer, 436

28 Cancers of the Central Nervous System, 458

29 Cancers of the Head and Neck, 470

30 Cancer of the Breast, 492

31 Cancer of the Lung, 507

Section 12 ■ *CANCERS OF THE LOWER BODY*

32 Cancers of the Abdomen, 516

33 Cancers of the Reproductive System, 532

34 Cancers of the Musculoskeletal System, 553

Section 13 ■ *HIV AND AIDS*

35 Living with HIV and AIDS, 565

CHAPTER 1

Understanding Chronic Illness and Disability

Sharron Guillett, PhD, RN

OBJECTIVES

After reading this chapter, you should be able to do the following:

- Define chronic illness or disability
- Locate chronic illness and disability within the context of personhood
- Discuss theories related to chronic illness and quality of life
- Describe the impact of chronic illness on individuals, families, and society at large
- Describe techniques for assessing and addressing the impact of chronic illness or disability on individuals, families, and society at large
- Recognize the importance of managing chronic pain effectively
- Identify a framework for organizing concepts related to caring for people with chronic illnesses or disabilities

Although managing chronic illness and disability is one of the biggest health care problems facing developed countries, the U.S. health care system is not yet positioned to provide optimal care for the more than 125 million individuals requiring that care. The over 7000 acute care hospitals operating in the United States today, which follow a predominantly curative medical model, give testament to the fact that the U.S. health care system is designed to provide care for people experiencing episodic or acute illnesses. Health care payment systems have also developed around this model of health care to help subscribers manage the costs of doctor visits for the purpose of treating illness, emergency care visits, and hospitalizations. The emphasis on acute care persists in spite of the fact that people with chronic illnesses constitute the largest group of health consumers. Projections indicate that by 2050 one in five Americans will have a chronic illness or disability, and associated medical costs will exceed $1 trillion (Merck Institute of Aging and Health, 2002). The U.S. Department of Health and Human Services (DHHS) has addressed the need for a systematic approach to managing chronic illness and improving the quality of life for people with disabilities in a set of objectives outlining national health goals entitled *Healthy People 2010* (DHHS,

2000). *Healthy People 2010* sets forth two overarching objectives: to eliminate disparities in health care delivery and to improve the length and quality of life. To accomplish these goals, the DHHS has identified 28 focus areas encompassing 247 objectives. Eleven of the 28 focus areas relate specifically to chronic illness and disability and are listed in Box 1-1. A concerned public as well as committed and knowledgeable professionals will be required to accomplish these goals.

Public interest in chronic care is increasing for a number of reasons, not the least of which is the fact that, because the baby boom generation is aging and living longer thanks to advances in health, nutrition, and technology, increasing numbers of them are living with chronic conditions. According to a study conducted by the Partnership for Solutions (2001), two thirds of Americans who do not have a chronic condition believe that they are likely to develop one and are concerned that they will not be able to obtain the care they need. Ninety percent of respondents felt that the government should intervene, and studies repeatedly report that persons with chronic conditions feel that they do not receive appropriate care from their providers.

Health care providers must be educated to recognize the special needs of the person with a chronic illness or disability and to organize, plan, and provide care to meet those needs. To appreciate the need for a specific, unique approach to

---

Box 1-1 *Healthy People 2010* **Focus Areas Related to Chronic Illness and Disability**

- Access to Quality Health Services
- Arthritis, Osteoporosis, and Chronic Back Conditions
- Cancer
- Chronic Kidney Disease
- Diabetes
- Disability and Secondary Conditions
- Heart Disease and Stroke
- HIV
- Mental Health and Mental Disorders
- Respiratory Diseases
- Vision and Hearing

planning and providing care for individuals with chronic illnesses and disabling conditions, providers must first understand the concepts of chronicity and disability.

CHRONICITY

Unlike acute illnesses, which are usually abrupt in onset and self-limiting (the illness is either resolved or death ensues), chronic illnesses may be abrupt or insidious in onset and by definition persist for an extended and indefinite period. Many definitions of chronic illness have been developed. However, all definitions include one or more of the characteristics first outlined by the Commission on Chronic Illness (1957). These characteristics include any impairment or deviation from normal that

- Is permanent
- Leaves a residual disability
- Is caused by a nonreversible pathologic condition
- Requires special training of the patient for rehabilitation
- Requires a long period of supervision, observation, or care

A significant consideration in attempting to define or understand any health-related condition is locating it within the experience of being human. It is important to recognize that the illness experience is just one aspect of being human. In fact, developing a chronic illness is the "norm" in an aging population. Emmanuel (1982) referred to life as "the accumulation of chronic illness [to] which we eventually succumb."

The most common chronic conditions in the United States across all age groups are arthritis, hypertension, orthopedic impairments, sinusitis, and hay fever. Diabetes is among the most common chronic conditions for people over the age of 45, and hearing impairments, heart disease, and cataracts are common among those over the age of 75. Prevalence of chronic conditions is also affected by race, gender, and income level. Lower income levels are associated with conditions that are more serious and costly (Merck Institute of Aging and Health, 2002).

Many chronic conditions have commonly expressed symptoms, such as the joint pain of arthritis; however, the manner in which a condition such as arthritis is experienced is variable and highly individualized. Health professionals must guard against adopting a "one size fits all" approach to caring for those in their practices.

People with chronic illnesses are often marginalized by society and viewed as "abnormal." This distinction may prevent persons from fully engaging in the rights and liberties enjoyed by so-called normal citizens. For example, people with human immunodeficiency virus (HIV) infection or acquired immunodeficiency syndrome (AIDS) may be denied employment or lose certain health care benefits. In addition, health care providers often develop paternalistic attitudes toward people with chronic conditions, which prevents them from fully participating in treatment and care planning.

The health care provider and the person with the chronic condition likely will have different perspectives about how to manage the condition and how well the treatment plan is working. Unlike acute illness, in which the experience is new to the individuals with the illness but may be commonplace to the health care provider, in chronic illness the experts in the experience of the illness are the individuals with the disorder. Therefore, their experiences and insights must be explored and valued.

DISABILITY

The Americans with Disabilities Act (ADA) was signed into law in 1990. This landmark legislation provides protection against discrimination for people with disabilities. Universally accepted, the ADA defines an individual as disabled if he or she has a physical or mental impairment that substantially limits one or more of his or her major life activities, has a record of such an impairment, or is regarded as having such an impairment.

As is the case with chronic illness, it is important to recognize that having a disability is just one of many variants of the normal human experience. One could assert that all individuals are only temporarily able-bodied and that at some point in life we will all experience some form of disability. It is essential to develop this level of awareness to avoid labeling groups of people in ways that might disenfranchise them.

Persons with disabilities, like people with chronic illnesses, are first and foremost people. They are not their illness or their disability. They are more than the sum of their parts and *should* be identified as such. A holistic, person-first approach that honors the shared experience of being human along with the uniqueness of the individual and recognizes strengths as well as impairments must form the basis for planning care that promotes health and positively affects the quality of life.

Furthermore, providers must offer interventions that address the need of persons with chronic illnesses or disabilities to develop personally within the context of that illness or disability. Too often providers focus on battling the condition or use a physical function frame of reference with populations for whom such battles and referents are inappropriate and demeaning (Nolan and Nolan, 1999).

PRACTICE MODELS

Several nursing theories have been used to develop greater understanding of the experience of chronic illness or disability. Parse's theory on human becoming (1981) and Watson's theory of human care (1999) are especially well suited for this undertaking. Parse's theory suggests that illness must be viewed from the individual's perspective and that health care providers need to ask "How is that for you?" rather than attach either positive or negative connotations to the illness experience. Watson goes further to state that living with difficulty and suffering opens up new opportunities for becoming fully human.

In addition to these nursing theories about quality of life, a number of conceptual frameworks and practice models have been developed to help health care professionals meet the needs of people with chronic illnesses and/or disabilities. The Canadian Centre for Health Promotion (CHP) quality-of-life model (Raeburn and Roth, 1996), the chronic illness model developed by Burks (1999), and Paterson's shifting perspectives model (2001) are particularly useful for guiding practice, research, and policy.

Canadian Centre for Health Promotion Model

The CHP model depicted in Figure 1-1 takes a holistic view of the person and represents quality of life as a multidimensional concept that includes health as a subelement. Quality of life is defined as the degree to which a person enjoys the important possibilities of his or her life. Possibilities refer to the restraints and opportunities present in one's life as well as the balance between them. These possibilities arise out of the ongoing interaction of person and environment and therefore are dynamic and fluid. Some determinants, such as race or gender, are the result of chance. Others are a result of choice and are therefore controllable to a certain extent by the individual. All individuals are confronted with many possibilities over the course of their lives. Some possibilities are acted upon and others are not depending on the importance ascribed to them.

Quality of life arises out of those possibilities that have become important for the way a person lives his or her life. The model focuses on the interplay between opportunities and constraints occurring both by choice and by chance that create what is possible in a person's life. The CHP framework depicts three fundamental aspects of life in which possibilities occur: being, belonging, and becoming. Being represents the most basic level of who a person is; belonging represents a person's connectedness; and becoming focuses on purposeful activities directed at achievement and actualization. Each of these three broad areas has subcomponents embodying different aspects of that area. For example, belonging can be considered from a social, community, or ecologic perspective. A strength of this model is that it depicts all domains of life as interconnected and as having both positive and negative aspects that contribute to overall life quality.

The model also illustrates that, although quality of life is a measure of the importance and enjoyment of the possibilities that arise out of the person-environment interaction, moderating factors must be considered.

Determinants are seen as long-term existential conditions, whereas moderating conditions are external factors that may alter these determinants. The model includes four moderating factors: resources, supports, control, and potential opportunities. One problem in segregating moderating factors from quality-of-life determinants is that the two may be difficult to differentiate in practice. However, separating the two groups of factors emphasizes the perspective that the effects of determinants such as disability on quality-of-life are not "pure" but can in fact be altered by the presence or absence of moderating factors.

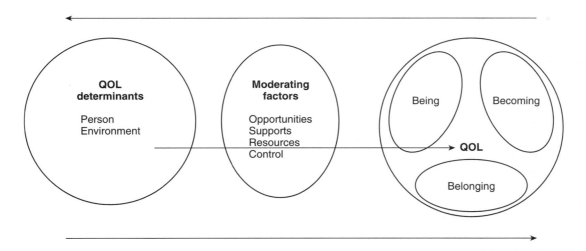

Figure 1-1 The Canadian Centre for Health Promotion model. *QOL,* Quality of life. (From Raeburn J, Rootman I: The centrality of life in health promotion and rehabilitation. In Renwick R, Brown I, Nagler M, editors: *Quality of life in health promotion and rehabilitation,* Thousand Oaks, Calif, 1996, Sage Publications.)

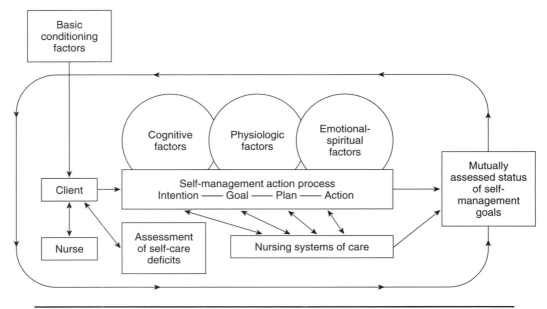

Figure 1-2 The nursing practice model. (From Burks KJ: A nursing practice model for chronic illness, *Rehabil Nurs* 24[5]:198, 1999.)

Nursing Practice Model

As the name implies, the nursing practice model (Figure 1-2) focuses on how nurses can assist people with chronic illnesses in promoting their own health through the development of self-management skills. Although designed with rehabilitation nurses in mind, the model can serve as a guide to all health care providers whose practices include the care of people with chronic illnesses and disabilities. The model is based on Orem's theory of self-care (2001), which portrays people as having the ability to take action. This ability is called *self-care agency*. When the work required for self-care exceeds one's self-care agency, a "self-care deficit" exists. It is in this area that health care professionals can intervene to restore effective self-care agency.

The nursing practice model focuses on intentional action and assumes that the individual is both capable and desirous of taking action. The first step of the action process is assessment. The health care provider works with the individual to assess self-care agency, identify self-care deficits, and develop a plan. The model depicts three domains surrounding the action process. These domains represent the cognitive, physiologic, and emotional-spiritual factors that influence the process. Health care providers take action related to each of these domains to enhance self-care agency. For example, the nurse might provide education about illness management, the physical therapist might provide information about exercises and teach energy management techniques, and the social worker might provide information about support groups. Development of knowledge, skills, and networks ultimately serves to enhance self-confidence, which further strengthens self-care agency.

The final step in the practice model is evaluation. Because chronic illness has an uncertain trajectory, any plan of care must be constantly evaluated. The individual and the health care provider assess how effective the self-management plan is and take steps to modify the plan if necessary. It is important to encourage the person with the illness to be involved in the evaluation process and to recognize the need for frequent reevaluation. The very act of assessing one's self-care management outcomes strengthens one's self-care agency.

A strength of this model is that it fosters collaboration between the health care professional and the individual with the chronic illness or disability. This collaboration can be empowering at each step of the action process. For this empowerment to be realized, however, the professional must resist the urge to act paternalistically, attend to the patient's experiences, and recognize the patient as both credible and knowledgeable.

Shifting Perspectives Model

The shifting perspectives model (Figure 1-3) portrays chronic illness as a state of being that has elements of both illness and wellness. Whether illness is in the foreground or the background is a matter of perspective. Davis and Magilvy (2000) define perspective as "representative of beliefs, perceptions, expectations, attitudes, and experiences about what it means to be a person with a chronic illness within a specific context ... [that] determine[s] how people respond to the disease, themselves, caregivers, and situations" (p. 23).

The model illustrates that perspectives are not static and suggests that understanding the individual's perspective at any given time enables health care providers to individual-

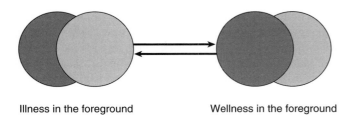

Illness in the foreground   Wellness in the foreground

Figure 1-3   The shifting perspectives model. (From Paterson B: The shifting perspectives model of chronic illness, *J Adv Nurs* 33[1]:21-6, 2001.)

ize care in a more meaningful way. For example, holding illness in the background, which has been traditionally viewed as a form of denial, may in fact be a mechanism that allows individuals with illness to experience a sense of well-being that permits them to live their lives as they choose. Rather than forming judgments about the person's perspective, nurses and other providers need to appreciate the perspective as reflecting the person's view of self. Providers need to ask "How is that for you?" rather than attaching positive or negative meanings to the perspective.

Wellness in the Foreground

When wellness is in the foreground, chronic illness and disability are seen as providing opportunities for personal growth and change. The self, not the illness or disability, is the person's source of identity. This allows people to rate their overall health as good or excellent even when physical functioning is significantly impaired. This view locates illness and disability outside of the "person." This view has led quality-of-life researchers to separate quality of life from health-related quality of life and underscores the difficulty of coming to a consistent understanding of either concept.

Unfortunately, keeping wellness in the foreground may prevent individuals from getting the services and/or attention they need. For example, ignoring symptoms may result in exacerbation or extension of the illness. More distressing is the fact that, to receive health care services or access resources, individuals are forced to focus on their limitations and weaknesses. This threatens the person's integrity and sense of self.

Illness in the Foreground

The perspective of illness in the foreground is one with which health care professionals are much more comfortable. People who place their illnesses in the foreground are typically overwhelmed by or absorbed with the illness. Nurses and other providers are exceptionally skilled at assisting these individuals in learning about and managing their illness or disability. The value of these efforts cannot be overstated. Although these skills are of tremendous value, they often foster dependency and serve to keep illness in the foreground. For example, providers frequently view their role as one of

helping people recognize and accept their limitations, which serves to emphasize the things the person cannot do rather than the possibilities for what they might do. To fully assist people, nurses and other providers must understand what function is served by the individual's particular perspective. People who choose to place their illness in the foreground may do so because it allows them to attend to the illness, because they receive secondary social gains such as attention or validation, or because focusing on the illness protects them from dwelling on other painful aspects of their lives.

The strength of this model is that it enables professionals to reframe their own perspectives on living with chronic illness and disability and to provide the appropriate care and support for individuals with either perspective.

Assumptions of the Practice Models

The assumptions of these practice models (Box 1-2) underpin each chapter of this text. They are guided by values and beliefs rooted in a knowledge base that focuses on human beings as irreducible wholes who are constantly in the process of becoming.

IMPACT OF CHRONIC ILLNESS AND DISABILITY

The impact of chronic illness and disability depends on both the nature of the illness or disability and the resources that the individual has to mitigate its effects. Therefore, the impact of chronic illness or disability on individuals and families is highly variable. Although the global impact of chronic illness and disability on society is less variable, significant differences are seen in the way various societies and cultures organize public and private sector resources to deal with the effects of these conditions.

Box 1-2   Assumptions of Conceptual Models

- Quality of life and health are multidimensional constructs.
- Every individual is biopsychosocial in nature and in continual interaction with the environment.
- Quality of life arises out of this person-environment interaction, and therefore a holistic approach is required to understand it.
- Chronic illness and disability, by themselves, do not necessarily lead to increased or decreased quality of life.
- The basic components of quality of life are common to all people and constitute the human condition.
- Even though the basic components of quality of life are the same for all people, the meaning attached to them varies based on the individual's culture, opportunities, and views of what is important to that individual.
- The perspectives of the individual are the most important consideration in determining health status or quality of life.

Impact on the Person

The impact of an illness or disability may be perceived as overwhelming, or it may be viewed merely as annoying if the person with the illness is able to carry out the normal activities of daily living and continue in normal roles. Research suggests that symptom experience has the most significant effect on reported quality of life, health status, and emotional health status (Haworth and Dluhy, 2001; Souza et al, 1999). For example, research involving HIV-infected women demonstrated that illness appraisal as a function of the symptom experience accounted for the greatest portion of variance in adjustment to the illness (Bova, 2001). Similarly, a study of 51- to 61-year-olds with chronic conditions indicated that this group was more likely than the general population to report their emotional health as fair or poor. This was particularly true of people with arthritis (Merck Institute of Aging and Health, 2002), a condition characterized by symptoms that produce pain and interfere with function.

At the point at which symptoms interfere with usual functions, people seek help and intervention. When function cannot be fully restored or roles cannot be continued at their previous level, the impact of the illness increases. Women with chronic illnesses report more symptoms and poorer health than their male counterparts (O'Neil and Morrow, 2001), which suggests that gender plays a role in symptom interpretation and management. The symptoms associated with illness and disability that produce the greatest amount of functional disruption are pain, immobility, and fatigue. These three factors significantly affect quality of life through their impact on the degree to which individuals are able to realize the important possibilities of their lives.

Chronic Pain

Chronic pain has been defined as "pain that persists for longer than the expected time frame for healing or pain associated with progressive, nonmalignant disease" (Ashburn and Staats, 1999). Chronic pain is disabling for many of the 34 million Americans who suffer from it (Bedard, 1997). Chronic pain depletes the individual's physiologic and emotional reserves, interfering with sleep, nutrition, motor function, and moods. Individuals find it difficult to carry out role functions and maintain relationships. People with chronic pain are often depressed, and undertreatment may provoke suicidal thoughts.

In spite of the amount of suffering and the more than $100 million spent annually on pain management, chronic pain remains undertreated (Bedard, 1997). This may be due to lack of knowledge on the part of both providers and the individuals they treat as well as a fear of addiction. Studies have shown that these fears are unfounded. Although a physical dependency may develop, addiction is rare.

Providers should assess the location and character of the pain following general pain assessment guidelines. Equally if not more important in the management of chronic pain is an assessment of aggravating and alleviating factors, and the effect of the pain on life quality. In addition, understanding what the client has already tried, with or without success, will lay a foundation for future interventions. Some current therapies for pain management are listed in Box 1-3.

Assessment of the family and support systems is also essential. Individuals with chronic pain often become isolated from friends and family because the pain becomes all encompassing.

Cultural Responses to Pain

Just as culture affects the meaning attached to illness and disability, culture plays a significant role in the way pain is managed, expressed, and discussed. People in some cultures do not talk about pain openly or feel that to discuss pain is to complain that the care provider is not doing a good job. Providers must let individuals know that talking about pain is helpful and appropriate.

It is important, however, not to stereotype individuals or assume that they will respond to pain based on culture. The provider must determine the extent to which the individual identifies with his or her cultural origins. The acronym FICA (faith/beliefs, importance/influence, community, address in care) has been used to describe a method of assessing spiritual beliefs and attitudes (Puchalski, Larson, and Post, 2000) and can be modified for cultural assessment by asking about cultural rather than spiritual beliefs (Box 1-4).

Specific interventions for managing pain are discussed as part of symptom management in subsequent chapters.

Effects Related to the Nature of the Illness or Disability

Chronic illness or disability also affects daily living in ways that are related to the nature of the illness or disability but may

---

Box 1-3   Pain Management Therapies

- Acupuncture
- Biofeedback
- Chiropractic
- Distraction
- Hypnosis
- Imagery
- Magnetic field therapy
- Massage
- Nerve block
- Opioid and nonopioid analgesics
- Physical therapy
- Reiki
- Therapeutic touch
- Transcutaneous electrical nerve stimulation

From Puchalski CM, Larson DB, Post SG: Physicians and patient spirituality, *Ann Intern Med* 133[9]:748-9, 2000.

Box 1-4   Cultural Assessment

F (C)   What are the individual's cultural beliefs?

I   How much do these cultural beliefs influence the individual's health management?

C   Is the individual a part of a cultural community and does the community provide care and support?

A   How would the individual like cultural beliefs to be addressed and incorporated into the plan of care?

Modified from Puchalski CM, Larson DB, Post SG: Physicians and patient spirituality, *Ann Intern Med* 133[9]:748-9, 2000.

not be connected to symptoms. Three concerns in particular are time management, social isolation, and self-identity.

Time Management

An often overlooked but very important effect of chronic illness and disability is the effect on time management. Activities that once were considered routine and required very little thought may now necessitate careful planning. The person with a chronic illness or disability must allow more time for bathing, dressing, grooming, and so on. If mobility aids are used, more time is required to get out of the house and into some form of transportation. There are no more quick trips to the store. Indeed, transportation itself may be an issue that requires thought and planning, especially if the individual relies on public transportation. Everything must be thought out in advance, which makes spontaneity virtually impossible. Time is also a critical factor in employability. In business markets speed is often valued more than quality, which makes it difficult for people with illnesses and disabilities to get or keep jobs.

Social Isolation

Social isolation is a negative or threatening state of aloneness experienced by an individual. It may be self-imposed or perceived as being imposed by others. It can occur even when people are living with and in contact with others. For example, many persons living in extended care facilities are surrounded by staff and other residents, yet they feel socially isolated. Characteristics of social isolation include having few contacts with peers, significant others, or the community; lacking support from significant others; and/or verbalizing feelings of rejection or unwanted aloneness.

People with chronic illnesses withdraw from social situations for many reasons. Very often the social gathering is in an environment that is difficult to navigate physically because of steps, clutter, narrow passageways, uneven ground surfaces, and so on. Sometimes the energy demands of managing the illness are substantial, and even climbing a few steps can become an obstacle that prevents someone from leaving home. A frequently cited reason for avoiding social outings is the need to be near bathroom facilities.

People with illnesses that cause incontinence are fearful of not reaching a bathroom in time, and individuals with a physical disability need bathroom facilities that have handrails and space to accommodate mobility aids. Another factor that prevents people with chronic illnesses from fully participating in society is their treatment schedule. Frequent hospitalizations, trips for therapies, or complex therapies such as dialysis performed in the home often make it difficult to maintain relationships outside of the family. Isolation also occurs as family members and friends begin to withdraw from the person with the illness or disability. People with chronic illnesses and disabilities come to see themselves as "different," and this separates them from others who either do not understand, fear, or simply reject that difference (Biordi, 2002). The withdrawal can occur slowly as friends begin to recognize that the person can no longer engage in shared activities at the same level or it can occur abruptly if the stigma associated with the illness is high, as in the case of people with HIV or AIDS.

Self-Identity

Chronic illness and disability alter many aspects of the self. These alterations require individuals to develop a new sense of self that incorporates the experience of the illness or disability and its management. Contrary to popular belief, these changes in the self may be either positive or negative. Body image may or may not be affected depending on whether or not the illness or disability affects the body's appearance.

Other aspects of self that are not as readily apparent may also be altered, including the sense of self as being in control and having power to conduct the business of living, the sense of self as a sexual being capable of enjoying intimacy and giving enjoyment, and the sense of self as purposeful and able to fulfill roles effectively.

Individuals with a chronic condition may experience feelings of hopelessness from time to time. It is important that providers listen attentively and recognize the validity of these feelings. Acknowledging the truth of the situation while encouraging the individual to find other areas in which realistic hope can be offered is useful. For example, a person who has no hope of walking should not be given false hope that with time and effort the situation will change. The provider should listen to the person's feelings about this, encourage expression related to the associated losses, and then encourage the individual to explore ways that life quality can be attained in view of the fact that walking is not a possibility.

When feelings of hopelessness and despair are expressed, the provider should listen carefully for any signs that the individual has suicidal thoughts. Referral to counselors and psychologists may be appropriate.

Positive effects related to personal and spiritual growth have been reported both by individuals with illness or disability and by those around them. A deeper appreciation for life and loved ones is frequently cited.

Impact on Families

All individuals are members of families, and what affects the individual ultimately will affect that individual's family. The extent to which the family's quality of life is affected depends on the structure of the family, as well as its resources, strengths, values, and beliefs. As with the individual, the level of impact will vary with the degree to which normal family activities and roles are disrupted by the illness or disability.

Although some individuals receive services from a personal assistant, use home health aides, or live in long-term care facilities, the majority of care is provided by families. Families, often supportive at the onset, may become exhausted by the demands of providing this care. Roles may be reversed, as when children become care providers for their parents. Sometimes new roles must be taken on and new skills developed. For example, when husbands assume care of their wives that includes bathing, dressing, grooming, and toileting, they must learn how to manipulate undergarments, apply makeup, and style hair. This can be disconcerting for both parties.

In addition, providing care may require someone in the family to reduce their work hours, change their shift, or give up work altogether, which can create financial stress as well as role stress. Faculty at the University of California conducted a study of persons with Alzheimer's disease in which they compared the costs and hours spent caring for these people at home with the costs and hours spent for care provided in nursing homes. Remarkably, the costs were virtually the same (about $47,000 per year) with families reporting spending an average of 286 hours per month giving care and 36 hours per month visiting the nursing home.

Tasks reported to be the most time consuming were giving emotional support, completing household chores, and providing transportation. The literature is replete with studies related to the "burden" of caregiving. Health care professionals must be careful, however, not to presume that all, or even most, families perceive giving care as burdensome. To assume that a burden exists is to assume that the individual being cared for does not contribute to the family in meaningful ways but rather just consumes resources. Providers should always assess for signs that caregiving tasks are overwhelming family members to the extent that their own needs are not being met but should not assume that this is the case. There is great joy and satisfaction in caring for others; otherwise the helping professions are misguided.

Family members frequently report positive outcomes as a result of living with and caring for someone with an illness or disability (National Family Caregivers Association, 2003). Aspects reported to be most difficult for family members include providing emotional support; managing behaviors such as irritability, confusion, moodiness, and so on; and dealing with communication difficulties.

Chronic Sorrow

Chronic sorrow can be described as periodic pervasive feelings of sadness or grief that are related to the disparities created by loss. Some people living with chronic illness or disability and their families experience ongoing losses with no predictable end. For these individuals, chronic sorrow is a normal response to the situation. Chronic sorrow is cyclical and interspersed with times of happiness, contentment, and even joy.

Grief-related feelings might be triggered by a missed developmental milestone or an anniversary of the date of the loss. Health care providers must recognize chronic sorrow as normal and encourage clients to share and explore their feelings so that coping strategies can be assessed and supported or modified if necessary.

Impact on Society

The number of people with chronic illnesses or disabilities is expected to reach 157 million by 2020. Direct medical costs associated with these conditions amounted to $510 billion in 2000 and are increasing faster than the prevalence rate (Partnership for Solutions, 2001). Financing chronic care as well as finding ways to decrease costs is a prominent part of the U.S. government's policy agenda. The health care sector is challenged to meet the needs of people with chronic illnesses or disabilities. Numerous studies indicate that people with chronic illnesses or disabilities are dissatisfied with the care they receive and believe that the government should do more to provide financial assistance. Health care systems and educational institutions are reorganizing the way health care is provided and learned. Health care agencies and third-party payers are emphasizing wellness and health promotion to prevent chronic conditions. Care is being moved out of acute care settings into community settings and homes to decrease costs and provide better outcomes. Universities are offering courses in chronic care management, and nursing programs are offering clinical experiences in nontraditional settings such as outpatient facilities, homes, and parishes.

Since the passage of the ADA, businesses and places of entertainment have had to reconfigure their physical plants and redesign the way work is accomplished to accommodate people with disabilities. Many facilities have followed the letter of the law (if not its intent) by creating spaces for wheelchair users, parking spaces for people who cannot walk great distances, bathroom stalls for people with disabilities, and so on. However, much remains to be done. Two wheelchair spaces in a theater that accommodates 200 people is insufficient. As the number of people requiring accommodation increases, society will have to respond to the need and demand for nondiscriminatory treatment.

One very important consequence of the increasing numbers of persons with chronic illnesses and disabilities is the shift in focus from life expectancy to life quality as a measure of how well we are doing as a nation. Quality of life has been referred to as one of the most influential concepts of the past decade and its predominant theme (Guillett, 1998), and improving quality of life is one of the two objectives of *Healthy People 2010* (DHHS, 2000).

Although this shift in focus has produced many positive outcomes, caution must be exercised to avoid disadvantaging people on the basis of some perceived or arbitrarily determined quality-of-life measurement. Consider what would happen if resources were allocated on the basis of quality-of-life expectations and potential for improvement. This is already happening in Europe. A measure has been developed called quality-of-life years (QALYs). QALYs are determined using matrices that factor in mobility, pain, and age. Resources are then allocated on the basis of a person's QALY score. Measuring quality of life and categorizing people according to that measure has associated risks. For example, if a health care provider believes that an individual's quality of life is poor and without hope for improvement, he or she may not provide the same level of services that would be given to others with more potential. There is also great risk when someone other than the individual living the life ascribes some value to that life. The euthanasia and sterilization programs conducted in this country in the earlier years of the twentieth century are examples of what can happen when society sets out to decide whose lives are worth living.

Health care providers must be concerned about enhancing quality of life, and valid tools must be available for measuring it. The key is to remember that quality of life is determined by the person living the life, and the criteria for measuring quality should originate with that person, not with the researcher. Factors that are important to the individual should be the standard by which quality of life is measured (Haas, 1999; LaPlege and Hunt, 1997).

Role of the Health Care Provider

The health care team works with individuals and families to meet the daily challenges of maintaining health and function and allowing individuals to lead productive, satisfying lives. Strategies and interventions vary based on the type of illness or disability and the strengths, abilities, and resources of the people involved. According to the literature the interventions that families and individuals cite as most helpful are those embodied in the roles of expert, teacher, and "caring professional" (Eaks, Burke, and Hainsworth, 1998). The task of the health care provider is to enhance the quality of life of individuals with chronic illnesses or disabilities as well as that of their families and their communities. To do this, providers must be sensitive to each individual's values and circumstances, recognizing that the individual may want to take, share, or relinquish control at any given time and respecting his or her desires. It is important to assess abilities and strengths as well as deficits. A simple strategy for accomplishing this work is to "think S for success" by focusing on symptoms, sequelae, safety, support/services, and satisfaction. Although each illness or disability has its own uniquely experienced myriad of symptoms and sequelae, the "think S for success" strategy addresses the major concerns in each situation. These six *S*'s serve as an organ-

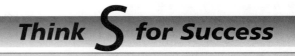

Think **S** for Success

Symptoms
■ What strategies can be used to manage the most common symptoms associated with the illness or disability being discussed, such as pain, stiffness, nausea, or fatigue?

Sequelae
■ What interventions should be undertaken to prevent common complications of the illness or disability, such as preventing skin breakdown, contractures, and social isolation?

Safety
■ What are the major safety issues and what measures should be taken to decrease risk?

Support/Services
■ What resources are available to assist individuals and families?

Satisfaction
■ What can be done to maintain or enhance quality of life?

izing framework for providing comprehensive holistic care and will be highlighted in each of the chapters of this text. See the accompanying box that identifies the type of information that falls under each heading.

Box 1-5   Caring for the Caregiver

■ Determine the caregiver's level of knowledge.
■ Teach strategies for providing care that conserve energy and avoid strain (e.g., body mechanics).
■ Determine the caregiver's attitude regarding the caregiving role.
■ Demonstrate acceptance of negative and/or ambivalent feelings.
■ Identify stressors and resources for managing them.
■ Teach stress management techniques.
■ Assess family strengths and weaknesses.
■ Teach the caregiver strategies for maintaining his or her own health.
■ Inform the caregiver of community resources that may be of assistance.
■ Assess for the presence of grieving or chronic sorrow.
■ Offer support and anticipatory guidance through the grieving process.
■ Encourage participation in support groups.
■ Encourage participation in social activities outside of the home.
■ Be vigilant for signs that the caregiver is overburdened and provide additional resources as needed (e.g., home care, Meals on Wheels, respite care).

Caring for the Caregiver

The level of informal caregiving being provided must be evaluated in terms of the level of engagement and the stress being experienced by the caregiver. Wrubel et al (2001) identified three categories of caregiver: those who are engaged, those who feel conflicted in attempting to provide care for their family member and to meet their own personal needs, and those who are distanced (want to provide support and comfort but not physical care). Understanding the needs of the caregiver and the point at which the caregiver needs the provider to take control is essential for developing therapeutic relationships and preserving the relationship between the individual with the illness or disability and the informal caregiver.

The needs most often mentioned by caregivers are instrumental support, emotional support, information, and social activities. Box 1-5 lists some interventions to support caregivers.

Internet and Other Resources

AARP: *http://www.aarp.org*
American Chronic Pain Association: *http://www.theacpa.org*
American Disability Association: *http://www.adanet.org*
Association of Rehabilitation Nurses: *http://www.rehabnurse.org*
Disability information: *http://www.disabilityinfo.gov*
Family Caregiver Alliance: *http://www.caregiver.org*
National Association of Area Agencies on Aging (for agencies throughout the United States): *http://www.n4a.org/locator.cfm*
National Association of Professional Geriatric Care Managers: *http://www.caremanager.org*
National Family Caregivers Association: *http://www.nfcacares.org*
National Institute on Disability Rehabilitation Research: *http://www.ed.gov/about/offices/list/osers/nidrr/index. html?src=mr*

REFERENCES

Ashburn M, Staats P: Management of chronic pain, *Lancet* 353(9167): 1865-9, 1999.

Bedard M: Fact sheet on chronic pain, retrieved from *http://www.cssa-inc.org/Articles/Chronic_Pain.htm* on Jan 23, 2003, 1997.

Biordi DL: Social isolation. In Lubkin I, Larsen P, editors: *Chronic illness,* ed 5, Boston, 2002, Jones and Bartlett.

Bova C: Adjustment to chronic illness among HIV infected women, *Image J Nurs Sch* 33(3):217-24, 2001.

Burks KJ: A nursing practice model for chronic illness, *Rehabil Nurs* 24(5):197-200, 1999.

Commission on Chronic Illness: Chronic illness in the United States. In Braslow L, editor: *Chronic illness in the United States,* vol 1, Cambridge Mass, 1957, Harvard University Press.

Department of Health and Human Services: Healthy people 2010, ed 2, Washington, DC, November 2000, US Government Printing Office, retrieved from *http://www.healthypeople.gov* on July 20, 2003.

Davis R, Magilvy JK: Quiet pride: the experience of chronic illness by rural older Americans, *Image J Nurs Sch* 32(4):385-90, 2000.

Eaks G, Burke M, Hainsworth M: Middle-range theory of chronic sorrow, *Image J Nurs Sch* 30(2):179-84, 1998.

Emmanuel E: We are all chronic patients, *J Chronic Dis* 3(7):501-2, 1982.

Guillett S: Quality of life among children with physical disabilities, doctoral dissertation, Fairfax, Va, 1998, George Mason University.

Haas BK: A multidisciplinary concept analysis of quality of care, *West J Nurs Res* 21(6):728-42, 1999.

Haworth SK, Dluhy NM: Holistic symptom management: modeling the interaction phase, *J Adv Nurs* 36(2):302-10, 2001.

LaPlege A, Hunt H: The problem of quality of life in medicine, *JAMA* 278(1):47-50, 1997.

Merck Institute on Aging and Health: The state of aging and health in America, 2002, retrieved from *http://www.agingsociety.org/aging society/publications. state/index.html.*

National Academy on an Aging Society: Chronic conditions: a challenge for the 21st century, 2002, retrieved from *http://www.agingsociety.org* on Jan 10, 2002.

National Family Caregivers Association: A profile of caregivers, 2003, retrieved from *http://www.nfcacares.org* on July 20, 2003.

Nolan M, Nolan J: Rehabilitation, chronic illness and disability: the missing elements in nurse education, *J Adv Nurs* 29(4):958-66, 1999.

O'Neil E, Morrow L: The symptom experience of women with chronic illness, *J Adv Nurs* 33(2):257-68, 2001.

Orem DE: Nursing: concepts of practice, ed 6, St Louis, 2001, Mosby.

Parse R: *Man-living-health: a theory of nursing,* New York, 1981, John Wiley and Sons.

Partnership for Solutions: Statistics and research, 2001, retrieved from *http://www.partnershipforsolutions.org/statistics/perceptions.cfm* on Jan 23, 2002.

Paterson B: The shifting perspectives model of chronic illness, *J Adv Nurs* 33(1):21-6, 2001.

Puchalski CM, Larson DB, Post SG: Physicians and patient spirituality, *Ann Intern Med* 133(9):748-9, 2000.

Raeburn J, Rootman I: Quality of life and health promotion. In Renwick R, Brown I, Nagler M, editors: *Quality of life in health promotion and rehabilitation: conceptual approaches, issues, and applications,* Thousand Oaks, Calif, 1996, Sage Publications.

Souza K et al: Dimensions of health related quality of life in persons living with HIV disease, *J Adv Nurs* 29(1):178-87, 1999.

Watson J: Human science and human care: a theory of nursing, Sudbury, Mass, 1999, Jones and Bartlett.

Wrubel J et al: Tacit definitions of informal caregiving, *J Adv Nurs* 33(2):175-81, 2001.

CHAPTER 2

Settings of Chronic Care

Leslie Jean Neal, PhD, RN, FNP-C

> ## OBJECTIVES
>
> After reading this chapter, you should be able to do the following:
>
> - Describe the settings in which persons with chronic illnesses or disabilities receive nursing care
> - Differentiate the care that is provided within these settings
> - Describe the roles of the interdisciplinary team members who care for persons in chronic care settings.

Individuals with chronic illnesses or disabilities are cared for in a variety of settings. When a person with a chronic illness or disability experiences an exacerbation or episode that alters the maintenance state of health that previously allowed the person to live in another setting, the hospital becomes the predominant site of care. Once the acute episode has been resolved, the individual may either move back to the previous care setting or move to another setting that can provide the new level of care required. For example, a person with a history of congestive heart failure who is living at home may experience an exacerbation, be admitted to the hospital, and eventually be discharged back home. However, the exacerbation may alter the person's level of functioning to a point that requires admission to a nursing home or skilled nursing facility (SNF) either temporarily or permanently.

Settings for persons with chronic illnesses or disabilities vary with regard to the services provided, the allowed length of stay, and the criteria for admission. The most common settings in which individuals receive skilled care include the SNF, the rehabilitation facility, the nursing home, and the individual's home with formal home care. Other settings, such as day care centers for persons with dementia or the frail elderly, do not typically provide skilled care. This chapter does not discuss the hospital setting because it is only a temporary setting for persons with chronic illnesses or disabilities. The goal is to return individuals to the community, preferably to the home setting.

Table 2-1 summarizes the different settings of care and indicates the typical patient each setting serves.

SUBACUTE CARE

Subacute care settings are inpatient facilities that are designed for persons who are not able or qualified to participate in intensive functional rehabilitation. The nursing care and rehabilitation services provided in subacute settings are generally less intensive than those provided in a hospital or rehabilitation facility (Quigley, 2000).

There are several types of subacute care settings. A transitional subacute care program is used when the length of stay will be shorter than 30 days and the person requires highly skilled nursing, rehabilitation, and pharmacologic services. Such a setting is a facility in which patients stay temporarily until they become able to move to another less acute care setting. General subacute care programs allow a stay of 10 to 40 days and include rehabilitation and nursing care. Chronic settings allow a length of stay of 60 to 90 days and are designed for persons with medical diseases who require long-term medical and nursing care. Long-term care settings allow a length of stay that averages 25 days or more (Quigley, 2000).

These various subacute care settings share some similarities in that they are inpatient facilities and typically offer nursing and rehabilitation care. However, the length of stay allowed differs, as does the severity of the illnesses of the residents. Long-term care settings, such as nursing homes, are designed for people who are not able to live at home independently and require some level of regular nursing care, whether it is temporary acute care for a longer time than is allowed in the hospital setting or care intended to maintain the person's current level of function. The phrase *long-term care* is sometimes applied to home health care. This can be a misnomer, however, because most formal home care is intermittent and temporary. High-technology home care may be considered long term because it can be provided in the patient's home until the patient recovers or expires.

LONG-TERM CARE

Long-term inpatient care settings include long-term acute care (LTAC) and long-term nonacute care (LTC). LTAC settings allow 30 days as an average length of stay and offer services that combine medical and nursing care and rehabilitation and respiratory care. LTC settings provide skilled

Table 2-1   Settings for Chronic Care

Setting	Purpose	Patient/Circumstance
Subacute care	To provide medical and nursing treatment to patients who are unable or unready to participate in acute rehabilitation	All ages, although facilities for pediatric patients are usually separate Typically used after neurologic trauma or disease
Long-term care	To provide care to people who are unable to live independently	Primarily geriatric patients but also younger people with chronic conditions Typically used in cases of neurologic, orthopedic, and autoimmune diseases or trauma
Rehabilitation (outpatient or inpatient)	To provide intensive rehabilitative care	All ages Typically used after neurologic or orthopedic trauma or disease
Home health care	To provide care in the home setting to restore maximal independence and self-care to the patient and family	All ages Used for temporary conditions such as recovery from surgery or fracture or for chronic conditions such as heart disease or wounds
Independent living	To provide individuals with a sense of control over their medical care, health, and decision making	Primarily adults Used after neurologic disease or trauma, or in advanced age

Adapted from Parker BJ: Community and family-centered rehabilitation nursing. In Edwards PA, editor: *The specialty practice of rehabilitation nursing: a core curriculum,* Glenview, Ill, 2000, Association of Rehabilitation Nurses, pp 17-31.

nursing care and attendant care for an extended period for people with chronic illnesses or disabilities. LTC settings include SNFs, residential facilities, long-term care hospitals, and transitional living centers (Figure 2-1) (Quigley, 2000).

Some nursing homes are trying to do away with the traditional idea of a standard mealtime, activity time, and bedtime for residents. The contention is that people do not do things in a standard way if they are living in their own homes and should not be expected to do so just because they must live in a nursing home. Other nursing homes have incorporated animals, plants, and children into daily life so that nursing home life is more like everyday life in the community (Baker, 2002). More innovative ideas likely will emerge as health care providers and business people recognize that there are better and more cost-effective ways to meet the needs of people with chronic illnesses or disabilities.

REHABILITATION FACILITY

The purpose of rehabilitation is to maximize the person's functional ability and to teach the individual and caregiver how to incorporate the chronic illness or disability into their way of life. Rehabilitation services may be provided in inpatient or outpatient settings. They may be freestanding or hospital-based programs. Inpatient facilities are for persons who have not regained enough functional ability or independence to be able to move back into the community. Individuals stay in inpatient rehabilitation facilities for varying lengths of time depending on their diagnosis and their insurance or ability to pay.

Inpatient rehabilitation facilities are designed to provide individuals with the security and skilled services they need while they and their caregivers learn to care for their needs and to incorporate the chronic illness or disability into

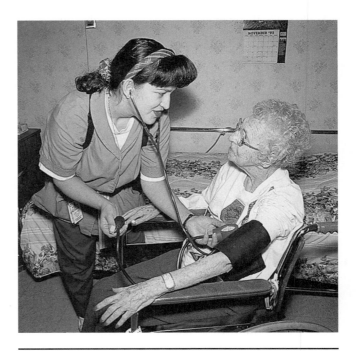

Figure 2-1   Nurse taking blood pressure for a patient in a long-term care setting. (From Potter PA, Perry AG: *Basic nursing: a critical thinking approach,* ed 4, St Louis, 1999, Mosby.)

their lifestyle. Consequently, these facilities are set up to resemble life in the community and often include a kitchen, mock supermarket, and vocational and occupational work areas so that individuals can regain or learn new life skills.

Patients are encouraged to dress in street clothes and to participate in their own care as much as possible. Caregivers and family members are included in every aspect of care so that they can learn to adjust to the lifestyle changes and assist the patient in the transition once the patient leaves the facility.

Sometimes individuals are discharged from the hospital directly into the community or indirectly via an SNF, nursing home, or inpatient rehabilitation facility. In any case, some individuals continue to require outpatient rehabilitation. The facilities providing this service may or may not be attached to the inpatient rehabilitation facility. Typically, individuals receive fairly intensive rehabilitation in which they spend half a day or more receiving physical, occupational, and/or speech therapy in the outpatient setting. Individuals are expected to practice the techniques they learn at home, because the length of time spent in outpatient therapy is limited by the payer.

SKILLED NURSING

SNFs are inpatient settings that provide skilled care while patients make the transition from the hospital to the community. Because managed care continues to foster discharge of the patient from the hospital before the patient is fully recovered from an illness or injury, SNFs are necessary to provide a supervised level of care to aid in the patient's recovery. Persons who have experienced a cerebral vascular accident, spinal cord injury, or total hip replacement, for example, may move from the hospital to the SNF to recover sufficiently to return home, where they will have less skilled supervision. SNFs typically provide nursing, physical, occupational, and speech therapy as well as social work assistance. Physicians provide on-site medical care.

COMMUNITY-BASED CARE

Persons with a chronic illness or disability who live in the community manage their day-to-day needs and activities independently or with the assistance of their family or hired caregiver. Community-based care involves a wide spectrum of options ranging from day treatment programs that include supervised care to formal home health care that includes visits from nurses, therapists, dietitians, and medical social workers.

In day care centers, individuals may participate in recreational activities and benefit from the opportunity to socialize in a supervised setting. Skilled care is not provided, but health care professionals may visit to furnish care or to teach participants about health-related topics.

Individuals who are able to live in independent living centers typically reside in their own apartments but have easy access to skilled nursing care. Skilled care is usually provided in a facility that is located on the grounds of the apartment complex so that persons who become ill can receive care there. Persons who are no longer able to live independently may then move to a different level of care.

In assisted living centers, nurses often administer medications to residents, and nurses and nurse's aides monitor the health and safety of the residents. Lately, more persons with dementia or Alzheimer's disease are living in assisted living facilities where they are able to participate in daily activities, wear their own clothes, and attend meals with other residents but are very closely supervised and cared for. Assisted living residents are expected to have a high level of physical function so that they do not require constant skilled nursing care. Frequently, visiting nurses from community agencies will call on assisted living residents to provide wound care or to change an indwelling catheter, for example. However, individuals for whom intermittent skilled care is inadequate to meet health care needs are not expected to continue living in an assisted living facility.

Rural outreach programs, nursing centers, senior citizen centers, and outpatient clinics are other community-based settings that persons with chronic illness or disability can access (Quigley, 2000).

Rural Outreach Programs

Individuals who live in rural areas may not have easy access to health care services. Rural outreach programs are designed to assist people in accessing services, and they often bring services directly to patients living in the community. One example of this kind of service is the traveling health care van. Nurses, nurse practitioners, therapists, dentists, and other health care professionals may staff the van and take turns traveling into rural areas to provide free or low-cost services to people with both acute and chronic health care needs. Otherwise, people living in rural areas must travel long distances to access health services.

Nursing Centers

Nursing centers may be facilities to which people come to receive blood pressure checks, foot care, health care teaching, or other assistance or they may be central locations from which nurses visit people in their homes to provide these services. Nursing centers are managed and staffed by nurses and seek to provide nursing care that does not require medical orders. Nurses may consult with the patient's physician or another member of the health care team to advocate for a referral or to attempt to obtain needed services for the patient. However, physicians are not typically on staff and are not required to supervise or order the care that is given.

Senior Citizen Centers

Senior citizen centers are locations at which relatively well, functional elderly persons can find social and recreational activities. Frequently, meals are offered for a fee and participants are free to come and go as they please. Health care providers may visit to educate participants about health care–related issues, but health care services are not standard.

Outpatient Clinics

Outpatient clinics may or may not be hospital based. They typically include nurses, physicians, and other health care providers depending on the size of the clinic. People may need to be referred elsewhere for therapy, nutrition services, or social work assistance. Outpatient clinics are intended for nonemergent situations. They provide care for acute illnesses such as colds, influenza, and muscle sprains but may or may not be able to manage on site cases such as fractures and those requiring minor surgery. In addition, they provide primary health care to the populations they serve.

PUBLIC HEALTH CARE

Public health care strives to provide primary prevention services, that is, to prevent disease and to enhance wellness. To that end, public health practitioners provide immunizations, health screening, well-woman services, antepartum and postpartum instruction and supervision, instruction and care for persons who have or who may be at risk for sexually transmitted diseases, and other types of care aimed at preventing illness and keeping people as well as possible. Public health agencies also provide systems-level care aimed at prevention of disease or injury for groups or populations of people, such as the underserved and the elderly.

Persons with chronic illnesses or disabilities may use public health resources in a number of ways. For example, people with chronic illnesses or disabilities are typically vulnerable to infection. They may obtain pneumonia and influenza vaccines through their public health departments. They can also learn good nutrition and energy conservation, and they may have the opportunity to participate in a support group that includes other people with a similar illness or disability.

A main focus of public health is teaching. Public health professionals usually do not provide hands-on care to their patients. They may perform blood pressure measurement or blood glucose screening but will not usually provide wound care or enteral feedings such as might be performed by a home health nurse.

HOSPICE CARE

Hospice services are available to people whose life expectancy is 6 months or less. Palliative care and social, spiritual, and emotional assistance are provided to people who have chosen to forego aggressive medical treatment but who want to die comfortably and peacefully. Hospice care may be provided in an inpatient setting or in the home setting via intermittent visits by nurses, chaplains, therapists, dietitians, social workers, physicians, and others.

Studies have shown that patients consider hospice services to be equal or superior to conventional end-of-life care (Naik and DeHaven, 2001). In addition, hospice services are significantly more cost effective in the last year of life than conventional medical care. Unfortunately, patients are typically admitted to hospice too late to receive more than a month of services (Naik and DeHaven, 2001).

HOME CARE

The term *home care* may be used to refer to care provided in the home by nursing assistants, companions, or housekeepers. The term may also be used to refer to formal home care. Formal home care includes the services of skilled health care professionals such as nurses, therapists, dietitians, and social workers. Currently, most of these skilled services are covered by Medicare and are covered by Medicaid in the majority of states. However, unskilled care that is provided without the supervision of a registered nurse (RN) or a therapist often is not covered by Medicare and may or may not be covered by Medicaid or private health insurance.

Patients and their caregivers may contact agencies or individuals to contract for the services of personal care attendants to bathe, dress, groom, and cook for the patient, for companions to sit with the patient while caregivers are away during the day or to watch the patient at night, or for housekeepers to clean the home. These services are considered unskilled but are extremely helpful to a person with a chronic illness or disability because they may make the difference between placing the person in an inpatient facility and permitting the person to remain at home.

Formal home care or intermittent skilled health care visits to persons in their homes is provided by freestanding or hospital-based home health agencies (HHA). The discharge planner from an inpatient facility, the patient or family, or the patient's physician or primary care provider may call the HHA to arrange for home care. In any case, the physician must give the HHA an order for home care services and must monitor the patient's progress through communications from the home health care providers. The physician may order nursing, physical therapy, occupational therapy, speech therapy, nurse's aide services, social work services, nutrition services, or other specialty services, or a combination of these. An RN or therapist must participate in the case for nurse's aide services to be ordered.

Persons receiving formal home care must be homebound (unable to leave the home without great difficulty or with an assistive device) and must require *skilled* care in order for the care to be reimbursable by Medicare and many private insurance plans. There are many people who are chronically ill or disabled who do not meet these criteria and may also be unable to afford skilled or unskilled care.

All of the patient's care is provided within the person's community setting, whether that setting is a street corner, mansion, assisted living facility, or day care center. Therapists and dietitians provide specialized services, whereas medical social workers assist patients in managing their finances so they can afford food *and* medicine, and assist and advise regarding occupational, vocational, sociological, and psychological issues. Licensed practical nurses (LPNs) and RNs perform wound care, instruct patients and caregivers regarding medications and diet, give injections and intravenous medications, monitor the patient's health status and specialized equipment that formerly was seen only in the hospital, and coordinate and reinforce the other services the patient is receiving (Figure 2-2). RNs perform care that is highly skilled and must be accomplished in the home with much creativity and flexibility because of the nature of the home setting. RNs and therapists may also manage the patient's case while the patient is on service. This involves coordinating all of the services, arranging case conferencing, communicating with the physician, garnering the resources needed for care, ensuring that the services provided are reimbursable and documented appropriately, and generally ascertaining that all services and documentation have been provided properly according to the guidelines of standards of care, of the insurers, and of the agency.

High-Technology Private Duty Care

Some individuals who require complex, high-technology skilled nursing services for a chronic illness or disability are able to receive those services within the home. The patient and family may prefer to pay the extra costs associated with this type of care so that the patient can remain at home rather than move into an LTC facility. In some circumstances, Medicaid or Medicare may reimburse for these services. Patients who use these services frequently require ventila-

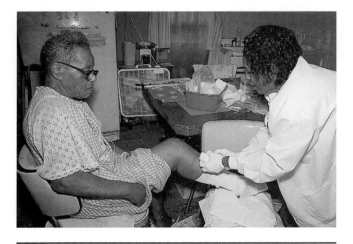

Figure 2-2　Physical therapist performing dressing change in the home. (From Potter PA, Perry AG: *Fundamentals of nursing: concepts, process, and practice,* ed 4, St Louis, 1997, Mosby.)

tory assistance or other complex treatments and procedures that must be monitored 24 hours a day.

Telehealth Care

Telehealth is becoming a more prevalent method of providing care to the chronically ill. Telehealth involves the use of computer technology to monitor the patient's status and to transfer health-related information between a remote location and the patient's home.

Telehealth makes the patient an active participant in care and allows the patient's status to be monitored more frequently than if one were to rely on intermittent home visits. Telehealth systems are typically used as a temporary measure to monitor a patient during an exacerbation period (Frantz, 2001).

INTERDISCIPLINARY TEAM

A particular characteristic of chronic care is the interdisciplinary team (IDT). Although acute care should likewise involve the IDT, in chronic care the IDT is critical to a high-quality outcome for the patient and family. The IDT forms the core from which extend branches that make chronic care holistic. Picture a wagon wheel in which the center is the IDT and the spokes individually and together reach out to the rim—the patient and the environment in which she or he resides and functions.

The IDT is not limited, so all disciplines that might be part of it could not possibly be discussed in this space. However, there are some core members of the team who are typically involved in chronic care. These members are supported intermittently by those in ancillary disciplines. This section of the chapter discusses the primary members of the IDT and describes how the team functions as a whole.

The term *interdisciplinary* is to be distinguished from *multidisciplinary*. Multidisciplinary teams are composed of personnel from many of the same disciplines as those who make up the IDT. However, the approach is to provide discipline-centered care. In other words, the physical therapist (PT) may give the patient exercises to perform, whereas the nurse may provide wound care to the patient. In multidisciplinary care, the nurse and therapist may confer, but they are largely independent and work on their own individual goals for the patient. In interdisciplinary care, the nurse and therapist confer frequently, reinforce each other's instructions and plans with the patient and family, and focus on reaching a mutually defined outcome.

Patient and Significant Others

The most important members of the IDT are the patient with the illness or disability and the people who are the most meaningful to that person. A distinction of chronic care is that care is directed by the patient and, by extension, by his or her significant others and those in the patient's environment. This core group should always be included in plans of care; in the design of goals, objectives of treatment, and interventions; and in the evaluation of care. The group should have a clear understanding of what is being done, why it is being done, and by whom.

The efforts and accomplishments of the IDT are greatly enhanced by the inclusion of the patient and the patient's family and friends, because chronic care is based on doing "with" the patient and not doing "to" the patient. A plan of care that is implemented without the active support of the core group will not succeed—chronic care requires and desires maximum patient and caregiver participation.

Physician or Nurse Practitioner

The physician is typically the primary care provider for the person with a chronic illness or disability. However, a nurse practitioner or physician's assistant may also perform this role. The primary care provider prescribes the care and writes orders allowing the involvement of the IDT members. The primary provider, as well as the specialty physician(s) who are typically involved, are kept informed and are consulted about changes in the patient's condition, particularly when new orders are required to assist the IDT to care for the patient.

The primary provider and specialty physician(s) may be involved to the extent that they attend case conferences and meetings of the IDT and see the patient frequently to monitor his or her condition. Alternatively, the primary and specialty providers may see the patient monthly or biannually and rely on telephone or paper communication from IDT members to obtain updates and provide consultation. When home health care is used after surgery, for example, the patient often sees the physician for a postoperative visit and then does not return for another 6 to 8 weeks. During that period, the rest of the IDT is caring for the patient and family and consults with the physician when there is a change in condition or a new order is needed. Similarly, in many LTC situations, the physician may see the patient only monthly or less frequently.

The physiatrist is a physician who specializes in rehabilitation care. The physician in this particular specialty focuses on helping the patient to achieve self-care and on monitoring the functioning of the IDT. Other specialty physicians who play an important role in handling the acute exacerbations experienced by the patient and in monitoring their chronic care include, but are not limited to, cardiologists, orthopedists, neurologists, pulmonologists, urologists, oncologists, and endocrinologists.

Registered Nurse

In many chronic care settings, the RN is the coordinator of care and therefore the coordinator of the IDT. All members play an equal role in the IDT. However, someone must make sure that everyone is staying on track and that members are communicating with one another. It may seem that this should be the primary care provider's role. In fact, in some

settings the nurse practitioner may coordinate the IDT. The primary care provider, however, rarely performs this task. In some settings, the PT or another provider, such as the physiatrist, may be the coordinator. In most settings in which an RN is part of the team, however, the RN coordinates the team.

The RN is typically the constant in patient care, whether the care is in the home setting or in a nursing home. For people who are living at home and are not receiving any skilled care, case management is performed by an independent case management agency or by the insurance case manager. The case manager has a function similar to that of the IDT coordinator. Case management is discussed later.

RNs provide skilled nursing care, such as the administration of medications, wound care, ventilatory care, and other services that RNs are educated and licensed to perform. The RN who works with the person with a chronic illness or disability must be a strong and autonomous critical thinker. The nurse who is new to chronic care, especially home health care, often lacks the experience needed for the autonomous decision making required in home care (Neal, 2001). Typically, nurses who function in community settings in particular do not have readily available resource people on whom to rely when a quick decision is needed. The community health nurse is often in the home setting assessing a patient's status. There are resources available by telephone should she or he have a question about what to do. Unlike in the inpatient setting, however, there is no one within the home to whom the RN can turn for advice and support. Consequently, the nurse must be very knowledgeable, possess excellent assessment skills, be flexible and creative, and know how to find out the information he or she needs to know (Neal, 2001).

The parish or congregational nurse should be mentioned before closing this section on the RN as a member of the IDT. The congregational nurse offers health education and counseling, referral, and health screening to people within her or his spiritual community. Hands-on care is not usually provided (Parker, 2000). The congregational nurse is the perfect liaison between the individual living independently in the community who may require only skilled supervision to maintain independence and the rest of the health care delivery system.

Physical Therapist

The PT is a health care provider who specializes in functional recovery and rehabilitation, particularly improvement of gross motor skills, balance, and gait. PTs evaluate the patient's impairments, functional limitations, and disabilities and develop intervention plans that use therapeutic exercise, manual techniques, functional training, physical agents, and orthotic devices to assist patients in moving toward maximal functional independence.

PTs recommend equipment and assistive devices such as wheelchairs, walkers, and canes to enable patients to navigate their environment with the least reliance on other people but with optimal safety. They usually prescribe a series of exercises carefully designed to assist the patient in improving strength, mobility, and function. PTs are especially important in chronic care programs, because persons with almost any chronic illness or disability can benefit from these services at some point during the course of the illness or disability.

Occupational Therapist

Occupational therapists (OT) often work very closely with PTs. OTs concentrate on enabling the individual to perform the activities of daily living (ADL) and instrumental activities of daily living (IADL) and on refining and enhancing fine motor skills. ADL include basic activities such as bathing, feeding, grooming, toileting, and transferring in and out of a wheelchair or bed. IADL include more advanced activities such as taking transportation, doing laundry, shopping, and telephoning.

OTs also recommend assistive devices and equipment that will help the patient function independently. For instance, they may suggest the use of plate guards so that the patient with hemiplegia can eat without the food sliding off the plate or use of a specialized computer device to assist the legally blind individual or the person with aphasia to communicate with others. OTs also work to strengthen the upper extremities so that the person with a chronic illness or disability is better able to perform ADL and IADL. Table 2-2 differentiates the roles of OTs, PTs, and nurses with regard to motor function.

Speech Pathologist

Speech pathologists or therapists (STs) specialize in speech, swallowing, and memory. Persons with dysphasia or dysphagia work with the ST, using exercises and devices to deal with speech and swallowing impairments that result from stroke, brain injury, or other neurologic or neuromuscular changes. STs also evaluate problems for which the patient

Table 2-2 Differentiation of Therapy and Nursing Roles

Factors Influencing Function	Occupational Therapy	Physical Therapy	Nursing
Sensorimotor function	Evaluation of sensorimotor processing	Evaluation of sensorimotor processing	Assessment of impact of sensorimotor impairments on routines and lifestyle
Neuromuscular function	Evaluation of muscle tone, reflexes, and ROM and their influence on ability to perform ADL and IADL Specialty: arm and hand function	Evaluation of muscle tone, reflexes, and ROM and their influence on performance of ADL and IADL Specialty: mobility and stability of back, hips, legs	Assessment of impact of medical status on movement, self-care, work and home activities
Motor function	Evaluation of gross and fine motor skills, impact of neurologic status on motor function Specialty: fine motor, eye-hand coordination, visual-motor function	Evaluation of gross and fine motor skills and impact of neurologic status on motor function Specialty: gross motor function, balance and equilibrium, coordination	Instruction in use of gross and fine motor skills during daily routines at home and at work
Adaptive equipment	Evaluation and recommendation of positioning equipment based on functional need Specialty: manufacture of hand splints, adaptation of feeding utensils and environment	Evaluation and recommendation of positioning equipment to prevent structural deformity Specialty: training in use of leg braces, orthotics	Instruction in use of positioning equipment at home and at work
Functional movement	Instruction in use of body for communication and self-care Specialty: feeding, toileting, dressing, grooming	Assistance in achieving mobility and walking Specialty: locomotion, walking, body mechanics, energy conservation	Assessment of impact of medical issues on movement at home and at work

Adapted from Hanft B, Sippel K, Pokorni J: *Case management for children with disabilities course,* Atlanta, Ga, May 17-19, 1994, Office of the Surgeon General, U.S. Army Medical Department.
ADL, Activities of daily living; *IADL,* instrumental activities of daily living; *ROM,* range of motion.

may need to be referred to other professionals for further testing and medical treatment.

STs work with people who have experienced memory loss, teaching them techniques such as the use of a memory book in which the person writes down what he or she is doing and what needs to be done so that the person can refer to it later. STs prescribe various exercises to help the person with a memory impairment to recover what is possible of lost memory and to retain what memory the person still has. Families and significant others are also taught how to cope with and best assist the patient with a memory, speech, or swallowing disorder. For example, people who are talking with someone who has a speech impairment have a tendency to try to finish sentences or to anticipate what the person with the impairment will say next. STs teach caregivers to be patient and to allow the person with the impairment plenty of time to speak for themselves.

Medical Social Worker

Medical social workers (MSWs) are professionals who, in the context of chronic care, assist people in managing their financial affairs, obtaining food and medicine, and connecting with community resources that can help them remain out of the hospital. In home health care, for instance, the MSW will become involved in a case if the nurse, therapist, or physician recognizes that the patient is not purchasing medicine because he or she cannot afford it or that the patient and family have complex psychosocial dynamics that are interfering with the effectiveness of care and the management of the patient's illness or disability.

MSWs are very knowledgeable and aware of community resources, such as meal programs and companion or housekeeping services, and work to help the patient and family to be proactive about hiring or using these services. MSWs are also highly trained mental health counselors who assist persons with chronic illnesses or disabilities and their loved ones in adjusting to the changes in lifestyle resulting from the illness or disability.

MSWs may work in the community in a variety of settings or within the inpatient setting. They are excellent discharge planners because they are able to appropriately match patients with a care setting and providers that will best meet the patient's needs. They are especially knowledgeable regarding payers and reimbursement for health care services. They help patients and families work out strategies and plans that will enable them to afford services, food, and medicine over the short and long term.

Dietitian

Dietitians are excellent resources for the other members of the IDT. They provide nutrition counseling to health care professionals, patients, and caregivers. Their recommendations regarding appropriate food and fluid intake are specific for the patient's illness, weight and size, preferences, lifestyle, and socioeconomic status. Nutrition is a highly specialized science and involves calculation of the proper amounts of nutrients for good health or for recovery of health. However, these health care professionals incorporate the person into the diet prescription, because the patient and family are the key members of the team and must adhere to the recommendations if nutritional status is to improve.

Registered dietitians provide consultation regarding enteral and parenteral nutrition as well as oral nutrition. They use various screening tools to identify patients at risk for poor nutrition and educate other health care professionals regarding dietary guidelines and methods of reinforcing good nutrition practices. This is particularly important for persons with a chronic illness, who may lack the ability to adequately process nutrients in food. In addition, because of the energy required to function with a chronic illness or disability, additional and often special food and fluid intake may be required. Registered dietitians prescribe diets that meet the specific needs of the person for healing and optimum energy (Andrews, Gibbons, and Neal, 2002).

Aides

Several types of aides assist health care professionals in providing chronic care. They are vital members of the IDT because they tend to have the most intimacy with the person with the chronic illness or disability. They are often underappreciated, but their care is priceless both to the patient and family and to the rest of the team. Frequently, patients and caregivers will tell aides things they will not tell the professional provider. This is most likely because the aide spends more time with them, and the time spent may involve very personal interactions.

Nurse's aides work under the supervision of the RN. They usually provide personal care, including bathing, grooming, dressing, toileting, and transferring the patient into and out of a wheelchair or bed. The patient tends to develop a close relationship with the nurse's aide over a long period of time. Often, other providers come and go and the patient's needs for skilled care change. However, as long as the patient needs personal care of the nature described, the aide will remain on the team.

PT assistants help PTs to provide PT care. PT assistants work under the supervision of the PT. They may work alone with the patient, but in doing so they carry out the prescribed orders of the PT.

Certified OT assistants help OTs to provide OT services. They reinforce what the OT has taught the patient and family and work under the supervision of the OT.

Pastor or Clergy

The spiritual needs of persons with chronic illness and their families must be considered. The clergy can provide comfort, counseling, leadership, teaching, and advocacy for the patient and family. The clergy may also serve as a source of support to the rest of the team as members struggle with feelings of helplessness and inadequacy. Sometimes, despite their best efforts, team members are unable to help the patient and family to a satisfactory quality of life, and clergy can offer comfort to the health care professionals as well as to nonprofessional caregivers (Easton and Andrews, 2000).

FUNCTION OF THE INTERDISCIPLINARY TEAM

The purpose of the IDT is to provide holistic, well-rounded care to and with the person with a chronic illness or disability. The member of each discipline involved in the case functions within his or her own specialty but confers regularly with the rest of the team, including the primary and specialty physician or nurse practitioner, the patient, and caregivers.

Telephone conversations and face-to-face case conferences and personal conversations are used to communicate the status of the patient from the perspective of each specialty area. The member of each discipline expects that the other team members will reinforce the care he or she has provided and that the goals of care will be mutually agreed upon and attained. As the patient's condition changes physically, emotionally, or environmentally, each team member is updated and, if necessary, goals are revised. Ideally, each team member has his or her own objectives for care that have been reached by consultation with the patient and caregivers. These objectives should fit the ultimate goals that have been designed by the entire team.

In the community setting, just as the primary care provider or specialty provider orders the addition of a new member to the team, the provider must approve the departure of a particular member from the team. Typically, the patient reaches a point at which he or she no longer needs a given service, such as that of the MSW (the financial situation may be stabilized and the patient may have made a connection with community resources). The MSW explains to the patient and caregivers that the objectives have been met and that MSW services are no longer needed and the MSW will discharge the patient from his or her care. The MSW advises the primary care provider and the rest of the team, particularly the team coordinator, that the social work objectives toward the common goals have been met and that the MSW plans to discharge the patient from social work services. Depending on the setting, the MSW may remain on the team only during the time that "skilled" services are provided. In the inpatient setting, such as in an LTC facility, the resident will continue to receive skilled or custodial care for the duration of stay.

CASE MANAGEMENT

This book does not describe case management in detail. Case management is an area of health care entirely unto itself, and many books and articles have been written about it. It is important to mention it here, however, because many people with chronic illnesses or disabilities use case management to great advantage. The function of the coordinator of the IDT is that of a case manager. The coordinator sees that the team members are working toward common goals, communicating frequently, and documenting their care to ensure that the care will be reimbursed by third parties. The coordinator is typically the last team member off the case, and the coordinator does not discharge the patient until he or she is sure that the patient and family have other resources once skilled care is no longer necessary.

Case managers may also work out of independent agencies or for insurance companies. Independent case managers act as advocates for people with illnesses or disabilities. They help people to navigate the health care delivery system and to get the best and most appropriate health care for their dollars. Insurance company case managers also strive to provide the best care for their patients but are expected to make recommendations that are the most cost effective for the insurance company. Health care providers or their agents must consult insurance company case managers to ensure that the care they are providing to patients is allowed and covered by the insurance plan so that patients are not billed for services for which they had not planned and which they cannot afford.

Case managers work tirelessly for their patients because they must constantly be up to date on the latest coverage, resources, and changes in the health care field in order to best advise their patients. They are a great resource both for the patient and family and for the members of the IDT.

●　　　　●　　　　●

This chapter has discussed the most common settings of care for persons with chronic illnesses or disabilities. As the population of people with chronic illness and disabilities increases, concepts for care settings that are the most comfortable and helpful for people are developing and evolving. Consequently, it is impossible to cover every setting one may encounter.

Throughout this book, the reader will find case studies and case conferences. These are intended to illustrate how the IDT works to assist the person with a chronic illness or disability in incorporating the change into his or her lifestyle. As the reader studies these case conferences, the roles and functions of the team members will become clearer.

REFERENCES

Andrews M, Gibbons R, Neal LJ: Nutrition. In Neal LJ, Rea K, Pearce L, editors: *Core curriculum for home health nursing,* Washington, DC, 2002, Home Health Nurses Association.

Baker B: Old age in brave new settings, *Washington Post*, pp F1, F6, July 16, 2002.

Frantz A: Telehealth. In Neal LJ, Madigan EA, editors: *Core curriculum for home health nursing,* Washington, DC, 2001, Home Health Nurses Association, pp 73-80.

Easton KL, Andrews JC: The roles of the pastor in the interdisciplinary rehabilitation team, *Rehabil Nurs* 25(1):10-2, 2000.

Naik A, DeHaven MJ: Short stays in hospice, *Caring* 20(2):10-3, 2001.

Neal LJ: *On becoming a home health nurse,* Washington, DC, 2001, Home Care University.

Parker BJ: Community and family-centered rehabilitation nursing. In Edwards PA, editor: *The specialty practice of rehabilitation nursing: a core curriculum,* Glenview, Ill, 2000, Association of Rehabilitation Nurses.

Quigley PA: Environment of care and service delivery. In Edwards PA, editor: *The specialty practice of rehabilitation nursing: a core curriculum,* ed 4, Glenview, Ill, 2000, Association of Rehabilitation Nurses, pp 342-9.

CHAPTER 3

Alternative Approaches and Therapies for Chronic Care

Theresa Perfetta Cappello, PhD, RN

OBJECTIVES

After reading this chapter, you should be able to do the following:

- Define complementary and alternative (CAT) therapy
- Describe the use of CAT
- Outline the credentialing and regulation of CAT
- Describe selected CAT modalities and their use in chronic care

In the last decade anecdotal information regarding the efficacy of alternative medicine has sparked immense media coverage in the United States. Prominent magazine stories herald the benefits and pitfalls of healing modalities described as alternative, complementary, integrative, self-help, and self-care, to name a few (Goldstein, 1999).

These stories are eclipsed by Eisenberg's landmark studies on the use of alternative medical therapies by Americans. Eisenberg et al (1998) reported that, in 1990, about one third of American adults had used some form of nontraditional medical care at an estimated cost of $13.7 billion and that visits to alternative practitioners far outnumbered visits to all primary care physicians. Even more startling, more than 70% of patients using nontraditional therapy never mentioned this to their physicians. By 1997, the total out-of-pocket expenditures for nonconventional therapies was estimated at $27 billion, considerably more than expenditures for conventional medical care.

In 1998, the U.S. Congress fully funded the National Center for Complementary and Alternative Medicine (NCCAM). NCCAM's mission is to support rigorous research on complementary and alternative medicine (CAM), to train researchers in CAM, and to disseminate information about which CAM modalities work, which do not, and why. NCCAM's research initiatives focus on clinical laboratory-based research trials and on training and career development for career researchers. NCCAM provides information through a clearinghouse and a website (*http://www.nccam.nih.gov*) in addition to sponsoring conferences and educational programs. NCCAM also publishes research results on CAM efficacy to integrate scientifically proven CAM practices into conventional medicine. The current top research priorities for NCCAM are listed in Box 3-1.

Since the nineteenth century, Western medicine has emphasized the physical aspects of disease. This separation of mind and body has been reinforced by the development of highly specialized and sophisticated techniques for the diagnosis and treatment of disease, the use of antibiotics, and advances in pharmacology, immunology, organ transplantation, and genetics. Western medicine emphasizes cure rather than prevention and is effective in treating acute illness. It is less successful in managing chronic diseases and conditions. Many individuals and families experiencing or living with those who have chronic or developmental disorders recognize that Western medicine is not resolving their health problems; therefore, they are increasingly seeking health care alternatives (Jonas and Levin, 1999).

The dominant Western approach to medicine taught in U.S. medical schools is termed *conventional, biomedical, traditional, allopathic,* or *contemporary* medicine (Hoeman, 2002). This type of medical practice generally uses an approach that reduces the body to its component parts. The body is healthy when the parts work well and unhealthy when the parts break down.

Nontraditional healing practices are called *complementary and alternative therapy (CAT)* or *CAM*. These healing practices come primarily from Eastern medical traditions and include cultural and spiritual practices. CAT is not commonly understood or accepted in Western conventional medicine. Until recently, CAT was not included in U.S. medical school curricula nor recognized by third-party payers in the United States. Many medical schools now offer CAT courses, however, and third-party reimbursement for selected CAT modalities is becoming more common.

The terms *complementary* and *alternative* have been used interchangeably. The confusion created by this mixed terminology has been complicated by the addition of the term *integrative*, coined by Dr. Andrew Weil. For the purposes of this text, *alternative therapy* refers to nontraditional modalities used *instead of* traditional Western medicine and

---

Box 3-1 NCCAM Research Priorities

ARTHRITIS

Studies of mechanisms of action and pharmacology of glucosamine and chondroitin sulfate

ASTHMA AND ALLERGY

Basic and clinical investigations of CAM approaches to treatment and prevention of asthma and allergy

CARDIOVASCULAR DISEASE

Approaches to management of hypertension, heart failure, stroke, and peripheral vascular disease, including studies of the biology of EDTA chelation therapy in animal models

CLIMACTERIC

Endocrinologic and symptomatic effects of popular CAM approaches to menopause and andropause

DIGESTIVE DISEASES

CAM approaches to management of chronic hepatitis, inflammatory bowel disease, and irritable bowel syndrome

IMMUNOLOGY

CAM approaches that purport to enhance or inhibit immune responses

INFECTIOUS DISEASES

Antimicrobial and palliative effects of CAM on infectious diseases, especially HIV infection and AIDS

AIDS, Acquired immunodeficiency syndrome; *CAM,* complementary and alternative medicine; *EDTA,* ethylenediaminetetraacetic acid; *HIV,* human immunodeficiency virus; *NCCAM,* National Center for Complementary and Alternative Medicine.

Box 3-2 Assessment Criteria for Evaluating CAT/CAM Practitioners

- Professional license or credentials
- Records of specific specialty training
- Eligibility for third-party payment
- Requisite years of experience
- Malpractice and liability coverage
- Passage of peer review of practitioner's application and related documents
- Appropriate recording and reporting capabilities
- Passage of on-site review of practitioner's office and operations

CAM, Complementary and alternative medicine; *CAT,* complementary and alternative therapy.

---

complementary therapy refers to nontraditional modalities used *with* traditional Western medicine. *Integrative therapy* refers to nontraditional modalities that are prescribed along with or *blended* with conventional Western medicine by health care practitioners to enhance treatment.

Many CAT providers are associated with organizations that support and credential their practices. Most consumers believe that the credentialing of CAT providers offers some level of assurance that the practitioners are competent and can be trusted to provide quality care. In reality, credentialing of CAT practitioners varies from organization to organization and is only as good as the standards established for the given credentialing process. There is no one credentialing body for CAT practices, and there are no uniform standards for evaluating CAT practitioners.

When a CAT credentialing program such as the National Certification Commission for Acupuncture and Oriental Medicine is assessed, it is important to consider the standards used to evaluate the practitioner. These generally include the optimal level of training and experience for each modality. This information can usually be obtained by contacting specific credentialing agencies. Box 3-2 lists some essential information and documents that can be used in the evaluation process.

Licensing for health care practitioners varies by state. Information on state requirements is usually available from the department of health or the department of public health in each state. Practitioners in some specialties do not need licenses but must have state certification. Professional organizations for specific specialists are excellent sources of information on standards of practice and certification (Box 3-3).

Licensing is important for professional recognition. State licensure instills consumer confidence in the practitioner, indicates a certain level of review, and verifies the training and quality of service of practitioners. Some states do not regulate CAT; however, every state has some educational and training requirements for health care practitioners (Table 3-1). A list of programs and institutions recognized by the state is available from the state specialty regulatory agency. Nationally recognized programs or institutions can be found by contacting the specialty organizations within the discipline. All practitioners should have some form of certification or registration.

The licensure of CAT providers has significantly increased the use of CAT in the United States (Sparber, 2001). Many boards of nursing have established CAT practice as congruent with nursing practice. The Louisiana Board of Nursing has defined CAT as "a broad domain of healing resources that allow registered nurses to promote and/or enhance care supportive to or restorative of life and well-being" (Sparber, 2001, p. 2).

In 2001, Sparber contacted the 53 boards of nursing in the United States, Puerto Rico, and the Virgin Islands to glean information regarding the boards' policies on CAT therapies and nursing practice. He found that 47% of boards of nursing had statements that included CAT. Of the remaining boards, 7 were in the process of developing language regarding CAT and 21 had not addressed the topic but did not discourage CAT practices (Table 3-2).

Box 3-3   Selected Certification and Professional Standards Organizations

- Academy for Guided Imagery (AGI)
- Accreditation Commission for Acupuncture and Oriental Medicine (ACAOM)
- Alternative Medicine Foundation
- American Association of Naturopathic Physicians (AANP)
- American Association of Oriental Medicine (AAOM)
- American Chiropractic Association (ACA)
- American Holistic Nurses Association (AHNA)
- American Massage Therapy Association (AMTA)
- American Naturopathic Medical Association (ANMA)
- American Naturopathic Medical Certification and Accreditation Board (ANMCAB)
- American Organization for Bodywork Therapies of Asia (AOBTA)
- Associated Bodywork and Massage Practitioners (ABMP)
- Ayurvedic Institute
- Council of Colleges of Acupuncture and Oriental Medicine (CCAOM)

- Council on Chiropractic Education (CCE) Commission on Accreditation
- European University of Chinese Medicine (EUCM)–North American College of Acupuncture
- Federation of Chiropractic Licensing Boards (FCLB)
- Healing Touch International
- National Board of Certification for Therapeutic Massage and Bodywork (NBCTMB)
- National Center for Homeopathy (NCH)
- National Certification Commission for Acupuncture and Oriental Medicine (NCCAOM)
- National College of Naturopathic Medicine (NCNM)
- Naturopathic Physicians Acupuncture Academy (NPAA)
- Northwest Institute of Acupuncture and Oriental Medicine (NIAOM)
- Oriental Healing Arts Institute (OHAI)

Nurses are nationally recognized as leaders and gate-keepers for consumers. Nurses working in states that include CAT in the scope of nursing practice are positioned to bridge the gap between traditional therapies and CAT, and to enhance safe and effective use of CAT (Sparber, 2001).

An analysis of CAT use by Eisenberg et al (1998) found that there are two distinct interest groups for CAT. The first group is made up of those proactive individuals who use CAT for prevention, health enhancement, self-help, and self-care. Some of the modalities used by this group include yoga, vitamin and herbal supplements, meditation, and exercise. The second group is composed of those who have chronic illnesses. CAM is used most frequently by this group to reduce symptoms as well as to relieve stress and pain. Reasons individuals choose CAM therapies are listed in Box 3-4.

COMPLEMENTARY THERAPY SYSTEMS
Homeopathy

The word *homeopathy* is derived from the Greek terms *omoios* meaning "the same" and *pathos* meaning "feeling." In the fourth century BC, Hippocrates declared that "through the like, disease is produced, and through the application of the like, it is cured" (Decker, 1999, p. 64). At the end of the eighteenth century, Samuel Hahnemann, a German physician, became known as the father of homeopathy when he began experiments to treat malaria with quinine-containing Peruvian bark. He subsequently experimented with plants, animal products, and minerals and found that they could treat the same symptoms that they caused. He carefully recorded a list of all medications and the indications for their use in the homeopathic *Materia Medica*.

Hahnemann believed that each person possesses a "vital force" that organizes, energizes, and enlivens to keep people healthy. The medicinal effect of homeopathic medicine is to arouse this vital force to eliminate symptoms and therefore effect healing. Homeopathic diagnosis focuses on symptoms that are thought to be the body's attempts to reach homeostasis in the face of illness or disease. Both acute and chronic conditions are treated by very individualized homeopathic treatment regimens. Treatment depends not on diagnosing disease but rather on paying particular attention to the patient's symptoms.

Homeopathic treatments are usually administered in the form of pills or liquids that are placed under the tongue. Preparation of homeopathic remedies requires repeated diluting and shaking of the substance until very little of the active ingredient remains. On evaluation, some homeopathic preparations have been found to contain no molecules of the original remedy. In theory, a person's vital force is sensitive to ultramolecular homeopathic remedies. Homeopathic remedies that are used in conventional medical practice today are nitroglycerin, colchicine, digitalis, and gold salts.

Ullman (2003) reviewed literature referenced in MEDLINE and in nonindexed homeopathic journals reporting clinical trials using homeopathic medications to treat people with acquired immunodeficiency syndrome (AIDS) and those infected with human immunodeficiency virus (HIV). This review concluded that homeopathic medicine is useful as an adjunctive therapy in treating drug-resistant HIV infection. Other researchers comparing homeopathic medicine and acetaminophen for pain control in patients with osteoarthritis found that homeopathic medicine was as effective as acetaminophen but did not have its potential adverse effects (Shealy et al, 1998).

Table 3-1　Health Professionals Regulated by State or Jurisdiction

State or Jurisdiction	Acupuncturists	Chiropractors	Dental Hygienists/Assistants	Dentists	Homeopaths	Medical Assistants	Naturopaths	Nurse Midwives	Dietitians	Optometrists	Pharmacists	Physical Therapists	Physicians—MDs	Physicians—DOs	Physician Assistants	Podiatrists	Practical/Vocational Nurses	Psychologists/Behavioral Therapists	Registered Nurses	Respiratory/Inhalation Therapists	Social Workers	Speech Pathologists
AL	2	2	2	2	—	—	—	2	—	2	2	2	1	1	1	2	2	2	2	2	2	—
AK	2	2	2	2	—	—	2	2	2	2	2	2	1	1	1	1	2	2	2	—	2	—
AZ	2	2	—	2	2	—	2	3	3	2	2	2	1	2	1	2	2	3	2	1	2	2
AR	3	2	2	2	—	—	—	2	—	2	2	2	1	1	1	2	2	2	2	1	2	2
CA	3	2	2	2	—	1	—	2	2	2	2	2	1	2	2	2	2	2	2	2	2	2
CO	3	2	2	2	2	—	2	2	—	2	2	3	1	1	1	2	2	2	2	1	2	—
CT	3	2	2	2	3	3	3	3	3	2	2	2	1	1	2	2	2	2	2	3	3	3
DE	1	2	2	2	—	—	2	2	3	2	2	2	1	1	1	2	2	2	2	1	2	2
DC	2	2	2	2	—	3	2	2	2	2	2	2	1	2	1	2	2	2	2	2	2	—
FL	1	2	2	2	—	—	—	2	1	2	2	2	1	1	1	2	2	2	2	2	2	—
GA	2	2	2	2	—	—	—	2	2	2	2	2	1	1	1	2	2	2	2	1	2	2
GU	2	2	2	2	—	—	2	2	2	2	2	2	1	1	1	1	2	2	2	2	—	2
HI	1	2	2	2	3	—	—	2	—	2	2	1	1	2	1	2	3	2	2	—	3	2
ID	1	1	2	2	3	—	—	2	2	2	2	2	1	1	2	2	2	2	2	1	2	2
IL	1	2	2	2	—	—	3	2	2	2	2	1	1	1	1	2	2	2	2	2	2	—
IN	3	2	2	2	—	2	3	2	2	2	2	1	1	1	1	1	2	2	2	1	2	2
IA	—	1	2	2	—	3	—	2	2	2	2	1	1	1	1	2	2	2	2	2	2	2
KS	3	—	2	2	—	3	—	2	—	2	2	1	1	1	—	2	3	2	2	1	2	2
KY	—	2	—	—	—	—	2	—	2	—	—	2	—	—	1	—	2	—	2	—	—	2
LA	1	2	2	2	—	—	—	2	2	1	2	2	1	1	1	1	2	2	2	1	2	2
ME	2	2	2	2	—	—	3	2	—	2	2	2	1	1	1	2	2	2	2	2	2	2
MD	2	2	2	2	3	—	—	2	—	2	2	1	1	1	1	2	2	2	2	1	2	2
MA	1	2	2	2	—	1	3	2	2	2	2	2	2	2	2	2	2	2	2	2	2	2
MI	—	2	2	2	—	—	—	2	2	2	2	1	1	1	1	1	2	2	2	—	2	2
MN	1	2	2	2	—	—	2	2	—	2	2	2	1	1	1	—	2	2	2	2	2	3
MS	—	2	—	—	—	—	—	2	2	2	2	—	1	1	—	—	2	2	2	2	2	2
MO	—	2	2	2	—	—	—	—	—	2	2	2	1	1	1	1	2	2	2	—	2	2
MT	1	2	2	2	2	—	—	2	—	2	2	2	1	1	1	1	2	2	2	2	—	—
NE	—	—	2	2	—	2	—	2	2	2	2	2	1	1	1	2	2	2	2	—	2	2
NV	—	2	2	2	2	—	2	—	2	2	2	2	1	2	2	2	2	2	2	2	2	2
NH	2	2	2	2	—	—	—	2	2	2	2	2	1	1	1	2	2	2	2	2	—	2

State																						
NJ	2	2	1	—	2	—	—	2	2	2	2	2	2	1	1	2	2	—	2	2	2	2
NM	2	2	2	—	2	—	2	2	2	1	2	2	2	2	2	2	2	—	2	2	2	2
NY	2	2	2	—	2	—	2	2	2	2	2	2	2	1	1	2	2	2	2	2	2	2
NC	—	—	—	—	—	—	—	—	—	—	—	—	—	—	—	—	—	—	—	—	—	—
ND	3	2	2	—	3	3	3	2	2	2	2	2	2	2	2	2	2	3	2	2	2	2
OH	1	2	2	—	—	—	—	2	2	2	2	1	1	2	2	2	2	—	2	1	2	2
OK	—	2	2	—	2	2	2	2	2	2	2	2	2	2	2	2	2	2	2	1	2	2
OR	1	2	2	—	2	2	2	2	2	2	2	1	1	1	1	2	2	2	2	2	1	2
PA	1	2	2	—	2	—	2	2	2	2	2	2	2	2	2	2	2	—	2	2	2	2
PR	1	2	2	—	2	—	—	—	2	2	2	2	2	2	2	2	2	2	2	2	2	2
RI	3	2	2	2	3	3	3	2	2	2	2	2	2	2	2	2	2	2	2	2	2	2
SC	1	2	2	—	2	—	—	2	2	2	2	2	2	2	2	2	1	2	2	1	2	2
SD	—	2	—	—	2	—	2	2	2	1	1	2	2	2	2	1	2	—	2	2	2	2
TN	—	2	2	—	2	3	3	2	2	2	2	1	1	2	2	2	2	—	2	3	2	2
TX	1	2	2	—	3	3	—	2	2	2	2	1	1	2	2	3	2	—	2	2	2	2
UT	2	2	2	—	2	2	—	2	2	2	2	2	2	2	2	2	2	—	2	2	2	2
VT	2	2	1	—	2	1	2	1	1	1	2	1	1	1	1	2	1	3	1	2	1	1
VA	1	1	—	—	2	—	—	—	1	1	1	1	1	1	1	2	1	—	1	2	1	2
VI	—	—	—	—	—	—	—	—	—	—	—	—	—	—	—	—	—	—	—	—	—	—
WA	2	2	2	—	2	3	3	2	2	2	2	2	2	2	2	2	2	3	2	3	3	3
WV	2	2	2	—	2	—	—	2	2	2	2	2	2	2	2	1	2	—	2	2	2	2
WI	3	2	2	—	2	—	—	2	2	2	2	2	2	1	2	2	2	—	2	1	2	2
WY	—	2	2	2	2	—	—	2	2	2	2	1	1	2	2	2	2	—	2	2	2	2

Adapted from Federation of State Medical Boards: Table 46: Health professions regulated by states, *The Exchange*, vol 3, pp 67-8, copyright 2003, the Federation of State Medical Boards of the United States.

1, Regulated by state medical board; 2, regulated by separate or other board; 3, regulated but under no board.

Table 3-2 Positions of State Boards of Nursing on CAT Therapies

Scope of Care Described	States
Permit practice	47% of boards of nursing (N = 25)
	AR, AZ, CA, CT, IA, IL, KS, LA, MA, MD, ME, MO, MS, NC, ND, NH, NV, NY, OH, OR, PA, SD, TX, VT, WV
Under discussion	13% of boards of nursing (N = 7)
	DC, DE, GA, MN, NJ, NM, WA
No formal position	40% of boards of nursing (N = 21)
	AK, AL, CO, FL, GA, HI, ID, IN, KY, MI, MT, OK, PR, RI, SC, TN, UT, VA, VI, WI, WY

From Sparber A: State boards of nursing and scope of practice of registered nurses performing complementary therapies, *Online J Issues Nurs* 6(3), ms 10, Aug 31, 2001, retrieved from *http://www.nursingworld.org/ojin/topic15/tpc15_6.htm* on July 13, 2003.
CAT, Complementary and alternative therapy.

Naturopathic Medicine

Naturopathic medicine is not a particular method of treatment but rather a philosophical approach that stresses health, disease prevention, and patient responsibility rather than disease and disease management. Benedict Lust founded the first school of naturopathic medicine in New York City around 1900. At the same time, James Foster established a similar school in Idaho.

Naturopathic medicine maintains that the body has an innate ability to heal itself and to ward off illness even in stressful environments. The treatment of disease is through the stimulation, enhancement, and support of the inherent healing capacity of each person. Health is believed to exist on a continuum with death at one end and optimal health at the other. The role of the naturopathic physician is to assist in the creation of a healthy internal and external environment that enables balancing of the whole person, including their physical, mental, emotional, and social aspects.

Naturopathic physicians emphasize the doctor-patient relationship, use the least invasive therapy possible, and specify lifestyle changes necessary for healing and health. Naturopathic physicians use clinical nutrition, minor surgery, and botanical, homeopathic, physical, Oriental, and psychological medicine. Principles of naturopathy are shown in Box 3-5.

Sarell, Cohen, and Kahan (2003) conducted a double-blind study involving 171 children 5 to 18 years old who had clinical findings of middle ear infection. Children were randomly assigned to receive treatment with Naturopathic Herbal Extract or anesthetic ear drops, with or without amoxicillin. The researchers found no significant differences between treatment groups in associated symptoms and severity of otitis media. However, pain control after 3 days was better in those treated with Naturopathic Herbal Extract.

Ayurveda

Ayurveda is an intricate system of healing that originated more than 6000 years ago with a group of holy men in India known as the Rishis. The Rishis compiled spiritual books called the *Vedas* or books of wisdom (Decker, 1999). The word *ayurveda* is derived from two Sanskrit words: *ayu* meaning "life" and *veda* meaning "knowledge of" (Bright, 2002). The principle of wholeness of mind, body, and soul is critical in ayurveda. The mind influences the body, and achieving awareness brings about a balance in the body that

---

Box 3-4 Reasons for Using Complementary and Alternative Medicine

■ Pursue therapeutic benefit
■ Seek a degree of wellness not supported in biomedicine
■ Improve quality of life
■ Increase high personal involvement in decision making
■ Believe conventional medicine treats symptoms not underlying cause
■ Believe conventional medical treatments are ineffective
■ Avoid toxicities and/or invasiveness of conventional interventions
■ Decrease use of prescribed healing system as part of cultural background

---

Box 3-5 Principles of Naturopathic Medicine

■ The body has an inherent ability to establish, maintain, and restore health.
■ Illness does not occur without a cause.
■ The cause of illness must be found and removed before a person can completely recover.
■ Therapeutic interventions should be complementary to and synergistic with the healing process. Symptoms should not be suppressed without removing the underlying cause.
■ The doctor-patient relationship has inherent therapeutic value. A major role is to educate and motivate responsibility for health.
■ Good health is created through education and healthy life habits. The ultimate goal is prevention.

creates freedom from illness. Lifestyle is integral to health; therefore, diet, herbs, exercise, sleep, meditation, yoga (Figure 3-1), and purification are important for prevention of disease and self-healing (Bright, 2002).

The five basic energies or elements in ayurveda are the following (Decker, 1999):

1. Ether *(akasha)*
2. Air *(vayu)*
3. Fire *(tejas)*
4. Water *(jala)*
5. Earth *(prthivi)*

Each individual is endowed with a unique pattern of these elements. The five elements are further organized in the body into three combinations of elements known as *doshas: vata* (earth and air), *pitta* (fire and water), and *kapha* (earth and water). Each person has a pattern of *doshas* that characterizes physiologic and psychological functions. A person may have a dominance of one *dosha*, or a combination of two or three *doshas*. The person with a *vata-pitta-kapha dosha* is the most balanced and in harmony with the environment. Optimal health is a state in which the individual finds harmony living with the inborn pattern. Disharmony with the inborn *dosha* causes stress that weakens the body's defenses and may lead

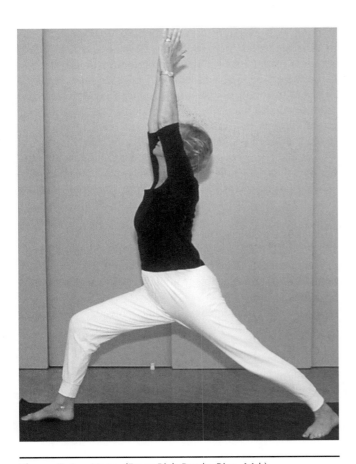

Figure 3-1 Yoga. (From Rick Brady, Riva, Md.)

to disease. The goal of ayurevedic therapy is to balance the *doshas* with the environment. Ayurvedic treatments include but are not limited to meditation, diet, self-massage, herbal therapy, fasting, and aromatherapy.

A review of clinical trials conducted using traditional Indian medicines yielded the following findings (Lodha and Bagga, 2000):

- Curcumin reduced inflammation and disability in patients with rheumatoid arthritis.
- *Pterocarpus marsupium* decreased blood glucose and glycosylated hemoglobin levels in patients with non–insulin dependent diabetes mellitus.
- *Bacopa monnieri* significantly improved short-term and long-term memory in children with mental retardation.

Traditional Chinese Medicine

Traditional Chinese medicine (TCM) is the oldest formalized coherent system of medicine practiced in the world. The Yellow Emperor, Huang Di, born in 2697 BC, is credited with being the father of TCM. His text the *Huang Di Nei Jing* is the first classic work on TCM. It is divided into two books: the *Simple Questions* describes medical theory, and the *Spiritual Axis* describes acupuncture, the use of needles on points of the body for pain relief and treatment of health conditions.

The fundamental concepts or basic theories of TCM begin with *yin* and *yang,* terms that express direct opposites but complementary phenomena in a state of equilibrium (Bright, 2002). Yin refers to dark, inactive, and cold, whereas yang refers to heat, movement, and external body. These opposites represent all things in nature and the body. Health in the body is assured only when yin and yang are in equilibrium. Yin and yang are not absolute but relative, exist in dependence on one another, and can transform into one another (Bright 2002; Jonas and Levin, 1999; Micozzi, 1996).

The five phases or five elements, *wu xing,* are based on the TCM concept that all in the universe consists of five elements: wood, fire, metal, water, and ether or earth. In TCM, the *wu xing* are in a dynamic relationship with the seasons, directions, weather, colors, tastes, and organs of the body, as well as the emotions and the voice.

The major components in TCM are *qi* (universal life energy), blood, body fluid, the internal organs, and the meridians, or pathways through which *qi* travels throughout the body. *Qi* has five general functions: to promote, warm, defend, govern, and transform. Within the body, blood and *qi* are closely related because blood is thought to contain *qi* and flows with it (Micozzi, 1996). *Qi* and blood are essential for life. Body fluids are the liquids produced by the body: saliva, urine, sweat, tears, and semen. Many organs are influential in the production and distribution of body fluids. The internal organs are the solid organs—heart, liver, spleen, lungs, and kidneys—and the hollow organs—stomach, gallbladder, large and small intestines, and urinary bladder. One organ, the triple burner, has a physiologic function in TCM but no physical form. The triple burner is thought to circulate and eliminate fluids.

In TCM the spirit encompasses both a healthy mind and physical function. The notion of a separation between mind and body does not exist in TCM. It is understood that what happens in the mind, or the emotions, is expressed in the body; for example, joy is related to the heart (Micozzi, 1996).

Illness is caused in the body by a disturbance of *qi*. Diseases are classified as due to internal imbalance, external imbalance, or neither internal nor external imbalance. There are six external factors: wind, cold, dryness, summer heat, dampness, and fire. The seven internal factors include anger, melancholy, worry, grief, fear, fright, and joy. The noninternal, nonexternal factors are dietary irregularities, excessive sexual activity, physical taxation or fatigue, trauma, and parasites. Any imbalance of these factors may cause disease.

In TCM diagnosis is made using the following:
- Inspection
- Listening and smelling
- Inquiry
- Palpation

Inspection includes visual inspection of the person's spirit through examination of the form and bearing of the head and face, the eyes, overall appearance, complexion, and quality of the voice (Micozzi, 1996). Another major component of inspection is observation of the tongue, including its color, shape, markings, moisture, and coating.

Listening and smelling involves odors of the breath, body, and excreta, including urine when warm and cold. The quality of the person's voice, speech, and breath are evaluated, as are any abnormal sounds such as wheezes or coughs.

A comprehensive medical history is taken and a thorough description of presenting symptoms is obtained. In addition, individuals are questioned about sleep, diet, bowel movements, urination, appetite, dreams, sensations of hot and cold, perspiration, hearing, thirst, status of the head and neck, status of the trunk and limbs, emotions, pain, exposure to cold, and headache.

Palpation includes general palpation of the body, the pulse, and the acupuncture points. Body palpation includes tactile sensing to evaluate heat, cold, hardness, tenderness, softness, masses, and other abnormalities. Pulse palpation can reveal a great deal about the person's condition. The practitioner places three fingers on the radial arteries on both the right and left wrists. Each hand has three pulse locations corresponding to particular organs of the body.

The most important principle of TCM is the prevention of disease. Once symptoms of disease appear, however, the goal is to treat the symptoms to head off disease. If a person has a serious or acute illness, the goal of treatment is to reduce or eliminate the symptoms and then to treat the underlying disease. The goal is to balance yin and yang, and to eliminate any blocks to the flow of *qi*.

After diagnosis, treatments may include acupuncture, Chinese herbs, massage, dietary therapy, and acupressure.

The NCCAM supports two specialty research centers at which scientists are investigating acupuncture therapy. Researchers at the University of Maryland in Baltimore found that patients treated with acupuncture after dental surgery had less pain than those who received a placebo. They also found that older patients with osteoarthritis experienced less pain when acupuncture was combined with conventional therapy.

A randomized, blinded study was conducted at the university hospital in Vienna, Austria, to determine the effects of auricular acupressure as a treatment for anxiety in patients transported to the hospital via ambulance. Patients in the acupressure group reported significantly less anxiety on arrival at the hospital, reported less pain, and were more positive about their treatment outcomes than those in the group receiving a sham acupressure procedure (Kober et al, 2002).

MIND-BODY THERAPY

For centuries Eastern philosophical medical traditions, steeped in holism, have noted the connection of mind, body, and spirit. Not until 1974, however, in a laboratory at the University of Rochester School of Medicine and Dentistry, did modern research on the mind-body connection begin with an accidental discovery. Robert Adler, conducting a classic pavlovian conditioning experiment to teach rats to respond with aversion to saccharine-flavored water, found that the immune system in the rats developed a conditioned response. Adler gave the rats saccharine-flavored water and at the same time injected them with a nausea-inducing drug. Just one injection of the drug produced conditioning. He then noted that the once-healthy young rats began dying. Examining his results, he found that the rats' immune systems had been suppressed—specifically, the number of T cells had been reduced—which rendered the rats vulnerable to infection. Adler successfully replicated the study, demonstrating the connection between the brain and the bone marrow manufacturing T cells (Goleman and Gurin, 1993). Adler's studies sparked the development of the new science of psychoneuroimmunology. The very complicated and not well understood connection between the mind and the neuroendocrine, hormonal, and immune systems is currently under investigation to identify how this connection functions.

Psychoneuroimmunology has the potential to improve health and quality of life. When used in conjunction with traditional allopathic treatments, the mind-body interventions such as meditation, prayer, relaxation techniques, social support groups, imagery, visualization, hypnotherapy, and humor have great potential to improve emotional and physical health.

Hypnotherapy was offered to 303 patients who complained of persistent asthma, chest pain and pressure, habitual cough, hyperventilation, shortness of breath, sighing, and vocal cord dysfunction. Patients were treated over a 30-month period at a pediatric pulmonary center. Hypnotherapy was associated with improvement of symptoms in 80% of cases. No patients developed new symptoms following hypnotherapy. The researcher concluded that this rapid improvement of symptoms in these patients was unlikely without hypnotherapy (Anbar, 2002).

Taylor and Ingleton (2003) investigated the use of hypnotherapy to treat the emotional distress associated with cancer. Their qualitative analysis of interviews with patients following 12 sessions of hypnotherapy demonstrated that patients had acquired skills necessary to cope with invasive medical procedures and other traumas they faced.

A pilot study of the efficacy of mindfulness-based stress reduction in improving quality of life for individuals suffering from traumatic brain injuries was reported in 2003. Researchers found that after 12 weeks of group sessions using insight meditation, breathing exercises, guided visualization, and group discussion, patients' mean quality-of-life scores improved, they experienced improvements in the cognitive-affective domain, and they reported less stress and depression (Bedard et al, 2003).

BIOLOGICAL- AND CHEMICAL-BASED THERAPY

Biological-based treatments arouse the most controversy among CAT modalities. These treatments use active biologic or chemical compounds that are promised to provide everything from weight loss to a cure for AIDS and cancer. These treatments are often invasive and may be given by intravenous (IV) injection, taken orally, or inhaled. There is considerable concern about the safety and efficacy of many of these treatments, because serious medical research to substantiate claims is lacking for most. Of particular concern is that persons suffering from serious illness may reject conventional medical treatments. NCCAM has funded studies of many promising biological-based treatments such as shark cartilage therapy.

Shark Cartilage Therapy

Shark cartilage is a dietary supplement used as a cancer treatment. Interest in shark cartilage was intensified when Lane and Cormac (1992) wrote *Sharks Don't Get Cancer.* Shark cartilage contains a substance that inhibits blood vessel growth and is thus believed to protect sharks from cancer. In reality, sharks do get cancer; however, the antiangiogenic properties of shark cartilage impair tumor growth. Given orally or by retention enema, shark cartilage does not inhibit the growth of normal cells. Although research by Feyzi, Hassan, and Mostafaie (2003) on the effects of shark cartilage on tumor immune response support continued investigation of the use of shark cartilage for cancer therapy, no definitive studies exist on the efficacy of shark cartilage in treating cancer. Concern regarding the purity of preparations, expense of the product, and difficulty in administration of large doses confounds its use.

Chelation Therapy

In chelation therapy the synthetic amino acid ethylenediaminetetraacetic acid (EDTA) is used to remove heavy metals such as lead, copper, mercury, iron, aluminum, and calcium from the body. EDTA was approved by the Food and Drug Administration in 1950 for the treatment of heavy metal poisoning. When given IV, the compound binds with the metal and is excreted through urine. CAT uses for EDTA were found when follow-up of individuals who had been treated for lead poisoning revealed improvement in angina and intermittent claudication as well as improved memory and problem-solving ability. Decker (1999) reported that patients with the circulatory problem of intermittent claudication showed marked improvement following chelation therapy. Although chelation therapy has been found to lower levels of lipids and triglycerides and to increase blood flow throughout the body, the Food and Drug Administration has not approved EDTA for uses other than treatment of heavy metal toxicity.

Chelation therapy requires IV infusions lasting 3 hours; approximately 30 treatments are needed over 3 to 5 months, at an average cost of $3000. A licensed physician must administer the therapy; however, a nurse may insert the peripheral venous line. Dosage and protocol for the administration is individualized with special consideration for age, sex, weight, and renal function (Decker, 1999). Most insurance companies deny reimbursement for EDTA therapy.

In patients with thalassemia major, long-term survival is limited because of cardiac complications of transfusional siderosis. In a study involving eight thalassemia major patients with cardiac complications, chelation therapy with deferoxamine was found to be successful in decreasing mean ferritin blood levels and resolving cardiac arrhythmias (Miskin et al, 2003).

Aromatherapy

Aromatherapy has been used for healing the mind, body, and spirit since ancient times. The first recorded uses of aromatherapy were in Egypt, Mesopotamia, and China around 3000 BC (Hill, 1997). Aromatherapy is the use of essential oils extracted from flowers, plants, and herbs for inhalation and direct application to the skin through massage, baths, compresses, salves, creams, and gels. Aromatherapy became popular in the 1930s when René-Maurice Gattefosse, a French chemist, began experimenting with the healing properties of essential oils. While working in his family's factory, Gattefosse burned his hand and immediately submerged it into lavender oil for relief. He found that his burn healed quickly and without scarring (*Nurse's handbook*, 1999).

Aromatic compounds are termed *essential* because the fragrance represents the plant's inner nature. Each essence is endowed with a unique property for assisting in the healing process. To render essential oils, the relevant parts of plants are distilled. Distillation captures the odoriferous substances that can be used for massage, worn as perfume, added to water in aromatic baths, inhaled, or diffused. Once in the body, essential oils may interact with hormones and enzymes to produce physiologic and psychological changes such as relaxation, decreased blood pressure, and slowed pulse.

The specific mechanism of action is not understood; however, activation of the olfactory nerve is thought to stimulate the limbic system, which communicates with the hypothalamus and pituitary gland to further stimulate the immune system.

Essential oils have many actions. For example, citronella repels bugs, and eucalyptus decreases sinus and lung congestion. Table 3-3 identifies specific effects associated with essential oils.

Several recent studies have concluded that aromatherapy is useful in the management of agitation in patients with dementia. In one study, aromatherapy with lavender oil was used to treat 15 patients meeting the International Classification of Diseases-10 diagnostic criteria for severe dementia. Results of this study showed an improvement in nine patients, a change in five patients, and worsening of symptoms in one patient (Holmes et al, 2002). In a second study, 72 patients with agitation of severe dementia were randomly assigned to aromatherapy with melissa essential oil or placebo. The researchers concluded that aromatherapy was effective in treating clinically significant agitation in people with severe dementia, with the additional benefit of improved quality of life (Ballard et al, 2002).

MANIPULATIVE AND BODY-BASED THERAPIES

CAT involving the use of hands on or above the body, also called manual therapy or biofield intervention, had its beginnings in ancient times. Manual therapies incorporate the holistic concepts of mind, body, and spirit and enhance health by promoting relaxation, soothing muscles, reducing pain, and stimulating circulation.

There are many body-based therapies, including movement repatterning techniques using Alexander, Feldenkrais and Trager methods; the adjustment-based techniques of applied kinesiology and chiropractic; the pressure-based techniques of massage, rolfing, and reflexology; and the energetic healing techniques of therapeutic touch, healing touch, acupuncture, acupressure, and reiki. Those covered here are the Alexander technique, reflexology, and reiki.

Table 3-3 Essential Oils and Their Effects

Oil	Promotes Relaxation	Promotes Concentration	Eases Depression	Increases Energy	Aids Insomnia	Promotes Immune Function	Eases Inflammation	Fights Colds	Eases Headache
Angelica		X							
Basil	X		X	X					X
Bergamot		X							
Black spruce									
Cardamom		X							
Chamomile	X		X		X		X		X
Cinnamon		X		X			X	X	
Clove		X					X	X	
Eucalyptus				X			X		
Frankincense	X		X						
Geranium									
Ginger		X							
Jasmine	X		X	X					
Lavender	X		X		X		X		X
Lemon			X		X	X			
Lemon grass			X	X					
Mandarin	X								
Neroli	X								
Orange			X		X	X		X	
Peppermint		X	X	X				X	X
Petit grain	X								
Rose	X								
Rosemary							X		
Sage		X							
Sandalwood	X								
Ylang-ylang					X				

Alexander Technique

The Alexander technique is defined as reeducation of the mind and body (Goldberg, 2002). It is a method for releasing unnecessary tension in the body by reeducating the interaction of the head, neck, and trunk. Habitually overtightened muscles are thought to cause distortion in the body leading to compression and imbalance. The Alexander technique focuses on improving awareness of movement and releasing unnecessary muscular tension in the head, neck, and back. Reducing tension reduces the pain and discomfort associated with habitual tightening of muscles.

Matthias Alexander, the father of the technique, was an actor in Australia in the late 1800s. Alexander frequently lost his voice during performances and was convinced that his problem was caused by the way he used his muscles. While experimenting with his own body, he found that contracting the muscles in his head and neck and down his back affected his voice. He began to use postures that relieved the muscular tension and his voice problems disappeared. With this personal success, he began teaching the Alexander technique as a method of vocal training for singers and actors of the time. His students found that Alexander's method of reeducation helped with their respiratory difficulties and other physical problems (Decker, 1999).

The Alexander technique is still popular with performing artists and is used primarily for prevention and relaxation to enhance posture and improve performance (*Nurse's handbook*, 1999). It is thought to be effective in chronic care for neck and back pain, breathing problems, anxiety, myalgia, and hypertension.

The effects of using the Alexander technique on the management of disability and feelings of depression in patients with Parkinson's disease were evaluated with four self-report questionnaires. The Beck Depression Inventory as well as questionnaires on activities of daily living, body concept, and social functioning disability were used. The findings of this study showed that patients with Parkinson's disease experienced significantly less depression, had a more positive body concept, and had less difficulty performing activities of daily living after studying the technique than before they learned the technique (Stallibrass, 1997).

Reflexology

The practice of reflexology can be traced to ancient Egypt, China, and India. The modern precursor to reflexology, zone theory, originated in the early 1900s with Dr. William Fitzgerald, an ear, nose, and throat specialist working in Boston and Connecticut. He found that applying pressure to terminal points of nerves achieved pain relief and analgesia. He further discovered that this same pressure relieved the underlying cause of the pain. In 1917, Fitzgerald and Dr. Edwin Bowers wrote *Relieving Pain at Home* describing zone therapy.

Bright (2002) defines reflexology as a massage technique that promotes unblocking of a terminal nerve reflex to improve function associated with that particular reflex pathway.

Fitzgerald worked closely with Eunice Ingham, a physical therapist who developed her foot reflex theory in 1930. Ingham determined that the reflexes on the hands and feet are mirror images of the organs and glands of the body and developed the present map showing the body parts associated with the various reflex areas on the hands and feet (Figure 3-2). In the 1970s Ingham's nephew, Dwight Byers, began working with her, and after her death, he consolidated her teaching through the International Institute of Reflexology.

The exact mechanism of action of reflexology is not known. Manipulation of the reflex zones is thought either to stimulate balance as occurs with acupuncture, or to reduce lactic acid in the feet and break up calcium crystals that accumulate on the nerve endings (Bright, 2002).

Offered in many health clubs and spas, reflexology is used to treat hypertension, muscle tension, premenstrual syndrome, anxiety, pain, eczema, gastrointestinal disorders, migraines, and asthma, and to promote relaxation.

Stephenson, Weinrich, and Tavokili (2000) studied the effects of reflexology on anxiety and pain in patients with breast and lung cancer. Thirty minutes of foot reflexology treatment was provided to 23 patients. This study found a significant decrease in anxiety in patients with breast and lung cancer following foot reflexology, and breast cancer patients experienced less pain following the treatment.

Reiki

Reiki is a Japanese word meaning "universal life energy." The use of energy to heal has been practiced throughout the ages. Chinese call this energy *qi*, Hawaiians *mana*, and Christians *breath of life;* in Sanskrit it is know as *prana*. Reiki can be traced to Japan and Tibetan *Sutras* and Buddhism. In the 1800s, Mikao Usui began searching for information about the healing ability of Jesus and Buddha. Mastering the ancient language of Sanskrit, he found information in the Tibetan Lotus *Sutras*. He took his healing ability to the slums of Kyoto, Japan, and spent the rest of his life healing and teaching reiki. On Usui's death, Dr. Chujiro Hayashi, a retired naval officer, established a reiki clinic in Japan. In 1935, a woman named Takata received treatment and attunement in reiki at the Hayashi clinic. She immigrated to the United States and passed on the reiki tradition to her granddaughter and others. Since that time, thousands of people have received training and attunement, and it is impossible to estimate the number of reiki masters in the United States

Reiki involves the "laying on of hands" and is used to connect the "universal life energy" with the body's innate power of healing (Rivera, 1999). The laying on of hands transfers life energy through the reiki master into the person being treated. The receiver of energy can never take in too

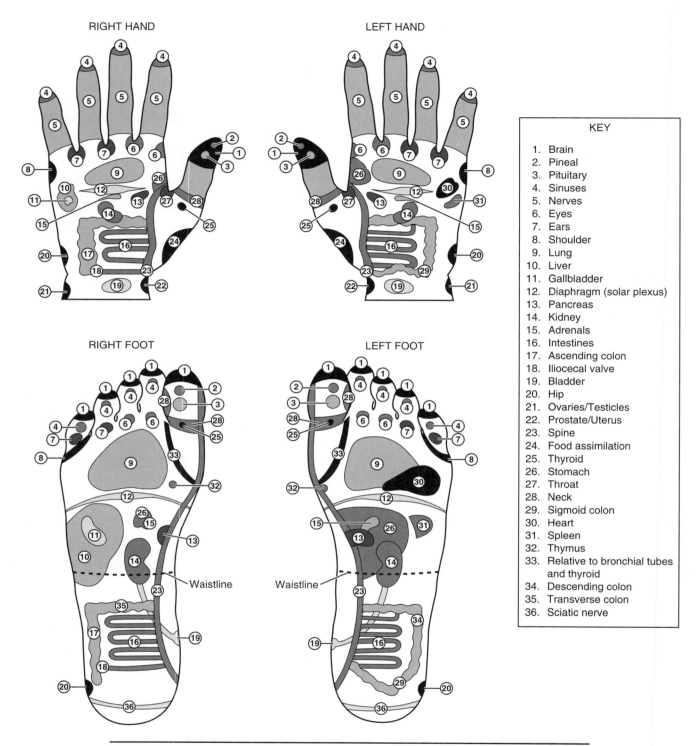

Figure 3-2 Reflexology maps.

much energy, and the practitioner never loses energy. Reiki energy goes to where it is needed in the receiver's body.

Reiki therapy is useful for promoting relaxation, overcoming fear, treating phobias, decreasing anxiety, promoting wound healing, reducing blood loss during surgery, improving postoperative recovery, and diminishing scar tissue. In chronic conditions, reiki is useful in treating headaches, colds and influenza, cancer, HIV and AIDS; in managing pain; and in helping the individual cope with the emotional stress of terminal illness. In everyday life, reiki is helpful in reducing tiredness and in increasing confidence and self-esteem.

The effects of reiki on stress and anxiety were studied in a convenience sample of 23 healthy subjects. Stress reduction was measured using a state anxiety scale, salivary immunoglobulin A levels, cortisol levels, blood pressure, galvanic skin response, muscle tension, and skin temperature. Researchers concluded that both biochemical and physiologic changes indicated stress reduction in these subjects in response to treatment (Wardell and Engebretson, 2001).

ETHICAL CONSIDERATIONS

Because of the limited number of studies to date related to complementary and alternative therapies and the fact that the findings of these studies are inconclusive, providers must carefully advise patients regarding these modalities. Providers must respect individual autonomy and cultural diversity and, at the same time, protect patients from harm as much as possible (Kaler and Ravella, 2002). Both traditional and nontraditional therapies can be harmful. The danger with CAM and CAT is potentially greater, however, because much of it is not regulated. Herbs, for example, are not controlled by the Food and Drug Administration, so individuals cannot be sure about the strength or purity of the substances they are taking. Furthermore, they are often unaware of the potential dangers associated with mixing herbs with traditional medications, and providers are unaware that herbs are being taken. The providers' ethical responsibility is to be aware of all the therapies, remedies, herbs, and medications being used by individuals under their care. Box 3-6 lists some common herbs and their potentially adverse effects.

Box 3-6   Potentially Adverse Effects of Common Herbs

HERBS THAT RAISE BLOOD PRESSURE
Bayberry, broom, cayenne, ephedra, ginger, ginseng, kola, licorice, St. John's wort

HERBS THAT LOWER BLOOD PRESSURE
Aconite, arnica, barberry, black cohosh, goldenseal, hawthorn, mistletoe, quinine, shepherd's purse

HERBS THAT CAUSE HYPOKALEMIA
Celery, dandelion, juniper, kava kava root, parsley

HERBS THAT ARE ANTICOAGULANTS
Alfalfa, angelica, anise, bilberry, birch, cat's claw, celery, coleus, fenugreek, feverfew, garlic, ginger, ginkgo, ginseng, green tea, red clover, turmeric, white willow

HERBS THAT ARE CARDIOTONIC
Dogbane, foxglove, ginseng, hawthorn, immortal, lily of the valley, lime, mistletoe, motherwort

---

IMPLICATIONS FOR PROVIDERS

Traditional Western medicine is grounded in an approach that separates body from mind. CAT follows a holistic paradigm. Both systems of thought have risks and benefits. Providers must become knowledgeable about CAT so that they can offer their patients the best care possible and help them make informed decisions. Providers should do the following:

- Become knowledgeable about the state of the science related to CAT
- Encourage patients to discuss all of their health care practices
- Ask what the patient believes the CAM treatments will do and how they will be helpful
- Remain nonjudgmental and open to new ideas
- Discuss the risks and benefits of traditional and nontraditional therapies
- Educate patients about the dangers involved in combining therapies and encourage them to inform their provider before doing so
- Advocate for reform in payment systems
- Advocate for practice standards for CAM and regulation of product manufacturing

Internet and Other Resources

Alternative Medicines (Federal Trade Commission): *http://www.ftc.gov/bcp/conline/pubs/health/whocares/altmeds.ht*
Clinical trials (National Institutes of Health): *http://clinicaltrials.gov/*
Cochrane Collaboration Complementary Medical Field Registry of Controlled Trials: *http://www.compmed.umm.edu/cochrane/Field.html*
Commission on Dietary Supplement Labels: *http://web.health.gov/dietsupp/*
Federation of State Medical Boards of the United States: *http://www.fsmb.org*
Healthology: *http://healthology.com/*
Herb Research Foundation: *http://www.herbs.org*
Homeopathic Educational Services: *http://www.homeopathic.com*
National Center for Complementary and Alternative Medicine (NCCAM): *http://nccam.nih.gov/*
Office of Cancer Complementary and Alternative Medicine: *http://www3.cancer.gov/occam/*
U.S. Food and Drug Administration: *http://www.fda.gov*

REFERENCES

Anbar RD: Hypnosis in pediatrics: application at a pediatric pulmonary center, *BMC Pediatr* 2(1):11, 2002.

Ballard CG et al: Aromatherapy as safe effective treatment for the management of agitation in severe dementia: the results of a double-blind, placebo-controlled trial with melissa, *J Clin Psychiatry* 63(7):553-8, 2002.

Bedard M et al: Pilot evaluation of a mindfulness-based intervention to improve quality of life among individuals who sustained traumatic brain injuries, *Disabil Rehabil* 25(13):722-31, 2003.

Bright MA: *Holistic health and healing*, Philadelphia, 2002, FA Davis.

Decker GM: *An introduction to complementary alternative therapies*, Pittsburgh, 1999, Oncology Nursing Press.

Eisenberg DM et al: Trends in alternative medicine use in the United States, 1990-1997, *JAMA* 280(18):1569-75, 1998.

Feyzi R, Hassan ZM, Mostafaie A: Modulation of CD4+ and CD8+ tumor infiltrating lymphocytes by a fraction isolated from shark cartilage: shark cartilage modulates anti-tumor immunity, *Int Immunopharmacol* 3(7):921-6, 2003.

Fitzgerald W, Brown E: *Zone therapy or relieving pain at home,* Whitehall, Mont, 2003, Kessler Publishing (originally published in 1917).

Goldberg M: The FM Alexander technique, 2002, retrieved from *www.alexandercenter.com/index.html#1Anchor* on Jan 25, 2004.

Goldstein MS: *Alternative health care: medical miracle or mirage,* Philadelphia, 1999, Temple University Press.

Goleman D, Gurin J: *Mind body medicine: how to use our mind for better health,* Yonkers, NY, 1993, Consumer Reports Books.

Hill C: *The ancient and healing art of aromatherapy,* Berkeley, Calif, 1997, Ulysses Press.

Hoeman SP: *Rehabilitation nursing: process application, and outcomes,* ed 3, St Louis, 2002, Mosby.

Holmes C et al: Lavender oil as a treatment for agitated behavior in severe dementia: a placebo controlled study, *Int J Geriatr Psychiatry* 17(4):305-8, 2002.

Jonas WB, Levin JS: *Essentials of complementary and alternative medicine,* Philadelphia, 1999, Lippincott, Williams & Wilkins.

Kaler M, Ravella P: Staying on the ethical high ground with complementary and alternative medicine, *Nurse Pract* 27(7):38-42, 2002.

Kober A et al: Prehospital analgesia with acupressure in victims of minor trauma: a prospective randomized, double-blinded, trial, *Anesth Analg* 95:723-7, 2002.

Lane IW, Cormac L: *Sharks don't get cancer,* Garden City Park, NY, 1992, Avery.

Lodha R, Bagga A: Traditional Indian systems of medicine, *Ann Acad Med Singapore* 29(1):37-41, 2000.

Micozzi MS: *Fundamentals of complementary and alternative medicine,* New York, 1996, Churchill Livingstone.

Miskin H et al: Reversal of cardiac complications in thalassemia major by long term intermittent daily intensive iron chelation, *Eur J Hematol* 70(6):398-403, 2003.

Nurse's handbook of alternative and complementary therapies, Springhouse, Pa, 1999, Springhouse Corp.

Rivera CR: Reiki therapy: a tool for wellness, *Imprint,* pp 31-3, Feb/March 1999.

Sarrell EM, Cohen HA, Kahan E: Naturopathic treatment of ear pain in children, *J Fam Pract* 52(9):673-6, 2003.

Shealy CN et al: Osteoarthritic pain: a comparison of homeopathy and acetaminophen, *Am J Pain Manage* 8:89-91, 1998.

Sparber A: State boards of nursing and scope of practice of registered nurses performing complementary therapies, *Online J Issues Nurs* 6(3), ms 10, Aug 31, 2001, retrieved from *http://www.nursingworld.org/ojin/topic15/tpc15_6.htm* on July 13, 2003.

Stallibrass C: An evaluation of the Alexander technique for the management of disability in Parkinson's disease—a preliminary study, *Clin Rehabil* 11(1):8-12, 1997.

Stephenson NL, Weinrich SP, Tavakoli AS: The effects of foot reflexology on anxiety and pain in patients with breast and lung cancer, *Oncol Nurs Forum* 27(1):67-72, 2000.

Taylor EE, Ingleton C: Hypnotherapy and cognitive-behavior therapy in cancer care: the patient's view, *Eur J Cancer Care* 12(2):137-42, 2003.

Ullman D: Controlled clinical trials evaluating homeopathic treatment of people with human immunodeficiency virus or acquired immune deficiency syndrome, *J Altern Complement Med* 9(1):133-41, 2003.

Wardell DW, Engebretson J: Biological correlates of reiki touch (sm) healing, *J Adv Nurs* 33(4):439-45, 2001.

CHAPTER **4**

Disorders of the Eyes

Sharron Guillett, PhD, RN

OBJECTIVES

After reading this chapter you should be able to do the following:

■ Describe the pathophysiology of age-related macular degeneration, cataracts, diabetic retinopathy, and glaucoma
■ Describe the clinical manifestations of age-related macular degeneration, cataracts, diabetic retinopathy, and glaucoma
■ Describe the functional health patterns affected by conditions that cause blindness or visual impairment
■ Describe the role of each member of the interdisciplinary team involved in the care of patients with blindness, low vision, and the specific chronic disorders of age-related macular degeneration, cataracts, diabetic retinopathy, and glaucoma
■ Describe the indications for use, side effects, and nursing considerations related to drugs commonly used to treat chronic disorders of the eye

Approximately 14 million Americans have some form of visual impairment. Of these, about half are elderly people living in nursing homes (American Foundation for the Blind, 2003). The number of people with low vision is expected to grow as the population ages. Close to 1.5 million people report being legally blind; about 10% of these are unable to perceive light.

Low vision is a term used to describe a condition in which the individual has some usable vision but a visual impairment exists that cannot be fully corrected by medical, surgical, or optical means. For the purposes of this chapter, the following definitions are used:

• Blindness—inability to perceive light
• Legal blindness—central visual acuity of 20/200 in the better eye with the best possible correction
• Visual impairment—functional limitation in seeing; in severe cases, inability to discern words or letters

Low vision can be caused by a number of conditions such as diabetes and stroke. It can also result from specific eye conditions such as glaucoma, macular degeneration, and cataracts.

The cost of providing care and services for people with impaired vision is over $20 billion per year. Aside from the financial costs, people with impaired vision report personal costs related to the physical, emotional, and social changes in their lives. Many of the causes of low vision can be treated so that maximal vision is retained. Health care providers who work with individuals to prevent vision loss and promote independence include ophthalmologists, optometrists, low vision specialists, orthoptists, visual rehabilitation therapists, occupational therapists, and nurses.

ASSESSMENT

Standard vision assessment includes a test of visual acuity as well as a general evaluation of eye structures and a funduscopic examination using an ophthalmoscope. Visual acuity is generally tested using the Snellen eye chart (Figure 4-1). If the patient being examined does not recognize standard English letters, then an "E" chart is used in which the E faces right, left, up, or down and the patient is asked to detect which way the E is pointing (Figure 4-2). If the patient is unable to see the chart, then the examiner asks the patient to count the number of fingers being held up. If the patient cannot count fingers, then the examiner waves a hand and asks the patient if he or she can detect hand motion. Visual acuity is recorded for each eye and is expressed as the number 20 (representing the distance [in feet] at which a normally sighted person sees the test types) over the distance the person being examined sees them. For example, 20/20 acuity means that the person can see at a distance of 20 ft what a normally sighted person can see at a distance of 20 ft. Acuity of 20/200 means that the individual can see at a distance of 20 ft what a normally sighted person can see at a distance of 200 ft. Therefore, the larger the bottom number, the worse the person's vision. In the medical record, visual acuity is written as:

$$Va < \frac{20/20}{20/40}$$

The upper set of numbers represents vision in the right eye, and the lower set of numbers represents vision in the left eye. An examination by an ophthalmologist generally includes measurement of intraocular pressure and may require the use of eye drops to dilate the pupil so that a thorough examination of the retina can be completed.

35

A number of systemic diseases and syndromes have ocular manifestations (Box 4-1). Health care providers should familiarize themselves with these manifestations and be certain to include an assessment of vision and ocular structures when patients come to them with these systemic conditions.

Not all ocular conditions or changes have associated visual deficits. For example, many changes associated with aging have no affect on vision (Box 4-2). Similarly, some

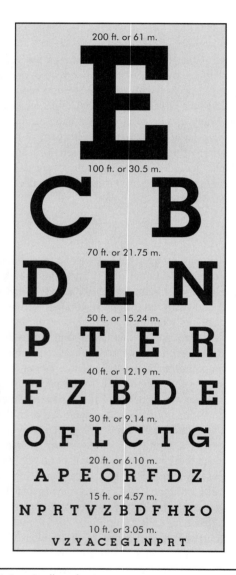

Figure 4-1 Snellen chart.

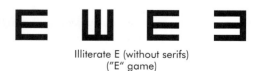

Illiterate E (without serifs)
("E" game)

Figure 4-2 Modified Snellen chart using an E without serifs.

patients with early diabetic retinopathy may not notice any visual changes. All functional health patterns are likely to be affected by an alteration in vision, however, and a focused assessment must be carefully completed, with screening for any deficits and evaluation of the impact of those deficits (Box 4-3). Depending on the level of visual impairment and degree of adjustment by the patient and family, home care services may or may not be necessary. Certainly, the individual who is newly impaired will need significant support, guidance, education, and home services. On the other hand, someone who has been blind or visually impaired for a number of years may function fairly independently at home.

DIAGNOSIS

Low vision is diagnosed based on patient report and visual acuity testing. Specific conditions such as cataracts, glaucoma, retinopathies, and macular degeneration are discovered during the ophthalmic examination. Cataracts can sometimes be seen by the naked eye as a white or cloudy area in the pupil. Ophthalmologists use a device called a slit lamp to examine the structures of the eye and with this device may be able to detect a cataract that is forming and is not yet visible to others. Retinopathies and macular degeneration are discovered while examining the fundus. A special procedure known as fluorescein angiography may be performed to visualize the retinal vasculature in more detail.

Glaucoma is detected by measuring intraocular pressure, which should be between 10 and 20 mm Hg. To determine how much or which portion of the visual field has been lost as a result of glaucoma, a visual field test may be performed using a device called a Goldman perimeter.

These tests, with the exception of angiography, are non-invasive and are well tolerated by most people.

CLINICAL MANIFESTATIONS

The clinical manifestations of low vision vary with the specific cause of the visual change, but certain general signs and symptoms indicate that an eye examination is warranted (Box 4-4).

Symptoms that require immediate attention are any sudden change in vision and eye pain, particularly if the pain is accompanied by nausea and vomiting. Pain accompanied by nausea and vomiting may indicate an acute glaucoma crisis. The crisis must be managed by lowering the intraocular pressure within 4 hours or the optic nerve will suffer irreparable damage.

INTERDISCIPLINARY CARE

Care of the patient with low vision is directed at preventing further visual loss and helping the individual maintain independence and a satisfactory quality of life. The specific measures taken vary based on the cause of visual impair-

Box 4-1 Systemic Diseases and Syndromes with Ocular Manifestations

ACQUIRED IMMUNODEFICIENCY SYNDROME
Keratitis, cytomegalovirus retinitis, Kaposi's sarcoma of the eyelids, endophthalmitis, cotton-wool spots, retinopathies

ALBINISM
Photophobia, nystagmus, decreased visual acuity

DIABETES
Cataracts, glaucoma, retinopathies, macular edema, visual disturbances

DOWN SYNDROME
Myopia, cataracts, nystagmus, strabismus, keratoconus

ENDOCARDITIS
Subconjunctival and/or retinal petechiae

HYPERTENSION
Cotton-wool spots, "silver wiring" of retinal vessels, tortuous retinal vessels

LYME DISEASE
Diplopia, conjunctivitis, keratitis, retinal detachment

MARFAN'S SYNDROME
Lens dislocation, myopia, keratoconus, retinal detachment

MYASTHENIA GRAVIS
Ptosis

RHEUMATOID ARTHRITIS
Dry eye syndrome, keratitis, scleritis

SYSTEMIC LUPUS ERYTHEMATOSUS
Dry eye syndrome, uveitis, scleritis

TEMPORAL ARTERITIS
Ptosis, vision loss, nystagmus, oculomotor disturbance

THYROID DISEASE
Lid retraction, lid lag, exophthalmos, dry eye, increased intraocular pressure

TUBERCULOSIS
Conjunctivitis, keratitis, uveitis

VITAMIN DEFICIENCIES
A—Night blindness
B—Optic neuropathies, retinal hemorrhage, nystagmus
C—Hemorrhage
D—Exophthalmos

Box 4-2 Ocular Changes Associated with Aging

COSMETIC CHANGES
- Eyebrows and eyelashes become thinner and gray.
- Muscle tone decreases, producing mild ptosis, entropion, ectropion, excessive eyelid skin.*
- Yellow pigmented spots (pingueculae) form on conjunctiva.
- Sclera take on yellow hue.
- White or yellow ring develops at periphery of cornea (arcus senilis).
- Iris loses pigment and changes color.

STRUCTURAL CHANGES
- Corneal sensitivity decreases.
- Tear production decreases.
- Rigidity of iris and lens increases.*
- Opacities develop in lens.*
- Number of retinal cones decreases.*
- Retinal arteries straighten and narrow.

VISUAL CHANGES
- Accommodation and near vision decrease.
- Color discrimination becomes difficult especially blues/blacks, blues/greens.
- Glare interferes with vision, especially at night.
- Cataracts diminish visual acuity.
- Macular degeneration interferes with central vision.

*Likely to produce some change in vision.

ment and the functional ability and visual acuity of the individual involved. Activities specific to a particular visual impairment are addressed in the section discussing that impairment. However, common strategies and interventions exist for improving performance of the activities of daily living (ADL) and instrumental activities of daily living (IADL) and ensuring safe navigation of the environment (Box 4-5).

Primary Provider (Physician/Nurse Practitioner)

Primary providers may or may not perform visual screening as part of a routine examination. A funduscopic examination is customary, however, especially for patients with glaucoma, diabetes, and hypertension. Changes in the optic disc or fundus are recorded, and the patient is referred to an ophthalmologist.

Nurse

The nurse evaluates the individual's functional ability and level of adjustment to the visual impairment and makes appropriate referrals to visual and occupational therapists, counselors, and medical social workers. In addition, the nurse makes the patient and family aware of the numerous agencies that provide information, assistance, and in some instances equipment for people with low vision, many of which are listed at the end of this chapter. The nurse also assesses the environment for hazards and educates the patient and family about safety. One area in which the nurse must be particularly vigilant is in following up on the success

---

Box 4-3   Functional Health Pattern Assessment for Alteration in Vision

HEALTH PERCEPTION/HEALTH MANAGEMENT

■ When was the patient's last eye examination? What type of provider was seen?

■ When was the last checkup for glaucoma?

■ What medications does the patient take for eye-related problems?

NUTRITION/METABOLISM

■ Is the patient on a diabetic diet or a salt-restricted diet for hypertension?

■ What is the patient's typical dietary intake (daily)?

■ Does the patient have difficulty shopping for or preparing meals?

ELIMINATION

■ Is there any difficulty urinating?

■ Does the patient strain at stool?

ACTIVITY/EXERCISE

■ Do the changes in vision limit the activities of daily living?

■ Do the changes in vision interfere with participation in sports or other leisure activities?

COGNITION/PERCEPTION

■ Has visual acuity (far or near) changed?

■ Are glasses or contact lenses worn?

■ Does the patient have difficulty seeing at night?

■ Does the patient experience problems with lighting?

■ Are colors difficult to discriminate?

■ Does the patient experience headaches or eye pain?

■ Are halos or floaters seen? Is the visual field diminished?

SELF-PERCEPTION/SELF-CONCEPT

■ How have the visual changes affected self-esteem?

ROLES/RELATIONSHIPS

■ What kind of work does the patient perform?

■ What changes in vision have interfered with job-related activities?

■ How have the visual changes affected family role and relationships with others?

■ How have the visual changes affected the patient's level of independence and driving?

SEXUALITY/REPRODUCTION

■ Is the patient sexually active?

■ Does the patient have concerns about sexual activity, now or after treatment?

COPING/STRESS TOLERANCE

■ Have changes in vision created additional stress?

■ How has the patient coped with this stress?

■ What resources are available to the patient?

VALUES/BELIEFS

■ What constitutes good quality of life for the patient?

■ What is important to the patient?

■ What are the patient's beliefs related to this condition?

■ To what extent do the patient's cultural/spiritual beliefs influence decision making related to this condition?

---

of the plan put in place to enhance vision, orientation, and mobility. All too often, people are given specialized equipment, assistive devices, and technologies without enough education to use them fully. Patients become frustrated because they have trouble using the new equipment or because they are not getting the results they hoped for, and they stop trying. This leads to depression and isolation. Furthermore, they are reluctant to try other strategies when the initial interventions are unsuccessful. Careful follow-up with patients about how the equipment is working, whether or not the strategies suggested have been implemented, and what their levels of satisfaction are with their ability to carry out ADL, IADL, and social interactions is important. Adjusting to a new way of living and developing the skill and confidence to move about safely takes many months.

Ophthalmologist

Ophthalmologists are physicians who have specialized education in conditions of the eye. They complete residencies in both medicine and surgery and therefore manage medical disorders of the eye and perform surgical procedures. They also measure visual acuity and correct refractive errors by prescribing corrective lenses.

Low Vision Specialist

Low vision specialists are either ophthalmologists or optometrists with specialized training in techniques and devices for treating those with low vision. They prescribe specialized eyewear such as telescopic lenses and prismatic glasses.

Occupational Therapist

The occupational therapist (OT) helps the patient with low vision adapt work and home environments so that employment and diversional activities can be maintained for as long as possible. The OT is familiar with a wide array of adaptive equipment that allows the individual to continue to perform work-related tasks and hobbies. Talking clocks, enhanced computer screens and keyboards, global positioning system (GPS) orientation devices, and computerized walking canes are examples of products being developed by the growing

---

Box 4-4   Symptoms of Low Vision

GENERAL
- Blurred or hazy vision
- Trouble seeing because the lights aren't bright enough
- Trouble recognizing colors, faces
- Trouble crossing the street or reading street signs

AGE-RELATED MACULAR DEGENERATION
- Loss of central vision

CATARACTS
- Cloudy or blurred vision
- Trouble with light
  Glare from lamps
  Halos around lights
  Car headlights seem too bright
- Faded appearance of colors
- Difficulty seeing at night
- Double vision
- Need for frequent changes in glasses or contact lens prescription

DIABETIC RETINOPATHY
- Changes in visual acuity
- Blurred or hazy vision
- Increased sensitivity to light
- Altered color vision
- Decreased ability to perceive light

GLAUCOMA
- Increased intraocular pressure on examination
- Decreased accommodation
- Loss of visual field
- Loss of visual acuity
- Halos around lights
- Headache, eye pain
- Changes in optic disc

Box 4-5   Strategies for Daily Living

- Teach others to identify themselves when entering or leaving the presence of person with low vision.
- Maintain a consistent environment. Do not move furniture or objects without informing patient.
- Paint stair treads different colors or apply contrasting tape so steps are clearly outlined.
- Color or otherwise label knobs and dials at reference points, for example:
  Oven dials at 350°, stove dials at Off
  Thermostat at 70°
  Washer or dryer at Start positions
- Fold denominations of paper money in different ways for easy identification.
- Place Velcro strips on walls near light switches and outlets.
- Ambulate by having person with low vision hold companion's elbow and walk a few paces behind.
- Use contrasting colors, for example, white dishes on dark-colored place mats.
- Use felt pens for writing.
- Use color film overlays to reduce glare when reading.
- Use audio tapes or large print books available from libraries.
- Use computer aids found in "Settings" menu of most computer programs and systems.
- Use clock-face system to orient individual to location of objects in work area or on table.

---

industry in assistive devices and technology for those with visual impairments.

Vision Therapist

Like the OT, the vision therapist (VT) assists the individual with low vision in maintaining quality of life by helping the person remain actively involved in work, family, and community activities. The VT advises the individual about the level of services and types of devices most appropriate for the patient's individual needs and provides support, education, and information related to travel, technology use, and vision maintenance and enhancement. Although the VT generally provides services for only a specified period of time, the VT too must be diligent in follow-up and make sure that the patient is able to successfully incorporate the techniques and strategies developed for the patient.

Medical Social Worker

The medical social worker may be involved in the care of the patient with low vision if assistance is needed in securing financial help, equipment, and/or services such as transportation or meals on wheels. In instances in which the person with low vision must be cared for in a long-term care facility, the medical social worker makes arrangements for placement.

FAMILY ISSUES AND CONCERNS

Involving the family in the education of and care planning for individuals with low vision is important. If the loss of vision has been gradual, family members very likely have already become involved in the care of the individual with the loss. Nevertheless, they can benefit from a frank discussion of the patient's condition, abilities, and needs. They may be unaware of the resources available to make their lives easier and allow the patient more independence. They may be fearful for the patient's safety or anxious about the future and can benefit greatly from participating in the planning and decision making regarding the patient's care. If the visual loss has been sudden, then both patient and family will have many adjustments to make emotionally, logistically, and psychologically. Health care providers must assess the family's response to the change in their loved one. The family must also be assessed for strengths, resources, level of knowledge, and areas of need. Some families are unable or unwilling to assume the care required, whereas others may try to do too much and create dependence that is unnecessary. It is essential to involve the family as part of the health care team to ensure that both patient and family adjust to the changes brought about by the patient's condition.

AGE-RELATED MACULAR DEGENERATION

Age-related macular degeneration (AMD) is a common cause of vision loss in people over the age of 60. Although it rarely causes blindness, AMD can severely affect a person's quality of life (O'Neill et al, 2001). AMD involves a loss of central vision, which makes it difficult for people to read, drive, sew, and in some instances perform their work duties.

Pathophysiology

The macula is in the center of the retina and is the area responsible for the sharpest vision. For unknown reasons, in AMD the cells in this area begin to break down. Two types of AMD are seen: wet AMD and dry AMD. Dry AMD is by far the most common and least destructive of the two types. In dry AMD cells deteriorate slowly and the disease may affect only one eye. People with monocular dry AMD may not notice any change in vision. Although only about 10% of people with AMD have the wet variety, it accounts for 90% of the vision loss associated with AMD (National Eye Institute [NEI], 2001). In wet AMD new blood vessels that are very fragile and leak blood and fluid grow toward the macula. This fluid causes edema of the macula, which distorts vision. Wet AMD is much more rapid in onset and can quickly cause irreversible damage.

Clinical Manifestations

Individuals with dry AMD most commonly experience blurred vision and difficulty recognizing faces unless people are close to them, and find that they need more light to read, sew, or do close work.

Individuals with wet AMD often think that straight lines look wavy. An easy test to detect this symptom is use of the Amsler grid (Figure 4-3). The individual covers one eye and stares at the center of the grid. If lines appear wavy or some lines seem to be missing, the person may have wet AMD. Rapid loss of central vision is another indication that the person has wet AMD. Neither form of AMD is painful. In both types of AMD, a blurred area is present in the center of the visual field that gets larger and darker as the disease progresses, and ultimately becomes a blind spot.

Interdisciplinary Care
Ophthalmologist

The ophthalmologist examines individuals with dry AMD at least annually to monitor the progression of the disease and

check for other eye conditions that may have developed. Individuals with wet AMD are treated with laser surgery to destroy leaking blood vessels. Neovascularization is common after laser surgery. Therefore, frequent follow-up care is necessary to check for new vessels and to be sure that leakage has been controlled. AMD cannot be cured, but additional vision loss can be avoided.

Low Vision Specialist

The low vision specialist recommends and prescribes assistive technologies and devices that allow individuals to carry out ADL, IADL, and work-related activities.

Nurse

The nurse provides education and support and refers patients and their families to agencies and organizations that provide services, financial support, and equipment to enhance and maintain quality of life. Interventions related to loss of vision are the same regardless of the cause. There is some evidence that smoking increases the likelihood that new blood vessels will develop after laser treatments. The nurse should encourage patients to stop smoking and provide information on smoking cessation programs. There is also some evidence that ingesting large amounts of zinc and antioxidants decreases the risk for advanced AMD (NEI, 2001). The nurse should review dietary intake with individuals and encourage healthy eating habits, including the use of multivitamins.

Vision Therapist

The vision rehabilitation therapist works with individuals with AMD to assess functional ability and develop individualized strategies to assist with mobility, orientation, grooming, travel, and employment.

CATARACTS

A cataract is an opacity of the normally crystalline lens of the eye. The lens refracts light rays so that they can be focused on the retina. Any opacity interferes with this function and distorts the retinal image. The amount of distortion depends on the density of the cataract as well as its location in the lens. For example, a central opacification presents more problems for a patient than does a peripheral opacity. Cataracts develop in approximately 5 million to 10 million people worldwide and in about half of all Americans over the age of 65 (NEI, 2001). Cataracts are classified either by their nature or by the time of onset. Age-related cataracts are the most common.

Pathophysiology

Cataracts result when proteins in the lens break down and form precipitates. No one knows for sure why this happens in some individuals and not in others, although some researchers believe that a link exists between cataract for-

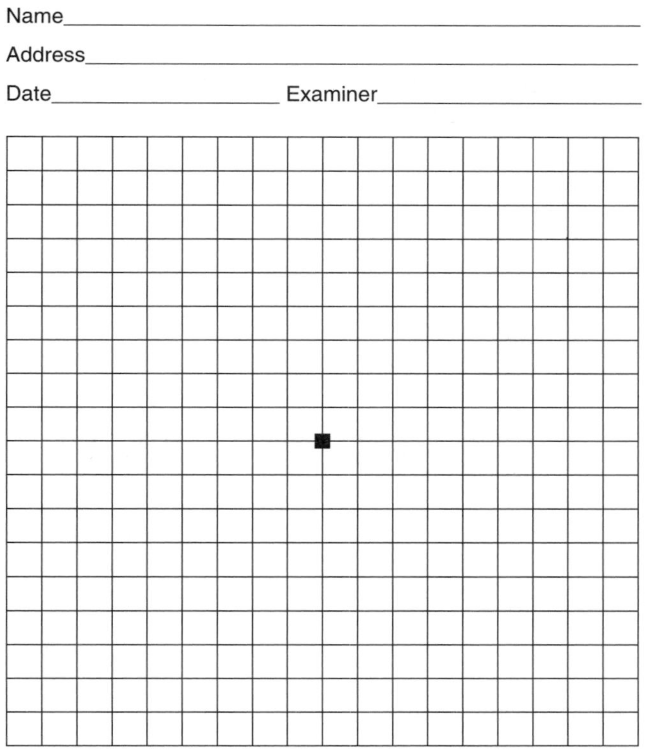

Name_____

Address_____

Date_____ Examiner_____

Figure 4-3 Amsler grid.

mation and smoking, diabetes, and exposure to sunlight. There is some evidence that a diet high in both vitamin A and vitamin C can protect against the development of cataracts (Eliopoulos, 1999).

Assessment

The standard assessment for visual acuity described earlier should be performed along with direct visualization of the lens using an ophthalmoscope. Not only can opacities in the lens be seen, but the examiner will also note difficulty in visualizing the retina through the opacity. As the cataract matures, the red reflex may be totally absent, which causes the pupil to appear white or, in some instances, brownish gray. Dark-colored cataracts are called morganian cataracts. A focused assessment of functional health patterns such as that outlined in Box 4-3 should be completed.

Clinical Manifestations

No visual changes may be noticed in the early stages of cataract development, and because cataracts grow slowly, visual changes are gradual. These changes include cloudy or blurred vision; the appearance of halos around lights; glare, especially at night; double vision; and changes in color vision.

Interdisciplinary Care
Ophthalmologist

The individual with a cataract should have regular checkups by an ophthalmologist, who will monitor the growth of the cataract and advise the patient regarding the need for surgical treatment. Cataracts are not removed unless they interfere with the treatment of another eye condition such as diabetic retinopathy or the patient's vision has deteriorated to the point that ability to perform ADL and life quality are severely limited. Until that time, decreased vision is managed using corrective lenses, magnifying glasses, glasses with pinholes, or stronger illumination.

If surgery is required, it is usually performed on an outpatient basis, and only one eye is treated at a time. Once the lens has been removed, the eye has lost its refractive power. Therefore, a small plastic intraocular lens is usually inserted at the time the cataract is removed. In some instances this implanted lens is designed to correct any refractive errors the patient had prior to surgery. However, most people will still need glasses for reading. Lenses that eliminate the need for glasses or contact lenses are under development.

Nurse

The primary responsibilities of the nurse are to promote safety, ensure that the individual is capable of performing ADL and IADL, and make families aware of the resources available to them. Postoperative instructions for the patient who has had cataract surgery are outlined in Box 4-6. Some patients experience a dramatic improvement in vision immediately, whereas others may become discouraged because visual acuity is not as good as they had hoped it would be. These individuals must be reminded that vision will continue to improve for 4 to 6 weeks after surgery and that glasses may be worn to correct accommodation and refractive errors.

DIABETIC RETINOPATHY

Diabetic retinopathy is a result of the microvascular changes that occur with diabetes. It is the leading cause of new cases of blindness among individuals between the ages of 20 and 75. As many as 40% of people with diabetes have some form of retinopathy, and the incidence increases with the duration of the diabetes so that 80% of those who have had diabetes for 15 years have retinal damage. The incidence is higher in people who have a fasting blood glucose level higher than 129 mg/dl or poorly controlled blood glucose levels. A 1% increase in total glycosylated hemoglobin level has been associated with a 10% increase in the incidence of retinopathy (Cohen et al, 1999). Because people who are Hispanic, Native American, or African American have a high risk of developing diabetes, individuals from these ethnic groups should have annual screening eye examinations.

Box 4-6   Postoperative Instructions for the Patient Undergoing Cataract Removal Surgery

REPORT SIGNS AND SYMPTOMS OF COMPLICATIONS

- Pain unrelieved by mild analgesics
- Sudden, sharp pain
- Headache accompanied by nausea and vomiting
- Bleeding or increasing discharge
- Changes in vision
  Flashes of lights, floating shapes, sense of a shade being pulled down

AVOID ACTIVITIES THAT INCREASE INTRAOCULAR PRESSURE

- Bending at the waist (teach to stoop to pick up objects)
- Sneezing, coughing, blowing the nose
- Straining at stool
- Sexual intercourse

RESUME NORMAL ACTIVITIES SLOWLY WITH DOCTOR'S PERMISSION

- Driving should be avoided for first few weeks.
- Patient may shower and wash hair with head tilted back (keep eye from getting wet).
- Perform light housework only; no vacuuming, scrubbing, etc.
- Do not participate in any sports activity without physician's approval.

PROTECT EYE

- Do not remove eye patch until directed to do so.
- Wear protective shield at night.
- Instill eye drops as directed. (Teach patient to place drops in lower conjunctiva using clean technique and to avoid pulling on upper lids.)

Think **S** *for Success*

Symptoms

- Preoperatively: visual changes; halos, blurring, glare, decreased night vision
- Postoperatively: decreased visual acuity, mild eye pain or headache

Sequelae

- Teach patient to avoid activities that raise intraocular pressure (see Box 4-6).

Safety

- Assess ability to move about in environment and carry out instrumental and other activities of daily living.
- Postoperatively: make patient and family aware of complications of surgery and need to seek immediate treatment for bleeding or pain that is unrelieved by medication or lasts more than 24 to 36 hours.
- Instruct patient not to remove eye patch until told to do so and to wear protective shield at night. If patch needs to be retaped or reinforced, care must be taken not to apply pressure to eye. Tape should be placed diagonally across outer edges of patch.

Support/Services

- Refer to low vision services as needed.

Satisfaction

- Assess the degree to which visual changes interfere with patient's quality of life and assist patient in enjoying self-identified important possibilities of his or her life.
- Remind patient that visual acuity will improve postoperatively.

Pathophysiology

Two types of diabetic retinopathy are seen: proliferative and nonproliferative (which is also referred to as background retinopathy). Both types begin with damage to the retinal capillaries caused by small vascular occlusions that lead to the formation of microaneurysms. In background retinopathy, these microaneurysms leak fluid into the retina, causing swelling and the formation of hard exudates and/or intraretinal hemorrhages. Proliferative retinopathy is the more severe form of diabetic retinopathy and involves both the vitreous body and the retina. In proliferative disease, new blood vessels grow in response to the occlusion of the retinal capillaries. These new vessels are very fragile and hemorrhage readily. The hemorrhages cause the vitreous humor to become clouded with blood so that light is prevented from reaching the retina. This may lead to vitreous contraction, which ultimately causes retinal holes, tears, and detachments.

Assessment

Vision should be evaluated using standard visual acuity measures as already outlined in this chapter. The most important assessment techniques are funduscopic examination and slit-lamp examination of the retina. Although any health care provider trained in the use of an ophthalmoscope can perform a fundus examination, the ophthalmologist is the provider best qualified to conduct the type of examination needed to ensure that the patient receives early appropriate treatment. On examination the fundus will show areas of neovascularization, "dot and blot" hemorrhages, and hard exudates (Figure 4-4). Examination by an ophthalmologist specializing in retinal diseases maybe required to evaluate

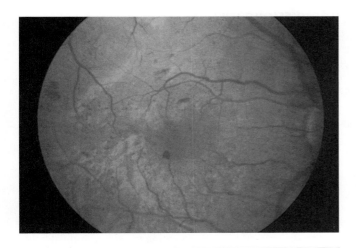

Figure 4-4   Optic fundus of a patient with diabetic retinopathy. (From Ignatavicius DD, Workman ML, editors: *Medical-surgical nursing: critical thinking for collaborative care*, Philadelphia, 2002, WB Saunders.)

retinal damage. A framework for the assessment of functional health patterns can be found in Box 4-3.

Clinical Manifestations

The individual may not notice any visual changes in the early stages of diabetic retinopathy unless the macula is involved. Some individuals report intermittent blurring of vision and indicate that this temporary change in vision is an indication that blood glucose levels are too high. As the disease progresses and retinal vessels are torn, individuals see red or black spots or lines. If vitreous hemorrhage occurs, the patient will report visual loss.

A complication of diabetes is retinal tearing and detachment. If the retina tears or detaches at the macula, there is sudden loss of vision. When other parts of the retina are involved, the individual may experience sudden flashes of light or the sensation of a curtain coming down or a window shade being pulled halfway down. Detachments are not painful because there are no pain fibers in the retina. A detachment requires immediate professional attention.

Interdisciplinary Care
Primary Provider (Physician/Nurse Practitioner)

The primary care provider assesses the patient's management of factors that precipitate microvascular changes, specifically hyperglycemia and hypertension. First-line therapy for patients with hypertension includes the use of angiotensin-converting enzyme inhibitors and maintenance of tight glycemic control (Bush, 2001). For individuals who cannot tolerate angiotensin-converting enzyme inhibitors, β-blockers and angiotensin receptor blockers may be used.

Nurse

The role of the nurse is primarily one of education and encouragement. It is essential that the individual recognize the importance of maintaining glycemic control, and the nurse must reinforce appropriate nutrition, exercise, and medical management.

When vision becomes impaired, the nurse must ensure the patient's safety and help the individual to stay as independent as possible. Box 4-5 outlines interventions for people with low vision.

Ophthalmologist

The individual with diabetic retinopathy should be examined regularly by an ophthalmologist who specializes in diabetes or diseases of the retina. In the early stages of the disease, leaking blood vessels can be treated with lasers to prevent further damage. The frequency of eye examinations depends on the type and degree of retinopathy present, but all diabetic patients should visit their ophthalmologists at least once every 6 months (Slawson, 2000).

If the retina detaches, surgery may be required to reattach the retina and anchor it in place. The surgery performed is called a scleral buckle. During the recovery phase, positioning of the patient is of utmost importance, because the pull of gravity can prevent the retina from attaching properly. The physician will explain the position desired based on the location of the detachment.

If the patient has repeated hemorrhages into the vitreous humor, a vitrectomy may be performed to improve vision and also to allow the physician to monitor changes in the retina.

Low Vision Specialist

The low vision specialist evaluates the individual regularly throughout the course of the illness, monitoring changes in vision and prescribing appropriate devices to enhance the patient's vision as the disease progresses.

Occupational Therapist and Vision Therapist

Therapists may become involved in the care of the patient when visual impairment is significant enough to interfere with daily routines and activities.

GLAUCOMA

Glaucoma affects more than 3 million Americans. It is the leading cause of blindness among African Americans and ranks third among causes of legal blindness among whites. It can occur in all races and age groups, but people over the age of 60, those with a family history of the disease, and African Americans are at higher risk than others.

Pathophysiology

Glaucoma is classified as either congenital, primary (either acute or chronic), secondary, or normal-tension glaucoma.

Regardless of the type of glaucoma, the blindness that occurs is the result of pressure on the optic nerve. The physiologic mechanisms that create this pressure are related to the flow of aqueous humor, which percolates between the anterior and posterior chambers of the eye at a relatively constant pressure (10 to 20 mm Hg). Aqueous humor is produced by the ciliary body of the eye and drains from the eye through the trabecular meshwork in a structure called the canal of Schlemm. When the flow of aqueous humor is blocked, as in the case of closed- or narrow-angle glaucoma, or too much aqueous is produced, the pressure in the eye increases. Left untreated, this pressure begins to destroy the optic nerve. Once the nerve is destroyed, it cannot regenerate. However, the progression of the damage can be halted by taking measures to maintain the intraocular pressure within normal limits.

Assessment

Glaucoma is detected by measuring the intraocular pressure, a process known as tonometry. A variety of tonometric techniques are available. The ophthalmologist generally uses an applanation tonometer affixed to a slit-lamp biomicroscope. The patient sits in a darkened room and places his or her chin in a rest on the examining microscope. The ophthalmologist positions a small cone-shaped tonometer on the cornea and exerts gentle pressure until the intraocular pressure is recorded. Other methods include the use of puffs of air to measure corneal resistance and the use of a Schiötz tonometer, a handheld device that works in much the same way as the applanation tonometer. Damage to the optic nerve can be assessed by directly visualizing the nerve head (the optic disc). As the nerve becomes damaged, the optic disc becomes smaller and appears cupped. Another way to assess the amount of damage sustained is to measure vision loss through visual field testing.

Clinical Manifestations

In most instances there are no early signs or symptoms of glaucoma. It has been called the "sneak thief" of sight because individuals are not aware that a problem exists until significant portions of the visual field have been lost. The first areas of the visual field to be affected are in the periphery, and the decline is so gradual that most people are not aware that vision has been lost. In some instances, when the angle of the eye (the space between the iris and the peripheral cornea) closes abruptly, as may be the case with injury or postoperative complications, the patient will experience severe pain in the affected eye along with headache, nausea and vomiting, and redness (injection) of the normally white sclera. This is a crisis situation and intervention must take place within 4 hours if vision is to be saved. Although abrupt angle closure is an acute manifestation of glaucoma, it is mentioned here because some chronic conditions of the eye may produce this condition, and the chronic care provider must be aware of its urgent nature.

Interdisciplinary Care
Ophthalmologist

The ophthalmologist is the primary physician involved in the management of glaucoma. Because of the insidious nature of the disease, all persons over the age of 35 should have an annual eye examination by an ophthalmologist. Optometrists often screen for glaucoma but are not qualified to treat it or to thoroughly evaluate the optic disc and fundus of the eye. Optometrists and low vision specialists can assist people by providing corrective lenses and vision-enhancing devices, but only ophthalmologists prescribe treatment in the form of medications or surgery.

Drug Therapy

The drugs used to treat glaucoma consist of topical solutions and oral preparations that either produce miosis (pupillary constriction) or interfere with the production of aqueous humor. They include cholinergics, β-blockers, and drugs that inhibit the enzyme carbonic anhydrase (Table 4-1).

The individual and his or her family must understand the proper technique for instilling eye drops as outlined in Box 4-7. It is interesting to note that the effectiveness of drugs used to produce miosis (and mydriasis) is often affected by eye color. In general, individuals with darker irises require more medication to produce either miosis or mydriasis and require a longer time for the effects of such drugs to wear off.

In some instances, very potent osmotic diuretics are used to lower intraocular pressure. These should be used with caution. Health care providers must be certain that the individual has good kidney function and is not in danger of developing congestive heart failure before these diuretics are given. Failure to do so can place the patient in a life-threatening situation.

Surgery

Laser surgery may be performed to scar down the trabecular meshwork and enlarge the openings that drain off aqueous humor. Other surgical procedures aimed at improving the outflow of aqueous humor include iridotomy, iridectomy, trabeculotomy, and the creation of scleral blebs.

Nurse

The nursing care of patients with chronic glaucoma involves primarily education of patients about the lifelong nature of treatment and the importance of adhering to medication regimens and undergoing annual follow-up examinations. Interventions related to vision loss are the same regardless of the cause.

CHRONIC CONDITIONS LESS FREQUENTLY ENCOUNTERED

The health care provider may encounter a number of other chronic eye conditions that, although bothersome for the

Table 4-1   Commonly Used Ophthalmic Medications

Drug	Side Effects	Nursing Considerations
Topical Anesthetics Proparacaine (Ophthaine, Ophthetic) Tetracaine (Pontocaine)		Anesthesia produces loss of blink reflex for up to 15 minutes; patch eye to protect cornea.
Antiinfectives *Antibacterial* Chloramphenicol (Chloromycetin) Ciprofloxacin (Ciloxan) Erythromycin (Romycin) Gentamicin (Garamycin) Norfloxacin (Noroxin) Tobramycin (Tobrex)		Although these are used primarily to treat acute infections, they are also used prophylactically to prevent postoperative complications following cataract or glaucoma surgery.
Antifungal Natamycin (Natacyn)	Stinging or blurred vision	
Antiviral Idoxuridine (Herplex Liquifilm) Trifluridine (Viroptic) Vidarabine (Vira-A)		Store in refrigerator.
Antiinflammatories Diclofenac (Voltaren) Dexamethasone (AK-Dex)	Decreased platelet aggregation Interaction with contact lens material	Monitor for bleeding. Instruct patient not to wear soft contact lenses. Steroidal preparations should be gradually reduced in dosage and should not be given for minor abrasions or wounds.
Flurbiprofen (Ocufen) Medrysone (HMS Liquifilm) Prednisolone acetate (Econopred) Prednisolone Na phosphate (Inflamase)	Increased risk of infection	Monitor for signs of infection. Steroidal preparations should be gradually reduced in dosage and should not be given for minor abrasions or wounds
Carbonic Anhydrase Inhibitors (CAIs) Acetazolamide (Diamox)	Drowsiness, lethargy, anorexia, dry mouth, nausea and vomiting, paresthesias, tinnitus	Monitor for dehydration and postural hypotension. Check K$^+$. Instruct patient to use good oral hygiene, increase fluids, use ice chips or sugarless gum for dry mouth. Patient should not operate hazardous machinery. Patient should not stop medication abruptly.
Brinzolamide ophthalmic solution 1% (Azopt)		Give topically.
Dichlorphenamide (Daranide)	Confusion, especially in the elderly	Given PO. Monitor for dehydration and postural hypotension. Check K$^+$ (see Diamox).
Dorzolamide (Trusopt)	Burning, stinging, bitter taste	Given topically. *Do not give with PO CAIs.*
Methazolamide (Neptazane)	Increased action of amphetamines, barbiturates, salicylates, and lithium	Given PO (see Diamox).

Continued

Table 4-1   Commonly Used Ophthalmic Medications—cont'd

Drug	Side Effects	Nursing Considerations
Lubricants Isopto Tears Tearisol Ultra Tears Lacri-Lube Tears Naturale Tears Plus	Allergic reaction to preservative	Generally purchased over the counter. Teach patient and family proper technique for instilling drops or applying ointment
Miotics *Cholinergics* Acetylcholine (Miochol) Carbachol (Miostat) Pilocarpine (Isopto Carpine) Echothiophate (Phospholine Iodide)	Headache, eye pain, brow pain, decreased vision, bloodshot eye Nausea and vomiting with systemic absorption Diarrhea, asthma, weakness, dyspnea	Avoid systemic absorption in patients with asthma, CAD, bowel obstruction. Monitor heart rate and blood pressure. Monitor lung sounds. Have atropine sulfate on hand in case of toxicity.
Cholinesterase inhibitors Physostigmine (Isopto Eserine) Demecarium (Humorsol)		
β-Blockers Betaxolol (Betoptic) Levobunolol (Betagan Liquifilm) Timolol (Timoptic)	Orthostatic hypotension, bradycardia, bronchospasm	Monitor vital signs, lung sounds. Instruct patient to avoid systemic absorption. Instruct patient not to stop drug abruptly.
Mydriatics* Dipivefrin (Propine) Epinephrine (Epifrin, Glaucon) Phenylephrine (AK-Dilate)	Headache, eye pain, brow pain, worsening of narrow angle glaucoma	Monitor IOP. Do not use in patients with narrow-angle glaucoma. Use with caution in the elderly and patients with Parkinson's disease. *Do not use* in patients who have arrhythmias or cerebral arteriosclerosis.
Osmotics Glycerin Isosorbide ophthalmic (Ismotic) Mannitol (Osmitrol) Urea (Ureaphil)	Hyperglycemia, nausea and vomiting, headache, disorientation Syncope, lethargy, irritability Pulmonary congestion	Use with caution in patients with diabetes. Monitor I&O, electrolyte levels. Monitor I&O, electrolyte levels. Assess for CHF prior to administering. Monitor I&O, electrolyte levels. Weigh daily. Do not use if patient is dehydrated or anuric. Monitor I&O, electrolyte levels. *Do not mix* with other medications or blood. Do not use in patients who are dehydrated or have intracranial bleeding.

Modified from Kee J, Hayes E: *Pharmacology. a nursing process approach,* ed 4, Philadelphia, 2003, WB Saunders.
CAD, Coronary artery disease; *CHF,* congestive heart failure; *I&O,* intake and output; *IOP,* intraocular pressure; *PO,* by mouth.
*Other mydriatics and cycloplegics used to dilate eye for examination include atropine (Isopto Atropine), homatropine (Isopto Homatropine), cyclopentolate (Cyclogyl), scopolamine, and tropicamide (Mydriacyl, Opticyl). These should not be used in the treatment of glaucoma.

Box 4-7 Instillation of Eye Drops

- Be sure to check the order and label for correct dose, correct drug, and correct eye (OD = right eye, OS = left eye, OU = both eyes).
- Determine if there are contraindications to the drug; for example, underlying conditions such as asthma or eye conditions such as lens implants or glaucoma.

  If systemic absorption is a concern, cover the puncta with a clean tissue while the drop is being administered.
- Check the type of container the eye drops are in.

  Some drops are contained in Ocumeter bottles. These bottles have an indentation on the bottom that, when pressed, delivers one drop of medication. Squeezing the sides of these bottles may deliver more than the desired amount.
- Steady the hand holding the eye dropper by gently resting the side of the hand on the patient's forehead above the eye into which the drop is to be instilled.
- Ask the patient to look up.
- Gently pull down on the lower eyelid. *Do not pull on upper eyelids.*
- Instill drop in lower conjunctival sac.
- Ask the patient to close eyelids gently to distribute the medication evenly. *Do not squeeze the lids together.*
- Note: If the patient has a problem with avoiding blinking, ask him or her to open the mouth. This sometimes prevents blinking.

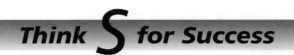
Think S for Success

Symptoms
- Gradual visual field loss

Sequelae
- Encourage annual eye examinations and compliance with medical regimen; be sure patient and family understand importance of taking medication as prescribed and instilling eye drops properly.

Safety
- Assess ability to move about in environment and carry out instrumental and other activities of daily living. Loss of peripheral vision greatly affects driving, and patient and family must be made aware of need to turn head laterally to scan environment for hazards when driving, crossing streets, walking in crowds, etc.

Support/Services
- Refer to low vision services as needed.

Satisfaction
- Assess the degree to which visual changes interfere with patient's quality of life.
- Assist patient in enjoying self-identified important possibilities of his or her life.

patient, require little more than monitoring and treatment of symptoms. Some of these conditions and their related treatments are listed in Table 4-2.

In rare instances, the entire globe must be removed. The procedure for removing the globe of the eye from its bony orbit is called enucleation. Once healing has taken place the patient is fitted for a prosthetic eye. The health care provider should know how to remove, replace, and care for the prosthesis (Box 4-8).

Table 4-2 Chronic Eye Conditions

Affected Area	Condition	Nursing Considerations
Lids/lashes	Blepharitis	Gently cleanse lids and lashes with baby shampoo to ease itching and burning and remove scales. Use over-the-counter drops with caution because preservative may make symptoms worse.
Cornea	Keratoconus	Monitor for thinning of cornea (may lead to perforation).
Lacrimal apparatus	Dry eye syndromes	If cause is related to gland dysfunction, warm compresses and gentle lid massage will help express tears. If tear production is inadequate, artificial tears can be used sparingly.
Retina	Retinitis pigmentosa	Teach and support use of low vision strategies and equipment.

Box 4-8   Care of Ocular Prosthesis

REMOVAL

■ Wash hands and put on gloves.

■ Ask the patient to tilt the head downward slightly.

■ Place one hand, palm side up, against the cheek under the prosthetic eye.

■ Using the other hand, gently pull the lower lid down and to the side, allowing the prosthesis to slide onto your palm.

■ If necessary, use a small suction-tipped appliance to remove the prosthesis.

INSERTION

■ Wash hands and put on gloves.

■ Ask the patient to tilt the head backward slightly.

■ Open the upper lid by applying upward pressure on the bony orbit under the eyebrow (Do not pull on the upper lids).

■ Insert top of the prosthesis under the upper lid.

■ Gently pull down the lower lid and apply light pressure on the prosthesis until it slides under the lower lid.

CARE AND CLEANING

■ Clean the prosthesis with mild soap and water and rinse thoroughly.

■ Store the prosthesis in a lined container so it does not become damaged.

Internet and Other Resources

American Council of the Blind: *http://www.acb.org* (information, services, advocacy)

American Foundation for the Blind: *http://www.afb.org* (information clearinghouse)

American Printing House for the Blind: *http://www.aph.org* (offers free magazine subscriptions on disposable audiocassettes)

Blinded Veterans Association: *http://www.bva.org* (links veterans with services, helps them find employment)

EyeCare America: *http://www.eyecareamerica.org* (information, sponsored by American Ophthalmology Association)

Guide Dogs for the Blind: *http://www.guidedogs.com*

Lighthouse National Center for Vision and Aging: *http:/lighthouse.org*

Low Vision Council: *http://www.lowvisioncouncil.org* (resources, information for people with low vision)

National Association for Visually Handicapped: *http://www.navh.org* (information and advocacy)

National Eye Institute: *http://www.nei.nih.gov* (information, research, treatment)

National Federation of the Blind: *http://www.nfb.org* (works with agencies and people with impairments to provide jobs and other services)

National Library Service for the Blind and Physically Handicapped: *http://Lcweb.loc.gov/nls*

Prevent Blindness America: *http://www.preventblindness.org*

CASE STUDY

Patient Data

Mrs. R. is an 83-year-old woman who lives alone and is in good health except for hypertension, which is controlled by the oral medications atenolol (Tenormin) and amlodipine (Norvasc), and osteoarthritis of the knees and ankles, for which she takes meloxicam (Mobic). During a routine examination Mrs. R. says she would like a referral for her arthritis and asks for the name of a doctor in her neighborhood because she drives only in her surrounding area. A discussion related to her driving reveals that she cannot read street signs or directional signs and is bothered by glare. She is unable to see well enough to drive at night and so runs errands only in the daytime in areas with which she is familiar. She wears bifocals for near vision only. Mrs. R. has a family history of glaucoma. Her mother, who is 108, is still living, as are 10 brothers and sisters. Her mother has lost her vision due to "old age."

Thinking It Through

■ What do you suspect is causing Mrs. R.'s visual disturbance?

■ What might you expect to find when you perform a funduscopic examination?

■ What types of assessment can you perform in the office to help you determine the nature of the problem?

Case Conference

Mrs. R. is referred to an ophthalmologist, who determines that Mrs. R. is developing bilateral cataracts and has elevated intraocular pressure. Because the cataracts are not yet mature, a conservative treatment plan is being developed. The ophthalmologist informs Mrs. R. that she would like to see Mrs. R. every 6 months to follow up the increased pressure and to monitor the development of the cataracts. She prescribes timolol maleate (Timoptic) eye drops for each eye to control the intraocular pressure. This ophthalmologist is not a low vision specialist and so provides Mrs. R. with the name of one who can help her enhance her vision until the cataracts are removed.

The nurse demonstrates how to instill the eye drops and watches Mrs. R. demonstrate in return. The nurse reminds Mrs. R. to keep her puncta covered when instilling the drops because she is taking atenolol and the eye drops could potentiate the action of that drug. Mrs. R. is asked to check her blood pressure and pulse daily for a couple of weeks and note if there is a change.

The occupational therapist schedules a visit to Mrs. R.'s home to see if there is a need to modify the environment or obtain any assistive devices to help Mrs. R. perform ADL and IADL.

The social worker informs Mrs. R. that she can use transportation services to ride to doctor's appointments so that she does not have to worry about driving, but Mrs. R. is reluctant to give up this piece of her independence and declines. The social worker gives Mrs. R. telephone numbers for the transportation service for future reference.

Mrs. R. states that she can get along just fine. She likes to garden and to write letters, and so far she can still do that. She does her own shopping and cooking. She agrees to have the occupational therapist come out to the house but she doesn't think she'll need much help.

■ Do you think Mrs. R. should continue driving?

■ What safety concerns should be considered?

■ What resources are available to help Mrs. R. with her ADL and IADL?

■ Why has the doctor chosen to wait to do surgery? Do you agree with this decision? Why or why not?

Resources for Rehabilitation: *http://www.rfr.org* (provides training programs and publications)

Visions: Services for the Blind and Visually Impaired: *http://www.visionsvcb.org* (free services to teens and adults over 55 with severe impairments)

REFERENCES

American Foundation for the Blind: Statistics and sources for professionals, 2003, retrieved from *http://afb.org/info_document_view.asp?documentid=1367* on June 22, 2003.

Bush M: Preventing microvascular complications: the essential therapeutic goal, *Fam Pract Recertification* 24(11):65-74, 2001.

Cohen RA et al: Determinants of retinopathy progression in type 1 diabetes mellitus, *Am J Med* 107(1):45-51, 1999.

Eliopoulos C: *Integrating conventional and alternative therapies: holistic care for chronic conditions,* St Louis, 1999, Mosby.

National Eye Institute: Frequently asked questions about low vision, August 2001, retrieved from *http://www.nei.nih.gov/nehep/faqs.htm* on June 22, 2003.

O'Neill C et al: Age-related macular degeneration: cost of illness, *Drugs Aging* 18(4):233-41, 2001.

Slawson D: How often should patients with type 2 diabetes be screened for retinopathy? *Evid Based Pract* 3(5):2-3, 2000.

CHAPTER 5

Disorders of the Ears

Sharron Guillett, PhD, RN

OBJECTIVES

After reading this chapter, you should be able to do the following:

- Describe the clinical manifestations of chronic disorders of the ears
- Describe the pathophysiology of hearing loss
- Describe the pathophysiology of vestibular disorders
- Describe the functional health patterns affected by chronic conditions of the ears
- Describe the role of each member of the interdisciplinary team involved in the care of patients with hearing loss and vestibular disorders
- Describe the indications for use, side effects and nursing considerations related to drugs commonly used to treat chronic disorders of the ear

Chronic conditions involving the ear include problems with hearing and balance as well as sensory disturbances such as vertigo and dizziness. These conditions, although not life threatening, have a profound impact on functional ability and quality of life. Hearing deficits can lead to confusion, anxiety, and social isolation. Disturbances in the vestibular system can interfere with mobility and activities of daily living and increase the risk of injury, particularly in the older population.

The signs and symptoms associated with chronic ear disorders include difficulty hearing sound, difficulty recognizing sound, difficulty recognizing speech, tinnitus, a feeling of fullness in the ear, alterations in gait, loss of balance, vertigo, dizziness, nausea, and vomiting. Many chronic ear conditions can be treated successfully so that individuals can enjoy their lives to the fullest. Early diagnosis, intervention, and follow-up by the interdisciplinary team is the key to success.

HEARING LOSS

The number of people with hearing impairments worldwide is estimated to be around 500 million (Better Hearing Institute, 2003). This number is expected to increase to more than 700 million by 2015 and to more than 900 million by 2025, primarily as a result of noisy surroundings and an aging population. Twenty-eight million (or roughly 1 in 10) people living in the United States and Canada report hearing loss, and 80% of these have irreversible hearing loss. In fact, hearing loss is one of the physical disabilities most frequently cited by Americans, on a par with arthritis (American Speech and Hearing Association, 2003). It is the third most common physical impairment in the older population. According to the National Center for Health Statistics (1995), 54% of the population over age 65 has hearing loss. There are, in all likelihood, many more individuals with unreported hearing loss, because the loss can be so gradual that many do not recognize that the problem exists.

The Better Hearing Institute (2003) estimates the annual costs of untreated hearing loss to be about $56 billion due to decreased productivity and the need for special education and health care. Beyond the financial costs, untreated hearing loss significantly affects quality of life. A survey by the National Council on Aging (1999) of people over the age of 50 suffering from hearing loss showed that those who were untreated were more likely to report depression, isolation, and anxiety, whereas those who were treated were more likely to report positive relationships with friends and family and greater independence leading to higher levels of self-esteem.

Assessment

Before hearing acuity is assessed, a generalized evaluation of the external and internal ear structures should be conducted. The external ears are assessed through direct observation and palpation. The internal ear structures are evaluated with the aid of an otoscope. The technique for using an otoscope is described in Box 5-1. Normal findings include a clear, intact tympanic membrane with visible landmarks and light reflex and the absence of tenderness and lesions.

The tympanic membrane is normally pearl gray, white, or pink. It may appear dusky in persons with dark skin coloration. The normal landmarks and the position of the light reflex are illustrated in Figures 5-1 and 5-2.

If the tympanic membrane is not visible because of the amount of cerumen in the ear canal, the ear can be gently irrigated with body-temperature water (Box 5-2). This procedure

Box 5-1   Otoscope Technique

1. Attach a speculum that is slightly smaller than the individual's ear canal to the otoscope.
2. Ask the patient to slightly tilt his or her head toward the opposite shoulder.
3. Gently pull the pinna up and back.
4. Hold the otoscope in the dominant hand and support the hand against the patient's head so that, if the patient moves, the otoscope will move with the patient.
5. Insert the speculum slowly at a slightly lateral angle. (The lateral wall of the ear canal is less sensitive than the medial wall).
6. Adjust the speculum so that the tympanic membrane is visible.

may cause pain and or dizziness, however, without successfully removing the cerumen. If the internal examination can be postponed, the patient should be advised to use lubricant drops to soften the cerumen and then return for cleansing and inspection.

A number of simple tests can be performed to determine if the patient has hearing loss. Perhaps the simplest test is the whisper test or voice test. In this test the examiner asks the individual to cover one ear and then, while standing about a foot away from the person, whispers a sentence and asks the patient to repeat it. A simple way to test for conductive hearing loss is through the use of a tuning fork. The examiner taps the tuning fork tines gently to start their vibration and then places the stem of the tuning fork in the center

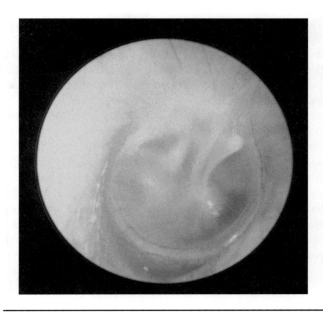

Figure 5-2   Otoscopic view of a normal tympanic membrane. (From Ignatavicius DD, Workman ML, editors: *Medical-surgical nursing: critical thinking for collaborative care,* ed 4, Philadelphia, 2002, WB Saunders.)

of the patient's skull or forehead. This test is called Weber's test and may also be performed by placing the tuning fork over the patient's teeth. This placement is very uncomfortable for most people, however, and is not used often. The patient is asked in which ear the sound is heard the loudest.

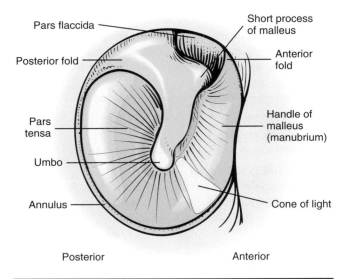

Figure 5-1   Drawing showing the normal landmarks of the right tympanic membrane as would be seen through an otoscope. (From Lewis SM, Heitkemper MM, Dirksen SR: *Medical-surgical nursing: assessment and management of clinical problems,* ed 6, St Louis, 2004, Mosby.)

Box 5-2   Ear Irrigation

1. Gather the necessary equipment and wash your hands.
2. Explain the procedure to the patient.
3. Examine the ear with the otoscope to confirm that the eardrum is intact and note location of cerumen.
4. Place a towel around the patient's neck and a basin under the ear to be irrigated.
5. Fill a syringe with water that has been warmed to body temperature.
6. Angle the syringe so that the fluid pushes against one side of the impaction.
7. Do not push fluid directly on the cerumen because this may force it further into the ear canal.
8. Allow fluid to drain from the ear and watch for the cerumen plug.
9. Continue to irrigate until 60 to 70 ml of fluid has been instilled. If there are no results, wait 10 minutes and repeat. (With older patients, never use more than 5 to 10 ml of water at a time.)
10. Monitor for pain, dizziness, and nausea and stop the procedure if present.

The sound should be heard equally in both ears. Lateralization of the sound (hearing the sound better in one ear than in the other) indicates either a conductive loss in the ear in which the sound is heard best or a sensorineural loss in the opposite ear. Another test using the tuning fork is the Rinne test. This test compares conduction of sound through bone and air. The stem of the vibrating tuning fork is placed on the mastoid bone and the patient is asked to say when he or she can no longer hear the sound. When the patient indicates that the sound is no longer heard, the tuning fork is quickly moved in front of the ear and again the patient is asked to indicate when the sound can no longer be heard. The examiner notes the length of time that the sound was heard for each placement. Normally, sound can be heard twice as long with air conduction. If the sound is heard longer with bone conduction, the patient may have conductive hearing loss. Tuning fork tests are very subjective and should be used with caution. If findings are abnormal, the patient's hearing should be evaluated using more sensitive audiometric methods.

Other diagnostic assessment methods include computed tomography; magnetic resonance imaging; auditory evoked potential testing, in which electrodes are placed on the scalp much as in electroencephalography and responses to auditory stimuli are evaluated; and auditory brainstem response testing, which measures electrical activity along the auditory pathway to the brain. In addition to diagnostic assessments, a functional health pattern assessment should be performed to determine whether the hearing loss is disrupting other aspects of the patient's life. A framework for a focused health assessment is presented in Box 5-3. If the patient is receiving home care, it is important to indicate what services might be required as a result of the hearing impairment.

Box 5-3   Functional Health Pattern Assessment for Ear Disorders

HEALTH PERCEPTION/HEALTH MANAGEMENT
- When and by whom was hearing loss first noted?
- What are the patient's personal practices to protect hearing, such as use of headphones or ear plugs?
- What medications does the patient take?

NUTRITION/METABOLISM
- Do symptoms worsen when certain foods are eaten?
- How much alcohol does the patient consume?
- Is the patient on a sodium-restricted diet? How much salt is used daily?
- What is the patient's typical dietary intake (daily)?
- Does the patient have difficulty chewing or swallowing?
- Does the patient experience nausea or vomiting associated with attacks of vertigo or dizziness?

ELIMINATION
- Does the patient strain at stool?

ACTIVITY/EXERCISE
- Does the patient swim? How often? In what kind of water?
- Do changes in hearing or balance interfere with participation in sports or other leisure activities?
- Has the patient experienced any falls? If so, how many? Has the patient had drop attacks?
- What specific activities cause dizziness or vertigo to worsen or improve?
- At what time of day is dizziness or vertigo worse?
- Is mobility or gait affected?

COGNITION/PERCEPTION
- What changes in hearing have occurred?
- Does the patient use hearing aids or other devices?
- Does the patient use lip reading or sign language?

- Is vertigo or dizziness present (have the patient describe it in his or her own words)?
- What are the duration, precipitating and alleviating factors, and frequency of attacks?

SELF-PERCEPTION/SELF-CONCEPT
- How have hearing changes, balance impairments, and/or vertigo affected self-concept and self-esteem?

ROLES/RELATIONSHIPS
- What kind of work does the patient perform?
- What changes in hearing or balance have interfered with job-related activities?
- How have hearing changes, balance impairments, and/or vertigo affected family roles or relationships with others?
- How have these changes affected the patient's level of independence and driving?
- How have these changes affected social life and activities?

SEXUALITY/REPRODUCTION
- Is the patient sexually active?
- Does the patient have concerns about sexual activity?

COPING/STRESS TOLERANCE
- Have changes in hearing and/or balance created additional stress?
- How has the patient coped with the stress?
- What resources are available to the patient?

VALUES/BELIEFS
- What are the patient's cultural beliefs related to communication?
- What constitutes good quality of life for the patient?
- What is important to the patient?
- What are the patient's beliefs related to this condition?
- To what extent do the patient's cultural/spiritual beliefs influence decision making related to this condition?

Pathophysiology

Hearing loss in adults may be the result of the aging process or it may be due to trauma, disease, infection, use of ototoxic drugs, or excessive noise. Hearing loss due to these many different causes is categorized into three types of impairment: sensorineural hearing loss, conductive hearing loss, and mixed conductive-sensorineural hearing loss. Mixed hearing loss, as the name implies, has components of both types of hearing loss and produces profound deficits.

Conductive hearing loss is caused by external or middle ear disorders that keep sound waves from reaching the inner ear. Infection, trauma, cerumen impaction (especially in the elderly), and otosclerosis are examples of conditions that block sound waves. Otosclerosis is a disease with autosomal dominant transmission that involves the middle ear capsule and specifically affects the movement of the stapes. An overgrowth of spongy bone originating in the labyrinth immobilizes the footplate of the stapes, fixing it to the oval window. The inability of the stapes to vibrate interferes with the transmission of sound waves to the inner ear. The ossification of the stapes is usually bilateral, although hearing loss may progress more rapidly in one ear. Individuals are not usually aware of the hearing loss until it interferes with communication. Left untreated, the hearing loss will escalate. Otosclerosis is more common among whites, who have twice the prevalence rate of African Americans.

Sensorineural hearing loss is caused by conditions that affect the cochlea and the eighth cranial nerve, and interfere with the transmission of nerve impulses to the brain. It can also result from damage to the brain itself. Conditions that produce sensorineural hearing loss include diabetes, infection, acoustic neuroma, Ménière's disease, exposure to ototoxic agents, prolonged exposure to loud noises, and presbycusis. Diabetes and infection accelerate degeneration of the cochlea. A more detailed discussion of the pathophysiology of the other conditions listed follows.

Acoustic Neuroma

An acoustic neuroma is a benign tumor that involves the eighth cranial nerve (acoustic nerve). Symptoms are related to compression and destruction of this nerve by the tumor. Early symptoms include decreased sensation of touch in the posterior ear canal and reduction of hearing in one ear accompanied by a feeling of fullness in the ear.

Ménière's Disease

Ménière's disease affects the membranous inner ear. For unknown reasons, endolymph, a fluid found in the membranous labyrinth, accumulates in excessive amounts until the membrane ruptures and endolymph mixes with the fluid of the bony labyrinth, the perilymph. This mixture causes the degeneration of the hair cells in both the cochlea and vestibular apparatus. Initially, hearing loss is related to the distortion of the inner ear canal and dilation of the cochlear duct and is therefore reversible. However, repeated attacks result in significant cochlear damage and permanent hearing loss. Hearing loss is usually unilateral. Care of the patient with Ménière's disease is discussed elsewhere in this chapter.

Exposure to Ototoxic Agents

Drugs used to manage some diseases are damaging to the auditory system (ototoxic) and may cause both transient and permanent hearing loss. In some cases the effect of the drug is dose related. For example, occasional use of salicylates for pain does not generally cause harm. However, salicylate toxicity has a profound effect on hearing. Drugs that are excreted by the kidney pose an additional risk, especially in the elderly, because failure to clear them from the system can result in drug levels that affect hearing even when these drugs are taken at fairly low dosages. Drugs known to be ototoxic are listed in Box 5-4.

Box 5-4   Ototoxic Drugs

ANTIBIOTICS
Aminoglycosides
- Amikacin (Amikin)
- Erythromycin (E-Mycin)
- Gentamycin (Garamycin)
- Kanamycin (Kantrex)
- Netilmicin (Netromycin)
- Neomycin (Muci-fradin)
- Streptomycin SO_4
- Tobramycin (Nebcin)
- Vancomycin (Vancocin, Lyphocin)

Unclassified
- Chloramphenicol (Chloromycetin)

NONSTEROIDAL ANTIINFLAMMATORY AGENTS
- Ibuprofen (Advil, Motrin)
- Indomethacin (Indocin)
- Naproxen (Aleve, Anaprox, Naprosyn)
- Salicylates (aspirin, Bufferin, Ascriptin)

LOOP DIURETICS
- Bumetanide (Bumex)
- Furosemide (Lasix)
- Ethacrynic acid (Edecrin)

CHEMOTHERAPEUTIC DRUGS
- Cisplatin (Platinol)
- Carboplatin (Paraplatin)
- Nitrogen mustards

MISCELLANEOUS
- Acetazolamide (Diamox)
- Carbamazepine (Tegretol)
- Quinine (Quinamm)
- Quinidine (Cardioquin)

Noise-Induced Hearing Loss

Hearing loss can be the result of a sudden loud noise such as an explosion. This acoustic trauma causes mechanical destruction of the organ of Corti. The individual who has sustained this type of trauma may recover some hearing within the first few weeks following the injury. The residual hearing loss is permanent.

Prolonged exposure to noise damages the hair cells in the cochlea and results in permanent hearing loss. This form of noise-induced hearing loss usually develops gradually and painlessly. Any activity that produces sound at levels above 65 dB can affect hearing if the exposure is continuous. Table 5-1 shows the decibel scale. The higher the decibel level, the shorter the exposure time required to produce hearing loss.

Presbycusis

Presbycusis is the gradual but progressive loss of hearing as a result of the aging process. High-frequency sounds, such as the consonant sounds *s* and *sh,* are affected first. Individuals with presbycusis often say that they can hear what you are saying but cannot understand what is being said. The degenerative changes responsible for this type of hearing loss include decreased blood supply, loss of inner ear hair cells, loss of neurons in the cochleae, and a decrease in the production of endolymph. Individuals may have one or more of the degenerative changes that cause presbycusis; the prognosis for improvement depends on which changes are present in that individual.

Clinical Manifestations

A number of behaviors are exhibited by individuals when hearing is impaired (Box 5-5). The individual may not be aware of these behaviors, and when they are pointed out by friends or family members, the individual may deny that a problem exists. Hearing loss may also be accompanied by symptoms of tinnitus, dizziness, and vertigo. Individuals are reluctant to admit hearing loss and frequently delay seeking treatment. The health care provider should continue to encourage patients to have their hearing tested by an audiologist, however, and any patient with a history of active drainage from the ear, pain or discomfort, facial paralysis, dizziness, or tinnitus should be referred to a physician or audiologist for follow-up as soon as possible.

Tinnitus

Tinnitus, commonly referred to as "ringing in the ears," is a noise in one's head when no such sound is present in the external environment. The sound is generally not heard by others, although a health care provider may be able to detect the sound by placing a stethoscope over the patient's jaw, temple, or ear. The sound may be like ringing or it may be perceived as roaring, pulsing, whooshing, chirping, or whistling. It has also been described as the sound of the ocean such as is heard when a seashell is held to the ear. Tinnitus can occur in one ear or both ears. It is reported to be worse at night, which is probably a function of the setting rather than any real change in the tinnitus. When the individual is distracted by work or other activities and the environment is noisy, the tinnitus is less apparent. Patients report that fatigue also seems to make tinnitus worse.

Dizziness and Vertigo

Dizziness and vertigo are almost entirely a result of disturbances in the vestibular system and therefore are discussed in more detail in the section on vestibular disorders.

Interdisciplinary Care
Primary Provider (Physician/Nurse Practitioner)

Because both hearing loss and tinnitus are symptoms, the first step should be to diagnose the underlying cause. The physician performs a comprehensive examination with special attention given to checking for systemic factors that may be responsible for the problem, such as high blood pressure, impaired kidney function, drug intake, improper

---

Table 5-1   Decibel Scale

Sound	Decibel Level	Listener's Perception
Whisper	10	Barely audible
Quiet conversation	30	Faintly heard
Average office	50	Moderate level
Summer nocturnal insects, sewing machine, normal conversation	60	Moderate level
Noisy restaurant, busy traffic	70	Loud
Heavy street traffic, factory noise	85	Very loud
Jackhammer, stereo headphones	100	Extremely loud
Jet aircraft taking off, thunderclap, rock band concert (near speakers)	120	Physical pain
Gunshot blast	140	
Rocket launch	180	

Box 5-5 Behaviors Associated with Hearing Loss

- Turning television, radio, or CD player abnormally loud
- Frequently asking to have speech repeated
- Failing to respond to speech
- Failing to respond to sounds in the environment
- Complaining that people don't speak clearly
- Favoring one ear or tilting one ear toward the sound or person speaking
- Responding or behaving inappropriately to comments or requests
- Speaking too loudly
- Avoiding conversation
- Withdrawing from social situations

diet, and allergies. Central nervous system conditions should also be ruled out. When systemic causes have been excluded, the physician generally refers the patient to an otolaryngologist or audiologist for further evaluation.

Nurse

The focus of nursing care is to assist the patient and family in adjusting to the changes created by the hearing deficit and coping with the tinnitus if it is present. Aiding adjustment to the hearing loss involves assisting with communication strategies or devices, alleviating anxiety, promoting safety, and preventing social isolation. The nurse must educate others that hearing loss is complex and involves speech recognition as well as sound detection. Speaking louder does not necessarily improve communication. In fact, speaking louder can create a barrier to communication if the deficit involves the frequency rather than the intensity of sound. Communication strategies for people with hearing deficits are listed in Box 5-6.

Another area in which careful instruction is essential is the care and use of hearing aids. Hearing aids are very expensive and must be handled carefully. In addition, time is required to adjust to hearing with a hearing aid. Patients are often frustrated by the squeaking or squealing sounds made by a hearing aid when the amplification is too high. All sound is amplified, and some patients have difficulty adjusting to the increased level of background noise. The nurse should advise the patient to get used to the hearing aid slowly by wearing it for short periods of time. Hearing with any new device takes practice, and patients should be advised to practice using their hearing aids at home by listening to television, radios, books on tape, and so on. Patients also must be taught how to preserve battery life and how to care for their hearing aids (Box 5-7).

Strategies for coping with tinnitus vary depending on the severity of the tinnitus and the characteristics of the individual experiencing it. Tinnitus maskers help some people cope with the tinnitus. Maskers are sound-producing devices that cover the unpleasant sound with a more tolerable sound, so-called white noise. White noise can be generated by a ceiling fan, by a sound machine that produces the sound of the ocean, a rain forest, and so on, or by a device worn much like a hearing aid. Some people just leave the television or radio on to create background noise. Self-help groups are available in many communities to offer support and provide information on coping strategies. Information on self-help groups is available from the American Tinnitus Association (*http://www.ata.org/*).

Audiologist

The audiologist diagnosis the type of hearing loss present, prescribes the appropriate hearing aid, and fits it to the patient. Audiologists often provide rehabilitation services to individuals and small groups. These services usually include educating patients and families about the hearing loss that the individual is experiencing and about ways of facilitating communication. Audiologists also teach

Box 5-6 Strategies for Improving Communication

STRATEGIES TO TEACH OTHERS
- Get the attention of the individual with the hearing impairment before speaking.
- Speak to the individual at close range.
- Speak slowly and clearly.
- Lower the tone of your voice; *don't shout.*
- Don't cover your mouth.
- Don't stand in front of a window.
- Reduce background noise.
- Avoid communicating in large group situations.
- Ask what you can do to make communicating easier.

STRATEGIES TO TEACH THE PERSON WITH THE IMPAIRMENT
- Ask people to rephrase rather than repeat themselves.
- Ask for clarification.
- Attend to facial expressions, gestures, and context to help understand what is being said.
- In restaurants, ask for a seat away from the kitchen.
- Rearrange furniture to promote easier conversation.
- Adjust lighting so the conversation partner's face can be seen.
- Use alerting devices that can identify when the doorbell rings.
- Investigate the use of TV listening devices, personal FM systems, conference microphones, and telephone amplifiers.

Box 5-7   Hearing Aid Care

USE
- Wear the hearing aid while awake only.
- Hearing aids that are worn in the ear, in the canal, or completely in the canal are coded red for the right ear. Check proper placement.
- Adjust the volume for maximum benefit; there should be no squeal when the device is in the user's ear.
- Some feedback is normal when an obstruction is placed close to the microphone.

CARE
- Keep the hearing aid in its container when not in use.
- When the hearing aid is not in use, open the battery compartment to break the contact and preserve battery life (a battery used 16 hours a day will last only 1 to 3 weeks)
- Clean daily with a soft cloth or tissue.
- Keep away from moisture, heat, and hairspray.

IF THE HEARING AID DOES NOT WORK
- Check the volume control.
- Check to be sure the receiver is not plugged with ear wax.
- Check the battery and connections.

IF THE HEARING AID SQUEALS
- Check fit and insertion.
- Check volume setting.
- Check for ear wax in ear canal.
- Check for obstruction of the microphone.

---

patients and families about the different kinds of hearing aids that are available and why a particular hearing aid was prescribed for the patient. Patients must understand that hearing aids are not interchangeable and that what works for one person may not work for another. How to take care of hearing aids and fix problems that may arise is also addressed.

Drug Therapy

Drug therapy is not used in the treatment of hearing loss. However, drugs are given to treat infections if they are present and to treat pain. Drug therapy is also useful as a coping strategy for patients for whom the tinnitus creates great emotional distress and anxiety or interferes with sleep. Table 5-2 lists drugs commonly used to treat symptoms associated with disorders of the ears.

Complementary and Alternative Therapies

Vitamin therapy, biofeedback, and hypnosis are interventions that have been used to treat tinnitus, but there is not sufficient evidence for any of these interventions to support their use in the population at large.

VESTIBULAR DISORDERS

The hallmark of vestibular disorders is vertigo, the ninth most common symptom reported by primary care patients, which affects more than 90 million Americans (Sandhaus, 2002). Most people use the terms *dizziness* and *vertigo* interchangeably, but vertigo is actually a very specific disorder characterized by the illusion of movement. Individuals may report the sensation that the world around them is spinning (objective vertigo) or that they are spinning (subjective vertigo). Others may complain of a sense of swaying or tilting, and of being off balance. The type of vertigo experienced has no diagnostic significance, but listening carefully to descriptions of dizziness can help providers determine whether or not the "dizziness" is truly vertigo and is related to the vestibular apparatus or is caused by some other systemic disorder such as syncope or orthostatic hypotension.

Vestibular disorders can be either central or peripheral in origin. Although approximately 85% of vestibular disorders are peripheral and therefore benign, a thorough history taking and neurologic examination is essential to rule out central nervous system disorders, which may be life threatening. Table 5-3 compares the clinical findings associated with each type of vertigo. In general, central nervous system lesions produce vertigo that is mild but long-lasting. Nystagmus is also more prominent in central nervous system disorders. The three most common peripheral vestibular disorders are Ménière's disease, labyrinthitis, and benign paroxysmal positional vertigo (BPPV). BPPV, the most commonly reported condition that produces vertigo, is also one of the most easily diagnosed and treated (Baloh, 2000; Touma and Hirsch, 2001).

Pathophysiology

The vestibular apparatus is located in the inner ear and consists of the semicircular canals and two sacs containing endolymph. These structures make up the membranous labyrinth, which is housed within the bony labyrinth. The bony labyrinth contains perilymphatic fluid to cushion the labyrinthine structures. The labyrinth also contains sensory neurons with cilia that respond to movement and transmit impulses to the eighth cranial nerve, which carries information to the brain.

Central Nervous System Disorders

Central nervous system lesions such as cerebellar neoplasms, acoustic neuromas, stroke, and multiple sclerosis interfere with transmission of impulses to the brain. In these conditions, vertigo is only one of many presenting symptoms and usually the least significant.

Peripheral Vestibular System Disorders

Benign Paroxysmal Positional Vertigo

The pathology associated with BPPV is related to the movement of small crystals of calcium carbonate called

Table 5-2   Drugs Commonly Used for Chronic Ear Disorders

Drug	Side Effects	Nursing Considerations
Ceruminolytics Boric acid (Ear-Dry) Carbamide peroxide (Debrox)		Hydrogen peroxide solution (3% diluted with water to half strength) is just as effective.
Antihistamines *Decongestants* Numerous over-the-counter drugs (Actifed, Allerest, Dimetapp, Triaminic)	Drowsiness, blurred vision, dry mouth, increased blood pressure	Instruct patient not to drive or operate machinery. Prescription drug may be needed if patient is hypertensive.
Antiemetics Dimenhydrinate (Calm-X, Dimetabs, Dramamine) Meclizine (Antivert, Bonine, Antrizine) Dramamine Less Drowsy	Drowsiness, blurred vision, dry mouth	Instruct patient not to drive or operate machinery. Can be purchased over the counter. Treats vertigo with less drowsiness, but patient should still be cautioned about safety.
Benzodiazepines Diazepam (Valium) Lorazepam (Ativan)	Syncope, confusion, drowsiness, blurred vision	Instruct patient not to drive or operate machinery. Use only as needed in acute attack of vertigo.

Think *S* for Success

Symptoms
- Teach patient how to cope with hearing loss and tinnitus. Teach family members to recognize signs that hearing is impaired.

Sequelae
- Assess and support self-esteem and positive self-image. Prevent social isolation by teaching communication strategies.

Safety
- Make sure patient can navigate in environment safely. Teach safe handling of hearing aids and batteries.

Support/Services
- Refer patient and family to support groups and agencies that can assist with hearing-related problems. Make sure patient is aware of assistive devices that can be used to enhance independence in work, school, and leisure activities.

Satisfaction
- Assist patient in identifying the important possibilities of his or her life and developing strategies for maintaining or enhancing quality of life.

canaliths. These canaliths are normally located in an area of the vestibule where they do not interfere with the fluid dynamics of the semicircular canals. In BPPV, however, certain movements cause these canaliths to float into the posterior semicircular canals, which causes disruption in neuronal receptors and produces momentary vertigo.

Ménière's Disease

Ménière's disease is thought to be related to an increase in the pressure of the endolymphatic fluid. The pressure increases until the membrane of the labyrinth ruptures, and endolymph and perilymph mix together. The increased fluid pressure (hydrops) often creates a sense of fullness in the ear. The reason for the increase in endolymphatic pressure is unknown.

Labyrinthitis and Vestibular Neuronitis

Labyrinthitis or vestibular neuronitis is caused by either an infection or an inflammation of the inner ear. Infection can enter the inner ear from the middle ear, the bloodstream, or the brain. Vestibular neuronitis may also follow a viral illness. Although labyrinthitis is an acute disorder, it may have long-lasting effects.

Table 5-3   Differentiating Characteristics of Vertigo

Characteristic	Central	Peripheral
Onset	Gradual	Sudden
Intensity	Mild	Severe
Positional	No	Yes
Nausea and vomiting	Rare	Severe
Hearing loss	Rare	Yes
Loss of balance	Severe	Mild
Lessening with time	No	Yes
Other accompanying neurologic deficits	Common	Rare

Adapted from Sandhaus S: Stop the spinning, *Nurse Pract* 27(8):11-23, 2002.

Assessment

Thorough assessment, beginning with history taking, is the key to diagnosis and treatment. The individual should always be asked to describe in his or her own words the unpleasant sensations being experienced. Descriptions that involve movement, either of the individual or his or her surroundings, indicate vertigo rather than dizziness. The patient should be asked about factors that precipitate the sensations, such as changing positions, bending over too fast, and looking up too quickly. Unlike the dizziness experienced with cardiac or neurologic conditions, vertigo is usually transient and related to changes in head position.

The severity and duration of the symptoms should be assessed. The duration of the vertigo is the most significant factor for differentiating between BPPV, Ménière's disease, and labyrinthitis (Sandhaus, 2002). BPPV episodes are frequent but last only 10 to 20 seconds, whereas symptoms of Ménière's disease last hours to days and recur several times a year. Labyrinthitis is acute in onset and lasts a week to 10 days.

In a number of cases, vertigo occurs in association with migraine headaches or cervical and shoulder pain (Bracher et al, 2000; Solomon, 2000). The provider should take care to question the patient about any pain or discomfort that accompanies or precedes the vertigo, even if it seems unrelated.

Along with the history, an assessment of functional health patterns is essential for developing a plan of care. This assessment should focus on the nature of the vertigo as well as its impact on daily living and quality of life (see Box 5-3).

The physical assessment should include an evaluation of the internal and external ear structures, a cardiovascular examination with auscultation for carotid bruits, and a neurologic examination focusing on the intactness of the cranial nerves, especially III through VIII. Other neurologic tests that should be performed are Romberg's test, heel-to-toe walking, and the finger-to-nose test. Normal proprioception and vibratory perception in the extremities should also be verified. Nystagmus, the only objective sign of vertigo, can be elicited by conducting the Dix-Hallpike test. In this test the patient is moved rapidly from a sitting position to a supine position with the head turned to one side and hang-

ing over the examination table (Box 5-8). This maneuver produces dizziness and nystagmus lasting 10 to 20 seconds in patients who have BPPV.

Many of the individuals seen in the primary care setting will require further diagnostic testing. Tests specific to the vestibular system are caloric testing and electronystagmography. In caloric testing, either warm or cold water is infused into the patient's ear. This produces vertigo and nystagmus within 20 to 30 seconds and may cause nausea and vomiting as well. Individuals with long-standing vertigo may have developed some compensatory mechanisms that interfere with the nystagmus. To prevent such interference, the patient is often asked to perform some mental task requiring concentration, such as counting backwards from 100 by 7, during the test. This keeps the individual from controlling the nystagmus. The caloric test is very uncomfortable for

---

Box 5-8   Dix-Hallpike Maneuver for Diagnosing Benign Paroxysmal Positional Vertigo

1. Place the patient in an upright sitting position on the examination table with feet and legs extended on the table.
2. Place your hands on the sides of the patient's head and rotate the head 45 degrees to the side that is believed to be unaffected.*
3. Keeping your hands on the patient's head, lower the patient to the supine position with the head hanging over the edge of the examination table.
4. Observe for nystagmus (absent on unaffected side).
5. Return the patient to the sitting position and repeat the procedure, turning the head to the side presumed to be affected.
6. Observe for nystagmus (starts within 1 to 5 seconds and lasts 10 to 20 seconds if patient has benign paroxysmal positional vertigo).

*Patients can usually indicate which head positions produce symptoms of vertigo.

patients. They should fast for several hours before the test and be supported throughout the procedure.

In electronystagmography, electrodes are placed near the eyes and nystagmus is provoked. Failure to elicit nystagmus with cerebral stimulation indicates a central lesion. Individuals must be made aware that caloric testing might be used to elicit the nystagmus. Other methods of eliciting nystagmus include changing head position and/or gaze position. Preparation for the examination is similar to that for caloric testing, but patients are also advised to avoid caffeine and alcohol.

Clinical Manifestations

Individuals with central disorders have a variety of signs and symptoms related to the nature of the central problem. For example, individuals with migraine may come to the physician with pain, photosensitivity, and nausea, whereas individuals with multiple sclerosis demonstrate weakness,

especially in the lower extremities, bowel and bladder problems, and visual disturbances. Box 5-9 lists clinical manifestations associated with various central and peripheral disorders that help in differentiating central vertigo from that related to ear conditions. Individuals with peripheral disorders also have vertigo but in addition may experience hearing loss, tinnitus, nausea, and vomiting. These symptoms, though benign, can be disabling depending on their duration, frequency, and severity. Ménière's disease, in particular, can be totally disabling during an attack, which may last for several days.

Interdisciplinary Care

Primary Provider (Physician/Nurse Practitioner)

The main role of the primary care provider is assessment and diagnosis. Correctly diagnosing BPPV, for example, can lead to a quick and effective cure in many cases. If BPPV is

---

Box 5-9 Clinical Manifestations of Disorders Associated with Vertigo

VERTIGO OF CENTRAL ORIGIN
- Cardiovascular disease
  Cardiac murmurs, dysrhythmias
  Carotid bruits
  Orthostatic hypotension
- Central nervous system lesions
  Severe imbalance
  Vertigo that is persistent and nonpositional
  Nystagmus that changes direction with gaze
- Disabling positional vertigo
  Vertigo that is positional but nonparoxysmal and does not lessen over time
  Hearing loss
  Tinnitus
- Migraine
  Vertigo that is variable but not positional and does not lessen over time
  Headache
  Sensitivity to light
  Nausea, vomiting
- Multiple sclerosis
  Diplopia
  Focal weakness
  Bowel and bladder dysfunction
- Psychogenic disorders
  Vertigo that is not positional and is described as light-headedness or a "woozy" sensation (Ask patient to hyperventilate for 2 minutes; if this produces vertigo, suspect psychogenic origin [Sandhaus, 2002])
  Depression, anxiety

- Syphilis
  Asymmetric hearing loss
  Positive results on VDRL test
- Vertebrobasilar insufficiency
  Visual disturbances
  Light-headedness, confusion, loss of consciousness
  Dysarthria, facial numbness
  Extremity weakness
  Vertigo that is not precipitated by changes in position

VERTIGO OF PERIPHERAL ORIGIN
- Benign paroxysmal positional vertigo
  Vertigo that is positional, episodic, and brief (10 to 20 seconds)
  Nausea and vomiting
  Nystagmus that is unidirectional in all fields of gaze
  Lessening of symptoms over time
- Ménière's disease
  Vertigo that is episodic but occurs in attacks lasting for hours to days
  Unilateral sensorineural hearing loss
  Tinnitus
  Drop attacks and disturbances in gait and balance during attacks of vertigo
  Nausea, vomiting
- Labyrinthitis
  Vertigo that is constant and lasts 7 to 10 days

diagnosed, the physician can perform canalith repositioning maneuvers to return canaliths to their appropriate place in the vestibule. Following the repositioning maneuvers, the patient is instructed to keep the head elevated for 24 to 48 hours. Epley (1992) reported an 80% success rate for the procedure, with a 30% recurrence rate after 30 months. More recent studies show a success rate between 40% and 90% with only a 15% incidence of recurrence (Froehling et al, 2000; Furman and Cass, 1999; Gans and Harrington-Gans, 2002).

If Ménière's disease is diagnosed, the practitioner will most likely attempt to manage the condition conservatively with diet and diuretics until the patient can no longer function effectively or has significant hearing loss. More aggressive treatments include endolymphatic decompression, vestibular resection, and labyrinthectomy. Endolymphatic decompression is a procedure in which the endolymph is drained from the endolymphatic sac. Some patients undergoing this procedure experience relief from the vertigo without further loss of hearing. More radical surgical treatments such as resecting the vestibular nerve or removing the labyrinth are controversial because the procedures result in hearing loss.

Nurse

Managing vertigo requires a three-pronged approach: control of symptoms, treatment of the underlying causes of vertigo, and rehabilitation to compensate for vestibular damage (Walling, 1999). The nurse focuses on assessment and diagnosis. The nurse practitioner is capable of performing repositioning maneuvers and, in some states, can prescribe appropriate medications. Medications treat symptoms and are not prophylactic; therefore, they should be prescribed only as needed and limited to a 2-week course of therapy. Furthermore, they cause sleepiness and lethargy, may increase the risk of falls in the elderly, and delay compensation by the central nervous system (Sandhaus, 2002).

A nurse who is not an advanced practitioner can assess the nature of the vertigo and make recommendations for follow-up based on their findings. The nurse refers patients to advanced practitioners for additional diagnostic studies or treatment, to the physical therapist for exercise and compensation maneuvers, and to the chiropractor for management of cervical conditions that may perpetuate vertigo.

Symptom management includes treating nausea and vomiting; treating tinnitus, if present, using the methods outlined earlier in this chapter; and calming the vertigo. Interventions that ease the symptom of vertigo call for the patient to lie down in a position that is comfortable. Very often the individual has a preferred head position that helps to control the sensation of spinning. This head position should be maintained, and the individual should be instructed to avoid any sudden shifts in position. The room should be quiet and darkened. The television set should be turned off. Taking antihistamine medications such as meclizine hydrochloride (Antivert) to treat the vertigo at the onset of an attack can shorten the duration of the attack and may have the benefit of producing sleep. Safety should be maintained. Once the attack has subsided, the patient should resume activities cautiously. Specific treatments include teaching individuals with Ménière's disease to restrict salt intake, avoid caffeine, and stop smoking. Rehabilitation measures include encouraging activity and supporting habituation therapy.

Chiropractor

The chiropractor is involved primarily in the treatment of vertigo related to chronic cervical and shoulder girdle dysfunction. A variety of treatments are performed including massage, spinal manipulation, electroanalgesic therapy, exercise, and surface electromyographic biofeedback. A study of 15 patients with cervically related vertigo by Bracher and colleagues (2001) found that symptoms improved with a combination of these conservative therapies.

Physical Therapist

The physical therapist works with patients who have BPPV to develop central compensation for vestibular damage. This is done through a series of exercises that put the patient in provocative positions until vertigo subsides. The patient is placed in a provocative position with the lateral aspect of the occiput resting on a therapy table or floor mat (bed or couch at home). Once the vertigo subsides, the patient returns to a sitting position for 30 seconds and then lies on the opposite side for 30 seconds. These steps are repeated until the vertigo is no longer provoked. The exercise is done every 3 hours while awake until the patient has 2 consecutive days without symptoms.

Drug Therapy

Drug therapy is aimed at controlling the vertigo, nausea, and vomiting. Ménière's disease is also treated with mild diuretics to reduce the amount of endolymph and with nicotinic acid to improve circulation. Antibiotics are added to the drug regimen for patients with labyrinthitis. Drugs commonly used to treat chronic ear disorders are listed in Table 5-2.

Complementary and Alternative Therapies

Some herbal remedies suggested for relief of vertigo are actually intended to treat motion sickness. They include ginger, ginkgo, celery seeds, and pumpkin seeds. Other Chinese remedies are aimed at clearing the ear canals and include Coix seed *(yi yi ren)*, magnolia flower *(xin yi hua)*, and Asarum leaf *(xi xin)*. Of these herbal remedies, only ginger has been found in scientific studies to be useful in the treatment of dizziness and nausea. A variety of herbal teas and remedies containing a combination of herbs are available for purchase. Patients should be cautioned to examine

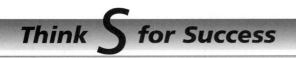

Think **S** *for Success*

Symptoms
- Manage vertigo by placing individual in quiet darkened room in a comfortable position and cautioning person to avoid position changes.
- Treat nausea and vomiting with antiemetics.

Sequelae
- Prevent repeated attacks by limiting intake of salt, fluids, and caffeine, and by refraining from smoking.

Safety
- Caution individuals taking antivertigo drugs not to drive or operate machinery.
- Place individual in a safe position during an attack. Perform fall risk assessment, especially for older patients.

Support/Services
- Refer individual and family members to organizations and agencies that can provide support.
- If vertigo becomes disabling, social services may need to provide assistance with financial and other resources.

Satisfaction
- Determine impact of episodes of vertigo on individual's ability to enjoy the important possibilities of his or her life.

such products carefully, identify all ingredients, and check to make sure that there are no contraindications for taking them, such as interactions with prescribed medications or harmful side effects like elevation of blood pressure.

FAMILY CONCERNS AND CONSIDERATIONS

Families are often frustrated by family members who have hearing loss. The need to repeat things many times can cause people to become impatient. Sometimes attempts at communication are reduced. Other family members may try to compensate in public places by answering for the family member with the hearing impairment, and the individual who does not hear well may feel excluded and lose interest in social events. Families benefit from education and participation in support groups.

ETHICAL CONCERNS

People who are hearing impaired are often prevented from participating fully in society, particularly in the area of employment. One dilemma that frequently arises is related to the health professions. Should a person with hearing loss be allowed to study medicine or nursing? The ethical issues surrounding this question involve a duty to the individual as well as to society. What ethical principles would you cite to support your point of view in this matter?

CASE STUDY

Patient Data

Ms. G. is a 54-year-old white woman who has a history of incapacitating attacks of vertigo. She states that she can feel the attacks coming on and can sometimes avoid them by taking meclizine hydrochloride (Antivert) or decongestants if her head feels congested. The attacks are sometimes brought on by changes in position, and when she feels dizzy she must keep her head position steady. If a full-blown attack occurs, then she must go to bed and lie quietly in the dark without moving until the attack subsides. Her husband cannot sleep beside her because the slightest motion of the bed intensifies the vertigo. She describes the sensations she experiences as a feeling of falling backward in space and spinning around. Although these attacks occur only three or four times a year, she has a history of having experienced "motion sickness" her entire life. She is unable to ride in the back seat of a car or sit in a swing or rocking chair, and states that flashing light patterns in her peripheral vision can provoke an attack. She denies having hearing loss or tinnitus. Nausea is severe during vertigo attacks but she reports no vomiting. Ms. G. underwent a variety of tests in her twenties including caloric testing, electronystagmography, visual evoked potential testing, auditory evoked potential testing, and electroencephalography. She says she was told that she had "motion sickness" and has just tried to live with it. Ms. G. met a physical therapist at a party recently who told her that her symptoms could be helped, and she is coming now for that assistance.

Other Medical History
- Migraine in her twenties and thirties
- Tonsillectomy at age 28
- Frequent sinus infections and congestion

Medications
- Atenolol 25 mg/day for systolic hypertension
- Premarin 0.625 mg/day after hysterectomy

Thinking It Through
- How would you classify Ms. G.'s vertigo?
- What diagnostic tests, if any, would you recommend?
- Do you think she is a good candidate for repositioning maneuvers?

Case Conference

Ms. G. is meeting with the rehabilitation team, which includes a physician, a nurse practitioner, and a physical therapist. After reviewing the case, the physician recommends a hearing test to be sure that no damage has occurred over the past 30 years and suggests that a Dix-Hallpike maneuver be performed to determine if components of Ms. G.'s vertigo originate in BPPV.

Ms. G. is reluctant because the vertigo she experiences is so severe she is afraid that she will be unable to tolerate the test, that the symptoms will persist, and that she will be unable to drive herself home. It is agreed that she will make an appointment to see the physician for follow-up testing.

Continued

CASE STUDY—cont'd
Case Conference

The nurse practitioner reviews Ms. G.'s health patterns, paying particular attention to diet and any factors that precipitate the vertigo. The nurse practitioner recommends that Ms. G. avoid caffeine (she currently drinks four or five cups of coffee and two colas daily) and cut back on the use of additional salt at meals and during cooking. When she inquires about Ms. G.'s use of decongestants, she learns that Ms. G. takes over-the-counter drugs containing pseudoephedrine hydrochloride (Sudafed). Pseudoephedrine hydrochloride is contraindicated for people with hypertension, so the nurse recommends that Ms. G. take guaifenesin instead and gives her a prescription for Humibid.

The physical therapist explains that there are a number of exercises that Ms. G. can do to decrease her short episodes of vertigo but that they may not have any effect on the longer attacks that she experiences several times a year. He warns her that these exercises will provoke vertigo at first but that the symptoms will lessen over time. They will begin the exercises in the physical therapy department initially and observe her responses. She will then continue the exercises at home. Before beginning, however, the physical therapist would like to know the results of the tests performed by the physician so he can choose the appropriate exercises.

Ms. G. agrees to return after visiting the physician and states that she will bring her husband with her so he can learn how to help her with her exercises and her symptoms.

■ Do you think Ms. G. will benefit from physical therapy?
■ Do you think Ms. G. would benefit from chiropractic interventions?
■ Who else should be part of the case conference?

Internet and Other Resources

Alexander Graham Bell Association for the Deaf and Hard of Hearing: *http://www.agbell.org*
American Speech-Language-Hearing Association: *http://www.asha.org*
American Tinnitus Association: *http://www.ata.org*
Cochlear Implant Association, Inc.: *http://www.cici.org*
National Association of the Deaf: *http://www.nad.org*
Self Help for Hard of Hearing People: *http://www.shhh.org*

REFERENCES

American Speech and Hearing Association: Prevalence and incidence of hearing loss in adults, 2004, retrieved from *http://www.asha.org/public/hearing/disorders/prevalence_adults.htm* on Jan 23, 2004.

Baloh RW: Treatment of the common causes of vertigo, *J Audiol Med* 9(3):135-59, 2000.

Better Hearing Institute: 500 hearing impaired people, 2003, retrieved from *http://www.hear-it.org/forside.dsp?forside=yes&area=34* on Jan 23, 2004.

Bracher E et al: A combined approach for the treatment of cervical vertigo, *J Manipulative Physiol Ther* 23(2):96-100, 2000.

Froehling DA et al: The canaliths repositioning procedure for the treatment of benign paroxysmal positional vertigo: a randomized controlled trial, *Mayo Clin Proc* 75(7):695-700, 2000.

Epley JM: The canalith repositioning procedure for treatment of benign paroxysmal positional vertigo, *Otolaryngol Head Neck Surg* 107(3):399-404, 1992.

Furman J, Cass S: Benign paroxysmal positional vertigo, *N Engl J Med* 341(21):1590-6, 1999.

Gans R, Harrington-Gans P: Treatment efficacy of benign paroxysmal positional vertigo (BPPV) with canalith repositioning maneuver and Semont Liberatory Maneuver, *Semin Hearing* 23(2):149-59, 2002.

National Center for Health Statistics: Current estimates from the National Health Interview Survey, 1995, retrieved from *http://www.cdc.gov/nchs/products/pubs/pubd/series/sr10_1999.htm* on Jan 23, 2004.

National Council on the Aging: Untreated hearing loss linked to depression, anxiety, social isolation in seniors, May 26, 1999, retrieved from *http://www.ncoa.org/content.cfm?sectionID=105&detail=46* on Jan 23, 2004.

Sandhaus S: Stop the spinning, *Nurse Pract* 27(8):11-23, 2002.

Solomon D: Distinguishing and treating causes of central vertigo, *Otolaryngol Clin North Am* 33(3):579-601, 2000.

Touma J, Hirsch B: Treating benign paroxysmal positional vertigo, *Emerg Med* 33(1):94-8, 101, 2001.

Walling A: Presentations of some common types of vertigo, *Am Fam Physician* 59(8):2318-19, 1999.

CHAPTER 6

Disorders of the Skin

Sharron Guillett, PhD, RN

OBJECTIVES

After reading this chapter, you should be able to do the following:

- Identify commonly occurring chronic conditions of the skin
- Describe chronic conditions of the skin associated with aging
- Describe clinical manifestations of commonly occurring chronic skin disorders
- Describe the functional health patterns affected by chronic skin disorders
- Describe the role of each member of the interdisciplinary team involved in the care of patients with chronic skin disorders
- Describe the indications for use, side affects, and nursing considerations related to drugs commonly used to treat chronic skin disorders

The skin is part of the integumentary system, the largest organ of the body. Other structures of the integumentary system—hair, nails, and glands—are not discussed in this chapter except as they contribute to chronic disorders of the skin. The skin has several important functions. Foremost among these is to serve as a protective barrier between an individual's internal and external environments. In addition, skin provides thermoregulation, absorbs ultraviolet light for production of vitamin D, provides sensory input and emotional feedback, and is increasingly used as a route for administering medications. Apart from showing one's emotional state to others, an individual's skin provides important clues about that person's health status. Therefore, it is essential that health care professionals become accustomed to assessing skin not only in individuals for whom the skin condition is the chief complaint but in all individuals with chronic illnesses and/or disabilities in order to enhance evaluation of the underlying physiologic condition. Table 6-1 lists common systemic disorders and the skin conditions associated with them.

The approach to managing chronic skin conditions is similar for all disorders. For example, assessment follows the same structure, many of the symptoms are identical, and the treatments are generally symptom focused. Therefore,

the format of this chapter is somewhat different in that the sections on assessment and interdisciplinary care are presented first, and these elements are presumed to be largely the same for all skin conditions. Specific chronic disorders of the skin are highlighted and their pathophysiology, clinical manifestations, and preferred treatment modalities are discussed.

Assessment

When assessing the skin, health care providers must differentiate between skin changes that are considered normal and related to the aging process (Batchelor and Remo, 1998), minor skin problems that may or may not be the reason for the patient's visit, and important lesions indicating that serious disease may be present. Box 6-1 lists skin changes that occur with aging.

The generalized assessment of the individual with a chronic skin disorder does not vary much from condition to condition (Box 6-2). Skin lesions themselves should be evaluated with regard to four characteristics: type, shape, arrangement, and distribution. Common types of lesions along with brief descriptions are presented in Table 6-2. When the type of lesion is described, the color should be noted as well as the consistency, depth, temperature, mobility, and tenderness of the lesion. Terms used to describe the shape of skin lesions include *round, oval, polygonal, polycyclic, annular, umbilicated,* and *serpentine* or *serpiginous.* Assessment of the arrangement and distribution of lesions in a skin disorder entails determining the pattern, location, and extent of involvement, and noting whether or not the lesions are grouped, discrete, or diffuse.

Health care providers are always on the alert for skin cancer and assess all moles or nevi using the ABCDE format. Moles that raise suspicion of cancer and need follow-up are **A**symmetrical, have irregular **B**orders, are dark in **C**olor, and have a **D**iameter greater than 6 mm (Figure 6-1) (Cuzzell, 2002). Two other characteristics that are indicative of melanoma are **E**levation and **E**nlargement. A history of increase in lesion size may be one of the most important indicators of malignant melanoma.

Diagnosis of chronic skin conditions is based on the findings of the history, physical assessment, laboratory tests, and sometimes biopsies and imaging studies.

Table 6-1 Skin Signs Associated with Systemic Conditions

Systemic Problem	Dermatologic Manifestations
Endocrine	
Hyperthyroidism	Increased sweating, warm skin with persistent flush, thin nails, vitiligo and alopecia, fine, soft hair
Hypothyroidism	Cold, dry, pale to yellow skin; slightly hyperkeratotic epidermis with follicular plugging; generalized nonpitting edema; dry, coarse, brittle hair; brittle, slow-growing nails
Glucocorticoid excess (Cushing's syndrome), induced endogenously or exogenously)	Atrophy; striae; epidermal thinning; telangiectasia; acne; decreased subcutaneous fat over extremities; thin, loose dermis; impaired wound healing; increased vascular fragility; mild hirsutism; excessive collection of fat over clavicles, back of neck, abdomen, and face; increased incidence of pyodermas
Addison's disease	Loss of body hair (especially axillary), generalized hyperpigmentation (especially in folds)
Androgen excess	Enlarged facial pores, male sexual characteristics, acne, acceleration of coarse hair growth
Androgen deficiency, after puberty	Development of sparse hair; marked reduction in sebum production
Hypoparathyroidism	Opaque, brittle nails with transverse ridges; coarse, sparse hair with patchy alopecia; eczematous and exfoliative dermatitis; hyperkeratotic and maculopapular eruptions
Hyperpituitarism (acromegaly)	Coarsened skin, deepened lines; increased oiliness and sweating; acne; increased number of nevi, hyperpigmentation; hypertrichosis
Hypopituitarism (Fröhlich's syndrome)	Smooth skin; scant hair growth; obesity; small, thin fingernails
Diabetes mellitus	Increased xanthomas and carotene, shin spots, necrobiosis lipoidica diabeticorum, delayed wound healing
Gastrointestinal	
Ulcerative colitis, Crohn's disease	Pyoderma gangrenosum, mouth ulcers
Liver disease and biliary tract obstruction	Jaundice, itching, pigmentary abnormalities, alterations in nails and hair, spider angiomas, telangiectasia
Deficiency of essential fatty acids	Scaly skin
Malabsorption syndrome	Acquired ichthyosis
Cystic fibrosis	Abnormal sweat gland function resulting in failure to convert sodium
Musculoskeletal and Connective Tissue	
Systemic lupus erythematosus	Maculopapular semiconfluent rash (butterfly rash)
Scleroderma	Leathery hardening and stiffness of skin
Dermatomyositis	Edema; purplish red upper eyelids; butterfly rash; scaly, macular erythema over knuckles; linear telangiectasia of posterior nail fold
Metabolic	
Lipidoses	Xanthomas
Vitamin A deficiency	Generalized dry hyperkeratosis
Hypervitaminosis A	Hair loss, dry skin
Vitamin B_1 (thiamine) deficiency	Edema, redness of soles of feet
Vitamin B_2 (riboflavin) deficiency	Red fissures at corner of mouth, glossitis
Nicotinic acid (niacin) deficiency	Pellagra; redness of exposed areas of hand or foot, face, or neck; infected dermatitis
Immune	
Drug sensitivity	Rash of any morphology
Serum sickness	Pruritus
Cancer of breast, stomach, lung, uterus, kidney, ovary, colon, bladder	Metastasis to skin
Hodgkin's disease	Pruritus and nonspecific erythemas
Lymphomas	Papules, nodules, plaques, pruritus

Table 6-1   Skin Signs Associated with Systemic Conditions—cont'd

Systemic Problem	Dermatologic Manifestations
Cardiovascular	
Arteriosclerosis	Decreased oxygenation leading to gangrene
Rheumatic heart disease	Petechiae, urticaria, rheumatoid nodules, erythema nodosum and multiforme
Periarteritis nodosa	Periarteritis nodules
Thromboangiitis obliterans (Buerger's disease)	Superficial migrating thrombophlebitis, pallor or cyanosis, gangrene, ulceration
Respiratory	
Inadequate oxygenation secondary to respiratory disease	Cyanosis
Hematologic	
Anemia	Pallor, hyperpigmentation, pale mucous membranes, hair loss, nail dystrophy
Clotting disorders	Purpura, petechiae, ecchymosis
Renal	
Chronic renal failure	Dry skin, pruritus, uremic frost, pallor, dry skin, bruises
Reproductive	
Primary syphilis	Chancre
Secondary syphilis	Generalized skin lesions
Late benign syphilis	Gummas
Paget's disease	Eczematous patch of nipple and areola
Neurologic	
Syringomyelia, chronic sensory polyneuropathies, spinal cord trauma	Trophic changes in skin resulting from sensory denervation, pressure ulcers, anesthesia, paresthesias

The majority of chronic skin disorders are not life threatening and create only mild physical discomfort for the individuals experiencing them. However, the psychosocial and emotional consequences of skin disorders cannot be overemphasized. A quote from a short story authored by John Updike (1963) about an artist with psoriasis captures the impact of skin disorders on a person's self-image and self-esteem: "Lusty, though we are loathsome to love. Keen sighted, though we hate to look upon ourselves. The name of the disease spiritually speaking, is Humiliation." The emotional impact of skin disorders can be much more significant and longer lasting than any of the physical symptoms encountered. It is therefore essential that the health care provider conduct a thorough assessment of functional health patterns to determine what effect this illness has had on the individual's everyday life and relationships. A framework for a functional health assessment appears in Box 6-3.

Interdisciplinary Care
Primary Provider (Physician/Nurse Practitioner)

The primary provider examines skin lesions through direct observation and prescribes treatment based on the findings. Simple rashes, skin ulcers, and wounds may be treated successfully in this manner. Frequently, the primary provider

---

Box 6-1   Skin Changes Related to Aging

- Skin is less elastic.
- Skin tears easily.
- Skin bruises easily.
- Skin and mucous membranes become drier.
- Senile lentigines (hyperpigmented macular lesions) develop on face and hands.
- Seborrheic keratoses and skin tags are common on neck and axilla and increase in numbers.
- Reddish brown discoloration of the neck (poikiloderma) is very common in women.
- Blackheads develop on the face lateral to the eyes.
- Bright red hemangiomas appear on the trunk.

refers the individual to a physician specializing in treatment of skin conditions, wounds, and skin cancer.

Nurse

The role of the nurse is primarily to promote skin health through education, to teach patients and families how to perform their own treatments and therapies, to assess therapeutic outcomes, and to support patients as they struggle with related psychosocial issues. In some cases, the nurse may be called upon to apply dressings or ointments, but for the most part treatments are carried out by the patients and or the patient's informal caregivers.

Health promotion includes encouraging good nutrition, adequate rest and exercise, good hygiene, and safety in exposure to ultraviolet light, either from the sun or from tanning devices.

Nutrition

Good nutrition involves eating a well-balanced diet to maintain a healthy weight and staying adequately hydrated. In general, patients should follow the recommended daily allowances for each of the five food groups and drink at least eight 10-oz glasses of water every day. Individuals who are trying to lose weight should eat smaller amounts of food and should not eliminate any of the recommended food groups. Protein is essential for cell growth and wound healing, and fatty acids maintain the integrity of the cell. Vitamins that are essential for healthy skin and wound healing are vitamins A, B, and C.

Exercise

Exercise is important for physical and emotional well-being. Exercising increases circulation, which nourishes skin cells and dilates blood vessels, giving the skin a healthy color. Exercise stimulates the release of endorphins, which improve mental well-being, and the effects of exercise on fitness, stamina, and appearance can be a boost to self-image and self-esteem. Sweating sometimes makes rashes and itching worse, however, and outdoor exercise may bring on problems related to exposure to wind, sun, heat, and cold. Therefore, as is true with any therapeutic plan, recommendations for exercise cannot be generalized but must be individualized to meet the patient's unique needs.

Skin Protection

Similarly, teaching regarding hygiene practices must be based on the type and condition of the patient's skin as well as the patient's work and leisure habits and cultural beliefs. Patients with oily skin should avoid using moisturizing soaps and creams, whereas patients with dry skin can benefit from them. Patients with dry skin should bathe less often, use warm rather than hot water, and dry the skin by patting rather than by rubbing. Moisturizers should be applied when the skin is still wet to seal in the moisture. Older patients, in particular, should avoid excessive bathing. Long-term care facilities very often have bathing schedules for residents, in part to protect the skin from overdrying. In between full baths, partial baths of the axillae and perianal area can be carried out as needed. Face and hands should be washed several times a day, but again, care should be taken to use mild soaps or moisturizing cleansers. Frequent hand washing itself can lead to dermatitis of the hands.

A very important area for teaching is the use of a sun block and avoidance of excessive exposure to the sun. The ultraviolet rays of the sun are believed to be the major cause of skin cancer. Therefore, patients should wear sun block every day or take measures to protect the skin with clothing, wear wide-brimmed hats, or use parasols. Women and men who use cosmetic products can purchase products with sun block as one of the ingredients. Generally, a sun block product with a sun protection factor (SPF) of 15 is acceptable. However, if an individual will spend prolonged periods of time in the sun—gardening, golfing, or swimming, for example—the SPF may need to be higher or the lotion applied more frequently. Swimmers and those who perspire freely should use waterproof sun block products. Individuals should be reminded that the most dangerous time of day for sun damage is between 10 AM and 2 PM standard time and

Table 6-2   Common Skin Lesions

Lesion	Description	Diagram
Macule	Circumscribed area of change in skin color (from the Latin word *macula,* which means "spot")	
Papule	Superficial solid lesion with well-defined borders, most of which is above the skin surface (from the Latin word *pupula,* which means "pimple")	
Plaque	Well-defined elevation with a width that is greater than its elevation	
Wheal	Rounded or flat-topped, pale papule or evanescent plaque that disappears in a matter of hours	
Nodule	Palpable, small, solid, round or elliptical lesion with more depth than a papule (from the Latin word *nodulus,* which means "small knot")	

Continued

Table 6-2   Common Skin Lesions—cont'd

Lesion	Description	Diagram
Pustule	Circumscribed, superficial cavity that contains a purulent exudate	
Vesicle	Circumscribed, elevated, superficial cavity less than 0.5 cm wide containing fluid } (from the Latin word *vesicula,* which means "little bladder")	
Bulla	Circumscribed, elevated superficial cavity more than 0.5 cm wide containing fluid (from the Latin word *bulla,* which means "bubble")	
Crust	Dried exudates (from the Latin word *crusta,* which means "rind," "bark," or "shell")	
Scale	Flake of skin that may be loose or adherent	

Table 6-2   Common Skin Lesions—cont'd

Lesion	Description	Diagram
Ulcer	Loss of epidermis and upper layer of dermis that always occurs in pathologically altered tissue, in contrast to wounds, which always occur in normal tissue (from the Latin word *ulcus,* which means "sore")	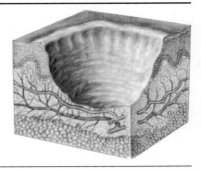

From Bryant R: *Acute and chronic wounds*, ed 2, St Louis, 2000, Mosby.

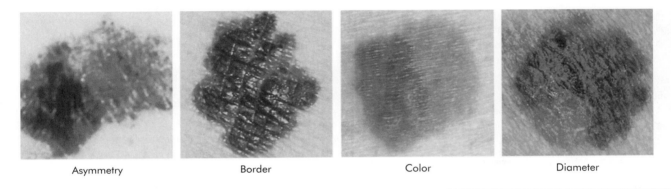

Asymmetry   Border   Color   Diameter

Figure 6-1   The ABCDs of skin cancer. **A,** Asymmetry: one half is unlike the other half. **B,** Border irregularity: edges are ragged, notched, or blurred. **C,** Color: varied pigmentation; shades of tan, brown, and black. **D,** Diameter: larger than 6 mm (diameter of a pencil eraser). (From Habif TP: *Clinical dermatology: a color guide to diagnosis and therapy,* ed 4, St Louis, 2004, Mosby.)

that ultraviolet rays are not blocked by clouds. People should also be cautioned to avoid using tanning beds. Individuals with specific skin conditions such as psoriasis may use ultraviolet light as part of their treatment, and these individuals must take special care to avoid additional exposure. Teaching about safe sun practices also involves discussing any medications that the patient is currently taking, because many medications make the patient more susceptible to sun damage. Drugs that cause photosensitivity are listed in Table 6-3.

One of the most important things the nurse can do is support and foster self-esteem (Weiss et al, 2002). It is important for the nurse to treat patients with dignity and respect and not to show any reaction to their appearance or reluctance to touch or be near them. Patients should be encouraged to discuss their feelings openly. The nurse should provide guidance and offer hope when realistic. Socialization should be encouraged and strategies for dealing with public reactions should be discussed. Ultimately the nurse may wish to consider referring a patient for psychological counseling if the individual continues to struggle with acceptance and self-esteem.

Dermatologist

The dermatologist uses specialized techniques to examine skin lesions, such as dermatoscopy, diascopy, acetowhitening, and patch testing. The dermatologist also performs biopsies, microscopic examinations, and minor surgical procedures in the office. Blood and urine samples useful in diagnosing systemic disorders may be collected in the physician's or dermatologist's office but are generally sent out for analysis. Based on the diagnosis, the physician prescribes medications and therapies to treat the lesions, provide comfort, and prevent disfigurement or further illness. Common methods for treating skin disorders are listed in Box 6-4.

Surgeon

A patient with basal or squamous cell skin cancer is often referred to a surgeon certified in microscopic surgery. Mohs

---

Box 6-3   Functional Health Pattern Assessment for Chronic Skin Conditions

HEALTH PERCEPTION/HEALTH MANAGEMENT
- What is the patient's perception of his or her overall health?
- What medications and therapies does the patient use, including over-the-counter drugs, herbals, and alternative therapies?
- How long has the skin condition been present?
- What remedies have been tried?
- Is there a family pattern or history of similar occurrences?
- Does the patient use sun protection measures?
- Does the patient have a history of severe sunburn as a child?
- Is the patient aware of the risk factors for skin cancer?
- How often does the patient check moles, freckles, etc.?

NUTRITION/METABOLISM
- What is the condition of the skin and mucous membranes?
- What is the daily intake of nutrients and vitamins?
- Does the patient have any food allergies?
- Does the patient have any systemic disorders that affect nutrition or metabolism, such as thyroid condition, diabetes, or irritable bowel syndrome?

ELIMINATION
- Have any changes occurred in bowel or bladder habits?
- Does the patient complain of perianal itching or discomfort?

ACTIVITY/EXERCISE
- What are the patient's regular exercise activities and recreational activities?
- Is the patient able to perform regular and instrumental activities of daily living?

SLEEP/REST
- How many hours of uninterrupted sleep does the patient get at night?
- What sleep aids are used?
- If itching is present, is it worse at night?

COGNITION/PERCEPTION
- What are the nature, character, location, and duration of the pain and/or itching?
- What factors aggravate and alleviate the pain and/or itching?

- How effective are pain and/or itch management strategies?
- What is the level of distress associated with the symptoms?

SELF-PERCEPTION/SELF-CONCEPT
- How does the patient describe himself or herself?
- How has the condition affected the patient's self-esteem?
- How has the condition changed the patient's body image?

ROLES/RELATIONSHIPS
- What kind of work does the patient perform?
- What role does the patient play in the home and family?
- What changes have occurred in the patient's ability to carry out role functions?
- How satisfied is the patient with his or her current roles and relationships?
- How has the condition affected the patient's spouse or significant other?

SEXUALITY/REPRODUCTION
- Is the patient sexually active?
- Is the patient satisfied with current sexual patterns?
- Does the patient use birth control pills?

COPING/STRESS TOLERANCE
- Has the condition caused or increased stress?
- What are the patient's coping strategies?
- What support systems are available to the patient?
- Can the patient manage the condition in the current setting?
- Is the patient with a terminal condition aware of hospice and palliative care options?

VALUES/BELIEFS
- What constitutes good quality of life for the patient?
- What is important to the patient?
- Does the patient express feelings of hopelessness?
- What are the patient's beliefs relating to the condition, the locus of control, end-of-life concerns, and do-not-resuscitate questions and decisions?
- To what extent do the patient's cultural/spiritual beliefs influence decision making related to this condition?

---

surgery, named after its inventor, Dr. Frederic Mohs, is a procedure in which the cancerous tissue is excised, sectioned horizontally, and divided into quarters; each section is then examined for cancerous roots and residue. Tissue surrounding the lesion continues to be excised and examined until clear margins are obtained. The procedure takes longer than routine excisions but produces higher cure rates and less disfigurement (American Society for Mohs Surgeons, 2003). The surgery requires specialized equipment and is performed only by physicians trained in the procedure.

Drug Therapy

Drugs used in the treatment of chronic skin conditions are primarily topical and locally applied (Table 6-4). They include medications designed to stop itching (antipruritics), remove skin layers (keratolytics), fight infections (antibiotics, antifungals, antivirals, antiseptics), soften skin surfaces (emollients), treat eczema, and suppress inflammation (corticosteroids). These drugs can be delivered by many routes and can be proprietary products or generic products mixed and prepared by the pharmacist according to the

Table 6-3   Drugs That Cause Photosensitivity

Drug Category	Examples
Antibiotics	Amoxicillin (Amoxil), ciprofloxacin (Cipro), doxycycline (Vibramycin), sulfonamides (Septra, Gantrisin), tetracycline (Achromycin)
Anticancer drugs	Dacarbazine (DTIC), fluorouracil (5FU), flutamide (Eulexin), methotrexate (MTX), vinblastine (Velban)
Antidepressants	Amitriptyline (Elavil), doxepin (Sinequan), phenelzine (Nardil), trazodone (Desyrel)
Antihistamines	Astemizole (Hismanal), cimetidine (Tagamet), diphenhydramine (Benadryl), ranitidine (Zantac)
Antihypertensives	β-Blockers (Tenormin), angiotensin-converting enzyme inhibitors (Capoten), diltiazem (Cardizem), methyldopa (Aldomet), minoxidil (Rogaine), nifedipine (Procardia)
Antiparasitics	Chloroquine (Aralen), quinine (Quinamm), thiabendazole (Mintezol)
Antipsychotics	Chlorpromazine (Thorazine), prochlorperazine (Compazine), thioridazine (Mellaril), haloperidol (Haldol), perphenazine (Trilafon)
Diuretics	Acetazolamide (Diamox), furosemide (Lasix), metolazone (Zaroxolyn), hydrochlorothiazide (Hydrodiuril), polythiazide (Renese-R)
Hypoglycemics	Acetohexamide (Dymelor), chlorpropamide (Diabinese), glipizide (Glucotrol), glyburide (Amaryl), tolazamide (Tolinase), tolbutamide (Orinase)
Nonsteroidal antiinflammatory drugs	Diflunisal (Dolobid), ibuprofen (Motrin), indomethacin (Indocin), naproxen (Naprosyn), phenylbutazone (Butazolidin)

Box 6-4   Common Treatment Modalities

■ Baths
■ Creams and ointments
■ Cryosurgery
■ Electrosurgery
■ Lotions
■ Oils and emulsions
■ Pastes
■ Powders
■ Soaps and shampoos
■ Tinctures and aqueous solutions
■ Ultraviolet light therapy
■ Ultraviolet light therapy combined with oral psoralen
■ Wet dressings and soaks

physician's orders. Numerous corticosteroid preparations are available. Box 6-5 lists them in order of potency.

Complementary and Alternative Therapies

A number of complementary therapies may be useful (Eliopoulos, 1999). For example, massage and touch therapy stimulate circulation, proper nutrition promotes healthy skin and wound healing, and a variety of essential oils and topical herbs can be used therapeutically for both comfort and healing (Box 6-6). Additional interventions include guided imagery, visualization, relaxation, distraction, and deep-breathing techniques.

The most important aspect of using any complementary therapy is ensuring that the provider is aware that these ther-apies are being used, so that he or she can determine if any potential for harm exists.

BENIGN SKIN CONDITIONS
Pruritus

Pruritus, or itching, is responsible for more visits to the physician than any other skin symptom. Persistent itching can be maddening, causing sleepless nights and interfering with the patient's ability to carry out the day-to-day business of living. Many skin diseases cause itching, as do many systemic disorders, but generalized pruritus can occur without diagnostic lesions or systemic disease.

Pathophysiology

Generalized pruritus is usually associated with winter dry skin or senile skin. Winter dry skin is the result of loss of humidification in the environment. Senile pruritus is thought to be related to a disorder of keratinization (Simandl, 2002).

Clinical Manifestations

Patients complain of sudden onset of severe itching, especially at night. The itching associated with senile pruritus occurs most commonly on the scalp, shoulders, sacrum, and legs. Winter itch is usually confined to the legs. The skin appears to have dry, curled plaques, and signs of excoriation are seen. Scratching usually makes the itch worse because it further damages the skin cells.

A common skin condition characterized by chronic patches of itching, thickened, scaly dry skin, called lichen simplex chronicus, is actually the result of scratching an itch. The itching leads to scratching, which creates itching,

Table 6-4   Drugs Commonly Used to Treat Chronic Skin Conditions

Drug	Route	Side Effects	Nursing Considerations
Antipruritics Menthol Phenol Camphor	Topical	Local reaction	Instruct patient to stop use if irritation occurs.
Antihistamines Astemizole (Hismanal) Cetirizine (Zyrtec) Loratadine (Claritin) Clemastine (Tavist) Hydroxyzine (Vistaril, Atarax) Diphenhydramine (Benadryl)	Oral Topical/oral	Drowsiness, dry mouth, hypotension	Take vital signs. Instruct patient to avoid alcohol or CNS depressants. Instruct patient to take care in driving or operating machinery.
Keratoplastics Salicylic acid 1-2%	Topical	Local reaction	Instruct patient to stop use if irritation occurs.
Keratolytics Adapalene (Differin) Azelaic acid (Azelex) Benzoyl peroxide (Benzac) Salicylic acid 4% (Sebulex) Resorcinol (Bicozene) Urea 20-40% Sulfur 4-10% Alpha hydroxyl acids 15-80%	Topical	Burning, itching, redness with frequent use Increased susceptibility to sunburn	Instruct patient to report side effects. Instruct patient to use sun block and other sun protection measures.
Antieczematous Agents Burow's solution Coal tar solution	Topical Topical	 Redness, staining	 Instruct patient to use care around clothing.
Antibacterials Bacitracin (Neosporin) Neomycin (Muci-fradin) Mupirocin (Bactroban)	Topical		
Antibiotics Tetracycline (Achromycin)	Topical/oral	Nausea and vomiting, diarrhea, rash, headache, heartburn, photosensitivity	Store away from light and heat. Instruct patient not to take with milk products. Instruct patient to take 1 hour before or 2 hours after meal. Instruct patient to use sun protection. Check laboratory test results for renal and liver function.
Erythromycin (E-Mycin, Emgel)	Topical/oral	Anorexia, nausea and vomiting, cramps, tinnitus, pruritus	Instruct patient to take 1 hour before or 2 hours after meal. Instruct patient to report any side effects.
Clindamycin (Cleocin)	Topical/oral	Anorexia, nausea and vomiting, cramps	Incompatible with phenytoin (Dilantin), amoxicillin (Amoxil), and aminophylline (Theo-Dur)

Table 6-4   Drugs Commonly Used to Treat Chronic Skin Conditions

Drug	Route	Side Effects	Nursing Considerations
Antivirals			
Acyclovir (Zovirax)	Topical/oral	Nausea and vomiting, diarrhea, headache	Check laboratory test results. Monitor intake and output.
Penciclovir (Denavir)	Topical	Lethargy, rash, pruritus, nephrotoxicity	Check laboratory test results Monitor intake and output.
Antipsoriatic Agents			
Anthralin (Anthra-Derm)	Topical	Redness, staining	Instruct patient to use care around clothing.
Calcipotriene (Dovonex)	Topical	Possible increase in serum calcium level	Check laboratory test results.
Coal tar (Estar, psoriGel)	Topical	Burning, staining	
Methoxsalen (Oxsoralen)	Topical/oral	Nausea, headache, vertigo, rash, burning, peeling	Use with ultraviolet light (UVL) to lower dosage.
Etretinate (Tegison)	Oral	Anorexia, nausea and vomiting, rash, bone and joint pain, burning, peeling, alopecia, hematuria, hepatitis	Use with UVL to lower dosage. Check laboratory test results.
Corticosteroids			
See Box 6-5	Topical/oral	Topical: skin atrophy with long-term use	Patient usually on short-term therapy.
		Oral: nausea, diarrhea, flushing, depression, mood changes, headache	Instruct patient to taper medication as directed and take with food.
Emollients			
Mineral oil	Topical	Possible plugging of pores	Instruct patient to cleanse skin with soap.
Petrolatum	Topical	Comedogenic	Instruct patient to cleanse skin with soap.
Nivea lotion	Topical		
Urea 5-10%	Topical		
Miscellaneous			
Metronidazole 0.75% (MetroGel)	Topical	Dry skin	May be used with emollients.
Tretinoin 0.025-0.1% (Retin-A)	Topical	Burning, blistering, peeling	Start with low dosages and increase gradually. Instruct patient to use sun protection.
Isotretinoin (Accutane)	Topical/oral	Nosebleeds, pruritus, eye irritation, hepatotoxicity, nausea and vomiting, anorexia, thrombocytopenia, photosensitivity, depression, Rare: suicidal ideation, suicide attempts, and suicide	Obtain laboratory test results prior to and during treatment.

Box 6-5   Commonly Used Corticosteroids in Order of Potency

HIGH POTENCY
- Temovate cream, ointment, gel 0.05%
- Diprolene ointment 0.05%
- Psorcon cream, ointment 0.05%
- Ultravate cream, ointment 0.05%
- Cyclocort ointment 0.1%
- Diprosone ointment 0.05%
- Topicort cream 0.025%
- Topicort gel 0.05%
- Topicort ointment 0.025%

MODERATE POTENCY
- Aristocort cream HP 0.5%
- Cyclocort cream, lotion 0.1%
- Diprosone cream 0.05%
- Florone cream 0.05%
- Halog ointment, solution 0.1%
- Cordran ointment, cream 0.05%
- Elocon cream, lotion 0.1%
- Kenalog cream, ointment 0.1%
- Valisone ointment 0.1%
- Synalar ointment 0.025%
- Lidex cream, gel 0.05%
- Valisone cream 0.1%
- Westcort cream 0.2%

LOW POTENCY
- Aclovate cream, ointment 0.05%
- Aristocort cream 0.1%
- DesOwen cream 0.05%
- Kenalog cream, lotion 0.025%
- Tridesilon cream 0.05%
- Dexamethasone cream 0.1%
- Hytone ointment 0.25% to 2.5%
- Cortef cream 0.25% to 2.5%
- Medrol ointment 0.25% to 1.0%

Box 6-6   Complementary and Alternative Therapies for Common Skin Disorders

AROMATHERAPY
- Treatment of psoriasis: bergamot, lavender

ESSENTIAL OILS
- Cellular regeneration: celery, rosemary
- Infection prevention: garlic, thyme
- Rejuvenation: neroli
- Relief of stings or bites: cinnamon, garlic, lavender, lemon, sage, thyme

HOMEOPATHIC REMEDIES (CONSULT WITH HOMEOPATHIC PROVIDER)
- Arsenicum album
- Calendula
- Cuprum metallicum
- Graphites
- Psorinum
- Sulfur

TOPICAL HERBS
- Antieczema: goldenseal, nettle
- Antiinflammatory: chamomile baths or soaks
- Antipruritic: peppermint
- Astringent: witch hazel
- Emollient: aloe vera
- Wound healing: St. John's wort

---

and so on, until a chronic dermatosis develops. This condition is sometime referred to as *neurodermatitis*.

Treatment

Generalized pruritus is treated with emollient lotions such as Eucerin and Lac-Hydrin, low-potency corticosteroid ointments, and oral antihistamines. Patients are instructed to bathe in cool water using as little soap as possible and to bathe less frequently. Mild soaps like Dove and Basis are recommended, and oils such as Alpha-Keri are added to the bath water. Patients must be reminded that, when oils are added to the water, extra precautions must be taken to avoid slipping and falling. Individuals with lichen simplex chronicus are given similar instructions and are told that the con-

dition is caused by scratching so that they must try to keep their hands off the affected area. The itching is treated with ice packs of Burow's solution and moderate-potency steroid ointments. The ointments can be applied and covered up with wraps overnight. This helps by treating the skin and preventing scratching. However, long-term use of occlusive steroidal dressings can lead to atrophy of the skin. If the patient still complains of itching, corticosteroids can be injected into the lesions themselves every 2 to 3 weeks until the lesions disappear, a short course of oral prednisone can be given, and if necessary tranquilizers can be prescribed.

Urticaria

The common term for urticaria is *hives*. Approximately 20% of the population has experienced urticaria at some point in their lives. Urticaria can be acute or chronic, with chronic urticaria defined as urticaria lasting more than 30 days. Acute urticaria usually has a known precipitating factor, whereas the cause of chronic urticaria is usually unknown.

Pathophysiology

Wheals are caused by a hypersensitivity response in which immunoglobulin E reacts to antigens and stimulates the release of histamine by mast cells, producing swelling and erythema.

Table 6-5 Common Types of Chronic Urticaria

Type of Urticaria	Age (yr)	Clinical Features
Chronic idiopathic	20-50	Generalized pale or pink edematous papules or wheals accompanied by itching
Cold	10-40	Itchy pale or red swelling where skin comes in contact with cold surfaces
Pressure	20-50	Large painful or itchy red swelling at pressure sites
Solar	20-50	Itchy pale or red swelling where skin is exposed to ultraviolet light
Cholinergic	10-50	Itchy, small, pale or pink wheals on trunk, neck, and limbs in response to stress, exercise, or a hot shower
Symptomatic dermatographic	20-50	Itchy linear wheals, red flare wherever skin is rubbed or scratched

Clinical Manifestations

The type of urticaria determines the signs and symptoms manifested. Table 6-5 lists the common types of chronic urticaria and their associated manifestations.

Treatment

Urticaria that lasts longer than 6 months is treated with oral antihistamines. Patients are asked to keep a diary of everything ingested, including food, medicines, breath mints, and so on. Patients are also encouraged to avoid foods known to provoke the condition, such as chocolate, strawberries, nuts, and seafood, and to limit consumption of coffee and tea. Corticosteroid therapy may be used in severe cases.

Dermatitis

Chronic dermatitis is classified as either contact dermatitis or atopic dermatitis. Contact dermatitis can be related to frequent contact with a chemical irritant or an antigen that elicits an allergic response and is generally confined to the areas of contact. Atopic dermatitis, commonly referred to as eczema, is an inherited condition associated with other allergic conditions such as hay fever. Either a personal or a family history of asthma, allergic rhinitis, or hay fever is noted in 66% of people reporting atopic dermatitis.

Pathophysiology

Allergic dermatitis is a delayed cell-mediated hypersensitivity reaction. The sensitizing antigen is taken up by epidermal cells and carried to the lymph nodes. T cells proliferate in the lymph nodes and enter systemic circulation, where they mediate the release of inflammatory agents such as cytokines. This process renders all the skin sensitive to the antigen. Toxic dermatitis is the classic defense mechanism in response to insult by a toxic substance.

Clinical Manifestations

Chronic Contact Dermatitis

The difference between toxic contact dermatitis and allergic contact dermatitis lies in the origin of the problem. In allergic dermatitis, the individual has a sensitivity to the substance in question. Therefore, reactions are not related to the concentration of the offending substance but to the degree of individual sensitivity. This is not true of toxic dermatitis, in which the causative agent is a substance that is toxic to all individuals. The reaction to the toxic substance varies with the concentration of that substance as well as the thickness and permeability of the individual's skin. The reaction in toxic dermatitis is confined to the area of exposure, and lesions do not spread beyond these margins. In contrast, the lesions associated with allergic dermatitis very often spread beyond the area of contact. The majority of industrial diseases are dermatoses related to contact with toxic substances, especially cutting oils and solvents (Hall, 2000). Over $100 million is spent annually in the United States as a result of occupational dermatitis. Some common contact allergens are listed in Box 6-7.

Contact dermatitis is treated with wet soaks and corticosteroid ointments. In cases that are resistant to treatment, sulfur or coal tar can be added to the ointment. In some cases a short course of oral steroids is beneficial. Patients should be taught that injured skin is sensitive long after the problem has been relieved and should be encouraged to use mild soaps and avoid continued contact with the irritant.

Atopic Dermatitis

The skin lesions of atopic dermatitis begin as poorly defined red patches, papules, and plaques that thicken over time. Painful cracks and fissures develop, especially in the palms, fingers, and soles. The lesions may be generalized

---

Box 6-7 Common Contact Allergens

- Chromates
- Cobalt sulfate
- Formalin
- Mercury
- Neomycin
- Nickel sulfate
- Procaine
- Sulfonamides
- Turpentine

---

but tend to occur in the flexures of arms, wrists, and knees, on the sides of the neck, and across the face, forehead, and eyelids. Because atopy is a generalized allergic reaction, individuals may also have sneezing, runny nose, congestion, and itchy, watery eyes. Cataracts may develop in young adults with severe atopy.

Acne

Acne is a common skin condition among young adults. Although the condition usually resolves by age 18 or 19, flare-ups can continue for years. In addition, if the acne creates scarring and pitting, self-esteem may be affected far into adulthood.

Pathophysiology

Acne lesions are caused by the interaction of hormones and bacteria. Androgens stimulate the release of sebum, and bacterial lipase converts lipid into fatty acids. The sebum and the fatty acids combine to create an inflammatory reaction that causes follicular walls to break down and spread irritants into the dermis, which provokes the foreign body response of papules and pustules.

Clinical Manifestations

Acne lesions are generally round comedones (blackheads or whiteheads), papules, pustules, nodules, or cysts. They can appear singly or nodules may coalesce. Pitting and scarring occur as secondary lesions. Outbreaks are worse in fall and winter and are more severe in men than in women.

Treatment

Mild acne is treated with topical antibiotics, retinoids, and benzoyl peroxide gels. Oral tetracyclines are added for cases of moderate acne. Oral antibiotics should be used in combination with topical treatments, however, and should not be the sole treatment method used. In women, birth control pills with high amounts of estrogen are very effective, but cardiovascular risks must be considered before selecting this treatment modality. For very severe acne, isotretinoin (Accutane) is used. Isotretinoin is teratogenic, so women of child-bearing age should use contraception if taking this drug. Isotretinoin

is also hepatotoxic and in some individuals causes a rise in lipid and triglyceride levels. Therefore laboratory tests should be done before initiating therapy and throughout the course of treatment. A rare side effect of isotretinoin therapy that warrants careful assessment is depression and suicidal ideation. The patient taking this agent should be questioned about changes in mood at every visit.

Rosacea

Rosacea is a chronic disorder of the sebaceous glands coupled with increased reactivity of capillaries. It was once referred to as acne rosacea, but there is no relationship between the two conditions other than the fact that many people who develop rosacea have a history of acne. Although physiologically benign, rosacea causes significant disfigurement, especially in males, who more commonly develop hyperplasia and telangiectasia of the nose. Rosacea usually develops in the third to fifth decades and is more common among women and people of Celtic descent.

Clinical Manifestations

The skin lesions associated with rosacea are round, dome-shaped papules and nodules without blackheads. The lesions are discrete and scattered across the face in a symmetrical pattern. Late in the disease swelling of the forehead, eyelids, ear lobes, or chin and marked enlargement of the nose may occur. The normally white sclera of the eyes may appear red due to conjunctivitis. (If any eye involvement is noted, the patient should be referred to an ophthalmologist, because corneal ulcers may develop.)

Rosacea progresses through four stages:

1. Episodic rosacea: The patient experiences episodes of erythema, especially in response to heat.
2. Stage 1: The erythema is persistent with telangiectases.
3. Stage 2: Stage 1 symptoms plus papules and pustules are present.
4. Stage 3: Erythema deepens and nodules develop, along with hyperplasia and lymphedema of central facial structures.

Treatment

Some individuals respond well simply to avoidance of external and internal heat. Keeping out of the sun, staying away from hot stoves or ovens, and eliminating hot beverages and alcohol is helpful in the episodic period. Topical creams and ointments are very effective, especially metronidazole (MetroGel) and erythromycin (Emgel). If topical treatments are unsuccessful, oral antibiotics are added to the regimen. Isotretinoin (Accutane) is prescribed for particularly resistant cases.

Perioral Dermatitis

Perioral dermatitis is a rosacea-like dermatitis that affects primarily women between the ages of 20 and 30.

Clinical Manifestations

Unlike rosacea, the rash of perioral dermatitis is pustular with confluent plaques. Papules are irregular and symmetrically grouped around the mouth and chin. The patient may also complain of a burning or itching sensation, which is not present in rosacea.

Treatment

Topical steroids should be avoided because they will only aggravate the condition. Treatment is the same as that for rosacea but is given for a shorter period of time because perioral dermatitis is less chronic in nature.

Psoriasis

The word *psoriasis* comes from a Greek word that means "itch." Psoriasis is a hereditary disorder that affects about 5 million people in the United States (Javitz et al, 2002). If one parent has psoriasis, there is less than a 10% chance that offspring will develop the condition. If both parents have psoriasis, however, the chances that the offspring will develop the disorder increase to over 40%. The incidence is equal in men and women, and onset is generally between the ages of 16 and 22, although at least one fourth of people with psoriasis develop the condition in their fifties (Fitzpatrick et al, 2001).

Research findings demonstrate that psoriasis has a profound effect on quality of life in terms of self-esteem, confidence, and physical functioning (Rapp et al, 1999; Weiss et al, 2002). In addition, the financial burden of the illness is staggering. In the United States the direct costs associated with managing psoriasis are estimated to be $650 million per year (Javitz et al, 2002).

Pathophysiology

Psoriasis is a scaling disorder characterized by abnormal proliferation of epidermal cells in which the rate of cell division is 6 to 10 times higher than normal. As a result, epidermal cells are produced at nearly 30 times the normal rate. The cause of the proliferation is not clear, but some evidence exists that psoriasis may be an immune disorder (Fitzpatrick et al, 2001). It is a lifelong disease with periods of exacerbation and remission. Flare-ups are thought to be provoked by trauma, infections, stress, and drugs. The symptoms are caused by the irritation of skin cells that are disrupted by the accelerated growth of epidermal cells.

Clinical Manifestations

The skin lesions of psoriasis are salmon pink papules and plaques that are sharply marginated and have silvery white scales (Figure 6-2). The lesions take many shapes and arrangements. The distribution pattern is bilateral but not symmetrical. Areas of involvement include the scalp, elbows, knees, palms, soles of the feet, lower back, folds of the buttocks, penis, and scrotum. Pruritus is common, especially with scalp and anogenital lesions. A rare form of pso-

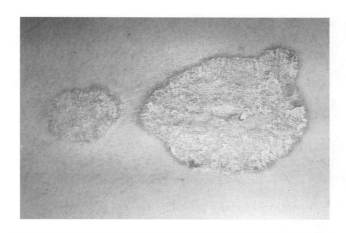

Figure 6-2 Psoriasis vulgaris in a patient. (From Ignatavicius DD, Workman ML, editors: *Medical-surgical nursing: critical thinking for collaborative care,* ed 4, Philadelphia, 2002, WB Saunders.)

riasis known as guttate psoriasis produces generalized discrete lesions over the entire surface of the body, although palms and soles are usually spared.

Some individuals with psoriasis may have joint pain and should be evaluated for psoriatic arthritis, the more severe form of which causes bone erosion.

Treatment

No cure exists for psoriasis, but a number of treatments can help to control this condition, including ultraviolet B (UVB) phototherapy. Patients may need as many as three full-body treatments a week for 10 weeks before a significant response is seen. A new procedure using the excimer laser is being tested for the treatment of psoriasis. Because this laser delivers more concentrated UVB light than the light used in other forms of phototherapy, it often has a greater effect on the treated area, so that treatment time is shortened and the amount of harmful exposure to UV rays is decreased (Feldman, 2002).

Treatment for psoriasis depends on the location of the lesions. For example, guttate psoriasis is treated with psoralen and ultraviolet A phototherapy (PUVA), whereas calcipotriene, a synthetic vitamin D now available in prescription form, is useful for management of localized psoriasis. Psoriasis of the scalp is treated with tar shampoo followed by the application of steroid lotions. Lotions and creams applied to the scalp are usually left on overnight covered by plastic wrap or a shower cap.

PUVA is used when psoriasis does not respond to other treatments or is widespread. With PUVA therapy approximately 30 to 40 treatments per year are required to keep the psoriasis under control. Because psoralen remains in the lens of the eye, patients must wear UVA-blocking eyeglasses when exposed to sunlight from the time of treatment until sunset of that day. Long-term treatment with PUVA increases the risk of skin aging, freckling, and skin cancer, and therefore treatment must be monitored very carefully.

Steroids may control the condition in many patients. Weaker preparations should be used on more sensitive areas of the body such as the genitals, groin, and face. Stronger preparations are usually required to control lesions on the scalp, elbow, knees, palms and soles, and parts of the torso, and may need to be applied under dressings. Side effects of the stronger cortisone preparations include thinning of the skin, dilation of blood vessels, bruising, and skin color changes.

People experiencing psoriatic flare-ups used to go to hospitals to receive concentrated treatment with ultraviolet light and tar applications. Today, these treatments are given in psoriasis day care centers. Individuals with psoriasis spend the day receiving the appropriate treatment along with others who share their situation and experience similar challenges. A definite benefit of these centers is the fact that informal support groups develop and social contacts increase.

Patients should be instructed not to stop steroid therapy abruptly because this may cause the condition to flare up and to avoid scratching the lesions because this only creates more lesions.

Pigmentation Disorders

Two common disorders of pigmentation are chloasma or hyperpigmentation, and vitiligo or hypopigmentation. The etiologies of both of these conditions are unknown, but chloasma appears to have hormonal associations, whereas vitiligo is thought to be an autoimmune disorder. Neither condition produces uncomfortable symptoms, nor is either life threatening. The problem is one of self-image and self-esteem. In addition, depigmented skin is sun sensitive and therefore at greater risk for the development of sunburns and skin cancer.

Clinical Manifestations

Chloasma lesions are irregular in shape and brown in color. They appear primarily on the face and forehead and are more obvious in summer months.

Vitiligo may appear as white patches of skin but these are, in reality, patches of depigmentation. They occur primarily on the face and hands but can appear anywhere.

Treatment

Treatment for chloasma includes use of a sun block and use of cosmetics in mild cases. If the chloasma occurs with pregnancy, the patient should be informed that the discolored areas will probably fade somewhat after delivery, although breast-feeding may delay that process.

Hydroquinone creams can be applied to help with fading and must be continued for a period of at least 3 months to be effective. Other creams that exfoliate, such as those containing retinoic acid or glycolic acid, may also be of benefit. Patients must be reminded that progress is slow.

Treatment for vitiligo can be cosmetic or much more radical. Corticosteroid creams can be used for early mild cases. Traditionally, vitiligo patients have been exposed to synthetic UVA light in an attempt to stimulate repigmentation. However, a minimum of 100 treatments, given 2 to 3 times a week, is necessary before any response is seen, and treatment is successful in fewer than 50% of individuals. In more difficult cases psoralen derivatives and PUVA therapy have been used with varying degrees of success.

The excimer laser may be useful in the treatment of vitiligo because of its ability to deliver UVB light with deep penetration, which stimulates the pigment-producing cells. Other procedures to which patients often resort include desquamation, skin grafting, and surgery. Support as the patient learns to accept and adjust to the changes in appearance is an essential part of any treatment plan.

PREMALIGNANT AND MALIGNANT SKIN CONDITIONS

Malignancies of the skin are usually slow growing and, with the exception of melanomas, are rarely fatal. Even the non-melanoma cancers can be locally invasive, however, and can produce significant disfigurement and disability. Two of the objectives of *Healthy People 2010* (US Department of Health and Human Services, 2000) are related to skin cancer. Objective 3.8 calls for a reduction of deaths related to melanoma. Objective 3.9 is aimed at increasing the proportion of persons who use protective measures that may reduce the risk of skin cancer. Data related to the use of protective measures are obtained through the National Health Information Survey. The questions that are related to protective measures are shown in Box 6-8. Respondents are considered to use protective measures if they answer "very likely" to any of the three questions.

Box 6-8   National Health Information Survey Questions on Sun Protection

■ If you were to go outside on a very sunny day for *more* than 1 hour, are you very likely, somewhat likely, or unlikely to wear protective clothing such as wide-brimmed hats or long-sleeved shirts?

■ If you were to go outside on a very sunny day for *more* than 1 hour, are you very likely, somewhat likely, or unlikely to avoid the sun by staying in the shade?

■ If you were to go outside on a very sunny day for *more* than 1 hour, are you very likely, somewhat likely, or unlikely to use sunscreen or sun block lotion?

Actinic Keratoses

Actinic keratoses are precancerous lesions seen in light-complexioned older adults and in younger persons who are frequent sunbathers or who work in jobs that require them to be outside most of the time, such as farmers, gardeners, and constructions workers. The lesions appear in areas exposed to the sun and are often called *solars*.

Clinical Manifestations

The lesions begin as faint red scaly patches that enlarge over several years. Patients often complain that the patches are tender or give rise to a burning sensation. The lesions are predominantly found on the face, ears, neck, and dorsal surfaces of the hands.

Treatment

Single lesions are usually removed by applying liquid nitrogen to the lesion. If multiple lesions are present, the patient is generally given fluorouracil cream to apply twice a day over 2 weeks. If the lesions are diffuse, a small area of skin is treated at a time.

Any patient with actinic keratoses should be taught the importance of using sun block every day and of seeing a dermatologist every 6 months.

Dysplastic Nevi Syndrome

Nevi are skin tumors that contain nevus cells and are commonly referred to as moles. They are present in all adults, can be pigmented or nonpigmented, hairy or nonhairy, elevated or flat, and are for the most part benign. However, several types of nevi can be precursors to malignant melanoma. Dysplastic nevi belong to this group of precancerous lesions. Because dysplastic nevi can progress to cancer, special care is called for when these lesions occur in a familial pattern or in a family with a history of melanoma. The nevi must be monitored carefully and frequently so as to detect the development of melanoma at the earliest possible time.

Clinical Manifestations

Dysplastic nevi are larger (5 mm to 15 mm) and more numerous than common nevi, and tend to show irregular borders and mixed coloration. Nevi are most prevalent on the head and neck but can appear anywhere. Nevi are not generally found on palms, soles, or genitalia. Nevi that occur in these areas are probably junctional nevi. Junctional nevi are benign active nevi that can become melanomas and thus require close scrutiny.

Treatment

Removal is indicated only when necessary for cosmetic reasons or when malignancy is suspected. All nevi that are excised should be biopsied regardless of the level of suspicion. Suspicious moles should be removed by surgical excision and not by electrosurgery or laser surgery.

Basal Cell Carcinoma

Basal cell carcinoma (BCC) is the most common type of skin cancer and usually involves epidermis that is capable of growing hair. Over 400,000 new cases of BCC are reported in the United States annually. BCC is aggressive and destructive, but its ability to metastasize is limited by its own lack of growth factors, so it is readily controlled by surgery or cryotherapy. BCC is invasive, however, and can cause deep, extensive destruction of muscle and bone. Serious complications can arise when BCC occurs around the eyes, ears, or nasolabial folds.

Clinical Manifestations

The skin lesions in BCC are usually pearly or translucent papules or nodules, or ulcers with rolled borders. occasionally the lesions are brown or black. Single lesions are usually round or oval with a depressed center.

Treatment

BCCs are removed surgically. Cryosurgery or electrosurgery can be used in some locations but should not be used in areas in which invasion presents serious concerns. In these areas, microscopic surgery (Mohs surgery) is recommended. Skin grafts may be required if damage to underlying structures is extensive.

Cryosurgery causes cellular death by freezing. Liquid nitrogen at a temperature of −200° C is applied to the lesion. Swelling and tenderness may occur after the procedure.

The patient is instructed to clean the area with hydrogen peroxide and apply a topical antibiotic once or twice daily.

Squamous Cell Carcinoma

Squamous cell carcinoma (SCC) is a malignant tumor of epithelial cells in the skin and mucous membranes that occurs in response to exposure to exogenous carcinogens such as radiation from the sun, ingested arsenic, ionizing radiation, and human papillomavirus. Although the incidence of SCC is only about 1 in 10,000, the incidence has risen steadily over the past decade. The incidence is particularly high in areas of the world where there are many days of sunshine annually, especially if the population in that area is fair skinned. For example, among white-skinned people, the incidence of SCC is six times higher in Hawaii than in the continental United States (Fitzpatrick et al, 2001).

Clinical Manifestations

SCC lesions are usually isolated, rapidly growing nodules that develop a central ulcer with surrounding redness. They are generally found in skin areas exposed to the sun, especially the face, lower lip, tops of the ears, and dorsal surfaces of the hands. They may also appear on the tongue if related to tobacco use.

Treatment

Treatment options for individuals with SCC are the same as those for individuals with BCC. Occasionally, topical fluorouracil cream is applied if there are multiple actinic keratoses (precursors of SCC).

Malignant Melanoma

The incidence of malignant melanoma, a tumor of the cells that produce melanin, is increasing faster than that of any other cancer (Hall, 2000). It is the most deadly form of skin cancer because it can metastasize to any body organ. The most common sites for metastasis are lung, liver, brain, and bowel. Although melanoma accounts for only 1% of all skin cancers, it is responsible for over 60% of skin cancer–related deaths. If the melanoma is localized to the skin, it is almost 100% curable by excision. If lymph nodes are involved, the 5-year survival rate drops to 50%, and if metastasis is present, the care is only palliative. The American Joint Committee on Cancer has identified six stages and substages of malignant melanoma (Box 6-9). The most important factor affecting prognosis in the cutaneous form of melanoma is the thickness of the lesion, which differentiates tumors in the first two stages.

Clinical Manifestations

The typical lesion is a black or purple nodule, but the color can vary from pink to tan to brown. Any change in the color, size, or character of any skin lesion should be investigated promptly. The site of the lesion varies with the type. There are four types of malignant melanoma that differ in terms of onset, course, distribution, and prognosis (Box 6-10).

Treatment

Malignant melanoma is treated with wide-excision, full-thickness removal of the lesion and surrounding tissue.

When metastasis is a possibility, wide excision may be accompanied by use of a recently developed method for identifying the lymph nodes at greatest risk for metastasis, known as lymphatic mapping and sentinel node biopsy. Lymphatic mapping is performed to determine the lymph nodes most likely to receive lymphatic drainage (and can-

---

> ### Box 6-9   American Joint Committee on Cancer Stages of Melanoma
>
> **Stage Ia:** localized skin involvement with thickness of ≤0.75 mm
> **Stage Ib:** localized skin involvement with thickness of 0.75 to 1.5 mm
> **Stage IIa:** localized skin involvement with thickness of 1.5 to 4.0 mm
> **Stage IIb:** localized skin involvement with thickness of ≥4.0 mm
> **Stage III:** regional lymph node involvement
> **Stage IV:** distant metastasis

> ### Box 6-10   Types of Malignant Melanoma
>
> **SUPERFICIAL SPREADING MELANOMA**
> - Most common, accounts for 70% of all melanomas
> - Grows slowly
> - Good prognosis
>
> **NODULAR MELANOMA**
> - Accounts for 16% of all melanomas
> - Grows rapidly
> - Poor prognosis
>
> **LENTIGO MALIGNA MELANOMA**
> - Accounts for 5% of all melanomas
> - Develops from lentigo maligna on the exposed body parts of the elderly
> - Grows slowly
> - Good prognosis
>
> **ACRAL LENTIGINOUS MELANOMA**
> - Least common of all melanomas
> - Most common melanoma in dark-skinned people
> - Occurs on the palms, soles, and nails, and periorally and perirectally
> - Metastasizes quickly
> - Poor prognosis

cerous cells) from the melanoma site and to identify the first lymph node to receive lymph draining from the melanoma site (the sentinel node). The sentinel node is removed surgically and analyzed for the presence of melanoma cells. If no melanoma cells are found, it is very unlikely that any melanoma cells have passed on to the next nodes in the drainage system. If melanoma cells are found in the sentinel node, then all of the nodes may be excised. The effect of performing this procedure on patient 5-year survival has not yet been determined.

T-Cell Lymphoma

T-cell lymphoma is a lymphoma that, except in rare instances, involves only the skin. The disease has three stages. The first two stages typically progress slowly over many years with exacerbations and remissions. The prognosis is poor, however, and when the tumor stage is reached, death is imminent.

Clinical Manifestations

Stage 1 lesions are red scaly patches that are sharply defined and produce severe itching. This stage is referred to as the erythematous stage. In stage 2, the plaque stage, the scaly patches become indurated and slightly elevated. The centers of the lesions heal somewhat, which produces a ringlike appearance. The third and terminal stage is the tumor stage. In this stage nodules and tumors grow from the plaques formed in stage 2. These tumors are prone to ulceration and secondary infection.

Treatment

Most providers treat symptoms only as they appear. Therefore early lesions are treated with tar preparations and corticosteroid creams. Ultraviolet light therapy is temporarily effective. Systemic corticosteroids are also given in the early stages. Radiation therapy is useful in treating superficial lesions, and sometime total-body radiation is prescribed late in the course of the disease. Chemotherapy is initiated in the second and third stages of the disease. The most common agents used are cyclophosphamide (Cytoxan), methotrexate (MTX), vincristine (Oncovin), and doxorubicin (Adriamycin) (see Table 27-3).

END-OF-LIFE CARE

The patient and family should be consulted about their wishes related to palliative and end-of-life care. Advanced directives should be discussed with all family members and appropriate documents prepared. See Chapter 27 for a more detailed discussion of care of the patient with cancer.

FAMILY AND CAREGIVER ISSUES

Roles, relationships, employment, patterns of interacting, and sexual intimacy are all affected by one's sense of self, which may be altered by a skin condition. Therefore, the families of individuals with skin conditions, whether benign or malignant, may find themselves adversely affected. Families may experience financial and social strains in addition to feeling concern for the family member. Providers should assess the responses to the skin condition and the way in which these responses affect family dynamics.

Think S for Success

Symptoms
- Assess for signs of self-esteem disturbance, hopelessness.
- Treat itching with the appropriate medications, baths, lotions, and so on.
- Treat skin lesions as indicated.

Sequelae
- Encourage patient to avoid scratching to prevent scarring and further irritation.
- Teach sun protection measures.
- Monitor use of creams, ointments, etc., and over-the-counter drugs to prevent overuse and interactions.

Safety
- Make sure drugs are labeled and patient understands not to ingest topical medications.
- Teach patient to check skin for suspicious lesions.
- Teach all patients sun safety.
- If patient uses bath emollients, teach to take care to avoid slipping and falling in tub and care in getting out of tub onto tile floor. If patient is undergoing ultraviolet light treatments, instruct to keep eyes covered during exposure.
- Monitor for signs of depression, mood swings, or suicidal ideation.
- Stress the importance of follow-up, especially if patient is taking medication that requires monitoring of renal or liver function.

Support/Services
- Inform patient of skin care centers, day care treatment centers, and support groups available in the community. Elderly patients may need assistance with treatments and, if eligible, can receive home care.

Satisfaction
- Encourage patient to openly discuss feelings about quality of life.
- Help patient attain or maintain optimal life quality as defined by patient.

CASE STUDY

Patient Data

Mr. B. is a 40-year-old man who has been bothered by psoriasis since he was in his twenties. It has not been too much of a problem because it flares up only occasionally, and he gets some cream from the drugstore to put on his knees and elbows that usually clears it up. He has recently moved to Michigan from Florida to start a new job and his psoriasis is "acting up." He says he cannot stop scratching his elbows and knees and that makes the sores bleed. He is uncomfortable at night and in his clothes, and he is afraid of what the people at his new place of work must be thinking about him.

Diagnostic Findings

Mr. B. is afebrile with blood pressure of 140/80, heart rate of 88 beats per minute, and respiration rate of 16 breaths per minute. Clusters of erythematous plaques with well-defined margins and silvery scales are noted bilaterally on elbows and knees. Plaques on elbows have small open cracks and areas of abrasion. A small amount of blood is evident on a 2 × 2 inch area when swabbed. Complete blood count is within normal limits.

Thinking It Through

- Why do you think Mr. B.'s psoriasis has suddenly gotten worse?
- From what type of treatment do you think he would benefit most?
- What effect does his new job have on his ability to manage a treatment regimen?

Case Conference

Mr. B. has come to the dermatologist's office alone. His wife and family are still in Florida.

The dermatologist explains to Mr. B. that there are many reasons why his psoriasis is flaring up. One important reason could be the change in the weather and lack of humidity; another could be the stress associated with a new job and with moving. One thing that is certainly keeping the psoriasis active is the scratching. The doctor explains that scratching leads to itching

and thickening of the lesions. He writes a prescription for a steroid cream to be applied every 8 hours to the lesions.

The nurse talks with Mr. B. about his current living arrangements and lifestyle and tries to determine how the psoriasis is affecting his other life patterns. Mr. B. is most concerned about his new job and the impression he is making. The nurse encourages Mr. B. to talk more about this, and they discuss ways that Mr. B. can dress to be more comfortable and prevent chafing of the psoriatic spots. The nurse asks if he has told his colleagues about his psoriasis and he says he has not. They discuss the pros and cons of sharing the information, and the nurse asks Mr. B. if having the psoriasis affects the way he feels about himself. He denies any effect on his self-esteem; he just does not want people to think he is going to be a problem or that he has got something "catching" because of the itching. The nurse explains how to reduce the itching by bathing less often, using mild soaps, and putting a humidifier in his bedroom at night and even a small one in his office.

The physician agrees to order an oral antihistamine to stop the itching as well as promote sleep. The nurse instructs Mr. B. not to drink alcohol while taking the antihistamine and to avoid over-the-counter drugs. She warns him that he may feel drowsy and instructs him to take the medication at night first to see how it will affect him and then to take care with driving or operating machinery when he takes the medicine again. Mr. B. is scheduled to return in 2 weeks, and the nurse will call to check on his progress in a few days.

The counselor has been listening and watching Mr. B.'s affect and feels that he is coping fairly well, all things considered. He says as much to Mr. B., but he tells Mr. B. that he understands that psoriasis is a chronic disorder and that there may be a time when he is feeling overwhelmed by it. He gives Mr. B. his business card and advises him to get in touch if he feels the need of some additional support. He also gives Mr. B. a list of telephone numbers and Internet sites for support groups.

- Do you agree with the treatment plan? Why or why not?
- What other strategies could have been explored?

Internet and Other Resources

American Academy of Dermatology: *http://www.aad.org*

American Cancer Society: *http://www.cancer.org*

American Society for Mohs Surgery: *http://www.mohssurgery.org*

International Psoriasis Community: *http://www.psoriasis support.org*

National Institutes of Health: *http://www.nlm.nih.gov/medlineplus/ psoriasis.html*

National Psoriasis Foundation: *www.psoriasis.org*

SKINCAREPHYSICIANS.com: *http://www.skincarephysicians. com*

REFERENCES

American Cancer Society: Cancer facts and figures—2003, retrieved from *http://www.cancer.org* on May 25, 2003.

American Society for Mohs Surgeons: Patient information brochure, 2003, retrieved from *http://www.mohssurgery.org/brochure/patient_brochure.htm* on June 1, 2003.

Batchelor N, Remo B: Normal changes of aging. In Luggen A, Travis S, Meiner S, editors: *NGNA core curriculum for gerontological advanced practice nurses,* Thousand Oaks, Calif, 1998, Sage Publications, pp 423-35.

Cuzzell J: Assessment of the skin, hair and nails. In Ignatavicius D, Workman M, editors: *Medical surgical nursing: critical thinking for collaborative care,* ed 4, Philadelphia, 2002, WB Saunders, pp 1495-1513.

Eliopoulos C: *Integrating conventional and alternative therapies: holistic care for chronic conditions,* St Louis, 1999, Mosby.

Feldman SR: Remissions of psoriasis with excimer laser treatment, *Dermatol Online J* 8(2):23, 2002; retrieved from *http://www.dermatology. cdlib.org/DOJvol8num2/correspondence/laser/laser.html* on Jan 24, 2004.

Fitzpatrick T et al: *Color atlas and synopsis of clinical dermatology: common and serious diseases,* New York, 2001, McGraw-Hill.

Hall J: *Sauer's manual of skin diseases,* ed 8, Philadelphia, 2000, Lippincott Williams & Wilkins.

Javitz H et al: The direct cost of care for psoriasis and psoriatic arthritis in the U.S., *J Am Acad Dermatol* 46(6):850-65, 2002.

Rapp S et al: Psoriasis causes as much disability as other major medical diseases, *J Am Acad Dermatol* 41(3):401-7, 1999.

Simandl G: Manifestations of skin disorders. In Porth C, editor: *Pathophysiology: concepts of altered health states,* ed 6, Philadelphia, 2002, Lippincott Williams & Wilkins, pp 1401-4.

Updike J: *The centaur,* New York, 1976, Knopf.

US Department of Health and Human Services: Healthy people 2010, ed 2, Washington, DC, November 2000, US Government Printing Office, retrieved from *http://www.healthypeople.gov* on July 20, 2003.

Weiss S et al: *J Am Acad Dermatol* 47(4):512-8, 2002.

CHAPTER 7

Wounds

Dot Goodman, BS, RN, WOCN

OBJECTIVES

After reading this chapter, you should be able to do the following:

- Describe the pathophysiology of pressure necrosis, venous stasis, arterial ulcers, and diabetic ulcers
- Describe the clinical manifestations of pressure necrosis, venous stasis, arterial ulcers, and diabetic ulcers
- Describe the functional health patterns affected by pressure necrosis, venous stasis, arterial ulcers, and diabetic ulcers
- Describe the role of each member of the interdisciplinary team involved in the care of patients with pressure necrosis, venous stasis, arterial ulcers, and diabetic ulcers
- Describe the treatments and interventions that are available and appropriate for the care of chronic wounds

During the last 15 years, a significant shift has occurred in the level of interest in chronic wound care. Three major factors have influenced this shift: an increase in the incidence of chronic wounds, a larger population of elderly people, and intensified medical practices that make it possible to live with chronic illnesses. Both the elderly and those who live with chronic disease are at increased risk for developing chronic wounds. Estimates are that during the next 15 years the population of those 65 years of age and over will double, whereas the population of those 85 years of age and over will quadruple (Kane, 2001). Further compounding an already complicated situation is a decrease in health care funding and a reduction in the length of care permitted by third-party payers. Therefore, early diagnosis, patient education, and state-of-the art treatment are critical for successful outcomes.

The U.S. Department of Health and Human Services estimated that in 1990 alone 2.1 million pressure ulcers occurred; the cost for treatment was $1.3 billion (Kane, 2001). A recent study found that 1 in 10 hospitalized patients develops pressure ulcers, which result in an increased cost of $10,000 to $20,000 per admission (Meraviglia et al, 2002). It is estimated that leg ulcers affect approximately 2.5 million people in the United States. Approximately 2 million workdays are lost annually in the United States because of leg ulcers (Hess, 2000).

A wound is a break in the continuity of the skin. Wounds can be either acute or chronic. Acute wounds progress from origin to healing in an orderly and timely manner. Surgical wounds, burns, and skin tears are all examples of acute wounds. Acute wounds heal when the host is healthy enough to provide the body with the nutrients and fluids it needs. The end result of healing is skin that closes with a strong enough base to stay closed. Conversely, chronic wounds do not proceed through a timely and orderly process. Chronic wounds do not reach a strong, lasting closure and the skin does not return to normal functioning; such wounds require extra time and extra help to heal. Chronic wounds occur because of an underlying disease process such as malnutrition, dehydration, autoimmune disease, diabetic pathology, arterial obstruction, and/or venous congestion.

Some of the earliest images of nurses show them caring for the wounded and preparing bandages. Although physicians established the original treatments, the care of wounds has always been the responsibility of nurses. The treatment choices were few and simple. There was little understanding of how wounds healed. Some people healed, some had their wounds for life, and others died from complications. Since those early days tremendous advances have been made. In fact, wound care has evolved into its own discipline supported by wound science. Now research provides a plethora of treatment choices based on the assessment of the individual patient and the wound tissue. Knowledge of the pathophysiology and the healing process of wounds is growing continuously. The role of the nurse has also evolved and now includes physical assessment and wound and skin evaluation based on knowledge of underlying disease processes, provision of referrals when indicated, and recommendation of treatments. Wounds and wound care may evoke a multitude of reactions from nurses, ranging from disgust and dread to excitement and challenge. It is therefore important for nurses to have the opportunity to explore their feelings and to receive peer and supervisory support. Nurses are involved in all aspects of chronic wound care, from prevention and early detection to leadership of a multidisciplinary team of wound care specialists.

This chapter discusses the most common chronic wounds: pressure ulcers and lower extremity wounds—diabetic foot ulcers, venous stasis, and arterial wounds. Chronic wounds significantly alter the functional health patterns of individuals who have developed a pressure ulcer or lower extremity wound. A guide for assessing functional health patterns is listed in Box 7-1.

PRESSURE ULCER
Overview

Pressure ulcer is the currently accepted term for wounds that occur when pressure is high enough and lasts long enough to cut off the supply of nutrients and oxygen to an area of the skin, causing cell death (necrosis). Historically, pressure ulcers were referred to as *bedsores* or *decubiti*. Pressure ulcers are a national problem. Currently there are federal standards for the prediction and prevention of pressure ulcers, as well as clinical practice guidelines for their care. The U.S. Department of Health and Human Services, Agency for Health Care Policy and Research (renamed Agency for Healthcare Research and Quality) published guidelines for prevention in 1992 and guidelines for treatment in 1994.

The high incidence and prevalence of pressure ulcers, coupled with the cost of treatment, has prompted increased attention. The cost of healing a single ulcer can range from $5000 to $65,000. More than 1 million adults in the United States are diagnosed with pressure ulcers, which puts the cost of care into the billions of dollars (Krasner, 1997). The prevalence of pressure ulcers (the number of patients with pressure ulcers on a given day) is 10.1% to 17% in acute care settings, 2.3% to 28% in long-term care facilities, and 0% to 29% in home care (Cuddigan, Berlowitz, and Ayello, 2001). These numbers do not capture any of the associated costs, such as the pain and suffering of patients and their caregivers, which result in loss of time at work and decrease in quality of life.

Box 7-1   Functional Health Pattern Assessment for Wound Management

HEALTH PERCEPTION/HEALTH MANAGEMENT
- How long has the wound been present?
- Does the patient have a history of other wounds?
- How is the patient's overall health?
- Does the patient use any other medications or treatments, including prescribed, over the counter, or alternative?

NUTRITION/METABOLISM
- Has the patient experienced recent weight gain or loss?
- Does the patient require a special diet?
- How much fluid does the patient consume?
- Does the patient use food supplements?
- How much protein does the patient consume daily?
- What is the patient's blood glucose history?
- What are the results of blood albumin, prealbumin, and creatinine tests?

ELIMINATION
- How is the patient's bowel and bladder function, especially with regard to continence and/or a training program?

ACTIVITY/EXERCISE
- Is the patient able to perform activities of daily living and instrumental activities of daily living, routine activity, and exercise?
- What is the patient's level of mobility? Does he or she require special supportive equipment? Observe ambulation.
- Is the patient able to reach affected areas?
- How is the patient's manual dexterity?

SLEEP/REST
- What are the patient's sleep patterns?
- What are the patient's day and night sleeping positions?
- Does the patient use a support surface?

COGNITION/PERCEPTION
- What is the nature, character, location, and duration of the pain?
- Does any activity or position increase or decrease the pain?
- How are the patient's orientation and cognitive abilities?
- Does the patient have any sensory deficits? Is the patient able to accurately describe pain and pressure on the feet, hands, and trunk? What is the patient's visual acuity?

SELF-PERCEPTION/SELF-CONCEPT
- How has the present health condition affected the patient's self-description, self-confidence, and body image?

ROLES/RELATIONSHIPS
- Has the present health issue altered the patient's ability to perform necessary tasks as an employee, family member, and caretaker?

COPING/STRESS TOLERANCE
- What activities, community resources, and significant others are available to support the patient's health goals?
- What coping strategies has the patient used in previous stressful situations?

SEXUALITY/REPRODUCTION
- How has the present condition affected the patient's sexual patterns, activities, and performance?
- Have there been any changes in the patient's menstrual cycle?

VALUES/BELIEFS
- What constitutes good quality of life for the patient?
- What is important to the patient?
- What are the patient's beliefs related to this condition?
- To what extent do the patient's cultural/spiritual beliefs influence decision making related to this condition?

Pathophysiology

Arterial capillaries supply the skin with oxygen and nutrients. These capillaries remain open for blood to flow to the muscles and subcutaneous tissues unless pressure constricts a vessel and decreases the blood flow. The amount of pressure required to cause constriction varies. The range of pressure required to close a capillary is 12 to 32 mm Hg. In healthy persons who sit on a hard surface, pressure as high as 300 mm Hg can be measured over the ischial bone. However, their skin is not likely to break down because of frequent shifts in weight and an intact pain sense that alerts them to tissue hypoxia. On the other hand, a person with diminished feeling, restricted movement, muscle wasting, or altered capillary flow requires a padded surface, proper weight distribution, frequent assisted movement, and trained surveillance for early signs of tissue hypoxia to avoid a pressure ulcer. Although pressure necrosis can occur on any part of the body, the tissue over a bony prominence is the most common site. This includes trunk sites—the sacrum, coccyx, greater trochanters, and ischial tuberosities—and the shoulders, scapula, and spine. The back of the head, elbows, knees, heels, and malleoli are other common sites of pressure damage. In addition, patients who have tubes, catheters, braces, and external equipment are prone to pressure necrosis where the equipment applies pressure to the skin (Figure 7-1).

Clinical Manifestations and Diagnosis

Pressure is not the only cause of necrosis. There are a host of other predisposing factors, of which immobility is the most obvious. Patients who are immobile include those who are bed or chair bound and those who require the assistance of another person or a device to move. Immobility is associated with friction and shear. Friction is the rubbing or scraping of the skin over a surface, which can result in damage to the epidermis and dermis that often resembles a burn. Shear is a scraping or tearing force that pulls the skin in one direction while the skeletal muscles and bones are pulled in the opposite direction. These opposing movements stretch and trap the blood vessels, which further decreases the vascular supply to the skin. Shearing occurs when the head of the bed is elevated while the person is lying flat. The skin remains stationary, but gravity forces the skeleton to fall toward the foot of the bed. It is believed that 40% of all so-called pressure wounds are actually shear wounds.

Moisture is another factor that contributes to skin breakdown. Macerated skin is easily damaged, and excess moisture serves as a medium for infection. Sources of skin moisture include wound drainage, perspiration, and urine and feces in incontinent individuals. Furthermore, urine and stool alter the pH and the bacterial balance of the epidermis.

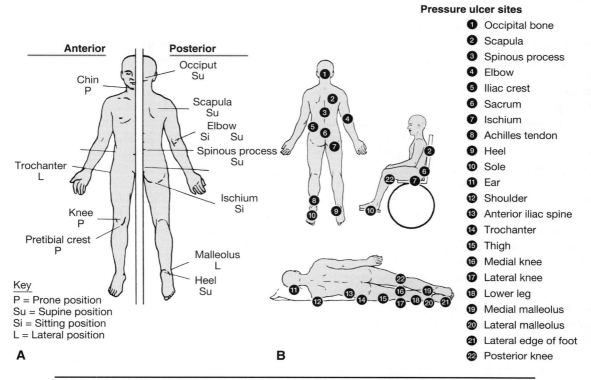

Figure 7-1 **A,** Bony prominences most frequently underlying pressure ulcers. **B,** Pressure ulcer sites. (From Trelease CC: Developing standards for wound care, *Ostomy Wound Manage* 20:46, 1988.)

Nutritional deficits are another leading cause of wounds and poor wound healing. Weight loss is associated with poor nutrition and may cause loss of muscle and fat pads, which allows bony prominences to be closer to skin level. In addition, without padding the risk of pressure and damage to the blood supply is increased. Persons with too much fat may also have nutritional deficits accompanied by poor muscle maintenance and altered blood flow, which creates weight over bony prominences that are without strength and protection. In a balanced nutritional state, intake of calories and nutrients is equal to the requirements of the body.

All adults need protein, carbohydrates, fats, vitamins, minerals, and adequate amounts of water. The required quantities of each shift with varying physical and mental conditions. Persons who are malnourished or dehydrated are at increased risk for skin changes, especially inflammation, infection, bleeding, and pressure necrosis. Once a person develops pressure necrosis, the required amounts of water, protein, and carbohydrate, the vitamins A, D, E, and C, and the minerals zinc, copper, and iron will increase.

Protein is essential to the immune system because the cells that fight infection need protein to develop. Collagen, which gives skin strength; elastin, which allows skin to stretch; and the cells that form the new blood supply are protein dependent. Vitamin C, iron, zinc, and copper promote wound healing by enhancing collagen formation and fibroblast function, which increases the response to infection.

The importance of optimal nutrition in both the prevention and treatment of pressure ulcers cannot be overemphasized. Malnutrition is directly associated with impaired wound healing, increased incidence of infection, longer hospitalizations, and even higher mortality rates. Hypermetabolism is the response of the body to the stress of ulcers; thus a previously sufficient diet may be profoundly inadequate to meet the needs of a hypermetabolic patient (Table 7-1).

One of the protections skin affords is the sensation of pain and pressure. Without these protections, skin is susceptible to damage, as is seen among patients with sensory perception impairment from diabetes, neurologic diseases, or spinal cord injuries. Other patients at increased risk for developing pressure necrosis are those with pain, those of advanced age, those with low blood pressure or elevated body temperature, and those who smoke or have dry skin.

When pressure ulcers are discussed, the first thing that should come to mind is prevention. It is imperative to assess the individual patient's risk for developing pressure necrosis and then to develop and implement an effective prevention plan (Box 7-2). Several nursing researchers and educators have created risk assessment tools that provide a uniform scientific approach. The two best assessment tools are the Norton scale and the Braden scale (Tables 7-2 and 7-3). The Braden scale is the most widely used and the most tested. Both tools are included in the guidelines of the Agency for Healthcare Research and Quality, and any facility that has a wound care program uses one of these tools. How often to

Table 7-1 Nutrients and Their Role in Wound Healing

Nutrient	Role in Healing
Protein	Fibroplasia, neogenesis, collagen formation, wound remodeling, maintenance of integrity of immune system
Carbohydrates	Energy supply, protein sparing
Fat	Cell walls, intracellular organelles, absorption of fat-soluble vitamins
Vitamin A	Epithelialization, wound closure, inflammatory response
B vitamins	Synthesis of protein, fat, and carbohydrate
Vitamin C	Collagen synthesis; promotion of capillary wall integrity, fibroblast function, immunologic function
Vitamin D	Calcium metabolism for building and maintaining bone
Vitamin E	Unknown
Vitamin K	Coagulation
Copper	Collagen cross-linking
Iron	Collagen formation
Magnesium	Protein synthesis
Zinc	Collagen formation and protein synthesis

From Bryant R, editor: *Acute and chronic wounds: nursing management,* ed 2, St Louis, 2000, Mosby.

conduct an assessment and what to do with the information are important concerns. The frequency of conducting a risk assessment depends on the setting. In general, an assessment is made within 24 hours of admission to a facility, daily in acute care settings, at each home care visit by a nurse, and once a week for 4 weeks and then quarterly in long-term care facilities (Braden, 2001).

Research shows that using a risk assessment tool is very effective for prevention and early intervention. Nevertheless, assessment tools are not perfect. There are times when a score is not consistent with nursing judgment or experience, and therefore the tool should not replace critical thinking.

After the determination of risk, the next step is the development of a care plan. The following must be considered: what type of surface is available for lying and sitting, what types of bathing products are being used, whether the person needs a continence program (bowel and/or bladder training), and whether an incontinence care program is appropriate.

Movements and shifts to different positions are the key to prevention and must occur every 2 hours. Some individuals show early signs of pressure and pain in 1 hour, and this fact must be taken into account in the care plan. Small shifts in body weight rather than a complete repositioning may be sufficient. Other measures include keeping the head of the bed 30 degrees or lower, making sure that a person is turned

---

Box 7-2   Prevention of Pressure Ulcers

- Inspect skin daily for erythema; specifically note pressure points and bony prominences. Do not massage. Remove thromboembolic hose. Check heels carefully.
- Encourage patient movement or do passive range-of-motion exercises every shift.
- Initiate rehabilitation efforts if the potential for improvement exists; request physical and occupational therapy consultation.
- Use proper positioning, transferring, and turning techniques to minimize skin injury due to friction and shear forces. Use lifting devices (e.g., trapeze or turning pad) to move rather than drag patients during transfers and position changes. Use a sliding board when transferring patients from bed to stretcher.
- Establish a turning and repositioning schedule of at least once every 2 hours for bed-bound patients and alter as needed. Use a written repositioning schedule. Modify this schedule if the patient has fewer than two turning surfaces.
- Avoid uninterrupted chair sitting by the patient. Shift the patient's position every hour.
- Place an at-risk patient on a pressure-reducing mattress or chair cushion. Do not use donut-type devices.
- Use pillows to keep bony prominences such as knees and ankles from direct contact with each other.

- Use pillows to relieve pressure on heels (e.g., place pillows under the calf to raise the heels off the bed). Use heel protectors to prevent friction.
- Avoid positioning directly on the trochanter (hip) by using the side-lying position (use the 30-degree lateral inclined position).
- Elevate the head of the bed as little as possible (maximum 30-degree angle) and for as short a time as possible.
- Use mild soap or bag bath and moisturizers for dry skin. Avoid hot water and excessive friction. Avoid massaging over bony prominences.
- Cleanse the skin at the time of soiling. Use incontinent care spray and moisture barrier cream on all incontinent patients. Use absorbent briefs and linen underpads. If appropriate, use external catheter or a fecal incontinent pouch.
- Change bed linens as needed for diaphoretic and incontinent patients.
- Identify and correct factors compromising protein and calorie intake.
- Encourage adequate fluid and nutritional intake.
- Initiate a nutritional consultation.
- Provide nutritional supplements or support for nutritionally depleted patients.

---

side to side before the head of the bed is rolled up (to prevent shear), and lifting the buttock up off the surface rather than sliding it (to decrease friction). The latter is best accomplished with the help of the patient, who bends the legs, or by using a lift sheet or other device. Turn the patient 20 to 30 degrees to the side to avoid too much pressure on the greater trochanter.

Most of the time pressure ulcers develop over a bony prominence. The first step in the assessment of a patient with an existing pressure ulcer is to establish the location of the ulcer. The next step is to determine why the ulcer is in that specific location. If the patient has a sacral coccyx wound and is receiving continuous tube feedings with the head up 45 degrees, a probable cause has been established. After the cause is determined, one must then decide what is required to remove the cause. Can the patient be given intermittent feedings and/or can some rest periods be instituted during which the head is lower than 45 degrees? What support surface and positioning will reduce the risk?

Classification of pressure ulcers is by depth. The four-stage classification system accepted by the Wound, Ostomy and Continence Nurses Society, the National Pressure Ulcer Advisory Panel, and the Agency for Healthcare Research and Quality is as follows:

Stage I: Nonblanchable erythema, a reddened area on the skin that remains red even after the pressure has been relieved for 20 minutes (the area does not become pale [blanch], it remains red). The affected area may be boggy or warmer, harder, or more painful than the surrounding skin.

Stage II: break in the skin, blister, or superficial opening of the dermis and epidermis

Stage III: wound that has penetrated through to the subcutaneous tissue, down to fascia

Stage IV: pressure necrosis involving tissue other than skin, such as ligament, muscle, or bone

Stages I and II are partial-thickness loss because only epidermis and dermis are involved. Removing the cause of pressure permits the epidermis to regenerate and the wound to heal. Stage III and IV wounds, on the other hand, are full-thickness loss involving deeper structures, as described. The difficulty, duration, and expense of healing are directly associated with the depth of a wound. Full-thickness wounds heal through the growth of new tissue called granulation tissue. Granulation fills in the area of tissue loss, up to the level of the epidermis. The wound contracts and then, if enough epidermis is available, it regenerates and closes the defect. If the defect is too large, however, a skin graft may be required (Figure 7-2).

Although the staging system has greatly improved, some problems nonetheless remain. For example, a wound filled with necrotic tissue is a full-thickness wound; however, until

Table 7-2 Braden Scale for Predicting Pressure Sore Risk

Sensory Perception Ability to respond to pressure-related discomfort	**1. Completely limited:** Unresponsive (does not moan, flinch, or grasp) to painful stimuli due to diminished level of consciousness or sedation. *Or* Limited ability to feel pain over most of body.	**2. Very limited:** Responds only to painful stimuli. Cannot communicate discomfort except by moaning or restlessness. *Or* Has a sensory impairment which limits the ability to feel pain or discomfort over one half of body.	**3. Slightly limited:** Responds to verbal commands but cannot always communicate discomfort or the need to be turned. *Or* Has some sensory impairment which limits ability to feel pain or discomfort in one or two extremities	**4. No impairment:** Responds to verbal commands, has no sensory deficit which would limit ability to feel or voice pain or discomfort.
Moisture Degree to which skin is exposed to moisture	**1. Constantly moist:** Skin is kept moist almost constantly by perspiration, urine, etc. Dampness is detected every time patient is moved or turned.	**2. Very moist:** Skin is often but not always moist. Linen must be changed at least once a shift.	**3. Occasionally moist:** Skin is occasionally moist, requiring an extra linen change approximately once a day.	**4. Rarely moist:** Skin is usually dry, linen only requires changing at routine intervals.
Activity Degree of physical activity	**1. Bedfast:** Confined to bed.	**2. Chairfast:** Ability to walk severely limited or nonexistent. Cannot bear own weight and/or must be assisted into chair or wheelchair.	**3. Walks occasionally:** Walks occasionally during the day, but for very short distances, with or without assistance. Spends majority of each shift in bed or chair.	**4. Walks frequently:** Walks outside room at least twice a day and inside room at least once every 2 hours during waking hours.
Mobility Ability to change and control body position	**1. Completely immobile:** Does not make even slight changes in body or extremity position without assistance.	**2. Very limited:** Makes occasional slight changes in body or extremity position, but unable to make frequent or significant changes independently.	**3. Slightly limited:** Makes frequent though slight changes in body or extremity position independently.	**4. No limitation:** Makes major and frequent changes in position without assistance.
Nutrition <u>Usual</u> food intake pattern	**1. Very poor:** Never eats a complete meal. Rarely eats more than one third of any food offered. Eats two servings or less of protein (meat or dairy products) per day. Takes fluids poorly. Does not take a liquid dietary supplement. *Or* Is NPO and/or maintained on clear liquids or IVs for more than 5 days	**2. Probably inadequate:** Rarely eats a complete meal and generally eats only about one half of any food offered. Protein intake includes only three servings of meat or dairy products per day. Occasionally will take a dietary supplement. *Or* Receives less than optimum amount of liquid diet or tube feeding.	**3. Adequate:** Eats over half of most meals. Eats a total of four servings of protein (meat, dairy products) per day. Occasionally will refuse a meal, but will usually take a dietary supplement when offered. *Or* Is on tube feeding or TPN regimen which probably meets most of nutritional needs.	**4. Excellent:** Eats most of every meal. Never refuses a meal. Usually eats a total of four or more servings of meat and dairy products. Occasionally eats between meals. Does not require supplementation.

Table 7-2 Braden Scale for Predicting Pressure Sore Risk—cont'd

Friction and Shear	**1. Problem:**	**2. Potential problem:**	**3. No apparent problem:**
	Requires moderate to maximum assistance in moving. Complete lifting without sliding against sheets is impossible. Frequently slides down in bed or chair, requiring frequent repositioning with maximum assistance. Spasticity, contractures, or agitation leads to almost constant friction.	Moves feebly or requires minimum assistance. During a move, skin probably slides to some extent against sheets, chair, restraints, or other devices. Maintains relatively good position in chair or bed most of the time, but occasionally slides down.	Moves in bed and in chair independently and has sufficient muscle strength to lift up completely during move. Maintains good position in bed or chair.

Select the one number in each category that best describes the patient's status. Add the numbers checked to obtain the total score. Implement appropriate skin care protocol accordingly.

Protocol for Identified Risk Factors

Low Risk (Score ≥15)	Moderate Risk (Score 12-14)	High Risk (Score ≤11)
Provide routine skin care. Encourage activity. Avoid massaging bony prominences.	Evaluate for use of pressure-reduction mattress (static air, low air loss, SPR Plus, Total Care, Dynamic Aire), critical care bed, therapeutic foam (not in hospitals). Follow preventive skin care protocol. Maintain head of bed 30 degrees or less unless contraindicated. Follow turning schedule with pillows. Float heels. Use incontinence barrier cream, underpads or briefs. Keep skin clean and dry. Use skin sealant for wound drainage. Use moisturizers on dry skin. Obtain nutrition consultation. Encourage activity; obtain physical therapy consult PRN.	Follow same protocol as for moderate risk plus the following: Consider other support surfaces (air-fluidized bed, ZoneAire). Notify WOCN for consultation. Request order for multivitamin, vitamin C, zinc (if skin breakdown is present).

IV, Intravenous; *NPO,* nothing by mouth; *PRN,* as needed; *TPN,* total parenteral nutrition; *WOCN,* wound, ostomy, and incontinence nurse.

Table 7-3 Norton Scale Risk Assessment Tool

Physical Condition	Mental Condition	Activity	Mobility	Incontinence	Total Score
4 Good	4 Alert	4 Ambulant	4 Full	4 Never	———
3 Fair	3 Apathetic	3 Ambulant with help	3 Slightly limited	3 Occasionally	———
2 Poor	2 Confused	2 Chair bound	2 Very limited	2 Usually/urine	———
1 Very bad	1 Stuporous	1 Bed bound	1 None	1 Urine and feces	———

From Norton D, McLaren R, Exton-Smith AN: *An investigation of geriatric nursing problems in the hospital,* London, 1962, National Corporation for the Care of Old People (now the Centre for Policy on Ageing).

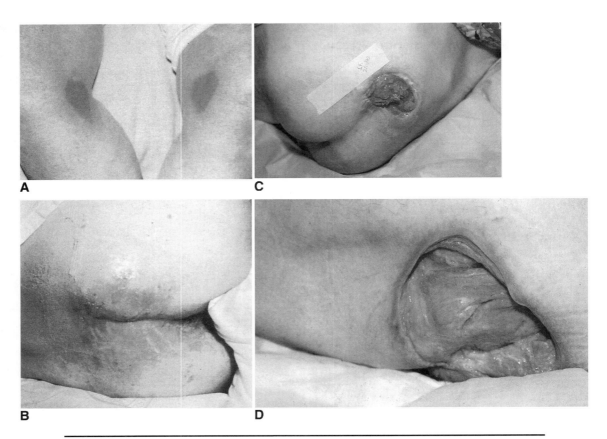

Figure 7-2 **A,** Stage I pressure ulcer. **B,** Stage II pressure ulcer. **C,** Stage III pressure ulcer. **D,** Stage IV pressure ulcer. (**A** and **B,** From Bryant R: *Acute and chronic wounds,* St Louis, 1992, Mosby. **C** and **D,** From Bryant R: *Acute and chronic wounds,* ed 2, St Louis, 2000, Mosby.)

the necrotic tissue is removed (débrided), the wound cannot be classified as either stage III or stage IV. Nevertheless, some state, federal, and private regulatory reimbursement systems require staging on initial assessment.

Another potential problem with staging is the inappropriate use of back staging. This occurs, for example, when a wound classified as a stage IV wound heals. Granulation replaces the damaged tissue, and the clinician reclassifies the wound as stage II. Reclassification is never correct and therefore should never be done. Despite replacement with granulation tissue, the tissue will never be as it was before the wound occurred.

Finally, a reddened area may be noted, the size documented, pressure relief initiated, nutritional deficits improved, moisture reduced, and a complete care plan put in place, and yet a stage I wound may progress to full-thickness necrosis. It is possible that the original red area was an early sign of a full-thickness loss and that the damage had been done. Thus, unlike in early detection of a stage I wound, reversal of the process is not possible.

As long as the limitations of the staging system are recognized and understood, staging remains the standard of care for assessment of pressure ulcer wounds.

The next phase of wound assessment is measurement. The length, width, and depth of the wound are measured. Such measurement should take place on initial assessment and once a week until the wound has healed. Centimeters should always be used in documenting wound size. Wound care experts are always searching for effective ways to determine wound healing. For the clinician working with one patient, the wound measurements, the observation of the tissue in the wound, and the outcome of closure are sufficient. For the researcher who wants to prove that treatment A is statistically better than treatment B, however, a subjective measurement system is not enough.

Length is measured in the direction from head to toe, width is measured from side to side, and depth is measured from the top of the skin to the base of the wound straight down. If there is undermining (skin around the wound with no tissue under the skin) or tunneling (opening from the wound edge inward in a specific direction), it should be measured separately and the direction noted. View a wound as a clock, with the head of the patient at 12 o'clock. Undermining may exist between 9 o'clock and 12 o'clock and may be 4 cm deep. A tunnel may be located at 5 o'clock and be 6 cm deep. The patient's position during measurement should be noted; for example, the patient is turned 60 degrees to his or her right, with the left leg bent 45 degrees and the right leg straight. For accuracy, any subsequent measurements must be made with the patient in the same position. The length exactly from head to toe may not be the longest dimension. Some experts take multiple measurements, whereas others make a tracing of the wound using a marker and transparency. Taking photographs with a grid film or measuring device in the picture is another alternative. In most clinical settings, reporting the longest length and the widest width is the accepted procedure.

The type of tissue in the wound is important for reaching a diagnosis and determining how much damage exists. Is the wound shallow with a moist red base, is the tissue yellow and stringy (slough), or is the wound covered with black necrotic tissue? Can one see or probe to a bone (if so, then osteomyelitis, or underlying bone infection, is present)? All of these observations affect the treatment choices.

The assessment is complete once the patient's current health status is determined, his or her medications are documented, the side effects are noted, and the risk factors for pressure necrosis, pressure relief measures, moisture control measures, turning schedule, and nutritional support are all recorded in the plan of care. Furthermore, a comprehensive assessment must include the staging and measurement of wounds, as well as a description of the amount, type, and odor of drainage and the condition of the surrounding skin.

Treatment

In 1962 the British physician Dr. George Winter demonstrated that wounds healed twice as fast in a moist wound environment (Brassard, 2001). Since then, there has been a surge of new products, some of which are designed to absorb excess moisture, débride necrotic tissue, and decrease the bacterial count (Table 7-4). As the science

Table 7-4 Wound Care Products

Category	Action	Product Name
Calcium alginate	Absorbs 20 times its weight; forms a gel when exposed to wound exudates; maintains moist wound environment; facilitates autolytic débridement; fills in dead space; requires a secondary dressing; is produced in sheets and ropes for packing wounds	Algicel AlgiDERM Curasorb Kalginate Kaltostat Maxsorb Sorbsan
Collagens	Absorb light-to-moderate drainage; maintain moist environment; conform to the wound surface; are nonadherent; require secondary dressing; are produced in sheets, pads, particles, and gels	Fibracol Kollagen-Medifil gel Kollagen-Medifil pads Kollagen-Medifil particles Kollagen-SkinTemp sheets
Contact layer	Is a woven, single-layer net; has low adherence; allows wound drainage to pass through to secondary dressing; protects wound bed from trauma during dressing changes; requires a secondary dressing	Comformant Dermanet Mepitel N-Terface Profore wound contact layer
Foams	Are nonadherent, resulting in nontraumatic removal and ease in application; absorb light-to-moderate drainage, should be changed when saturated to prevent periwound maceration; are produced with adhesive border or require secondary dressing	Allevyn Biatin Hydrasorb Hydrocell Lyofoam Mepilex Otifoam Sof-Foam
Hydrocolloids	Are occlusive; are impermeable to water vapor, oxygen, bacteria, and other contaminants; adhere to surrounding skin but not to wound bed; provide moist wound healing and autolytic débridement, absorb light-to-moderate drainage; do not require secondary dressing; require knowledge and skill for application and removal; are produced in many sizes and shapes	Comfeel Duoderm Exuderm Restore Signal Dress Tegasorb

Continued

Table 7-4 Wound Care Products—cont'd

Category	Action	Product Name
Hydrogels	Maintain moist environment to promote granulation and epithelialization and to facilitate autolytic débridement; are soothing and reduce pain; rehydrate wound bed; provide minimal absorption; offer ease of removal and application; require secondary dressing; are produced in sheets, amorphous gel, and as impregnated gauze	Aquasorb Biolex Carasyn Curasol Elastogel Intrasite Safgel Skintegrity Vigilon
Transparent dressings	Are waterproof and semipermeable (transfer vapor out but are impermeable to bacteria and other contaminants); retain moisture; facilitate autolytic débridement; allow wound observation; do not absorb exudate; do not require secondary dressing	Bioclusive CarraFilm Mefilm OpSite Polyskin Tegaderm
Silver dressings	Contain timed-release silver ions that are antimicrobial; decrease the bacteria count; maintain moisture and promote a healing environment; are produced as film, wound filler, powder, pad, and rope	Acticote Argles Aquacel Ag
Débriding agents	Chemical use of enzymes that interact with necrotic tissue, digesting the nonviable tissue but causing no harm to healthy granulation; maintain moist environment; prescription required	Accuzyme Gladase
	Hypertonic dressings that remove wound edema and loosen necrotic tissue	Mesalt Hypergel
Absorbent dressings	Do not adhere to wound bed; absorb moderate-to-large amounts of drainage away from wound; maintain moist wound environment	Aquacel Pad Aquacel Rope Exu-Dry SofSorb
Pharmaceuticals	Iodine copolymers absorb wound exudate and decrease the bacteria count	Iodoflex Pad Iodosorb
	Displays biologic activity similar to that of growth factors; promotes the chemical activity that stimulates production of granulation tissue	Regranex
	Débrides; promotes granulation; controls inflammation; reduces odor; maintains moist wound environment	Panafil
Other	Provides negative pressure to the wound, which removes edema and promotes growth of granulation tissue; has a closed system that protects wound from contamination; requires skill and knowledge of precautions and contraindications	Vacuum-assisted closure device (e.g., KCI Wound V.A.C.)
	Warms wounds to promote vasodilation, increasing oxygen and growth factors to wound bed	Warm-up therapy
	Stimulates migration of cells to the wound; improves blood flow; is probably bacteriostatic; is not approved for wound care; is not reimbursed for wound care	Electrical stimulation

expands, so does the development of products. Currently more than 2000 wound care products are on the market (Hess, 2001). This variety allows wound care to be individualized for each patient but can be overwhelming for the professional who is recommending the care.

Moist wound healing creates an atmosphere that allows the body's healing process to thrive. Wound healing involves the migration of cells to fight infection and rid the wound of devitalized tissue, biologic production of new tissue, and chemical removal of waste or by-products.

This living, active process is inhibited or halted by a dry environment.

Wound care products can be categorized into several groups: transparent films, hydrocolloids, calcium alginates, foams, hydrogels, collagens, antimicrobials, débriding enzymes, impregnated gauze, and products providing adjunctive therapy. An understanding of the properties of each category, coupled with an assessment of the patient and his or her wound, makes the choice more manageable (Table 7-5). For example, consider a patient who has pressure necrosis on the ischial tuberosity. The wound has been surgically débrided and the overgrowth of bacteria has been treated both topically and systemically. The wound is clean but deep and thus needs to be packed, and enough drainage occurs to macerate the wound edges and create a periwound environment that is susceptible to fungal infection. A check of the product formulary reveals that calcium alginate rope (for packing) can absorb 15 to 20 times its weight in fluid, whereas hydrofiber rope can absorb 30 times its weight. Depending on the amount of drainage and the frequency with which the dressing will be changed, one of these could be the dressing choice.

The assessment of the patient and evaluation of the wound give the clinician information to establish the goal of the wound treatment and the necessary interventions to reach that goal. A topical wound treatment must follow these principles (Doughty, 1990):

■ Remove necrotic tissue—Any tissue in a wound that is not alive, has no blood supply, and is a medium for bacterial growth should be removed.

■ Identify and treat infection—Infection may manifest as indurations, increased exudates, odor, and pain. The infection may be more silent, as in a diabetic patient who comes to the health care provider with increased blood glucose level and retarded or regressed wound healing. If bone is exposed in a wound, it is generally accepted that osteomyelitis is present. Topical treatments alone cannot address wound infections; rather, they augment systemic treatment and decrease bacterial count in patients at risk.

■ Obliterate the dead space—The dead space is the area in the wound that is empty or devoid of tissue. To avoid premature closing of the epidermis before the base is filled with granulation tissue, the area must be gently packed. In addition, any excess drainage must be directed from inside to outside the wound to prevent abscess formation.

■ Absorb exudates—Excess moisture is a risk factor for infection and maceration of the surrounding tissue. Any damage to the surrounding tissue can cause the wound to enlarge.

■ Maintain moisture—Cells grow in a moist environment; thus wound healing takes place in a moist environment.

■ Insulate—Wounds heal at body temperature. If a wound is too cold, cell activity will slow or stop. Opening wounds to air more than every 12 hours reduces temperature and impedes wound healing.

■ Protect—Prevent further trauma by determining if the initial cause of the trauma is eliminated or reduced. Assess whether the irritant or microbe has been contained or treated.

Interdisciplinary Care

The goal of the care of a patient with pressure necrosis is to provide the optimum environment for the wound to heal while preventing further pressure necrosis during the healing and in the future.

Primary Provider (Physician/Nurse Practitioner)

Several medical specialists are involved in the healing of pressure necrosis, including medical physicians who treat the underlying medical problems that perpetuate pressure necrosis (diabetes, neuromuscular diseases, cardiac problems, gastrointestinal disorders, pulmonary problems) and surgical physicians who diagnose, surgically débride, and reconstruct wounds as necessary. Doctors who specialize in infectious diseases very often are involved in treating chronic wounds, especially when osteomyelitis is present. Infection of wounds is so common that the infectious disease specialist is sometimes the primary medical professional directing the care in conjunction with the wound care nurse specialist. Most often, however, multidisciplinary wound care clinics are directed by a plastic surgeon or a wound, ostomy, and continence nurse (WOCN), and all the aforementioned specialists, as well as a vascular surgeon, podiatrist, physiatrist, hyperbaric specialist, and radiologist, are involved.

Wound, Ostomy, and Continence Nurse

The WOCN works closely with the physicians. The WOCN is often the first member of the team to assess a wound, recommend dressings or other wound care modalities, provide débridement if needed, and amend the care plan to match progression of the individual wound. The nurse who is a wound specialist has the opportunity to help care for patients who have wounds resulting from conditions other than pressure. Because of this experience, the wound specialist nurse is often the professional at the bedside who suggests the possible differential diagnosis, proposes the tests to be performed to make the diagnosis, and recommends the most knowledgeable specialists in the area. The WOCN partners with the primary nurse in the hospital, in long-term care and rehabilitation centers, and in home care to provide state-of-the-art wound care. The nurse initiates the process of care with the nursing assessment and prepares the patient and family for the laboratory studies and consultations. The nurse also develops a plan of care individualized for each patient. What setting is best for this patient? What equipment will

Table 7-5   Seven Steps in Wound Care with Product Examples

Function*	Transparent Film Dressings	Hydrocolloids	Hydrogels	Foams	Alginates	Debriding Agents	Other	Absorbent Products	Biosynthetics/ Skin Substitutes	Contact Layers	Antimicrobials
Remove necrotic tissue	X	X	X	X	Minimal	X		X			X
Infection control/ protect	X	X		X	X	X	VAC X	X	X		X
Obliterate dead space		Minimal	Minimal		X	X	VAC X	X	X		X
Absorb exudates		X	Minimal	X	X	X	VAC X	X	Minimal	X	X
Maintain moist environment	X	X	X	X	X	X	VAC X	X	X	X	X
Insulate	Minimal	X	X	X	Minimal	X	VAC X	X	X	X	X
Protect	X	X	X	X	X	X	VAC X	X	X	X	X
Product examples	Bioclusive CarraFilm Mefilm OpSite Polyskin Tegaderm	Comfeel DuoDERM Exuderm Restore Signal-Dress Tegasorb	Aquasorb Biolex Carrasyn Curasol Elasto-Gel IntraSite Safgel Skintegrity Vigilon	Allevyn Biatin Hydrasorb Hydrocell Lyofoam Mepilex Otifoam Sof-Foam	Algicel AlgiDERM Curasorb Kalginate Kaltostat Maxsorb Sorbsan	Accuzyme Dakins Santyl Mesalt Panafil Gladase Hypergel	Electrical stimulation VAC Warm-up therapy	Aquacel Pad Aquacel Rope Exu-Dry SofSorb	Biobrane Fibracol Medifil Mediskin Panafil Regranex Silon Skin Temp	DermaNet Conformant 2 Mepitel N-Terface Pro-Force Tegapore	Acticote Aquacel Ag Argles Iodoflex Iodosorb

Modified from Chameleon Healthcare™, 1994, Linda Dunham and Janice Mentz. Revised 2003 by Pamela W. Cox.
VAC, Vacuum-assisted closure.
*Acronym to aid memory: **R**ick **I**s **O**n **A** **M**ountain **I**n **P**eru.

this patient need? Who must learn the care and how will the nurse teach the caregiver? When is it appropriate to change the care plan? What is the patient's response to the plan of care and how can this be improved? The WOCN and the primary nurse are the team leaders who will implement the recommendations obtained from the aforementioned consultants.

Physical Therapist

The physical therapist is an integral part of the team caring for a patient with pressure necrosis. After an extensive assessment, the physical therapist establishes a program that will move the patient from the current functional state to the preillness level or to a level that is reasonable to the patient and the care team. For the patient with pressure necrosis, this usually means establishing a program that will help the patient to become strong enough to independently change or assist in changing positions. Accomplishing this goal allows the patient and family to limit pressure on bony prominences that are healing or at risk. The physical therapist is involved in and often directs the seating evaluation for a patient who uses a wheelchair for mobility. This is an essential intervention that can prevent a patient from experiencing seating pressure necrosis. A seating evaluation is individualized for the given patient. Choice of a wheelchair, a pressure-reduction chair cushion, and a method of in-chair pressure relief depends on the patient's height, weight, strength, and occupation, on the caregiver's ability, and on skin and wound condition. The physical therapist also instructs caregivers and family members in the proper methods of moving the patient to prevent injury to the patient as well as to the caregivers. The physical therapist may also instruct the team in the use of equipment for transfers, such as the Hoyer lift. Physical therapy modalities for wound care include whirlpool baths, pulse lavage, sharp débridement, vacuum-assisted closure, and electrical stimulation. Physical therapy, like nursing, is both an art and a science. The physical therapist can instill confidence in a patient who is frightened and hopeless about returning to independent, pain-free mobility.

Dietitian

Every person who is at risk for pressure necrosis or who has a chronic wound should have a nutrition assessment. The nurse, the physician, or the dietitian can initiate this assessment. The evaluation includes an analysis of general appearance: Is the person cachectic or obese? Is the individual's weight stable or has he or she lost weight? Does the patient have conditions or take medications that require changes in "normal" dietary intake? What is normal and is that adequate for the specific patient? Does the patient have the ability and means to purchase and prepare meals? Can the patient feed himself or herself? Has appetite changed? Have changes in psychological health occurred? If any one of these conditions exists, then a nutrition professional should be part of the team.

The dietitian evaluates the patient's current nutritional status, including body weight, muscle mass, fat stores, and laboratory data. What food is taken in, how it is digested, and how the body metabolizes the nutrients can be revealed by the appropriate laboratory tests. Low serum protein level is a major indicator of malnutrition. The serum albumin level indicates the patient's protein intake and absorption during the previous month. The prealbumin level is an indicator of protein intake and absorption during the previous few days. The patient's hydration status and renal function can alter both of these results. The dietitian also looks at levels of electrolytes, especially creatinine, and at the results of a complete blood count. The complete blood count includes lymphocyte count. Lymphocytes are an indicator of the immune state of the patient, and the immune system is sensitive to changes in the protein level.

Before making recommendations for oral diets, supplements, tube feeding, or parenteral nutrition, the dietitian reviews the results of the physical assessment, laboratory data, a list of previous and current medications, and the state of current wounds or sites from which the patient is losing fluids and electrolytes. Fluid loss is assessed for protein, carbohydrates, fats, vitamins, minerals, amino acids, and antioxidants. The required levels change as the patient's physical and emotional needs progress. The dietitian is an essential member of any team that prevents and treats chronic wounds.

Medical Social Worker

In some institutions the social worker may be a permanent member of the team and in other settings the social worker is hired as a consultant. The social worker is the team member who will assist in the psychosocial evaluation of the patient to determine the patient's needs for support while in acute care and/or the level of care needed after discharge. The social worker knows how to obtain financial support for necessary equipment, food, and ongoing care.

The social worker meets with the nurse, doctor, patient, and patient's family. The social worker's communication skills and understanding of social systems allows him or her to gather information about the patient so that realistic goals can be set. The social worker ascertains what the previous social situation of the patient was and what can be expected of the patient and his or her social system in the future.

LOWER EXTREMITY ULCERS
Overview

Lower extremity ulcers fall into three major categories: arterial, venous, and neuropathic. Each type has a different incidence, prevalence, pathophysiology, and treatment. What all three have in common is chronicity, pain, forced lifestyle change, and difficult healing process. Lower extremity wounds have been the precursor to amputation in persons with diabetes and vascular problems. Only in the recent past have limb salvage clinics replaced the amputation clinics that existed for so many years. Limb salvage clinics have arisen because leg and foot ulcers are considered serious problems. Today differential diagnosis is better, treatments with topical wound care and antibiotics are more sophisticated, and there are professionals who are interested and specialize in the area of lower extremity wounds. Most of the wound centers in the country have large populations of patients with lower extremity wounds. Although lower extremity wounds have many causes, it is beyond the scope of this chapter to address more than the three most common of these.

Venous Stasis Disease

The most common cause of leg ulcers is venous insufficiency. Approximately 1% of the general population and 3.5% of people over age 65 have venous ulcers. The prevalence is rising as the population ages. The recurrence rate of venous ulcers approaches 70%. The estimated cost of care can exceed $40,000 per individual. Approximately 2 million workdays per calendar year are lost due to chronic venous ulcers (Hess, 2000).

Pathophysiology

The best way to explain venous stasis disease is to begin with a description of the venous system in the lower extremity. There are deep veins (femoral, popliteal, and tibial veins), superficial veins (greater and lesser saphenous veins), and veins that connect the deep and superficial veins, referred to as connector or perforator veins. One-way valves allow the blood to flow in the direction from superficial to deep but prevent backflow. If the system is functioning, the superficial veins collect the blood used by the tissues in metabolism. This blood passes from the superficial vein through the connector vein and into the deep vein to return to the inferior vena cava and back to the heart. When a person walks, the calf muscle pumps the blood from the leg to the heart. When the person stops walking, the pump stops but the one-way valve between the connector and the deep veins closes and prevents the blood from flowing in reverse. If these valves are damaged or the forward flow is inhibited, the blood returns to the superficial veins. The backflow increases the pressure on the veins, and eventually the veins will leak the fluid and metabolic waste into the subcutaneous tissue, and the tissue will be damaged. The extent of damage can range from dermatitis to ulceration and cellulitis. The return of metabolized fluid from the leg to the heart involves the calf muscle, the valves in the veins, and the pathway of the veins. The venous pathway can be damaged by deep vein thrombosis, joint replacement or traumatic injury, and by vein harvest for cardiac bypass surgery. Valvular dysfunction can occur because of hereditary or congenital problems, thrombophlebitis, trauma, or infection. A decrease in activity, paralysis, or ankle injury may negatively affect the calf muscle pump.

Clinical Manifestations and Diagnosis

Obesity, multiple pregnancies, congestive heart failure (CHF), occupations that involve prolonged standing or sitting, traumatic limb injuries, joint replacement, and paralysis or immobility are predisposing factors to venous stasis disease.

People who have venous stasis disease have increased venous pressure. The increased pressure causes the capillaries in the lower extremities to dilate and the fluid to accumulate, which leads to edema. If the pressure is not relieved, the fluid will seep out into the surrounding tissue. Hemosiderin is released when red blood cells in the fluid break down. Hemosiderin stains the skin, and its brownish color is present in the gaiter region of the legs (ankle to below the knee). This is a classic sign of venous stasis. As the condition progresses, the skin develops scales and erythema. This condition is known as venous stasis dermatitis (Figure 7-3). During this period, the patient has an increased sensitivity to external substances and thus is at increased risk for developing contact dermatitis (Figure 7-4). The combination of edema and inflammation often leads to weeping and itching. Ulcerations occur from scratching, mild trauma, and open blisters. Any opening in the skin can lead to bacterial invasion, as is often noted by the medical professionals who first see patients with cellulitis in the emergency department. Untreated cellulitis is both limb threatening and life threatening (Figure 7-5). Repeated bouts of cellulitis weaken the immune system and create resistance to antibiotic therapy.

CHF is a predisposing factor in venous stasis disease. Both patients with CHF and those with venous stasis can show pitting edema in the early stages. Therefore, it is important to know the history and duration of the edema before treatment is begun. With CHF, the edema is always bilateral and will respond to diuretic therapy. Edema associated with venous stasis disease, on the other hand, can be unilateral or bilateral. Diuretics alone will not resolve the edema of venous stasis disease because the fluid is no longer moving toward the heart and kidney. The cornerstone of

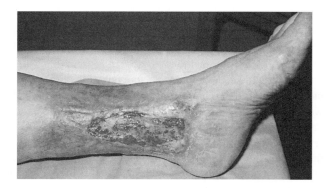

Figure 7-3 Classic venous ulceration in the malleolar region. (From Belch JFF et al, *Color atlas of peripheral vascular diseases,* ed 2, London 1996, Mosby-Wolfe.)

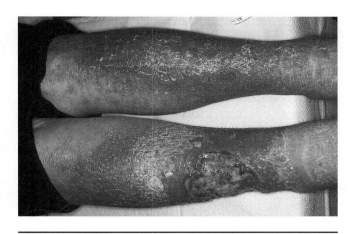

Figure 7-4 Venous stasis dermatitis of the legs. (From Bryant R: *Acute and chronic wounds,* ed 2, St Louis, 2000, Mosby.)

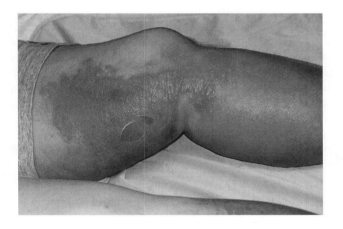

Figure 7-5 Cellulitis in a patient with long-standing diabetes and stasis dermatitis. (From Black JM, Hawks JH, Keene AM: *Medical-surgical nursing: clinical management for positive outcomes,* ed 6, Philadelphia, 2001, WB Saunders.)

treatment for venous stasis is to elevate the legs and to add compression. It is critical that precautions be taken when mobilizing the fluid from edematous extremities of patients diagnosed with CHF. Elevation and compression can actually cause an episode of CHF. Thus, this treatment is best carried out in an acute care setting for a fragile patient. In this situation diuretics are appropriate adjuncts in the treatment of venous stasis edema.

Venous stasis disease is most commonly diagnosed by history and physical examination. In making a diagnosis, the following should be addressed: Does the edema and discomfort or pain increase at the end of the day? Does leg elevation relieve the pain? Is skin staining present in the gaiter region of the leg?

Swelling, redness, and pain in one lower extremity can also be the symptoms of a deep vein thrombosis. Deep vein thrombosis should be ruled out by noninvasive scans and Doppler imaging before treatment is initiated.

Arterial disease should also be ruled out before treatment is initiated for venous stasis. Compression is contraindicated for persons with arterial disease. A comprehensive discussion of arterial disease is presented in the next section. Ankle-brachial pressure index (ABI) is one of the measures to assess for arterial disease. ABI compares blood pressure at the arm with blood pressure at the ankle. A Doppler device is used to determine ABI. Blood pressure is taken in both arms and both legs. The highest ankle pressure is divided by the highest brachial pressure to derive ABI. A normal result is 0.9 to 1.0. Most clinicians will not use compression if the ABI is 0.8 or lower.

If the ABI is between 0.5 and 0.8, the patient probably has both arterial and venous disease, and a vascular consultation is advisable. The vascular specialist may approve mild compression with close follow-up. When the ABI is below 0.5, an evaluation for arterial vascular surgery generally begins. Compression should never be used if the ABI is 0.5 or lower (Table 7-6).

Table 7-6 Ankle-Brachial Index (ABI)

ABI Value	Interpretation/Clinical Significance
0.95-1.3	Normal range
0.5-0.95	Mild to moderate peripheral arterial disease: 0.5-0.8
	Associated with intermittent claudication
	Ability to heal wound usually maintained
<0.5	Severe arterial insufficiency; wound healing unlikely unless revascularization can be done
>1.3	Abnormally high range, typically because of calcification of the vessel wall in patients with diabetes
	Renders ABI test invalid as measure of peripheral perfusion

From Bryant RA, editor: *Acute & chronic wounds: nursing management,* ed 2, St Louis, 2000, Mosby. Data from Cantwell-Gab K: Identifying chronic peripheral arterial disease, *Am J Nurs* 96(7):40, 1996; McGee S, Boyko D: Physical examination and chronic lower-extremity ischemia: a critical review, *Arch Intern Med* 158(12):1357, 1998; Rockson S, Cooke J: Peripheral arterial insufficiency: mechanisms, natural history, and therapeutic options, *Adv Intern Med* 43:253, 1998.

Treatment

The most important aspect of treating a venous stasis wound is controlling the edema. Elevation, compression, and ambulation are the three components of edema control. The feet and legs should be elevated 4 to 6 inches above the heart. Placing blocks under the foot of the bed or elevating the mattress above the box spring is an effective means of accomplishing the desired elevation. Placing pillows under the legs and feet is effective only for a short period. The person should elevate the legs above the heart all night and for two half-hour periods during the day.

The patient should be instructed to avoid prolonged sitting or standing. If standing is necessary, weight should be shifted from one foot to the other and ankle flexion exercises should be performed to promote venous return. Frequent rest periods with elevation of the legs above heart level are recommended. In addition, the feet should always be elevated when the patient sits.

Compression therapy involves the application of external wraps or stockings that create sustained compression of 20 mm Hg or higher. Compression should be applied only after the legs have been elevated for at least 2 hours. This will ensure that gravity has drained some of the excess fluid from the area and decreased pressure. Compression usually begins with short stretch wraps and progresses to stockings

fitted for the person's legs only after optimal edema control has been reached. It is important that the compression do no harm. The bony prominences (ankles and shins) should be protected from pressure and friction with padding. The compression should be comfortable. The patient's adherence is essential for the successful treatment of venous stasis disease. When the patient is included in the decision making regarding care, he or she is more likely to accept the plan. Fortunately, many forms of compression are available (Table 7-7). The patient should be given a choice, and the choice must be comfortable. The patient will have to use some form of compression for the rest of his or her life. The patient's acceptance of this fact is the first hurdle.

Normal ambulation (heel-to-toe stride) activates the calf muscle pump and allows the compression to move the fluid from the legs to the heart. Exercises that mimic the calf muscle pump are effective for patients who do not have a normal gait or do not ambulate at all. Thromboembolic disease (TED) stockings are not appropriate for controlling the edema associated with venous stasis. TED stockings are not strong enough to keep the fluid out of the tissue; therefore, as the leg swells, the stocking will act as a tourniquet. Ace bandages do not provide sustained pressure when the person walks and do not help move the fluid upward. Compression

Table 7-7 Comparison of Types of Compression Therapy

Type of Compression Therapy	Mechanism of Action	Advantages	Disadvantages	Comments
Therapeutic support stockings: Static, short stretch (Biersdorf-Jobst)	Support calf muscle pump with ambulation Compress superficial system to minimize edema	Available in varying degrees of compression at the ankle Custom fit for different types of legs Can be removed frequently for wound care and assessments Patient or caregiver can apply	Difficult to apply and remove; stocking donners and slickers are available Success heavily dependent on adherence, which cannot be closely monitored	Must be premeasured Must be replaced at appropriate intervals Available in variable levels of compression: Light: 14-17 mm Hg Medium: 25-35 mm Hg Strong: 25-35 mm Hg
Orthotic device: Static, inelastic (CircAid [CircAid Medical Products], Thera-Boot [Coloplast Corp.])	Supports calf muscle pump with ambulation Provides sustained compression	Very easy for patient to apply Custom fit Easy removal for wound care and assessments Sustained pressures Can be adjusted for patient comfort and as edema decreases Good patient adherence because patient has some control over adjustment of Velcro closures for comfort	Somewhat bulky with multiple Velcro closure straps	Must be premeasured

Table 7-7 Comparison of Types of Compression Therapy—cont'd

Type of Compression Therapy	Mechanism of Action	Advantages	Disadvantages	Comments
Zinc paste bandage: Static, inelastic (Unna boot, Dome paste bandage)	Supports calf muscle pump Prevents edema buildup	Comfortable and soothing to skin Provides protection from scratching Serves as a dressing in addition to providing compression	Some dressing components known to cause allergic reaction May not accommodate highly exudative wounds Change in pressure over time as edema decreases	Can add a self-adherent elastic wrap to continue providing active compression as leg size changes Outer wrap required to protect clothing from moist dressing Must be applied by trained physician, nurse, or physical therapist
Multilayer bandage system: Four-layer bandage system Static layers 1 and 2 inelastic; layers 3 and 4 elastic (Profore [T.J. Smith and Nephew, Ltd.]) (Dyna-Flex [Johnson & Johnson Medical] Three-layer bandage system: layer 1 inelastic; layers 2 and 3 elastic	Provides support for calf muscle pump with ambulation Provides continuous compression during rest to increase interstitial tissue pressures and partially collapse superficial venous system	Provides sustained pressure for up to 1 week Good for highly exudative wounds Very comfortable Profore 4-layer system provides a wide range of safe and therapeutic compression at variable stretch (40% to 70%)	Somewhat bulky and hot Can be adjusted to leg shape with additional padding	Must be applied by trained physician, nurse, or physical therapist
Limited-stretch wrap: Static, elastic (Comprilan [Biersdorf-Jobst], Setopress [ConvaTec])	Supports calf muscle pump Prevents edema buildup	Markers indicate correct degree of stretch Can be washed and reused multiple times Can be applied by caregiver with appropriate training	Sometimes difficult to keep on because of decreased elasticity Potential risk for moisture maceration Potential risk for pressure necrosis May not be effective in a nonambulatory patient	Can add a self-adherent elastic wrap to secure in place May need to add an absorbent dressing for a highly exudative wound
Compression pumps: Dynamic Intermittent pneumatic compression (IPC) Sequential compression (A-V Impulse [Kendall])	Enhance venous return by propelling and/ or milking blood out of lower extremity	Good for patients unable to tolerate static devices IPC shown to stimulate fibrinolysis A-V impulse can be used safely in patients with arterial ischemia Allow treatments to be done in home setting Calf pump function not necessary Promotes lymphatic flow	Daily rental charge that may become expensive Requires 2 to 4 hours per day of immobility during treatments	Close monitoring for acute pulmonary edema required

From Bryant R, editor: *Acute and chronic wounds: nursing management,* ed 2, St Louis, 2000, Mosby.

is an essential component of treatment; however, if it is performed by someone not properly trained, compression may result in further damage to the skin and limb. A professional who is experienced in the management of venous stasis disease and compression should be involved in the patient's treatment until the leg ulcer is healed and/or until the patient or the patient's caretaker can demonstrate knowledge of safe use of compression.

Choose the topical treatment for a specific wound by considering the wound characteristics as described earlier in the section on assessment (Table 7-5).

Untreated, venous stasis often leads to venous stasis dermatitis. The leg should be kept dry and skin protection ointment should be used to prevent weeping from causing dermatitis. Often, the leg appears indurated and the skin scaly and weeping, and the patient may have pruritus and burning. Venous stasis dermatitis should be treated with topical steroid cream or ointment. Patients with venous stasis are also sensitive to topical cleansers and ingredients, especially lanolin, neomycin, bacitracin, latex, chemical perfumes, and preservatives. It is best to clean the legs with white vinegar or apple cider vinegar and water, 1 part vinegar to 5 to 10 parts water. The vinegar will remove the debris left behind by topical agents and drainage. The vinegar will also return the skin to its natural acid pH, which helps prevent infection. Vinegar has proven to be so soothing that some patients report using it as part of their on-going leg care.

Cellulitis is a serious consequence of untreated venous stasis disease. Cellulitis and venous stasis dermatitis are often confused. They both manifest with indurations, weeping, swelling, and pain. Skin temperature may also be increased, which can be assessed with a skin thermometer. Cellulitis is well demarcated and involves the full thickness of the skin, whereas venous stasis dermatitis is generalized and superficial. Hospitalization for a course of intravenous antibiotics is recommended for those with cellulitis. Dermatitis can be treated on an outpatient basis. The person with cellulitis should have the legs elevated, but compression should be withheld until the antibiotics have reached a therapeutic blood level. Before discharge from the hospital, the patient should undergo the necessary testing to diagnosis venous stasis. If the patient does have venous stasis disease, then a long-term treatment plan that includes exercise, compression, and patient education and referral to outpatient follow-up should be initiated.

Finally, of all the manifestations of venous stasis disease, ulcers or open wounds can be the most upsetting. They are painful, irregular in shape, superficial, coated with yellow slough, and wet. Venous stasis ulcers are found on the lower calf and involve the medial malleolus in particular. Patients with venous stasis disease who have trauma or an animal bite to or infection of the calf may develop venous ulcers at the site. Venous stasis ulcers of the lower extremity can drain large amounts of fluid. Patients are often confined to one or two rooms because nothing contains the drainage and their legs are constantly weeping. These patients are not comfortable lying down, so they spend all day and all night sitting in a chair with their legs in a dependent position. This prevents return of this fluid to the vascular system, where it is usually eliminated. Patients in this condition do not walk because their legs are heavy and they cannot get shoes on their feet. This decreases the opportunity for calf muscle pumping action. The longer the wounds are present, the larger they become and the more difficult they are to heal. Some patients will admit to having had an ulcer for 20 years. It is difficult to get a person to believe in a treatment plan if the person has lived with a wound for a long time and has had multiple failed treatments. In addition, if the person does heal, he or she needs support and understanding, because the person must adjust to the change of not having a wound. Although the new situation is healthier, there is often ambivalence and always the need for adjustment. Some patients' social contacts are built around their ulcers. Without support and recognition of their possible ambivalence, some patients have sabotaged the final steps of healing and/or prevention. Seventy percent of patients with venous stasis ulcers have a recurrent ulcer. Most often, the patient stopped using compression or did not replace worn-out compression stockings. The leg edema returns, the compression sleeve is then too tight, the swelling progresses, and the cycle begins again.

If the patient's edema is worse at night than in the morning and the edema resolves with elevation, controlling the edema will be less difficult. If the person has had swelling for a long time and it does not resolve with elevation, involves the feet, and is hard rather then pitting, the individual may have lymphedema. This is a more difficult and serious problem. The lymphatic system works with the arterial and venous systems to keep the correct plasma balance in various locations. When plasma leaves the arterial or venous system, the lymph system rescues what it can and returns the plasma to the circulation. The lymphocytes that are circulating in the lymph system can pick up bacteria, toxins, and malignant cells and therefore play a role in defending the body against infection, poisons, and cancer. The lymph system mobilizes 2000 to 4000 ml of fluid a day. If there is too much lymph fluid (excess production) or a blockage occurs in the flow, the lymph system will shut down and the patient will develop lymphedema. Lymphedema is progressive and results in changes in the appearance and shape of the skin and the ability to fight infection. A leg or arm with lymphedema can become infected and develop cellulitis after even a minor trauma or scratch. Patient education is essential for patients who have lymphedema. In particular, the patient must be taught what the early signs and symptoms of infection are and how to protect the area from injury. Exercise, elevation, and compression are helpful treatments for patients with lymphedema, as for patients with venous stasis disease.

However, many times the area is so blocked off that the fluid must be mobilized by manual lymphedema massage. Lymphedema massage is performed by trained therapists to drain the entire lymphatic system. A patient with leg involvement will have the chest, abdomen, groin, and leg massaged. It is intense therapy, performed once or twice a day for 3 to 6 weeks. Compression is also used, and the patient or caregiver is instructed in techniques to maintain the affected area.

Interdisciplinary Care

The goals of care for a person with venous stasis disease include healing and preventing leg ulcers, dermatitis, and cellulitis, and providing the tools and skills that will allow the patient to succeed in prevention.

Primary Provider (Physician/Nurse Practitioner)

Physicians of many specialties participate in the care of the patient with venous stasis disease. The primary care physician, vascular surgeon, plastic surgeon, infectious disease specialist, and dermatologist may all be involved in the diagnosis and treatment of venous stasis.

Wound, Ostomy, and Continence Nurse

The WOCN works closely with physicians. The WOCN is often the first member of the team to assess a wound, recommend dressings or other wound care modalities, provide débridement if needed, and amend the care plan to match the progression of the individual wound.

Nurses play many roles in the care of the person with venous stasis disease. They serve as advocates in diagnosis, treatment, and follow-up, especially for a patient who has had two or three admissions to the same unit for cellulitis.

The WOCN serves as a change agent to engage the patient in playing an active role in prevention. The WOCN acts as a counselor to help the patient accept this chronic condition, an educator who can teach the patient and family about wound care and compression, and a facilitator for referrals to occupational therapists, physical therapists, medical social workers, a home care team, wound care centers, and compression aid fitters.

Physical and Occupational Therapists

The physical therapist plans a program to improve or maximize mobility, especially when ambulation is altered. Whirlpool treatments and lymphedema massage are physical therapy modalities used to treat and prevent edema and leg ulcers.

The occupational therapist is instrumental in assessing the patient's ability to use compression independently. The occupational therapist works closely with the nurse and the physical therapist to choose the best form of compression for the individual patient. The occupational therapist helps adapt the necessary equipment and/or teach the patient to use the tools that can assist a patient with disabilities.

Medical Social Worker

The medical social worker is the patient's and family's guide to community resources and source for referrals, and provides support and information if alternative living arrangements are indicated.

Arterial Ulcers

As many as 10 million people in the United States may have peripheral vascular disease. It is estimated that 4 million of those suffer leg pain symptoms. At the highest risk are those who are older than 50 years of age, are smokers, or are diabetic, overweight, hypertensive, or hyperlipidemic.

Pathophysiology

Arterial leg ulcers or ischemic ulcers are the result of altered arterial flow to the bone, muscle, connective tissue, and skin in the lower extremity. This decreased flow is associated with arteriosclerosis and atherosclerosis. Arteriosclerosis causes the walls of the arteries to become thick and less supple, whereas atherosclerosis is characterized by a buildup of residue on the inner walls of the arteries, which narrows the lumen. Both conditions lead to a decrease or stoppage in the flow of oxygenated blood to the leg. This is a progressive disease; the amount of damage depends on the timeliness of diagnosis and treatment. Left untreated, the condition can progress to gangrene of the lower extremity, which is limb and life threatening.

Clinical Manifestations

Patients who complain of pain during ambulation (claudication) should be taken seriously. This could be the first reported symptom of arterial insufficiency in the lower extremity. A patient will state, for example, that every time he or she reaches the corner, the pain begins. Ambulation increases the demand for oxygen to the muscle. Other symptoms include an absence of palpable or Doppler ultrasonography–sensed pulses in the leg, capillary refill time of longer than 3 seconds, skin that is pale and cool to the touch, absence of hair below the occlusion, shiny or taut epidermis, atrophy of subcutaneous tissue, and delayed venous filling. A patient with such symptoms should be referred to a vascular surgeon. Unfortunately, patients often come to the health care provider in the later stages of the disease. Patients who complain that they have pain at rest have 90% occlusion of an area. They may complain that they are in pain at night when lying in bed and state that to relieve the pain they drop the foot off the bed, sit up, or just sleep sitting up in a chair. Often patients come to a private medical doctor or emergency department with a foot ulcer. Arterial ulcers are usually located on the distal area of the lower extremity. Arterial ulcers are dry, black, and painful, and if gangrene is present, they have a strong, unpleasant odor.

Treatment

The treatment of choice is to open up the artery or bypass the artery that is occluded. Some of the interventions, such as balloon angioplasty and stent placement, can be carried out without going to the operating room. Surgery is performed only after testing to determine in what artery and at what level the occlusion occurs and after any infection is treated, the wound is débrided, and other medical conditions are stabilized. Débridement is never done on dry gangrene; it is performed only when fluid is trapped under the skin. If the patient had an ulcer before the surgery, the wound most often will still be present after the procedure. After surgery, however, there is a chance that the wound can heal because of the improved blood supply. Healing will still depend on good nutrition, abstinence from smoking and caffeine, pain control, control of edema, maintenance of a stable blood glucose level, appropriate wound care, and patient education. Surgery will improve the circulation to the affected location, but it will not cure the disease. Peripheral vascular arterial disease is a chronic progressive disease with no cure; however, behavior changes and medications can control or slow its progress. The patient should be made aware that the feet should be kept warm and protected. Any trauma will create another opportunity for gangrene. Tight-fitting garments, including girdles, garters, or any items that cut into the lower leg, should not be worn.

Smoking decreases the flow of blood to the peripheral vessels and the supply of oxygen from the lungs to the blood. Smoking is so damaging to these patients that some vascular surgeons will not attempt to operate on a patient unless he or she agrees to stop smoking. Lowering stress in the patient's life is another way to decrease the demand for blood. Optimal skin and nail care of the feet should be maintained, with daily inspection, cleansing, lubrication, use of supportive footwear, and podiatrist oversight of nails and calluses (Figures 7-6 and 7-7).

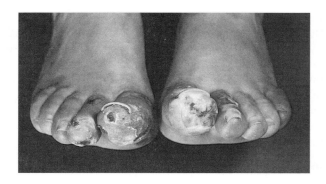

Figure 7-7 Diabetic foot ulcers, an example of a wound with yellow, soft slough that needs cleaning. (From Black JM, Hawks JH, Keene AM: *Medical-surgical nursing: clinical management for positive outcomes*, ed 6, Philadelphia, 2001, WB Saunders.)

Drug Therapy

The most common use of drugs in patients with peripheral vascular disease is treatment of the pain. All three categories of pain medication must be used to relieve the pain: nonsteroidal antiinflammatory drugs, narcotics, and drugs for nerve pain. All attempts to use systemic medications to improve circulation have been either ineffective or detrimental.

Nutritional Care

Patients who can stabilize their blood glucose levels and control hypertension, edema, cholesterol, and triglyceride levels do the best in preventing disease, which may progress to limb loss. A dietitian who can work out a meal plan that provides a low-sodium, low-fat, low-cholesterol, diabetic diet and that also meets the patient's cultural needs and satisfies the taste buds is invaluable.

Interdisciplinary Care

Primary Provider (Physician/Nurse Practitioner)

The vascular surgeon, private medical doctor, diabetologist, radiologist, interventional radiologist, plastic surgeon, and pain control specialist are a part of the team from diagnosis to wound closure.

Nurses

The WOCN, diabetic nurse, pain control specialist, hospital, and home care nurses assume the roles of teacher, caregiver, patient advocate, and coach. The WOCN is often instrumental in referring the patient to the appropriate physician specialist, especially if the patient seeks treatment for a wound. The WOCN also assesses the wound, recommends changes in wound care modalities, and provides débridement if needed until the wound heals. The diabetic nurse specialist assesses the patient and his or her insulin needs and directs instruction of the patient and the nurses who provide primary care to the patient. The nurses who specialize in pain control assist the primary care team in optimizing the patient's pain

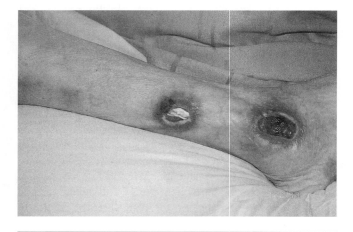

Figure 7-6 Arterial ulcers of the lateral malleolus and distal lateral portion of the leg. Note round, smooth shape. (From Black JM, Hawks JH, Keene AM: *Medical-surgical nursing: clinical management for positive outcomes*, ed 6, Philadelphia, 2001, WB Saunders.)

control. The hospital nurse and the home care nurse lead the team along with the patient until the goals are attained and the patient has the necessary skill to assume control.

Podiatrist and Orthotist

As noted earlier, the podiatrist recommends proper protective footwear and provides nail care, whereas the orthotist builds or alters foot support as prescribed.

Physical and Occupational Therapists

The physical therapist and occupational therapist work together to return the patient to exercise and self-care. They may use special equipment to observe and care for the feet and legs, and to increase activity to healthy tolerance.

Medical Social Worker

Because of all the necessary behavioral changes and the fear associated with the possibility of limb loss, the social worker can be a support to patient, family, and nursing staff. Often the patient's disease leaves the individual in a state of dependence, and the patient cannot return to his or her home or needs organized community support to be safe. The social worker is instrumental in guiding the patient to accept referrals and can access community resources.

Diabetic Foot Ulcer

Approximately 16 million people are diagnosed with diabetes in the United States. Twenty-five percent of them will develop a foot ulcer, and 15% of patients with foot ulcers will require an amputation. Approximately 67,000 diabetes-related amputations are performed each year in the United States (Orsted and Inlow, 2001). Many factors predispose the diabetic patient to a foot ulcer and an amputation. Identifying the risk factors, educating the patient and family to recognize the early signs of problems, and knowing how to prevent ulcers is the most effective limb-saving approach. Once a patient has developed an ulcer, a multidisciplinary team of knowledgeable professionals must work with the patient to prevent amputation.

Pathophysiology and Assessment

The damage to the diabetic foot occurs because of neuropathy and peripheral vascular disease. The neuropathy is sensory, motor, and autonomic, and the peripheral vascular disease affects the small vessels. The effects of sensory neuropathy are seen when the patient cannot distinguish pain, pressure, or temperature changes on the extremities. Neuropathy predisposes the patient to undetected structural, thermal, or chemical injury. There are degrees of loss of sensation, and this loss is monitored to determine appropriate preventive measures.

The motor neuropathy affects the innervations to the ligaments and muscles of the feet. Without proper movement of the ligaments and muscles, the foot becomes deformed with hammer toes, claw foot, or Charcot's foot. The fat pads are redistributed and the bones often collapse. Just the pressure of walking or standing on a foot with this type of dam-

age can cause an ulcer. An early sign of pressure is a callus. If the callus is not removed, it continues to enlarge and will compress the skin to the bone and cause an ulcer in a poorly vascularized, dry, contaminated area. Eventually bone will be involved. Because of the sensory neuropathy, the patient cannot feel the pain or pressure from this injury.

Autonomic neuropathy affects the innervations to the areas that are automatically controlled by the body: sweat glands, blood vessels, and sebaceous glands. Autonomic neuropathy results in dry and cracked skin, which opens an area for bacteria to enter. This can result in an infection, which can lead to a foot wound and then to amputation. Bacteria will enter a fissure in a diabetic foot and cause an infection. The patient does not have enough sensation to feel the effects of the foot infection and there is not enough peripheral circulation to bring defensive cells to the area. Because of this altered flow and the diabetic patient's immune-suppressed state, the usual response to infection—which produces an area that is red, hot, and swollen—will not occur. The diabetic patient can have a raging infection that is silent and painless. Often the only signs are an unexplained increase in blood glucose level and necrosis. The effects of glucose on the cells that fight infection are similar to those of alcohol on the body. The cells become slow moving, ineffective, and uncommitted to their purpose. If the patient also has visual impairment and does not closely monitor blood glucose level, he or she can appear for treatment with a wound that is limb threatening and a systemic infection that is life threatening (Figure 7-8).

Every patient with diabetes must have his or her feet assessed. The evaluation includes visual inspection of the entire foot, including the area in between the toes, which is a common site for fungal infections as well as cracks and ulcers. Sensory neuropathy should be assessed using a Semmes-Weinstein monofilament instrument. This fine wire is placed on the skin and enough pressure is applied to bend the filament into a C shape. If the patient cannot feel the pressure of the filament, neuropathy is present, and the patient should be placed in the appropriate care track to monitor for and prevent wounds. Measures may include inspection every 1 to 3 months by a trained professional, use of special shoes or orthotics for reducing pressure, and increased patient and family surveillance. Diabetic patients must be taught what steps to take to prevent foot ulcers and what to do if a foot wound is present. This information is a part of the teaching programs, which include information on nutrition, exercise, medications, eye care, weight control, and smoking cessation.

Diabetes predisposes the patient to atherosclerosis. In the diabetic patient, the atherosclerosis is diffuse. In the nondiabetic patient, the atherosclerosis may affect the major vessels of one limb, whereas in the diabetic patient the small vessels of both legs will be involved. The diabetic patient can come for treatment with a wound and a strong pedal pulse but a low skin oxygen level. Transcutaneous partial

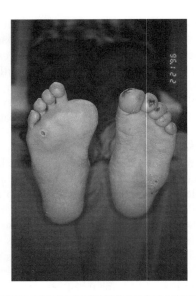

Figure 7-8 Neuropathic foot with claw toes on right foot and ulcers on tips of claw toes. Note deformation of lateral plantar surface of the patient's left foot and amputated toe on the patient's right foot. (From Bryant R, editor: *Acute and chronic wounds: nursing management,* ed 2, St Louis, 2000, Mosby.)

pressure of oxygen (tcPo$_2$) can be measured in a vascular laboratory and is important information to consider during the development of a treatment plan for a patient with a foot ulcer. For a wound to heal, a tcPo$_2$ of at least 30 mm Hg is required (normal value is 55 mm Hg).

Clinical Manifestations and Treatment

When the patient with diabetes comes for treatment with a foot wound, the initial assessment includes a vascular evaluation with Doppler ultrasonography to measure pulses and determination of tcPo$_2$ to ensure that blood supply is adequate to heal the wound. Every foot wound in a diabetic patient is infected, and the patient should be treated systemically with antibiotics. If it is possible to probe to bone, then osteomyelitis is present. In this case, the treatment for infection is altered and lengthened, and removal of the bone is indicated. If blood supply is adequate, then the wound is débrided. If there is a callous, it is removed to assess what is under the callous. The patient is expected to be non–weight bearing if the wound is on the heel or the bottom of the foot. If the wound is on the tip of the toe or the side of the foot, then the patient's footwear is replaced to better accommodate the area and eliminate pressure. Diabetic patients with foot ulcers often must undergo a revascularization procedure before any orthopedic or plastic reconstruction and/or aggressive wound care can begin. Even black eschar that is locked to the skin edges and does not have surrounding erythema is left intact until a limb has been revascularized. Once adequate blood flow has been restored, then débridement of the wound, bone removal, and reconstruction and

wound closure can be initiated. This often requires several trips to the operating room, support from the medical team for glucose control and antibiotic therapy, and wound treatment that provides the correct environment to prevent infection and damage of new tissue.

Interdisciplinary Care

The goal of the care of the diabetic patient with a foot wound is to save the limb. When this is not possible, then the goal is to preserve enough of the limb to allow the patient to return to everyday life with the tools to protect the other limb from injury. Care of the diabetic patient with a wound requires the expertise of each member of the interdisciplinary specialty team working together toward this goal.

Primary Provider (Physician/Nurse Practitioner)

The vascular surgeon, plastic surgeon, and orthopedic surgeon evaluate the patient concurrently, and each may perform surgery before the treatment is completed. The diabetologist, hyperbaric specialist, and infectious disease specialist are intervening at the same time. In different settings, a different specialist is the team leader. In limb salvage centers a designated primary care nurse or doctor usually leads the team.

Nurses

The diabetic nurse, WOCN, hospital nurse, clinic nurse, and home care nurse work to help the family and patient learn about their roles in maintaining blood glucose levels, the action and side effects of medications, and the *do*s and *don't*s of diabetic foot care. They also demonstrate and instruct in proper wound care.

The diabetic nurse specialist is an invaluable member of the team. This nurse has an in-depth understanding of the effects of diabetes on the entire body and mind. He or she is knowledgeable about current best practices in nutrition, exercise, and medication to treat diabetes. The diabetic nurse works with the patient to support and educate him or her in the lifestyle changes necessary to return to optimum health.

The WOCN is most often involved in care of the diabetic patient who has a foot wound. The WOCN may be the first wound specialist to intervene and therefore may be the member who initiates referrals to the other members who are essential for the wound healing and limb salvage care. The WOCN may also be the wound specialist who follows the patient to healing. The WOCN has first-hand experience of how difficult it is to heal a diabetic foot ulcer. This nurse has taken an active role in teaching primary care nurses and physicians how to assess the feet of the diabetic patient to prevent injury. WOCN education programs offer special modules in nail care and callous removal.

Nurses in all settings and all specialties care for diabetic patients. They can often be the change agents for the patient and family. Nurses play the pivotal role in influencing care, advocating for the best practice, and supporting the patient with his or her response to treatment.

Dietitian

The dietitian adapts the diet program to the patient's tastes, preferences, needs, and cultural habits so that glucose level is controlled, activity is resumed, and adequate nutrition for healing is provided. This takes several initial sessions and then ongoing adjustment. All the assessment skills and teaching tools available for the nutritional education of the patient and family are used with the diabetic patient. The information about wound healing presented in the section on pressure necrosis applies here. The patient with diabetes is immunocompromised by the disease. The diabetic patient has significantly less chance of healing and a much greater chance of infection. The best treatment known for a diabetic patient is a diet that controls blood glucose and cholesterol levels. The dietitian working with a diabetic patient at any level has a major role in that person's care

Podiatrist and Orthotist

The podiatrist and orthotist must assess the patient's foot so that the correct support is prescribed, built, and adapted, and must reassess this support to make sure there are no pressure points during and after healing. The podiatrist evaluates the patient's gait with and without assistive devices. He or she looks at the changes in the structure of the feet. If abnormal pressure is being placed on a poorly padded area, the podiatrist builds more padding or shifts the weight with an orthotic or a total contact cast. A total contact cast is cast material applied to a foot and leg to redistribute the weight. The patient with an insensate foot who has an ulcer on the heel or plantar region of that foot cannot shift the weight. The cast can alter the gait so that the patient can ambulate with minimal pressure on the affected area. This cast is often applied after the callus has been removed, the wound has been débrided, the edema and drainage are minimal, and no cellulitis or tracts are present in the wound. The cast is left in place for 3 to 7 days. Only a skilled professional should apply a hard material to a deformed, insensate foot that already has a limb-threatening ulcer. In the hands of a skilled professional, the contact cast is an excellent adjunct to the treatment of the diabetic foot wound.

For the diabetic patient, a foot assessment, nail care, foot skin care, and appropriate shoes can be a matter of limb or life without a limb.

Physical and Occupational Therapists

The physical therapist and occupational therapist teach the patient how to resume activity while using protective footwear or remaining non–weight bearing. (The modalities described in the pressure necrosis section are all applicable to the diabetic patient.) The physical therapist creates an exercise program that uses the rest of the body for strengthening and mobility. Physical therapists are sometimes trained in applying total contact casts.

The occupational therapist has his or her own thorough evaluation system that helps the therapist decide what assistive devices the patient requires. The occupational therapist is the expert in enabling the patient to perform the activities of daily living independently in spite of his or her disabilities in mobility, strength, vision, and cognition. The diabetic patient with low vision and limited flexibility must inspect the feet each day. The occupational therapist provides the patient with a lighted magnifying mirror with a long, flexible handle and then tests the patient's ability to use the device effectively and safely. The patient, the nurses, the physical therapist, and the physicians provide information to the occupational therapist. Each member of the team will have a need or will have a task for the patient to accomplish. The occupational therapist is the team member who recommends equipment that will help the patient regain independence in these tasks and instructs the patient in its use. The occupational therapist is knowledgeable about commercially available equipment that can augment the patient's performance.

Pharmacist

The pharmacist provides education about and oversight of the many pharmaceuticals prescribed by multiple specialists. The pharmacist is a constant professional in the diabetic patient's life. The pharmacist often knows the latest developments in medications and medication administration. The pharmacist can influence the care of the diabetic patient by providing education and state-of-the-art information to the entire team.

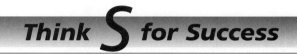

Think **S** *for Success*

Symptoms
■ Manage the four major symptoms of wounds—pain, swelling, drainage, and odor—with the appropriate medications and treatment.

Sequelae
■ Take measures to prevent infection and premature wound closure.

Safety
■ Educate patient/caretaker in the proper technique to prevent wound infection and to recognize early signs and symptoms of infection for early intervention.

Support/Services
■ Educate the patient/caretaker in the care of the wound.
■ Refer to professionals in the appropriate setting when the wound cannot be managed by the patient or caretaker because of complexity or location.
■ Refer patient to rehabilitation team dietitian, and equipment specialist as needed.

Satisfaction
■ Determine the lifestyle changes the patient requires to meet the goal of healthy skin.
■ Determine the degree to which wounds interfere with important aspects of patient's life and develop a plan to maintain quality of life.

REFERENCES

Agency for Health Care Policy and Research: Pressure ulcers in adults: prediction and prevention, Public Health Service Pub No 9200047, Rockville, Md, 1992, Department of Health and Human Services.

Agency for Health Care Policy and Research: Treatment of pressure ulcers, Public Health Services Pub No 95-0652, Rockville, Md, 1994, Department of Health and Human Services.

Braden B: Risk assessment in pressure ulcer prevention. In Krasner DL, Rodeheaver GT, editors: *Chronic wound care: a clinical source book for health professionals,* ed 3, Wayne, Pa, 2001, HMP Communications.

Brassard A: Wound care: putting theory into practice in Canada. In Krasner DL, Rodeheaver GT, editors: *Chronic wound care: a clinical source book for health professionals,* ed 3, Wayne, Pa, 2001, HMP Communications.

Cuddigan J, Berlowitz D, Ayello E: Pressure ulcers in America: prevalence, incidence, and implications for the future, *Adv Skin Wound Care* 14(4): 208-15, 2001.

Doughty D: The process of wound healing: a nursing perspective, *Progressions* 2(1):3-12, 1990., 1990.

Hess CT: Management of the patient with a venous ulcer, *Adv Skin Wound Care* 13(2):79-83, 2000.

Hess CT: *Wound care,* ed 4, Springhouse, Pa, 2001, Springhouse Corp.

Kane DP: Chronic wound healing and chronic wound management. In Krasner DL, Rodeheaver GT, editors: *Chronic wound care: a clinical source book for health professionals,* ed 3, Wayne, Pa, 2001, HMP Communications.

Krasner D: Pressure ulcer: assessment, classification, and management. In Krasner D, Kane D, editors: *Chronic wound care,* ed 2, Wayne, Pa, 1997, Health Management Publications, pp 152-7.

Meraviglia M et al: Maintenance of skin integrity as a clinical indicator of nursing care, *Adv Skin Wound Care* 15(1):24-9, 2002.

Orsted H, Inlow S: The team approach to treating ulcers in people with diabetes. In Krasner DL, Rodeheaver GT, editors: *Chronic wound care: a clinical source book for health professionals,* ed 3, Wayne, Pa, 2001, HMP Communications.

CHAPTER 8

Obstructive Airway Disease

Helen Mautner, MS, RN

OBJECTIVES

After reading this chapter, you should be able to do the following:

- Describe the pathophysiology of chronic obstructive airway disease
- Describe the clinical manifestations of chronic obstructive airway disease
- Describe the functional health patterns affected by chronic obstructive airway disease
- Describe the role of each member of the interdisciplinary team involved in the care of patients with chronic obstructive airway disease
- Compare and contrast the progression and management of chronic obstructive pulmonary disease and asthma
- Describe the indications for use, side effects, and nursing considerations related to the drugs commonly used to treat chronic obstructive airway disease

OVERVIEW OF OBSTRUCTIVE AIRWAY DISEASE

Chronic conditions of the lower respiratory tract are the fourth leading cause of adult deaths in the United States (Minino and Smith, 2001). Airway obstruction is a defining characteristic of several diseases in this category. The irreversibility of the airway obstruction in chronic obstructive pulmonary disease (COPD) is what distinguishes it from asthma, in which the airway obstruction is reversible. Chronic bronchitis and emphysema, which often coexist, have been included under the umbrella term of COPD. However, only certain subsets of these conditions and certain subsets of asthma meet the criteria for chronic obstructive airflow disease. Spirometric data and presenting symptoms provide the diagnostic data to determine the presence of COPD and to assign a severity classification of COPD (Table 8-1).

In 2001, the World Health Organization and the National Heart, Lung, and Blood Institute developed comprehensive guidelines for the management of COPD. In their consensus workshop report titled "Global Strategy for the Diagnosis, Management, and Prevention of Chronic Obstructive Pulmonary Disease," COPD is defined as a progressive inflammatory condition of the lungs characterized by airflow obstruction that is not fully reversible (National Heart, Lung, and Blood Institute, 2000). Because of the chronic nature of these conditions, they often result in the frequent and costly use of the health care system, with some estimates of expenditures exceeding $30 billion annually.

Regardless of the underlying pathology, persons with COPD share many of the same symptoms and experience similar challenges in daily living. This chapter describes the broad category of COPD and the differences between chronic bronchitis, emphysema, and chronic asthma. It also presents the therapeutic interventions and symptom management techniques that are common to these conditions.

ASSESSMENT

Varying degrees of dyspnea and activity intolerance are common in all persons with chronic airway obstruction, regardless of the underlying cause, and must be considered in the assessment. Other items suggested for inclusion in the

Table 8-1 Classification of Severity of Chronic Obstructive Pulmonary Disease (COPD)

Stage 0: At risk	Normal spirometry results
	Chronic cough or sputum production
	Minimal impact on quality of life
Stage 1: Mild COPD	Spirometry results showing mild airflow limitation with or without chronic symptoms
Stage 2: Moderate COPD	Worsening airflow limitation
	Progression of symptoms
	Shortness of breath with exertion
	Possible repeated exacerbations
Stage 3: Severe COPD	Severe airflow limitation or presence of respiratory failure or clinical signs of right-sided heart failure.
	Impaired quality of life
	Possible critical exacerbations

Adapted from National Heart, Lung, and Blood Institute: Global initiative for chronic obstructive lung disease, 2000, retrieved from *http://www.goldcopd.com* on Nov 8, 2002.

Box 8-1   Functional Health Pattern Assessment for Chronic Airway Obstruction

HEALTH PERCEPTION/HEALTH MAINTENANCE
- Is the patient exposed to tobacco smoke and/or other inhaled irritants?
- At what age did the patient start smoking? What are the patient's total pack-years of smoking?
- What is the patient's past medical history, including respiratory infections, asthma, allergies, α_1-antitrypsin deficiency, immunizations?
- What is the patient's general perception of his or her health?

NUTRITION/METABOLISM
- Have there been any recent unexplained changes in weight?
- Does the patient have anorexia related to dyspnea or sputum production?
- Is the patient nutritionally depleted?
- What are the patient's diet history, meal patterns, and supplement use?
- Does the patient experience bloating?
- Is there early satiety due to pressure on the diaphragm?
- Are meals interrupted by cough attacks or dyspnea?
- What foods affect sputum production?

ELIMINATION
- Does the patient have difficulty getting to the bathroom because of dyspnea?
- Is there constipation related to inactivity?

ACTIVITY/EXERCISE
- Does the patient have a chronic cough? How frequent is the coughing? Does it occur during the day? at night?
- How much sputum is produced?
- Can the patient perform instrumental activities of daily living?
- Does the patient experience dyspnea? Is it persistent? Does it worsen over time? Does it occur only on exertion?
- Is there edema of the lower extremities?
- How many steps are in the home?

SLEEP/REST
- Does the patient complain of sleepiness or daytime drowsiness?
- Does the patient have difficulty sleeping?
- How many pillows are used?
- Does the patient sleep in a chair instead of the bed?
- Does the patient complain of increased fatigue?

- Is there a persistent lack of energy?
- Does the patient experience nocturnal dyspnea?

COGNITION/PERCEPTION
- Does the patient show forgetfulness or confusion?
- Does the patient report chest or abdominal discomfort related to coughing?

SELF-PERCEPTION/SELF-CONCEPT
- How has the condition affected the patient's self-image?
- What life changes have been or will become necessary because of the condition?
- How does the patient feel about oxygen use?

ROLES/RELATIONSHIPS
- How has the condition affected daily living, normal activities, and work?
- What is the economic impact of the condition on the patient and family?
- Does the patient have adequate social and family support?

SEXUALITY-REPRODUCTION
- Does the patient experience a lack of sexual drive?
- How does dyspnea affect the patient's sexual activity?
- Is the patient interested in learning ways to decrease dyspnea during sexual activity?

COPING/STRESS TOLERANCE
- What coping strategies does the patient use?
- How does stress affect breathing?
- Is the patient interested in joining a support group or pulmonary rehabilitation program?

VALUES/BELIEFS
- Is the patient satisfied with the current treatment plan?
- Is the patient interested in exploring alternative therapies to supplement medical interventions?
- What are the patient's beliefs related to this condition?
- What are the patient's health beliefs regarding long-term mechanical ventilation?
- What constitutes good quality of life for the patient?
- What is important to the patient?
- To what extent do the patient's cultural/spiritual beliefs influence decision making related to this condition?

---

initial assessment and organized according to functional health patterns are presented in Box 8-1.

Many assessment tools have been developed for further evaluation of chronic airway obstruction and its impacts, some of which are listed in Box 8-2. In the assessment of chronic airway obstruction, an instrument that measures the impact of the respiratory symptom on the quality of life is very useful. The combination of a subjective instrument and an objective pulmonary measurement tool should be consid-

ered. Data obtained with these assessment tools provide a starting point for the generation of an individualized plan of care that is tailored to the person's physiologic, psychological, and social needs.

Ethnic Variations

Case rates of COPD are higher among white Americans than among African or Hispanic Americans (American Lung Association, 2002b). The opposite is true for asthma,

Box 8-2   Instruments for Assessment of Chronic Airway Obstruction

Asthma Quality of Life Questionnaire
Baseline Dyspnea Index
Borg Dyspnea Scale
Chronic Respiratory Disease Questionnaire
Functional Performance Inventory
Oxygen Cost Diagram
Pulmonary Functional Status and Dyspnea Questionnaire
Respiratory Illness Quality of Life Questionnaire
Saint George Respiratory Questionnaire
Short Form 12 (SF-12) Health Survey
Short Form 36 (SF-36) Health Survey
Sickness Impact Profile
Six Minute Pulmonary Distance Walk
Transition Dyspnea Index
Visual Analog Dyspnea Scale

however, for which the case rates for African Americans are slightly higher than those for white Americans. In addition, the case rates for hospitalizations and deaths from asthma are almost three times higher for African Americans than for whites (American Lung Association, 2002a).

CHRONIC OBSTRUCTIVE PULMONARY DISEASE

As stated earlier, COPD is a broad term that includes chronic bronchitis and emphysema. Irreversible airway obstruction is the common denominator in these disorders. Estimates are that at least 10 million Americans have some type of COPD, including more than 8 million with chronic bronchitis and more than 2 million with emphysema (American Lung Association, 2002b). Asthma is often a component of these conditions.

Symptoms of COPD usually appear during the middle or later adult years. In the past, occurrences were higher in men than in women, but the gap is narrowing because more women now smoke. Cigarette smoking is clearly the most significant contributing factor in the development of COPD. Other inhaled irritants that promote the development of COPD include air pollutants, occupational pollutants, and second-hand smoke. These irritants impair the protective function of the cilia, causing chronic inflammation of the airways. Smoking cessation or the elimination of the irritant is essential to slow the process and improve long-term outcomes. Many programs and strategies are available to assist with smoking cessation. Nicotine replacement therapies, either over the counter or prescribed, are helpful in the management of withdrawal symptoms such as irritability and restlessness. Success is often achieved when nicotine

replacement is combined with structured support in a group setting or on an individual basis.

The initial pathophysiology and clinical manifestations of chronic bronchitis and emphysema differ and are addressed separately. However, both conditions lead eventually to chronic airway obstruction as depicted in Figure 8-1. Once irreversible damage to the airways occurs, the pharmacologic and therapeutic interventions are similar and these are discussed together.

Chronic Bronchitis

The American Thoracic Society (1995) defines chronic bronchitis as the presence of a chronic cough with sputum production for three consecutive months in at least two consecutive years. Other causes of chronic cough are assumed to have been considered and excluded. Chronic bronchitis is more common in middle-aged men, and cigarette smoking remains the most significant etiologic factor.

Pathophysiology

Physiologic changes in chronic bronchitis include inflammation, edema, and the eventual scarring of the bronchial airways. Progression of the disease varies, based on host

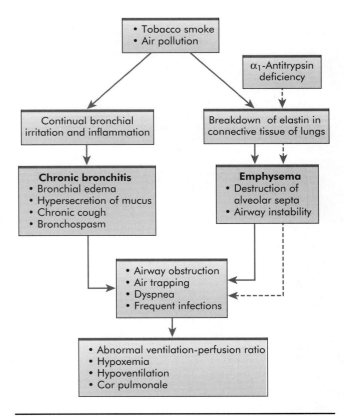

Figure 8-1 Pathophysiology of chronic bronchitis and emphysema. (From Lewis SM, Heitkemper MM, Dirksen SR: *Medical-surgical nursing: assessment and management of clinical problems,* ed 6, St Louis, 2004, Mosby.)

factors and environmental exposures. The noxious effects of smoking or inhalation of other irritants contribute to the activation of the inflammatory process in the airways with the release of macrophages and eosinophils. Inflammatory mediators are released and the inflammatory process continues, possibly causing additional inflammation.

The enlargement of the bronchial mucus glands and the increase in the number of goblet cells cause an increase in the production of mucus and mucus plugging. When smoking is a contributing factor, the damage to the cilia that line the airways limits effective airway clearance, which further contributes to the accumulation of mucus.

All of these changes cause a narrowing of the central airways and subsequent hypoventilation and impaired gas exchange. The chronic hypoxemia and acidosis that are often associated with chronic bronchitis may result in constriction of the pulmonary vasculature and initiation of a cascade of events leading to increased pulmonary pressures and eventual right ventricular hypertrophy or cor pulmonale (Figure 8-2). The compromise of right ventricular function is sometimes associated with venous stasis, thrombosis, and an increased risk of pulmonary embolism (National Heart, Lung, and Blood Institute, 2000). The management of cor pulmonale requires the use of supplemental oxygen and continued treatment of the underlying pulmonary condition.

Clinical Manifestations

The person with chronic bronchitis, sometimes referred to as a "blue bloater," is often obese. The physical appearance is dramatically different from that of a person with emphysema. Other clinical differences between the two conditions are described in Table 8-2.

The most common presenting symptoms are chronic cough and sputum production. In fact, the diagnosis of chronic bronchitis is based in part on the evaluation of sputum production and the frequency of symptoms. Many persons with chronic bronchitis report frequent upper respiratory tract infections accompanied by purulent sputum and dyspnea.

The American Thoracic Society (1998) defines dyspnea as the subjective experience of breathing discomfort. The dyspnea associated with chronic bronchitis is often variable and not as profound as the dyspnea described in emphysema. As the condition progresses, however, reports of activity intolerance and dyspnea become more frequent and severe as a result of impaired gas exchange.

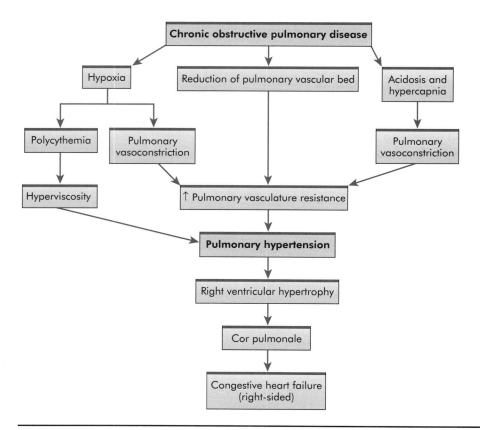

Figure 8-2   Mechanisms involved in the pathophysiology of cor pulmonale secondary to chronic obstructive pulmonary disease. ↑, Increased. (From Lewis SM, Heitkemper MM, Dirksen SR: *Medical-surgical nursing: assessment and management of clinical problems*, ed 6 , St Louis, 2004, Mosby.)

Table 8-2   Distinguishing Characteristics of Chronic Bronchitis and Emphysema

Characteristic	Emphysema	Chronic Bronchitis
Descriptive term for patient	"Pink puffer"	"Blue bloater"
Skin and nail color	Pink	Cyanotic
Body build	Thin, frail	Often overweight
Cough	Minimal	Chronic
Sputum production	Minimal	Excessive
Breathing pattern	Prolonged expiration	Variable
Cor pulmonale	Rare	Frequent episodes
Dyspnea	Progressive, often disabling	Variable

Inspiratory and expiratory wheezes may be audible to auscultation, especially if some component of asthma is present. Other possible clinical manifestations are weight loss and anorexia caused in part by frequent coughing spells, which can also lead to rib fractures. In the presence of cor pulmonale, peripheral edema may also be present.

Emphysema

The term *emphysema*, derived from a Greek word meaning "blown up," describes a chronic pulmonary condition characterized by the enlargement and eventual destruction of the alveoli of the lungs. The loss of alveolar elasticity causes air trapping and overinflation of the lung. Smoking is the primary contributing factor in emphysema, which affects approximately 2 million adults in America. The incidence is higher among males. The condition usually manifests in the middle adult years.

Premature development of emphysema can also be precipitated by a rare genetic deficiency of α_1-antitrypsin, a protein necessary for the protection of lung tissue. This predisposition is most common in persons of northern American descent and affects young adults 20 to 40 years of age. Emphysemic changes in this group can begin even earlier in those with a history of smoking.

Emphysema is classified into two main groups depending on the site of pulmonary involvement. Centrilobular emphysema, which usually affects the upper lung zones, is often associated with chronic bronchitis and is rarely seen in nonsmokers. It is the most common type of emphysema. Panlobular emphysema is less common and occurs most often in persons with α_1-antitrypsin deficiency. Both types result in an alteration in the normal structure of the alveoli and impairment of gas exchange.

Pathophysiology

Inflammation of lung tissue as a result of exposure to cigarette smoke or other inhaled irritants leads to the release of proteolytic enzymes that cause direct damage to alveolar tissue. Usually these enzymes are kept in check by the protective enzyme α_1-antitrypsin. Destruction of alveolar tissue occurs when this protective enzyme is inactivated by smoking or is absent due to a genetic deficiency. As damage to alveolar tissue continues, further inflammation and permanent lung injury result.

The lung damage in emphysema is seen in the air spaces that are distal to the terminal bronchioles where the functional units of the lung are located. Alveolar walls lose their elastic recoil, which results in increased lung compliance and hyperinflation of the lung. In addition, as alveolar walls are destroyed, the surface area available for gas exchange is decreased, which causes ventilation-perfusion abnormalities and subsequent hypoxemia. Attempts to compensate by increasing the respiratory rate are effective initially, but the chronic hypoxemia often leads to the need for supplemental oxygen.

Clinical Manifestations

In contrast to the individual with chronic bronchitis, the person with emphysema, sometimes called a "pink puffer," appears frail and underweight. This is likely due to the increased energy required for the work of breathing. Dyspnea is the major symptom in emphysema, but it may not be present until considerable alveolar destruction has occurred. In advanced stages, a forward-leaning position is adopted to help relieve the dyspnea. Diaphragm motion is compromised as a result of the hyperinflation of the lung, and accessory muscles of respiration are often recruited. Lung hyperinflation also results in an increase in the anterior-posterior diameter of the chest wall and the typical barrel-chested appearance of the person with emphysema. Coughing and sputum production are usually minimal unless some component of chronic bronchitis is present.

Diagnosis

The diagnosis of COPD is based partly on the presenting symptoms described earlier and is confirmed by the results of pulmonary function tests. Spirometry is essential in the diagnosis of any chronic obstructive airflow disease to determine the presence of airflow limitation, assess the reversibility of obstruction through the use of bronchodilators, and judge the severity of the condition. This testing is also strongly recommended for persons at risk for the development of COPD, although in the early stages of the disease pulmonary function test results may be normal (Petty, 2001).

Specific anatomical changes may be evident on the chest radiograph in severe COPD, reflecting distention of the lungs and pulmonary hypertension. If pulmonary hypertension is present, the electrocardiogram will show changes that indicate right ventricular hypertrophy. Arterial blood gas analysis is another diagnostic test that quantifies levels of hypoxemia and hypercarbia in advanced stages of COPD.

Interdisciplinary Care

Interdisciplinary care for the person with COPD is focused on the management of symptoms, the prevention of respiratory infections, and the proper combination and use of pharmacologic interventions. Either a primary care physician or a pulmonologist directs medical management, depending on the severity and complexity of the condition. Nurse practitioners often assist in the management of care. Other members of the team include nurses, respiratory therapists, physical and occupational therapists, and dietitians. Medical social workers and psychologists also provide valuable therapeutic interventions in many cases.

As in the management of other chronic conditions, there are no clear boundaries between disciplines. The roles of team members and the choice of services are guided by the individual needs of the person receiving care.

Primary Provider (Physician/Nurse Practitioner)

The primary provider is often the first to identify stage I or stage II COPD. Interventions at this stage are focused on symptom management and risk reduction, and specifically include smoking cessation strategies. As the severity of the condition progresses to stage III, the expertise of a pulmonary specialist is often required, especially if the person is prone to frequent episodes of exacerbation. At each encounter with the patient with COPD, the provider should question the person regarding continued exposure to risk factors and the status of symptoms, and should conduct a comprehensive review of current medications. Comorbidities should also be monitored carefully, with special attention to the use of medications that may interfere with COPD therapies.

Many pulmonary specialists and primary care groups use pulmonary nurse practitioners to assist in the management of persons with respiratory conditions. This specially trained nurse is in a unique position to make appropriate adjustments to the pharmacologic regimen, to educate the person with COPD on management of the activities of daily living and symptom control, and to develop a practical plan of action for emergencies. The pulmonary nurse practitioner may also act as the liaison between specialists in other disciplines, making referrals as needed.

Living with a chronic condition requires a partnership between the physician, the other members of the health care team, and the person with COPD. Each person with COPD must be acutely aware of his or her own particular symptoms and accept an active role in self-monitoring, including knowing the baseline status and identifying changes that warrant a call to the physician. All team members should educate the person with COPD that early identification and reporting of symptoms may avoid emergency office or hospital visits.

Nurse

Nursing support for the person with COPD begins with a careful assessment of functional status (Box 8-1). Subjective and objective information provides the foundation for an individualized plan of care that helps determine which disciplines should be actively involved. The nurse often assumes a team leadership role, coordinating and integrating the interdisciplinary interventions.

Each person with COPD has different motivations and desired outcomes. The nurse must take the time to discover the desired end point to ensure the cooperation of the person and acceptance of the care plan. The teaching plan that the nurse develops should cover the following topics:

- Correct use and administration of prescribed medication(s)
- Knowledge of what the signs and symptoms of exacerbations are and when to seek help
- Need for early identification of signs and symptoms of respiratory infection
- Energy conservation techniques
- Breathing exercises and effective coughing techniques
- Need for annual influenza immunization and pneumonia immunization every 5 years
- Nutritional needs
- Safe use of supplemental oxygen
- Management of secretions
- Need to maintain a careful balance between activity and rest
- Advance directives and end-of-life decisions

Careful adherence to the interdisciplinary plan of care is helpful in avoiding episodes of acute exacerbation, which can often last several weeks. The nurse who is actively involved with the person with COPD is in a position to detect subtle changes in clinical symptoms that suggest a possible exacerbation of the condition. Upper respiratory tract infections often are the precipitating factor in an exacerbation, and the nurse should collaborate with the physician or nurse practitioner to develop a plan for early intervention. Home management of an exacerbation includes increasing the dose or administration frequency of the inhaled bronchodilator. The nurse should evaluate for clinical signs of infection such as an increase in the amount of sputum, change in the color of sputum, or fever, which indicate the need for antibiotic therapy. Corticosteroids may be added if more conservative interventions are unsuccessful.

For persons with stage III COPD, home management of exacerbations is difficult because such exacerbations often lead to acute respiratory failure and the need for intubation and mechanical ventilation. No matter what intervention is prescribed, close monitoring of symptoms by both the nurse and the person with COPD is extremely important, because each exacerbation causes further decline in functional status and quality of life (Agency for Healthcare Research and Quality, 2000).

Drug Therapy

The long-term decline in lung function associated with COPD cannot be reversed by pharmacologic interventions. However, symptoms can be managed and the frequency and severity of exacerbations can be reduced by the use of inhaled bronchodilator therapy. This intervention is used more for maintenance than for management of acute attacks. The choice of drug therapy for COPD is based on individual symptoms, response to treatment, and consideration of any comorbid conditions present. Drug selection involves a stepwise approach that encourages the active participation of the person with COPD.

The three classes of bronchodilator used in the treatment of COPD are β-agonists, anticholinergics, and xanthine derivatives. Combination therapy is not uncommon and may produce more sustained relief of symptoms. However, the anticholinergic class of bronchodilator, specifically ipratropium, is the first-line maintenance drug used for COPD (Pauwels et al, 2001). Slow-release theophylline preparations have also been shown to be effective, especially when used in combination with other bronchodilators (Pauwels et al, 2001). Education on the correct use of inhalers and nebulizers is essential for patients to derive the full benefit of the inhaled bronchodilators.

Use of corticosteroids for the treatment of COPD remains controversial. In the small percentage of persons with COPD who respond to inhaled or oral corticosteroids, some component of asthma most likely is present. The benefits of steroid therapy are often outweighed by the side effect of muscle weakness, which further compromises respiratory function. This class of drug should be employed with caution, and its use should be based on improvement in spirometric measurements.

Other medications that may be used intermittently include mucolytic expectorants, antibiotics to treat infectious exacerbations of the condition, and cardiac drugs to treat right-sided heart failure if present. Some of the medications used in the treatment of obstructive airway disease are listed in Table 8-3.

Pulmonary Rehabilitation

Many factors contribute to the cascade of events leading to disability from chronic obstructive airway disease. Nutritional depletion, age-related muscle loss, and muscle weakness related to steroid therapy are just a few. Although no evidence exists that pulmonary rehabilitation programs improve lung function, the literature is replete with reports showing that these programs provide motivation and support to those living with this chronic condition. The major components of a pulmonary rehabilitation program include education and coaching on all topics related to the condition, which bring together the skills and knowledge of all members of the interdisciplinary team.

Physical Therapy

Evidence is growing that COPD is a multisystem disease (American Thoracic Society, 1999). Specifically, skeletal muscles do not function normally, which adds to activity intolerance and the subsequent decline in quality of life. In addition, reduced muscle mass, impaired oxygen uptake, and nutritional depletion result in further compromise of muscle function and exercise capacity.

Although all members of the interdisciplinary team work toward general muscle reconditioning, the physical therapy interventions are more focused on the rebuilding of specific muscles. Lower extremity exercises usually include walking, treadmill, or stationary cycling exercises. Upper extremity exercise is also an important component of the physical therapy plan because the muscles of the upper extremities support the work of respiration. Upper extremity exercises can include supported arm exercise with ergometry or unsupported arm exercises using free weights or stretching bands. The desired outcome of each individualized plan is improved activity tolerance.

Occupational Therapy

Energy conservation techniques and strategies are important to the person living with COPD, who must consider the energy expenditure of every activity. Chronic fatigue and activity intolerance often cause the person with COPD to become isolated and depressed.

Upper extremity use is limited secondary to the disease process. Some persons with COPD may be able to walk a considerable distance yet be unable to brush their hair or put on a sweater without feelings of dyspnea. The occupational therapist helps the individual deal with such challenges and develop individual strategies and adjustments in daily living that will shortcut certain activities to prevent unnecessary fatigue. A list of some energy-saving suggestions is presented in Box 8-3.

Oxygen Therapy

The decision to supply supplemental oxygen is based partly on the severity of the dyspnea. However, objective measures of hypoxia provide additional support for the use of oxygen and fulfill the criteria that must be met for insurance reimbursement. Supplemental oxygen may be used continuously, at night, or with activity. For many persons with COPD, hypoxemia is the stimulus to breathe, so high levels of oxygen may suppress respiration and must be used with caution.

Table 8-3 Drugs Used in the Treatment of Chronic Obstructive Airway Disease

Drug	Side Effects	Nursing Considerations/Teaching
Bronchodilators *β-Agonists*	Tremors, nervousness, tachycardia and other arrhythmias	Provide rapid relief of acute asthma attack.
Short acting Albuterol (Proventil, Ventolin) Metaproterenol (Alupent) Pirbuterol (Maxair) Terbutaline (Brethine)		Maintenance drug for COPD. Not always the best choice for routine use in emphysema. Most effective method of administration is inhalation.
Long acting Formoterol (Foradil) Salmeterol (Serevent)		Salmeterol and formoterol have delayed onset of action and should not be used for acute attacks. Use of spacer may improve administration and decrease side effects.
Anticholinergics Atropine (Atro-Pen) Ipratropium (Atrovent) Oxitropium (Oxivent) Tiotropium (Spiriva)	Dry mouth, coughing, headache Possible exacerbation of urinary retention and angle-closure glaucoma	Maintenance drugs of choice for COPD. Less effective for asthma. Tiotropium provides once-daily maintenance dose.
Xanthine Derivatives Theophylline (Theo-Dur, Aerolate)	Nausea, vomiting, anxiety, restlessness	Theophylline clearance is altered by many drugs; medical literature should be consulted. Plasma theophylline levels should be monitored. Has moderate benefit in chronic asthma. Smokers require higher dosages. Drug should be taken at same time each day.
Corticosteroids Flunisolide (AeroBid) Beclomethasone (Beclovent) Budesonide (Rhinocort) Cortisone (Cortone) Fluticasone (Flonase) Hydrocortisone (Cortaid) Methylprednisolone (Solu-Medrol) Prednisone (Deltasone) Triamcinolone (Aristocort)	Oral candidiasis Steroid myopathy	Inhaled method used for prophylactic treatment of asthma. Used in COPD only to treat exacerbations. Inhaled method safer than oral administration Use spacer for inhaled administration. Patient should rinse mouth or gargle after each dose. Inhaler tip should be rinsed and air-dried after each dose. Inhaler should be stored in reclosable plastic bag when patient is away from home.
Mast Cell Stabilizers Cromolyn (Crolom) Nedocromil (Tilade)	Throat irritation, unpleasant taste	Used for prophylactic treatment of asthma. For routine use, not for acute attack.

Table 8-3   Drugs Used in the Treatment of Chronic Obstructive Airway Disease—cont'd

Drug	Side Effects	Nursing Considerations/Teaching
Leukotriene Modifiers Montelukast (Singular) Zafirlukast (Accolate) Zileuton (Zyflo)	Headache	Used as oral prophylaxis and chronic treatment for asthma. Not for acute asthma attacks. Evening administration recommended.
Antibiotics		Use empirically for persons with purulent infections. Used for early treatment of upper respiratory tract infections.
Protease Inhibitors α_1-Antitrypsin		Used for persons with deficiency of this specific glycoprotein.
Antismoking Medications Nicotine products: gum, inhaler, nasal spray, patch Antidepressant: Bupropion (Wellbutrin)	Insomnia, headache, tachycardia Agitation, headache, tremors	Encourage participation in smoking cessation program. Smoking should be stopped during second week of therapy.

Box 8-3   Energy Conservation Techniques for the Person with Chronic Obstructive Pulmonary Disease

- Make half the bed while still in it.
- Eliminate unnecessary decorative bedding.
- Organize drawers and shelves to decrease the need for bending or reaching.
- Facilitate morning routine by leaving clothes at bedside.
- Select slip-on shoes and nonrestrictive garments.
- Use a shower chair to facilitate bathing.
- Bathe at the sink on days when fatigued.
- Use a long terry-cloth robe to replace toweling.
- Keep frequently used items, including a cordless telephone, nearby.
- Keep frequently used telephone numbers taped to the telephone.
- Use a small utility cart to move items from one room to another.
- If stairs must be climbed, rest at intervals, especially when carrying items.
- Use pick-up tongs to help in retrieving items.
- Select foods that are easy to prepare.
- Divide food preparation jobs into manageable segments.

Respiratory Therapy

The respiratory therapist makes a valuable contribution to the plan of care for the person with COPD. The use of supplemental oxygen requires specific patient education regarding the types of equipment available (Tables 8-4 and 8-5), the care of delivery devices (Box 8-4), and the safety issues associated with oxygen therapy (Box 8-5). The respiratory therapist is the prime resource for this part of the plan of care.

The respiratory therapist also performs many of the assessment tests that measure the effectiveness of current therapies. Secretion management is a significant challenge in some types of COPD, and instruction by a respiratory therapist in effective cough techniques offers a planned approach to address this quality-of-life issue. Chest physical therapy and postural drainage is an additional method used for secretion management. Pursed-lip breathing and diaphragmatic breathing techniques are other strategies that will maximize air exchange in this population, especially for those whose primary symptom is dyspnea.

Use of home mechanical ventilation is becoming more popular as an alternative to prolonged hospitalization. Development of smaller, more mobile units makes this a viable option. Noninvasive positive pressure ventilation may be another option for certain subgroups of COPD sufferers to avert the need for intubation. Newer noninvasive positive pressure ventilation devices have been developed that reduce

Table 8-4 Oxygen Administration Devices

Device	Advantages	Disadvantages	Considerations
Nasal cannula	Safe, simple to use Comfortable Allows patient to eat, talk, cough easily Can be used for low-flow oxygen	Can be easily dislodged	Usual flow rate for COPD is 2 L/min
Simple mask	Provides oxygen concentration of 35-50% with flow rates of 6-12 L/min Provides adequate humidification	May not be well tolerated Uncomfortable because of need for tight seal Poses risk for skin breakdown Must be removed for eating	Area under mask must be washed and dried frequently
Oxygen-conserving cannula	Has built-in reservoir that increases oxygen concentration and allows lower flow rate More comfortable, less costly than regular cannula	Cannula cannot be cleaned Needs to be replaced frequently	Useful in home situations "Moustache" or "pendant" type may be used
Transtracheal tube	Less visible Has low flow rate so oxygen source lasts longer Causes less nasal irritation	Tracheal stoma care must be learned Invasive Placement procedure increases oxygen therapy cost	Not effective for those with excessive secretions due to risk of clogging

COPD, Chronic obstructive pulmonary disease.

the leakage of air through the face or nasal mask. However, this treatment is not recommended for patients with acute respiratory failure (National Heart, Lung, and Blood Institute, 2000). Because of the complexity of care and the increased burden on the family, there must be consensus among all participants whenever home ventilation is used.

Dietitian

Nutritional status is an important indicator of the severity of symptoms and the level of potential disability associated with COPD. In fact, the summary report from the Global Initiative for Chronic Obstructive Lung Disease identified a reduction in body mass as an independent risk factor for

Table 8-5 Oxygen Delivery Methods

Oxygen Source	Advantages	Disadvantages
Oxygen concentrator	Less costly Extracts oxygen from room air Plugs into existing electrical outlet Resupply unnecessary Small portable systems available	Backup oxygen source needed in case of power failure Takes up space Increases electrical bill Noisy
Compressed gas	Oxygen-conserving device available Small portable tanks available	Large tanks are heavy and only for stationary use
Liquid oxygen	Light in weight Can be used with adapted oxygen-conserving device Takes up less space Can be transferred into smaller portable containers	More expensive than other methods

---

Box 8-4   General Guidelines for Care of Oxygen Equipment

- Wash nasal prongs at least one or two times per week with liquid soap and water; rinse and dry thoroughly.
- Replace nasal prongs as needed and at least every 2-4 weeks.
- Replace nasal prongs after each upper respiratory tract infection.
- Wash humidifier bottles with soap and warm water between each refill.
- Unplug concentrator daily and wash down with damp cloth.
- Clean air filter of concentrator at least twice per week.

---

mortality in COPD (National Heart, Lung, and Blood Institute, 2000). The special skills of the registered dietitian can help to modify this risk factor, beginning with an assessment of body weight, muscle mass, and nutritional habits. An obese condition further increases the workload of the heart and lungs, whereas an underweight condition further accelerates muscle wasting.

The act of breathing creates an increased energy requirement for the person with COPD and the act of eating and digesting increases oxygen demands. Symptoms such as dyspnea and excess sputum production often interfere with adequate nutritional intake, however. The challenge for the registered dietitian and the person with COPD is to select foods that are easy to prepare and easy to digest, and provide calories of high nutritional value.

Adherence to good dietary habits that will allow the patient to achieve or maintain ideal body weight should be emphasized. In some cases, ingestion of carbohydrates in excess of nutritional needs can cause additional stress on the respiratory system, because carbohydrates produce more carbon dioxide than other energy sources. Some suggestions for maximizing nutritional balance while minimizing oxygen consumption are listed in Box 8-6.

Complementary and Alternative Therapies

The use of nontraditional, alternative therapies can be helpful in the management of the anxiety and panic related to dyspnea. Many people are receptive to the breathing and flexibility techniques practiced in yoga and other movement therapies. Although no compelling scientific evidence exists to support the use of complementary therapy in COPD, interventions such as relaxation training, guided imagery, reiki, massage, reflexology, and hypnosis should be explored and considered in an individualized plan of care.

Persons with COPD should feel comfortable speaking of these options with members of their health care team. Physicians and nurse practitioners should be aware of any herbal medicines the patient is considering or using in conjunction with pharmaceuticals. For example, some compounds found in botanical medicines can interfere with theophylline absorption (Brinker, 2001).

Box 8-5   General Safety Tips for Oxygen Use

- Post "No Smoking" signs in the home.
- Stand at least 5 feet away from an open source of flame.
- Secure cylinder tanks in a stand.
- Keep the liquid oxygen vessel upright to prevent skin damage caused by the very cold liquid.
- Notify the fire department that oxygen is being used in the home.
- Avoid use of extension cords.
- Keep the telephone number of the oxygen supplier and the product procedure guidelines available in case of technical problems.
- Do not change the flow rate except at the direction of a physician.
- Avoid the use of alcohol or sedating drugs that may cause respiratory depression.
- Order oxygen in a timely manner to ensure that enough is on hand.
- Use water-based lubricants rather than oil-based products on the nose and lips.
- Place soft gauze under the nasal cannula tubing to prevent skin irritation.
- Time any outings to ensure that enough portable oxygen is available.

Box 8-6   Tips for Ensuring Nutritional Balance

- Eat four to six light meals per day that provide adequate nutrition.
- Avoid foods with little nutritional value.
- Maintain adequate fluid intake to keep secretions thin.
- Avoid caffeine, which may interfere with some medications or cause nervousness.
- Eliminate foods such as gas-forming foods that cause distention, which may limit movement of the diaphragm.
- Prevent constipation, which can cause bloating and dyspnea.
- Collaborate with a clinical dietitian to determine necessary amounts and sources of calories, protein, and other nutrients.
- Choose foods that do not require extensive preparation or extensive chewing.
- Eat in a relaxed environment.
- Postpone activity for 1 hour after eating to allow for the increased oxygen demands of digestion, but do not lie down.

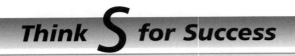

Think S for Success

Symptoms
- Manage secretions with coughing exercises
- Manage dyspnea with medication, energy conservation, and controlled breathing.
- Educate patient regarding signs of exacerbation: increased sputum production, purulence of sputum, increased tenacity of sputum.

Sequelae
- Caution patient to avoid exposure to viral or bacterial infections, especially in winter, as these can often lead to exacerbations and hospitalizations.
- Ensure annual influenza immunization and pneumonia immunization every 5 years.
- Monitor closely for signs of right-sided heart failure.

Safety
- Instruct patient in safe use of oxygen equipment.
- Instruct patient in proper use of inhaled medications.

Support/Services
- Assist with referral and/or funding for pulmonary rehabilitation, oxygen therapy, and local support groups.

Satisfaction
- Determine the degree to which COPD interferes with important aspects of patient's life and develop a plan to maintain quality of life.

CHRONIC ASTHMA

Asthma is a chronic inflammatory condition of the airways that is characterized by airway hyperresponsiveness and airflow limitation, which cause acute exacerbations of symptoms. Some symptoms suggestive of asthma are listed in Box 8-7.

The condition is usually precipitated by exposure to a trigger. Triggers include a wide range of airway irritants as well as respiratory infections, exercise, medications, food products, and emotional stress. Table 8-6 presents many of

---

Box 8-7   Symptoms Suggestive of Asthma

- Recurrent episodes of wheezing
- Persistent cough, particularly at night or early morning
- Interruption of sleep by coughing or breathing difficulty
- Persistent cough precipitated by physical activity or exercise
- Seasonal symptoms
- Symptoms related to particular allergens or irritants
- Upper respiratory tract infections that last longer than 10 days
- Interruption of conversation due to breathlessness

---

the common triggers and suggests interventions to minimize exposure.

Unlike chronic bronchitis and emphysema, asthma is reversible, either spontaneously or with treatment. Chronic inflammation of the airways, however, can cause permanent scarring leading to irreversible obstruction. Causes of asthma are unknown, but host factors exist that increase the risk for developing asthma. Atopy, an inherited family tendency toward allergic reactions, is an example of a genetic predisposition to this condition.

The prevalence of asthma in the United States is estimated to be 14 million cases. Annual direct health care costs for asthma are estimated at $8 billion, an estimate that does not include the indirect costs of lost work and productivity (American Lung Association, 2002a).

Pathophysiology

Exposure to a trigger initiates the complex inflammatory process characteristic of asthma (Figure 8-3). Immunoglobulin E is a plasma protein that attaches to mast cells and plays an important part in the allergic response. The response to an antigen mediated by immunoglobulin E and mast cells stimulates the release of mediator substances such as histamine, leukotrienes, and prostaglandins. Initial clinical responses include airway narrowing, bronchial edema, and an increase in respiratory secretions. Treatment with an inhaled bronchodilator is usually effective in relieving the initial bronchoconstriction.

The initial response is followed about 6 hours later by a second inflammatory response that is often more difficult to treat. A damaging process continues as neutrophils, eosinophils, and other inflammatory cells infiltrate the airway epithelium, which results in more edema, mucus production, and airway hyperresponsiveness. Repeated episodes or exacerbations of acute asthma can lead to permanent airway injury and remodeling, as the subepithelial layers of the airway thicken (National Institutes of Health, 2002). It is remodeling that most likely contributes to residual airway obstruction despite treatment with inhaled steroids (National Institutes of Health, 2002).

Clinical Manifestations

Wheezing, a musical sound produced by the vibration in narrowed airways, is a common symptom of asthma. It is often accompanied by dyspnea, chest tightness, and the production of thick, tenacious sputum. Although audible wheezing can be dramatic, it is not the best indicator of airway blockage. In severe asthma attacks, airway obstruction is so great that air cannot move with enough force to create a wheezing sound. Individual peak flow measurement is the most reliable indicator of airflow movement.

Use of accessory muscles of respiration, significantly reduced breath sounds, and orthopnea are additional manifestations in severe cases and are hallmarks of impending respiratory failure. Early signs of associated hypoxemia

Table 8-6 Common Asthma Triggers and Suggested Interventions to Minimize Exposure

Trigger	Intervention
Airway irritants	Eliminate carpets, rugs, draperies, and other furnishings that collect dust.
Dust, dust mites	Avoid chores that require extensive dusting.
Roaches	Protect mattress with dust-proof cover.
Mold	Put pillows in protective cover.
	Use vacuum with special filter.
	Store foods in sealable containers, clean up clutter where roaches hide.
	Choose pesticide carefully.
Animal dander	Eliminate trigger. If not possible, keep animals out of bedroom. Bathe pet weekly.
Smoke (cigarette or fire)	Eliminate exposure to smoke.
	Enroll in smoking cessation program.
	Avoid wood stoves and fireplaces.
	Be assertive with family and friends.
Aerosol products, cleaning products	Avoid intense odors.
	Avoid use of strong cleaning products.
	Use nonaerosolized products.
Pollen, mold, spores	Consider use of air conditioner that will allow windows to remain closed.
	Consider use of dehumidifier, especially in basements. Change water regularly to prevent mildew.
Medical conditions	Obtain influenza immunization annually.
Upper respiratory tract infections	Treat underlying condition.
Gastroesophageal reflux disease	
Medications	Avoid aspirin and other nonsteroidal drugs that may cause exacerbation.
Aspirin	Read all product inserts.
Food products	Avoid known food triggers.
Nuts	Read all labels carefully.
Chocolate	Make appropriate inquiries when eating away from home.
Eggs	
Shellfish	
Sulfites	
Emotional stress	Use alternative therapies to deal with stressful conditions.
Physical exercise	Use inhaled β-agonist prior to planned physical exercise.

include tachypnea, restlessness, and confusion, and immediate emergency intervention is required.

Diagnosis

Any person with symptoms of episodic dyspnea, wheezing, chest tightness, and cough should be evaluated for asthma. In many people coughing is the only presenting complaint, and symptoms are often mistaken for upper respiratory tract infections. Spirometry, an essential assessment tool in the diagnosis of asthma, measures multiple pulmonary functions, including the forced volume of air that can be expired in 1 second (FEV_1) and the forced vital capacity (FVC). These measures give the best assessment of airflow limitation (Petty, 2001).

Peak flow meters provide an alternative measure of airflow limitation that can be used by the person with airflow obstruction as a daily indicator of changes in the airway. Peak flow readings can serve as an early indicator of worsening airway obstruction and can provide an evaluative

measure of treatment effectiveness. Both the FEV and the peak flow measurements provide objective criteria for classifying the severity of asthma as detailed in Table 8-7.

Interdisciplinary Care

As in the care of other chronic conditions, successful team management depends on the ability of members to overlap roles into another discipline to provide the service needed to achieve desired outcomes. Each encounter of the patient with a health care team member should be regarded as an opportunity to reinforce asthma education.

The interdisciplinary team members involved in the care of the person with asthma include the physician, the nurse, the respiratory therapist, and the dietitian. In many cases, especially those in which a component of chronic bronchitis or emphysema is present, the special skills of the physical therapist and occupational therapist are helpful in promoting upper body muscle strengthening and energy conservation.

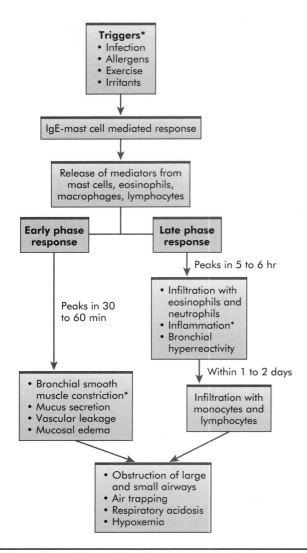

Figure 8-3 Early- and late-phase responses of asthma. Items with an asterisk (*) are primary processes. *IgE,* Immunoglobulin E. (From Lewis SM, Heitkemper MM, Dirksen SR: *Medical-surgical nursing: assessment and management of clinical problems,* ed 6, St Louis, 2004, Mosby.)

Primary Provider (Physician/Nurse Practitioner)

The primary provider usually makes the initial diagnosis of asthma. The severity of the condition, based on spirometric measurements, guides the provider in determining the medication treatment plan. Current guidelines provide additional support for an individualized treatment plan.

In more complex cases, a pulmonologist and pulmonary nurse practitioner are added to the team. Regardless of who is directing the medical care, management of chronic asthma should include ongoing spirometric readings. Adjustments in the medication regimen should be based on these objective measures as well as reports from the person with asthma.

Nurse

Symptom control and the monitoring of medications are primary nursing goals in the care of a person with chronic asthma. Efforts are aimed at helping the person achieve normal activity levels, including exercise. The number of times a rescue medication is required can indicate how well the asthma is controlled. It is important for the nurse to teach the person with asthma to monitor and record this information, because a change in the frequency of symptoms may indicate a need for a change in therapy. Guided self-management gives the person with chronic asthma the ability to manage symptoms and to recognize early changes in airway limitation, so that acute attacks can be prevented. The zone system is one of the frequently used tools for asthma self-management (Figure 8-4).

Respiratory tract infections can often precipitate an acute asthma episode. As with other chronic respiratory conditions, the nurse should advise against unnecessary exposure to those with respiratory tract infections, especially during the winter months. An annual influenza immunization and a pneumonia immunization every 5 years are also recommended. Physical exercise is another potential trigger for an asthma attack; pretreatment with an inhaled β-agonist can prevent an attack.

Elements of a teaching plan for a person with asthma include but are not limited to the following:

- Explanation of the condition
- Roles of asthma medications
- Inhaler and spacer technique
- Method for monitoring the amount of medication left in the canister (Figure 8-5)
- Use of peak flow meters
- Review of potential triggers and measures to avoid exposure
- A written action plan that has received medical approval
- Interventions to decrease asthma attacks
- Indications of the need for immediate medical care (Box 8-8)

Development of a therapeutic relationship with the person with asthma is another important nursing role. Adequate time must be allowed for the person with asthma to discuss fears and concerns regarding the condition. The plan of care must be adjusted as much as possible to fit the person's lifestyle and cultural beliefs.

Drug Therapy

Pharmacologic interventions for asthma are aimed at maintenance and symptomatic control in an attempt to suppress airway inflammation and avoid subsequent irreversible damage. The antiinflammatory effect of inhaled corticosteroids provides the most effective treatment for asthma (National Institutes of Health, 2002). Regular use of inhaled corticosteroids limits the exacerbation of symptoms and prevents the chronic overuse of rescue bronchodilators. To achieve desired outcomes with the least possible medica-

Table 8-7 Classification of Severity of Asthma by Clinical Features Before Treatment

Step	Classification	Symptoms
Step 1	Intermittent	Symptoms less than once a week Brief exacerbations Nocturnal symptoms no more than twice a month FEV_1 or PEF ≥80% of predicted PEF or FEV_1 variability <20%
Step 2	Mild persistent	Symptoms more than once a week but less than once a day Exacerbations that may affect activity and sleep Nocturnal symptoms more than twice a month FEV_1 or PEF ≥80% of predicted PEF or FEV_1 variability 20-30%
Step 3	Moderate persistent	Symptoms daily Exacerbations may affect activity and sleep Nocturnal symptoms more than once a week Daily use of inhaled short-acting β_2-agonist FEV_1 or PEF 60-80% of predicted PEF or FEV_1 variability >30%
Step 4	Severe persistent	Symptoms daily Frequent exacerbations Frequent nocturnal asthma symptoms Limitation of physical activities FEV_1 or PEF ≤60% of predicted PEF or FEV_1 variability >30%

Adapted from National Institutes of Health: Global strategy for asthma management and prevention. NIH Pub No 02-3659, Bethesda, Md, 2002, The Institutes.

FEV_1, Forced expiratory volume in 1 sec; *PEV,* pulmonary extravascular volume.

tion, a stepwise approach is recommended in which treatment is stepped up when symptoms are not well suppressed and stepped down when symptoms are under control. Spirometry is critical in guiding individual therapy. New technology is being tested that may offer more assistance in the monitoring and management of asthma, including a portable pulmonary testing device with a built-in modem that can send spirometric data to a physician within minutes via fax or the Internet.

The addition of long-acting β-agonists, mast cell stabilizers, and leukotriene modifiers completes the initial drug treatment plan. Multiple administrations of rapid-acting β-agonists and early treatment with systemic corticosteroids are recommended for management of exacerbations. Table 8-3 lists many of the drugs used for the treatment of chronic asthma.

Respiratory Therapist

The respiratory therapist makes a valuable contribution to the success of asthma management. Education on the correct use and care of inhalation medication equipment is critical to ensure that the medication is administered as prescribed (Box 8-9). The respiratory therapist is also involved in the spirometric testing and other pulmonary

function testing necessary for the diagnosis and management of asthma.

Dietitian

Because food allergies are often a factor in asthma, the registered dietitian is an important member of the interdisciplinary team. Special dietary restrictions may have to be implemented for certain persons, and the dietitian can assist in development of an individualized diet plan that provides adequate nutrition.

Complementary and Alternative Therapies

The efficacy of alternative methods of treatment for asthma has not been established. Some methods, such as the use of herbal comfrey products and the use of ionizers, can be potentially dangerous. However, the therapeutic effects of other complementary interventions such as reiki, yoga, massage, and breathing exercises used as an adjunct to standard asthma medications should be explored by the health care team. The pursuit of additional research on this subject is one of the recommendations of the recently published global initiative for asthma (National Institutes of Health, 2002). Individual preferences and cultural variations should be explored and considered in the development of a plan of care.

NAME	PERSONAL BEST PEAK FLOW	DATE

Green—GO
- Breathing is good
- No coughing, wheezing, chest tightness, or shortness of breath
- No problems talking or walking

> **Peak Flow Number:**
> _____ to _____
> (80%–100% of Best)

PLAN A: Continue regular medicines. Use **preventer** medicines all the time.
Bronchodilator Inhaler (**Quick Reliever**): _____
Steroid Inhaler (**Preventer/Controller**): _____
Other Inhaler/Nebs: _____
Additional Instructions:
- At the first sign of a cold, you may double the dose of the steroid inhaler *until the cold subsides.* Then resume usual dose.
- Monitor your peak flows daily. When exposed to triggers or when you have a cold, monitor your peak flows at least 2 times/day or more.
- Use quick reliever medicine 10 minutes before exercise if you have exercise-induced asthma.

Yellow—CAUTION
- Mild to moderate symptoms
- Coughing, wheezing, chest tightness, or shortness of breath
- No problems talking or walking but may feel anxious
- Unable to sleep because of asthma symptoms

> **Peak Flow Number:**
> _____ to _____
> (50%–80% of Best)

PLAN B: Continue Plan A and add quick reliever medicine.
❶ Immediately take 2-4 puffs or quick reliever _____ or by nebulizer treatment.
❷ Wait 20 minutes.
  - If peak flow returns to Green Zone or asthma symptoms subside, follow Green Zone plan.
  - If peak flow remains in the Yellow Zone and/or symptoms do not improve, repeat ❶ and ❷. You may repeat this a third time if still not improved.
❸ If still in the Yellow Zone after _____ hours and/or symptoms do not improve, _____ or begin prednisone (Deltasone) or Medrol on the following schedule: _____

WARNING: If at any time you progress to the Red Zone, proceed to Plan C.

Red—STOP—Danger
Severe Symptoms
- Continuous coughing, wheezing, chest tightness, or shortness of breath
- Able to speak in short sentences only but feel very anxious
- Lips and nails still pink color

> **Peak Flow Number:**
> _____ to _____
> (0%–50% of Best)

Very Severe Symptoms →
- Severe chest tightness, struggling to breathe, hunching over, chest pulled or sucked in with each breath
- Having trouble walking and talking
- Must stop activity you are doing and cannot start again
- Lips and nails may be blue

PLAN C: This is the **DANGER ZONE!** Act immediately.
❶ Immediately take 2-6 puffs of quick reliever or nebulizer treatment _____
❷ If you are still in the Red Zone in 10-20 minutes, begin prednisone (Deltasone) or Medrol in the following schedule, if instructed to do so: _____
❸ Repeat ❶ and ❷ for a total of three times in 1 hour if asthma symptoms persist.
❹ Call your health care provider if you do not have instructions to begin prednisone (Deltasone) or Medrol or if your symptoms do not improve.

STOP

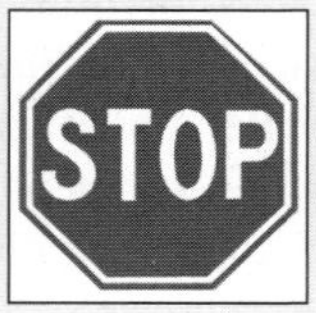

PLAN D: Call 911 immediately to be taken to the emergency room.
- Take 6 puffs of beta bronchodilator (quick reliever) inhaler every 5-10 minutes OR take a continuous nebulizer treatment while waiting or in route.
- If you have prednisone, take 40 mg immediately.

Any time you are having an asthma episode, **STAY CALM.** Breathe out slowly through pursed lips. If possible, identify the specific trigger for this episode and try to avoid it. If you need help, call your health care provider.

_____   _____
Provider Signature   *Patient Signature*

Source: Lovelace Health Systems Adult Asthma Program, Albuquerque, N.M.

Figure 8-4 Asthma management plan. (From Lovelace Health Systems Adult Asthma Program, Albuquerque, N Mex.)

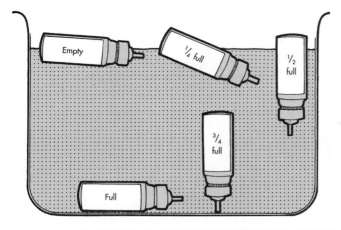

Figure 8-5 A simple method of estimating the amount remaining in an inhalant canister by placing in a container of water. (From Perry AG, Potter PA: *Clinical nursing skills and techniques,* ed 5, St Louis, 2004, Mosby.)

Think **S** for Success

Symptoms
- Suggest journaling to provide a record of symptoms and interventions.

Sequelae
- Prevent respiratory decompensation.

Safety
- Instruct patient in proper use of inhaled medications.
- Teach patient and family to recognize signs and symptoms indicating need for emergency medical treatment.

Support/Services
- Provide referrals to group education or individual counseling.

Satisfaction
- Assess how condition is affecting quality of life and incorporate coping strategies into plan of care.

Box 8-8   Indications for Immediate Medical Care

- Dyspnea at rest
- Inability to speak in sentences
- Loud or absent wheeze
- Pulse rate >120 beats per minute
- Peak expiratory flow rate ≤50% of predicted personal best even after treatment

---

Box 8-9   Procedure for Effective Use of Inhalers

1. Administer bronchodilator before an inhaled steroid.
2. Take a sip of water to moisten throat.
3. Remove cap.
4. Shake canister for 5-10 seconds.
5. Tilt head back slightly.
6. Exhale normally.
7. Administer medication at beginning of next inhalation using a spacer.
8. Slowly inhale (over 3-5 seconds) through the mouth.
9. Hold the breath for up to 10 seconds.
10. Exhale through pursed lips.
11. Wait a minimum of 30-60 seconds before inhaling a second puff.
12. Rinse and gargle with warm water. Do not swallow. This is especially important with inhaled steroids to prevent oropharyngeal thrush.

FAMILY AND CAREGIVER ISSUES

Lifestyle changes associated with COPD and chronic asthma often produce a strain on personal relationships, and the nurse should encourage expression of these concerns and address them in the plan of care. Family members need to provide emotional and physical support to the person with COPD, but this support should be balanced with promotion of independence.

Families must be knowledgeable about the medication regimen and administration techniques, because their support may be needed in an emergency. Family members and caregivers also should know how to recognize the signs and symptoms of deterioration and how to activate emergency treatment.

END-OF-LIFE ISSUES AND PALLIATIVE CARE

Acute respiratory failure is a complication of chronic airway obstruction despite the best care and interventions. In many cases, intubation and mechanical ventilation are the only medical treatment options left. It is important that the person with COPD discuss his or her desired management of this complication with family members and the health care team. One of the greatest fears of a person with end-stage COPD is experiencing the acute breathlessness associated with respiratory failure. Assuring that end-of-life comfort measures will be taken is an important part of the discussion. Adopting a proactive approach will help to avoid any unwanted end-of-life interventions, which often place an additional burden on family members during a medical crisis.

All members of the health care team must be aware of the patient's end-of-life choices and support this difficult decision. It is sometimes up to the team members to initiate this conversation and to educate the person and the family about the durable power of attorney for health care or other legal documents that will support the patient's decision. Care must be taken to respect ethnic and cultural variations, however, because the plan must be consistent with the person's values and beliefs. The end-of-life decisions that are made must be communicated to all members of the health care team.

CASE STUDY

Patient Data
Mrs. C. is a 68-year-old retired secretary. She is a widow with three adult children. Mrs. C. lives independently in a three-level town home. She is active in several bridge clubs and plays four or five times a week.

After smoking a pack of cigarettes a day for 40 years, Mrs. C. stopped smoking 3 years ago. At present, she suffers from a chronic cough and frequent upper respiratory tract infections, especially during the winter months, at which time she seeks medical care from her family physician. Hospitalization was required on two separate occasions in the past year. Mrs. C. refused discharge planning recommendations for rehabilitation services on both occasions. Since her last hospitalization, Mrs. C. has been reluctant to seek medical help because "they will try to put me back in the hospital."

Recently she has been suffering from increasing shortness of breath, which is usually relieved by her "breathing medicine." She admits to spending almost all of her time on the main level of her town home, sleeping in the recliner. In addition, Mrs. C. admits to canceling many of her bridge activities and isolating herself more over the past 6 months. Mrs. C.'s oldest daughter, who lives locally, has become increasingly concerned about her mother's decreased activity and dyspnea and suggests a visit to her doctor. After the office visit, the family physician recommends the addition of a pulmonary specialist to the health care team. Mrs. C. agrees and the physician makes a referral to a pulmonologist for evaluation and treatment.

Diagnostic Findings
- Laboratory test results
  - White blood count: 9700/mm^3
  - Hemoglobin level: 17.2 g/dl
  - Hematocrit: 53.5%
- Pulmonary function test results
  - FEV$_1$: 1.32 (45% of predicted value)
  - FVC: 3.11 (88% of predicted value)
  - FEV$_1$/FVC: 43%
- Arterial blood gas values on room air
  - pH: 7.37
  - Pco$_2$: 44 mm Hg
  - Po$_2$: 64 mm Hg
- Chest radiograph: Suggestive of slight cardiomegaly

Thinking It Through
- What nursing diagnoses are most appropriate for Mrs. C. at this time?
- How would the nursing interventions for Mrs. C. differ from those for a person with asthma?
- What quality-of-life issues are surfacing at this time and how can the health care team intervene?
- Why do you think Mrs. C. is afraid of hospitalization?
- What family issues are likely to arise?

Case Conference
Based on the objective data and examination of Mrs. C., the pulmonologist makes a diagnosis of COPD with components of both chronic bronchitis and emphysema. The pulmonary nurse case manager plans a case conference for Mrs. C. and her daughter to meet with the health care team, including the pulmonologist, the respiratory therapist, the physical therapist, the occupational therapist, and the clinical dietitian.

Mrs. C. openly states that she "does not need all this attention" and that her daughter is just "worrying too much." This prompts her daughter to describe her concerns about her mother's increased shortness of breath and inactivity, her difficulty managing secretions, and the coughing and shortness-of-breath episodes that interfere with almost every meal. The clinical dietitian takes this opportunity to instruct Mrs. C. about strategies and menu choices that can maximize nutritional intake and minimize the metabolic cost of eating. Mrs. C. admits to making poor choices, eating many things that are easy to prepare but have little nutritional value. Mrs. C.'s daughter offers to prepare single-sized meal servings that can be frozen for individual use. The clinical dietitian agrees to give Mrs. C.'s daughter some menu selections that would provide the nutrients to maintain muscle strength.

The mention of muscle strength leads to a discussion by the physical therapist on the importance of maintaining upper body strength, and the therapist demonstrates simple exercises that Mrs. C. can do independently. Mrs. C. says that she is hesitant to do any exercises because she becomes so short of breath with activity. The occupational therapist acknowledges this concern but tells Mrs. C. that there are daily living strategies that can be implemented to conserve energy so that oxygen is available for desired activities, such as her bridge clubs.

The pulmonologist notes that he will be adding some supplemental oxygen to the treatment plan, which will help with Mrs. C.'s oxygen deficit. Mrs. C's daughter seems concerned about this intervention, reminding the team of Mrs. C.'s limited resources. The respiratory therapist reassures her that Mrs. C. meets the criteria for reimbursement for this treatment. The respiratory therapist also offers to provide the necessary instruction regarding oxygen therapy as well as instruction on the proper use of inhalers, because new maintenance bronchodilators have been prescribed. The pulmonary nurse case manager promises to explore financial entitlements that will link Mrs. C. to community programs such as pulmonary rehabilitation.

Recognizing Mrs. C.'s fatigue, the pulmonary nurse case manager closes the conference with a promise to follow up by telephone with Mrs. C. and her daughter on the following day, once they have had time to absorb all of the new information. Continued telephone contact by the pulmonary nurse case manager will be important to the success of the plan.

Internet and Other Resources

American Lung Association (ALA): *http://www.lungusa.org;* telephone 800-LUNG-USA

American Thoracic Society (ATS): *http://www.thoracic.org;* telephone 212-315-8600

National Center for Chronic Disease Prevention and Health Promotion (NCCDPHP): *http://www.cdc.gov/nccdphp;* telephone 770-488-5401

National Heart, Lung, and Blood Institute (NHLBI): *http://www.nhlbi.nih.gov;* telephone 301-592-8573

National Institute of Allergy and Infectious Disease (NIAID): *http://www.niaid.nih.gov;* telephone 301-496-5717

National Institutes of Health (NIH): *http://www.nih.gov;* telephone 301-496-4000

National Jewish Medical and Research Center: *http://www.njc.org;* telephone 800-222-5864

REFERENCES

Agency for Healthcare Research and Quality: Management of acute exacerbations of chronic obstructive pulmonary disease, Evidence Report/Technology Assessment No 19, AHRQ Pub No 00-E020, Rockville, Md, 2000, The Agency, retrieved from *http://www.ahcpr.gov/clinic/epcsums/copdsum.htm* on Oct 28, 2002.

American Lung Association: Trends in asthma: morbidity and mortality, New York, 2002a, American Lung Association, Epidemiology and Statistics Unit.

American Lung Association: Trends in chronic bronchitis and emphysema: morbidity and mortality, New York, 2002b, American Lung Association, Epidemiology and Statistics Unit.

American Thoracic Society: Standards for the diagnosis and care of patients with chronic obstructive pulmonary disease, *Am J Respir Crit Care Med* 152:S77-S120, 1995.

American Thoracic Society: Dyspnea: mechanisms, assessment, and management: a consensus statement, *Am J Respir Crit Care Med* 159:321-40, 1998.

American Thoracic Society: Skeletal muscle dysfunction in chronic obstructive pulmonary disease, *Am J Respir Crit Care Med* 159:S1-S40, 1999.

Brinker F: Interactions of pharmaceutical and botanical medicines. In Faass N, editor: *Integrating complementary medicine into health systems,* Gaithersburg, Md, 2001, Aspen Publishers.

Minino A, Smith B: Deaths: preliminary data for 2000, *Natl Vital Stat Rep* 49(12):1-40, 2001.

National Heart, Lung, and Blood Institute: Global initiative for chronic obstructive lung disease, 2000, retrieved from *http://www.goldcopd.com* on Nov 8, 2002.

National Institutes of Health: Global strategy for asthma management and prevention, NIH Pub No. 02-3659, Bethesda, Md, 2002, The Institutes.

Pauwels R et al: Global strategy for the diagnosis , management, and prevention of chronic obstructive pulmonary disease, *Am J Respir Crit Care Med* 163:1256-76, 2001.

Petty T: The national lung health education program and managed care, *Dis Manag Health Outcomes* 9(5):249-54, 2001.

CHAPTER 9

Tuberculosis

Helen Mautner, MS, RN

OBJECTIVES

After reading this chapter, you should be able to do the following:

- Describe the pathophysiology of tuberculosis (TB)
- Describe the clinical manifestations of TB
- Describe the functional health patterns affected by TB
- Describe the role of each member of the interdisciplinary team involved in the care of patients with TB
- Describe the progression and management of TB
- Describe the indications for use, side effects, and nursing considerations related to the drugs commonly used to treat TB

OVERVIEW OF TUBERCULOSIS

Tuberculosis (TB) is an infectious disease caused by the *Mycobacterium tuberculosis* bacillus (MTB). After a period of decline, the incidence of TB worldwide has increased, and it is a major international disease that kills more than 2 million people each year (World Health Organization, 2000). Efforts in the United States to control the spread of the disease have been effective, and the American Lung Association (2001) cited a 39% decrease in the number of reported TB cases between 1992 and 2000. Many states reported case rates that were less than or equal to the target of 3.5 per 100,000 population set by *Healthy People 2000* (1991). Even with this downward trend, estimated direct and indirect costs of the disease exceed $1 billion (American Lung Association, 2001). Although TB rates are decreasing, the presence of human immunodeficiency virus (HIV) infection, the outbreak of resistant organisms, the immigration of persons from areas with high rates of the disease, and the uncertain numbers of persons with latent, untreated TB make the disease a significant threat in the United States.

The American Thoracic Society (ATS), in collaboration with the Centers for Disease Control and Prevention (CDC) (2000), developed standards for the diagnosis and classification of TB. Classification categories for persons exposed to or infected with MTB are presented in Box 9-1. The classification system offers an operational framework to guide the health care team in the assessment of the infection and the active disease. Although the TB bacillus can infect or reside in other organs, the discussion in this chapter is limited to pulmonary TB.

ASSESSMENT

Many factors must be considered in the assessment of a person with TB. Because of the complex issues associated with the condition, it is essential to complete a detailed social assessment that covers living and working conditions, potential exposures and contacts, and current access to health care. Other risk factors that must be considered are listed in Box 9-2. Confidentiality must be respected during the assessment, because some persons may feel that there is a stigma attached to an infectious disease diagnosis.

Successful treatment of active and latent TB requires strict adherence to the medication treatment regimen and, for this reason, an initial encounter should include an assessment of the individual's understanding of infectious disease and the person's ability to follow treatment guidelines. These assessment findings provide the baseline for the teaching component of the individualized plan of care. Other areas of focus in the assessment of a person with TB are shown in the functional health pattern framework presented in Box 9-3. Some assessment tools that are related to functional health and are specific for respiratory function are listed in Box 9-4.

Ethnic Variations

The rate of new cases of TB is significantly higher among minorities than among non-Hispanic whites. In fact, in the year 2000, minorities accounted for more than 75% of new TB cases (American Lung Association, 2001). These minority groups included Pacific Asians, non-Hispanic blacks, Native Americans, and Native Alaskans.

In addition, TB case rates are more than 7% higher among persons born outside the United States. Some of the countries with higher case rates include Mexico, the Philippines, Vietnam, India, China, Haiti, and Korea. These patterns play an important role in the initial assessment of a suspected TB case, the evaluation of a positive TB skin test result, and the therapy choices for latent TB infection.

Box 9-1   Classification of Tuberculosis

0   No tuberculosis exposure, not infected
1   Tuberculosis exposure, no evidence of infection
2   Latent tuberculosis infection, no disease
3   Tuberculosis, clinically active
4   Tuberculosis, not clinically active
5   Tuberculosis suspected, diagnosis pending

Adapted from American Thoracic Society, Centers for Disease Control and Prevention: Diagnostic standards and classification of tuberculosis in adults and children, *Am J Respir Crit Care Med* 161(4):1376-95, 2000.

Box 9-2   Risk Factors for Tuberculosis

■ Exposure to *Mycobacterium tuberculosis* bacillus
■ Immunocompromised state (cancer, acquired immunodeficiency syndrome, chronic steroid use)
■ Institutional living (long-term care facilities, mental health facilities, prisons)
■ Substance abuse (intravenous drug use, alcohol abuse)
■ Crowded, substandard living conditions
■ Low socioeconomic status (homelessness, impoverishment)
■ Immigration from country with high incidence of tuberculosis
■ Chronic medical condition
■ Health care occupation in high-risk area

Box 9-3   Functional Health Pattern Assessment for Tuberculosis

HEALTH PERCEPTION/HEALTH MANAGEMENT
■ What are the patient's symptoms?
■ Does the patient have any self-care deficits?
■ Is there a history of other chronic conditions, especially conditions that result in immunosuppression?
■ What precautions have been taken to avoid transmission?
■ What is the patient's exposure and contact history?
■ What is the patient's health adherence history?
■ Does the patient smoke or have a history of smoking?
■ Does the patient use alcohol or recreational drugs?

NUTRITION/METABOLISM
■ Has there been recent unexplained weight loss?
■ How is the patient's appetite?
■ Does the patient have anorexia related to sputum production?
■ What are the patient's food preferences?
■ What is the patient's typical dietary intake (daily)?
■ Does the patient take supplements?
■ Does the patient have food restrictions related to other conditions?
■ What foods affect sputum production?
■ What is the patient's food budget?

ELIMINATION
■ Have any changes occurred in bowel or bladder habits?

ACTIVITY/EXERCISE
■ Does the patient complain of fatigue?
■ Does the patient experience dyspnea at rest or with activity?
■ Is there a productive or nonproductive cough?
■ Is temperature elevated in the afternoon?

SLEEP/REST
■ What are the patient's sleeping patterns?
■ How effective is the patient's sleep?
■ Does the patient experience night sweats? Do they affect the sleep pattern?

COGNITION/PERCEPTION
■ Are visual deficits present?
■ When was the last eye examination?
■ Has the patient experienced any changes in color discrimination?
■ Is there pain? If so, where is it located and how does the patient describe it?

SELF-PERCEPTION/SELF-CONCEPT
■ How does the patient describe himself or herself?
■ How has the condition affected the patient's self-concept?

ROLES/RELATIONSHIPS
■ What is the patient's role in the home and family?
■ How have the patient's role functions changed because of the condition
■ What are the patient's current family, social, and work relationships?

SEXUALITY/REPRODUCTION
■ Is the patient sexually active?
■ Does the patient take birth control pills?

COPING/STRESS TOLERANCE
■ What stressors are associated with the patient's condition?
■ What are the patient's coping strategies?
■ What support systems are available to the patient?

VALUES/BELIEFS
■ What are the patient's health beliefs and spiritual and cultural values?
■ What constitutes good quality of life for the patient?
■ What is important to the patient?
■ What are the patient's beliefs related to this condition?
■ To what extent do the patient's cultural/spiritual beliefs influence decision making related to this condition?

Box 9-4   Instruments for Assessment of Tuberculosis

- Baseline Dyspnea Index
- Borg Dyspnea Scale
- Chronic Respiratory Disease Questionnaire
- Functional Performance Inventory
- Respiratory Illness Quality of Life Questionnaire
- Short Form 12 (SF-12) Health Survey
- Short Form 36 (SF-36) Health Survey
- Sickness Impact Profile

PATHOPHYSIOLOGY

Initial infection with MTB results from inhalation of droplet nuclei containing the organism, which are sneezed or coughed into the air by a person whose sputum contains the tubercle bacillus (Figure 9-1). Invasion of the lung tissue by the bacillus initiates the infectious process and the inflammatory response. MTB infection is unique in that no early immune response to the organism occurs. Instead, there is a delayed cell-mediated response that can take 2 to 12 weeks to develop, during which time the organism can invade the lymphatic system and spread to other sites. Other favorable locations for organism growth include the brain, kidneys, and bones, where oxygen content is high and favors growth of the organism (ATS and CDC, 2000).

The immune response of the host, the virulence of the organism, and the extent of exposure are important factors influencing the progression of the infection. The small percentage of individuals who develop clinically active TB (classification 3) will do so within weeks or months of exposure.

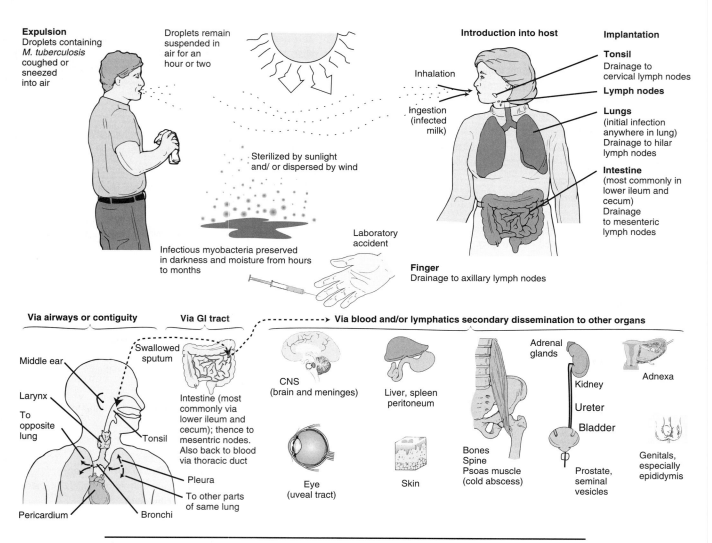

Figure 9-1   Dissemination of tuberculosis. *CNS*, Central nervous system. (From McKenry LM, Salerno E: *Mosby's pharmacology in nursing*, ed 21, St Louis, 2003, Mosby.)

Latent Tuberculosis Infection

A great number of infected persons never become clinically ill but are infectious during the initial phase. They carry the infection but may remain disease free indefinitely (classification 2). In other cases, the disease reactivates at a later time, possibly after some disturbance in immune function. Reactivation TB is often more difficult to treat because of the decreased defense mechanisms of the host. Targeted testing and treatment regimens for latent tuberculosis infection (LTBI) have been developed by the ATS and the CDC (2000) in an effort to prevent the conversion from latent to active TB. A comparison of active disease and LTBI is presented in Table 9-1.

Human Immunodeficiency Virus Coinfection

The progressive immunosuppression associated with HIV infection increases susceptibility to lung infections, including TB. Moreover, the response of the person with HIV to an additional infection with MTB has the potential to accelerate the HIV infection.

Data related to coinfection with MTB and HIV are limited, partly because of the incomplete reports of HIV status of TB patients. It is clear, however, that the elimination of TB in the United States must include efforts to identify and aggressively treat HIV-infected persons with latent TB.

Miliary Tuberculosis

In some severe cases, the tubercle bacilli infiltrate the bloodstream, so that the organisms are carried throughout the body. The organisms continue to grow and cause disease in multiple sites. A common presenting symptom is a fever, which often precedes other symptoms. This systemic disease is called *miliary TB* because of the appearance of the chest radiograph, which shows fine, evenly distributed nodules in the lung that resemble millet seeds.

CLINICAL MANIFESTATIONS

The clinical manifestations of TB are variable, and the development of clinically active disease depends on many risk fac-

Table 9-1 Comparison of Active and Latent Tuberculosis (TB)

Active TB Disease	Latent TB Infection
Symptoms of active disease	No clinical symptoms
Infectious	Not infectious
Positive skin test	Usually positive skin test
Usually positive findings on chest radiograph	Usually normal chest radiograph
Positive sputum smear or culture	Sputum culture negative
Reportable TB case	Not a reportable case

tors (Box 9-2). The very young and the very old are at highest risk for clinical illness. Presenting symptoms reflect the ongoing infectious and inflammatory process and include fever, night sweats, unexplained weight loss, anorexia, and fatigue. A productive or nonproductive cough lasting more than 2 weeks is a common presenting symptom.

In advanced disease, hemoptysis, pleuritic pain, dyspnea, and respiratory failure may be present. Often, symptoms may be difficult to quantify, especially in the presence of other chronic conditions. TB infection may also cause hematologic responses, including leukocytosis or leukopenia, anemia, and eosinophilia.

DIAGNOSIS

Suspicion of TB should be high when a patient comes to the physician with pulmonary symptoms and a marked unexplained weight loss. Cell-mediated response following exposure to MTB can be measured by the Mantoux (tuberculin) test, in which a small amount of purified protein derivative (PPD) is injected on the inside of the forearm. A positive PPD test indicates MTB exposure but not necessarily active disease. The appearance of an induration of 15 mm is considered a positive result for most of the population. However, smaller indurations of 5 or 10 mm may be considered positive for high-risk or immunosuppressed groups.

A smear of a specimen, usually sputum, that tests positive for acid-fast bacilli provides preliminary evidence of TB. However, a specimen culture that is positive for MTB provides a definitive diagnosis of pulmonary TB. Obtaining culture and drug sensitivity results can often take several weeks, but treatment should not be delayed if other positive indications of TB are found. The drug regimen is adjusted once the sensitivity results are available. A final diagnostic tool is the chest radiograph, which may show upper lobe lesions.

INTERDISCIPLINARY CARE

Support for the person with TB challenges the skills of the interdisciplinary team, which usually includes a physician, a nurse, a pharmacist, a medical social worker, a registered dietitian, and sometimes physical and occupational therapists. All team members must understand the infectious process of TB and must know local and state reporting procedures. All states require that cases of active TB be reported to the CDC.

The complexity of the drug regimen, the cost of the medications, and lack of knowledge of the disease are only some of the factors that interfere with the effectiveness of treatment and that require the attention of the team. An important first step in a successful treatment plan is to engage the person with TB as an active participant in the program. This requires the development of a collaborative, individualized plan that will work, especially with regard to adherence to the medication regimen. Team members may want to consider use of a written contract that details the plan and the time line for completion. Directly observed therapy (DOT), an intervention that is essential for effective treatment, is discussed in detail in a later section. Other team strategies include providing regular reinforcements for positive behaviors. Many health departments have developed innovative incentives for adherence to the plan, for example, distribution of food coupons and public transportation passes.

Drug Therapy
Active Tuberculosis

A joint position statement of the ATS and the CDC (1994) have provided the foundation for the treatment of active and latent TB for the past several years, and subsequent statements have built on those recommendations. The treatment regimen must be individualized and must be based on clinical history and local reports of drug resistance. Recent guidelines from the CDC (2000) for the pharmacologic treatment of active TB recommend a multiple-drug regimen of four anti-TB drugs, at least until after the susceptibility results are available. A four-drug regimen is always recommended for those living in areas where TB caused by multidrug-resistant MTB organisms (MDR MTB) is prevalent. Table 9-2 delineates the recommended first-line drug regimen for the treatment of TB disease. The initial treatment continues for at least 2 months, and completion of the entire regimen may take 9 months to 2 years.

MTB is slow growing and requires treatment over a long period. Failure of patients to complete the full drug regimen is one of the major reasons for the development of resistant forms of the organism and the subsequent failure to eradicate TB in the United States. The CDC (2000) defines multidrug resistance of MTB as resistance to at least isoniazid (isonicotinic acid hydrazide, or INH) and rifampin. The number of cases caused by MDR organisms has decreased from 1993 to the present, but infection with MDR MTB is still of great concern, especially among foreign-born persons residing in the United States. TB caused by MDR MTB is much more challenging to treat, because second-line drugs (Table 9-3) are not as effective as first-line drugs, and the more aggressive drug therapy causes additional side effects and presents new challenges in compliance with the medication regimen.

Some combination drugs such as Rifater, which combines isoniazid, rifampin, and pyrazinamide, offer the benefit of decreasing the number of pills and eliminating the danger that MDR MTB will arise because the person takes only one of the prescribed drugs. Other options include rifabutin (for MTB-HIV coinfection) and rifapentine, which may be taken only once a week in the final 4 months of treatment instead of twice a week as for some other drugs.

The vaccine against TB is still controversial and is currently being used only in developing countries where there is a high incidence of TB.

Latent Tuberculosis Infection

Treatment with isoniazid for 6 to 12 months has been the standard therapy for LTBI for many years, and a 9-month course of isoniazid is still the preferred treatment for LTBI.

Table 9-2   First-Line Drug Therapy Used in Tuberculosis

Drug	Mechanism of Action	Side Effects	Considerations
Isoniazid (INH, Lanizid, Nydrazid)	Tuberculocidal	Hepatitis Peripheral neuropathy	Liver function test results should be monitored. Pyridoxine supplements should be considered to correct peripheral neuropathy. Inhibits metabolism of phenytoin (Dilantin).
Rifampin (RIF) (other rifamycins include rifabutin [Mycobutin], rifapentine [Priftin])	Tuberculocidal	Hepatitis Nausea and vomiting Fever, flulike symptoms	Liver function test results should be monitored. May color secretions red or orange. Can discolor contact lenses; glasses should be worn during treatment period. May suppress effect of birth control pills; different form of birth control should be selected. May decrease effectiveness of β-blockers, oral anticoagulants, digoxin, quinidine, and corticosteroids.
Pyrazinamide (PZA)	Tuberculocidal	Hyperuricemia Hepatitis	Uric acid levels should be monitored. Liver function test results should be monitored.
Ethambutol [Myambutol]	Tuberculostatic	Optic neuritis	Regular vision screening should be provided.
Streptomycin	Tuberculocidal	Eighth cranial nerve damage Nephrotoxicity	Periodic hearing examinations should be provided. Renal function should be monitored.

Table 9-3 Second-Line Drug Therapy Used in Tuberculosis

Drug	Mechanism of Action	Side Effects	Considerations

Aminoglycosides
  Kanamycin (Kantrex)
  Amikacin (Amikin)
  Capreomycin (Capastat
  Sulfate)
	Antiinfectives	Auditory toxicity
		Renal toxicity
			Assess hearing function prior to and during therapy.
			Monitor renal function during treatment.

Fluoroquinolones
  Ciprofloxacin (Cipro)
  Ofloxacin (Floxin)
  Levofloxacin (Levaquin)
	Antiinfectives	Gastrointestinal upset
		Dizziness
		Headache
		Restlessness
			Antacids and other products containing iron or zinc will decrease absorption and should not be taken within 2 hours.

However, recent trials have shown that a 2-month course of rifampin and pyrazinamide administered weekly with DOT is just as effective as a 12-month course of isoniazid (ATS and CDC, 2000). This offers an effective alternative to those persons who cannot tolerate isoniazid. The shorter duration of therapy is a distinct advantage of this treatment option.

Tuberculosis with Human Immunodeficiency Virus Coinfection

The challenge of pharmacologic treatment of TB with HIV coinfection is to provide a plan that will effectively treat the TB without interfering with the treatment of HIV. Concurrent treatment with anti-TB and antiretroviral drugs is not uncommon but requires special consideration. Antiretroviral drugs have been found to interact with the rifamycins and rifampin, in particular. For this reason, current guidelines recommend the use of rifabutin for those persons with TB who are also being treated with antiretroviral therapy (CDC, 1998). All drug therapy for persons with TB and HIV coinfection must be administered by DOT.

Primary Provider (Physician/Nurse Practitioner)

Medical management of persons with MTB infection or disease presents a challenge to the physician because other conditions such as immunocompromise, nutritional depletion, substance abuse, and other chronic disorders are often present. These other conditions may contribute to an altered response to the prescribed drug regimen, necessitating reduced or increased dosages of TB drugs. Recognizing the complexity of TB medical management, the Infectious Disease Society of America has issued practice guidelines offering recommendations to the physician for the treatment of TB disease and LTBI (Horsburgh, Feldman, and Ridzon, 2000).

The provider, in collaboration with other members of the health care team, is required by law to submit to the local health department a specific treatment plan within 1 week of a diagnosis of suspected TB. The plan the provider develops should include the drug regimen prescribed, the proposed methods of ensuring compliance, and the plan for monitoring the drug side effects.

Follow-up visits to the physician should include an evaluation of adherence to the treatment plan. In some cases, urine tests are performed to detect the presence of drug metabolites. The physician also evaluates response to treatment by monitoring the conversion of sputum cultures from positive to negative.

Nurse

The nurse, in the role of case manager, carries the responsibility for detecting active TB cases and monitoring treatment as well as identifying cases and testing for confirmation of LTBI. This is accomplished through collaboration with other members of the health care team who contribute to the development and implementation of a plan of care for management of the disease. In many areas, the number of trained specialists available for TB management is limited, and many interventions must be delegated to other members of the team. To lead the interdisciplinary team, the TB nurse case manager must possess extensive knowledge of the disease process, the clinical manifestations of the disease, and the challenges of effective drug therapy.

As stated earlier, failure of the patient to complete the full course of drug therapy is one of the major causes of reactivation TB and TB due to MDR MTB. For this reason, DOT is an efficient intervention that can help ensure proper completion of the drug regimen. Direct observation of drug ingestion should be incorporated into the plan of care and can be accomplished at a health clinic or by arranged visits to the person's home or workplace. It is the recommended method of medication administration, especially for regimens in which drugs are taken two or three times a week (CDC, 2000). Although this intervention is costly and labor intensive, the prevention of treatment failures and the reduction in the development of resistant MTB strains far outweigh the costs of DOT. Another benefit of DOT is the acceleration in the rate of recovery, which may allow a reduction in the dose or frequency of medications. It also allows the nurse to regularly monitor the effectiveness of the therapy, make early interventions to treat side effects, and provide early identification of disease reactivation. All of the information obtained through daily contact is important to the physician to determine if the drug treatment is effective.

If DOT is not possible, the nurse case manager should work closely with the patient and family to develop alternative ways for the patient to remember to take the medicine as prescribed. Some suggestions include taking the medicine at the same time every day, asking a family member or friend for a daily reminder, using a calendar to mark off each day, and using a weekly pill dispenser.

Depending on the prescribed drug regimen, the nurse case manager or other team member must carefully monitor for signs of drug side effects. Special attention to detect signs of hepatotoxicity is indicated, because many of the drugs are metabolized by the liver.

Elements of a teaching plan for the person with TB include the following:

- Explanation of disease process
- Medication regimen
- Reportable side effects: nausea, anorexia, vomiting, persistent dark urine, jaundice, unexplained fever, abdominal pain
- Importance of adherence to treatment regimen
- DOT procedure
- Need for hand washing and pulmonary hygiene
- Contact investigation
- Need for personal protective equipment during the infectious period
- Need for adequate rest and nutrition

Dietitian

Persons with TB are often nutritionally depleted secondary to the disease process, the side effects of medication, anorexia, and fatigue related to coughing, chest discomfort, or sputum production. Weight loss is often already present, and steps must be taken to avoid additional weight loss. Consumption of frequent small meals should be suggested, as well as consumption of nutritional supplements to meet caloric needs. The registered dietitian, working collaboratively with the person with TB and the interdisciplinary team, develops a reasonable and viable plan for adequate nutrition. If resources are limited, the medical social worker and the dietitian can provide information on valuable community resources for access to nutritious meals. The dietitian may also suggest recipes to increase caloric intake even with limited resources.

Use of supplemental vitamins, particularly vitamin B_6 to avoid neuropathy secondary to isoniazid therapy, should be considered. Also, foods containing tyramine and histamine, such as tuna, aged cheese, and red wine, should be avoided when taking isoniazid because they may cause headache, diaphoresis, chills, and itching. Because of the risk of hepatic dysfunction, avoidance of alcohol is imperative when anti-TB medication is being taken. Inability to adhere to this restriction is often a contributing factor in treatment failure. In some cases, the patient must be referred to an alcohol treatment program.

Medical Social Worker

The social component of this disease is considerable, partly due to the high incidence among the homeless and those living in crowded conditions. Many patients are malnourished and already have compromised health. The contributions of the medical social worker and his or her large network of community resources make the social worker an integral part of the health care team caring for the person with TB.

Social workers often help in the contact investigation process, identifying those who have been exposed to TB and should be tested or treated. Most health departments have extensive assessment tools that guide this process. It is in this role that the social worker frequently identifies situations that must be considered in the treatment plan, for example, immigration status.

Physical and Occupational Therapists

The increased metabolic needs of those with TB result in fatigue and complaints of lack of energy to maintain daily activities. Physical therapy interventions aimed at strengthening both the lower and the upper extremities help to improve endurance and relieve the feeling of dyspnea. The

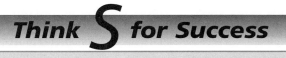

SYMPTOMS
- Manage dyspnea, fatigue, anorexia, paced breathing.

SEQUELAE
- Prevent further infection. Report all cases.
- Follow procedure for contact investigation.
- Evaluate home and social setting to identify contacts.
- Ensure that patient keeps scheduled appointments with primary care provider.
- Provide regular physical examinations with special attention to liver, kidney, and vision function.

SAFETY
- Stress infection-control precautions.
- Educate regarding hygiene for sneezing, coughing, and disposal of tissues.
- Educate regarding hand washing to prevent secondary infection.

SUPPORT/SERVICES
- Consider finances, referrals, and community resources.

SATISFACTION
- Provide special support during period of isolation.
- Assist with return to normal activities as soon as possible.
- Offer support and interventions for medication side effects.

person with TB can also be coached by the occupational therapist in energy conservation techniques that promote self-care and independence. Some of the suggestions already mentioned in the previous chapter may also be helpful in relieving symptoms. A list of energy-conserving activities is presented in Box 8-3.

FAMILY AND CAREGIVER ISSUES

A diagnosis of TB affects the entire family unit, whether the diagnosis is TB exposure, infection, or active disease. Prevention of further transmission of infection requires the attention of all family members and caregivers. The required identification of all contacts often creates stressful situations for family members and their social network. All specialists on the health care team, especially the medical social worker, must be aware of this stressor and assist the family in coping with it.

Adherence to the treatment plan is essential, and family support can make this difficult period less stressful. Family members can help the person with TB keep to the medication schedule by offering daily reminders. Families and caregivers also need to be able to recognize the signs of disease reactivation and drug toxicity. The health care team must identify key family members and include them in the ongoing education regarding the disease and the treatment plan.

ETHICAL CONSIDERATIONS

Cases of active TB must be reported to the local health department, whose case workers will assist in the effective management of the disease. They will also initiate an epidemiologic evaluation of contacts and sources. Failure to be forthcoming with information places society at risk for disease proliferation. For example, a recent immigrant to the United States feels fortunate to have a position as a mother's helper for a wealthy family in the suburbs. The family likes her very much and provides generous compensation for her work. She has recently been diagnosed with active TB. Because she is concerned about her position and is fearful of alarming her employers, she considers withholding their names as contacts. What would be the consequences of this decision? What strategies can a case manager use to ensure that a complete contact list is compiled? The case manager must impress upon each person with TB the importance of identifying, testing, and treating all contacts to protect the well-being of the person's family and friends. Knowledge of the consequences can help the person make an informed decision.

CASE STUDY

Patient Data

Mr. M. is a 24-year-old resident alien who immigrated to the United States with his family 2 years ago from a Central American country. He is employed by a construction company for which he works 40 hours a week. He lives in a two-bedroom apartment with his parents. He has two brothers who live in the next town. His father has been out of work for the past 6 months due to a back injury, and the adult children have been providing support for the family. All members of the family speak some English but prefer to speak Spanish.

Mr. M. came to the community clinic 3 days ago with complaints of a chronic, sometimes productive cough over the past 2 months. He also mentioned unusual fatigue that he attributed to frequent overtime hours. When questioned about his weight, he admitted to an unexplained loss of 10 lb in the last several weeks. A PPD skin test was administered and a sputum specimen was obtained. Additional diagnostic tests were completed at that time and consent was obtained for HIV testing.

Mr. M. was referred to a nurse case manager, who was able to meet with him that day. The nurse case manager advised him at that time to stay at home for the next few days and avoid close contact with others. He was also cautioned to be especially careful to cover his mouth and nose with tissues whenever he coughed or sneezed, disposing of tissues in a paper bag. He was instructed to return to the clinic in 72 hours to have his PPD test read and to discuss the results of his sputum smear analysis.

Diagnostic Findings
■ PPD test: 15 mm induration
■ Sputum smear: positive for acid-fast bacilli
■ Sputum culture and sensitivity: results pending
■ HIV test: negative

■ White blood count: 8000/mm^3
■ Chest radiograph: right upper lobe infiltrate
■ Liver function tests: normal values

Thinking It Through
■ What nursing diagnoses are most appropriate for Mr. M. at this time?
■ What are some of the legal and administrative issues that the nurse case manager must consider regarding this case?
■ How will the results of Mr. M.'s test affect his family?
■ What are some of the possible fears that Mr. M. may be experiencing and how can the health care team intervene?

Case Conference
When Mr. M. returns to the clinic, he is told that his test results are suspicious for TB and that the clinic physician has prescribed a four-drug regimen with DOT that is to begin immediately. The TB nurse case manager schedules a team visit to Mr. M.'s home for the following day.

Mr. M.'s parents are at home and Mr. M. requests that they be present for the meeting. Initial assessment reveals a very close, hard-working family. The TB nurse case manager introduces herself and the medical social worker to the family, explaining that the social worker speaks Spanish and will help interpret any information they do not understand. In an effort to provide the most appropriate information, the TB nurse case manager asks some questions to evaluate the family members' level of understanding of TB. All seem to comprehend the infectious nature of the condition, and Mr. M. acknowledges that this is of great concern to him. The nurse assures Mr. M. that a person is usually noninfectious within weeks of starting therapy and that his adherence to the medication regimen will help protect his family and friends. DOT will ensure completion of the treatment. Mr. M.'s mother asks what DOT is, and the nurse case

CASE STUDY—cont'd

manager explains that a member of the team will observe administration of each dose of medication and that arrangements will be made with Mr. M. regarding the details of DOT.

She also begins the education regarding the TB medications that have been prescribed and their potential side effects, and presents a TB patient teaching guide in Spanish for Mr. M. to use as a reference. The nurse case manager continues her assessment by asking Mr. M. about any medical conditions that might interfere with the effectiveness of the medications, which he denies. He also denies any use of alcohol, at which point his father reminds him that he stopped drinking several weeks ago when he began feeling ill. Both the nurse and the social worker stress the importance of avoiding alcohol while taking TB medication because of the added risk of liver damage.

The social worker continues the discussion of the infectious process by explaining the need to identify, test, and possibly treat all close contacts. Mr. M. says that his only close contacts are his parents and his brothers. Because he works so many hours, he has little time for a social life. His mother reminds him of the girl he dated the previous weekend. The social worker makes note of this and communicates the sense of urgency with regard to contact identification and notification. Mr. M.'s father asks how this will affect the family. He is told that all family members will need to have a TB skin test and, because of their recent close contact with Mr. M., will probably need to be treated with an antitubercular drug even if their initial PPD reading is negative.

While the social worker continues to work with Mr. M. on a list of contacts, the nurse answers Mr. M.'s mother's question about the need for special linens and dishes. She reassures Mr. M.'s mother that MTB is an airborne organism and cannot be transmitted through objects like dishes or clothing. However, living in close contact with an infected person does create considerable

risk. She suggests that Mr. M. sleep in a separate room or at least by an open window. His mother also expresses concern over Mr. M.'s lack of appetite and apparent weight loss. The nurse assures her that the dietitian who is a member of the team will meet with them to discuss strategies for providing high-calorie meals in light of Mr. M's anorexia, and she makes a note to provide this referral. Recognizing Mr. M.'s fatigue and shortness of breath, she suggests that he may also benefit from a consultation with an occupational therapist to help with energy conservation techniques and makes a note to initiate that referral as well.

Mr. M. asks about going back to work and the social worker tells him that he must have three consecutive negative sputum smears before he is allowed to return. Recognizing that Mr. M. is a major financial contributor to the family, she offers to investigate public services for which the family may be eligible.

The nurse case manager acknowledges that a considerable amount of information has been shared and that Mr. M. and his family will have many questions. She makes arrangements with Mr. M. for DOT in his home at least until he is able to return to work and leaves instructions for the family to be tested as soon as possible. The social worker reminds Mr. M. to contact her if he remembers any other close contacts. The initial conference has ended, but DOT will provide daily encounters with Mr. M. and the opportunity to identify problems and potential medication side effects.

Returning to the clinic, the nurse and the medical social worker meet to discuss this case and their approach to the plan of care.
- What new information was obtained as a result of the meeting with Mr. M. and his parents?
- What strengths did Mr. M. demonstrate? What strengths did his parents demonstrate?
- What barriers to learning were identified?
- List two collaborative problems that were identified as a result of the meeting.

Internet and Other Resources

American Lung Association (ALA): *http://www.lungusa.org;* telephone 800-LUNG-USA

American Thoracic Society (ATS): *http://www.thoracic.org;* telephone 212-315-8600

Centers for Disease Control and Prevention (CDC): *http://www.cdc.gov;* telephone 800-311-3435

National Center for Chronic Disease Prevention and Health Promotion (NCCDPHP): *http://www.cdc.gov/nccdphp;* telephone 770-488-5401

National Heart, Lung, and Blood Institute (NHLBI): *http://www.nhlbi.nih.gov;* telephone 301-592-8573

National Institute of Allergy and Infectious Disease (NIAID): *http://www.niaid.nih.gov;* telephone 301-496-5717

National Institutes of Health (NIH): *http://www.nih.gov;* telephone 301-496-4000

National Jewish Medical and Research Center: *http://www.njc.org;* telephone 800-222-5864

New Jersey Medical School National Tuberculosis Center: *http://www.umdnj.edu/ntbcweb;* telephone 800-482-3627

REFERENCES

American Lung Association: Trends in tuberculosis morbidity and mortality, Best Practices and Program Services, New York, December 2001, The Association.

American Thoracic Society: Targeted tuberculin testing and treatment of latent tuberculosis infection, *Am J Respir Crit Care Med* 161(4): S221-S247, 2000.

American Thoracic Society, Centers for Disease Control and Prevention: Treatment of tuberculosis and tuberculosis infection in adults and children, *Am J Respir Crit Care Med* 149:1359-74, 1994.

American Thoracic Society, Centers for Disease Control and Prevention: Diagnostic standards and classification of tuberculosis in adults and children, *Am J Respir Crit Care Med* 161(4):1376-95, 2000.

Centers for Disease Control and Prevention: Prevention and treatment of tuberculosis among patients infected with human immunodeficiency virus: principles of therapy and revised recommendations, *MMWR Morb Mortal Wkly Rep* 47(RR 20):1-51, 1998.

Centers for Disease Control and Prevention: *Core curriculum on tuberculosis: what the clinician should know,* ed 4, Washington, DC, 2000, US Department of Health and Human Services.

Horsburgh R, Feldman S, Ridzon R: Practice guidelines for the treatment of tuberculosis, *Clin Infect Dis* 31:633-9, 2000.

US Department of Health and Human Services, Healthy people 2000: national health promotion and disease prevention objectives, Washington, DC, 1991, US Government Printing Office.

World Health Organization: Tuberculosis, Fact Sheet No 104, Geneva, 2000, The Organization.

CHAPTER 10

Disorders of the Blood

Leslie Jean Neal, PhD, RN, FNP-C

OBJECTIVES

After reading this chapter, you should be able to do the following:

■ Describe the pathophysiology of anemia, thalassemia, polycythemia, sickle cell anemia, hemophilia, and hemochromatosis

■ Describe the clinical manifestations of anemia, thalassemia, polycythemia, sickle cell anemia, hemophilia, and hemochromatosis

■ Describe the functional health patterns affected by anemia, thalassemia, polycythemia, sickle cell anemia, hemophilia, and hemochromatosis

■ Describe the role of each member of the interdisciplinary team involved in the care of patients with anemia, thalassemia, polycythemia, sickle cell anemia, hemophilia, and hemochromatosis

■ Describe the indications for use, side effects, and nursing considerations related to drugs commonly used to treat anemia, thalassemia, polycythemia, sickle cell anemia, hemophilia, and hemochromatosis

OVERVIEW OF BLOOD DISORDERS

Blood cells (red blood cells or RBCs, white blood cells, and platelets) are produced in the bone marrow (see Figure 11-1). Through a process called hematopoiesis, blood cells develop from stem cells. Erythropoietin is a hormone that stimulates the production of RBCs or erythrocytes. Although blood cells are normally produced in the bone marrow, extramedullary production occurs in diseases such as pernicious anemia, sickle cell disease, thalassemias, and certain leukemias. Normal RBCs develop from immature cells called erythroblasts or normoblasts. When the cell is abnormal, it is called a megaloblast. Erythropoietin stimulates certain selected cells to become erythroblasts. Hemoglobin is the vital component of mature RBCs. Hemoglobin allows the RBCs to carry oxygen to the tissues. It is comprised of globins and heme (iron). Proteins, of which intrinsic factor is one, are necessary for erythropoietin production and absorption of vitamin B_{12}. Erythropoiesis cannot take place without the presence of vitamin B_{12}, folate, and some other nutrients (McCance, 2002).

Approximately 3.5 million Americans have anemia (Life Extension Foundation, 2003). There are many different types of anemia, and it is often an indicator of underlying disease (Montoya, Wink, and Sole, 2002). The most common forms of anemia are those resulting from hemolysis, blood loss, or a deficiency in an essential dietary nutrient.

Hemochromatosis is a hereditary blood disorder affecting iron storage. An estimated 1 in 250 to 300 whites has the disorder; 1 person in 10 is a carrier of the mutated gene that causes the disease. Hemochromatosis is considered to be the most common inherited single-gene disorder among people of northern European decent (Brandhagen, Fairbanks, and Baldus, 2002).

Polycythemia is characterized by an excess of RBCs and is categorized into two types: relative and absolute. Relative polycythemia occurs because of changes in the body associated with dehydration and is easily remedied by rehydration. Absolute polycythemia affects people who live at high altitudes or who have certain chronic diseases (Mansen and McCance, 2002).

Sickle cell anemia is a congenital form of anemia that affects approximately 70,000 Americans (Platt et al, 2002) and millions worldwide, especially people who live in Sub-Saharan Africa, Spanish-speaking countries, Saudi Arabia, India, and Mediterranean countries.

Hemophilia occurs in three major forms: hemophilia A, hemophilia B, and von Willebrand's disease. Estimated incidence is 1 in every 5000 males born alive for hemophilia A and 1 in 30,000 for hemophilia B. In contrast, von Willebrand's disease affects approximately 1 in 1000 persons (Mannucci and Tuddenham, 2001) or 2.6 million people in the United States (Pavlovich-Danis, 2001).

Box 10-1 indicates the ethnic groups disproportionately affected by selected blood disorders.

ASSESSMENT

Assessment of persons with chronic blood disorders differs according to the specific disease. However, the functional health patterns affected by chronic blood diseases are largely the same for all of these disorders. Box 10-2 provides a framework for assessing changes in functional health patterns.

ANEMIA

Pathophysiology

Anemia is characterized by a lack of RBCs and hemoglobin (Blackwell and Hendrix, 2001). In adults, anemia is defined as a hematocrit of less than 41% or a hemoglobin level of less than 13.5 g/dl for males and a hematocrit of 37% or a hemoglobin level of less than 12 g/dl in females. Personal and family history suggest congenital anemia. Causes of anemia include loss of blood, excessive RBC destruction, and deficient RBC production (Blackwell and Hendrix, 2001).

Several forms of anemia occur. They can be categorized according to underlying cause, basic effect (reduced production or excessive loss of RBCs), hemoglobin content, and cell size. The term *cytic* refers to cell size and the term *chromic* refers to the hemoglobin content of the RBC. Hence, hypochromic microcytic anemia is characterized by small RBCs with abnormal hemoglobin content. Normochromic macrocytic anemia is characterized by abnormally large RBCs with normal hemoglobin content. Normochromic normocytic anemia is characterized by a reduction in normal-sized RBCs with normal hemoglobin content (Mansen and

McCance, 2002). The categories of microcytic anemia include iron deficiency anemia, anemia of chronic disease, and thalassemia. Macrocytic anemias include the megaloblastic anemias (characterized by deficiency of vitamin B_{12} or folate) and nonmegaloblastic anemia (Linker, 2001). Because screening for anemia is not usually performed unless the patient is symptomatic, pregnant, or 50 years of age or older, anemia is frequently discovered incidentally (Montoya, Wink, and Sole, 2002). Figure 10-1 shows the progression and manifestations of anemia.

Microcytic Anemia

Iron deficiency anemia is very common worldwide, affecting approximately half a billion people. Twenty percent of females of child-bearing age and 2% of adult males in the United States are iron deficient (Blackwell and Hendrix, 2001). The most common causes of iron deficiency anemia are iron sequestration; hemoglobinuria; dietary deficiency (of iron and zinc); blood loss associated with menstruation, blood donation, or gastrointestinal illness; decreased absorption of iron in the blood; and unmet increased requirements for iron, such as during pregnancy and lactation (Linker, 2001). Medications such as tetracyclines, antacids, proton pump inhibitors, and histamine receptor blockers can reduce the absorption of iron, as can the tannins in tea (Holcomb, 2001).

Anemia is associated with several chronic diseases such as chronic infection or inflammation, renal disease, thyroiditis, rheumatoid arthritis, liver disease, and cancer. Acquired anemia of chronic disease may be normochromic normocytic or normochromic microcytic.

In renal failure, the source of the anemia is a reduction of erythropoietin, the hormone that stimulates production of RBCs. In other chronic diseases, the cause of anemia is typically a reduction in RBC survival and inadequate compensation by the bone marrow to produce more RBCs. Sequestration of iron is usually the cause of inadequate RBC production (Linker, 2001). Chemotherapy for cancer contributes to bone marrow suppression, which is responsible for the fatigue experienced by cancer patients (Boyer, 2000).

Thalassemias are hereditary forms of microcytic anemia and are characterized by the presence of fewer α or β globin chains than are necessary for hemoglobin synthesis. The form α-thalassemia results from a reduction in α globin chains, and β-thalassemia results from a reduction in or elimination of β globin chains. The disorder α-thalassemia major may result in poor oxygen delivery to the tissues. In β-thalassemia major, a reduction in β chains causes α chains to be unstable and RBC membranes to become damaged. Hemolysis occurs within the bone marrow and in the peripheral blood, and ineffective erythropoiesis results. This leads ultimately to pathologic fractures, bone deformities, and osteopenia (Linker, 2001). Both α-thalassemia minor and β-thalassemia minor (or α-thalassemia trait) are likely to be asymptomatic, and either disease may be discovered

Box 10-2   Functional Health Pattern Assessment for Chronic Blood Disorders

HEALTH PERCEPTION/HEALTH MANAGEMENT

■ Is there a family history of blood disorders?

■ What is the patient's perception of his or her overall health?

■ What medications, including over-the-counter drugs, does the patient take?

■ What alternative therapies does the patient use?

NUTRITION/METABOLISM

■ Is there a deficiency of iron, folate, and/or vitamin B_{12}?

■ Is iron intake excessive or has the patient undergone multiple transfusions?

■ What is the patient's current weight?

■ What is the condition of the skin and mucous membranes?

■ Does the patient have a history of peptic ulcer or gastrointestinal bleeding?

ELIMINATION

■ Have any changes occurred in bowel or bladder habits?

■ Has the patient experienced rectal or urinary bleeding?

ACTIVITY/EXERCISE

■ Does the patient experience fatigue or malaise?

■ Is the patient unable to perform instrumental and other activities of daily living without rest periods?

SLEEP/REST

■ How many hours of uninterrupted sleep does the patient get at night?

■ Does the patient take naps or rest periods?

■ What sleep aids does the patient use?

COGNITION/PERCEPTION

■ What is the nature and location of the pain?

■ What factors aggravate and alleviate the pain?

SELF-PERCEPTION/SELF-CONCEPT

■ How does the patient describe himself or herself?

■ How has the condition affected the patient's self-esteem?

■ How has the condition changed the patient's body image?

ROLES/RELATIONSHIPS

■ How has the condition affected the patient's ability to carry out vocational and occupational functions?

■ What changes have occurred in the patient's roles among and relationships with family and friends?

■ How satisfied is the patient with his or her current roles and relationships?

■ What are the effects of the patient's condition on others?

SEXUALITY/REPRODUCTION

■ Is the patient sexually active?

■ Has the patient experienced changes in menstrual bleeding?

■ Has the condition affected fertility?

■ Is the patient satisfied with current sexual patterns?

■ Has the patient undergone genetic counseling?

■ Is the patient pregnant?

COPING/STRESS TOLERANCE

■ What are the patient's coping strategies?

■ What support systems are available?

■ How able is the patient to manage the condition?

■ Is the patient concerned about a genetic predisposition to disease or the possibility of passing on a disease?

■ Does the patient show concern about life expectancy or anxiety in anticipation of feeling sick?

VALUES/BELIEFS

■ What constitutes quality of life for the patient?

■ What is important to the patient?

■ What are the patient's spiritual beliefs, health beliefs, cultural practices, and feelings about locus of control?

■ To what extent do the patient's cultural/spiritual beliefs influence decision making related to this condition?

---

serendipitously or when a family member has been found to have a blood disease. Both α-thalassemia major and β-thalassemia major may produce organomegaly, bone changes, and possibly mental retardation. Severe, untreated thalassemia major has high mortality and morbidity rates, but with treatment some patients do fairly well.

Macrocytic Anemia

The term *macrocytic* refers to large cells, and the RBCs in macrocytic anemias are abnormally large. The cells develop abnormally because of defects in DNA, protein synthesis, or RNA (Blackwell and Hendrix, 2001). Folic acid deficiency is one cause of macrocytic anemia. Citrus fruit and green leafy vegetables are especially high in folic acid, although most fruits and vegetables are rich in folic acid. The daily requirement for adults is 50 to 100 μg, and total body stor-

age of folate is estimated to be 5000 μg. Inadequate dietary intake of folic acid is the most common cause of this type of anemia (Linker, 2001).

Anemia caused by vitamin B_{12} (cobalamin) deficiency is the other most common form of macrocytic anemia. Although various elements contribute to this type of anemia, a lack of intrinsic factor, which allows the stomach to absorb vitamin B_{12} from food, is the most common cause. The deficiency of intrinsic factor is thought to be due to autoimmune dysfunction, and the resulting anemia is known as pernicious anemia. Ileal resection, tapeworm infestation, and gastrectomy affect the absorption of vitamin B_{12} and therefore can precipitate the onset of pernicious anemia.

Lack of sufficient vitamin B_{12} in the diet in the presence of adequate intrinsic factor can also cause vitamin B_{12} deficiency anemia (which is different from pernicious anemia).

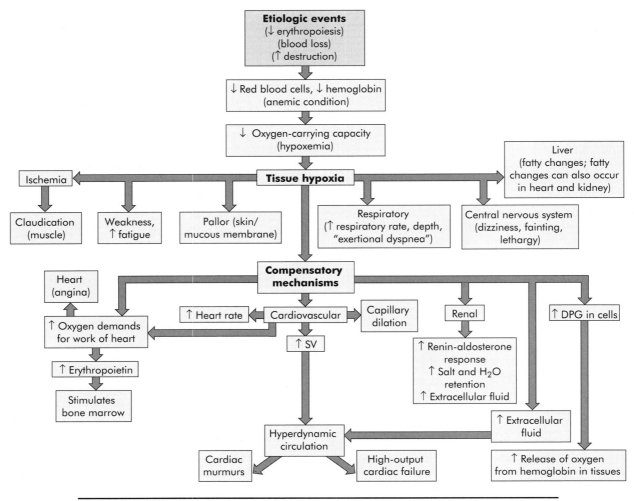

Figure 10-1 Progression and manifestations of anemia. ↑, Increased; ↓, decreased; *DPG,* diphosphatidylglycerol; *SV,* stroke volume. (From McCance KL, Huether SE: *Pathophysiology: the biologic basis for disease in adults and children,* ed 4, St Louis, 2002, Mosby, p 848.)

Crohn's disease (an inflammatory bowel disorder), chemotherapy, use of proton pump inhibitors, nutritional deficiency, adherence to a strict vegetarian diet, and a familial trait of selective malabsorption can also cause the disease. The body can store as much as 5 years' worth of vitamin B_{12}, so the deficiency frequently does not become apparent until it has continued for several years (Holcomb, 2001).

Clinical Manifestations

The person with anemia may be asymptomatic. However, chronic anemia is characterized by symptoms that include easy fatigability, palpitations, tachycardia, and tachypnea on exertion. Skin and mucosal changes may occur, depending on the severity of the anemia (Linker, 2001). The patient may feel dizzy, listless, anorexic, light-headed, or unable to concentrate, or have headaches and dyspnea. The elderly may demonstrate confusion with a tendency to feel faint or to fall (Huffstutler, 2000). Persons with iron deficiency ane-

mia may have pica, or an unnatural craving for specific non–iron rich foods, such as clay or ice.

The person with anemia may appear pale, with pale conjunctiva, rigid nails that are concave or spoon shaped, tongue atrophy, cheilosis, or glossitis. Anemia that is related to hypothyroidism may manifest with skin dryness and hoarseness (Huffstutler, 2000). Clinical manifestations of anemia are present especially during exertion but may be seen at rest depending on the severity of illness and the patient's overall health status.

Persons with α-thalassemia may have pallor and splenomegaly but tend to have a normal life expectancy. Persons with homozygous β-thalassemia develop severe anemia in the first year of life. Consequently, there is growth retardation with frequent jaundice, hepatosplenomegaly, bony deformities of the face, and pathologic fractures. Treatment with transfusions often modifies the clinical course. However, multiple transfusions can lead to an overload of iron that results in heart, liver, and endocrine abnormalities. In severe cases, heart failure can cause death in the second or third decade of life. Some persons have a milder form of this disease that does not require transfusion except during periods of high stress. They tend to survive into adulthood but can also experience complications of iron overload from transfusions. Heterozygous β-thalassemia causes the development of mild microcytic anemia without clinically significant symptomatology (Linker, 2001).

Vitamin B_{12} deficiency is significant because it leads to neurologic changes, particularly in the peripheral nerves, that result in paresthesias and numbness. If the condition is untreated, ataxia and mental status changes may appear, and Romberg and Babinski signs may be present. Folic acid deficiency may lead to mild confusion, loss of intellectual ability, apathy, and depression, but does not usually cause other neurologic changes (Montoya, Wink, and Sole, 2002). Box 10-3 lists signs and symptoms indicative of anemia.

Diagnosis

Several tests are used to diagnose the anemias. Table 10-1 lists these tests and results that indicate anemia.

Treatment and Care

Iron deficiency anemia is treated with dietary changes, iron replacement therapy, and elimination of the cause of the

---

Box 10-3 Signs and Symptoms of Anemia

- Weakness
- Fatigue
- Tinnitus
- Exertional dyspnea
- Mood disturbances
- Loss of libido
- Sleep disturbances
- Dizziness
- Headaches
- Altered mental status
- Venous hum
- Glossitis (vitamin B_{12}, folate, and iron deficiency anemias)
- Pallor
- Orthostatic hypotension
- Tachycardia
- Peripheral edema
- Retinal hemorrhages
- Jaundice (hemolytic anemia)
- Neurologic findings (vitamin B_{12} deficiency anemia)
- Splenomegaly
- Systolic ejection murmur
- Tachypnea

From Blackwell S, Hendrix PC: Common anemias, *Clin Rev* 11(3):53-62, 2001.

---

anemia. Ferrous sulfate in a dosage of 325 mg 3 times a day is standard. The count of reticulocytes (an immature type of RBC whose increase is indicative of increased RBC production) is checked in 1 week, the hemoglobin level (an indicator of RBC normalization) is measured in 1 month, and the ferritin level (indicative of adequacy of iron stores) is checked in 3 months after initiation of treatment. Iron replacement continues for 3 to 6 months following normalization of laboratory values. Normalization should occur within 2 months of initiation of treatment. If it does not, then parenteral iron treatments may be ordered and the cause of the iron deficiency anemia evaluated further. The patient may experience side effects of iron replacement therapy, including abdominal pain, nausea, diarrhea, and constipation, most of which can be minimized by taking the iron with food. Some foods may reduce iron absorption. However, vitamin C or foods such as citrus fruits may improve iron absorption (Holcomb, 2001).

For many patients with anemia of chronic disease, no specific treatment is required. If the person is symptomatic, then RBC transfusions may be given. RBC transfusion may be recommended when the hematocrit is below 25%. However, in cases of concomitant cardiovascular disease and advanced age, transfusion may be considered before the hematocrit falls that low (Diamond and Julian, 2001). Anemia related to cancer, inflammation (e.g., rheumatoid arthritis), or renal failure may require treatment with purified recombinant erythropoietin. Patients with anemia related to renal failure need adequate renal dialysis to optimize the effect of erythropoietin replacement. Epoetin alfa is the commercial preparation and is given by subcutaneous injection at least 3 times per week in doses of 10,000 U. Epoetin alfa is very expensive, and its use should be considered only when the patients is dependent on transfusions or when quality of life is significantly affected by the anemia (Linker, 2001). Adverse effects of epoetin alfa therapy include diarrhea and edema (Boyer, 2000).

Intravenous iron dextran has been given successfully to patients with iron deficiency anemia and normal renal function who cannot be treated with oral iron because of gastrointestinal symptoms, severe anemia, nonadherence to the medication regimen, or an inadequate hematologic response to oral iron supplementation (Barton et al, 2000).

Thalassemia minor (silent carrier status) does not require treatment unless the person develops symptoms. Thalassemia major is treated with blood transfusions, iron chelation therapy, and sometimes splenectomy. Neither type of thalassemia is curable (Kline, 2002).

Folic acid deficiency is initially treated by oral intake of 1 mg of folic acid daily for 4 months. If the anemia does not respond to therapy or a corrected dietary intake of folic acid, then 0.4 mg of folate supplementation should be continued daily. Replacement doses in excess of 1 mg/day may mask vitamin B_{12} deficiency. Rapid reticulocytosis and increased hematocrit and hemoglobin levels are indicators of improved

Table 10-1 Laboratory Tests Used to Diagnose Anemias

Test	Type of Anemia	Result Indicative of Anemia
Serum ferritin level	Iron deficiency anemia	<30 µg/dl (low)
	Anemia of chronic disease	Normal or increased
	Vitamin B_{12} deficiency anemia	High
	Folic acid deficiency anemia	High
Serum total iron-binding capacity	Iron deficiency anemia	Increased
	Anemia of chronic disease	Low
	Vitamin B_{12} deficiency anemia	Normal
	Folic acid deficiency anemia	Normal
Transferrin saturation	Iron deficiency anemia	<15%
	Anemia of chronic disease	Extremely low
Serum iron level	Iron deficiency anemia	Low
	Anemia of chronic disease	Low
	Vitamin B_{12} deficiency anemia	High
	Folic acid deficiency anemia	High
Serum folic acid level	Folic acid deficiency anemia	Low
	Anemia of chronic disease	Probably low
	Iron deficiency anemia	Normal
	Vitamin B_{12} deficiency anemia	Normal or decreased
Hematocrit	Iron deficiency anemia	Low in severe disease
	Renal failure	Low
	α-Thalassemia	Mildly reduced
	Vitamin B_{12} deficiency anemia	Low
	Folic acid deficiency anemia	Low
Hemoglobin level	Iron deficiency anemia	Low
	Vitamin B_{12} deficiency anemia	Low
	Folic acid deficiency anemia	Low
Mean corpuscular volume	α-Thalassemia	Extremely low
	Iron deficiency anemia	Low
	Vitamin B_{12} deficiency anemia	High
	Folic acid deficiency anemia	High
Red blood cell count	α-Thalassemia	Normal or increased
Reticulocyte count	α-Thalassemia	Normal
	Iron deficiency anemia	Decreased initially
	Vitamin B_{12} deficiency anemia	Normal or decreased
	Folic acid deficiency anemia	Normal or decreased
Peripheral blood smear	Thalassemia	Microcytes
	Iron deficiency anemia	Hypochromic cells
	Vitamin B_{12} deficiency anemia	Cabot's ring bodies
	Folic acid deficiency anemia	Howell-Jolly bodies and hypersegmented neutrophils
Serum cobalamin level	Vitamin B_{12} deficiency anemia	<250 pg/ml
	Iron deficiency anemia	Normal
	Folic acid deficiency anemia	Normal
Schilling test (24-hr urine)	Vitamin B_{12} deficiency anemia	Excretion of <8% of administered dose of tagged cyanocobalamin
Hemoglobin electrophoresis	Thalassemia	Decreased α or β chains
Fetal DNA test	α-Thalassemia	Decreased α chains

status. Supplementation may be needed during pregnancy and lactation, disease, growth spurts, and chemotherapy. Persons on fad diets and alcoholics should be encouraged to eat a diet rich in green leafy vegetables, yeast, nuts, dried beans, bran, and fruit and to abstain from alcohol (Montoya, Wink, and Sole, 2002).

Vitamin B_{12} deficiency anemia is treated with replacement vitamin B_{12} given intramuscularly, orally, or intranasally. Initiation of therapy for all patients with vitamin B_{12} deficiency usually includes intramuscular injections of 100 µg of cobalamin daily for 7 days, followed by weekly injections for 1 month. Monthly injections may be required for life if the patient has a deficiency of intrinsic factor. If not, then an alternative treatment of daily oral doses of 1000 to 2000 µg of vitamin B$_{12}$ may be given for up to 2 weeks followed by 25 to 100 µg daily for maintenance. An intranasal gel may be used for maintenance therapy and is given once per week in doses of 500 µg. Foods enriched with vitamin B$_{12}$ and oral vitamin supplements are helpful for patients without intrinsic factor deficiency (Montoya, Wink, and Sole, 2002).

Persons with anemia should be encouraged to participate in self-care and to be their own advocates. Some of the self-care practices of which patients and families should be aware are the following (Boyer, 2000):
■ Assess fatigue level.
■ Understand the possible causes of the fatigue.
■ Manage the fatigue using the following:
  ■ Relaxation exercises
  ■ Balancing energy and activity
  ■ Dietary modifications
  ■ Physical exercise
  ■ Energy conservation strategies
  ■ Assistive devices
  ■ Pharmaceutical interventions

Complementary and Alternative Therapies

Alternative therapies are especially useful for managing the fatigue associated with many blood disorders. A consistent and healthful diet and exercise program with periods of rest may help restore energy to a level high enough to allow the person to perform instrumental and other activities of daily living. Adequate fluid intake and avoidance of caffeinated beverages, fried foods, and sugar along with increased fiber intake promote energy and prevent fatigue. Various herbs have been recommended to combat fatigue. However, these should be used only in consultation with a physician or advanced practice nurse (APN) to avoid interaction with medications the patient may be taking and to avoid an increase in the tendency to bleed.

POLYCYTHEMIA
Pathophysiology

Whereas anemia may be characterized by a deficiency of RBCs, polycythemia is distinguished by an excess of RBCs. Exogenous causes such as exposure to radiation or drugs and endogenous causes such as immune defects or the body's compensatory physiologic response to an event may result in an excess of erythrocytes.

Relative polycythemia occurs when dehydration results in hypovolemia and a relative excess of RBCs. This condition is corrected with adequate rehydration. Absolute polycythemia can be primary or secondary. Primary polycythemia, or polycythemia vera (PV), is chronic and can result in splenomegaly. In many patients, white blood cell and platelet counts are also elevated. The disease is associated with stem cell neoplasias but is rare and occurs primarily in individuals over 60 years of age. The onset of PV is gradual as abnormal stem cells and RBCs proliferate. Erythropoietin levels may be normal or decreased, yet RBCs proliferate abnormally for unknown reasons (Mansen and McCance, 2002).

Secondary polycythemia is more common than PV and is a compensatory response to reduced oxygen levels. Erythropoietin secretion is increased in response to hypoxia. High altitude, smoking, and chronic hypoxia such as occurs in chronic obstructive pulmonary disease or in congestive heart failure can cause the body to produce massive quantities of RBCs to compensate for decreased oxygen levels. Persons with abnormal hemoglobin and with tumors such as renal cell carcinoma may also develop secondary polycythemia (Mansen and McCance, 2002).

Clinical Manifestations

Increased blood viscosity and blood volume are responsible for the symptoms associated with polycythemia. Thrombi and occlusions of blood vessels can result in tissue or organ ischemia or infarction. Persons with this disease develop a ruddy complexion, and the mucous membranes and skin become reddened, especially in the extremities. Eye and cerebral blood vessels may become engorged. Table 10-2 lists common clinical manifestations of polycythemia.

Table 10-2 Clinical Manifestations of Polycythemia

System	Manifestation
Skin	Ruddy or reddened
	Painful itching
Neurologic	Headache
	Drowsiness
	Visual changes
	Delirium
	Mania
	Psychotic depression
	Chorea
	Cerebral thrombosis
Cardiovascular	Elevated blood pressure
	Angina
	Raynaud's phenomenon
	Thromboangiitis obliterans
Gastrointestinal	Thrombosis
	Hemorrhaging
	Splenomegaly
	Hepatomegaly
	Portal hypertension
Respiratory	Thrombosis
	Emboli

Adapted from Mansen TJ, McCance KL: Alterations of erythrocyte function. In McCance KL, Huether SE, editors: *Pathophysiology: the biologic basis for disease in adults and children*, ed 4, St Louis, 2002, Mosby.

Diagnosis

Laboratory findings that are diagnostic of polycythemia include an absolute rise in RBCs, hematocrit levels above 51% for males and above 48% for females, sustained increase in hemoglobin level to greater than 18 g/dl, and an RBC count of 6 million/mm^3 (Schneider, 2002). Absolute total blood volume rises, and leukocyte and platelet counts may also be increased. Erythrocytes typically have normal morphology (Mansen and McCance, 2002).

Treatment and Care

Phlebotomy is used to reduce the blood volume. Blood may be drawn up to three times per week in quantities of 300 to 500 ml on each draw. Frequency of phlebotomy may decrease to quarterly intervals. As the volume of RBCs decreases, so does the quantity of iron in the blood, which leads to iron deficiency anemia. Iron deficiency anemia reduces erythropoiesis, however, and thus decreases the phlebotomy requirement. Radioactive phosphorus may be given at 18-month intervals to suppress erythropoiesis. Anemia, thrombocytopenia, leukemia, or leukopenia may result because of the suppression of hematopoietic processes. Hydroxyurea, a chemotherapeutic drug, is most commonly used because it suppresses the bone marrow. This treatment reduces the possibility of thrombosis and the occurrence of leukemia. Interferon is a relatively new treatment for PV. Patients with polycythemia who do not receive treatment have a 50% risk of dying within a year and a half of the onset of symptoms. Hemorrhage or thrombosis results in death. Conversion to acute myelogenous leukemia occurs in 10% of patients and does not usually respond to treatment. Most persons with PV survive for 10 to 15 years after diagnosis (Mansen and McCance, 2002). Smokers who have polycythemia should quit smoking, and those with chronic obstructive pulmonary disease or congestive heart failure should be treated appropriately.

SICKLE CELL ANEMIA

Pathophysiology

Sickle cell syndromes result from a genetic mutation of the β globulin gene. The genetic abnormality causes the membrane of the RBC to stiffen, increases blood viscosity, and leads to dehydration because potassium leaks into the cell and calcium moves out. In this genetic defect, valine is substituted for the glutamic acid normally present on the β globin chain. Sickle hemoglobin (hemoglobin S) is formed instead of normal hemoglobin. The sickle shape that characterizes the cells prevents the RBCs from moving freely through the blood vessels. Vasoocclusion and hemolytic anemia (destruction of RBCs) occur. The spleen destroys the abnormal RBCs, and the abnormal cells, which are sticky, adhere to the walls of the blood vessels and cause clogging. Tissue ischemia, end-organ damage, and severe pain result. Persons with sickle cell trait carry about 55% hemoglobin A

(normal hemoglobin) and 45% hemoglobin S in their RBCs (Platt et al, 2002). These individuals may experience painless hematuria but otherwise show no significant clinical manifestations (Benz, 2001).

The disease shows an autosomal recessive pattern and is inherited from both parents. Although there are various forms of the disease, homozygous sickle cell disease is the most common and is characterized by inheritance of the hemoglobin S gene from both parents (Gailliard and Hall, 2000).

Clinical Manifestations

Periods of acute pain from ischemia, known as crises, as well as dysfunction or infarction of the spleen, lungs, liver, bones, kidneys, and central nervous system are common manifestations of the disease. In addition to acute pain from ischemia (which may occur anywhere in the body), tenderness, anxiety, fever, and tachycardia are seen intermittently during crises. There is much individual variability in the frequency and duration of painful crises. However, the occurrence of more than three crises per year presage reduced survival because of the likelihood of end-organ damage. Hypoxia, exposure to hypertonic dyes, strenuous exercise, fever, anxiety, infection, and abrupt changes in temperature can provoke a crisis (Benz, 2001).

A splenectomy may be necessary by as early as 3 years of age due to repeated microinfarction. After splenectomy, resistance to infection, especially from pneumococci, is decreased, so that vaccination is required every 3 to 5 years. Eventually, occlusion of retinal and renal blood vessels may occur, causing hemorrhage or detachment of retinal vessels and necrosis of renal vessels. The femoral and humeral heads may develop aseptic necrosis accompanied by chronic arthropathy and a predisposition to osteomyelitis. Chronic lower leg ulcers may also arise due to vascular occlusion. Acute chest syndrome may develop as evidenced by arterial oxygen desaturation, chest pain, fever, tachypnea, and cough. The syndrome is probably caused by sickling in the pulmonary tissue. Pneumonia and pulmonary infarction may also occur. Repeated crises signify decreased survival and complications of cor pulmonale and pulmonary hypertension that ultimately lead to death (Benz, 2001).

Diagnosis

Hemoglobin electrophoresis and sickling solubility tests confirm the diagnosis of sickle cell disease. However, the presence of hemolytic anemia and the characteristic RBC morphology, and periodic episodes of ischemic pain raise suspicion of the disease. A comprehensive hemoglobin analysis must be performed to differentiate sickle cell anemia from sickle thalassemia or hemoglobin SC disease, variants of the disorder. Chorionic villus sampling and amniotic fluid analysis help in reaching a prenatal diagnosis, and newborn screening is standard (Kline, 2002). Typically, sickle cell anemia is diagnosed in childhood. However, symptoms may not appear until adolescence with the onset of puberty or in early adulthood with pregnancy. More than three crises per year, more than one episode of acute chest syndrome, chronic neutrophilia, cerebrovascular accidents, and a history of splenic sequestration or hand-and-foot syndrome are associated with increased morbidity and mortality (Benz, 2001).

Treatment and Care

Genetic counseling is important for patients with sickle cell disease and for those with many of the other blood disorders discussed in this chapter because many of these disorders are inherited. The recognition of the pattern of disease as it applies to the individual is an important preventive measure, as are retinal examinations, antibiotic prophylaxis, immunizations, adequate oral hydration, and avoidance of abrupt temperature changes, stress, and infection. Avoidance of fever, dehydration, infection, exposure to cold, and constriction by clothing are supportive measures. Supportive care helps to improve quality of life and prognosis (Kline, 2002). Table 10-3 lists the treatments provided to individuals with sickle cell anemia in response to various manifestations.

HEMOPHILIA

Hemophilia results from deficiencies in clotting factors. Gene deletions and mutations characterize the hereditary defects that cause hemophilia. There are four major categories of hemophilia: hemophilia A, hemophilia B, hemophilia C, and von Willebrand's disease. The disorder may manifest in mild, moderate, or severe forms (Mannucci and Tuddenham, 2001). New techniques are being used to diagnose the genetic defects that cause hemophilia, so that carriers can be identified and alerted to the possibility of the disease in their offspring before children are conceived. Table 10-4 lists the different types of hemophilia and outlines the pathophysiology, clinical manifestations, diagnostic tools, and treatment. Table 10-5 provides information on the specific drugs used to treat hemophilia.

Persons with hemophilia should be instructed regarding lifestyle changes that can improve quality of life and psychosocial outlook. Patients should be encouraged to do the following (Pavlovich-Danis, 2001):

- Join a support group in person or via the Internet
- Engage in moderate physical exercise to increase and maintain mobility and strength
- Avoid high-risk activities, such as contact sports
- Use protective equipment when engaged in physical activity
- Avoid the use of aspirin and other nonsteroidal antiinflammatory medications
- Become empowered and informed about the disease
- Learn to treat bleeding incidents at home
- Learn how to assess the severity of bleeding
- Know when to seek medical treatment
- Wear identification jewelry (such as a Medic Alert bracelet) in case of emergency
- Carry a letter from the health care provider explaining the disease and its treatment
- Ask the health care provider about proper prophylaxis before invasive procedures are performed
- Avoid scheduling surgical procedures during the menstrual cycle or during ovulation
- Carry Gelfoam or medications to treat small lacerations and abrasions

Table 10-3 Treatment of Sickle Cell Anemia

Disease Manifestation	Treatment/Care
Acute crisis	Vigorous hydration
	Evaluation and treatment of underlying cause
	Narcotic analgesia
	Nasal oxygen as needed
	Blood transfusion as needed
Sickle cell arthropathy	Nonsteroidal antiinflammatory drugs
Acute chest syndrome (medical emergency)	Hydration
	Oxygen
	Evaluation and treatment of pneumonia and pulmonary embolism
	Transfusion
Repeated episodes of acute chest syndrome or more than three crises per year	Hydroxyurea (Hydrea) (10 to 30 mg/kg/day)
Repeated crises early in life, high neutrophil count, hand-and-foot syndromes	Bone marrow transplantation

Adapted from Benz EJ Jr: Hemoglobinopathies. In Braunwald E et al, editors: *Harrison's principles of internal medicine,* ed 15, New York, 2001, McGraw-Hill, pp 666-74.

HEMOCHROMATOSIS
Pathophysiology

Hereditary hemochromatosis (HH) is a disease with an autosomal recessive pattern of transmission. Iron is deposited in organs as a result of an increase in intestinal iron absorption. The disorder is associated with a mutation of the HFE gene in which cysteine is replaced with tyrosine and results in the specific mutation C282Y. HH is a disease of iron overload as opposed to iron deficiency. The disorder is often overlooked because it may have no clinical manifestations and health care providers do not routinely screen for it (Brandhagen, Fairbanks, and Baldus, 2002).

Iron overload may be caused by other disorders such as excess iron supplementation, multiple or large transfusions, chronic anemia, alcoholism, and chronic liver disease. In HH, the iron accumulates in the hepatocytes, unlike in secondary

Table 10-4   The Hemophilias

Type	Pathophysiology	Clinical Manifestations	Diagnostic Tests	Treatment
Hemophilia A (classic)	Inherited X-linked recessive Primarily affects males Transmitted by females Deficiency in factor VIII	Easy bruising Easy bleeding Hemorrhage into joints Spontaneous hematuria, epistaxis Phases/cycles of spontaneous bleeding Coinfection with HIV, hepatitis B or C if treated with blood products	Thrombin time PT (if prolonged, deficiency in factors II, V, VII, and/or X) Activated PTT (tests factors XII, XI, IX, VII) Prothrombin consumption time Thromboplastin generation test (identifies deficiencies in factors VIII and IX)	Recombinant antihemophilic factors, plasma-derived factors, somatic gene therapy (use of each depends on cost, availability, and safety) Prophylaxis Treatment of symptoms
Hemophilia B (Christmas disease)	Deficiency in factor IX X-linked recessive trait	Same as for hemophilia A	Same as for hemophilia A	Same as for hemophilia A
Hemophilia C	Deficiency in factor XI Autosomal recessive Affects males and females	Bleeding less severe than in hemophilia A or B	Same as for hemophilia A	Same as for hemophilia A
Von Willebrand's disease	Most common genetic bleeding disorder Defect in VWF (necessary for the adhesion of platelets and carrier and protector of factor XIII) Autosomal dominant Classified as type I, II, or III based on amount of VWF present Carriers may be symptomatic Affects males and females	Inadequate platelet plug and prolonged bleeding Same signs and symptoms as in hemophilia A Menorrhagia or metrorrhagia Pain with intercourse	Same as for hemophilia A: PT normal PTT occasionally prolonged Bleeding time normal or prolonged activity VWF antigen Ristocetin cofactor activity VWF multimers	Treatment of symptoms Amicar (fibrinolytic agent to keep clots from dissolving) Desmopressin (DDAVP) (causes release of body's VWF and factor VIII), clotting factor concentrates, cryoprecipitate

Adapted from Pavlovich-Danis SJ: Update on von Willebrand's disease, *Clin Advisor* pp 28-39, Nov/Dec 2001.
HIV, Human immunodeficiency virus; *PT,* prothrombin time; *PTT,* partial thromboplastin time; *VWF,* von Willebrand's factor.

disorders of iron overload in which the iron accumulates in Kupffer's cells (Brandhagen, Fairbanks, and Baldus, 2002).

Excess iron is absorbed through the small intestine. It is thought that the mutated HFE gene causes incorrect sensing of the body's iron status, which leads to increased absorption. The iron generates free radicals, which result in lipid peroxidation, and causes alterations in protein structure and DNA. Iron also appears to promote fibrogenesis in the liver. HH affects the liver, endocrine system, musculoskeletal system, pancreas, heart, pituitary gland, and reticuloendothelial immune system (Vautier, Murray, and Olynyk, 2001).

Clinical Manifestations

Persons with HH tend to have vague, nonspecific symptoms including fatigue and arthralgia. Family screening and incidental abnormal liver laboratory test results may initially reveal the disease. Persons with type 2 diabetes mellitus, congestive heart failure, cardiac arrhythmias, cardiomyopathy, peripheral arthropathy, and impotence or infertility should be suspected of having HH (Vautier, Murray, and Olynyk, 2001).

Typically, clinical manifestations of the disease appear after age 40, because it takes a long time for body iron stores to reach a level high enough to cause symptoms (15 to 40 g). A normal iron level is approximately 4 g. Men and women

Table 10-5   Drugs Used to Treat Hemophilia

Drug	Action/Indication	Dosage	Side effects
Aminocaproic acid (Amicar)	Adjunctive fibrinolytic agent, keeps formed clots from dissolving		
Desmopressin (DDAVP) infusion or Stimate nasal spray	Causes body to release own VWF and factor VIII, shortens PTT, reduces bleeding times	SQ or IV 0.3 µg/kg Intranasally 150 µg once during 24-hr period for maximum of 3 consecutive days	Fluid retention, seizures, hyponatremia, facial flushing, drowsiness, headache
Recombinant monoclonal factors	Ineffective with VWD Stops spontaneous hemorrhages and prevents excessive bleeding	Approximately 90 µg/kg of body weight every 2-3 hr	Possible anaphylaxis
Cryoprecipitate	Used in life-threatening situations in which there is risk of hepatitis and HIV	Depends on individual	Acquisition of HIV, hepatitis

Adapted from Pavlovich-Danis SJ: Update on von Willebrand's disease, *Clin Advisor* pp 28-39, Nov/Dec 2001.
HIV, Human immunodeficiency virus; *IV,* intravenous; *PTT,* partial thromboplastin time; *SQ,* subcutaneously; *VWD,* von Willebrand's disease; *VWF,* von Willebrand's factor.

are homozygous for HH with equal frequency. However, men are more likely to manifest the disease because of their higher incidence of alcohol abuse and hepatitis C. The point at which the disease becomes manifested may be affected by pregnancy, menstrual blood loss, dietary iron, age, and gender. Previously HH was classically diagnosed in a patient with liver cirrhosis who had diabetes mellitus and hyperpigmentation of the skin. The increased likelihood of detecting abnormal iron levels through laboratory testing and increased awareness of the disease among health care providers have promoted earlier, presymptomatic diagnosis (Brandhagen, Fairbanks, and Baldus, 2002).

Persons with HH are more likely to die from the complications of untreated HH than from the initial iron overload.

Hepatocellular carcinoma is 200 times more frequent in persons with HH than in the general population. Also, individuals with HH are more likely to die of cirrhosis, cardiomyopathy, and diabetes mellitus than are those in the population at large (Laudicina and Legrys, 2001).

Diagnosis

Diagnosis of HH is based on several different factors, including clinical, pathological, and laboratory findings. Table 10-6 lists the criteria used for diagnosis of HH. In addition to the studies indicated, a liver biopsy is performed to reach a definitive diagnosis. Liver biopsy is done for patients who have a serum ferritin level above 1000 µg/L, hepatomegaly, or abnormal aminotransferase levels, or are

Table 10-6   Criteria for Diagnosis of Hereditary Hemochromatosis (HH)

Test	Normal Range	Level in HH
Serum transferrin saturation	14-50%	>50%
Serum iron concentration	Males: 50-150 µg/dl	151-250 µg/dl
	Females: 35-145 µg/dl	
Total iron-binding capacity	250-400 µg/dl	200-300 µg/dl
Aspartate aminotransferase level	8-50 U/L	High or normal depending on extent of liver disease
Alanine aminotransferase level	0-50 U/L	High or normal depending on extent of liver disease
Glucose level	60-110 mg/dl	High or normal depending on involvement of pancreas
Testosterone level	Males: 300-800 ng/dl	Low or normal depending on involvement of pituitary
	Females: 25-100 ng/dl	
Hepatic iron concentration	100-2200 µg/g	5000-30,000 µg/g
Complete blood count with differential	Various normal levels	May or may not be elevated

Adapted from Brandhagen DJ, Fairbanks VF, Baldus W: Recognition and management of hereditary hemochromatosis, *Am Fam Physician* 65(5): 853-60, 2002; and Dolbey CH: Hemochromatosis: a review, *Clin J Oncol Nurs* 5(6):257-60, 2001.

over 45 years of age. Magnetic resonance imaging may be used in some cases to detect abnormal liver iron levels and liver fibrosis (Vautier, Murray, and Olynyk, 2001).

Treatment and Care

Phlebotomy, as described earlier in the discussion of polycythemia, is used to treat HH. The patient's body mass determines the frequency of blood draws and the quantity of blood removed. Treatment should continue until the transferrin saturation level is reduced to less than 50% and the serum ferritin level is less than 50 µg/L or the hemoglobin level is normal. Blood draws typically occur weekly at first; once normal levels are attained, 3 to 8 U of blood is drawn each year. Conditions associated with excess body iron stores, such as cardiac, liver, and musculoskeletal disorders, should be treated as if they were primary disorders (Vautier, Murray, and Olynyk, 2001).

Genetic testing may eliminate the need for liver biopsy, especially in young patients with iron overload who are not yet symptomatic. Screening for the disease is optimally done between ages 18 and 30 years. General screening of the population has been advocated by scientists, but screening has not yet been recommended by governmental public health organizations except for persons who meet specific criteria (Brandhagen, Fairbanks, and Baldus, 2002; Vautier, Murray, and Olynyk, 2001). The Centers for Disease Control and Prevention recommends testing for iron overload in people who have a close blood relative with HH, have a significant risk of developing complications, and are members of an ideal target group for preventive interventions. In addition, the Centers for Disease Control recommends testing of persons with diabetes mellitus and unexplained symptoms that characterize HH (Reyes, Blanck, and Khoury, 2003).

The primary care physician, registered nurse (RN), APN, or physician assistant is the most likely professional to suspect initially that an individual has HH. The RN and APN will be involved in the care of the person with HH as they assist with laboratory and biopsy testing and genetic screening. The patient and family should be reassured that, although the disease is genetic and family members should be tested, early detection of the disease prevents its complications. The dietitian is an important member of the health care team for a person with HH because dietary changes are recommended. The following are lifestyle and dietary changes that the interdisciplinary team should teach the person with HH (Laudicina and Legrys, 2001):

- Do not take iron supplements or vitamins with iron.
- Minimize intake of red meat.
- Minimize alcohol intake.
- Do not eat raw shellfish because of the increased risk of infection (Information from your family doctor, 2002).
- Avoid use of cast iron pots and pans.
- Avoid vitamin C intake with meals (enhances iron absorption) and vitamin C supplements.

- Avoid tobacco because of its high iron content.
- Discuss with a health care provider whether to drink more tea, take calcium carbonate, and eat more fiber to block iron absorption.

INTERDISCIPLINARY CARE

The primary health care provider (physician, physician assistant, or APN) is likely to be the first provider to suspect any of the disorders discussed in this chapter. Routine blood work or incidental findings from laboratory studies performed because of an unrelated chief complaint may indicate various abnormalities that must be further researched. The RN assists in performing venipuncture for laboratory studies and in administering transfusions and medications when required. Nurses as well as the other members of the team instruct the patient and family about the course of the disease, treatment, follow-up, and genetic testing and screening.

The dietitian is a key player because all of these disorders require dietary modification. In addition, other specialists may become involved if there is difficulty reaching a diagnosis or if and when complications arise. The neurologist may be consulted if the person with vitamin B_{12} deficiency is not diagnosed before neurologic changes occur or the anemic patient is an elderly person who is confused and falls frequently. The cardiologist, endocrinologist, and gastrointestinal specialist may also be added to the team if complications develop from any of these blood disorders or if the

---

Think S for Success

SYMPTOMS
- Manage fatigue, pain, and causes and complications of disease with medication, rest, and self-care.

SEQUELAE
- Prevent complications by ensuring regular checkups and compliance with treatment and dietary modifications.
- Encourage family members to undergo genetic screening.

SAFETY
- Instruct patient to avoid high-risk activity, wear protective equipment during physical activity, learn self-care and bleeding management strategies.

SUPPORT/SERVICES
- Help patient obtain assistance with finances (medications can be costly) if necessary.
- Refer patient to specialist if necessary.

SATISFACTION
- Determine degree to which blood disorder is interfering with patient's life and develop a plan to help patient reach or maintain desired quality of life.

nervous system, heart, endocrine system (particularly hypothyroidism), or gastrointestinal system is implicated in the cause of the disorder. The orthopedist, physiatrist, or physical therapist may become involved if the patient is confused or otherwise at high risk of falling. In addition, the physical therapist may provide strengthening exercises to improve activity tolerance.

ETHICAL CONSIDERATIONS

Patients may have religious and/or ethical, fear-based, or medically based objections to blood transfusions or to pharmacologic treatment. The patient or family member may prefer not to undergo genetic screening and to remain ignorant of disease status and prognosis. Patients may have concerns about possible discrimination based on genetic predisposition.

FAMILY AND CAREGIVER ISSUES

The family or caregiver should be taught strategies to support the patient, especially when fatigue is overwhelming to the patient. Reassure the family or caregiver that the patient's energy level will return to normal once treatment is initiated and if complications are prevented. The family or caregiver should receive instruction regarding dietary modifications, especially if the family member or caregiver is the cook in the home. Family members should be encouraged to undergo genetic testing and routine laboratory screening.

LONG-TERM CARE

Persons with any of the diseases discussed here except sickle cell anemia are not likely to be treated with formal home care or in a long-term care facility unless they have comorbidities or complications develop. Persons with sickle cell anemia may require formal home care or nursing home placement if skilled care becomes necessary on a frequent basis.

END-OF-LIFE ISSUES

The patient and family should be assisted in adjusting to the diagnosis. The patient and family should be told that, if the disease is not treated and monitored, serious life-threatening complications may develop. If the disease or its sequelae become terminal, the patient and family should be supported and assisted in finding and using hospice services. The health care provider should serve as an advocate for the patient and family.

CASE STUDY*

Patient Data

Mrs. S. is a 60-year-old white female who visits her nurse practitioner for her annual physical examination. Although she says that she feels in generally good health, she describes feeling fatigued and mildly depressed, and complains of joint pain that has persisted for several months. She is a full-time homemaker. She has had hormone replacement therapy for 10 years and has delivered three healthy children, who are now adults. She drinks alcohol once or twice a week and occasionally takes ibuprofen to relieve her joint pain and vitamin supplements. She claims no use of other over-the-counter medications.

Mrs. S. states that her father died of liver disease but that her mother is alive and well, as is her brother. Her sister has diabetes mellitus type 2.

Physical Examination and Diagnostic Data

Mrs. S. is a well-nourished, well-appearing female with vital signs within the normal ranges. She has mild hepatomegaly and joint tenderness. The following are the findings from her laboratory studies:

Test	Finding
Glucose level	High normal
Blood urea nitrogen level	Normal
Aspartate aminotransferase and alanine aminotransferase level	Elevated
γ-Glutamyltransferase level	High normal
Cholesterol	High normal
High-density lipoprotein level	Normal
Triglyceride levels	Elevated

Test	Finding
Serum iron level	High
Total iron-binding capacity	Low normal
Serum transferrin saturation	Elevated
Serum ferritin level	Elevated
Erythrocyte sedimentation rate	Elevated
Rheumatoid factor	Negative
Antinuclear antibodies	Negative

Results of the complete blood count with differential are all within the normal ranges. Because the serum transferrin saturation and serum ferritin levels are elevated, DNA tests are ordered to detect genetic mutations. Mrs. S. is found to have a genetic mutation homozygous for C282Y and is referred to a gastroenterologist for evaluation of liver complications.

Thinking It Through

■ What blood disorder does Mrs. S. have?
■ What nursing diagnoses apply to Mrs. S.?
■ Will the care and teaching of Mrs. S. differ from that of a patient with anemia, hemophilia, or polycythemia?
■ How can the health care team contribute to the quality of life of Mrs. S.?
■ What are Mrs. S.'s concerns likely to be?
■ What are the family's concerns likely to be?

Case Conference

This particular case conference takes place approximately 1 year after the diagnosis.

The health care providers involved in the treatment and care of Mrs. S. are logistically unable to meet in one setting. Consequently,

*Adapted from Laudicina RJ, Legrys VA: Hereditary hemochromatosis: a case study and review, Clin Lab Sci 14(3):196-208, 2001.

CASE STUDY—cont'd

Mrs. and Mr. S., her children, the RN, physical therapist, and APN discuss the case and consult with the gastroenterologist and dietitian by telephone.

The gastroenterologist has reported that Mrs. S. declined a liver biopsy and he is aware that she has had weekly phlebotomy treatments at the outpatient clinic at the local hospital. Although she has had 50 weeks of treatments and her serum ferritin level has dropped to 175 mg/L, she is still having minor joint pain and fatigue. The RN explains that Mrs. S. has told her that the fatigue lasts for 1 or 2 days after each blood draw and that Mrs. S. occasionally misses work. The RN goes on to say that the phlebotomist has told her that Mrs. S. is "a hard stick" and that Mrs. S. has expressed a desire to donate her blood.

The physical therapist states that she began to work with Mrs. S. several weeks ago when the APN referred the patient to her. She has taught Mrs. S. and her family about energy conservation techniques and activities to be avoided. She has also offered Mrs. S. a walker or a cane to use until her energy is restored.

The dietitian explains that he also met with Mrs. S. and her family early in her treatment and explained the dietary changes that would be helpful to her. Mrs. S. comments that the physical therapy strategies and the dietary changes have helped reduce her fatigue and joint pain.

The APN notes that she has referred the family to a genetic counselor and has explained that it is possible that Mrs. S.'s father had hemochromatosis and developed liver disease as a complication. Mrs. S. laments that her brother has refused genetic counseling because of the potential problems with employment and health insurance should test results be positive.

■ What new information was gathered that would assist the nurse in developing a plan of care?

■ What alternative therapies or strategies could be used to minimize the fatigue and joint pain Mrs. S. is experiencing?

Internet and Other Resources

American Hemochromatosis Society: *http://www.americanhs.org;* telephone 407-829-4488 or 888-655-IRON

American Sickle Cell Anemia Association: *http://www.ascaa.org;* telephone 216-229-8600

Cleveland Clinic Journal of Medicine: telephone 216-444-2661 (for patient handouts on hemochromatosis)

Iron Overload Diseases Association: *http://www.ironoverload.org;* telephone 561-840-8512

National Center for Biotechnology Information—OMIM (Von Willebrand Disease): *http://www.ncbi.nlm.nih.gov/htbin-post/ Omim/ dispmim?193400*

National Hemophilia Foundation information service (HANDI): E-mail *HANDI@hemophilia.org;* telephone 800-42-HANDI

REFERENCES

Barton JC et al: Intravenous iron dextran therapy in patients with iron deficiency and normal renal function who failed to respond to or did not tolerate oral iron supplementation, *Am J Med* 109:27-32, 2000.

Benz EJ Jr: Hemoglobinopathies. In Braunwald E et al, editors: *Harrison's principles of internal medicine,* ed 15, New York, 2001, McGraw-Hill, pp 666-74.

Blackwell S, Hendrix PC: Common anemias, *Clin rev* 11(3):53-62, 2001.

Boyer CG: Chemotherapy-related anemia and fatigue in home care patients, *Home Healthc Nurse* 18(4 suppl T0):3-15, 2000.

Brandhagen DJ, Fairbanks VF, Baldus W: Recognition and management of hereditary hemochromatosis, *Am Fam Physician* 65(5):853-60, 2002.

Diamond PT, Julian DM: Practice trends in the management of low hematocrit in the acute rehabilitation setting, *Am J Phys Med Rehabil* 80(11):816-20, 2001.

Gailliard T, Hall D: Living with adult sickle cell disease, *Adv Nurses,* pp 21-2, May 22, 2000.

Holcomb SS: Anemia, *Nursing 2001* 31(7):36-42, 2001.

Huffstutler SY: Adult anemia, *Adv Nurse Pract* 8(3):89-92, 2000.

Information from your family doctor: hereditary hemochromatosis, *Am Fam Physician* 65(5):865-6, 2002.

Kline NE: Alterations of hematology function in children. In McCance KL, Huether SE, editors: *Pathophysiology: the biologic basis for disease in adults and children,* ed 4, St Louis, 2002, Mosby, pp 900-29.

Laudicina RJ, Legrys VA: Hereditary hemochromatosis: a case study and review, *Clin Lab Sci* 14(3):196-208, 2001.

Life Extension Foundation: Anemia-thrombocytopenia-leukopenia, May 27, 2003, retrieved from *http://www.lef.org/protocols/prtcl-009.shtml#ane* on Jan 21, 2004.

Linker CA: Blood. In Tierney LM, McPhee SJ, Papadakis MA, editors: *Current medical diagnosis and treatment,* New York, 2001, Lange Medical Books/McGraw-Hill, pp 499-575.

Mannucci PM, Tuddenham EGD: The hemophiliac—from royal genes to gene therapy, *N Engl J Med* 344(23):1773-9, 2001.

Mansen TJ, McCance KL: Alterations in erythrocyte function. In McCance KL, Huether SE, editors: *Pathophysiology: the biologic basis for disease in adults and children,* ed 4, St Louis, 2002, Mosby, pp 843-64.

McCance KL: Structure and function of the hematologic system. In McCance KL, Huether SE, editors: *Pathophysiology: the biologic basis for disease in adults and children,* 4 ed, St Louis, 2002, Mosby, pp 811-42.

Montoya VL, Wink D, Sole ML: Adult anemia: determine clinical significance, *Nurse Pract* 27(3):38-53, 2002.

Pavlovich-Danis SJ: Update on von Willebrand's disease, *Clin Advisor,* pp 28-39, Nov/Dec 2001.

Platt A et al: Sickle cell disease: pain management, *Adv Nurses,* pp 32-4, Feb 4, 2002.

Reyes M, Blanck HM, Khoury M: Screening for iron overload due to hereditary hemochromatosis [Centers for Disease Control and Prevention, National Center for Chronic Disease Prevention and Health Promotion, Nutrition & Physical Activity web page], 2003, retrieved from *http://www.cdc.gov/nccdphp/dnpa/hemochromatosis/ screening.htm* on Dec 19, 2003.

Schneider SM: Interventions for clients with hematologic problems. In Ignatavicius DD, Workman ML, editors: *Medical surgical nursing: critical thinking for collaborative care,* ed 4, Philadelphia, 2002, WB Saunders, pp 836-68.

Vautier G, Murray M, Olynyk J: Hereditary hemochromatosis: detection and management, *Med J Aust* 175(8):418-21, 2001.

CHAPTER 11

Malignancies of the Blood

Leslie Jean Neal, PhD, RN, FNP-C

OBJECTIVES

After reading this chapter, you should be able to do the following:

- Describe the pathophysiology of chronic leukemia, lymphoma, and multiple myeloma
- Describe the clinical manifestations of leukemia, lymphoma, and multiple myeloma
- Describe the functional health patterns affected by leukemia, lymphoma, and multiple myeloma
- Describe the role of each member of the interdisciplinary team involved in the care of patients with leukemia, lymphoma, and multiple myeloma
- Describe the indications for use, side effects, and nursing considerations related to drugs commonly used to treat leukemia, lymphoma, and multiple myeloma

OVERVIEW OF BLOOD MALIGNANCIES

The stem cell is the precursor of all of the blood cells in the human body. Stem cells differentiate into myeloid and lymphoid cells. Myeloid cells further differentiate into erythrocytes, macrophages, platelets, neutrophils, basophils, and eosinophils. Lymphoid cells further differentiate into T or B cells. T cells interact directly with invading foreign cells. An antibody-antigen reaction is required to initiate the maturation of B cells into plasma cells. The mature plasma cells form the immunoglobulins needed to mount an immune response (Barrick and Mitchell, 2001) (Figure 11-1).

Leukemias involve both the myeloid and lymphoid blood cells and have traditionally been divided into acute and chronic leukemias according to the average rates of survival. Only the chronic forms of leukemia are discussed in this chapter. Chronic lymphocytic leukemia (CLL) has been found to be a spectrum of diseases and is the most common form of leukemia in the Western world. It is very rare in children and most prevalent in older adults. The majority of cases occur in adults older than age 50. In the United States, approximately 13,000 people are newly diagnosed with CLL each year. Persons with CLL have long-term survival, so many more people than this are living with CLL (Armitage and Longo, 2001). Chronic myeloid leukemia (CML) affects

1.3 persons of every 100,000 per year. Incidence increases gradually with age until middle age and then rises rapidly.

Lymphomas are divided into non-Hodgkin's and Hodgkin's lymphomas. Hodgkin's lymphoma is defined by the presence of Reed-Sternberg cells. Non-Hodgkin's lymphomas include all tumors of either B or T lymphocytes. Approximately 8000 new cases of Hodgkin's disease are diagnosed each year in the United States. Ages of peak incidence are during the twenties and during the eighties. The frequency of non-Hodgkin's lymphoma is increasing by 4% per year in the United States. Approximately 60,000 cases are diagnosed per year, and the disease is more common in elderly persons and in men (Longo, 2001).

Multiple myeloma, a cancer of plasma cells, is newly diagnosed in approximately 13,200 individuals per year. Approximately 11,000 people die yearly from the disease. The average age of diagnosis is 68 years, and the disorder rarely occurs in those younger than age 40. The incidence of multiple myeloma yearly is 4 per 100,000 in the United States as well as around the world.

Ethnic Variations

CLL is most common in males and in whites. It is very uncommon among Asians (Armitage and Longo, 2001). Hodgkin's disease is more prevalent in whites than in blacks and in men than in women. The United States, Denmark, and the Netherlands have the highest incidence of Hodgkin's disease, whereas Japan and Australia have the lowest incidence (Mansen and McCance, 2002). The incidence of non-Hodgkin's disease varies geographically according to subtype. T-cell lymphomas are less prevalent in Western countries than in Asia, although some B-cell lymphomas are more common in Western countries. Multiple myeloma affects more males than females and twice as many blacks as whites. The disease is responsible for approximately 15% of all malignancies in whites and 2% of all malignancies in blacks, and accounts for 13% of blood cancers in whites and 33% in blacks (Longo, 2001).

ASSESSMENT

The major chronic blood diseases discussed in this chapter share many symptoms, and diagnostic methods are similar.

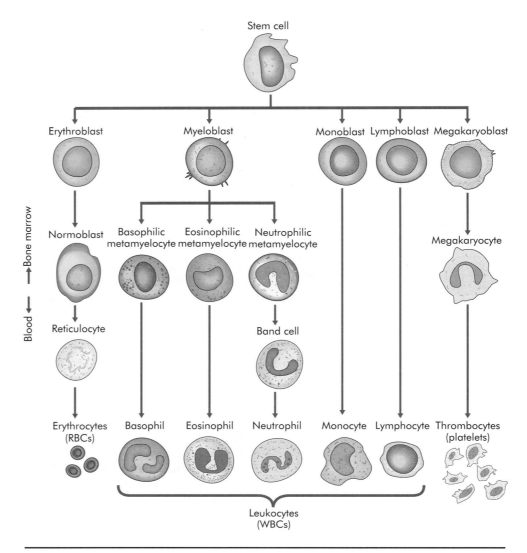

Figure 11-1 Development of blood cells. *RBCs,* Red blood cells; *WBCs,* white blood cells. (From Lewis SM, Heitkemper MM, Dirksen SR: *Medical-surgical nursing: assessment and management of clinical problems,* ed 6, St Louis, 2004, Mosby.)

Furthermore, because the associated symptoms and sequelae are similar for these diseases, the functional health patterns affected are largely the same. Box 11-1 provides a framework for assessing the effects of these disorders on functional health patterns.

CHRONIC MYELOGENOUS LEUKEMIA
Pathophysiology

CML is characterized by an excessive proliferation of myeloid cells. As long as bone marrow function remains normal, the disease is stable. During this time, the myeloid cells continue to be able to differentiate, and the neutrophils continue to fight infection. Over time, however, the disease transforms into malignancy, and eventually a crisis is reached. Because there is an abnormal proliferation of myeloid cells, the bone marrow becomes unable to produce red blood cells, platelets, and other mature leukocytes. Consequently, leukopenia of unaffected white blood cells, anemia, and thrombocytopenia develop. The presence of the Philadelphia chromosome in cultured leukocytes differentiates CML from other forms of leukemia, although this marker is absent in 5% of cases (Ignatavicius and Workman, 2002; Linker, 2000).

No clear connections exist between risk factors such as exposure to cytotoxic drugs or viruses and CML. However, smoking has been shown to accelerate the progression to blast crisis, and exposure to large doses of radiation is thought to be correlated with the disease (Wetzler, Byrd, and Bloomfield, 2001).

Box 11-1 Functional Health Pattern Assessment for Malignancies of the Blood

HEALTH PERCEPTION/HEALTH MANAGEMENT
- Is there a family history of blood disease?
- What is the patient's perception of his or her overall health?
- What medications, including over-the-counter drugs, does the patient take?
- What alternative therapies does the patient use?

NUTRITION/METABOLISM
- What is the patient's current weight? Has the patient experienced a recent unexplained weight loss?
- Is the patient on any special diet?
- What is the patient's typical dietary intake (daily)? Is it less than body requirements?
- What is the condition of the skin and mucous membranes? Is there stomatitis or mucositis?
- Is there a history of bleeding?

ELIMINATION
- Has the patient had any changes in bowel or bladder habits?

ACTIVITY/EXERCISE
- Does the patient experience difficulty walking, fatigue, or malaise?
- Does the patient require mobility aids?
- Is the patient able to perform instrumental and other activities of daily living?
- In what rest and recreational activities does the patient engage?

SLEEP/REST
- How many hours of uninterrupted sleep does the patient get? Does the patient take naps or rest periods?
- What sleep aids does the patient use?
- Does the patient experience fatigue or lethargy?

COGNITION/PERCEPTION
- What are the nature, character, duration, and location of pain?
- What factors aggravate and alleviate pain?
- What treatments have been tried and how effective were they?

SELF-PERCEPTION/SELF-CONCEPT
- How has the condition affected the patient's self-esteem?
- How does the patient describe himself or herself?

- How has the condition changed the patient's body image?
- How has the condition affected the patient's sense of self?

ROLES/RELATIONSHIPS
- Is the patient employed? What kind of work does the patient perform?
- What roles does the patient play in the home, family, and workplace?
- What changes have occurred in the patient's ability to carry out normal roles and functions?
- Is the patient satisfied with his or her current roles and relationships?
- How has the condition affected the patient and others?

SEXUALITY/REPRODUCTION
- Is the patient sexually active?
- Has the patient experienced any changes in the menstrual cycle?
- Have changes occurred in the patient's sexual performance? Is the patient satisfied with current sexual patterns?

COPING/STRESS TOLERANCE
- What are the patient's coping strategies?
- What support systems are available to the patient?
- Can the patient manage the condition in the current setting?
- Does the patient experience anxiety related to a fear of death?
- Does the patient experience a feeling of powerlessness or depression?

VALUES/BELIEFS
- What constitutes quality of life to the patient?
- What is important to the patient?
- What are the patient's spiritual beliefs, health beliefs, cultural beliefs, and feelings about locus of control?
- To what extent do the patient's cultural/spiritual beliefs influence decision making related to this condition?

Clinical Manifestations

The average age of presentation with CML is 42 years. Typical manifestations at presentation include low-grade fever, fatigue, and night sweats. The patient may complain of abdominal fullness related to splenomegaly, and in rare cases respiratory distress is present. Complications include cerebrovascular accident, myocardial infarction, and blurred vision related to leukostasis. Also, there may be infection, bleeding, or thrombosis caused by the dysfunction of platelets or granulocytes. Sometimes, the increase in white blood cell count (usually higher than 500,000/µl) is found accidentally, because patients are asymptomatic for a long period. As CML progresses, symptoms worsen. Weight loss, fever, bone and joint pain, infections, thrombosis, or bleeding may occur.

A focused history taking is helpful in diagnosing CML. Reports of bleeding episodes, easy bruising, epistaxis, increased menstrual flow, rectal bleeding or hematuria, and bleeding from the gums warrant laboratory testing. Indications of weakness or fatigue resulting from anemia may be revealed by asking about weight loss, headaches, increased fatigue, lethargy or weakness, decreased concentration or alertness, somnolence, or decreased attention span (Ignatavicius and Workman, 2002).

On examination, individuals may have petechiae, infected sores, ecchymoses, signs of decreased blood circulation, splenomegaly, hepatomegaly, weight loss, anorexia, hematuria or rectal bleeding, tachycardia or palpitations, dyspnea, fatigue, fever, or bone or joint pain or swelling. There may be additional gastrointestinal complaints such as nausea, abdominal pain, constipation, and decreased bowel sounds (Ignatavicius and Workman, 2002).

Diagnosis

Box 11-2 lists common findings in patients with CML.

Treatment

The goal of therapy for CML is to achieve hematopoiesis that does not involve malignant clones and is durable, and thus to achieve a cure. Recombinant interferon alpha is the current treatment of choice during the chronic phase of CML. The medication prolongs the chronic phase and lengthens survival. Interferon may be combined with low doses of cytarabine for increased effectiveness. Interferon must be given by injection, is expensive, and produces side effects, including anorexia, myalgias, and fatigue. The constitutional symptoms may prevent treatment with the optimal dose, which is 5×10^6 U/m^2/day for 5 years followed by continued treatment at a lower dosage. Patients who will benefit from interferon therapy will produce Philadelphia chromosome–negative leukocyte clones in 6 to 18 months. Among patients in whom a complete response is achieved, as indicated by the absence of the Philadelphia chromosome, rates of survival beyond 5 years are more than 90%. Among those who show a response level of fewer than 35% Philadelphia chromosome–positive clones, a 5-year survival rate of more than 60% is typically achieved.

Hydroxyurea is often given initially to control symptoms rapidly. It quickly decreases the white blood cell count, reduces the size of the spleen, and eliminates symptoms. The initial dose is 1 to 4 g/day, and the dosage is reduced by half each time a 50% reduction in the leukocyte count occurs. Hydroxyurea is less expensive than interferon, is taken by mouth, and has fewer side effects. It must be taken without interruption (Armitage and Longo, 2001; Linker, 2000).

The only curative treatment is allogenic bone marrow transplantation. This treatment is offered to patients who are younger than 60 years of age and who have HLA-matched siblings. Among adults, 60% are cured following transplantation. The highest success rates (70% to 80%) are seen in patients who receive a transplant within 1 year of diagnosis. Among persons who receive transplants from HLA-matched nonsiblings, the typical cure rate is 40% to 60%. Following transplantation, patients who relapse may go into remission after infusion with T lymphocytes from a bone marrow donor (Linker, 2000).

With treatment, the chronic phase typically lasts approximately 3 years. Without treatment, the disease may progress to an accelerated phase that is more symptomatic than the chronic phase. The accelerated phase ends in a brief blast crisis. After transformation to the accelerated or blastic phase, the disease may not respond to therapy (O'Mara and Whedon, 2000). During a blast crisis (in which the chronic form of the disease transforms into the acute phase), chemotherapy can be more effective and less toxic. Treatment with daunorubicin, prednisone, and vincristine leads to a short-lived remission in 70% of cases. Once the patient is in the blastic (acute) phase, survival is a period of months (Linker, 2000). During the blastic phase, the number of myeloblasts increases in the bone marrow and in the blood.

Imatinib (Gleevec) is a relatively new oral treatment for persons with CML who have not responded to interferon therapy. Imatinib inhibits the enzyme that causes the massive proliferation of white blood cells. The medication is given daily in 400-mg doses for patients in the chronic

---

Box 11-2   Common Findings at Diagnosis of Chronic Myelogenous Leukemia and with Disease Progression

LABORATORY FINDINGS
- Elevated white blood cell counts with variability in maturity of granulocytes
- Elevated platelet counts
- Mild normochromic normocytic anemia
- Low leukocyte alkaline phosphatase level
- Elevated serum levels of vitamin B$_{12}$ and B$_{12}$ binding proteins
- Increased histamine level later in disease
- Altered myeloid to erythroid ratio (due to increased myeloid cells)
- Basophilia, eosinophilia, and monocytosis
- With disease acceleration:
  Increasing degrees of anemia
  Blood or marrow blasts 10-20%
  Blood or marrow basophils more than 20%
  Platelet count less than 100,000/μl

PHYSICAL EXAMINATION FINDINGS
- Minimal to moderate splenomegaly
- Possible mild hepatomegaly
- With disease acceleration:
  Persistent splenomegaly despite therapy
  Lymphadenopathy and extramedullary myeloid tumors (indicate poor prognosis)

CHROMOSOMAL FINDINGS
- Gene fusion: T(9;22)(q34;q11)
- Philadelphia chromosome arising from 9;22 translocation

Adapted from Armitage JO, Longo DL: In Braunwald E et al, editors: *Harrison's principles of internal medicine,* ed 15, New York, 2001, McGraw-Hill, pp 715-27.

phase of CML and in 600-mg doses for persons in blast crisis or the accelerated phase of the disease. Side effects include nausea, diarrhea, muscle cramps, fluid retention, hemorrhage, fatigue, musculoskeletal pain, skin rash, and headache. Neutropenia, hepatotoxicity, and thrombocytopenia may also accompany use of the drug (Lobert, 2001). Refer to Chapter 27 for a detailed discussion of cancer therapy.

CHRONIC LYMPHOCYTIC LEUKEMIA
Pathophysiology

CLL is distinguished from CML by the type of leukocyte that begins to proliferate abnormally. As with CML, the cause of this abnormal proliferation is unknown. Lymphoid, erythroid, and myeloid cells, monocytes, and megakaryocytes arise from a common progenitor. The cell initially becomes lymphoid and then differentiates into a B or T cell. Malignancies of any type of lymphoid cell are associated with recurrent genetic abnormalities.

CLL is characterized by the abnormal proliferation of mature B cells (or rarely T cells) and manifests as either a leukemia or a lymphoma. It is distinguished by lymphocytosis (more than 5000 lymphocytes/μl), the appearance of mature lymphocytes, and coexpression of CD19 and CD5 antigens. The disease is slowly progressive and results in an accumulation of small lymphocytes.

Clinical Manifestations

Frequently, patients are found incidentally to have lymphocytosis. Approximately 80% have lymphadenopathy and 50% have splenomegaly or hepatomegaly. Patients may complain of fatigue or recurrent infections. CLL has been associated with autoimmune hemolytic anemia, autoimmune thrombocytopenia, and red cell aplasia. When the disease manifests as a lymphoma, the patient will most likely have asymptomatic lymphadenopathy.

The Rai staging system for CLL is used in determining prognosis (Linker, 2000; Wetzler, Byrd, and Bloomfield, 2001):

Stage 0: Lymphocytosis only in blood and marrow
Stage I: Lymphocytosis plus lymphadenopathy
Stage II: Lymphocytosis, lymphadenopathy, and organomegaly
Stage III: Lymphocytosis and anemia
Stage IV: Thrombocytopenia
The Binet staging system is also used:
A: Fewer than three areas of lymphadenopathy, no thrombocytopenia or anemia
B: Three or more involved areas of lymphadenopathy without anemia or thrombocytopenia
C: Hemoglobin level less than or equal to 10 g/dl and/or platelet count lower than 100,000/μl
Stage A is associated with a survival time of longer than 10 years; stage B, with a survival time of approximately 7 years; and stage C, with a survival time of approximately 2 years (Armitage and Longo, 2001).

Patients with stage 0 disease are at low risk and have a median life expectancy of more than 10 years after diagnosis. For those with stage I or II disease (intermediate risk), the median decreases to 7 years, and for those with stage III or IV disease (high risk), the median survival time is 1.5 years.

The disease is manifested by organ infiltration with immunodeficient lymphocytes, immunosuppression, and bone marrow failure. Clinical manifestations are typically related to these factors (Linker, 2000).

Diagnosis

Typical B-cell CLL is diagnosed when there is an increase in circulating lymphocytes (more than 4×10^9/L) that are monoclonal B cells displaying the CD5 antigen. Bone marrow infiltration by these cells confirms the diagnosis. If the patient has lymphadenopathy, lymph node biopsy specimens show small-lymphocyte lymphoma.

Typical B-cell CLL may be identified during a routine complete blood count. The white blood cell count is typically more than 20,000/μl, and the majority of those are lymphocytes. The lymphocytes are small and immature and may infiltrate the bone marrow as well. Hematocrit and platelet counts are typically normal initially.

Treatment

Most cases of CLL are identified at stage 0 and do not require treatment. If sufficient normal blood cells are present and the patient is asymptomatic, no treatment is generally required in the intermediate stages. Patients with stages III or IV disease have bone marrow failure and need treatment.

The most commonly used treatment is chlorambucil 0.6 to 1.0 mg/kg orally every 3 weeks for 6 months. It is usually effective and has minimal side effects. Alternatively, fludarabine is given intravenously; it is associated with complete remission but causes immune suppression. Fludarabine is commonly used in young patients and as a second-line treatment in elderly patients. Individuals with lymphoma may be given chemotherapy: cyclophosphamide, vincristine, and prednisone. Young patients may also be treated with allogenic bone marrow transplant, although the procedure carries significant risk (Armitage and Longo, 2001). Refer to Chapter 27 for a discussion of the details of cancer treatment.

LYMPHOMA
Pathophysiology

Lymphomas are characterized by the massive proliferation of lymphocytes, histiocytes, and their precursors and derivatives. The three primary types of lymphomas are B-cell and T-cell lymphomas (non-Hodgkin's disease) and Hodgkin's disease. Subtypes of these are categorized into prognostic groups (Mansen and McCance, 2002).

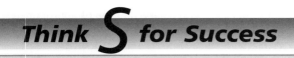

Hodgkin's Disease

The cell from which Hodgkin's disease originates is uncertain. However, most likely it is the B cell. Hodgkin's lymphoma is a group of cancers that are distinguished by the presence of Reed-Sternberg cells among benign host inflammatory cells. Ages of peak incidence of Hodgkin's disease are the twenties and the eighties. In the United States, those in the younger age group typically have nodular sclerosing Hodgkin's disease. Older patients, people living in Third World countries, and those with human immunodeficiency virus infection usually have mixed-cell Hodgkin's disease or lymphocyte-depleted Hodgkin's disease. Correlations have been made between infection with human immunodeficiency virus or Epstein-Barr virus and the development of Hodgkin's disease. Patients with primary or secondary immunodeficiency are predisposed to acquiring the disease (Armitage and Longo, 2001).

Non-Hodgkin's Disease

Non-Hodgkin's lymphoma is a term given to a group of cancers that are highly variable in course and presentation but that do not display Reed-Sternberg cells. Several environmental factors have been associated with non-Hodgkin's disease, such as chemical and infectious agents and medical treatments. Agricultural chemicals and treatment for Hodgkin's disease are associated with development of non-Hodgkin's lymphoma (Armitage and Longo, 2001).

Clinical Manifestations

The course and clinical presentation of lymphomas are highly variable. Patients whose disease takes an indolent (but incur-

able) course have isolated or widespread painless lymphadenopathy. Bone marrow involvement is typically high, and the disease is disseminated throughout the body. Persons with intermediate- and high-grade lymphomas often have weight loss, drenching night sweats, fever in the absence of infection, adenopathy, and possibly pruritus. There may be splenomegaly and/or an abdominal mass. Lymphadenopathy may be extranodal or isolated. In Hodgkin's lymphoma, a unique symptom is lymph node tenderness after ingestion of alcohol (Linker, 2000).

In Hodgkin's lymphoma, the disease tends to disseminate in a systematic fashion to contiguous areas of lymph nodes and widespread invasion occurs late in the disease course. The patient may come to the health care provider with a large, painless (but occasionally painful) mass in the neck. A mediastinal mass may be apparent on radiography.

Individuals with non-Hodgkin's lymphoma typically have painless generalized or local lymphadenopathy, most frequently in the cervical, femoral, inguinal, or axillary regions. Extranodal sites include soft tissue, testes, nasopharynx, thyroid, gastrointestinal tract, and bone. Patients may complain of abdominal fullness, ascites, leg swelling, and back pain related to abdominal or retroperitoneal masses. Table 11-1 lists the clinical differences between Hodgkin's and non-Hodgkin's lymphomas.

Diagnosis

As with any lymphoid malignancy, the importance of a careful history taking and physical examination cannot be overstated. The history and physical examination significantly aid in determining the diagnosis, cause, and stage of the lymphoma. A complete blood count; blood chemistry studies; erythrocyte sedimentation rate; computed tomographic scans of the chest, pelvis, and abdomen; and lymph node and bone marrow biopsies are typical tests performed to diagnose Hodgkin's and non-Hodgkin's disease. In addition, in cases of suspected non-Hodgkin's disease, serum levels of lactate dehydrogenase and β_2-microglobulin are measured and serum protein electrophoresis is performed. Laboratory findings indicate thrombocytosis, leukocytosis, eosinophilia, an elevated erythrocyte sedimentation rate, and an elevated alkaline phosphatase level. A gallium scan may be used at the completion of therapy to detect abnormalities, assist in assigning an anatomic stage, and aid in the planning of continued treatment.

The Ann Arbor staging system (Box 11-3) is used to stage both non-Hodgkin's and Hodgkin's lymphomas. The prognosis of non-Hodgkin's lymphoma is determined by calculating the International Prognostic Index in Box 11-4.

Treatment
Hodgkin's Disease

Radiation treatment is the initial therapy for persons with low-risk stage IA and stage IIA Hodgkin's lymphoma. Most

Table 11-1   Clinical Differences Between Non-Hodgkin's and Hodgkin's Disease

Characteristic	Non-Hodgkin's	Hodgkin's
Nodal involvement	Multiple peripheral nodes Mesenteric nodes and Waldeyer's ring commonly involved	Localized to single axial group of nodes (i.e., cervical, mediastinal, paraaortic) Mesenteric nodes and Waldeyer's ring rarely involved
Spread	Noncontiguous	Orderly spread by contiguity
B symptoms*	Uncommon	Common
Extranodal involvement	Common	Rare
Extent of disease	Rarely localized	Often localized

From McCance KL, Huether SE: *Pathophysiology: the biologic basis for disease in adults and children,* ed 4, St Louis, 2002, Mosby.
*Fever, weight loss, night sweats.

patients (including those with stage IIIB and stage IV disease) are treated with chemotherapy (doxorubicin [Adriamycin], bleomycin, vincristine, and dacarbazine).

The prognosis for persons with either localized or disseminated disease is good. Patients with stage IA or IIA disease who receive radiation therapy have an excellent prognosis, and 10-year survival rates are higher than 80%. Persons with stages IIIB or IV disease have 5-year survival rates of 50% to 60%. Patients who are older have poorer prognoses. Patients who experience a recurrence of the disease after initial chemotherapy receive high-dose chemotherapy and autolo-

gous stem cell transplantation, which yields a 35% to 50% cure rate (Linker, 2000).

Non-Hodgkin's Disease

The indolent lymphomas are typically incurable, and patients are offered palliative treatment. Because most patients are asymptomatic, treatment may not be necessary for 1 to 3 years until the disease progresses. Initially, chlorambucil is given alone or in combination with cyclophosphamide, vincristine, and prednisone. Administration of an antibody against the B-cell surface antigen (CD20 rituximab) is effective for treatment of recurrent follicular lymphoma (22% of non-Hodgkin's lymphoma) (Wetzler, Byrd, and Bloomfield, 2001). Allogenic transplantation is sometimes used as a treatment for younger patients.

Box 11-3   Ann Arbor Staging System for Lymphoma

Stage I: Involvement of one lymph node region or lymphoid structure

Stage II: Involvement of two or more lymph node regions on same side of the diaphragm

Stage III: Involvement of lymphoid regions or structures on both sides of the diaphragm

Stage III1:   Subdiaphragmatic involvement limited to spleen, portal nodes, splenic hilar nodes, or celiac nodes

Stage III2:   Subdiaphragmatic involvement of paraaortic, mesenteric, or iliac nodes including structures in stage III

Stage IV: Involvement of extranodal site(s) beyond those designated as "E"; more than one extranodal deposit in any location; any involvement of liver or bone marrow

Stage A: No symptoms

Stage B: Unexplained weight loss of >10% body weight during 6 months prior to staging; unexplained, persistent, or recurrent fever with temperatures >38° C during previous month; recurrent drenching night sweats during the previous month

Stage E: Localized, solitary involvement of extralymphatic tissue, excluding liver and bone marrow

---

Box 11-4   International Prognostic Index for Non-Hodgkin's Lymphoma

■ Five clinical risk factors are identified.
 1. Age ≥60 years
 2. Elevated serum lactate dehydrogenase levels
 3. Ann Arbor stage III or IV
 4. Performance status ≥2 (ECOG) or ≤70 (Karnofsky index)
 5. More than one site of extranodal involvement
■ A number is tallied for each risk factor.
■ Patients are grouped based on type of lymphoma.
■ For diffuse large B-cell lymphoma:
 0 or 1 factor: low risk, 35% of cases; 5-year survival, 73%
 2 factors: low, intermediate risk, 27% of cases; 5-year survival, 51%
 3 factors: high, intermediate risk, 22% of cases; 5-year survival, 43%
 4 or 5 factors: high risk, 16% of cases; 5-year survival, 26%

Adapted from Armitage JO, Longo DL: In Braunwald E et al, editors: *Harrison's principles of internal medicine,* ed 15, New York, 2001, McGraw-Hill, pp 715-27.

Median survival of patients with indolent lymphoma is 6 to 8 years, because the disease ultimately becomes unresponsive to chemotherapy. Age over 60 years, increased serum lactate dehydrogenase level, advanced stage (III or IV), and poor performance status are associated with a poor prognosis (Linker, 2000).

Think S for Success

Symptoms
■ Manage constitutional symptoms as they arise and manage symptoms associated with chemotherapy, radiation, and bone marrow transplantation.

Sequelae
■ Prepare patient and family for prognosis and provide palliative care when appropriate.

Safety
■ Educate patient and family regarding susceptibility to infection and bleeding tendency.

Support/Services
■ Instruct patient and family regarding community resources and interpret tests and laboratory findings in an understandable way.

Satisfaction
■ Determine degree to which lymphoma is interfering with important aspects of patient's life and work with patient and family to develop a plan to maximize quality of life.
■ Assist patient, when appropriate, to prepare for impending death.

MULTIPLE MYELOMA
Pathophysiology

Multiple myeloma (MM) is characterized by the presence of clones of malignant plasma cells in the bone marrow, which results in dysfunctional immunoglobulin. The mature B cell or plasma cell becomes malignant and releases unusual amounts of immunoglobulin (typically immunoglobulin G and immunoglobulin A). Replacement of bone marrow with malignant plasma cells leads to anemia and bone marrow destruction, and consequently to bone pain and pathologic fractures. Hypercalcemia is usually present, and tumors of plasma cells may form and compress the spinal cord. Renal failure may also occur because of high paraprotein levels (immunoglobulin G, M, or A). Recurrent infections are common and can be associated with neutropenia and immunosuppression caused by chemotherapy (Linker, 2000).

There is speculation that exposure to heavy metal, rubber, textiles, petroleum, radiation, or chemicals may cause genetic damage that alters cell replication and allows uncontrolled cell growth. Viruses, other infectious agents, and drugs that stimulate chronic antigen reactions may affect and alter the immune response and cause the development of a malignant clone of plasma cells (Barrick and Mitchell, 2001).

The infiltration of bone marrow by malignant cells, the weakening of the bone structure by the production of M protein, and the release of osteoclast activating factor result in skeletal damage. Osteoclast activating factor causes bone damage and produces lytic lesions, hypercalcemia, and pathologic fractures. The ribs and back are commonly affected (Barrick and Mitchell, 2001).

Erythrocyte production decreases because of the proliferation of plasma cells in the bone marrow and a decrease in erythropoietin production related to renal insufficiency. Hyperviscosity syndrome occurs because plasma cell proteins coat red blood cells and cause them to move slowly and sluggishly. The patient may experience headaches, blurred vision, irritability, confusion, and drowsiness because of circulatory congestion (Barrick and Mitchell, 2001).

Excess plasma proteins, hyperviscosity, and hypercalcemia damage kidney function. The kidney is unable to adequately filter the excess of proteins, which causes inflammation, obstruction, fibrosis, and ultimately renal failure (Barrick and Mitchell, 2001).

Clinical Manifestations

MM typically occurs in adults in their 60s. Patients come to the health care provider with pallor, infection, anemia, soft tissue masses, and bone pain, especially in the ribs or back. Sometimes, the individual has a pathologic fracture. Hyperviscosity syndrome (mental status changes, visual changes, mucosal bleeding, vertigo, and nausea), renal failure, or spinal cord compression may be evident on presentation (Linker, 2000). Neurologic changes related to spinal cord compression or neuropathy may be present, and there may be indications of congestive heart failure or hepatomegaly.

Diagnosis

Routine determination of calcium and protein levels indicates hypercalcemia and proteinuria. Erythrocyte sedimentation rate may also be elevated (Linker, 2000). Bence Jones proteins appear in the urine in most patients with MM (Barrick and Mitchell, 2001). Red blood cell morphology is normal, as are platelet and neutrophil counts. The finding of a paraprotein on serum protein electrophoresis is characteristic of MM. Myeloma is distinguished by spikes in immunoglobulin G level of more than 3.5 g/dl and in immunoglobulin A level of more than 2 g/dl. Withholding treatment initially to determine whether the paraproteinemia is benign or malignant may be helpful and is not detrimental to the patient (Linker, 2000). Box 11-5 lists tests used in the diagnosis of MM.

The bone marrow is infiltrated by plasma cells, which may or may not appear abnormal. Bone radiographs show lytic lesions in the spine, proximal long bones, and skull, or generalized osteoporosis (Linker, 2000). Box 11-6 presents the myeloma staging system.

Box 11-5   Diagnostic Tests for Multiple Myeloma

- Complete blood count with differential
- Platelet count
- Comprehensive metabolic panel
- Quantitative immunoglobulin levels
- Serum protein electrophoresis
- Immunofixation and quantification of M protein
- 24-hour urine collection for urine protein electrophoresis
- Plasma cell labeling index
- B$_2$-microglobulin level
- C-reactive protein level
- Bone marrow aspiration and biopsy
- Skeletal survey
- Computed tomography to evaluate for bone involvement

Adapted from Barrick MC, Mitchell SA: Multiple myeloma, *Am J Nurs* (suppl):6-12, 2001.

Box 11-6   Myeloma Staging System

STAGE I
- All of the following criteria are present:
  Hemoglobin level >10 g/dl
  Serum calcium level normal, <12 mg/dl
  Normal bone structure with or without solitary bone plasmacytoma
  Low M protein production rates
  Immunoglobulin G <5 g/dl
  Immunoglobulin A <3 g/dl
  Urine light-chain M protein component on electrophoresis <4 g/24 hr

STAGE II
- Fits neither criteria stage I nor stage III criteria

STAGE III
- One or more of the following is present:
  Hemoglobin level <8.5 g/dl
  Serum calcium level >12 g/dl
  High M protein production rates
- Immunoglobulin G >7 g/dl
- Immunoglobulin A >5 g/dl
- Urine light-chain M protein component on electrophoresis >12 g/24 hr

SUBCLASSIFICATION A
- Relatively normal renal function; serum creatinine level <2.0 mg/dl

SUBCLASSIFICATION B
- Abnormal renal function; serum creatinine level >2.0 mg/dl

Adapted from Salmon SE et al: Plasma cell neoplasms. In DeVita VT, editor: *Cancer principles and practice of oncology*, ed 5, Philadelphia, 1997, Lippincott, pp 1984-2013.

Treatment

The treatment goal for MM is to provide palliative and supportive care. Observation without treatment is frequently the choice in cases with minimal involvement or a questionable diagnosis. However, bone pain and other symptoms often require treatment on presentation. Clinical trials have established that high-dose chemotherapy and autologous stem cell transplantation is more effective than conventional therapy (Zaidi and Vesole, 2001). This treatment may also be used in patients who have experienced a relapse. A marker for the effectiveness of therapy is the height of the paraprotein spike seen in serum protein electrophoresis. Ancillary treatment includes radiation to palliate bone pain or to destroy a tumor that is contributing to pathologic fracture (Linker, 2000).

Chemotherapy is used to treat older patients, those who are symptomatic, and those with stage II or III disease. Melphalan and prednisone (orally) or vincristine, doxorubicin, and dexamethasone (central line administration) may be given. Autologous or allogenic transplant of stem cells accompanied by high-dose chemotherapy holds promise for achieving long-term remission. Other therapies that are undergoing testing are interferon alpha and thalidomide as an adjunct to chemotherapy (Barrick and Mitchell, 2001). Currently, the median survival rate for persons with MM is 3 years (Linker, 2000). A study of patients with MM of the spine found that surgical treatment significantly increased neurologic function and quality of life in the cases studied (Durr et al, 2002). Refer to Chapter 27 for a detailed discussion of cancer therapy.

Think S for Success

Symptoms
- Manage bone pain and symptoms associated with anemia with medication, rest, and protection (to avoid pathologic fracture and bleeding).

Sequelae
- Prevent pathologic fracture, infections, and bleeding by protecting bones and avoiding exposure to infection.

Safety
- Teach family how to move patient to avoid fracture.

Support/Services
- Provide palliative care and assist patient and family to use financial, medical, and community resources to maximize quality of care and life quality.

Satisfaction
- Assist patient and family in prioritizing activities that are meaningful to them and in developing a plan to attain optimal quality of life despite limitations of the disease.

INTERDISCIPLINARY CARE

Interdisciplinary care for persons with leukemia, lymphoma, and MM is largely the same. Most of the medical literature regarding these diseases focuses on drug therapy and transplantation. Consequently, the nurse's role is evident. Literature regarding the role of therapists and other health care providers, however, is not as easy to find. Specialists in all of the disciplines involved should work together toward a common goal of achieving and maintaining an optimal and maximal quality of life for the patient and family. Refer to Chapter 27 for a discussion of the management of fatigue, a common symptom experienced by persons with a chronic blood disease.

Nurse

The nurse not only provides direct care to the patient but also provides supportive care to the patient and family (Box 11-7). The nurse may be the first-line health care provider to identify that the individual has a chronic blood disease. In addition, the nurse carries out the treatment of the patient and observes for and reports complications. Most persons with chronic blood diseases are immunosuppressed because of pancytopenia. The nurse observes for signs and symptoms of infection, treats infection, and educates patients and families about preventing unnecessary exposure to infection. The nurse becomes involved if the patient experiences renal dysfunction or failure and needs hydration, electrolyte replacement, or dialysis.

In addition, the nurse is involved in pain management for individuals with leukemia, lymphoma, or myeloma. Development of pain varies according to the disease and its course. Correct use of analgesics and other pain management strategies is taught to the patient and family. Transplantation surgery requires preoperative, perioperative, and postoperative nursing care (Barrick and Mitchell, 2001).

In the home setting, the nurse assists the caregiver in maintaining and using central venous catheters and administering hyperalimentation infusions. The nurse may transfuse platelets or blood in the home setting. Chemotherapy and epoetin alfa (Epogen) injections may also be provided in the home (Ignatavicius and Workman, 2002). Refer to Chapter 27 for other aspects of nursing care for patients with cancer.

Primary Provider (Physician/Nurse Practitioner)

The physician, physician assistant, and advanced practice nurse are involved in many facets of patient care. They diagnose the disease and prescribe treatment and may be involved in research on the pathophysiology, etiology, and treatment of chronic blood diseases. Blood work and other laboratory studies are performed periodically to ascertain if the disease has progressed and guide changes in therapy as needed.

Physical and Occupational Therapists

Fatigue is a major symptom of chronic blood diseases. Physical and occupational therapists provide exercises for the patient to increase strength and maximize endurance. They educate the patient, family, and caregivers about how to assist the patient during functional activities to prevent pathologic fractures. Prescription and fitting of orthotics and assistive or adaptive devices may be needed to relieve bone pain and pain associated with vertebral collapse. In addition, therapists teach the patient energy conservation measures and techniques to optimize physical safety and quality of life.

Dietitian

The dietitian helps the patient to maximize energy by educating the patient about high-protein diets (unless the patient is in renal failure) that are rich in folic acid and vitamins. An anemic patient may need to incorporate more iron into the diet. In addition, the dietitian can help the family design a diet plan that includes foods that will stimulate the patient's appetite to prevent weight loss and to enhance quality of life.

Medical Social Worker and Psychologist

The medical social worker (MSW) or psychologist may provide counseling to the patient and family, especially when the disease reaches a stage during which only palliative care is offered and cure is unlikely. The MSW may assist the patient and family to work through potential ethical issues relevant to the disease (Box 11-8). The patient and family members may become depressed and suicidal because of hopelessness. The patient may feel that the pain cannot be relieved adequately, and quality of life and the will to live may sharply decline. The MSW or psychologist helps the patient to deal with changes in role, self-image,

---

Box 11-7   Family and Caregiver Issues

■ Acceptance that patient has less energy than previously
■ Adaptation to changing role of patient in family or system
■ Adaptation to change in relationship with patient as patient becomes more ill
■ Definition of family and/or caregiver role in patient care
■ Need for respite from caregiving role

Box 11-8   Ethical Issues

■ Treatment versus palliative care
■ Participation in experimental treatment
■ Allogenic versus autologous transplant

and lifestyle and helps the patient and family to cope with the patient's impending death from the disease (Box 11-9).

In addition, the MSW assists the patient in finding resources to allow the patient to remain in his or her home as long as possible or in making a transition to a long-term care facility. The MSW may locate resources for skilled home care services, food, and medicine.

Box 11-9   End-of-Life Issues

■ Readiness of patient and family to accept incurability of disease
■ Preparation for death of patient by patient and family
■ Preparation of advance directive
■ Use of hospice services

CASE STUDY*

Patient Data

Mrs. W. is a 36-year-old elementary school teacher. She comes to the outpatient clinic with complaints of worsening fatigue, easy satiety, a loss of 10 lb during the last 2 months, and left upper quadrant abdominal fullness. Her medical history is not remarkable. She reports no nausea, vomiting, diarrhea, fever, hematemesis, or night sweats. She does not take any medications. She has a history of regular menses with bleeding that is not excessive. Her maternal grandfather had diabetes mellitus, but otherwise her family medical history is not significant. Mrs. W. is married, has three healthy children, and works full time. She does not smoke or use alcohol, and reports no recent travel.

Physical Examination

■ Vital signs are within normal limits.
■ No acute distress is present.
■ No thyromegaly is present.
■ Lungs are clear.
■ Cardiac examination is normal.
■ Abdomen is normal without hepatomegaly, tenderness, or rigidity. The spleen is palpable 9 cm below the costal margin.
■ There is no lymphadenopathy.
■ No lower extremity edema is noted.
■ Skin is warm and moist.
■ Neurologic examination shows no focal deficits, cranial nerves are all grossly intact, and there is normal musculoskeletal strength.

Laboratory Findings

■ White blood count: 120,000/mm^3
■ Hemoglobin: 11 g/dl
■ Platelet count: 473,000/mm^3
■ Serum electrolyte levels: urea, creatinine levels normal
■ Lactate dehydrogenase and uric acid levels: normal
■ Vitamin B$_{12}$ and leukocyte alkaline phosphatase levels: normal
■ Peripheral blood smear: granulocytic cells at various stages of maturation
■ Karyotype from bone marrow biopsy: translocation between chromosomes 9 and 22 (Philadelphia chromosome)

Thinking It Through

■ Based on these data, what is the medical diagnosis?
■ What nursing diagnoses apply to Mrs. W.'s condition as she appears today?
■ How can the health care team contribute to Mrs. W.'s quality of life?
■ What are Mrs. W.'s concerns likely to be? How would you address them?
■ What can you tell Mrs. W. about her prognosis and the possible effects of the illness on her lifestyle?

Case Conference

The interdisciplinary team has gathered to discuss Mrs. W.'s case. The team consists of Mr. and Mrs. W., the family nurse practitioner (FNP), the registered nurse (RN), the MSW, and the hematologist. The FNP explains that, once she had performed the physical examination and obtained Mrs. W.'s preliminary laboratory results she deduced that leukemia might be a likely diagnosis and referred Mrs. W. to the hematologist. Although Mrs. W. will see the hematologist for monitoring and treatment for the CML, Mrs. W. will still be a patient of the clinic and the FNP will remain her primary care provider.

The hematologist explains that he ordered the peripheral blood immunophenotyping, the bone marrow biopsy, and cytogenic analysis to determine exactly what type of leukemia Mrs. W. has. Based on the results, he has concluded that she has chronic myelogenous leukemia (CML). Mrs. W. had come to the clinic in the chronic phase but with symptoms of abdominal fullness, fatigue, early satiety, anorexia, and weight loss with left upper quadrant discomfort. The splenomegaly, he explains, is a hallmark finding of CML. Because Mrs. W. does not have lymphadenopathy, she is not in the blastic phase (acute) of the disease.

The RN comments that she had been reading about CML and found out that the chronic phase typically lasts 4 to 5 years before the disease becomes more aggressive and eventually transforms into the blastic phase. The hematologist agrees and explains that the goal of treatment during the chronic phase is to control the progression of the disease and its symptoms. This is done with selected medications. However, Mrs. W. may be a candidate for bone marrow transplantation. Mr. W. immediately remarks, "I will donate my bone marrow right now. Let's do it!" The hematologist explains that attempts must first be made to find a matched sibling before nonblood relatives will be considered.

The MSW asks the W.'s if they feel that they could use some counseling to help them deal with the diagnosis and to help them decide whether they want to pursue the transplant option. She also states that she can help them find child care and people to help around the house until Mrs. W. feels better. She tells them that the entire team understands that this is a lot of information to digest. She encourages them to think about what has been said and to write down any questions that arise after the conference is over, and says that she will help make sure the questions get answered.

The nurse asks the W.'s if they have any questions now. Mrs. W. begins to cry and says that she feels "overwhelmed." The nurse puts an arm around her and gives her a tissue and repeats that there are several possible courses of action for treatment of

*Adapted from Archer TP, Kourlas PJ, Mazzaferri EL: Fatigue and abdominal fullness in a 36-year-old woman, *Hosp Pract* 33(3):141-2, 144-6, 1998.

CASE STUDY—cont'd

the disease. She suggests that she help Mrs. W. set up her next appointment to meet with the hematologist to discuss the possibility of transplantation in more detail.

■ Which details about CML should be discussed with the W.'s at this initial team meeting and which should be reserved for another time?

■ What are most likely to be the W.'s concerns in order of priority?

■ What kinds of resources can the team assist the W.'s in finding and using?

■ What barriers to care might exist?

■ Identify two collaborative problems that the plan of care should address.

Internet and Other Resources

Leukemia & Lymphoma Society: *www. leukemia.org;* telephone 800-955-4572; 1311 Mamaroneck Avenue, White Plains, NY 10605

Leukemia Research Foundation: *http://www.leukemia-research. org;* telephone 847-424-0600; 820 Davis St, Suite 420, Evanston, IL 60201

National Cancer Institute: *http://www.cancer.gov;* telephone 800-422-6237; Building 31, Room 10A24, Bethesda, MD 20892

REFERENCES

Armitage JO, Longo DL: Malignancies of lymphoid cells. In Braunwald E et al, editors: *Harrison's principles of internal medicine,* ed 15, New York, 2001, McGraw-Hill, pp 7215-727.

Barrick MC, Mitchell SA: Multiple myeloma, *Am J Nurs* (suppl):6-12, 2001.

Durr HR et al: Multiple myeloma: surgery of the spine, *Spine* 27(3):320-6, 2002.

Ignatavicius DD, Workman ML, editors: *Medical surgical nursing: critical thinking for collaborative care,* ed 4, Philadelphia, 2002, WB Saunders.

Linker CA: Blood. In Tierney LM, McPhee SJ, Papadakis MA, editors: *Current medical diagnosis and treatment,* New York, 2000, Lange Medical Books/McGraw-Hill, pp 499-552.

Lobert S: Research highlights: novel agents, *Oncol Nurs Forum* 28(10):1511, 2001.

Longo DL: Plasma cell disorders. In Braunwald E et al, editors: *Harrison's principles of internal medicine,* ed 15, New York, 2001, McGraw-Hill, pp 727-33.

Mansen TJ, McCance KL: Alterations of leukocyte, lymphoid, and hemostatic function. In McCance KL, Huether SE, editors: *Pathophysiology: the biologic basis for disease in adults and children,* ed 4, St Louis, 2002, Mosby, pp 865-99.

O'Mara AM, Whedon MB: Hematologic problems. In Lewis SM, Heitkemper MM, Dirksen SR, editors: *Medical-surgical nursing,* ed 5, St Louis, 2000, Mosby, pp 736-89.

Wetzler M, Byrd JC, Bloomfield CD: Acute and chronic myeloid leukemia. In Braunwald E et al, editors: *Harrison's principles of internal medicine,* ed 15, New York, 2001, McGraw-Hill, pp 706-27.

Zaidi AA, Vesole DH: Multiple myeloma: an old disease with new hope for the future, *CA Cancer J Clin* 51:273-85, 2001.

CHAPTER 12

Disorders of the Heart

Maryellen Zarnik Silva, MS, RN, CRNP

OBJECTIVES

After reading this chapter, you should be able to do the following:

- Describe the pathophysiology of angina, coronary artery disease (CAD), congestive heart failure (CHF), atrial fibrillation (AF), and valvular heart disease.
- Describe the clinical manifestations of angina, CAD, CHF, AF, and valvular heart disease.
- Describe the diagnostic testing associated with angina, CAD, CHF, AF, and valvular heart disease.
- Describe the indications for use, nursing considerations, and common side effects of medications used to treat angina, CAD, CHF, AF, and valvular heart disease.
- Describe the functional health patterns affected by angina, CAD, CHF, AF, and valvular heart disease.
- Describe the impact on the family and/or caregiver of the patient's angina, CAD, CHF, AF, or valvular heart disease.
- Describe the role of each member of the interdisciplinary team involved in the care of patients with disorders of the heart.
- Describe the ethical considerations and end-of-life issues associated with angina, CAD, CHF, AF, and valvular heart disease.

The chronic cardiac disorders discussed in this chapter are angina, coronary artery disease (CAD), congestive heart failure (CHF), atrial fibrillation (AF), and valvular heart disease. A comprehensive approach is used in examining each disorder. This information covers the pathophysiology, clinical manifestations, diagnostic testing, pharmacologic management, assessment of functional health patterns, impact of chronic cardiac disorders on the family and/or caregiver, and ethical considerations. An interdisciplinary case study is presented.

Chronic cardiac disorders develop from varying pathologic processes that affect the balance of oxygen supply and demand in the heart. The primary impact of these processes is seen throughout the structures of the heart.

ASSESSMENT

Not all patients with chronic cardiac disorders show the same clinical manifestations. Therefore, more than just the physical examination findings is required to determine the severity of the chronic cardiac disease with which the patient is diagnosed. The characteristic according to which all patients can be evaluated is the degree to which they can continue in their current functional health patterns. Box 12-1 is a framework for assessing functional health patterns for cardiac disorders.

ISCHEMIC HEART DISEASE

Despite a 26% decline in the incidence of ischemic heart disease (IHD) over the past 20 years, it remains the leading cause of death among men and women in every ethnic group (American Heart Association, 2003). IHD is responsible for approximately 1 million deaths each year. The annual costs associated with this disease are $51.6 billion (Gislason, 2002). The prevalence of IHD increases as age increases. Among those older than 60 years of age, 25% of all deaths of both men and women are attributed to IHD (Uphold and Graham, 1999). Box 12-2 describes ethnic differences in heart disease.

Pathophysiology

IHD is caused by decreased blood and oxygen supply to the heart muscle as a result of atherosclerotic plaque formation within the coronary arteries. Atherosclerotic plaque develops over many years through a process of lipid deposition within the blood vessels. The plaque creates a blockage within the coronary artery and results in ischemia. Ischemia leads to myocardial muscle cell damage that is reversible. However, there is a cascading effect on the heart from this process over time that can ultimately lead to myocardial infarction (MI), which results in irreversible myocardial muscle cell damage.

Atherosclerotic plaque narrows the coronary arteries. When diagnosed, this condition is referred to as CAD. A number of risk factors are associated with CAD. The modifiable risk factors include smoking, hypertension, obesity, diabetes mellitus, sedentary lifestyle, stress, and hypercholesterolemia. The nonmodifiable risk factors include age, gender (men are affected more than women until 60 years of age), race (African Americans are affected more than whites), and genetic predisposition (Lewis et al, 2002).

Box 12-1 Functional Health Pattern Assessment for Chronic Cardiac Disorders

HEALTH PERCEPTION/HEALTH MANAGEMENT
- Does the patient have a family history of ischemic heart disease?
- What is the patient's perception of his or her overall health?
- What medications, including over-the-counter drugs, does the patient take?
- What alternative therapies does the patient use?

NUTRITION/METABOLISM
- What is the patient's current weight? What is the patient's goal weight? Has there been a recent gain or loss of weight?
- Does the patient understand the diet appropriate for management of coronary artery disease (CAD)?
- What is the general condition of the skin?
- Is peripheral edema present?

ELIMINATION
- Have any changes occurred in bowel or bladder habits?
- Is the patient aware of the increased risk of incontinence because of the diuretic effects of selected cardiac medications?
- Does the patient experience periods of insomnia related to nocturia?

ACTIVITY/EXERCISE
- Does the patient experience shortness of breath or chest pain with exertion or increased fatigue after physical activity?
- Can the patient perform activities of daily living without experiencing symptoms?
- Can the patient function at work and remain symptom free?

SLEEP/REST
- How many hours of uninterrupted sleep does the patient get at night?
- How frequently does the patient take rest periods during daytime hours?
- What techniques does the patient use to decrease shortness of breath while in the supine position?
- Does the patient report awakening with chest pain or pressure?

COGNITION/PERCEPTION
- How does the patient describe the quality of CAD symptoms, including chest pain or pressure, shortness of breath, and diaphoresis? Where is the pain located? How long do the symptoms last?
- What actions does the patient take to alleviate symptoms?

SELF-PERCEPTION/SELF-CONCEPT
- What are the effects of CAD on body image?
- Does the patient have feelings of fear or loss of control related to ischemic heart disease?
- Does the patient experience depression related to the diagnosis?

ROLES/RELATIONSHIPS
- Is the patient employed?
- Does the patient have difficulty fulfilling responsibilities at home?
- How has the diagnosis of CAD affected the patient's family and/or caregivers?

SEXUALITY/REPRODUCTION
- Does the patient have concerns regarding sexual performance?
- Is the patient sexually active?
- Does the patient understand the effects of medications on libido?

COPING/STRESS TOLERANCE
- What support systems are available to the patient?
- Has the patient developed new strategies for coping with stress?
- Is the patient able to manage ischemic heart disease in the current living situation?

VALUES/BELIEFS
- What is important to the patient?
- What constitutes good quality of life for the patient?
- What are the patient's beliefs related to this condition?
- What are the patient's spiritual and cultural beliefs?
- To what extent do the patient's cultural/spiritual beliefs influence decision making related to this condition?

Box 12-2 Ethnic Differences in Coronary Artery Disease

- White middle-aged males have the highest incidence of CAD.
- African Americans have onset of CAD at an early age.
- African American women have a higher incidence of CAD than white women.
- African Americans have more severe CAD than whites.
- Native Americans younger than 35 years of age have heart disease mortality rates that are twice as high as those for other Americans.
- Hispanics have lower death rates from heart disease than non-Hispanics.
- Major modifiable cardiovascular risk factors for Native Americans are obesity and diabetes mellitus.

Clinical Manifestations

One of the most prominent symptoms associated with CAD is angina pectoris, which means "chest pain." Angina is intermittent, can be brought on by physical overexertion, is described by patients as a "tightness" or "pressure," can last from 3 to 5 minutes, and is generally relieved by rest or sublingual administration of nitroglycerin.

There are three types of angina. Stable angina most often occurs as a result of physical exertion. It is predictable and always shows the same pattern of symptoms, severity, and duration. The second type of angina is progressive angina. It is unpredictable and may occur at rest, and generally the patient experiences increasingly frequent episodes.

The third type of angina is referred to as Prinzmetal's angina, also known as variant angina. This type has a higher incidence in Japanese patients. Prinzmetal's angina was found in 20% to 30% of the Japanese population undergoing angiography for complaints of chest pain, whereas it was found in only 2% to 3% of the U.S. population undergoing cardiac catheterization for complaints of chest pain. Therefore, the patient's ethnic background should be considered in diagnosing the type of angina present.

Prinzmetal's angina occurs primarily at rest. The pathophysiology of this type of angina involves a coronary artery spasm in response to increased myocardial oxygen demand rather than an occlusion of the coronary artery from atherosclerotic plaque formation. A patient diagnosed with Prinzmetal's angina typically describes being awakened from sleep with chest tightness. The pain may even be relieved with physical movement.

Symptoms that may accompany any form of angina include diaphoresis; nausea; pain or sensations of pressure that radiate down the arms, up to the neck or jaw, or between the shoulder blades; shortness of breath; anxiety; and weakness.

Diagnosis

A decision to pursue diagnostic testing of a patient with suspected CAD is based on information obtained through a thorough history taking and physical examination. Significant findings in the patient's history include hyperlipidemia, hypertension, family history of lipid disorders or premature cardiovascular disease, tobacco usage, diabetes, sedentary lifestyle, and poor dietary choices. Based on the patient's responses and the findings of the physical examination, a series of diagnostic tests will be ordered by the physician. Table 12-1 lists diagnostic studies for CAD.

Table 12-1 Diagnostic Studies for Coronary Artery Disease

Study	Description and Purpose	Nursing Responsibility
Imaging Studies		
Chest radiograph	Patient is placed in two upright positions to examine the lung fields and size of the heart. The two common positions are posteroanterior and lateral. Heart size and contour in relation to the individual's age, sex, and size are noted.	Inquire about frequency of radiography in recent past and possibility of pregnancy. Provide lead shielding to areas not being viewed. Have patient remove any jewelry or metal objects that may obstruct the view of the heart and lungs
Electrocardiogram (ECG)	Electrodes are placed on the chest and extremities, allowing the ECG machine to record cardiac electrical activity from different views. ECG can reveal heart rhythm, activity of pacemaker, conduction abnormalities, position of heart, size of atria and ventricles, presence of injury, and previous myocardial infarction.	Inform patient that no discomfort is involved. Instruct patient to avoid moving to decrease motion artifact.
Holter monitoring	ECG rhythm is recorded for 24-48 hr and then rhythm changes are correlated with symptoms recorded in diary. Normal patient activity is encouraged to simulate conditions that produce symptoms. Electrodes are placed on chest and a recorder is used to store information until it is recalled, printed, and analyzed for any rhythm disturbance. Procedure can be performed on an inpatient or outpatient basis.	Prepare skin and apply electrodes and leads. Explain importance of keeping an accurate diary of activities and symptoms. Tell patient that no bath or shower can be taken during monitoring. Skin irritation may develop from electrodes.
Exercise treadmill test	Various protocols are used to evaluate the effect of exercise tolerance on myocardial function. A common protocol uses 3-min segments at set speeds and elevations of the treadmill belt. Continual monitoring of vital signs and ECG rhythms for ischemic changes are important in the diagnosis of left ventricular function and coronary artery disease. An exercise bike may be used if the patient is unable to walk on the treadmill.	Instruct patient to wear comfortable clothes and shoes that can be used for walking and running. Instruct patient about procedure and lead placement. Monitor vital signs and obtain 12-lead ECG before exercise and until all vital signs and ECG changes have returned to normal. Monitor patient's symptoms throughout procedure.

Continued

Table 12-1   Diagnostic Studies for Coronary Artery Disease—cont'd

Study	Description and Purpose	Nursing Responsibility
Imaging Studies—cont'd		
Two-dimensional echocardiogram	Transducer that emits and receives ultrasonic waves is placed in four positions on the chest above the heart. Transducer records sound waves that are bounced off the heart. It also records direction and flow of blood through the heart and transforms it to audio and graphic data to measure valvular abnormalities, congenital cardiac defects, wall motion, and cardiac function.	Place patient in a supine position on left side facing equipment. Instruct family and patient about procedure and sensations (pressure and mechanical movement from head of transducer). No contraindications to procedure exist.
Nuclear cardiology	Thallium imaging, most often combined with exercise testing, involves IV injection of a radioactive isotope. Radioactive uptake of the isotope is measured over the heart by scintillation camera. The test supplies information about myocardial contractility, myocardial perfusion, and acute cell injury.	Explain procedure to patient. Establish IV line for injection of isotope. Explain that radioactive isotope used is a small, diagnostic amount and will lose most of its radioactivity in a few hours. Inform patient that he or she will be lying still on back with arms extended overhead for 20 min. Repeat scans are performed within a few minutes to hours after the injection.
Cardiac catheterization	Catheter is inserted into heart. Information can be obtained about O_2 saturation and pressure readings can be taken within chambers. Contrast medium is injected to assist in examining structure and motion of heart. Procedure is done by insertion of catheter into a vein (for right side of heart) or an artery (for left side of heart).	Before procedure, obtain written permission. Check for iodine sensitivity. Withhold food and fluids for 6-18 hr before procedure. Give sedative, if ordered. Inform patient about use of local anesthesia, insertion of catheter, and feeling of warmth and fluttering sensation of heart as catheter is passed. Note that patient may be instructed to cough or take a deep breath when catheter is inserted and that patient is monitored by ECG throughout procedure.
Laboratory Studies		
Complete blood count	Helpful in diagnosing infectious heart disease and myocardial infarction Normal RBCs: 4.7-6.1 million/mm³ (men); 4.2-5.4 million/mm³ (women) Normal WBCs: 5000-10,000/mm³	RBCs are increased with inadequate tissue oxygenation, decreased in subacute endocarditis and in some congenital heart disease with right-to-left shunt. WBCs are increased in acute and chronic heart inflammations and in acute myocardial infarction.
Comprehensive metabolic profile	A group of 14 tests that gauge the current status of kidney and liver, and electrolyte and acid-base balance as well as blood glucose and blood protein levels. Used in combination with other specific tests to confirm or rule out a diagnosis and to monitor known conditions.	Fasting 10-12 hr before the test is preferred.
Cholesterol profile	Cholesterol is a blood lipid. Elevated cholesterol level is considered a risk factor for atherosclerotic heart disease.	Explain procedure to patient. Cholesterol levels can be obtained in a nonfasting state, but for triglyceride levels and lipoproteins, fasting for at least 12 hr (except for water) is necessary, and no alcohol intake is allowed for 24 hr before testing.

Table 12-1   Diagnostic Studies for Coronary Artery Disease—cont'd

Study	Description and Purpose	Nursing Responsibility
Laboratory Studies—cont'd Cholesterol profile—cont'd	Level can be measured at any time of day in a nonfasting state. Normal: 140-200 mg/dl (3.62-5.17 mmol/L); level varies with age and sex. Triglycerides are mixtures of fatty acids. Elevations are associated with cardiovascular cardiovascular disease. Normal: 40-190 mg/dl (0.45-2.15 mmol/L); level varies with age) Lipoproteins are separated by electrophoresis into HDLs, LDLs, and VLDLs and chylomicrons. Marked day-to-day fluctuations are seen in serum lipid levels. More than one determination is needed for accurate diagnosis and treatment. Normal: varies with age. Desirable LDL is <130 mg/dl. Desirable HDL is 37-70 mg/dl (men) and 40-88 mg/dl (women).	Cardiac risk is assessed by dividing the total cholesterol level by the HDL level.
Thyroid-stimulating hormone level	Test used to rule out symptoms of thyroid disorder.	
Homocysteine level	Homocysteine is an amino acid produced by the normal breakdown of proteins in the body. Test is used to assess risk of heart disease, stroke, and reduced blood flow to the hands and feet.	
High-sensitivity C-reactive protein level	Test is used to predict risk of heart disease.	Level may be measured in apparently healthy patients to determine if they are at risk for a coronary event, even if lipid levels are normal or borderline elevated.

HDL, High-density lipoprotein; *IV,* intravenous; *LDL,* low-density lipoprotein; *RBC,* red blood cell; *VLDL,* very low density lipoprotein; *WBC,* white blood cell.

Interdisciplinary Care

The goals of care for patients diagnosed with cardiac disease are to achieve lifestyle and risk factor modification, to ensure adherence to the prescribed medication regimen, to ensure adequate patient knowledge regarding disease progression, and to eliminate pain. These goals are complex and can be overwhelming to the patient and caregivers alike. To provide more comprehensive management of cardiac disease, a teaching approach should be used. Because the interdisciplinary care is similar for all cardiac disorders, the team will be similar to that for cardiac rehabilitation as described later in the chapter. In the community the team may include the primary physician, cardiologist, pharmacist, office nursing staff, skilled nursing staff for home visits, case managers, social workers, specialists in behavioral interventions, and respiratory therapists.

The case manager is the coordinator for the interdisciplinary team. Frequently the case manager is employed by the insurance company to ensure comprehensive, cost-effective care. The case manager may arrange for therapies to take place in the home or in an outpatient setting, approve home care equipment and services, and monitor the patient's progress. The case manager is also responsible for patient education and maintenance of communication among the multiple providers caring for the patient. In the absence of a case manager, the primary care provider, a nurse, or a family member may take on the role of coordinating the patient's many services.

The respiratory therapist determines the most appropriate form of oxygen delivery based on consumption and tolerance for various delivery methods. As cardiac disease progresses or improves, the oxygen requirements change and require reevaluation.

Drug interactions are frequent, and therapeutic ranges and tolerances can be narrow, especially in the elderly. Pharmacists are frequently involved in titrating medications or making recommendations for alternate medications.

The primary care provider oversees the well-being of the whole patient by coordinating treatment by multiple specialists, monitoring laboratory results, initiating referrals to the cardiologist, and writing orders for various services such as nursing, respiratory therapy, and occupational therapy. The cardiologist is primarily responsible for prescribing cardiac medications, monitoring cardiac function, ordering specific cardiac tests, and coordinating with other specialists as required.

Because the interdisciplinary team is similar for all cardiac disorders, a comprehensive look at the contributions of the different specialties to cardiac care is reserved for the section on cardiac rehabilitation at the end of the chapter (see p. 177).

Drug Therapy

A multidrug regimen best serves the patient with CAD. Long-acting nitrates such as the nitroglycerin patch provide vasodilation to the coronary arteries. During acute anginal attacks, patients use various formulations of short-acting nitrates such as sublingual nitroglycerin. The β-blockers are efficacious in preventing angina as well as in decreasing the heart rate to reduce cardiac workload. Calcium channel blockers also produce coronary artery vasodilation, decrease the heart rate, and aid in the prevention of coronary artery vasospasm.

Antiplatelet medications are the mainstay of treatment for patients with CAD. Aspirin prevents platelet plug formation in the arteries. Its use is indicated for CAD because it decreases the viscosity of blood, and as a result the blood is less likely to form a clot. The side effects of aspirin are the potential for bleeding, bruising, nausea, and gastrointestinal upset. Nursing considerations include teaching the patient to monitor for large areas of bruising, to be aware of the risk for injury in using sharp objects, and to consult a physician before taking over-the-counter analgesics.

Angiotensin-converting enzyme (ACE) inhibitors are in the forefront of treatment for CAD, specifically for patients who have experienced an acute MI. ACE inhibitors prevent ventricular remodeling and slow the progression of late heart failure (Lewis, Collier, and Heitkemper, 2002). ACE inhibitors are effective in reducing the risk of renal failure for patients with hypertension, kidney disease, and diabetes mellitus.

The remaining category of medications used in the treatment of chronic CAD is the antihyperlipidemic agents. The most commonly prescribed drugs in this category are β-hydroxy-β-methylglutaryl–coenzyme A reductase inhibitors. These medications help to reduce the total cholesterol and low-density lipoprotein levels and prevent the formation of atherosclerotic plaque (Deedy, 2002).

Drugs in this category are detoxified in the liver. As a result, liver function studies must be performed frequently.

The side effects of this class of drug are gastrointestinal upset, headaches, rash, and generalized pruritus. Nursing considerations include teaching the patient to take this medication at night, monitoring the frequency of liver function testing, and inquiring as to side-effect tolerance.

Nitrates, β-blockers, calcium channel blockers, and ACE inhibitors are used in treating CAD and also in the management of hypertension. Refer to Table 13-3 for the mechanisms of action, side effects, and nursing considerations for these medications.

Risk Factor Modification

Diabetes, hypertension, stress, obesity, and smoking can contribute the development of IHD. The first four of these risk factors can best be controlled through an appropriate diet, exercise, weight loss, adherence to medication regimen, and timely follow-up with the physician. Table 12-2 provides a detailed outline for dietary management of CAD.

Smoking cessation is difficult for almost all patients. Pharmaceutical measures are available that can contribute to the success of smoking cessation; however, it is the nurse's role to educate the patient regarding the effects of smoking on the development of IHD. Research has also shown that those who join a support group for smoking cessation are more likely to succeed in this venture (Deedy, 2002).

Nursing Considerations

Chronic home management of the patient with CAD or angina, or after MI is multifactorial. The primary role of the nurse is twofold: to assess and to educate the patient. The nursing assessment of a patient living with chronic CAD focuses on the patient's adjustment to the home environment and his or her ability to function. Initially, a nurse should assess what knowledge the patient has gained regarding the diagnosis of IHD. Then the nurse can target teaching to specific areas in which better comprehension is needed.

Nurses monitor the actions of medications and any adverse reactions to them, assist in developing a medication administration plan to promote better adherence, evaluate signs and symptoms of disease progression, and coordinate help from those in other medical disciplines, such as physical therapy, to aid in holistic care as needed.

Another important aspect to consider before educating the patient is the psychological impact that IHD can have on the patient. Patients experience a vast array of emotions when diagnosed with CAD. Feelings experienced by men with IHD start with disbelief and fear about the diagnosis, and progress to awareness of mortality, a feeling of loss of control of self, and heightened awareness of belief in a higher power. As men undergo treatment for IHD, they start to resign themselves to acceptance of necessary changes and ultimately view themselves as receiving a second chance (Keaton and Pierce, 2000).

Some evidence suggests that women experience cardiac symptoms differently from men. Women are less likely to seek assistance when first experiencing symptoms. They are less likely to receive assistance after being diagnosed with MI. They also experience different psychological consequences. Women are more concerned with who will provide care for their families. According to the American Heart Association's 2003 Statistical Fact Sheet, a greater percentage

Table 12-2 Dietary Recommendations for Coronary Artery Disease

Comparison of Step 1 Low-Fat Diet and Step 2 Low-Fat Diet

Principles of Step 1 Diet

8% to 10% of total calories come from saturated fat; ≤30% of total calories come from fat.

- Visible fat (e.g., butter, cream, margarine, salad dressing, cooking oil) is restricted to 1 tsp per meal.
- Unsaturated vegetable oils should be used.
- Only lean meats, skim milk or 1% milk, and no more than 3 egg yolks per week are used.
- High-fat foods (e.g., avocados, fat, meat, olives, nuts) are avoided.
- Cooking methods such as steaming, baking, broiling, grilling, or stir-frying in small amounts of fat are recommended.

Principles of Step 2 Diet

<7% of total calories come from saturated fat; ≤30% of total calories come from fat.

- Only the leanest cuts of meat are allowed.
- Organ meats and shrimp are restricted because they are high in cholesterol although low in total fat.
- Only 1 egg yolk per week is used because egg yolk is high in cholesterol. Egg whites or egg substitutes may be used as desired.
- Vegetable oils are used in cooking and food preparation. Coconut and palm oils are not allowed because of their high content of saturated fat. Margarine that contains ≤2 g of saturated fat per tablespoon is used.
- Skim milk is highly recommended. Low-fat yogurt and low-fat cheeses may be used. Low-fat ice milk or frozen yogurt or sherbet is allowed.

Sample Menus

Nutritional Exchange	Step 1			Step 2		
	Sample Meal 1	Sample Meal 2	Sample Meal 3	Sample Meal 1	Sample Meal 2	Sample Meal 3
Breakfast						
1 fruit	½ cup orange juice	1 banana	¼ cantaloupe	½ cup orange juice	1 banana	¼ cantaloupe
1 starch	¾ cup dry cereal	½ cup corn meal mush	½ cup corn meal mush	¾ cup dry cereal	½ cup oatmeal	½ cup corn meal mush
3 eggs/wk	1 poached egg	1 flour tortilla	1 scrambled egg	Low-cholesterol egg	1 corn tortilla with	1 slice toast with
1 fat	1 slice toast with	1 cup skim milk	1 slice toast with	1 slice toast with	1 tsp special	1 tsp special
1 skim milk	1 tsp butter or	Coffee with 1 tsp	1 tsp butter or	1 tsp special	vegetable oil	vegetable
	margarine	cream	margarine	vegetable oil	margarine	oil margarine
	1 cup skim milk		1 cup skim milk	margarine	1 cup skim milk	1 cup skim milk
	Coffee with sugar		Coffee with sugar	1 cup skim milk	Coffee with sugar	Coffee with sugar
				Coffee with sugar		

Continued

Table 12-2 Dietary Recommendations for Coronary Artery Disease—cont'd

Sample Menus—cont'd

Nutritional Exchange	Step 1			Step 2		
	Sample Meal 1	Sample Meal 2	Sample Meal 3	Sample Meal 1	Sample Meal 2	Sample Meal 3
Lunch						
2 meat	2 oz baked chicken	3 oz lean hamburger	2 oz baked fish	3 oz baked chicken (skinless)	¾ cup dry cottage cheese with peach slices	4 oz baked fish
2 starch	Mashed potato	Hamburger bun	Baked potato	Mashed potato with 1 tsp special vegetable oil margarine	Saltine crackers	Fried potatoes (cooked with allowed oils)
1 vegetable	Tossed salad with vinegar, lemon juice	Lettuce, tomato, pickle,	Zucchini	Tossed salad with vinegar, vegetable oil	Cucumber and tomato slices	Zucchini
1 starch	1 slice bread with	1 tsp mustard	1 slice bread with	Angel food cake	1 tsp special vegetable oil	1 slice cornbread (made with allowed oils)
1 fat	1 tsp margarine or butter	Sherbet	1 tsp butter or margarine	Iced tea with sugar and lemon	Sherbet	Gelatin dessert
1 dessert	Angel food cake	Carbonated beverage	Gelatin dessert		Carbonated beverage	Lemonade
	Iced tea with sugar and lemon		Lemonade			
Dinner						
2 meat	2 oz lean roast beef	Green chili stew (made with 2 oz lean beef cubes, potato slices, tomato, chili)	2 oz lean pork chop	2 oz lean roast beef	Green chili stew (made with 2 oz lean beef cubes, potato slices, tomato, chili)	3 oz breaded lean pork chop
2 starch	Rice	1 flour tortilla	Okra	Rice with 1 tsp special vegetable oil margarine	1 corn tortilla with	Corn on the cob with 1 tsp special vegetable oil margarine
1 vegetable	Green beans	Pudding (made from skim milk and egg whites)	Corn on the cob	Green beans	1 tsp special vegetable oil margarine	Okra
1 fat	Dinner roll with 1 tsp butter or margarine	Fruit punch	1 slice bread with 1 tsp margarine or butter	Dinner roll with 1 tsp special vegetable oil margarine	Pudding (made from skim milk and egg whites)	Biscuit (made with allowed oils)
1 fruit	Canned peach		Watermelon slice	Canned peach	Fruit punch	Watermelon slice
1 skim milk	1 cup skim milk		Buttermilk	1 cup skim milk		Buttermilk

of women have angina than men, and the death rate for females from cardiovascular disease exceeds that for males. In addition, 63% of women who died suddenly from coronary heart disease had no prior symptoms.

Educational information should be presented in small sections during each patient encounter. A teaching plan for the patient with CAD should include the following (Lewis, Collier, and Heitkemper, 2002):

- Anatomy and physiology of the heart and vessels
- Cause and effect of atherosclerosis
- Definition of terms (e.g., CAD, angina, MI)
- Signs and symptoms of IHD
- Healing after MI
- Identification of risk factors
- Discussion of diagnostic testing, monitoring, diet, and medication
- Discussion of expectations of recovery and cardiac rehabilitation programs
- Measures to promote recovery and health
- Importance of slow progression and resumption of regular activity

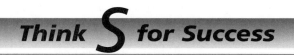

Think S _for Success_

Symptoms
- Monitor for recurrence of coronary artery disease (CAD) symptoms: chest pressure, shortness of breath, activity intolerance.

Sequelae
- Prevent disability associated with heart muscle reinjury by teaching patient to recognize when to seek medical treatment.

Safety
- Provide patient teaching regarding definition of ischemic heart disease, signs and symptoms of CAD and importance of complying with medication regimen, following diet and exercise routine, and monitoring tolerance of exercise and performance of activities of daily living.

Support/Services
- Provide access to medical social worker for assistance with finances and transportation, and psychological support.

Satisfaction
- Determine patient's degree of success in resuming prediagnosis routines (e.g., job, exercise) and performing activities important to patient.
- Develop a plan to maintain quality of life.

CONGESTIVE HEART FAILURE

CHF is one of the most frequent reasons for hospitalization in the United States. Part of the reason for the rise in CHF

hospitalizations is that patients are living longer and better because of the newer treatments available for the disease. Some 500,000 new cases of CHF are diagnosed annually. Over 5 million Americans currently suffer from CHF. The number of deaths associated with CHF have increased 115% since 1979, and hospitalizations for CHF have increased 70% since 1983, with the majority of patients 75 years of age or older (Capriotti, 2002).

Pathophysiology

CHF is not considered a disease. CHF is a symptom associated with a specific medical condition. Acute causes of CHF are acute MI, mitral or aortic regurgitation, endocarditis, and ruptured heart valve leaflets. Chronic causes of CHF symptomatology are CAD, anemia, hypertension, valvular heart disease, and cardiomyopathy.

The symptoms produced in CHF result from the heart's inability to pump an appropriate amount of blood to meet the increased cellular demands of the body's organs and tissues. Cardiac output decreases and peripheral tissue perfusion declines as a result of heart failure.

To improve cardiac output, five compensatory mechanisms are initiated: increased heart rate, improved stroke volume, arterial vasoconstriction, sodium and water retention, and myocardial hypertrophy.

As the heart rate increases, cardiac output rapidly improves. This compensatory mechanism has limited capabilities, however, because the increased heart rate may lead to increased myocardial oxygen demands.

Stroke volume is improved as the sympathetic system increases venous return to the heart. This has a limited ability to improve cardiac output because long-term over-stretching of the myocardial fibers leads to muscle thickening and impaired cardiac function. Arterial vasoconstriction also results from sympathetic stimulation. This vasoconstriction helps support the blood pressure but in turn also increases the systemic vascular resistance. The result is long-term increases in systemic vascular resistance with decreased cardiac output.

As a result of decreased perfusion to the kidneys, the angiotensin-aldosterone system is activated. This creates sodium and water retention to produce more blood volume returning to the heart.

The last compensatory mechanism for heart failure is myocardial hypertrophy. The heart muscle walls become thicker to create more forceful contractions and possibly to increase cardiac output.

All of these compensatory mechanisms lead to increased myocardial oxygen consumption. As this process progresses, the heart fails and the symptoms of CHF are revealed.

There are three categories of heart failure: heart failure related to systolic dysfunction, which is the most common; diastolic dysfunction; and mixed systolic and diastolic dysfunction. CHF is also further differentiated into right-sided and left sided ventricular failure.

Clinical Manifestations

The clinical manifestations of left-sided heart failure include crackles and cough on pulmonary examination, and dyspnea on exertion, which typically progresses to orthopnea, then to paroxysmal nocturnal dyspnea, and in end-stage CHF to dyspnea at rest. The clinical manifestations of right-sided heart failure are dependent peripheral edema, weight gain, ascites, abdominal pain, nausea, jugular venous distension, and hepatomegaly. A patient may have signs and symptoms of both right-sided and left-sided heart failure simultaneously.

Diagnosis

In addition to obtaining a thorough medical history and performing a physical examination, the clinician can order multiple diagnostic tests to confirm the diagnosis of CHF and determine the origin of the problem. The purpose of diagnostic testing is to evaluate the patient for alternative diagnoses, obtain a baseline of information before initiating therapy, determine the type of cardiac dysfunction present, and ascertain the degree of ventricular impairment and prognosis (Uphold and Graham, 1999).

An echocardiogram can reveal the size of the ventricular chambers and the thickness of the heart muscle, detect valvular defects, and gauge ventricular wall mobility and overall ejection fraction. An electrocardiogram can help in determining whether the patient has had any S-T wave changes and evaluate for the presence of arrhythmias. A chest radiograph reveals the degree of pulmonary congestion and uncovers possible infectious processes, and also gives the physician an overall picture of the size of the heart as it sits in the chest cavity. Blood tests consisting of a complete blood count, comprehensive metabolic panel, free thyroxine level, and thyroid-stimulating hormone level, as well as a urinalysis must be included in the diagnostic workup of CHF. Specialists such as cardiologists often perform various types of stress testing of the patient's heart as well as invasive cardiac catheterizations to evaluate the coronary arteries for atherosclerosis.

After a patient is diagnosed with CHF, he or she is classified according to and treatment recommendations are based on the level of disability. The New York Heart Association Functional Classification (NYHA-FC) system has long been the gold standard for staging the severity of CHF (Caboral and Mitchell, 2003). The most recent classification system for CHF, devised in 2002, was developed through the combined efforts of the American College of Cardiology and the American Heart Association to complement the NYHA-FC and focuses on the progressive nature of heart failure (Caboral and Mitchell, 2003). Table 12-3 presents these heart failure classifications and recommendations for treatment.

Interdisciplinary Care

The interdisciplinary team members are the same for all cardiac disorders. The goals for this team in the management of CHF are to improve the patient's quality of life, reduce the number of hospitalizations, and adequately control symptoms. Both the patient and family must be given a great deal of education regarding how to monitor the patient's disease and how to recognize when to seek medical treatment for disease progression.

Drug Therapy

The triad of medications used to treat CHF consists of diuretics, digoxin, and ACE inhibitors. ACE inhibitors decrease the systemic vascular resistance and, as a result, increase cardiac output. Digoxin is a drug that exerts inotropic action on the heart. The strength of contractility improves and the heart rate decreases, which reduces the cardiac workload. This drug has a narrow therapeutic window, and serum digoxin levels must be measured so that the patient's dosage can be adjusted if necessary. Because of the potential for toxicity in the elderly, monitoring is important. Digoxin toxicity is characterized by confusion, vomiting, and visual disturbances. A nursing consideration is to measure the apical heart rate for one full minute prior to drug administration. Because of the side effect of bradycardia, medication may have to be withheld. Primary physicians and cardiologists often provide written instructions specifying heart rate values at which the medication should not be given.

Diuretics have a role in the management of CHF by stimulating excretion of sodium and water and decreasing preload, which improves cardiac output. Recent studies have shown that the use of β-blockers leads to lower mortality rates and reduced hospitalization rates in patients diagnosed with NYHA-FC class II and class III heart failure (Hoyt and Bowling, 2001).

Drug classes to be avoided include antiarrhythmics, calcium channel blockers, and nonsteroidal antiinflammatory drugs.

New treatments for CHF are cardiac synchronization therapy, aldosterone inhibition, and exercise training. In selected patients, surgical revascularization, valvular repair, or valve replacement might also be appropriate.

For details on the mechanism of action and side effects of diuretics and ACE inhibitors, as well as associated nursing considerations, refer to Table 13-3.

Diet

For patients diagnosed with CHF, decreasing the sodium intake is crucial. Sodium causes fluid retention and therefore exacerbates the symptoms associated with CHF. Table 12-4 includes a list of high-sodium foods about which patients must be educated. In addition, patients who need to lose weight also require nursing and dietary help to plan meals that are low in fat and cholesterol and high in fiber.

Nursing Considerations

Initially, a patient should understand that CHF can be managed successfully in order to accept the diagnosis. Nurses

Table 12-3 Patient Classification and Treatment Recommendations for Heart Failure (HF)

New York Heart Association Classification	American College of Cardiology and American Heart Association Classification	Recommendations
	Stage A. People at high risk for developing HF but without structural heart disease or symptoms of congestive heart failure	Treat diabetes, hypertension, hyperlipidemia. Encourage patient to stop smoking and exercise regularly. Discourage use of alcohol and drugs. Give ACE inhibitor if indicated.
Class I. Patients with cardiac disease without limitations of physical activity. Ordinary physical activity does not cause undue fatigue, palpitations, dyspnea, or anginal pain.	Stage B. People who have structural heart disease but no symptoms of HF	All stage A therapies. Give ACE inhibitor unless contraindicated. Give β-blocker unless contraindicated.
Class II. Patients with cardiac disease who have slight limitations of physical activity. Patients are comfortable at rest. Ordinary physical activity results in fatigue, palpitations, dyspnea, or anginal pain.	Stage C. People who have structural heart disease with current or prior symptoms of HF	All stage A and B therapies. Prescribe sodium-restricted diet. Give diuretics. Give digoxin. Avoid or withdraw antiarrhythmic agents, most calcium channel blockers, and NSAIDs. Consider aldosterone antagonist, angiotensin receptor blockers, hydralazine, and nitrates.
Class III. Patients with cardiac disease who have marked limitations of physical activity. Patients are comfortable at rest. Less than ordinary physical activity causes fatigue, palpitations, dyspnea, or anginal pain		
Class IV. Patients with cardiac disease who cannot carry out any physical activity without discomfort. Symptoms of cardiac insufficiency or of the anginal syndrome may be present even at rest. Any physical activity increases discomfort.	Stage D. People with refractory HF that requires specialized interventions	All therapies for stages A, B, and C. Provide mechanical assistance such as biventricular pacemaker or left ventricular assist device. Give continuous inotropic therapy. Provide hospice care.

ACE, Angiotensin-converting enzyme; *NSAIDs,* nonsteroidal antiinflammatory drugs.

can play a vital role in this process. Educating the patient as early as possible regarding the diagnosis is helpful to the patient and family, who must make adjustments to their new lifestyle.

An area of difficulty nurses face in the management of this disease is the inability of many patients to implement the regimen prescribed by the physician. Failure to maintain a low-sodium diet or to comply with medication regimens and decreased self-awareness of a worsening condition promote unnecessary hospitalizations caused by acute exacerbations of symptoms. Home care nurses play a pivotal role in detecting the signs and symptoms of a patient's progress or decline by monitoring vital signs, evaluating the patient's response to medications, and communicating the patient's overall status to both family and physicians. Nurses can

intervene before the patient's condition potentially requires hospitalization. Box 12-3 provides a comprehensive list of topics to be covered in education and counseling of CHF patients (Jaarsna et al, 1997).

ATRIAL FIBRILLATION

AF is a serious cardiac disorder in both the acute and chronic phases because it puts the patient at significant risk for developing a stroke. According to the American Heart Association, one quarter of strokes, or 75,000 strokes per year, in the United States are related to AF. Up to 23% of these patients die and 43% experience permanent neurologic deficits. AF affects 2 million people in the United States over age 60 (Kennedy, 2002).

Table 12-4   High-Sodium Foods

Food	Examples
Beverages	Mineral water, club soda, Dutch-processed cocoa
Breads	Saltines, baking powder biscuits, muffins, biscuit mix, pretzels, salted snack crackers and chips, quick breads such as cornbread and nut bread, pancakes, waffles (including mixes)
Cereals	Instant cooked cereal, processed bran cereal, commercial granola
Dairy	Commercial buttermilk, regular cheese
Desserts	Commercial baked products, baked products and puddings made from mixes
Fats	Bacon fat, salted nuts or seeds, commercial dips (e.g., containing sour cream), regular salad dressings, mayonnaise
Juices	Tomato juice, V-8 juice, Clamato juice, Bloody Mary mixes
Meat	Smoked or cured products: bacon, ham, sausage, salt pork, hot dogs, lunch meat, corned or chipped beef; organ meats, shellfish, sardines, herring, anchovies, caviar, kosher meats, canned tuna fish and salmon, mackerel
Potato or substitute	Salted potato chips, salted French fries, instant potatoes, rice mixes, noodle mixes
Seasonings	Salt; excessive amounts of baking powder or baking soda; celery, onion, and garlic salt and other seasoned salts and peppers; meat tenderizers, Accent, monosodium glutamate, Worcestershire sauce, soy sauce, mustard, catsup, horseradish, chili sauce, tomato sauce, barbecue sauce, steak sauce
Soup	Commercial soups, bouillon cubes, powdered dehydrated soups
Vegetables	Sauerkraut, vegetables in creamed or seasoned sauces, frozen vegetables processed with salt or sodium
Miscellaneous	Olives; pickles; salted popcorn; commercially prepared, frozen, or canned entrees (e.g., pot pies, TV dinners); Mexican, Italian, Asian dishes as ordinarily prepared

From Lewis SM, Heitkemper SR, Dirksen SR: *Medical-surgical nursing: assessment and management of clinical problems,* ed 6, St Louis, 2004, Mosby.

Box 12-3   Educational Topics for Patients with Congestive Heart Failure

GENERAL COUNSELING
■ Explanation of heart failure
■ Explanation of the reason for dyspnea, thirst, diuresis, fatigue
■ Importance of monitoring weight daily
■ Importance of alerting the primary care physician in case of weight gain
■ Symptoms of worsening heart failure
■ Steps to take if symptoms worsen
■ Expected symptoms
■ Explanation of treatment/care plan
■ Role of family members
■ Support groups available
■ Classification of patient's and family's responsibilities
■ Importance of smoking cessation
■ Community services available
■ Role of stress
■ Prevention of hazards (e.g., pressure sores, dehydration)
■ Prevention of influenza and colds
■ Importance of obtaining immunizations against influenza and pneumococcal disease

PROGNOSIS
■ Life expectancy
■ Expectations for the future (progression and prognosis)
■ Advance directives
■ Advice for family members in the event of sudden death

ACTIVITY/REST
■ Recommended recreational, leisure, and work activity
■ Need to recognize activity limitations
■ Importance of engaging in regular physical activity and exercise
■ Need to prevent exhaustion
■ Importance of resting after heavy meals
■ Need to conserve energy
■ Need to avoid temperature extremes
■ Possibility of entering a rehabilitation program
■ Possible sexual difficulties and coping strategies
■ Proper positioning (Fowler position, elevation of legs when sitting down)
■ Use of elastic stockings
■ Need to plan rest during the day
■ Importance of maintaining a balance between activity and rest

DIET
Food
■ Sodium-restricted diet
■ Identification of high- and low-sodium foods
■ Importance of reading labels of food, over-the-counter medication
■ Need to choose restaurants with low-sodium dishes
■ Potassium-enhanced diet (if required)
■ Fiber-rich diet (to prevent constipation)
■ Healthy diet to provide minimal required metabolic needs (calories, proteins)

Box 12-3 Educational Topics for Patients with Congestive Heart Failure—cont'd

DIET—cont'd

Fluids

- Balance between fluid intake and output
- Minimal and maximal fluid intake
- Need to avoid excessive fluid intake
- Fluid restriction (if required)
- Alcohol restriction/abstinence

MEDICATION

- Benefits of medication for quality of life and survival

- Dosing
- Adverse effects and what to do if they occur
- Coping mechanisms for complicated therapeutic regimens
- Availability of lower-cost medication or financial assistance
- Signs of (digitalis) intoxication
- Signs of hyperkalemia

ADHERENCE

- Expected side medication effects

From Jaarsna T et al: Maintaining the balance: nursing care of patients with congestive heart failure, *Int J Nurs Stud* 34(3):213-21, 1997.

Think S for Success

Symptoms
- Observe for exacerbation of congestive heart failure (CHF) symptoms.

Sequelae
- Prevent unnecessary hospitalization by monitoring signs and symptoms of CHF.

Safety
- Teach patient and caregiver the significance of the following:
  Adhering to medication regimen
  Complying with low-sodium diet
  Watching out for increases in weight
  Participating in a prescribed exercise program

Support/Services
- Incorporate multidisciplinary team for maximum input to help patient manage disease.

Satisfaction
- Establish level to which CHF is impeding patient's quality of life and create a care plan incorporating necessary lifestyle changes.

Pathophysiology

The pathophysiology of AF is described as total disorganization of electrical activity from the atria that results in ineffective contractility. AF is often prompted by a premature atrial contraction that leads to a reentry-type rhythm, and at times the atrial rate can be 300 to 600 beats per minute. As these chaotic impulses are sent to the atrioventricular node, the impulses are picked up more slowly than they were sent, which results in an irregular display of atrial and ventricular complexes. AF may be episodic or chronic in nature. The associated risk factors for the development of AF are age over 60 years, hypertension, CAD, mitral valve prolapse, CHF, chronic lung disease, hyperthyroidism, alcoholism, congenital heart defect, and the use of stimulant substances.

As a result of AF, the patient is at risk for developing blood clots that can ultimately cause an embolic stroke as well as decreased cardiac output.

Clinical Manifestations

Many patients come to their primary care physicians for a physical examination and are found to have asymptomatic AF. However, there are also patients who come to their primary care physicians or to emergency departments with an array of symptoms. These include dizziness, chest pain, dyspnea, fatigue, fullness in the neck region, near syncope, and palpitations.

Diagnosis

As with any cardiac disorder, a thorough medical history taking and physical examination of the patient must performed in addition to diagnostic testing. Diagnostic tests include 12-lead electrocardiography to assess the rhythm for the absence of the p-wave complex in addition to an irregular presentation, serum thyroid function tests to evaluate for hyperthyroidism, an echocardiogram to detect valvular heart abnormalities, and a chest radiograph to look for cardiomegaly.

Interdisciplinary Care

The goals for the treatment of AF are to slow the rapid ventricular response, prevent the formation of blood clots, and convert the rhythm to normal sinus rhythm if possible. Whether the patient has acute or chronic AF, the goals remain the same. The first step in treating AF is to look for the cause of this arrhythmia and to correct it.

Drug Therapy

In addressing the goals of treatment, initially the patient is prescribed a medication to control the ventricular response. Examples are digoxin, β-blockers, and calcium channel blockers. Antiarrhythmics to help in converting to normal sinus rhythm are procainamide and amiodarone. These medications act by blocking the channels for ions such as sodium and potassium. Approximately 50% of the time, these medications will convert the rhythm. The prevention of blood clots and stroke is addressed with the use of anticoagulants. Unless a contraindication exists, warfarin (Coumadin), the most commonly used medication for thinning the blood, is prescribed. Warfarin works by blocking the synthesis of vitamin K, which is responsible for the formation of clotting factor II, otherwise known as prothrombin (Beers and Berkow, 1999). The conversion of fibrinogen to fibrin in the development of blood clots is delayed with warfarin. Aspirin is used to prevent clot formation by blocking the process of platelet aggregation. A dosage of 325 mg daily is sufficient.

Diet

Diet and certain medications can alter the effect of warfarin in the blood. A diet that is high in vitamin K can decrease the effectiveness of warfarin. Table 12-5 includes a complete list of foods to avoid while taking warfarin.

Nursing Considerations

Educating the patient with regard to the diagnosis of AF begins with a review of the symptoms. The nurse can teach the patient to take a radial pulse reading when the patient experiences palpitations, dyspnea, chest pain, and other symptoms that can occur in association with rapid ventricular response. Not only must the patient monitor for a rapid pulse, but the patient must understand that the medications prescribed to control the ventricular response can produce bradycardia (heart rate lower than 60 beats per minute) and that he or she must also monitor the pulse for rates below this level. For patients taking warfarin, the nurse should instruct the patient to consume a diet low in vitamin K. At the beginning of treatment, laboratory testing of prothrombin time (PT) and international normalized ratio (INR) is performed every 2 weeks until the values are stabilized. Therapeutic laboratory values of PT range from 1.5 to 2 times the patient's control value. INR readings between 2.0 and 3.0 are considered thera-

Table 12-5 Foods Containing High Amounts of Vitamin K

Food	Portion Size	Vitamin K Content*
Fats and Oils		
Mayonnaise	7 tbsp	High
Soybean oil	1 tbsp	High
Canola and salad oil	7 tbsp	High
Meats		
Beef liver	4 oz	High
Pork liver	4 oz	High
Vegetables		
Broccoli	½ cup	High
Brussels sprouts	½ cup	Very high
Chickpeas	½ cup, dry	High
Kale	½ cup, raw	High
Spinach	1 cup, raw	High
Turnip greens	½ cup, cooked	High
Cabbage, green (fresh or boiled)	1½ cups	High
Watercress	3 cups, chopped, raw	High
Lettuce (raw, bibb, red)	1 ¾ cups	High
Parsley (raw and cooked)	1½ cups	High
Collard greens	½ cup	High
Beverages		
Brewed green tea	1 cup	Insignificant interaction
Herbal teas with tonka beans, melilot (sweet clover), or sweet woodruff	1 cup	*Avoid;* significant interaction

Adapted from DuPont Pharmaceuticals: A patient's guide to using Coumadin® (2001), *Nutritive Value of Food, Home & Garden Bulletin,* 1998, US Department of Agriculture.
*High content indicates greater than 150 μg.

peutic. Once the INR is stabilized, the patient is scheduled for evaluation of PT and INR once a month unless bleeding or complications are noted.

Patients prescribed antiarrhythmic medications to control the rapid ventricular response associated with AF must undergo serum liver function testing every 3 to 6 weeks initially and then every 3 to 6 months thereafter.

For patients taking anticoagulants, nurses address other areas relating to safety. The patient is taught to use an electric razor to shave rather than a straight-edged razor, to use extra caution when cutting with a knife, and to be aware that, if the patient falls, excessive bruising may occur and the patient should be evaluated by a physician.

There are many different drugs that interact adversely with warfarin in particular. These are the nonsteroidal antiinflammatory drugs (including aspirin), antacids, carbamazepine, selective serotonin reuptake inhibitors, rifampin, and antihistamines (Uphold and Graham, 1999).

Think **S** for Success

Symptoms
- Monitor for episodes of rapid ventricular response with atrial fibrillation (AF).

Sequelae
- Ensure that patient avoids unnecessary hospitalization for uncontrolled AF by following prescribed medication regimen.

Safety
- Instruct patient and caregiver in need for and method of monitoring radial pulse.
- Instruct patient and caregiver regarding side effects of digoxin to prevent toxicity.
- Instruct patient and caregiver in need for monitoring through serum liver function testing.

Support/Services
- Patient may experience anxiety during episodic rapid ventricular response. Encourage patient and caregiver to contact physician when radial pulse is higher than 100 beats per minute.

Satisfaction
- Ascertain the level to which the patient and caregiver have adjusted to lifestyle changes, medication regimen, and frequency of blood testing.
- Develop a plan that allows patient to incorporate these changes and maintain prediagnosis level of functioning and quality of life.

VALVULAR HEART DISEASE

According to the American Heart Association's 2001 Heart and Stroke Statistical Update, valvular heart disorders are the cause of more than 18,500 deaths per year in the United States (Shappell, 2002). It is also a contributing factor in 38,000 deaths each year. The majority of patients with valvular heart disorders suffer from aortic valve dysfunction primarily and mitral valve dysfunction secondarily. Tricuspid and pulmonic valve disease is rare and contributes to only 3% of deaths (Shappell, 2002).

Pathophysiology

Mitral valve disorders and then aortic valve disorders are discussed. These disorders can be categorized according to the valve affected and the type of dysfunction present. Heart valve abnormalities are stenotic or regurgitant in origin. In a stenotic valve, the valve orifice is restricted. This restriction impedes the forward blood flow and creates a pressure gradient across an open valve. In a regurgitant valve, closure of the valve leaflets is incomplete and blood flows backward.

The most common cause of mitral valve stenosis is rheumatic heart disease. Mitral valve stenosis creates a narrowing of the circulatory outflow path from the left ventricle (Figure 12-1). The mitral valve becomes thickened and shortened, and develops a funnel shape. The resulting obstruction of blood flow increases left atrial pressure and pulmonary congestion.

Mitral valve regurgitation is caused by infective endocarditis, ischemic papillary muscle dysfunction, rheumatic heart disease, and ruptured chordae tendineae. The backward flow of blood as a result of mitral valve regurgitation causes fluid volume overload in the left ventricle, left atrium, and pulmonary vasculature.

The cause of mitral valve prolapse is unknown. Mitral valve prolapse is a structural disorder in which one or both of the valve leaflets is too large, which results in an uneven

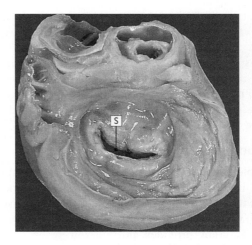

Figure 12-1 Aortic stenosis *(S)* with classic "fish mouth" orifice caused by chronic rheumatic heart disease. (Courtesy Dr. I. Leach, Department of Histopathology, University of Nottingham. From Stevens A, Lowe J: *Pathology,* ed 2, St Louis, 2000, Mosby.)

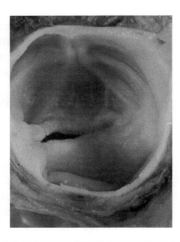

Figure 12-2 Mitral stenosis. Mild stenosis in valve leaflets of a young adult. (From Damjanov I, Linder J: *Pathology: a color atlas,* St Louis, 2000, Mosby.)

closure. The oversized valve leaflet prolapses back into the left atrium, causing leakage of blood.

Aortic valve stenosis creates an obstruction of blood flow from the left ventricle into the aorta during systole (Figure 12-2). The long-term effects are left ventricular hypertrophy and increased myocardial oxygen consumption.

Aortic valve regurgitation results in backward flow of blood from the aorta into the left ventricle. This fluid volume overload causes left ventricular hypertrophy and dilation, which leads to increased blood volume in the left atrium and pulmonary vasculature.

Clinical Manifestations

Signs and symptoms of mitral valve stenosis are dyspnea, fatigue, palpitations, and a diastolic murmur. Clinical manifestations of mitral valve regurgitation mimic those of mitral valve stenosis except that a systolic murmur is present.

Signs and symptoms of aortic stenosis are angina pectoris, syncope, symptoms of CHF, and a systolic murmur. Clinical manifestations of aortic regurgitation are exertional dyspnea, orthopnea, water hammer pulse, and a diastolic murmur.

Diagnosis

A complete medical history is taken and a physical examination is performed. The two-dimensional echocardiogram is the most accurate diagnostic tool to establish what type of valvular heart disease a patient may have. The echocardiogram provides information regarding valve function and overall configuration. Other helpful diagnostic tests are a chest radiograph to determine heart size and an electrocardiogram to assess any arrhythmias or chamber growth.

Interdisciplinary Care

The health care team members are the same for all the cardiac disorders. The goals in the management of valvular heart disease are to ensure patient understanding of the symptoms and disease progression so the patient will know when to seek additional treatment, to enable the patient to perform normal daily activities without exertional dyspnea, and to achieve prediagnosis heart function through medication or surgical intervention.

Surgical Treatment and Drug Therapy

Surgical treatment consists of valvular repair, valve replacement, or balloon valvuloplasty. Medications for the treatment of valvular heart disease include diuretics to diminish the exacerbation of CHF symptoms, β-blockers to help with palpitations, digoxin to treat any arrhythmias that occur (such as AF), oral nitrates to counter the vasodilatory effects of the pressure caused by stenotic valves, and oral anticoagulants to prevent blood clots. The mechanisms of action, side effects, and nursing considerations for nitrates, diuretics, and β-blockers are covered in Table 13-3.

Patients with valvular heart disease, in particular, should receive prophylactic antibiotics before any invasive procedure because they are susceptible to developing infective endocarditis.

Diet

Following a low-sodium diet regimen will help prevent exacerbations of CHF. These patients must avoid the use of caffeine and stimulants because these can contribute to the development of arrhythmias and increase palpitations.

Nursing Considerations

Management of chronic valvular disease starts with the nurse's education of the patient and caregivers about the disorder, including the pathophysiology of the disease, symptoms, medication regimen and side effects, acceptable activities, and circumstances under which to seek medical help for exacerbations.

A patient prescribed diuretics must to be taught the importance of keeping track of changes in weight daily. The patient must be aware of the potential for bleeding associated with anticoagulant usage. Monitoring the radial pulse for readings lower than 60 beats per minute is imperative when β-blockers and digoxin are taken. The patient must be taught the importance of taking prophylactic antibiotics prior to undergoing invasive procedures.

In planning activities for the patient with valvular heart disease, one must determine what level of activity the patient can tolerate without the development of symptoms. When that level is ascertained, the patient should be taught to plan for rest periods between activities to build up endurance slowly.

Think S for Success

Symptoms
- Ensure that patient keeps symptoms under control by following prescribed medication regimen, activity regimen, and diet, and undergoes appropriate medical follow-up.

Sequelae
- Assess patient in the home environment regularly for disease progression.

Safety
- Ensure that patient does not develop exacerbation of symptoms through proper teaching as outlined.

Support/Services
- Caregiver and/or patient may need to express fears associated with progression of the disease. Make referrals to medical social work as necessary.

Satisfaction
- Ascertain the plan of care patient has chosen to follow and help patient make adjustments to improve the quality of life.

CARDIAC REHABILITATION

The health benefits of physical conditioning for patients with CAD are reduction in mortality and cardiac events, improvement in symptoms, increased exercise tolerance, improvement in serum lipid levels, and improved psychological well being (Barker, Burton, and Zieve, 1999). The cardiac rehabilitation team may include cardiologists and physiatrists or other exercise providers, physical therapists, occupational therapists, registered dietitians, medical social workers, nurses, physiologists, and ancillary staff.

Cardiac rehabilitation may take place in an inpatient rehabilitation facility but is increasingly provided on an outpatient basis. After the initial phase of cardiac rehabilitation is completed, ongoing supervised community programs may continue to support the patient until he or she reaches a maintenance level. Total mortality and cardiac mortality are reduced for patients who participate in multifactorial cardiac rehabilitation exercise training (Agency for Healthcare Research and Quality, 1995).

Physical Therapy

Physical and occupational therapists may treat cardiac patients during the acute hospital stay if these specialties are part of a clinical pathway system. However, because these services are not directly reimbursed through diagnosis-related group billing, physical and occupational therapists are more likely to provide care in inpatient rehabilitation facilities or participate in outpatient rehabilitation in the community.

During the hospitalization phase physical therapists, together with nurses and other staff, assess the patient's functional abilities and endurance and make recommendations for exercises to improve endurance. They may also make recommendations for adaptive equipment to improve mobility and function, both while the patient is in the hospital and when the patient returns to the community after discharge. The assessment may indicate that the patient has stairs and will need a stair glide or should limit trips up and down the steps to once in the morning and once in the afternoon. If the bathroom is on the second floor and the kitchen is on the main floor, the therapist will make recommendations for accommodations. Symptoms related to CAD that occur while the patient is performing activities of daily living should be assessed. For example, at first the patient can simply wash the hands and face, which requires less energy expenditure and therefore should be tolerated better than showering, which requires a higher level of energy expenditure.

In cardiac rehabilitation, physical therapists are part of a comprehensive team that assesses the patient's exercise tolerance and develops a comprehensive treatment plan to help the patient maximize function. Physical therapists may provide exertion testing, evaluate metabolic function, and develop a plan to improve exercise endurance and maintain or improve existing function. Exercise rehabilitation is recommended for patients after MI and/or coronary artery bypass graft, for patients with stable angina if they have limiting symptoms, and for patients with symptoms of decreased left ventricular systolic dysfunction (Scottish Intercollegiate Guidelines Network, 2002). Continued exercise is required to sustain improved exercise tolerance. Exercise may also be a component of improved psychological functioning in cardiac patients.

In the home environment, cardiac conditioning begins with consideration of the appropriate type, intensity, duration, and frequency of exercise. The exercise should include repetitive motion activities such as walking and swimming. Intensity of exercise is individualized for each patient based on the individual's baseline heart rate and exercise tolerance, with the goal of maximizing functional abilities. At the beginning of rehabilitation, resting heart rate is measured. The maximum heart rate is determined by subtracting the patient's age from 220. Target heart rate is calculated from maximal heart rate and is generally considered to be 60% to 80% of the maximum heart rate. Patients are instructed in taking the pulse, usually radial or carotid. Intensity and duration of exercise are advanced based on exercise tolerance and ability to attain the target heart rate. Patients start slowly and build up gradually to 20 or more minutes of exercise per day. The goal is to maintain 20 to 30 minutes of exercise 3 to 6 days per week. The patient should continue to monitor radial pulse during exercise and stop exercising if the heart rate is too high or symptoms occur. All patients, including elderly patients of both genders, benefit from exercise-based cardiac rehabilitation, although elderly female patients are much less likely to be referred for rehabilitation (Agency for Healthcare Research and Quality, 1995).

Occupational Therapy

Occupational therapists may provide a psychosocial assessment and education in stress reduction techniques. A cognitive assessment may be indicated if there is evidence of cognitive damage from prolonged lack of oxygenation, either during cardiac arrest or during surgery that involved circulation of blood outside the body. Educational and occupational assessments are part of the occupational therapist's responsibility. Skill training for a new occupation may be included if the cardiac illness precludes resumption of the patient's previous work. Together with the medical social worker, the occupational therapist may recommend vocational rehabilitation. Lifestyle education addresses adaptations for daily function and may also support smoking cessation through stress reduction. It may include use of adaptive equipment such as computers or mnemonics to aid memory (Lubkin and Larsen, 1998).

Dietary Interventions

Dietitians provide nutrition education for both the patient and family. Consideration of the family's lifestyle and cultural values is necessary if healthy nutritional habits are to be incorporated into the patient's daily routine; therefore, the dietary education and assessment includes both the patient and the individual who has primary responsibility for shopping and preparing meals. For patients with cardiac disease, nutritional assessment and education focus on sodium, saturated fat, and caffeine intake. Weight control is also important. All hypertensive individuals need education regarding the use of processed foods and addition of table salt; however, hypertensive individuals who are African American and older patients are more sensitive to sodium intake than other populations. High potassium intake is inversely related to blood pressure and is generally encouraged, but in individuals taking potassium-sparing diuretics, ACE inhibitors, or nonsteroidal antiinflammatory drugs, or in those with chronic renal failure, high-potassium diets can be dangerous (Institute for Clinical Systems Improvement, 2002). Alcohol consumption should be limited to no more than 1 oz per day for men or 0.5 oz per day for women. Adequate dietary intake of potassium, calcium, and magnesium is best achieved by consumption of fresh fruits and vegetables. A heart-healthy diet such as the Dietary Approaches to Stop Hypertension (DASH) diet is recommended (US Department of Veteran's Affairs, 2001). The National Institutes of Health (2003) fact sheet regarding the DASH eating plan can be accessed online (see reference list for website).

To promote weight reduction or maintenance of appropriate weight, the dietitian may calculate an appropriate number of calories per day based on the metabolic rate determined during metabolic studies performed by the occupational or physical therapist. The multifaceted approach of dietary education, counseling, and behavioral intervention is most likely to help patients lose weight. Elderly patients may initially require consumption of concentrated calories because of decreased appetite and poor baseline nutrition. The dietitian may also calculate hydration requirements for patients with CHF, for whom a careful balance must be achieved to ensure adequate hydration while avoiding fluid overload.

Behavioral Interventions

The psychologist and/or medical social worker may suggest behavioral interventions for smoking cessation or eating disorders that contribute to cardiac disease. They may also teach stress reduction techniques. Cardiac patients often suffer from depression and anxiety. The social worker or psychologist may initiate counseling for these behavioral disorders. Cardiac patients are often concerned about sexual functioning after an acute cardiac event. Cardiac diseases alter independence in many ways. The social worker also assists the patient in problem solving and facilitates the patient's independence. For example, the patient's driving should be limited if the patient suffers from symptoms of heart failure at rest or angina at rest, or if the blood pressure consistently exceeds 180 systolic and/or 100 diastolic; for patients who drive commercial vehicles or who drive vehicles with many passengers, additional restrictions apply (European Society of Cardiology, 1998). These driving restrictions have many implications. They may affect the individual's ability to work, to buy groceries, or to keep doctor's appointments. They may also isolate the patient from his or her social contacts in the community. The social worker has knowledge of community resources and can identify alternative transportation services or vocational retraining resources. The social worker may also assist the patient in identifying existing social supports. Access to parking for the handicapped might be arranged, which would allow the patient to drive independently but prevent the exertion of carrying heavy groceries across a parking lot. Meals could be delivered, or the patient might be able to use special transportation services in the community. There may be neighbors or family or community members available to transport the patient. Although the social worker may provide initial assistance to establish such services, the patient's wishes guide these choices, and the goal is to teach the patient to access these services independently after they are set up. The social worker may also be instrumental in initiating benefits related to public entitlements programs such as Social Security Disability, Medicare, and Medicaid.

ALTERNATIVE THERAPIES

Over 40% of all Americans have used some form of alternative medicine. The number may be even higher among those with chronic disease. Alternative therapies have proven therapeutic effects in several areas of heart disease. Smoking cessation is frequently an area that receives attention from alternative therapies. A recent Cochrane review found no significant improvement in cessation from acupuncture treatment (White, Rampes, and Ernst, 2003). However, hypnosis has proven to facilitate smoking cessation (Green and Lynn, 2000).

Herbal medicines have demonstrated some positive effects as well. Garlic has been shown in multiple studies to help reduce blood pressure. Ginkgo biloba has antioxidative properties and also inhibits platelet aggregation (Zbinden and Seiler, 2002). The most common form of alternative medicine use reported to health care providers is the use of herbal supplements, but many patients do not tell their providers about their use of herbal products. It is essential for the interdisciplinary team to be aware of the use of herbal supplements by cardiac patients, because significant interactions occur between traditional prescription medicines and herbal products.

Ma huang, or ephedra, is an herb used in herbal decongestants, cold preparations, and weight loss formulations. It is a stimulant and should not be used by individuals with cardiac disease. Red clover, ginger, garlic, and various forms of ginseng may interact with warfarin products. The potential for hypokalemia as a result of diuretic therapy may be more pronounced with the use of licorice, dandelion, ginkgo biloba, gravelroot, horsetail, juniper, and uva ursi (Christopher, 2003). New information is becoming available about interactions between herbal products and prescription medicines. The patient should be counseled to check with the pharmacist before beginning any new herbal supplement if he or she is taking any prescription medications.

ETHICAL CONSIDERATIONS

Ethical considerations concerning end-of-life questions are encountered in cases of chronic cardiac disease. This is particularly true when the disease has advanced to the level of CHF and the issue of prolonging death versus prolonging life arises. Whom should the nurse support when the patient expresses the feeling that he or she has had enough yet the family is not ready to let go? Heart transplantation is the only cure for many patients with coronary disease. The question of who gets a heart transplant presents other ethical issues. Should an older man who smokes but has a family be given precedence over a young man who has rheumatic valvular disease but no family?

CASE STUDY
Patient Data

Mr. B. is a 60-year-old man who is retired from the landscaping business. He is used to being physically active without any difficulty. He is married and has three children ranging in age from 25 to 38 years old. He has no history of prior medical problems. He takes no prescribed medications. He occasionally takes an over-the-counter cough medicine for a cough he developed approximately 2 weeks ago. He drinks alcohol socially and admits to smoking a half pack of cigarettes per day. He was mowing his lawn when one of his children came to visit and observed him with severe shortness of breath, pallor, and seemingly greater fatigue than in the past when he had mowed the lawn. Mr. B. stopped mowing the lawn and went inside his home to rest. Approximately 2 days later he awaked from sleep with chest tightness and coughing, and complaining of being "unable to catch his breath." These symptoms lasted for an hour or so, and then he went to sleep in a recliner chair. The next morning, Mr. B. was unable to eat breakfast due to severe nausea, abdominal pain, and a feeling of being "bloated" all over. Mr. B. comes to the office of his primary care physician that afternoon. Shortly after being examined, he is admitted to the hospital for additional workup.

Physical Examination and Diagnostic Findings
- Blood pressure: 170/100
- Pulse rate: 110 beats per minute
- Respiration rate: 26 breaths per minute
- Skin color: pale
- Neck: jugular venous distension present
- Lungs: crackles at both bases
- Heart sounds: S_1 and S_2 normal with a systolic murmur noted
- Abdomen: mild distension and tenderness on palpation
- Extremities: +2 pedal edema bilaterally
- Chest radiograph: cardiomegaly with pulmonary effusion evident

- Hemoglobin level: 10 g/dl
- Hematocrit: 30%
- Blood urea nitrogen level: 45 mg/dl
- Creatinine level: 1.5 mg/dl
- Thyroid stimulating hormone level: 1.8 μIU/ml

Thinking It Through
- Based on the information given, from what cardiac condition is Mr. B. suffering?
- Categorize the signs and symptoms presented in the case study.
- What are the three most important nursing diagnoses regarding this condition?
- What two major concerns will Mr. B. potentially have regarding these new diagnoses? What interventions can you, as the nurse, perform to help him with these concerns?
- What educational topics should be discussed with Mr. and Mrs. B.?

Case Conference

As Mr. B. nears discharge from the hospital, the interdisciplinary team meets to discuss the home plan of care. The members of the interdisciplinary team consist of Mr. and Mrs. B, the primary care nurse, the cardiologist, a member of the cardiac rehabilitation team, and a dietitian.

As the team is seated to start the discussion, Mrs. B. immediately exclaims with tearful eyes and a shaky voice, "My husband is going to die, isn't he?" Mr. B. answers, "Listen, honey, it's not that bad, there's just a little too much fluid in my body. I'm better now."

The cardiologist takes over by acknowledging that Mr. B. has been diagnosed with CHF, most likely due to chronic undiagnosed and untreated hypertension. As a result of the hypertension, Mr. B. has also developed renal insufficiency and anemia. The physician reassures Mr. B. that all of these disorders have

Continued

CASE STUDY—cont'd

been known to be asymptomatic and therefore do not become diagnosed until the patient experiences a crisis as he did. Medication prescriptions are written and given to the nurse to go over with the patient and family.

Mr. B. has been in the hospital for 5 days and is being discharged the next day. He has been evaluated by the dietitian and staff of the cardiac rehabilitation program, and the primary care nurse has been educating him and his family regarding the diagnosis, symptoms, medications, and circumstances under which to seek medical attention for an exacerbation of CHF.

The primary care nurse begins a discussion with Mr. and Mrs. B. by asking them what knowledge have they gained over the 5 days of hospital stay for the treatment of CHF. In addition, she asks them to express any fears they have regarding this condition and to ask any questions regarding the information she has covered over the past 5 days.

Mr. B. asks, "Will I need to take these medications for the rest of my life?" He expresses concern that "one of these pills makes me urinate a lot. I won't be able to leave the house. I feel tired most of the time now."

Mrs. B. is quiet and states, "I have already mentioned my one concern."

The nurse recommends that a referral be made to the medical social worker for Mr. and Mrs. B. so that they will be able to talk about their anxieties in adjusting to the new diagnosis. The nurse then addresses Mr. B. and reminds him that following the prescribed medication regimen will prevent him from experiencing further flare-ups of CHF. She also explains in more detail how to take the diuretic with consideration for the daily activities planned.

The exercise physiologist from the cardiac rehabilitation department points out that slowly increasing his daily activity will help to strengthen Mr. B.'s heart muscle and provide Mr. B. with more energy so that he can participate in the activities he chooses. The physiologist then displays the cardiac rehabilitation outpatient program schedule and suggests that they discuss when Mr. B.'s first appointment can be made, which should be within 7 days of discharge assuming that his symptoms are under control and he is cleared to join the program.

The dietitian brings up the need to follow a diet that is not only low in sodium but also low in fat. She provides a handout listing all foods that are high in sodium and fat. She gives Mr. and Mrs. B. a list of all local restaurants and indicates the items on their menus that would be acceptable for Mr. B.'s new diet plan. Mrs. B. pays close attention to this information and says, "Well, at least I can do something to help him."

REFERENCES

Agency for Healthcare Research and Quality: Cardiac rehabilitation, Clinical Practice Guideline No. 17, Rockville, Md, 1995, US Department of Health and Human Services, Public Health Service.

American Heart Association: Statistical fact sheet, 2003, available online at www.americanheart.org/ presenter.jhtml?identifier=2007.

Barker L, Burton J, Zieve P: *Principles of ambulatory medicine,* ed 5, Baltimore, Md, 1999, Williams & Wilkins.

Beers M, Berkow R: *The Merck manual of diagnosis and therapy*, ed 17, Whitehouse Station, NJ, 1999, Merck and Co.

Caboral M, Mitchell J: New guidelines for heart failure focus on prevention, *Nurse Pract* 28(1):13-23, 2003.

Capriotti T: Current concepts and pharmacologic treatment of heart failure, *Medsurg Nurs* 11(2):71-83, 2002.

Christopher JR: LifeBalm.com: Drug/herb interaction chart, retrieved from *http://www.lifebalm.com/ page.cgi?drug_herb1* on July 5, 2003.

Deedy M: Coronary artery disease [Cleveland Clinic Foundation website], retrieved from *http:// www.clevelandclinicmeded.com/diseasemanagement/cardiology/ cad* on Nov 9, 2002.

European Society of Cardiology: Driving and heart disease, *Eur Heart J* 19(8):1165-77, 1998.

Gislason S: The book of arterial disease, retrieved from *http://www.nutramed.com/publishing/arteriestext.htm* in Dec 2002.

Green JP, Lynn SJ: Hypnosis and suggestions-based approaches to smoking cessation: an examination of the evidence, *Int J Clin Exp Hypn* 48(2):195-224, 2000.

Hoyt R, Bowling L: Reducing readmissions for congestive heart failure, *Am Fam Physician* 63(8):1593-8, 2001.

Institute for Clinical Systems Improvement: *Hypertension diagnosis and treatment*, Bloomington, Minn, 2002, The Institute.

Jaarsna T et al: Maintaining the balance—nursing care of patients with congestive heart failure, *Int J Nurs Stud* 34(3):213-21, 1997.

Keaton K, Pierce L: Cardiac therapy for men with coronary artery disease, *J Holist Nurs* 18(1):63-85, 2000.

Kennedy R: Atrial fibrillation, retrieved from *http://www.medical-library.net/sites/_atrial_fibrillation.html* on Nov 29, 2002.

Lewis S, Collier I, Heitkemper M: *Medical surgical nursing,* ed 5, St Louis, 2002, Mosby.

Lubkin IM, Larsen PD, editors: *Chronic illness: impact and interventions,* ed 4, Sudbury, Mass, 1998, Jones and Bartlett.

National Institutes of Health, National Heart, Blood, and Lung Institute: Facts about the DASH eating plan, 2003, retrieved from *http://www.nhlbi.nih.gov/health/public/heart/hbp/dash/new_dash.pdf* on Dec 26, 2003.

Scottish Intercollegiate Guidelines Network: Cardiac rehabilitation: a national clinical guideline, Scottish Intercollegiate Guidelines Network Pub No. 57, Edinburgh, 2002, Scottish Intercollegiate Guidelines Network.

Shappell S: Valvular heart disease overview [HeartCenterOnline for Patients website], retrieved from *http://www.heartcenteronline.com/myheartdr/common/articles.cfm?ARTID=187* on Nov 30, 2002.

Uphold C, Graham M: *Clinical guideline in adult health,* ed 2, Gainesville, Fl, 1999, Barmarrae Books.

US Department of Veterans Affairs: Diagnosis and management of hypertension in the primary care setting, Washington, DC, 2001, Veterans Health Administration.

White AR, Rampes H, Ernst E: Acupuncture for smoking cessation (Cochrane Review). In *Cochrane Library,* issue 2, 2003, Oxford: Update Software, retrieved from *http:// www.medscape.com/viewarticle/453716,* on July 5, 2003.

Zbinden S, Seiler C: Phytotherapy in cardiovascular medicine, *Ther Umsch* 59(6):301-6, 2002.

CHAPTER 13

Disorders of the Vasculature

Maryellen Zarnik Silva, MS, RN, CRNP

The chronic vascular disorders discussed in this chapter are hypertension (HTN), chronic arterial occlusive disease (CAOD), Buerger's disease, Raynaud's phenomenon, and varicose veins. A comprehensive approach is used in examining each disorder. The information provided includes pathophysiology, clinical manifestations, diagnostic testing, pharmacologic management, assessment of functional health patterns, interdisciplinary care plan, impact of chronic vascular disorders on the family and/or caregiver, and ethical considerations.

Vascular disorders range from conditions as simple as varicose veins to those as life threatening and complex as an aortic aneurysm. The root of all vascular disorders is compromised venous or arterial blood flow.

ASSESSMENT

To assess the patient with a chronic vascular disorder, one must consider the specific diagnosis of that patient, because no generalizations can be drawn regarding all chronic vascular disorders.

Patients with HTN may be asymptomatic or may have a myriad of symptoms. Patients diagnosed with CAOD most frequently come to the physician complaining of pain in the lower extremities and digits of the hands or feet. The primary concern for patients with HTN is the prevention of target end-organ damage. The focus for patients with CAOD is controlling pain and enabling the patient to maintain daily activities. A framework for assessing the effects of vascular disorders on functional health patterns is presented in Box 13-1.

HYPERTENSION

According to the Centers for Disease Control and Prevention, the number of reported cases of HTN rose from 22.9% of the population in 1991 to 24.9% in 1999. The increases were virtually equal for all races, genders, ethnic groups, and educational levels except among those 22 to 40 years of age. HTN is responsible for approximately 43,000 deaths per year and is a contributing factor in the deaths of 227,000 persons annually (Centers for Disease Control and Prevention, 2002). High blood pressure increases the risk for cerebrovascular accident, heart disease, and kidney failure. High blood pressure is defined as a systolic pressure reading of 140 mm Hg or greater and a diastolic pressure reading of 90 mm Hg or greater. The ideal reading is systolic pressure of 120 mm Hg and diastolic pressure of 80 mm Hg.

Pathophysiology

HTN occurs when the systemic vascular resistance (SVR) or cardiac output increases. SVR pertains to the vasomotor tone of the peripheral blood vessels and is the force required to push the blood through the vessels. The most common cause of heightened SVR is atherosclerosis. Atherosclerosis

---

Box 13-1   Functional Health Pattern Assessment for Vascular Disorders

HEALTH PERCEPTION/HEALTH MANAGEMENT
- Is there a family history of chronic arterial occlusive disease (CAOD)?
- Does the patient understand his or her overall condition of health?
- What medications, including over-the-counter drugs, does the patient take?
- What alternative therapies does the patient use?
- Does the patient measure blood pressure weekly or as directed by the physician? Does the patient know what constitutes abnormally high or low readings?

NUTRITION/METABOLISM
- What is the patient's current weight? What is the patient's target weight? Has there been a recent gain or loss of weight?
- Does the patient understand what daily dietary intake is normal and what diet is appropriate for management of hypertension?
- What is the general condition of the skin?
- Is peripheral edema present?
- Are there skin color changes associated with progressive CAOD?

ELIMINATION
- Have any changes occurred in bowel or bladder habits?
- Is the patient aware of the increased risk of incontinence due to the diuretic effects of some cardiac medications?
- Does the patient experience periods of insomnia related to leg cramps?

ACTIVITY/EXERCISE
- Does the patient experience shortness of breath or chest pain on exertion?
- Does the patient experience increased fatigue after physical activity?
- Can the patient perform the activities of daily living without experiencing CAOD symptoms?
- Can the patient function at work and remain symptom free?
- What is the patient's stair-climbing tolerance? Does the patient have leg cramps associated with walking?

SLEEP/REST
- How many hours of uninterrupted sleep does the patient get at night?
- How frequently does the patient take rest periods during the day?

- What techniques does the patient use to decrease leg cramps while in the supine position?
- Is the patient aware of awakening with chest pain or pressure?

COGNITION/PERCEPTION
- What is the quality of the CAOD symptoms, including hand, finger, or toe pain and skin color changes?
- How long do the symptoms last and what does the patient do to alleviate them?
- Does the patient experience occipital headaches or headaches during the morning hours?

SELF-PERCEPTION/SELF-CONCEPT
- What are the effects of CAOD on body image?
- Does the patient experience feelings of fear or loss of control related to CAOD?
- Is the patient depressed?

ROLES/RELATIONSHIPS
- What kind of work does the patient perform?
- Does the patient have difficulty fulfilling responsibilities at home?
- How has the diagnosis of a chronic vascular disorder affected the patient's family and/or caregivers?

SEXUALITY/REPRODUCTION
- Is the patient sexually active?
- Is the patient satisfied with current sexual patterns?
- Does the patient understand the effects of medications on libido?

COPING/STRESS TOLERANCE
- What support systems are available to the patient?
- Has the patient developed new strategies for coping with stress?
- Can the patient manage the chronic vascular disease in the current living situation?

VALUES/BELIEFS
- What is important to the patient?
- What constitutes good quality of life for the patient?
- What are the patient's beliefs related to this condition?
- What are the patient's spiritual and cultural beliefs?
- To what extent do the patient's cultural/spiritual beliefs influence decision making related to this condition?

---

is an insidious process that changes the diameter of the vessels. As vessel diameter becomes increasingly smaller, it becomes more and more difficult for blood to flow through the vessels. Figure 13-1 summarizes the pathophysiology of HTN.

Cardiac output is calculated as the heart rate in beats per minute multiplied by the stroke volume. Stroke volume is the amount of blood pumped from the left ventricle per heartbeat.

Three systems regulate blood pressure: the renal, endocrine, and nervous systems. The kidneys participate in the regulation of blood pressure through the action of the renin-angiotensin-aldosterone system. Renin is secreted by the kidney in response to low blood pressure and increased urinary sodium concentration. Renin then converts the plasma protein angiotensinogen to angiotensin I. The lungs release angiotensin-converting enzyme, which converts angiotensin I to angiotensin II. Angiotensin II acts as a

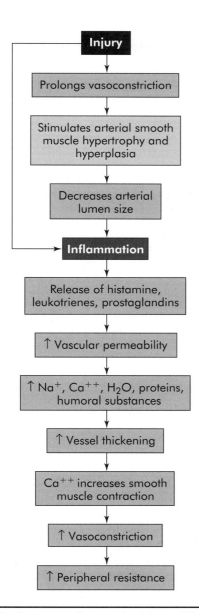

Figure 13-1 Summary of pathophysiology of hypertension. ↑, Increased. (From McCance KL, Huether SE: *Pathophysiology: the biologic basis for disease in adults and children,* ed 4, St Louis, 2002, Mosby.)

potent vasoconstrictor and also stimulates the release of aldosterone. Aldosterone promotes water and sodium retention, which results in an increase in blood pressure.

The nervous system controls blood pressure through the release of epinephrine and norepinephrine. As blood pressure decreases, norepinephrine is released by the sympathetic nervous system. In addition, when blood pressure drops, epinephrine and norepinephrine are secreted by the adrenal medulla. These substances are potent vasoconstrictors that lead to an increase in heart rate, cardiac output, and force of myocardial contractility, so that the blood pressure rises.

The endocrine system acts to control blood pressure by the release of multiple agents such as aldosterone and antidiuretic hormone. Angiotensin II stimulates the adrenal cortex to release aldosterone. Aldosterone causes the kidneys to retain sodium and water. As a result of increased sodium levels, the posterior pituitary then releases antidiuretic hormone, which raises extracellular fluid volume and blood pressure.

The three categories of HTN are primary (essential) HTN, secondary HTN, and isolated systolic HTN. The most common of the three is essential HTN.

Heredity and environmental factors are the best current explanation for this disease. Multiple risk factors contribute to the development of HTN. These are tobacco smoking, obesity, sedentary lifestyle, stress, increased dietary sodium intake, excessive alcohol consumption, advanced age, male gender, and African American race.

Secondary HTN develops as a result of another condition, such as renal artery stenosis, pheochromocytoma, pregnancy, brain neoplasm, or use of certain medications. Secondary HTN accounts for only 5% of cases of HTN. The physiologic result of secondary causes of HTN is either vasoconstriction or increased fluid volume. The primary problem must be corrected to improve the outcome of the secondary HTN.

Isolated systolic HTN is present when the systolic blood pressure is higher than 160 mm Hg and the diastolic blood pressure is lower than 85 mm Hg. This occurs more often in women than in men and more often in those older than 65 years of age. Isolated systolic HTN is a result of decreased elasticity of the larger arteries caused by atherosclerosis, as explained in Chapter 12.

Table 13-1 shows the categories of HTN as defined by the National Institutes of Health's Joint National Committee of Prevention, Detection, Evaluation and Treatment of Hypertension, which were released in May 2003.

Clinical Manifestations

A large percentage of patients with HTN are asymptomatic until HTN reaches a life-threatening stage and provokes a cerebrovascular accident. The degree of target end-organ

Table 13-1 National Institutes of Health Classification of Blood Pressure for Adults Aged 18 Years and Older

Category	Systolic (mm Hg)		Diastolic (mm Hg)
Optimal	<120	and	<80
Normal	<130	and	<85
High normal	130-139	or	85-89
Hypertension			
Stage 1	140-159	or	90-99
Stage 2	160-179	or	100-109
Stage 3	180-209	or	110-119
Stage 4	>210	or	>120

damage depends on multiple factors such as the severity of the HTN and the presence of comorbidities such as diabetes mellitus. Therefore, nurses must know what to look for when evaluating an asymptomatic patient with HTN. Because HTN affects the kidneys, the blood urea nitrogen and creatinine levels will be elevated. The ophthalmologic effects of HTN may include papilledema and blurred vision, and the patient may experience severe headaches.

When the medical history of a patient with HTN is taken, the patient may be found to have neurologic symptoms of a transient ischemic attack, which is a precursor to cerebrovascular accident. The patient may complain of slurred speech, unilateral weakness in the upper and lower extremities, and memory loss. All of these symptoms are brief and resolve completely.

The patient should be questioned about abdominal pain that radiates to the back because this may be an indication of aortic disease or cardiac disease that needs further diagnostic workup. Symptoms of dizziness, palpitations, and diaphoresis may indicate a secondary cause of HTN such as valvular heart disease or coronary artery disease.

Further investigation for other disorders that may be causing HTN may reveal symptoms of lower leg pain that is brought on by activity and relieved by rest, which indicate CAOD.

Diagnosis

The primary diagnostic test for HTN is to obtain blood pressure readings at two separate times. If the systolic blood pressure is higher than 140 mm Hg or the diastolic blood pressure is higher than 90 mm Hg during both testing periods, a diagnosis of HTN can be made.

Ninety-five percent of HTN is classified as essential HTN, and diagnostic testing for further causes is not routinely performed. If the patient's age or family history, the severity of the HTN, or findings of the physical examination suggest another cause for the HTN, then an additional diagnostic workup may be indicated. Table 13-2 lists the diagnostic and laboratory studies generally performed for a patient with essential HTN.

Interdisciplinary Care

The interdisciplinary team should include nurses, the patient, primary caregivers (physicians and/or nurse practitioners and physician assistants), a registered dietitian, and a medical social worker. The goals of treatment are to prevent target end-organ damage associated with HTN, ensure adherence to the medication regimen, promote compliance with necessary lifestyle modifications, and reduce blood pressure. Refer to Chapter 12 for specific cardiac rehabilitation interventions.

Drug Therapy

Seven different classes of medication are used in the treatment of HTN. Table 13-3 provides a complete list of medications and the mechanism of action, side effects, and nursing considerations for each.

Antihypertensive medications may decrease SVR, decrease fluid volume, or both.

Diet

Restriction of dietary sodium benefits all patients diagnosed with HTN. In particular, the elderly and African American persons are sensitive to the effects of sodium intake. Refer to Chapter 12, Table 12-4, for a list of high-sodium foods to be avoided. For patients diagnosed with coronary artery disease, choosing foods that have a lower fat content and lower cholesterol helps reduce atherosclerotic plaque formation and assist in the necessary weight reduction required by patients with HTN.

Nursing Considerations

A study published in 2001 (Aminoff and Kjellgren) examined the role of the nurse in the management of HTN. The purpose of the study was to assess differences in the communication between patients and different types of health care practitioner concerning HTN. These communications took place during follow-up appointments for patients with HTN. Topics discussed by the patients during these visits were lifestyle changes, review of new or changed medications, and stress. Mid-level providers were often asked by patients to clarify information presented to them by physicians at a prior visit. The results of the study were revealing. All nurses addressed the risk factors related to HTN and the behavioral modifications necessary to change those risk factors. Physicians spent more time discussing the medications and the disease prognosis with patients. The study

Text continues on p. 189.

Table 13-2 Diagnostic Studies for Hypertension

Study	Purpose
History	Ascertain risk factors.
Physical examination	Assess for target end-organ damage.
Serum electrolyte levels	Detect hyperaldosteronism (indicated by decreased potassium levels).
Serum glucose level	Detect diabetes or Cushing's disease.
Blood urea nitrogen and creatinine levels	Determine effects on kidneys.
Urinalysis, catecholamine levels	Determine effects on kidneys and detect pheochromocytoma.
Lipid profile	Ascertain additional risk factors.
Chest radiograph	Assess size of the heart, detect abnormalities of aorta.
Electrocardiogram	Indicate baseline cardiac status.

Table 13-3   Medications for the Treatment of Hypertension

Drug	Mechanism of Action	Side Effects and Adverse Effects	Nursing Considerations
Diuretics			
Thiazide and Related Diuretics			
Bendroflumethiazide (Naturetin) Benzthiazide (Aquatab, Exna) Chlorothiazide (Diuril) Chlorthalidone (Hygroton) Hydrochlorothiazide (Esidrix, HydroDIURIL, Oretic) Metolazone (Zaroxolyn) Methyclothiazide (Enduron) Trichlormethiazide (Metahydrin, Naqua)	Inhibit NaCl reabsorption in the distal convoluted tubule; increase excretion of Na^+ and Cl^-. Initial decrease in ECF; sustained decrease in SVR. Lower BP moderately in 2-4 wk.	Fluid and electrolyte imbalances (volume depletion, hypokalemia, hyponatremia, hypochloremia, hypomagnesemia, hypercalcemia, hyperuricemia, metabolic alkalosis); CNS effects (vertigo, headache, weakness); GI effects (anorexia, nausea, vomiting, diarrhea, constipation, pancreatitis); sexual problems (impotence and decreased libido); blood dyscrasias; and dermatologic effects (photosensitivity, skin rash). Decreased glucose tolerance.	Monitor for orthostatic hypotension, hypokalemia, and alkalosis. Thiazides may potentiate cardiotoxicity of digoxin by producing hypokalemia. Dietary sodium restriction reduces risk of hypokalemia. NSAIDs can decrease diuretic and antihypertensive effect of thiazide diuretics. Advise patient to supplement with potassium-rich foods. Current doses are lower than previously recommended.
Loop Diuretics			
Bumetanide (Bumex) Ethacrynic acid (Edecrin) Furosemide (Lasix) Torsemide (Demadex)	Inhibit NaCl reabsorption in the thick ascending limb of the loop of Henle. Increase excretion of Na^+ and Cl^-. More potent diuretic effect that thiazides, but shorter duration of action, less effective for hypertension.	Fluid electrolyte imbalance as with thiazides, except no hypercalcemia. Ototoxicity (hearing impairment, deafness, vertigo) that is usually reversible. Metabolic effects, including hyperuricemia, hyperglycemia, increased LDL cholesterol and triglycerides with decreased HDL cholesterol.	Monitor for orthostatic hypotension and electrolyte abnormalities. Loop diuretics remain effective even with renal insufficiency. Diuretic effect of drug increases at higher doses.
Potassium-Sparing Diuretics			
Amiloride (Midamor) Triamterene (Dyrenium)	Reduce K^+ and Na^+ exchange in the distal and collecting tubules. Reduces excretion of K^+, H^+, Ca^{2+}, and Mg^{2+}.	Hyperkalemia, nausea, vomiting, diarrhea, headache, leg cramps, and dizziness.	Monitor for orthostatic hypotension and hyperkalemia. Use of potassium-sparing diuretics is contraindicated in patients with renal failure and should be used with caution in patients on angiotensin-converting enzyme inhibitors or angiotensin II blockers. Avoid potassium supplements.
Spironolactone (Aldactone) Eplerenone (Inspra)	Inhibit the Na^+-retaining and K^+-excreting effects of aldosterone in the distal and collecting tubules.	Same as amiloride and triamterene; may cause gynecomastia, impotence, decreased libido, and menstrual irregularities.	
Adrenergic Inhibitors			
Central-Acting Adrenergic Antagonists			
Clonidine (Catapres)	Reduces sympathetic outflow from CNS. Reduces peripheral sympathetic tone, produces vasodilation; decreases SVR and BP.	Dry mouth, sedation, impotence, nausea, dizziness, sleep disturbance, nightmares, restlessness, and depression. Symptomatic bradycardia in patients with conduction disorder.	Sudden discontinuation may cause withdrawal syndrome, including rebound hypertension, tachycardia, headache, tremors, apprehension, and sweating. Chewing gum or hard candy may relieve dry mouth. Alcohol and sedatives increase sedation. May be given transdermally with fewer side effects and better compliance.

Continued

Table 13-3 Medications for the Treatment of Hypertension—cont'd

Drug	Mechanism of Action	Side Effects and Adverse Effects	Nursing Considerations
Adrenergic Inhibitors—cont'd			
Central-Acting Adrenergic Antagonists—cont'd			
Guanabenz (Wytensin)	Same as for clonidine.	Same as for clonidine.	Same as for clonidine, but not available in transdermal formulation.
Guanfacine (Tenex)	Same as for clonidine.	Same as for clonidine.	Same as for clonidine, but not available in transdermal formulation.
Methyldopa (Aldomet)	Same as for clonidine.	Sedation, fatigue, orthostatic hypotension, decreased libido, impotence, dry mouth, hemolytic anemia, hepatotoxicity, sodium and water retention, depression.	Instruct patient about daytime sedation and avoidance of hazardous activities. Administration of a single daily dose at bedtime minimizes sedative effect.
Peripheral-Acting Adrenergic Antagonists			
Guanethidine (Ismelin)	Prevents peripheral release of norepinephrine, which results in vasodilation; lowers CO and reduces SBP more that DBP.	Marked orthostatic hypotension, diarrhea, cramps, bradycardia, retrograde or delayed ejaculation, sodium and water retention.	May cause severe postural hypotension; not recommended for use in patients with cerebrovascular or coronary insufficiency or in older adults; advise patient to rise slowly and wear support stockings. Hypotensive effect is delayed for 2-3 days and lasts 7-10 days after withdrawal. Once-daily dosing.
Guanadrel sulfate (Hylorel)	Same as for guanethidine.	Similar to those for guanethidine.	Must be given twice daily.
Reserpine (Serpasil)	Depletes central and peripheral stores of norepinephrine; results in peripheral vasodilation (decreases SVR and BP).	Sedation and inability to concentrate; depression; nasal stuffiness.	Use contraindicated in patients with history of depression. Monitor mood and mental status regularly. Advise patient to avoid barbiturates, alcohol, and narcotics.
α_1-Adrenergic Blockers			
Doxazosin (Cardura) Prazosin (Minipress) Terazosin (Hytrin)	Block α_1-adrenergic effects, which produces peripheral vasodilation (decreases SVR and BP).	Variable amount of postural hypotension depending on the plasma volume. Possible profound orthostatic hypotension with syncope within 90 min after initial dose. Retention of salt and water.	Reduced resistance to the outflow of urine is seen in benign prostate hyperplasia. Taking drug at bedtime reduces risks associated with orthostatic hypotension. Has beneficial effects on lipid profile.
Phentolamine (Regitine)	Blocks α_1-adrenergic receptors, which results in peripheral vasodilation (decreases SVR and BP).	Acute, prolonged hypotension, cardiac arrhythmias, tachycardia, weakness, flushing. Abdominal pain, nausea, and exacerbation of peptic ulcer.	Used in short-term management of pheochromocytoma. Also used locally to prevent necrosis of skin and subcutaneous tissue after extravasation of an α-adrenergic drug. No oral formulation.
β-Adrenergic Blockers			
Acebutolol (Sectral) Atenolol (Tenormin) Betaxolol (Kerlone) Bisoprolol (Zebeta) Carteolol (Cartol) Carvedilol (Coreg) Metoprolol (Lopressor) Nadolol (Corgard) Penbutolol (Levatol)	Reduce BP by antagonizing β-adrenergic effects. Decrease CO and reduce sympathetic vasoconstriction tone. Decrease renin secretion by kidney.	Bronchospasm, atrioventricular conduction block, impaired peripheral circulation. Nightmares, depression, weakness, reduced exercise capacity. May induce or exacerbate heart failure in susceptible patients. Sudden withdrawal of β-adrenergic	β-Adrenergic blockers vary in lipid solubility, selectivity, and presence of partial sympathomimetic effect, which explains different therapeutic and side effect profiles of specific agents. Monitor pulse regularly. Use caution in patients with

Table 13-3 Medications for the Treatment of Hypertension—cont'd

Drug	Mechanism of Action	Side Effects and Adverse Effects	Nursing Considerations
Adrenergic Inhibitors—cont'd **β-Adrenergic Blockers—cont'd**			
Pindolol (Visken) Propranolol (Inderal) Timolol (Blocadren)		blockers may cause rebound hypertension and exacerbate symptoms of ischemic heart failure.	diabetes mellitus because drug may mask signs of hypoglycemia.
Esmolol (Brevibloc)	Reduces BP by antagonizing β$_1$-adrenergic effects.		IV administration; rapid onset and very short duration of action.
Combined α- and β-Adrenergic Blocker			
Labetalol (Normodyne, Trandate)	Has α$_1$-, β$_1$-, and β$_2$-adrenergic blocking properties producing peripheral vasodilation and decreased heart rate. Reduces CO, SVR, and BP.	Dizziness, fatigue, nausea, vomiting, dyspepsia, paresthesia, nasal stuffiness, impotence, edema. Hepatic toxicity.	Same as for β-adrenergic blockers. IV form available for hypertensive crisis in hospitalized patients. Patients must be kept supine during VI administration. Assess patient tolerance of upright position (severe postural hypotension may occur) before allowing upright activities (e.g., commode use).
Direct Vasodilators			
Diazoxide (Hyperstat)	Reduces SVR and BP by direct arterial vasodilation.	Reflex sympathetic activation producing increased HR, CO, and salt and water retention. Hyperglycemia, especially in patients with type 2 diabetes.	IV use only for hypertensive crisis in hospitalized patients. Administer only into peripheral vein.
Hydralazine (Apresoline)	Reduces SVR and BP by direct arterial vasodilation.	Headache, nausea, flushing, palpitation, tachycardia, dizziness, and angina. Hemolytic anemia, vasculitis, and rapidly progressive glomerulonephritis.	IV use for hypertensive crisis in hospitalized patients. Twice-daily oral dosing. Not used as monotherapy because of side effects. Use contraindicated in patients with coronary artery disease; used with caution in patients older than 40 years of age.
Minoxidil (Loniten)	Reduces SVR and BP by direct arterial vasodilation.	Reflex tachycardia, marked sodium and fluid retention (may require loop diuretics for control), and hirsutism. May cause ECG changes (flattened and inverted T waves) not related to ischemia.	Reserved for treatment of severe hypertension associated with renal failure and resistant to other therapy. Once- or twice-daily dosing.
Nitroglycerin (Tridil)	Relaxes arterial and venous smooth muscles, which reduces preload and SVR. At low dosage, venous dilation predominates; at higher dosage arterial dilation is present.	Hypotension, headache, vomiting, flushing.	IV use for hypertensive crisis in hospitalized patients with myocardial ischemia. Administered by continuous IV infusion with pump or control device.
Sodium nitroprusside (Nipride)	Produces direct arterial vasodilation reducing SVR and BP.	Acute hypotension, nausea, vomiting, muscle twitching. Signs of thiocyanate toxicity include anorexia, nausea, fatigue, and disorientation.	IV use for hypertensive crisis in hospitalized patients. Administered by continuous IV infusion with pump or control device. Use intra-arterial monitoring of BP. Light-resistant bags, bottles, and administration sets must be used; stable for 24 hr. Monitor thiocyanate levels with prolonged use (≥24-48 hr).

Continued

Table 13-3   Medications for the Treatment of Hypertension—cont'd

Drug	Mechanism of Action	Side Effects and Adverse Effects	Nursing Considerations
Ganglionic Blockers			
Trimethaphan (Arfonad)	Interrupts adrenergic control of arteries, results in vasodilation, and reduces SVR and BP.	Visual disturbance, dilated pupils, dry mouth, urinary hesitancy, subjective chilliness.	IV use for initial control of BP in patients with dissecting aortic aneurysm. Administered by continuous IV infusion with pump or control device.
Angiotensin Inhibitors			
Angiotensin-Converting Enzyme Inhibitors			
Benazepril (Lotensin) Captopril (Capoten) Enalapril (Vasotec) Fosinopril (Monopril) Lisinopril (Prinivil, Zestril) Moexipril (Univasc) Perindopril (Aceon) Quinapril (Accupril) Ramipril (Altace) Trandolapril (Mavik)	Inhibit angiotensin-converting enzyme; reduce conversion of angiotensin I to angiotensin II; prevent angiotensin II–mediated vasoconstriction.	Hypotension, loss of taste, cough, hyperkalemia, acute renal failure, skin rash, angioneurotic edema.	Aspirin and NSAIDs may reduce drug effectiveness. Addition of diuretic enhances drug effect. Should not be used with potassium-sparing diuretics. Can cause fetal morbidity or mortality. Captopril may be given orally for hypertensive crisis.
Enalaprilat (Vasotec Injection)	Inhibits angiotensin-converting enzyme when oral agents not appropriate.	Same as for oral administration.	Given IV over 5 min; may be given every 6 hr.
Angiotensin II Receptor Blockers			
Candesartan (Atacand) Eprosartan (Teveten) Irbesartan (Avapro) Iosartan (Cozaar) Olmesartan (Benicar) Telmisartan (Micardis) Tasosartan (Veridia) Valsartan (Diovan)	Prevent action of angiotensin II and produce vasodilation and increased salt and water excretion.	Hyperkalemia, decreased renal function.	Full effect on BP may not be seen for 3-6 wk.
Calcium Channel Blockers			
Amlodipine (Norvasc) Diltiazem (Cardizem) Felodipine (Plendil) Isradipine (DynaCirc) Mibefradil (Posicor) Nicardipine (Cardene) Nifedipine (Procardia) Nisoldipine (Sular) Verapamil (Isoptin)	Block movement of extracellular calcium into cells, causing vasodilation and decreased SVR.	Nausea, headache, dizziness, peripheral edema. Reflex tachycardia (with dihydropyridines). Reflex decrease HR (with diltiazem); constipation (with verapamil).	Use with caution in patients with heart failure. Contraindicated in patients with second- or third-degree heart block. IV nicardipine available for hypertensive crisis in hospitalized patients. Sustained-release formulations available for some drugs. Avoid grapefruit when on nifedipine.

From Lewis SM, Heitkemper MM, Dirksen SR: *Medical-surgical nursing: assessment and management of clinical problems,* ed 6, St Louis, 2004, Mosby.
BP, Blood pressure; *CNS,* central nervous system; *CO,* cardiac output; *DBP,* diastolic blood pressure; *ECF,* extracellular fluid; *ECG,* electrocardiogram; *GI,* gastrointestinal; *HDL,* high-density lipoproteins; *HR,* heart rate; *IV,* intravenous; *LDL,* low-density lipoproteins; *NSAIDs,* nonsteroidal antiinflammatory drugs; *SBP,* systolic blood pressure; *SVR,* systemic vascular resistance.

demonstrated that different types of health care providers play pivotal yet different roles in a comprehensive approach to the management of HTN.

Nursing interventions for long-term management of HTN begin with patient education. To assist the patient in making lifestyle modifications, the nurse can provide a list of foods high in sodium that the patient should avoid, give the patient information about smoking cessation programs, outline a simple daily plan of exercise, assess for lack of adherence to the medication regimen, and provide alternatives for coping with side effects of medications. Nurses can encourage the patient to monitor blood pressure at home with a pressure-measuring device and provide specific instructions on when to seek medical help based on systolic and diastolic measurements. One of the most important considerations in establishing a plan of care for a patient with HTN is ensuring that the patient participates actively in decision making.

Think S for Success

Symptoms
- Manage blood pressure by ensuring compliance with medication regimen.

Sequelae
- Prevent target end-organ damage by addressing necessary lifestyle changes.

Safety
- Teach patient need for home blood pressure monitoring, follow-up appointments, compliance with medication regimen, and behavior modification.

Support/Services
- Give patient and primary caregiver referrals for dietary consultation regarding low-sodium foods and meal preparation.
- Assist patient in formulating a care plan that helps patient manage side effects of medication.

Satisfaction
- Determine the degree to which blood pressure management interferes with important aspects of patient's life and maintain quality of life.

CHRONIC ARTERIAL OCCLUSIVE DISEASE

CAOD is caused by atherosclerosis and is a risk factor for early death. This disease affects 10% of individuals over 70 years of age, but it can also have an impact on performance of the activities of daily living among younger patients aged 35 to 69 years who are diagnosed with comorbid conditions such as diabetes or who smoke tobacco, are obese, and have a sedentary lifestyle (Bryant and Turkoski, 1999). This disorder affects men more frequently than women and there is a strong hereditary component.

Pathophysiology

Atherosclerosis is the primary cause of CAOD. The disease can affect any arterial blood vessel. This section addresses only CAOD of the lower extremities. The larger vessels primarily involved in lower extremity CAOD are the aortoiliac, femoral, popliteal, and tibial arteries.

The process of atherosclerotic plaque formation is insidious and causes narrowing of the arterial vessels, which can eventually lead to complete occlusion. This obstruction creates a decreased blood supply to and inadequate oxygenation of the tissues. As a result, the patient with CAOD experiences ischemic pain. The pain produced by ischemia leads to the accumulation of end products of anaerobic metabolism, including lactic acid and other metabolites.

The risk factors associated with the development of CAOD are smoking, diabetes, sedentary lifestyle, obesity, hyperlipidemia, HTN, and a family history of the disease.

Nicotine inhaled during tobacco use has a vasoconstrictive effect on the arterial vessels due to the release of norepinephrine and epinephrine. These catecholamines increase the heart rate and blood pressure and thus increase the workload of the heart. Accumulation of fat deposits associated with atherosclerosis narrows the vessels and reduces vessel elasticity. Uncontrolled HTN causes increased SVR, and thus blood flow to the peripheral vessels is reduced.

Clinical Manifestations

Intermittent claudication is the term used to describe lower extremity calf pain or cramping during walking that is relieved by rest. Pain may occur while the patient is performing the activities of daily living or during any other type of simple physical exertion. The decreased blood and oxygen supply leads to ischemic muscle pain. Approximately half of all persons in whom the arteries have narrowed by about 65% experience intermittent claudication (Bryant and Turkoski, 1999). Continued leg pain at complete rest is a sign that the disease has progressed to the most severe stage. The pain may vary from patient to patient and from day to day for a given patient.

Additional symptoms may be decreased sensation and paresthesias in the feet or toes. The skin over the affected extremity is shiny, without hair growth, and the color can range from pale to red to dusky blue. The lower extremity may be cool to the touch. The femoral, popliteal, tibial, and pedal pulses may be diminished or absent depending on the extent of the disease.

A complication that may develop as a result of compromised arterial blood flow and slight trauma is that of a skin ulceration over a bony prominence such as the ankle. Chronic ischemia produces atrophy of the skin, which contributes to poor healing of the skin, infection, and ultimately gangrene of the most distal part of the extremity on which the ulcer is found. These end-stage complications of CAOD may result in the need for amputation of the lower extremity.

Diagnosis

In CAOD, as in any disease, the history reported by the patient and the physical examination are crucial in the diagnosis. Questions regarding the type of pain, location of pain, onset of symptoms, duration of symptoms, and any factors that alleviate the pain can elicit the most helpful information. Significant findings for the diagnosis of CAOD are outlined in the section on clinical manifestations.

Noninvasive diagnostic Doppler ultrasonography can indicate the velocity of blood flow through an affected artery by the reflection of audible sound waves. When the blood flow through a section of the artery is diminished, the velocity increases.

Once the physician has determined that the patient with significant CAOD requires further interventions for management, such as surgery, invasive diagnostic arteriography is performed to ascertain the location and extent of the obstruction.

Interdisciplinary Care

The members of the interdisciplinary team are the primary nurse, physician, registered dietitian, endocrinologist, dermatologist, and patient and family and/or caregivers. The goals for the team members caring for the patient with CAOD are to provide pain relief, improve blood flow to the muscles of the lower extremity, improve the patient's tolerance of exercise, and prevent skin ulceration.

Medications that inhibit platelet aggregation have been shown to help the patient with CAOD walk greater distances and reduce pain. No other classes of medication are available to treat CAOD. The side effects of platelet aggregation–inhibiting medications are headache, diarrhea, and palpitations. Nursing considerations include educating the patient about the actions of the medication and their benefit to the patient as well as the importance of adherence to the medication regimen and awareness of side effects. If the patient with CAOD has other comorbid conditions, continued adherence to additional medication regimens must be addressed.

Nonpharmacologic management consists of a carefully developed exercise program, which is discussed in more detail in the section on physical therapy, and control of predisposing risk factors associated with chronic cardiac diseases, particularly hyperlipidemia and smoking, as discussed in Chapter 12.

Nursing Considerations

The mainstay of nursing care in any disease is education of the patient. The patient with CAOD should understand the significant detrimental impact of tobacco use. Smoking not only increases the viscosity of the blood but also decreases the amount of oxygen available to the tissues.

Educating the patient with regard to dietary intake consists of identifying foods that are low in fat and cholesterol.

If the patient suffers from HTN, it is important that the patient adhere to a low-sodium diet. Further consultation with a dietitian is advised to promote patient compliance with the dietary regimen.

The patient must be taught proper foot care to prevent skin ulcerations. A teaching plan for foot care should include educating the patient to use a mirror to view the plantar surface of the feet and to inspect the skin for calluses, scabs, or open wounds as well as to observe the color and temperature of the affected extremity. The patient should be instructed to wash the feet daily, dry them thoroughly, and use proper supportive footwear. Trimming the nails before they become ingrown is important in the prevention of skin breakdown.

Physical Therapy

Limitations in mobility can decrease the quality of life for a patient with CAOD. When the patient follows a regular supervised walking program, collateral blood vessels develop to help improve circulation to the lower extremity. Walking is the standard treatment for intermittent claudication to promote the development of collateral blood vessels.

Supervised walking programs start out slowly, with the patient walking only until symptoms are experienced. At that point, the patient stops walking until the pain is relieved. The initial goal may be only 10 minutes of walking. The walking exercise resumes until the pain reoccurs. This type of exercise is gradually increased until the patient can tolerate walking for a total of 35 minutes out of a 50-minute period (Uphold and Graham, 1999). There should be 5-minute warm-up and cooldown periods in which the large muscle groups are stretched to help provide the flexibility required for walking.

Think S for Success

Symptoms
■ Manage pain related to intermittent claudication with a walking program.

Sequelae
■ Prevent possible disability by instructing patient on modification of risk factors.

Safety
■ Encourage patient to participate in supervised walking program, inspect feet and skin every day, and report any signs of further disease progression.

Support/Services
■ Refer to community resources, such as dietitian, physical therapist, and smoking cessation programs, as necessary

Satisfaction
■ Assess the impact of chronic arterial occlusive disease on the patient's quality of life and develop a plan to reach goals.

BUERGER'S DISEASE
Pathophysiology

Thromboangiitis obliterans, also known as Buerger's disease, fits within the category of CAOD except that this disease affects the small and medium-sized arteries of the extremities. Buerger's disease is seen most often in men between the ages of 20 and 40 years. The effects of the disease are caused by a thrombotic process. The exact cause of this disorder is not known; however, research has shown it to be strongly associated with tobacco use in any form. There may be some ethnic predisposition to the disorder, because it is more prevalent in Asian countries and less prevalent in North America. Arsenic exposure has also been implicated, and in one study a factor V gene mutation was associated with increased risk (Watts and Scott, 2003). The presence of hyperlipidemia, diabetes, or HTN is not associated with the development of Buerger's disease, as is the case with CAOD. Buerger's disease can affect the upper and lower extremities.

Clinical Manifestations

The symptoms of Buerger's disease are insidious and are similar to those of CAOD. The toes are the first areas to be affected. The symptoms include decreased sensation of the lower extremity, tingling, coldness, and a heightened sensitivity to pain in the toe or foot. One or more wounds may be present. Unlike pressure ulcers, these wounds typically occur on the dorsum of the toes or foot, between the toes, or on the lateral malleolus. Because there is little circulation to the area, the wounds are dry instead of moist, with atrophic skin and sparse hair growth in the area (Lubisch, 2001). Dependent rubor with pallor on elevation may also provide evidence of poor circulation to the area. Additional symptoms include skin color changes, painful ulcerations, and the potential for gangrene (Lewis, Collier, and Heitkemper, 2002). An ominous sign and indication of a pregangrenous condition is pain in the extremity at rest.

Diagnosis

No formal set of diagnostic studies exists to determine if a patient has Buerger's disease. It can be considered a diagnosis of exclusion after a complete history taking and physical examination have been performed. The health care provider requests the patient to stop smoking for a trial period. During that time, the patient is asked to assess the return and/or frequency of the symptoms. If the patient has stopped smoking and the symptoms have not reappeared, then the diagnosis of Buerger's disease can be made.

Treatment and Nursing Considerations

No medication is available to treat or minimize the effects of the disease. Treatment focuses on education regarding the avoidance of agents or situations that can cause a compromise in blood flow. Smoking cessation is the most important element in halting the disease process.

The four most common reasons why patients smoke tobacco are the relief of tension, the stimulation gained from the nicotine, fear of quitting because of the potential for gaining weight, and the occurrence of withdrawal symptoms, including headaches, inability to concentrate, and insomnia.

The nurse's role in the treatment of Buerger's disease is to provide appropriate community and medical resources for smoking cessation. In addition, the nurse must continue to educate the patient about the signs and symptoms of disease progression so that the patient will obtain appropriate medical care.

Factors that help prevent the restriction of blood supply to the extremities are avoidance of extremes of heat or cold, prevention of injury, wearing of loose-fitting clothes, use of appropriate footwear, avoidance of prolonged periods of standing, and avoidance of walking barefoot (Funk, 2001).

Physical Therapy

The physical therapist promotes healing through débridement and wound care and through rehabilitation for individuals after amputation. Wound care may involve the use of whirlpool baths (Lubisch, 2003). Extremes of heat and cold are to be avoided because they contribute to tissue injury. Because a minor injury is frequently a site of major infection due to poor perfusion to the repair site, secondary infection of ulcerations is a significant risk (Vascular Associates of Bangalore, 2000).

Medical Social Work

Buerger's disease is more frequently seen in individuals who work outdoors or do manual labor. Therefore, amputations present a serious risk of loss of income. The medical social worker may participate in care by identifying training in alternative work and providing counseling for the patient and family regarding economic concerns and loss of self-esteem related to poor body image and inability to provide for the family. In cultures in which the male is the primary source of income, loss of the ability to work may be especially problematic. Secondary infection or amputation may also be associated with chronic pain. Treatment referral for substance abuse or addiction may be needed if the patient has attempted to self-medicate to control pain.

End-of-Life Issues

In one study of individuals with Buerger's disease, continuous follow-up indicated that all individuals had experienced gangrene. Many had multiple limb involvement. If revascularization is successful, healing proceeds well after amputation to remove gangrenous tissue, and successive amputations may be avoided. One study indicated that life expectancy is normal for individuals who stop smoking (Vascular Associates of Bangalore, 2001). In another study, however, the 5-year survival rate for all patients undergoing an amputation of a lower extremity (including those with diabetes) was less than 50% (Davidson, 1999).

For these individuals, life becomes a series of amputations. Amputees who walk with prostheses have an unsteady gait and are more likely to fall. Approximately half of all amputees who suffer fractures as a result of a fall remain wheelchair bound (Davidson, 1999). Buerger's disease has the potential to become a significant life-limiting illness, with sequential amputation and infection potentially resulting in death.

Family and Caregiver Issues

Lifestyle may be changed as a result of loss of income and repeated illness that leads to permanent disability. Alterations to the home to improve mobility and accommodate a wheelchair may be necessary. Caregivers must learn to change dressings and may need to assist the patient with daily foot checks. Some caregivers may resent providing this kind of care. The environment must be kept free of obstacles that may lead to lower extremity injuries. Caregivers may need to assist the patient in the use of smoking cessation techniques and endure the difficulties of the patient's cessation efforts.

Ethical Considerations

Ethical considerations relate to the patient's autonomy, especially a patient's desire to continue smoking in spite of the fact it will most likely result in continued gangrenous lesions that lead to amputations. The patient's desire for autonomy must be balanced against the cost to the patient's family and/or society in paying for this largely self-inflicted disability.

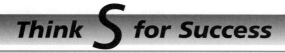

Think S for Success

Symptoms
- Help patient to recognize need for smoking cessation.

Sequelae
- Prevent disability associated with extremity amputation by assessing patient frequently and referring for additional medical care in a timely fashion to avoid need for amputation.

Safety
- Educate patient regarding proper clothing and footwear, and impart necessary knowledge concerning items and situations that promote decreased blood flow to extremities.

Support/Services
- Make referrals for and provide encouragement to patient participating in smoking cessation program.

Satisfaction
- Continue to show patient that overall health has improved as a result of ceasing tobacco use.
- Develop a plan to maintain quality of life.

RAYNAUD'S PHENOMENON
Pathophysiology

Raynaud's phenomenon is a vascular disorder that is episodic and affects primarily the toes and fingers. Estimates are that 5% to 10% of the general population in the United States has this disorder. Women between 15 and 40 years of age are affected more often than are men (Medical College of Wisconsin, 2000). The disorder is classified into primary and secondary Raynaud's phenomenon. The majority of persons are diagnosed with primary Raynaud's phenomenon. Secondary Raynaud's phenomenon can be associated with collagen vascular diseases such as scleroderma, Sjögren's syndrome, and rheumatoid arthritis.

The cause of Raynaud's phenomenon is not known. The disorder is characterized by spasms of the small cutaneous arteries of the toes and fingers (Lewis, Collier, and Heitkemper, 2002). When the patient with Raynaud's phenomenon is exposed to cold, experiences an emotional upset, or uses caffeine or tobacco, the cutaneous arteries constrict and the symptoms are produced.

Clinical Manifestations

As a result of the decreased blood supply to the fingers and toes during vessel constriction, skin color changes and alterations in sensation occur. The skin color changes with the onset of an episode of Raynaud's phenomenon progress from white to blue to red. White coloring signifies the initial response to the collapse of the digital arteries. A bluish color occurs next as a result of decreased oxygen supply to the fingers or toes. During this time, the patient may complain of pain and numbness in the affected digits. As the arterioles recover, the digits turn red because of the dilation of the vessels as appropriate blood supply is restored. The patient may also experience aching and swelling as the episode comes to an end. An attack of Raynaud's phenomenon can last from 1 minute to 2 hours.

Diagnosis

Table 13-4 lists criteria established by the National Institutes of Health to aid in the diagnosis of this disease.

Treatment and Nursing Considerations

The treatment of Raynaud's phenomenon is commonly supportive. The goals of treatment are to prevent tissue damage of the fingers and toes and to reduce the frequency of episodes (O'Connor, 2001). No specific protocol has been established for the treatment of this disease because of the variability in severity.

Education is the primary tool used in treatment of Raynaud's phenomenon. Informing the patient about the potential triggers of an episode is the initial step. The patient should wear gloves when handling cold items in a refrigerator or freezer. When going outside, the patient should wear multilayered loose-fitting socks, hats, and gloves. In addi-

Table 13-4 Diagnostic Criteria for Raynaud's Phenomenon

Primary Raynaud's	Secondary Raynaud's
Periodic vasospastic episodes of pallor or cyanosis	Periodic vasospastic episodes of pallor and cyanosis
Normal nail-fold capillary pattern	Abnormal nail-fold capillary pattern
Absence of antinuclear antibodies	Presence of antinuclear antibodies
Normal erythrocyte sedimentation rate	Abnormal erythrocyte sedimentation rate
Absence of pitting scars, gangrene, ulcers on fingers and/or toes	Presence of pitting scars, gangrene, ulcers on fingers and/or toes

tion, commercial pocket warmers can be placed in shoes or gloves for extra warmth. An important point that is sometimes missed when a patient is educated about this disease is the fact that air conditioning can also trigger an episode of Raynaud's phenomenon.

As for all the chronic vascular disorders, smoking cessation is essential to decrease the frequency of attacks and prevent tissue damage caused by vasoconstriction of peripheral vessels associated with nicotine use.

Helping the patient identify stressful situations and learn to avoid them can also assist in preventing these episodes. Patient referral to practitioners of alternative therapies for stress reduction may prove beneficial.

During an attack of Raynaud's, warming the affected area with warm water can decrease the vasospastic action of the disease.

Pharmaceutical approaches to treatment of this disorder include calcium channel blockers and aspirin. The vasodilatory effect of calcium channel blockers can help relax smooth muscles and dilate small vessels and thus decrease the frequency of attacks. Adverse reactions to calcium channel blockers are dizziness, constipation, and headache. The use of antiplatelet medications can increase blood flow.

If the episodes are frequent and long lasting, skin integrity can be compromised. Thus skin ulcerations may form. Regular examination of the fingers and toes can help prevent further breakdown by alerting the patient to seek medical attention sooner.

Physical and Occupational Therapy

Physical and occupational therapy are not routinely prescribed for patients with Raynaud's phenomenon. When such therapy is indicated, the assessment is usually performed by an occupational therapist, because the hands are most likely to be involved. Exercises to promote flexibility and improve circulation may be prescribed. Because tem-

perature extremes may exacerbate symptoms, therapeutic modalities involving heat or cold are used cautiously. When Raynaud's phenomenon is associated with scleroderma, additional therapies may be required to maintain flexibility because of the presence of fibrosis throughout the body.

Medical Social Work

The prognosis for Raynaud's phenomenon varies with the cause. The degree of social work involvement in patient care also varies. Raynaud's phenomenon primarily affects females, and it may be difficult for some male caregivers to take on the additional role of family caregiver and to perform household chores. Loss of income due to repeated work absences or the inability to perform jobs requiring fine motor coordination with the hands is another concern. The medical social worker may assist the family in identifying volunteers who can provide support by supplying household help. As with other disabilities, the social worker may also provide assistance in identifying alternative vocational settings. In addition, determination of disability status can be facilitated by the social worker.

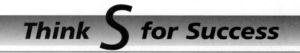

Think S for Success

Symptoms
- Decrease frequency of episodes by teaching patient to avoid triggering situations.

Sequelae
- Avert disability in affected digits by encouraging patient to take prescribed medication, stop smoking, avoid exposure to cold, and avoid stressful environments.

Safety
- Teach patient and caregiver importance of dressing with multiple loose-fitting layers on extremities, placing affected digit in warm water during an attack, and evaluating skin regularly for occurrence of ulceration .

Support/Services
- Refer patient to smoking cessation group, stress management program, and physical therapy as warranted to develop regular exercise routine.

Satisfaction
- Ascertain the level of impact of Raynaud's phenomenon on patient's ability to perform activities of daily living and on overall quality of life.

VARICOSE VEINS
Pathophysiology

Blood flows in subcutaneous veins through a series of one-way valves within the vessels. When a valve becomes incompetent, blood backs up and over time the vein becomes dilated and tortuous. As the backup of blood increases and less blood is returned to the heart via the venous system, the increased pressure is transmitted to the capillary bed and edema can develop.

Such distended veins may develop in the esophagus, in the rectal area in the form of a hemorrhoid, and wherever arteriovenous connections are made throughout the body. The most common site for the development of these varicosities is the saphenous vein of the lower extremity (Lewis, Collier, and Heitkemper, 2002).

The exact cause of varicose veins is unknown, but the risk factors have been identified and include work in an occupation that requires prolonged periods of standing, excessive weight, inadequate exercise, chronic straining with constipation, pregnancy, and use of contraceptive drugs (Chaitow, 2001).

Clinical Manifestations

The most common symptoms include aching pain, pressure, itching over the site of the varicose vein, discoloration of the tissues, and nighttime cramping and swelling of the affected extremity. This disorder develops bilaterally.

Diagnosis

Radiologic examination can be performed to determine if the varicosity is associated with the development of a deep vein thrombosis. Otherwise, a thorough physical examination of the patient in conjunction with the report given by the patient during history taking can determine the diagnosis of a varicose vein.

Treatment and Nursing Considerations

Surgery is used to remove unsightly varicose veins by stripping them out or by tying them off. This surgical intervention allows collateral vessels to develop and assist in the circulation of blood. When a patient develops chronic thrombophlebitis, a surgical intervention may be performed to prevent additional complications.

Venous stasis ulcers of the lower extremities and superficial thrombophlebitis may develop. Therefore, careful inspection of the skin over the lower extremities is of the utmost importance. Nonsurgical interventions include the use of support stockings while ambulating, elevation of the lower extremities, avoidance of tight, restrictive clothing, and participation in a regular exercise program prescribed by the health care provider.

Overweight individuals must be taught about appropriate foods to assist in weight loss. Increasing the amount of fiber in the diet may help a patient who suffers from constipation and reduce the frequency of episodes of straining with bowel movements.

The recipe for "power pudding" (Neal, 1995) to aid the patient with bowel management is provided in Box 13-2.

> **Box 13-2   Power Pudding**
>
> ½ cup stewed prunes
> ½ cup applesauce
> ½ cup yogurt or whipped cream
> ½ cup wheat bran
> Add small amount of prune juice for blending purposes.
> Mix ingredients and store in airtight container in refrigerator for up to 1 week.
> Eat ½ cup every morning to assist in softening stool.

From Neal LJ: Power pudding: natural laxative therapy for the elderly who are homebound, *Home Healthc Nurse* 13(3):66-71, 1995.

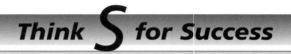

Think S for Success

Symptoms
- Manage the symptom of pain over varicose vein with use of elastic support stockings.

Sequelae
- Teach patient to prevent development of venous stasis ulcer by carefully inspecting skin and seeking medical treatment promptly when necessary.

Safety
- Instruct patient about the risk factors for the development of varicose veins:
  Obesity
  Sedentary lifestyle
  Chronic straining because of constipation
  Use of contraceptive drugs

Support/Services
- Refer patient for physical therapy if needed to develop exercise regimen.
- Provide instruction regarding calcium channel blocker medication.

Satisfaction
- Ascertain patient's degree of satisfaction in ability to perform activities of daily living, engage in exercise, and pursue physical activities that lead to desired quality of life.

COMPLEMENTARY AND ALTERNATIVE THERAPIES

Alternative therapies have proven therapeutic effects in managing several types of vascular disease. In particular, yoga, visualization, meditation, and biofeedback have been shown to reduce blood pressure. Herbal supplements such as St. John's wort, yohimbine, garlic, and licorice can adversely affect the patient already diagnosed with HTN (Mansor, 2001; Christopher 2003).

Massage therapy is effective in relieving stress and therefore HTN. Massage of the extremities toward the heart is generally to be avoided if there is any concern that a throm-bus may have formed in the veins and could potentially be dislodged and carried to the heart.

Little evidence exists to suggest the effectiveness of alternative remedies in the treatment of other forms of vascular disease. Some success has been reported in the use of Chinese herbal medicine to treat Raynaud's phenomenon (Zhang, Chen, and Liu, 2001).

CASE STUDY

Patient Data

Mrs. V. is a 64-year-old female who has been working full time as an assistant to three different teachers in a preschool facility for the past 24 years. She enjoys working with the 5-year-old children. She is married with two children aged 30 and 36. Her husband is 68 years old, and his health has been failing for the past 5 years as he struggles with recurrent cancer. She is worried about him and has decreased her work time to 30 hours a week. Her family experienced some financial difficulties 10 years ago but circumstances are now more stable. She has not been diagnosed with any medical problems thus far. She takes no medications. Mrs. V. drinks alcohol socially on Friday and Saturday nights only and admits to smoking cigarettes once every few days. She used to smoke every day.

While Mrs. V. was at work, one of the teachers noticed that Mrs. V. had been bringing a chair out to the playground every day for the past few weeks and sitting more than she used to. When Mrs. V. was asked why she needed the chair, she replied, "I haven't been getting enough sleep because I worry about my husband so much and I'm tired." One of the children saw Mrs. V. walk down the long hallway of the school, stop, hold onto the back of her left calf, and limp to sit down in a chair. Finally, more and more people started to notice this repeated behavior and told Mrs. V. she had to be evaluated by a doctor in order to return to work. Mrs. V. walked out of the preschool crying, "I can't go to the doctors until I turn 65 years old."

Mrs. V. reluctantly comes to be evaluated by the doctor the next day. Based on the history given by Mrs. V. and the physical examination findings, the doctor asks her to undergo a noninvasive radiologic test and blood work.

Physical Examination and Diagnostic Findings

- Height: 5 ft 2 inches
- Weight: 200 lb
- Blood pressure: 168/94
- Pulse: 88 beats per minute
- Respiratory rate: 24 breaths per minute
- Lungs: clear to auscultation bilaterally
- Heart sounds: S_1 and S_2 normal with no murmurs
- Abdomen: obese, soft, nontender
- Left lower extremity: diminished pulse +1, pallor at midcalf, dusky blue distal portion, shiny appearance, loss of hair, cool to touch
- Right lower extremity: diminished pulse +2, pallor from midcalf to distal portion, hair present, lukewarm to touch
- Hemoglobin level: 11 g/dl
- Hematocrit: 33%
- Fasting blood glucose level: 175 mg/dl
- Total cholesterol level: 262 mg/dl
- High-density lipoprotein level: 30 mg/dl
- Low-density lipoprotein level: 180 mg/dl
- Blood urea nitrogen level: 37 mg/dl
- Creatinine level: 1.2 mg/dl

- Doppler ultrasonography: decreased blood flow over left femoral, popliteal, and tibial arteries

On receiving all the significant diagnostic results, the doctor notifies Mrs. V. of the need for hospitalization to address her multiple medical problems. Mrs. V. cries as she listens to the doctor and says, "Going into the hospital will ruin all the plans I have, but I'll do it anyway." She is admitted to the medical-surgical unit.

Thinking It Through

- Based on the information provided, give the diagnosis for Mrs. V.'s vascular disorder.
- Categorize the symptoms and signs presented in the patient data as well as the physical examination and diagnostic findings.
- What are the educational topics that should be discussed with Mrs. V.?
- What is the best nonsurgical approach to helping Mrs. V. live with her diagnosis?
- Hypothesize as to why Mrs. V. is so upset about seeing a doctor and being hospitalized.

Case Conference

After a 5-day hospitalization, Mrs. V. is ready to be discharged. Her diagnoses are CAOD that developed as a result of uncontrolled HTN, hyperlipidemia, and adult-onset diabetes. The interdisciplinary team members are Mrs. V., the primary nurse, the primary care physician, an endocrinologist, Mrs. V.'s two children and spouse, a dietitian, a medical social worker, and a physical therapist.

The primary care physician begins the discussion by asking Mrs. V., "What is your understanding of the medical problems you have been diagnosed with during this hospitalization?" With tears in her eyes, Mrs. V. replies, "My whole life has to change. I can't eat good-tasting food, I have to take medicine, and most importantly I will not have enough money to retire because I was going to have to work for 6 more months before I would be eligible for a full pension."

The primary nurse hands out four separate one-page fact sheets pertaining to the diagnoses for Mrs. V. to refer to during the meeting. The endocrinologist leads the discussion by acknowledging that diabetes, HTN, and hyperlipidemia are often medical problems that do not have any obvious symptoms until a complication arises. The result of all of these disorders is the decreased blood flow to the leg that ultimately produced enough signs for others to notice despite the fact that Mrs. V. wanted to wait to seek medical attention until she was ready to retire in 6 months. The endocrinologist remarks that he will be addressing the issues associated with her diabetes.

The primary physician notes that her role will be to help Mrs. V. manage her hyperlipidemia and HTN with medications and to monitor the progression of her CAOD. The physician also comments on the need for frequent follow-up office visits to monitor for possible progression of renal insufficiency because the blood urea nitrogen and creatinine values are near the high-normal range. Prescriptions are written not only for medications

Continued

CASE STUDY—cont'd

but also for purchase of a home glucose-monitoring machine. They are given to the primary nurse to discuss with Mrs. V. and the family members.

The medical social worker adds, "Mrs. V., you appear very overwhelmed not only with all the medical problems you are facing but also with the potential disappointment about your retirement and future pension." The social worker informs Mrs. V. that he has set up frequent visits by a home care nurse to get treatment started and that he will be making home visits to assess the need for referrals regarding financial matters and assistance in coping with psychological issues.

The dietitian remarks, "Mrs. V., I want you to come up with a list of your favorite foods so I can help you incorporate them differently into the dietary program necessary to improve your multiple medical problems." When Mrs. V. completes the list, the dietitian explains how food choices affect diabetes, HTN, and hyperlipidemia. The primary focus of the dietitian is to ensure that Mrs. V. will be able to manage all these dietary changes with

the dietitian's assistance and will realize that consuming smaller portions of food at mealtime is very important.

Mrs. V. asks, "When can I go back to work? Will I ever be able to walk without pain in my leg?" The physical therapist who has been working with Mrs. V. during the last 2 days explains that he has established a walking program that will gradually allow her more walking to help build up collateral circulation. When this occurs, she will experience less leg pain. A physical therapist will also make home visits to continue to evaluate Mrs. V.'s strength and mobility, monitor progress in the walking program, and provide support for Mrs. V. as she returns to work.

The primary nurse provides Mrs. V. and her family with education pertaining to medications, follow-up appointments with the physicians, the need to balance daily activities with periods of rest, symptoms of disease progression, and the circumstances under which she should seek additional medical attention. She also answers their questions.

REFERENCES

Aminoff V, Kjellgren K: The nurse—a resource in hypertension care, *J Adv Nurs* 35(4):582-9, 2001.

Bryant J, Turkoski B: Relieving intermittent claudication: a nursing approach, *J Vasc Nurs* 17:81-5, 1999.

Centers for Disease Control and Prevention, High blood pressure fact sheet, retrieved from *http://www.cdc.gov/cvh/library/fs_bloodpressure.htm* on Dec 5, 2002.

Chaitow L: Varicose veins and hemorrhoids: prevention and treatment [HealthWorld Online website], 2001, retrieved from *http://www.healthy. net/asp/templates/article.asp?ID=500* on Nov 15, 2002.

Christopher JR: LifeBalm.com: Drug/herb interaction chart, retrieved from *http://www.lifebalm.com/page.cgi?drug_herb1* on July 5, 2003.

Davidson T: Amputation [Blueprint for Health website], July 14, 1999, retrieved from *http://www.blueprint.bluecrossmn.com/topic/topic 100586422* on Dec 28, 2003.

Funk SG et al, editors: *Key aspects of preventing and managing chronic illness,* New York, 2001, Springer.

Lewis S, Collier I, Heitkemper M: *Medical surgical nursing,* ed 5, St Louis, 2002, Mosby.

Lubisch K: Wound care, management of peripheral vascular disease and pressure ulcers, 2001, retrieved from *http://www.nursingceu.com/ NCEU/courses/woundkl/index.htm* on Dec 28, 2003.

Mansor GA: Herbs and alternative therapies in the hypertension clinic, *Am J Hypertens* 14(9 pt 1):971-5, 2001.

Medical College of Wisconsin: Raynaud's phenomenon, 2000, retrieved from *http://www.healthlink.mcw.edu/article/926055412.html* on Nov 9, 2002.

Navarro F: Peripheral arterial disease [Cleveland Clinic Center for Continuing Education website], 2002, retrieved from *http://www. clevelandclinicmeded.com/diseasemanagement/cardiology/pad/pad.htm* on Nov 9, 2002.

Neal LJ: Power pudding: natural laxative therapy for the elderly who are homebound, *Home Healthc Nurse* 13(3):66-71, 1995.

O'Connor C: Raynaud's phenomenon, *J Vasc Nurs* 19(3):87-93, 2001.

Uphold C, Graham M: *Clinical guidelines in adult health,* ed 2, Gainesville, Fl, 1999, Barmarrae Books.

US Department of Health and Human Services, National Heart, Lung, and Blood Institute: The Seventh Report of the Joint National Committee on Prevention, Detection, Evaluation, and Treatment of Hypertension, retrieved from *http://www.nhlbi.nih.gov/guidelines/hypertension* in May 2003.

Vascular Associates of Bangalore: Buerger's disease, Vascular Update, 3, 2000, retrieved from *http://www.indiandoctors.com* on Dec 27, 2002.

Vascular Associates of Bangalore: Thromboangiitis obliterans, *Vascular Update,* Feb 1, 2001, retrieved from *http://www.indiandoctors.com/ vasupdt/updtfeb1.htm* on Dec 28, 2003.

Watts RA, Scott DGI: Epidemiology of the vasculitides, *Curr Opin Rheumatol* 15(1):11-6, 2003.

Zbinden S, Seiler C: Phytotherapy in cardiovascular medicine, *Ther Umsch* 59(6):301-6, 2002.

Zhang Y, Chen Z, Liu, Y: Treating principles and methods of Chinese medicine in treatment of peripheral vascular disease, *J Tradit Chin Med* 21(2):130-3, 2001.

CHAPTER 14

Nutritional and Eating Disorders

Loretta Normile, PhD, RN

OBJECTIVES

After reading this chapter, you should be able to do the following:

- Describe the detection, prevention, and screening methodologies for anorexia nervosa, bulimia and purging, binge eating, nutritional anemia, undernutrition, and obesity.
- Identify the clinical manifestations of anorexia nervosa, bulimia and purging, obesity, binge eating, nutritional anemia, and undernutrition.
- Explain the pathophysiology of anorexia nervosa, bulimia and purging, obesity, binge eating, nutritional anemia, and undernutrition.
- Summarize the therapeutic strategies and nursing management for anorexia nervosa, bulimia and purging, obesity, binge eating, nutritional anemia, and undernutrition.
- Discuss the role of each member of the interdisciplinary team involved in the care of patients with chronic eating disorders.
- Identify community resources available for the patient with a chronic eating disorder and his or her family.
- Evaluate the psychosocial care requirements for patients with anorexia nervosa, bulimia and purging, obesity, binge eating, nutritional anemia, and undernutrition.

The amount and kinds of food eaten are basic determinants of overall health. Both underconsumption and overconsumption of food precipitate nutritional disorders that may result in medical complications leading to chronic illness or death. Nearly 13% of Americans have the eating disorders anorexia nervosa (AN), bulimia nervosa (BN), and binge eating (National Institute of Mental Health [NIMH], 2001).

Eating disorders involve physiological changes as well as a number of emotional and cognitive changes that affect the way a person perceives and experiences his or her body. These disorders are considered psychiatric illnesses that affect the body and are associated with a 5% to 15% mortality rate (Mahan and Escott-Stump, 2000).

Overconsumption of food has led to an epidemic of obesity in the United States. Today's affluent society offers a greater variety of foods, wide availability of fast food, and excessive accessibility of snack foods with little nutritional value. In addition, socialization to consume high-calorie snack foods and high-calorie beverages is commonplace in the American culture. At the same time, contemporary lifestyles present fewer opportunities in daily life to burn calories.

According to the Centers for Disease Control and Prevention (Mokdad et al, 1999), this mounting obesity epidemic threatens the health of millions of Americans. During the past decade, the number of overweight and obese people has increased by 33% (Koplan and Dietz, 1999). More than 50% of the adults in our country can be categorized as overweight or obese. Having a body weight 20% above the norm is a risk factor for comorbid conditions such as hypertension, hyperlipidemia, diabetes mellitus, joint disease, sleep apnea, and perhaps an early death (Mahan and Escott-Stump, 2000). In the United States overweight and physical inactivity account for more than 300,000 premature deaths annually (US Department of Health and Human Services, 2001).

Underconsumption often is the result of a simple diet or a weight loss program gone awry. In addition, demographic characteristics play a significant role in the development and incidence of eating disorders (Box 14-1).

NUTRITIONAL ASSESSMENT

American interest in being trim and fit, and the widespread practice of dieting, can sometimes make it difficult to tell where normal eating stops and a nutritional disorder begins. Assessment begins with a thorough history taking, a physical examination, and a nutritional assessment that includes a diet history. An evaluation of eating habits, attitudes, behaviors, and preferences may reveal food aversions as well as ritualistic or unusual eating patterns. Assessment of functional health patterns (Box 14-2) highlights areas that may be negatively affected by poor nutrition and alerts the provider to the possibility of an eating disorder.

Anthropometric measurements such as height in relation to total body weight help determine the association between relative body weight and a variety of other health conditions, principally, undernutrition or overnutrition.

Box 14-1 Demographic Differences in the Incidence of Nutritional and Eating Disorders

ANOREXIA NERVOSA
- More common in adolescent and young adult females
- More prevalent in Western societies where being thin is valued
- Less frequent in older women and males

BINGE EATING DISORDER
- Three women affected for every two men
- Affects African Americans as often as whites
- Seems to occur more in overweight and obese individuals

BULIMIA NERVOSA
- More common in adolescent and young adult females
- Less common in males
- May be linked to cultural overemphasis on physical appearance

NUTRITIONAL ANEMIA
- More likely in children; women of child-bearing age, especially teenagers; and the elderly
- Iron deficiency anemia more likely in athletes, especially female cross-country runners

UNDERNUTRITION/MALNUTRITION
- Elderly persons especially susceptible because of numerous sociocultural factors, including low income, polypharmacy, depression, and social isolation

---

Muscle mass (midarm circumference), triceps skin thickness, and dietary calorie count should be recorded. Patients should always be weighed and measured by health care providers to avoid errors from self-report. Individuals experiencing a 20% weight gain or loss may be at risk for a nutritional disorder.

Laboratory studies such as nitrogen or protein balance testing show net total body protein. The creatinine level–height index is used in the determination of lean body mass and protein calorie deficiency. Blood tests, which include a complete blood count (to detect anemia and decreased white cell count) and serum chemistry panels, may show decreased levels of albumin (a protein), transferrin, iron, folic acid and other B vitamins, β-lipoprotein, amino acids, and insulin. Guidelines for nutritional assessment are listed in Box 14-3.

EATING DISORDERS
Diagnosis

Diagnostic studies may include a chest radiograph, stool fat analysis, antigen skin testing, and a variety of blood tests. Diagnosis of eating disorders is made based on the presence of criteria developed by the American Psychiatric Association (APA). Examples of these criteria are listed in Box 14-4.

Anorexia Nervosa

Anorexia nervosa (AN) is a chronic eating disorder characterized by a distorted perception of the appearance and size of the body along with refusal to maintain a minimally normal body weight (APA, 2000). It is widely believed that the practice of excessive dieting and extreme regulation of weight provides a sense of control to individuals with AN. This disorder may have its roots in childhood and may persist to middle and old age. It occurs most often in females (90% of cases) but can also affect males. The onset is typically in puberty or young adulthood. However, research among fourth-graders revealed that 40% dieted either "very often" or "sometimes" (Gustafson-Larson and Terry, 1992).

The disorder is more common among girls whose sisters or mothers experienced AN (APA, 2000). Although the disorder may be mild or moderate and may be temporary, it is not unusual for AN to become long-standing and severe. AN is a very serious nutritional disorder that may lead to delayed psychosexual and physical sexual development, starvation, and death. The chance of death is 12 times higher for young women with AN than for women without AN (Sullivan, 1995).

Pathophysiology

The exact cause of AN remains unknown. Social attitudes, emotional factors, and familial predisposition may be contributing factors. Pathophysiologic changes in chronic and severe AN can affect every organ system. The most important and life-threatening changes are related to electrolyte imbalances and cardiac function (Beers and Berkow, 1999). Induced vomiting, diuretic use, and laxative use may seriously lower potassium levels and cause dehydration and metabolic alkalosis. Cardiotoxicity may result in tachyarrhythmias. Ventricular tachyarrhythmias, in particular, may cause sudden death. Dehydration leads to prolonged QT intervals. Enlargement of the cardiac muscles and heart chambers decreases cardiac output. Renal failure may occur. Physical examination often reveals bradycardia and low blood pressure, edema, and hypothermia. Laboratory tests may demonstrate endocrine changes such as low levels of thyroxin and triiodothyronine, and increased cortisol secretions (Beers and Berkow, 1999). Depression is also commonly seen.

Clinical Manifestations

Individuals with AN become intensely preoccupied with becoming obese. They may starve themselves, or eat excessively and then overexercise; purge with diuretics, laxatives, or enemas; and vomit food immediately after eating. Ipecac may be used to induce vomiting. Many individuals with AN already have extreme weight loss by the time they appear at the health clinic or facility. They also are emaciated, pale, and lethargic. Typical characteristics are listed in Box 14-5.

Box 14-2   Functional Health Pattern Assessment for Nutritional and Eating Disorders

HEALTH PERCEPTION/HEALTH MANAGEMENT
- What is the patient's perception of his or her overall health?
- What medications, including over-the-counter drugs, does the patient take?
- What alternative therapies does the patient use?
- Does the patient use alcohol?
- Does the patient have food security?
- Is the patient able to pay for health care?

NUTRITION/METABOLISM
- What is the patient's current weight? Has there been any recent unexplained weight gain or loss?
- Is the patient on any special diet?
- What is the condition of the skin and mucous membranes?
- Is saliva production adequate? Does the patient have any difficulty swallowing? Does the patient have loose or missing teeth, or mouth sores?
- What is the patient's typical dietary intake (daily)? Does the patient have nausea and/or vomiting?
- What are the patient's attitudes about eating? Are there any foods the patient avoids?

ELIMINATION
- Have any changes occurred in bowel or bladder habits?
- What are the color, frequency, and caliber of stool? Does the patient have a history of irritable bowel disease? Does the patient experience tenesmus?
- What is the character of the urine? Is dysuria or hematuria present?

ACTIVITY/EXERCISE
- Does the patient experience difficulty walking or fatigue?
- Does the patient experience dyspnea on exertion? What dyspnea management strategies does the patient use?
- What are the patient's regular exercise activities? In what recreational activities does the patient engage?
- Does the patient use mobility aids?
- Is the patient able to perform instrumental and other activities of daily living?
- Does the patient use supplemental oxygen?

SLEEP/REST
- How many hours of uninterrupted sleep does the patient get each night? Does the patient take naps or rest periods?
- What sleep aids does the patient use?
- Is fatigue relieved by sleep?

COGNITION/PERCEPTION
- What are the nature, location, and duration of pain? What factors aggravate and alleviate the pain?
- Is there bone involvement?
- Does the patient have paresthesias?

- How effective are pain management strategies?
- What is the level of distress associated with the symptoms?
- Has there been any change in mentation or level of consciousness?
- Does the patient experience depression or mood swings?
- Have any changes occurred in taste, smell, sight, or hearing, or in speech and communication patterns?

SELF-PERCEPTION/SELF-CONCEPT
- How does the patient describe himself or herself?
- How has the condition affected the patient's self-esteem?
- How has the condition changed the patient's body image?
- How has the condition affected the patient's sense of self?

ROLES/RELATIONSHIPS
- What kind of work does the patient perform?
- What role does the patient play in the home and family?
- Has the patient's ability to carry out role functions changed?
- How satisfied is the patient with his or her current roles and relationships?
- How has the condition affected family members and/or caregivers?
- Have there been changes in family organization or function?
- Who is the primary caregiver? How is this person involved in the patient's care?
- Who is the decision maker in the family?

SEXUALITY/REPRODUCTION
- Is the patient sexually active?
- Have any changes occurred in the menstrual cycle?
- Have there been any changes in sexual performance?
- Is the patient satisfied with current sexual patterns?
- Does the patient have concerns about potential changes in sexual performance or sexuality

COPING/STRESS TOLERANCE
- What are the patient's coping strategies?
- What support systems are available to the patient?
- Can the patient manage the condition in the current setting?
- What is the level of hopefulness or despair exhibited by the patient?
- What does the patient and/or family find comforting?

VALUES/BELIEFS
- What constitutes quality of life for the patient? What does the patient consider important?
- What are the patient's spiritual beliefs? What are the patient's health beliefs, including beliefs about the use of medications? What are the patient's beliefs about locus of control?
- What are the patient's cultural beliefs about food? To what degree does the patient participate in cultural traditions and the cultural community?

Box 14-3 Guidelines for Nutritional Assessment

- Measurements
  - Height to the nearest inch
  - Weight to the nearest pound or kilogram
  - Determination of body mass index
  - Anthropometric dimensions
- Laboratory studies
  - Complete blood count
  - Creatinine-height index
  - Folic acid level
  - Nitrogen balance
  - Serum albumin level
  - Serum cholesterol level
  - Transferrin level
- Drug use
- Clinical presentation
- Eating habits
- Living environment
- Functional health patterns
- Mental-cognitive status

Adapted from Nutrition Screening Initiative, a project of the American Academy of Family Physicians, American Dietetic Association, and National Council on Aging, Inc., and funded in part by a grant from Ross Products Division, Abbott Laboratories.

Box 14-4 Criteria for Diagnosing Eating Disorders

- Refusal to maintain body weight at or above a minimally normal weight for age and height
- Body image disturbance
- Preoccupation with weight
- Absence of several consecutive menstrual cycles
- Recurrent episodes of binge eating
- Use of inappropriate compensatory behaviors to prevent weight gain, including:
  Self-induced vomiting
  Misuse of laxatives
  Fasting
  Excessive exercise

Diagnosis

The diagnosis of AN is made by recognition of the group of described symptoms. The loss of more than 15% of body weight along with the presence of amenorrhea in an otherwise healthy individual suggests a diagnosis of AN. The individual's expression of fears related to obesity supports the diagnosis.

Interdisciplinary Care

Primary Provider (Physician/Nurse Practitioner)

The primary care provider may be the first to suspect AN. The primary care provider may begin medical treatment and/or refer the patient to other health professionals such as a psychiatrist specializing in eating disorders and a dietitian for treatment and counseling. The goal is to correct starvation, promote weight gain, and control the individual's compulsive and dangerous behaviors.

There are two phases to treatment of the anorexic patient. Short-term treatment is needed to sustain life and return the patient to a normal body weight. Long-term therapy is required to restore healthy psychological function and avoid future relapses. Inpatient hospitalization may be required if outpatient care is not successful. Inpatient hospitalization is necessary to begin refeeding the person with AN if the

weight has fallen below 75% of the ideal weight (Beers and Berkow, 1999). Ongoing therapy must address troubled interactions and/or unresolved family issues. This will require family as well as individual therapy for the patient and family members.

Nurse

The nursing interventions in AN include assessment, monitoring, prevention, and education (Box 14-6). When weighing the individual, the nurse should ensure that he or she is wearing the same type of clothing worn during previous weight measurements. Weight should always be measured at the same time of day. Vital signs and intake and output should be monitored. Food and beverages should be offered frequently and in small portions. Nutritionally complete beverages are a good alternative. Food should always be discussed in a matter-of-fact manner.

The individual should be allowed to feel in control and to assert himself or herself. The individual may need encouragement to accept his or her own feelings as valid. Family interactions should be observed and discussed with the

---

Box 14-5 Characteristics of Anorexia Nervosa

- Body mass index of less than 17.5 or a loss of more than 15% of body weight
- Greatly distorted body image
- Extreme fear of gaining weight or becoming obese even though underweight
- Inability to acknowledge the seriousness of the weight loss
- Presence of amenorrhea if female

Box 14-6 Selected Nursing Interventions for Management of Eating Disorders

- Confer with the team and the patient to set a target weight if the patient is not within a recommended weight range for age and body frame.
- Establish the amount of daily weight gain that is desired.
- Confer with the dietitian to determine the daily caloric intake necessary to attain and/or maintain target weight.
- Encourage the patient to discuss food preferences with the dietitian.
- Monitor physiologic parameters (vital signs, electrolyte levels) as needed.
- Weigh patient on a routine basis (e.g., at same time of day and after patient voids).
- Monitor daily caloric intake.
- Encourage patient self-monitoring of daily food intake and weight gain or maintenance, as appropriate.
- Establish expectations for appropriate eating behaviors, intake of food and fluid, and amount of physical activity.
- Use behavioral contracting with the patient to elicit desired weight gain or maintenance behaviors.
- Restrict food availability to scheduled, pre-served meals and snacks.
- Observe the patient during and after meals and snacks to ensure that adequate intake is achieved and maintained.
- Accompany the patient to the bathroom during designated observation times following meals or snacks.
- Limit the time the patient spends in the bathroom during periods when the patient is not under observation.
- Provide reinforcement for weight gain and behaviors that promote weight gain.
- Provide support (e.g., relaxation therapy, desensitization exercises, opportunities to talk about feelings) as the patient integrates new eating behaviors, changing body image, and lifestyle changes.
- Encourage the patient to use daily logs to record feelings as well as the circumstances surrounding the urge to purge, vomit, and overexercise.
- Provide a supervised exercise program when appropriate.
- Allow the opportunity to make limited choices about eating and exercise as weight gain progresses in a desirable manner.
- Assist the patient (and family or significant others as appropriate) to examine and resolve personal issues that may contribute to the eating disorder.
- Help the patient to develop self-esteem that is compatible with a healthy body weight.

From McCloskey JC, Bulechek GM: *Nursing interventions classification (NIC),* ed 3, St Louis, 2000, Mosby, pp 266-7.

---

interdisciplinary team. The entire family may need to be encouraged to obtain and continue therapy.

The patient and family need an opportunity to practice any procedures that involve special feeding measures such as tube feedings or parenteral nutrition. Health education should also include an explanation of laboratory test results and the fact that adequate nutrition can correct abnormal laboratory values.

Behaviors, especially ritualistic behaviors concerning eating, must be observed carefully. The patient may have distorted thinking and irrational beliefs about eating certain foods that must be corrected. Frequently, the patient has aversions to red meat, fried foods, and/or any dessert foods. These distorted thoughts, aversions, and irrational beliefs should be explored and discussed. Topics for education are listed in Box 14-7.

Drug Therapy

Although they are not effective in the acute phase of treatment, selective serotonin reuptake inhibitors (SSRIs) such as fluoxetine (Prozac), imipramine (Tofranil), and amitriptyline (Elavil) have been found to be useful after the patient's condition has been stabilized. The ineffectiveness of fluoxetine in the acute stage is due to the fact that protein is needed for metabolism of SSRIs (Strober et al, 1999), and individuals with AN have very low protein stores. Olanzapine (Zyprexa) is used in severe AN. It seems to

---

Box 14-7 Topics for Education in Anorexia Nervosa

- Impact of malnutrition on body systems
- Impact of exercise on caloric expenditure
- Impact of metabolic adaptation to vomiting
- Food Guide Pyramid (see Figures 14-1 and 14-2)
- Cues for hunger and satiety
- Long-term weight management
- Nutrition information

---

reduce agitation and promotes weight gain. Vitamins, minerals, and iron supplements are also prescribed.

Dietitian

The role of the dietitian is crucial in AN. In addition to performing a thorough and careful evaluation including a comprehensive assessment of nutrient intake, the dietitian will calculate a caloric prescription for weight gain in keeping with the guidelines for diet therapy in AN (Mahan and Escott-Stump, 2000).

Counselor/Medical Social Worker

Different forms of mental health counseling and therapy have been used with variable success. Many AN patients come to treatment with psychological, sociocultural, and family difficulties. Any prescribed therapy should address the individual's problems of low self-esteem, depression, ineffective coping, and basic family communication conflicts (Boyd, 2002). A referral should be made to an organization for anorexia and related disorders.

Bulimia Nervosa and Purging

Bulimia nervosa (BN) is characterized by recurrent and episodic binge eating and/or purging along with an inability to stop the behaviors (APA, 2000). There are two types of bulimia: the purging type and the nonpurging type. Although most individuals with BN are female, it is believed that between 10% and 15% of those diagnosed with BN are male (Andersen and Holman, 1997). Bulimia commonly manifests in adolescence and may continue for months or even years. The term *purging* refers to induction of vomiting and the use of diuretics, purgatives, and/or laxatives.

Pathophysiology

The pathophysiologic changes in bulimia and/or purging result chiefly from weight control practices and altered energy intake. Some of these changes, such as tooth erosion from exposure to gastrointestinal juices, are minor. Others, such as esophageal tears from frequent vomiting and electrolyte imbalances, have the potential to cause death.

Think S for Success

Symptoms
■ Manage symptoms with medical, nutritional supervision, and ongoing therapy.

Sequelae
■ Prevent exacerbations by avoidance of trigger foods and continued counseling and therapy.

Safety
■ Teach patient and family complications of anorexia nervosa. Reinforce that the disorder can cause death.

Support/Services
■ Ensure that patient obtains the necessary assistance. The extreme dieting and starvation-like eating patterns of anorexia nervosa provide a sense of control and gratification, and this disordered eating pattern is therefore very difficult to break. Normal eating habits may take years to achieve. Only half of those with anorexia or bulimia make a full recovery.

Satisfaction
■ Determine the extent to which the illness is interfering with quality of life for patient and family members.

Cardiac arrest from potassium imbalance and consequent arrhythmias is not altogether uncommon.

Clinical Manifestations

Bulimia is manifested by chronic ingestion of high-calorie foods with textures that allow rapid swallowing. Large quantities of food may be consumed in a highly secretive manner during times when the individual can eat unnoticed, such as late at night or when alone. Moving from binging to fasting over short periods of time is common. Bingeing may also be followed by compensatory behaviors such as vomiting. Patients with BN are likely to abuse diuretics, laxatives, and purgatives. After a heavy eating episode the individual with bulimia is likely to feel abdominal pain and the need to vomit. Vomiting usually relieves the pain and helps the individual to feel more in control of his or her life. Periods of normal eating between episodes of binging and/or purging are common. Individuals with BN may be normal weight to slightly underweight. Telltale findings may be scars on the dorsum of the hand used to induce vomiting, a "moth-eaten" appearance to the teeth from loss of dental enamel, and menstrual irregularities.

Diagnosis

Although this chronic disorder has the potential to cause serious medical complications, it is most commonly viewed as a psychiatric condition. The key to the diagnosis of bulimia is not the vomiting but the binge eating. Individuals report consumption of a large amount of food in less than 2 hours followed by a compensatory behavior such as vomiting, purging, laxative or diuretic use, and/or strenuous exercise to avoid weight gain. Along with the binge eating and inappropriate compensatory behavior, patients often show a great concern over body weight and overall appearance.

Interdisciplinary Care

Primary Provider (Physician/Nurse Practitioner)

The primary care provider may suspect BN and purging when telltale signs are identified during routine examination. A recent survey of adolescents (Klein and Wilson, 2002) pointed out that providers are not maximizing their opportunities to discuss risk behaviors, including binging and purging. Teens who had time alone with their health care providers were more likely to discuss their problems.

The patient with BN may exhibit few outward signs because the patient binges and purges secretly. Routine laboratory studies may reveal electrolyte imbalances and mildly elevated serum amylase levels. These findings warrant further exploration by the primary care provider.

If the condition diagnosed is believed to be mild, the primary care provider may treat and follow the patient. If the disorder is deemed moderate to severe, the individual will be referred to other health care providers such as a psychiatrist or psychologist who specializes in eating disorders.

The goals in treatment of BN and purging are to stabilize the weight without the use of binging and purging, and to change eating patterns. Treatment uses primarily two modalities: cognitive-behavioral therapy and antidepressant medications. Usually 4 to 6 months of therapy is required for both short- and long-term effects. Families must be included in all therapies if possible.

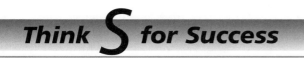

Think S for Success

Symptoms
- Manage periods of eating large amounts of high-calorie foods and purging.

Sequelae
- Prevent exacerbations by teaching patient to avoid triggers for bulimia and purging such as the following:
  Overeating
  Eating in response to emotion
  Wide weight fluctuations
  Inactivity and lack of exercise
  Negative mood
  Alcohol and/or drug use

Safety
- Teach patient and family about the importance of the following:
  Benefits of keeping a journal of foods eaten before, during, and after binging and/or purging behaviors
  Role of deprivation in binging
  Need to avoid unrealistic self-expectations

Support/Services
- Arrange for some type of long-term follow-up, because at least half of all bulimics make only a partial recovery or have insignificant improvement.

Satisfaction
- Determine the extent to which bulimia and purging are affecting healthy coping behaviors and quality of life.

Binge Eating Disorder

Binge eating disorder is a relatively recently documented condition that is believed to affect about 1 million to 2 million Americans (Boyd, 2002). Individuals with binge eating disorders frequently consume huge amounts of food and have no control over their eating. This chronic disorder is not the same as binge-purge syndrome (BN); individuals with binge eating disorders usually do not practice purging behaviors such as vomiting or laxative use after eating and do not use diuretics to reduce weight. Binge eating disorder is defined in the *Diagnostic and Statistical Manual of Mental Disorders* as recurrent episodes of binge eating in

the absence of compensatory behaviors (APA, 2000). It is probably America's most common eating disorder. Binge eating is characterized by the occurrence of binge eating episodes at least twice a week for 6 months (Shebendach and Reichert-Anderson, 2000). It is seen in both men and women, although it occurs slightly more often in women. More than likely, the individual who engages in binge eating is overweight and may even be obese. At least 15% to 20% of individuals in weight loss programs are thought to engage in binge eating (Shebendach and Reichert-Anderson, 2000).

Pathophysiology

Although the causes of binge eating disorder are largely unknown, up to half of all individuals with the disorder have a history of depression. The role of dieting and its consequences in binge eating is still undefined. Although findings vary, early studies reported that about half of all people with binge eating disorder had binge episodes before they started to diet. Nevertheless, strict dieting may worsen binge eating in some people (Healthier You, 2003).

Although binge eating disorder is classified as a psychiatric disorder, pathophysiologic changes from increased energy intake and weight gain occur over a period of time. Pathologic alterations such as elevated blood urea nitrogen levels, ketonuria, edema, dysrhythmias, gastric dyspepsia, and gallstones may have long-term health consequences. The medical complications of binge eating disorders are the diseases of obesity: diabetes, high blood pressure, high cholesterol levels, gallbladder disease, heart disease, and joint disorders. Certain types of cancer, including breast, uterine, ovarian, and prostate cancer, are also linked to excessive caloric intake and obesity.

Clinical Manifestations

Most people with chronic binge eating problems are distraught about their binge eating. Most have tried to control it on their own but do not succeed for very long. It is common for a binge eater to arrange his or her day around the binge eating. Binge eating behaviors can affect work, school, and social activities. Obese people with binge eating disorder often feel terrible about themselves, are particularly self-conscious about their appearance, and may avoid social contacts. Many times close family members and friends are unaware of the binge eating because it is done in an almost secretive manner.

The chronic binge eater experiences recurrent episodes of eating what others would consider an abnormally large amount of food and recurrent thoughts of what is to be eaten. The individual is unable to control what is eaten or how much is eaten. The chronic binge eater eats very quickly, consumes large amounts of food even when not hungry, and/or is unable to stop eating until he or she is painfully or uncomfortably full. The individual eats alone because of shame at the quantity of food being consumed and feels guilty and depressed after overeating. Obese individuals with binge eating disorder often became overweight at a younger age than those without the disorder.

Diagnosis

Health professionals are still debating the best ways to determine if an individual has binge eating disorder, because consuming large amounts of food does not, in itself, indicate that such a disorder is present. The occurrence of binge episodes at least twice a week for 6 months (Shebendach and Reichert-Anderson, 2000) in the absence of inappropriate compensatory behaviors such as induced vomiting, misuse of laxatives, and excessive exercise is the criterion used for diagnosis (APA, 2000).

Interdisciplinary Care

Primary Provider (Physician/Nurse Practitioner)

The primary care provider may find it a challenge to diagnose binge eating disorder, because a physical examination usually reveals a patient who is overweight but not necessarily obese. A careful history must be taken to learn that the patient sometimes ingests huge amounts of food or eats until uncomfortably full. The provider develops a treatment plan based on the individual's degree of overweight. Interventions are similar to those for BN.

Nurse

The role of the nurse who cares for an individual who binges is initially one of gaining trust. The goal of nursing is to bring the individual who binges to take responsibility for his or her own behavior. A kind, firm, consistent manner within a collaborative relationship is the best approach. Refer to Box 14-6.

Drug Therapy

Current treatments for binge eating disorder include pharmacotherapy with antidepressants, commonly the SSRIs such as fluoxetine, and appetite suppressants. Antidepressants are effective in treating this disorder even in the absence of depression. Both sertraline (Zoloft) and topiramate (Topamax) are being studied for their effectiveness in reducing binge eating (Shapira, Goldsmith, and McElroy, 2000).

Counselor/Medical Social Worker

Ongoing counseling and psychotherapy is required. The purpose of this therapy is to lessen the impact of guilt, disgust, and depression, which are common during binging. The focus of counseling, however, is usually self-control and self-esteem.

Many etiologic models of binge eating disorder have been developed, including addiction models, family dynamic models, sociocultural models, and psychodynamic models. In treatment applications, the most successful of these is the psychodynamic model, which focuses on helping the individual to avoid and control distressing feelings (Mahan and Escott-Stump, 2000). To date, cognitive therapy does not seem to be effective in treating the disorder (Boyd, 2002).

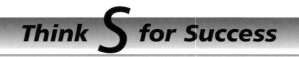

Think S for Success

Symptoms
■ Assist patient in managing painful feelings and binging episodes.

Sequelae
■ Prevent complications by monitoring for increasing frequency of binging.

Safety
■ Teach appropriate strategies such as exercise and dieting to achieve target weight.

Support/Services
■ If necessary, provide assistance in locating support groups and therapy. Patient will need encouragement to continue with psychotherapy and nutritional counseling, education, and/or self-help groups.

Satisfaction
■ Assess the impact of binging and depressive symptoms on quality of life.

Family and Caregiver Issues Associated with Eating Disorders

The patient's family and first-degree relatives influence values, eating patterns, and personal standards. The support of family members and friends is critical in the treatment of eating disorders. Because of the chronic nature of these disorders, the entire family often must engage in therapy.

Education about nutrition and eating disorders is essential to promote understanding of the family member's or friend's disorder and to help prevent relapses. Individuals frequently struggle with significant emotional distress, including low self-esteem, depression, and self-disgust. Eating disorders often occur in response to stressful events within the home, and an assessment of family dynamics may be helpful in the overall treatment.

NUTRITIONAL DISORDERS
Nutritional Anemia

Nutritional anemia is a broad diagnostic term for a decrease in the function or number of erythrocytes (red blood cells, or RBCs). Nutritional anemia is classified according to the cause of the erythrocyte change. Nutritional anemias include anemias due to iron, vitamin B_{12} (cobalamin), and folic acid deficiencies.

In the United States, poor and elderly persons are especially susceptible to iron deficiency anemia because of sociocultural factors. The poor as well as the elderly, who also tend to have a low income, are more likely to consume a poor diet and/or use multiple drugs because of poor health.

Menstruating females, particularly adolescents with poor iron consumption, are also at risk. For a detailed discussion of nutritional anemias, see Chapter 10.

Undernourishment and Malnutrition

Undernourishment and malnutrition are still prevalent to some extent in the United States. Any health problem, surgical procedure, or medical condition that increases protein and calorie requirements has the potential to cause negative nitrogen balance and to result in catabolism (Box 14-8). Socioeconomic condition and mental illness may be risk factors for undernourishment and malnutrition. Undernutrition is seen most often in the lower socioeconomic groups, particularly in high-risk groups such as the elderly, and individuals who have inadequate body reserves are especially susceptible to development of malnutrition.

Food security is a term used to describe the state of having physical and economic access to nutritious food. The prevalence of food insecurity with hunger in the United States is 3.1%, or 1 in every 10 households, or 8.5 million persons (USDA, 2002).

Pathophysiology

The most common form of malnutrition is protein-calorie malnutrition (PCM). PCM results from gastrointestinal absorption problems, trauma that increases the body's protein and calorie demands (e.g., severe burns), or a disease state such as cancer, and can occur secondary to a metabolic disorder. It may also follow a period of starvation.

When essential nutrients are not consumed or transported to the body's cells, serious pathophysiologic cellular effects occur. Proteins (amino acids) are the main structural units of cells. When cells are deprived of essential amino acids, enzymatic and hormonal functions are altered. This results in a decrease in intestinal mucosal mass and decreased absorption. The pancreas is affected, which leads to reduced exocrine activity. This lowers plasma protein levels, which causes fluid to move into the interstitium. If the body cannot obtain glucose from carbohydrate breakdown, the body compensates by metabolizing fats (lipids). As lipid levels become greatly altered, fatty acids are mobilized from the adipose tissue. This increases the production and circulation of ketones, acidic by-products of lipid metabolism. Ketone body excretion causes the loss of electrolytes and water and results in dehydration. Ketoacidosis, coma, and death may result. An increase in the level of lipoproteins in the blood results in deposition of fat in major organs such as the heart and liver.

Any disruption in nutrition will result in an imbalance of essential micronutrients such as vitamins and minerals. A lack of or excess in these valuable nutritional elements leads to problems in plasma membrane function, wound healing, and metabolism.

Physiologic functions of vitamins include cell differentiation, blood clotting, metabolism, and production of various coenzymes (Krause, 2000). Minerals are structural elements of many body tissues such as teeth and bone. Moreover, they help regulate acid-base balance and osmotic pressure in the body. A lack or excess of these essential micronutrients results in serious toxicities and/or dysfunction of major body systems (Krause, 2000).

Clinical Manifestations

Individuals who are chronically undernourished or malnourished have a gaunt appearance and lack adipose tissue. The skin is dry, the hair may be dull and sparse, and energy level is very low. Mental status is apathetic and mood is irritable. Individuals with PCM also have a decreased susceptibility to infection because the immune system becomes less efficient.

Assessment

Assessment tools such as measurement of body mass index (BMI), weight, and complete blood count provide information about the presence and degree of malnutrition. They are generally used once a state of malnutrition is suspected. Instruments that screen for malnutrition should also be used, especially in vulnerable populations. The Nutrition Screening Initiative (1991) recommends the use of the mnemonic "DETERMINE" to remind providers of the warning signs of malnutrition: **D**isease, **E**ating poorly, **T**ooth loss, **E**conomic hardship, **R**educed socialization, **M**any medications, **I**nvoluntary weight loss or gain, **N**eeds assistance with activities of daily living, **E**lder years above age 80.

Diagnosis

Clinical appearance alone is a very striking indicator for a diagnosis of PCM. A dietary history and anthropometric examination reveal a BMI lower than 18.5 and below-

---

Box 14-8   Risk Factors for Malnutrition in the United States

- Chronic illnesses or conditions such as the following:
  Severe burns
  Cancer
  Diabetes mellitus
  Infectious diseases such as acquired immunodeficiency syndrome and tuberculosis
  Major surgery
  Hyperthyroidism
  Trauma
  Malabsorption syndrome
  Renal disease
- Dementia
- Mental illness
- Poor dentition
- Poverty
- Radiation therapy
- Chemotherapy

standard arm circumference and triceps skin-fold measurements. Laboratory findings that confirm PCM are serum albumin level below 2.8 g/dl and abnormal 24-hour creatinine excretion for creatinine-height index.

Interdisciplinary Care

The goals of interdisciplinary treatment include bringing the individual to within 90% of his or her normal weight and maintaining this weight. Protein, calories, and other nutrients should be provided by whatever means is necessary. This may include enteral nutritional supplements as well as total parenteral nutrition.

Primary Provider (Physician/Nurse Practitioner)

The primary care provider first determines the cause of the malnutrition or underweight condition and then develops a treatment plan to correct the causative factor(s) and restore the patient to normal weight. A nutrient-dense diet is prescribed or referral may be made to a dietitian, who will develop a diet prescription.

Fluid and electrolyte levels must be restored parentally before any other nutritional intervention is attempted. Supplemental feedings through nasogastric or percutaneous endoscopic gastrostomy tube may be needed. Nutritional treatment must be proceed cautiously to avoid causing complications of overload in an individual with a compromised metabolic system.

Nurse

Careful nursing assessment is always required with attention to possible causes of undernutrition, especially in the elderly. Physical factors such as the use of many drugs (polypharmacy) and interactions between drugs and nutrients contribute to PCM in the elderly. This is especially likely in the presence of disorders that cause appetite loss. Other contributing factors include tooth and gum disease, swallowing difficulties, substance abuse, and depression. The nurse must collaborate very closely with the dietitian and monitor intake.

The nurse should offer continuous encouragement to consume as much nutrient-dense, appealing, high-calorie food and beverages possible, as well as assistance with eating if required. If total parenteral nutrition is given, strict adherence to aseptic technique should be practiced. Nurses should be alert to the nutritional intake of individuals who are hospitalized for a long period or are experiencing other chronic illnesses. Careful recording of intake and output is essential.

Nurses also educate individuals and families about good nutrition and provide them with information on how to overcome barriers to obtaining nutritious food.

Many factors influence the type and degree of health teaching offered. Nutritional health education is highly dependent on the cause(s) of the undernutrition or malnutrition, the presence of comorbidities such as acquired immunodeficiency syndrome or cancer, and socioeconomic factors such as poverty.

Individuals should be taught to use the Food Guide Pyramid (Figures 14-1 and 14-2), in conjunction with the dietary guidelines of the U.S. Department of Agriculture (USDA) (2000), as a template for daily food choices. Menu planning with nutrient-dense foods is important. Providing information on food selection and nutrient-dense foods is not enough. Many persons simply may not have the money for nor access to these foods, nor knowledge of resources to assist in obtaining them. Many programs of the USDA and U.S. Department of Health and Human Services (USD HHS), such as the Food Stamp Program, the School Lunch Program, Senior Adult Meals, and the Women, Infants and Children (WIC) Program, can provide nutrition to various segments of the undernourished or malnourished population from infants to the elderly (USDA, 1999). Patients should be given information on these programs as well as the locations of any local food banks and community resources.

Drug Therapy

Dronabinol (Marinol), a central nervous system agent, antiemetic, and cannabinoid, has been used successfully to stimulate appetite and/or to treat nausea and vomiting that do not respond to other antiemetics. Extended use beyond the time needed for appetite stimulation may cause accumulation of toxic levels of the drug and metabolites. Physical dependence may also result from long-term use.

Many health professionals recommend that elderly persons, even the healthy elderly, take a low-dose multivitamin. Some studies indicate that close to 70% of the elderly take higher levels of vitamins than recommended and may be at risk for toxicities (Chandra, 1991).

Dietitian

The dietitian plays a critical role in the treatment and rehabilitation of the undernourished or malnourished individual. A comprehensive nutritional assessment is completed; physical examination, anthropometric, and laboratory data are interpreted; a nutrient intake analysis is performed; and food diaries are kept. From these data, the dietitian develops and implements a detailed nutritional plan for optimal health. The nutritional plan is tailored to correct imbalances or deficiencies or excesses. It also provides the information for necessary nutritional education and counseling.

Counselor/Medical Social Worker

Psychosocial factors such as loneliness, depression, isolation, decreased mobility, and loss of independence may greatly affect appetite and the will to eat. The counselor or medical social worker can aid in providing counseling and family therapy relating to these matters. Moreover, when financial status is compromised the social worker can provide information and access community-sponsored nutrition programs.

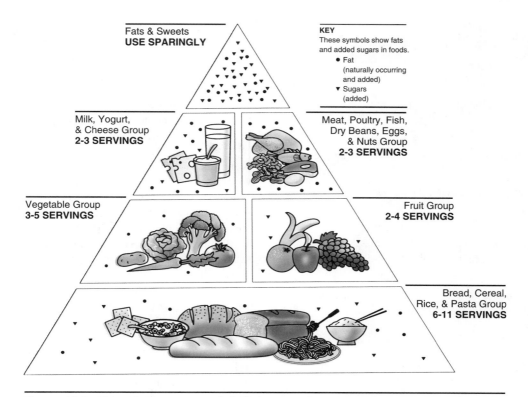

Figure 14-1 The U.S. Department of Agriculture Food Guide Pyramid.

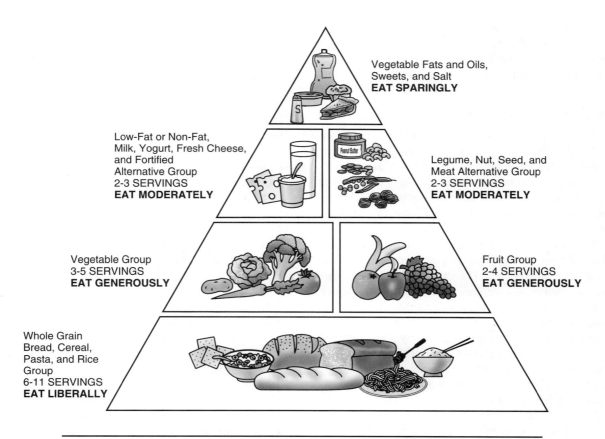

Figure 14-2 Food pyramid for a vegetarian diet. (Courtesy The Health Connection.)

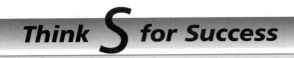

Think **S** *for Success*

Symptoms
■ Manage symptoms of nutritional anemia through diet and medication if applicable.

Sequelae
■ Prevent relapse and weight loss by monitoring dietary intake.

Safety
■ Teach patient the importance of eating a balanced diet.

Support/Services
■ Availability of food may be an issue. Inform about resources, services, and programs to obtain food and assist patient in accessing these resources if needed.

Satisfaction
■ Determine the degree to which undernourishment and malnutrition affect performance of the activities of daily living and quality of life.

Family and Caregiver Issues

Isolation and loneliness can greatly affect a person's desire to eat. The presence of others during meals may encourage food intake. Encouragement and assistance to eat may also be helpful. The individual's mood state and physical surroundings can be important factors influencing when, where, why, and how much a person partakes of food.

Overweight and Obesity

"The problem keeps getting worse," said USDHHS Secretary Tommy G. Thompson. "We've seen virtually a doubling in the number of obese persons over the past two decades and this has profound health implications. Obesity increases a person's risk for a number of serious conditions, including diabetes, heart disease, stroke, high blood pressure, and some types of cancer" (USDHHS, 2000).

Recent studies indicate that more than half of the adults in the United States are either overweight or obese (50.7% of women and 59.4% of men) (Flegal et al, 1998). The age-adjusted prevalence of combined overweight and obesity among minority women of color is generally higher than that among whites in the United States (Flegal et al, 1998).

The conditions of overweight and obesity are associated with a multitude of health problems, including diabetes, gallstones, hypertension, and heart disease. Obesity is also associated with colorectal cancer as well as with breast, uterine, and ovarian cancer in women and prostate cancer in men.

The definition of obesity has changed in recent years. According to the current definition, obesity is a BMI of 30.0 to 30.9 (Laquatra, 2000). In the past, obesity was defined as a weight 20% or more above an optimal weight for height derived from actuarial statistics that correlated with the lowest death rates. Today, some health experts argue that the weight-for-height yardstick is both inaccurate and rigid. Figure 14-3 shows the current guidelines for determining proper weight and degree of obesity.

Pathophysiology

A number of genetic mechanisms may influence body weight, among them genes that predetermine metabolism and appetite. Fat cells empty directly into the general circulation, and the fatty acid contents of abdominal fat cells pass on to the liver, by way of the portal vein, before being circulated to the muscles. The pancreas secretes more insulin in response to increased fat in the blood. Then the autonomic nervous system, which controls heart rate, blood pressure, and other vital functions, produces norepinephrine, which raises blood pressure. The heart enlarges to accommodate the increased demand. Hypercholesterolemia and heart disease eventually occur. Adipose tissue overlying the ribcage may impair pulmonary function. Gas exchange, expiratory volume, and vital capacity are decreased. The result is low oxygen tension and rising levels of carbon dioxide. Sleep apnea may occur as a result of these changes.

Clinical Manifestations

Development of an obese condition is an insidious and subtle process. The most basic manifestation of overweight and obesity is an increase in body mass to 20% above the ideal body weight. Rolls of subcutaneous adipose tissue are observed on the person.

Diagnosis

Most obese persons have primary obesity. BMI, commonly expressed as weight (in kilograms) divided by the square of height (in meters) is used to determine overweight (BMI of 25.0 to 29.9) and obesity (BMI of 30.0 or higher). Obesity can also be defined as a weight of 20% to 30% above the ideal or standard weight as indicated on height-weight charts. Simple observation is highly accurate in determining overweight and obesity. If a person appears fat, then he or she is overweight and may even be obese.

Interdisciplinary Care

Primary Provider (Physician/Nurse Practitioner)

The overall goal for overweight or obese individuals is to lose weight and maintain weight loss. Both clinical and nonclinical programs are available to accomplish weight loss. These programs stress appropriate selections of food along with meal planning, exercise, and behavioral change. Behavioral change must occur first, however.

The primary care provider prescribes a balanced low-calorie diet and an exercise plan to produce weight loss. Concurrent medical problems such as hypertension and

Height*

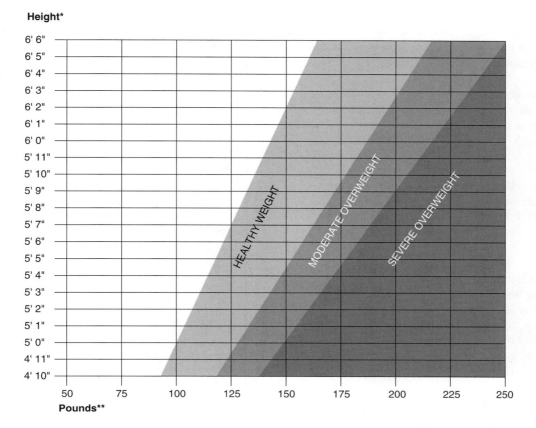

* Without shoes.
** Without clothes. The higher weights apply to people with more
   muscle and bone, such as many men.

Figure 14-3 The U.S. Department of Agriculture and U.S. Department of Health and Human Services guidelines for determining proper weight or degree of obesity. (Redrawn from *http://www.nalusda.gov/fnic/Dietary/9dietgui.htm.*)

increased cholesterol levels are treated. Medications and surgical procedures to promote weight loss are valid treatment and management options, especially for those with extreme or morbid obesity. Referral may be made to other health professionals, including a dietitian and/or psychologist.

Nurse

The role of the nurse is to assess, teach, encourage, and make referrals. Weekly assessment of baseline weight, instruction in nutritional self-care, nutritional evaluation, and assessment of activity patterns, degree of body image disturbance, and adherence to the treatment regimen should be ongoing activities. The overweight or obese individual should be taught basic nutritional information if necessary, including the Food Guide Pyramid, the caloric content of foods, selection of appropriate foods and menu planning, the way to read food labels, and the consequences of long-term

overweight. Encouragement from the nurse is needed to ensure that the individual consults a physician before beginning any exercise program. The patient may find it helpful to keep a diet journal and to set realistic goals for any weight loss program. Referral should be made to a physician if needed, to a dietitian, and to weight loss support groups.

Surgeon

Surgical options are available for persons with a BMI above 40 (severe obesity) or with life-threatening complications. Gastric procedures radically reduce stomach volume through surgical development of a pouch holding no more than 25 ml. The most common procedures are vertical banded gastroplasty and gastric bypass. Weight loss is rapid at first and then proceeds more slowly. These interventions have produced remarkable improvements in medical conditions. They also alter overweight appearance and provide relief from body image disturbances, increase activity levels, and improve overall interpersonal effectiveness. The mortality rate is less than 1%. Complications occur in fewer than 10% of cases (Beers and Berkow, 1999).

Drug Therapy

Use of medications for weight loss is recommended only for those obese individuals who are at increased risk for morbidity. Such medications are recommended only for short-term use.

The most common medications for weight loss are appetite suppressants. Use of some antidepressants, such as the SSRIs, will produce a small weight loss, but it is not lasting. Table 14-1 lists the drugs used most frequently for weight loss.

Dietitian

Use of the traditional very low calorie diet is no longer considered the best method for altering eating patterns. Safe, sensible, and gradual changes in eating patterns are recommended. The newer dietary recommendations call for increased intake of complex carbohydrates such as fruits and vegetables, and a decrease in the amount of simple carbohydrates and fats in the diet.

Complementary and Alternative Therapies
Exercise

No weight loss program can be effective without exercise. The merits of exercise cannot be overstated. Many studies have documented its health effects. Physical activity prevents a wide range of chronic disorders, in addition to controlling weight and obesity. Well-designed studies have detailed the benefits of exercise as a strategy for achieving weight reduction and overall general health effects such as reduced loss of calcium from the bone. Both aerobic and anaerobic exercise of at least 15 minutes per day is beneficial because such exercise contributes more directly to cardiovascular fitness and physical endurance. Moderate anaerobic exercise contributes to maintaining and building muscle mass and strength. Exercise should be incorporated into the individual's lifestyle. In *Healthy People 2010* (USDHHS, 2000), the objective related to exercise is to increase the proportion of adults who engage regularly in moderate physical activity. Many overweight individuals are either sedentary or elderly and may have undiagnosed heart disease. For that reason, these adults should consult with their health care providers before undertaking any exercise program. The general guideline is to participate in some form of exercise for 20 minutes at least three or four times a week.

Nontraditional Therapies

Hypnotism has been used to control overeating with varying degrees of success. Meditation, yoga, and programs focusing on nourishing the spiritual self have also been used in conjunction with traditional therapies. Providers should ask whether patients are using any of these therapies.

Other behaviors that should be explored with the patient are fasting and following fad diets, including those that encourage drinking tonics designed to cleanse, purify, or purge the body of toxins. It is important to remain nonjudgmental during this assessment and to correct any mistaken information the patient may have about the safety and usefulness of all therapeutic approaches, whether traditional or nontraditional.

Table 14-1 Prescription Weight Loss Medications

Generic Name	Trade Name
Diethylpropion	Tenuate, Tenuate Dospan
Mazindol	Sanorex, Mazanor
Orlistat	Xenical
Phendimetrazine	Bontril, Plegine, Prelu-2, X-Trozine
Phentermine	Adipex-P, Fastin, Ionamin, Oby-trim
Sibutramine	Meridia

Adapted from National Institute of Diabetes and Digestive and Kidney Diseases, National Institutes of Health, Bethesda, Md.

Think S for Success

Symptoms
■ Manage symptoms by helping patient to achieve weight loss.

Sequelae
■ Help patient to increase physical activity and reduce caloric intake, which for sedentary individuals can greatly lower the risk of many disorders.

Safety
■ Teach importance of weight loss by reviewing the many deleterious consequences of overweight.
■ Teach about the relationship of overweight or obesity to life expectancy and about major factors affecting adherence to a treatment plan.

Support/Services
■ Support services for weight loss are plentiful. Many times such services are free. Explore community resources, Internet resources, and health care resources and facilities.
■ Availability of food may be an issue. Inform about resources, services, and programs to obtain a balanced diet and assist patient in accessing these resources if needed.

Satisfaction
■ Determine the degree to which chronic overweight and obesity affect important aspects of the patient's life.

CASE STUDY
Patient Data
Ms. E. is a 24-year-old elementary school teacher who is 67 inches tall and weighs 132 pounds. Ms. E. has always been dissatisfied with her weight and tried a variety of fad diets throughout high school and college. She would lose some weight but always regained it. About 2 years ago, Ms. E. began to engage in binge eating. She now binges three or four times a week and usually consumes about 2000 to 3000 calories in a matter of just 2 hours. During her binges, Ms. E. eats cookies, cakes, ice cream, and chocolate. Following a binge, Ms. E. feels extremely guilty and immediately rushes off to a bathroom to induce vomiting. She literally starves herself over the next day or two to make up for the binge eating. During these times, she resorts to a liquid diet of about 500 calories. Ms. E. exercises by running 2 miles and then performing 75 pushups and 75 sit-ups three times a week. She has admitted using over-the-counter laxatives and sneaking her grandmother's hydrochlorothiazide tablets.

Ms. E. comes from a large middle class family with a domineering mother. She always felt tightly controlled while living at home. She has now been on her own for several years, but she continues to binge and purge.

Diagnostic Findings
- Albumin level: 4.1 g/dl
- Blood glucose level: 78 mg/dl
- Cholesterol level: 177 mg/dl
- Potassium level: 2.6 mmol/L
- Anthropometric circumference measurements: triceps, 19 mm; biceps, 7 mm; subscapular, 9.3 mm; suprailiac, 13 mm; midarm, 26.5 cm; midarm muscle, 20.3 cm

Thinking It Through
- Is Ms. E. susceptible to any medical complications as a result of her binge eating and fasting behaviors? What are they?
- Discuss Ms. E.'s laboratory values. What can you expect them to be after Ms. E. undergoes treatment?
- Determine Ms. E.'s ideal weight.
- How can Ms. E. control her vomiting episodes? What about her use of laxatives and diuretics?
- What can you tell Ms. E. about the foods she considers trigger foods?
- Discuss approaches to the teaching and learning process in chronic disease. What adjustments and adaptations should be considered for Ms. E.?

Case Conference
Ms. E. has increased binging and purging activities over the last week. This behavior is now complicated by the development of hypokalemia.

Ms. E. discusses her eating patterns over the last week, including the number of times she has binged and purged. She admits feeling great pressure in her job over the last month. She has also felt obliged to spend more time with her mother lately because her mother has been depressed.

The dietitian draws conclusions based on dietary indexes such as biochemical, metabolic, and anthropometric findings. She determines total energy consumption during binges and the degree of controlled eating between binges. She encourages Ms. E. to maintain a prescribed daily caloric intake while decreasing the number of purging episodes.

The nurse provides health instruction in dehydration and electrolyte imbalance, especially potassium depletion. She advises Ms. E. to be sure to include in her diet foods that are high in potassium and to be aware of any abnormal sensations such as tingling.

The counselor helps Ms. E. work on cue elimination and self-monitoring by daily journal writing. The counselor will continue to provide cognitive behavioral therapy to help Ms. E. address distorted thinking processes, which are believed to be causing the binging and purging behavior.

Ms. E.'s mother agrees to participate in family therapy and individual therapy.
- What strategies would you suggest to help Ms. E. modify her behaviors?

Internet and Other Resources
American Obesity Association: *http://www.obesity.org/*
Anorexia Nervosa and Related Eating Disorders, Inc. (ANRED): *http://www.anred.com/*
National Association of Anorexia Nervosa and Associated Disorders (ANAD): *http://www.anad.org/*
National Eating Disorders Association: *http://www.National EatingDisorders.org*
National Heart, Lung, and Blood Institute (NHLBI): *http://www.nhlbi.nih.gov/guidelines/obesity/ob_home.htm;* Clinical Guidelines on the Identification, Evaluation, and Treatment of Overweight and Obesity in Adults
National Hunger Clearinghouse Search Directory: *http://www.worldhungeryear.org/nhc_data/nhc_01.asp*
National Institute of Diabetes and Digestive and Kidney Diseases (NIDDK): *http://www.niddk.nih.gov/health/nutrition.htm;* health information: weight loss and control research, table summarizing long-term studies of pharmacotherapy for the management of obesity, statistics
North American Association for the Study of Obesity: *http://www.obesityresearch.org/*

Obesity Online: *http://www.obesity-online.com/;* a multidisciplinary forum for research on and treatment of massive obesity, including plastics, psychiatry, endocrinology, nutrition, nursing
Office of the Surgeon General: *http://www.surgeongeneral.gov/topics/obesity;* Overweight and Obesity: The Surgeon General's Call to Action to Prevent and Decrease Overweight and Obesity
Royal College of Psychiatrists: *http://www.rcpsych.ac.uk/info/help/anor/;* information on anorexia and bulimia

REFERENCES
American Psychiatric Association: *Diagnostic and statistical manual of mental disorders: DSM-IV-TR,* ed 4, text rev, Washington, DC, 2000, The Association.
Andersen AE, Holman JE: Males with eating disorders: challenges for treatment and research, *Psychopharmacol Bull* 33(3):391-7, 1997.
Beers MH, Berkow R: *The Merck manual of diagnosis and therapy,* ed 17, Whitehouse Station, NJ, 1999, Merck and Co.
Boyd MA: *Psychiatric nursing: contemporary practice,* ed 2, Lippincott, 2002, Philadelphia.
Chandra RK: Nutrition of the elderly, *Can Med Assoc J* 145:1475, 1991.

Gustafson-Larson A, Terry RD: Weight-related behaviors and concerns of fourth-grade children, *J Am Diet Assoc* 92:818-22, 1992.

Healthier You: Binge eating disorder, 2003, retrieved from *http://www. healthieryou.com/binge.html* on Dec 31, 2003.

Klein JD, Wilson KM: Delivering quality care: adolescents' discussion of health risk with their providers, *J Adolesc Health Care* 30(3):190-5, 2002.

Koplan O, Dietz WH: Caloric imbalance and public health policy, *JAMA.* 282(16):1579-81, 1999.

Laquatra I: Nutrition for weight management. In Mahan LK, Escott-Stump SE, editors: *Krause's food, nutrition and diet therapy,* ed 10, Philadelphia, 2000, WB Saunders.

Mahan LK, Escott-Stump, editors: *Krause's food, nutrition and diet therapy,* ed 10, Philadelphia, 2000, WB Saunders.

Mokdad AH et al: The spread of the obesity epidemic in the United States, 1991-1998, *JAMA* 282(16):1519-22, 1999.

National Institute of Mental Health: *Eating disorders: facts about eating disorders and the search for solutions,* NIH Pub No. 01-4901, Washington DC, 2001, US Government Printing Office.

Nutrition Screening Initiative: Determine your nutritional health, 1991, retrieved from *www.aafp.org/PreBuilt/NSI_DETERMINE.pdf* on Jan 25, 2004.

Shapira NA, Goldsmith TD, McElroy SL: Treatment of binge eating disorder with topiramate: a clinical case series, *J Clin Psychiatry* 61(5): 368-72, 2000.

Shebendach J, Reichert-Anderson P: Nutrition in eating disorders. In Mahan LK, Escott-Stump, editors: *Krause's food, nutrition and diet therapy,* ed 10, Philadelphia, 2000, WB Saunders.

Strober M et al: No effect of adjunctive fluoxetine on eating behavior or weight phobia during inpatient treatment in anorexia nervosa: a historical case controlled study, *J Child Adolesc Psychopharmacol* 9(3):195-201, 1999.

Sullivan PF: Mortality in anorexia nervosa, *Am J Psychiatry* 152(7):1073-4, 1995.

US Department of Agriculture: Dietary guidelines for Americans, ed 5, Washington, DC, 2000, US Government Printing Office.

US Department of Agriculture: Nutrition program facts, 1999, retrieved from *http://www.fns.usda.gov/nutritionlink/Partnerships/NGO.html* on Jan 25, 2004.

US Department of Health and Human Services: Healthy people 2010, vol II, ed 2, Washington, DC, November 2000, US Government Printing Office.

CHAPTER **15**

Disorders of the Esophagus, Diaphragm, and Stomach

Karen Rea, MSN, RN, BC

OBJECTIVES

After reading this chapter, you should be able to do the following:

- Describe the pathophysiology of gastroesophageal reflux disease (GERD), hiatal hernia, and peptic ulcer disease.
- Describe the clinical manifestations of GERD, hiatal hernia, and peptic ulcer disease
- Describe the functional health patterns affected by GERD, hiatal hernia, and peptic ulcer disease.
- Compare and contrast the progression and management of GERD and peptic ulcer disease.
- Describe the role of each member of the interdisciplinary team involved in the care of patients with disorders of the esophagus, diaphragm, and stomach.
- Describe the indications for use, side effects, and nursing considerations related to drugs commonly used to treat GERD, hiatal hernia, and peptic ulcer disease.

Chronic disorders of the esophagus, diaphragm, and stomach are classified as acid peptic disorders and are among the most common gastrointestinal problems treated today. Estimates are that the health care costs of these disorders in the United States total more than $20 million per year (Fennerty, 2001a). Treatment options have greatly expanded over the past two decades and include new classes of drugs and new minimally invasive surgical options. However, large numbers of people with these disorders still self-manage their diseases with over-the-counter medications and delay seeking appropriate medical care. This chapter focuses on the management of gastroesophageal reflux disease (GERD), hiatal hernia, and peptic ulcer disease. Table 15-1 identifies ethnic differences in the patterns of these disorders. Because these conditions generally are not life threatening, this chapter does not include a discussion of ethical or end-of-life issues.

ASSESSMENT

Because GERD, hiatal hernia, and peptic ulcer disease have similar manifestations, the questions and techniques used in assessment are the same for all three. The most valuable assessment tool is a thorough history of the problem. The most common manifestation of these upper gastrointestinal tract disorders is heartburn. It is important to determine when the heartburn occurs, what its relationship to eating is, and what makes it better. Is there a particular pattern to the heartburn? Are additional symptoms present with the heartburn? How does it affect activities of daily living and sleeping? Are there problems with nausea, vomiting, or diarrhea? Has there been any weight loss? The answers to these questions help the health care professional narrow down the potential source of the problem. Physical examination findings are generally nonspecific, although palpation over the epigastric area may reveal some tenderness. A framework for functional health pattern assessment is presented in Box 15-1.

GASTROESOPHAGEAL REFLUX DISEASE

GERD is a chronic disorder. Although it seldom causes death, it does produce significant morbidity. Many health care dollars are spent on over-the-counter preparations such as antacids and acid reducers.

Pathophysiology

Gastroesophageal reflux is a normal physiologic process that occurs regularly in most individuals. Gastric contents reflux, or splash back, into the esophagus many times throughout the day, and this generally causes no symptoms. When symptoms or tissue damage do occur, GERD is said to be present. GERD is the most common of the upper gastrointestinal tract disorders. Approximately 7% of Americans experience heartburn, the chief symptom, daily, and 40% experience it monthly. Among those with no symptoms, approximately 7% show signs of esophageal tissue damage on endoscopic examination. GERD is uncommon in African Americans but is very common in whites (Orlando, 1999). It is less common in Asians (Kang and Ho, 1999).

esophageal pH monitoring may be performed to quantify the degree of reflux and length of time the esophageal lining is exposed to gastric acids. Esophageal endoscopy may be carried out to detect the presence of inflammation or of Barrett's esophagus, as well as to obtain tissue biopsy specimens to evaluate for adenocarcinoma. However, endoscopy fails to reveal any abnormalities in about half of those who have symptoms of GERD (Kaynard and Flora, 2001). Barium swallow testing may show evidence of esophageal stricture, hiatal hernia, or tissue erosion. However, it will not detect tissue changes in mild or early GERD. Esophageal manometry may be performed to measure pressures within the esophagus as swallowing occurs and to determine how well substances are transported from the pharynx to the stomach (Jackson Gastroenterology, 2002). Perhaps the easiest and least invasive means of diagnosing GERD is to begin a trial of high-dose proton pump inhibitor (PPI) therapy. If symptoms are relieved by PPI therapy, it is assumed that GERD is present and is responding to the treatment (Kaynard and Flora, 2001).

Interdisciplinary Care

The primary members of the interdisciplinary team are the primary care provider and the nurse, although occasionally a dietitian may join the team. Therapy for GERD focuses on reducing contact between acidic gastric contents and the esophageal lining. A two-pronged approach is generally taken: drug therapy and lifestyle modifications. Surgical interventions may be performed if these methods are not successful.

Drug Therapy

The most commonly used medications are outlined in Table 15-2. These consist mainly of over-the-counter antacids, histamine 2 (H_2) blockers, and PPIs. All act either to neutralize or to decrease production of gastric acids. According to the American College of Gastroenterology, the use of antacids and over-the-counter H_2 receptor blockers is appropriate initial therapy for relief of symptoms (DeVault, Castrell, and the Practice Parameters Committee, 1999). If these are not effective, however, or if symptoms persist for a prolonged period, stronger therapy is needed. Two approaches are used in providing stronger medication: the "step-up" approach and the "step-down" approach. In the "step-up" approach, the person with GERD is given antacids and H_2 receptor blockers. If symptoms are not relieved within 1 to 4 weeks, the dosage of H_2 receptor blockers is increased. If relief is still not obtained, PPIs are prescribed. The step-up approach has the advantage of being less expensive initially and safer in the long term than prolonged PPI therapy. However, only about 50% of those with GERD respond favorably to this method. In the step-down approach, PPI therapy is given for

Table 15-2 Drugs Commonly Used to Treat Gastroesophageal Reflux Disease and Peptic Ulcer Disease

Category/Action	Drug and Dosage	Patient Education
Antacids Neutralize gastric acids and delay gastric emptying	Aluminum hydroxide (ALternaGEL, Amphojel): 5-10 ml PO PC and HS Aluminum hydroxide/magnesium hydroxide (Maalox, Mylanta): 10-20 ml PO PC and HS	Report any unusual reactions (e.g., constipation, intestinal obstruction, bone pain, muscle weakness). Shake liquid well before using.
	Bismuth subsalicylate (Pepto-Bismol): 524 mg PO every ½ hr, max. 4.2 mg/24 hr	Report any unusual reactions (e.g., confusion, increased bleeding time, tinnitus, metallic taste, black tongue [with chewable tablets], black stools). Shake liquid well before using. Chew tablets; do not swallow whole. Avoid concurrent use of other salicylates. Do not give to children under age 18 because of possibility of Reye's syndrome with use of salicylates.
	Calcium carbonate (Rolaids, Titralac, Tums): 359 mg to 1.5 g PO PC and HS	Report any unusual reactions (e.g., constipation, nausea, vomiting, headache, disorientation). Shake liquid well before using. Chew tablets; do not swallow whole.

Table 15-2   Drugs Commonly Used to Treat Gastroesophageal Reflux Disease and Peptic Ulcer Disease—cont'd

Category/Action	Drug and Dosage	Patient Education
H₂ receptor blockers Inhibit histamine at the H₂ receptor of the gastric parietal cells, which results in less gastric acid production	Ranitidine (Zantac): 75 mg PO BID (OTC), 150 mg PO BID, or 300 mg PO QHS Cimetidine (Tagamet): 200 mg PO QID (OTC), 400 mg PO BID, or 800 mg PO QHS Famotidine (Pepcid): 10 mg PO 1 hr AC (OTC), 20 mg PO BID, or 40 mg PO HS Nizatidine (Axid): 75 mg PO BID (OTC), 150 mg PO BID or 300 mg PO QHS	Report any unusual reactions (e.g., headache, dizziness, confusion, nausea and vomiting, headache). This drug class may cause bone marrow suppression. Ranitidine may cause hepatotoxicity. Cimetidine may cause convulsions, jaundice. Famotidine may cause seizures, bronchospasm. Nizatidine may cause hepatitis, cardiac arrest. Take all medication as prescribed; do not stop early if symptoms abate.
Proton pump inhibitors Block the final step in the production of gastric acid	Esomeprazole (Nexium): 40 mg PO QD Lansoprazole (Prevacid): 30 mg PO BID Omeprazole (Prilosec): 20 mg PO BID Pantoprazole (Protonix): 40 mg PO BID Rabeprazole (Aciphex): 20 mg PO BID Ranitidine bismuth citrate (Tritec): 400 mg PO BID	Report any unusual reactions (e.g., nausea and vomiting, diarrhea, constipation, rash, headaches, dizziness, cough, epistaxis, taste changes, tinnitus, insomnia, dream abnormalities). Lansoprazole may cause chest pain, hematuria. Omeprazole may cause proteinuria, back pain, bone marrow suppression. Avoid use in pregnancy and lactation. Take before meals, and do not chew or crush. Take all medication as prescribed; do not stop early if symptoms abate.
Prokinetic agent Speeds up gastric emptying	Metoclopramide (Reglan): 10 mg PO AC and HS	Report any unusual reaction (e.g., muscle tremors, agitation, insomnia, tardive dyskinesia). Take all medication as prescribed; do not stop early if symptoms abate.

Adapted from DeVault KR, Castrell DO, the Practice Parameters Committee of the American College of Gastroenterology: Updated guidelines for the diagnosis and treatment of gastroesophageal reflux disease, *Am J Gastroenterol* 94(6):1434-42, 1999; and Skidmore-Roth L: *Mosby's 2003 nursing drug reference,* St Louis, 2002, Mosby.
AC, Before meals; *BID,* twice a day; *HS,* at bedtime; *OTC,* over-the-counter strength; *PC,* after meals; *PO,* by mouth; *QD,* everyday; *QHS,* each bedtime; *QID,* four times a day.

6 to 8 weeks, then changed to H₂ receptor blocker therapy once symptoms have been controlled. The advantage of this approach is more rapid relief of symptoms. However, the treatment costs more initially, and the long-term safety of PPI therapy is unknown at this time (Mullick and Richter,

2000; Orlando, 1999). In some cases a prokinetic agent (metoclopramide) may be added to accelerate gastric emptying and thus decrease the length of time irritating gastric contents are in the stomach and esophagus. Many of those with GERD require a long-term maintenance therapy to control their symptoms. Generally the maintenance therapy dosage is the same as that used for treatment of active disease (DeVault, Castrell, and the Practice Parameters Committee, 1999).

Nurse

Nursing care of the person with GERD centers on education (Table 15-3). Recognition of the manifestations of the disease is very important. This is especially true if the major symptoms have been pulmonary instead of gastric. Of special importance is teaching the patient how to differentiate between heartburn and chest pain of cardiac origin, and what actions to take if a myocardial infarction is suspected. Medication management is another key area of education, as medications are the cornerstone of medical therapy. Because many of the medications are available over the counter and because GERD is a chronic disorder, the person with GERD must know how to use these drugs appropriately. Regardless of the type of medication being used, the person with GERD must understand the different mechanisms of action of the various classes of medication, the appropriate times to take them, the way to judge whether they are working, and potential complications for which to be alert.

Lifestyle modifications and surgical options are also important areas for education.

Education in Lifestyle Modifications

Lifestyle modifications are key to successful GERD therapy. The major modifications are dietary changes and care in positioning. Table 15-4 lists foods known to exacerbate GERD symptoms. Counseling by the nurse or dietitian helps the person with GERD identify those foods that are particularly bothersome and adjust the diet accordingly. Eating smaller but more frequent meals helps to minimize gastric distention. Because a feeling of satiety typically does not occur for 15 to 20 minutes after eating, it is especially important to identify cues to being full to avoid overdistention. Abstention from eating for 2 to 3 hours before going to bed is strongly recommended. This allows time for gastric emptying to occur and decreases the amount of gastric secretions in the stomach during the night. In addition, those with GERD are encouraged to avoid lying down immediately after eating during the day.

A standard lifestyle modification for GERD is to elevate the head of the bed for sleeping. This allows gravity to assist in preventing reflux while the patient sleeps. The bed can be elevated by placing blocks under the legs at the head of the bed. Such blocks are readily available for sale and can be easily improvised using thick telephone books or other large books. This method of elevation is not very practical for the long term, however. With the entire bed angled in this way, the occupants will slide to the bottom of the bed during the night because of gravity. An alternative means of elevating the head is to use a foam wedge with pillows on top to elevate the upper half of the body while the rest of the bed remains flat. This keeps the stomach lower than the esophagus during the night. Placement of pillows alone is not sufficient, because the esophagus will not be raised high enough to remain above the level of the stomach. The use of a wedge may be problematical for those who have arthritis of the neck or back as well as GERD, because it is difficult to assume a side-lying position with the head and trunk elevated. One small research study has indicated that, for those who cannot tolerate sleeping with a wedge or with the head of the bed elevated, lying on the left side to sleep results in fewer episodes of reflux during the night (Khoury et al, 1999). Alternatively, it is possible to purchase queen- and king-sized beds that have

---

Table 15-3 ■ Patient and Family Education on Upper Gastrointestinal Tract Disorders

Topic	Teaching Points
Disease process	Etiology of specific disorder: gastroesophageal reflux disease (GERD), hiatal hernia, and/or peptic ulcer disease
	Possible complications of specific disorder
	Signs and symptoms to report to health care provider
Medication management	Name, dosage, route, and frequency of medications
	Importance of taking all medication exactly as prescribed
	Expected effects of the medications
	Possible side effects and adverse reactions to report to health care provider
	Possible interactions with other medications and/or foods
Dietary modifications	Avoidance of foods that create gastric distress
	With GERD, avoidance of foods that lower tone of lower esophageal sphincter
	Weight loss methods if appropriate
Lifestyle modifications (with GERD)	Need to remain upright for 2-3 hr after eating
	Need to sleep with head of bed elevated
	Avoidance of tight-fitting clothing
	Avoidance of extremely large meals

Table 15-4   Foods and Medications That Predispose to Gastroesophageal Reflux

Mechanism	Food	Medication
Decrease lower esophageal pressure	Fatty foods Chocolate Carminatives (spearmint, peppermint) Alcohol	Anticholinergics Benzodiazepines Calcium channel blockers Opioids Progesterone-containing medications Xanthines
Irritate esophageal mucosa	Citrus fruit and juices Tomato-based products Coffee, both caffeinated and caffeine free Cola beverages	Alendronate sodium (Fosamax) Nonsteroidal antiinflammatory drugs, including aspirin Iron and potassium preparations Quinidine derivatives Tetracycline derivatives

Adapted from Fisher RS: Treatment of gastroesophageal reflux disease. In Wolfe M, editor: *Therapy of digestive disorder,* Philadelphia, 2000, WB Saunders; and National Institute of Diabetes & Digestive & Kidney Diseases: Heartburn, hiatal hernia, and gastroesophageal reflux disease (GERD), 2001, retrieved from *http://digestive.niddk.nih. gov/diseases/pubs/gerd/index.htm* on Nov 15, 2002.

electronic controls to elevate the head of the bed and allow each side of the bed to be operated independently. Such a bed may be more comfortable than the use of either elevating blocks or a wedge and pillows.

Several other lifestyle recommendations are standard for patients with GERD. An important one is smoking cessation, because nicotine is thought to decrease LES pressure (Mullick and Richter, 2000). Strict abstinence from alcohol is also important, because it can exacerbate GERD. Losing weight is also advised. Avoidance of tight-fitting clothing (especially belts and girdles or corsets) helps prevent pressure on the stomach.

Preparation for Surgical Intervention

For the person who has significant GERD symptoms unrelieved by medication and lifestyle modifications, surgical intervention may be required. The person with GERD must learn about the various options available, and the advantages and disadvantages of each. The newest option is the Enteryx procedure (Enteric Medical Technologies, 2003; US Food and Drug Administration, 2003), approved for use in April 2003. During endoscopy, a liquid material is injected into the LES muscle. The injected material forms a spongy implant within the muscle and thus helps the muscle to prevent reflux more effectively. The need for medication was eliminated in a higher percentage of those who underwent the Enteryx procedure than of those who underwent traditional surgical correction. Currently, three main types of surgery are used: Nissen fundoplication, the Stretta procedure, and the Bard EndoCinch System of suturing. Nissen fundoplication (Figure 15-1) is generally performed laparoscopically and involves tightening the LES by suturing a portion of the stomach around the esophagus. In the Stretta procedure, radiofrequency technology is used to tighten

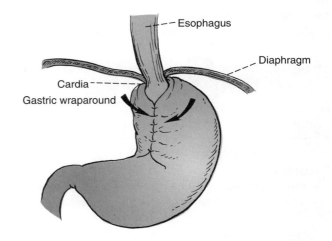

Figure 15-1 Nissen fundoplication procedure. The gastric fundus is wrapped around the distal esophagus and sutured to itself. (From Black JM, Hawks JH, Keene AM: *Medical-surgical nursing,* ed 6, Philadelphia, 2001, WB Saunders.)

the esophageal tissue around the gastroesophageal junction by creating scar tissue. This surgery is performed endoscopically as an outpatient procedure. The third surgical option is the EndoCinch suturing system, which creates "pleats" in the esophageal tissue and thus tightens the LES. This procedure is also performed endoscopically (Kaynard and Flora, 2001). These surgeries are generally performed on younger persons with GERD who have been unable to control their symptoms with medications and lifestyle changes. Undergoing the surgery does not guarantee that medications for GERD will not continue to be required. The nurse can educate the individual about the risks of surgery and serve as a sounding board in discussions of if and when surgery is to be considered.

Primary Provider (Physician/Nurse Practitioner)

The primary care provider may be a physician, adult nurse practitioner, or physician assistant. The initial evaluation will most likely be performed by a gastroenterologist. However, an otolaryngologist may be the first physician to identify the presence of GERD if the affected individual's chief complaints have been a chronic cough and globus. Once the diagnosis has been made, the adult nurse practitioner or physician assistant may be the appropriate clinician to provide long-term assessment and monitoring.

Dietitian

The dietitian is an important member of the interdisciplinary team if the affected individual is overweight and needs assistance with a weight loss program. He or she may offer nutritional education and counseling to assist the patient in identifying foods that exacerbate the reflux and in establishing a realistic diet for weight loss.

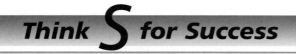

Think S for Success

Symptoms
- Manage gastric distress with appropriate medications, dietary modifications, and lifestyle modifications.

Sequelae
- Provide appropriate assessment to detect the development of chronic esophagitis, Barrett's esophagus, and esophageal cancer.
- Provide early intervention when appropriate to prevent sequelae.

Safety
- Teach about appropriate drug therapy to prevent disease deterioration and complications.
- Teach recognition of potential adverse reactions.
- Teach patient to differentiate substernal pain caused by gastroesophageal reflux disease (GERD) from that of cardiac origin.

Support/Services
- Provide support for patient and family in adhering to lifestyle modifications, dietary changes, and long-term medication regimen.

Satisfaction
- Determine the degree to which GERD interferes with patient's ability to participate in daily activities and discuss methods of adjusting lifestyle to achieve desired quality of life.
- Assess degree to which lifestyle modifications are acceptable to the affected individual and family.

HIATAL HERNIA

In hiatal hernia, the stomach moves up through the diaphragm into the chest cavity. In a sliding hiatal hernia, the more common type, the esophagus slides upward along with the stomach into the thoracic cavity. In a rolling hiatal hernia, a portion of the stomach herniates through the diaphragm alongside the esophagus (Figure 15-2). The latter type carries a higher risk for strangulation of the hernia. Because the LES remains in its normal location, however, a rolling hiatal hernia does not lead to reflux symptoms (Murphy-Blake, 2001). The cause of hiatal hernias is unknown, although incidence increases with age. Many times the hernia is completely asymptomatic. When symptoms do occur, they are very similar to those of GERD, with heartburn being the most common one. The method of diagnosis, pharmacologic therapy, and nursing care for hiatal hernia are the same as for GERD. Additional information should be given to the patient regarding how to recognize the symptoms of a strangulated hernia. These symptoms include abdominal pain and nausea and vomiting. In severe cases surgery is indicated to correct the hernia.

PEPTIC ULCER DISEASE

Approximately 11% to 14% of Americans will experience a peptic ulcer at some point in their lives, with the incidence slightly higher in men than in women (Del Valle et al, 1999). Significant health care dollars are spent on the treatment of peptic ulcer disease. The Centers for Disease Control and Prevention (1998) estimates that nearly $6 billion dollars are spent annually in hospitalizations, physician office visits, and lost productivity as a result of this disorder. In addition, a significant percentage of the population regularly uses nonsteroidal antiinflammatory drugs (NSAIDs), which puts them at high risk for development of ulcers. Many people spend much time, money, and energy in self-treating peptic ulcer disease before seeking appropriate health care.

Pathophysiology

Peptic ulcer disease includes gastric and duodenal ulcers. These ulcerations form in the mucosal lining of the stomach and duodenum, and may be symptomatic or asymptomatic. The chief causes are infection with *Helicobacter pylori* and the use of NSAIDs (Boxes 15-3 through 15-5). *H. pylori* infection is very common throughout the world, and NSAIDs are among the most commonly used over-the-counter medications. Both create a high risk for the development of ulcers because they lead to destruction of a focal area of the gastric or duodenal mucosa. *H. pylori* is a bacterium that damages the epithelial cells in the stomach and duodenum, elevates gastrin levels, and alters the permeability of the mucosa to hydrogen ions (Knigge, 2001). NSAID-induced peptic ulcers result from inhibition of prostaglandin production (Fennerty, 2001b). Prostaglandins are important in providing protection to the gastric and duodenal mucosa.

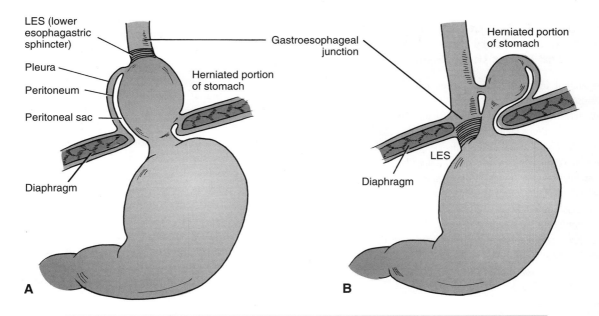

Figure 15-2 Types of hiatal hernia. **A,** Sliding hiatal hernia. The lower esophageal sphincter (LES) and a portion of the stomach protrude through the diaphragm into the thoracic cavity. **B,** Rolling hiatal hernia. A portion of the stomach protrudes through the diaphragm alongside the esophagus, with the LES remaining in the abdominal cavity. (From Black JM, Hawks JH, Keene AM: *Medical-surgical nursing,* ed 6, Philadelphia, 2001, WB Saunders.)

The major complications from peptic ulcers are bleeding, perforation, and gastric outlet obstruction. In some cases, the first sign of an ulcer is frank gastrointestinal hemorrhaging. Anemia may arise from chronic microscopic bleeding secondary to the gastritis. A history of previous ulcer disease increases the risk of complications, as does the use of corticosteroids along with NSAIDs. Advanced age is accompanied by a significantly higher risk of dying from upper gastrointestinal tract hemorrhaging (Wolfe, 2000).

Smoking is also a risk factor, because it increases the acidity of the duodenum.

Clinical Manifestations

The chief symptom of peptic ulcer disease is epigastric distress. This is generally experienced as heartburn or as a

---

Box 15-3　Epidemiology of Peptic Ulcer Disease

■ Peptic ulcer disease affects approximately 4.5 million people annually.
■ Twenty million people in the United States will have an ulcer at some point in their lifetime.
■ Peptic ulcer disease affects 11% to 14% of men and 8% to 11% women in the United States.
■ The rate of duodenal ulcers in men, but not in women, has decreased over the past 20 years.

Adapted from Knigge KL: The role of *H. pylori* in gastrointestinal disease: a guide to identification and eradication, *Postgrad Med* 110(3):71-82, 2001; and Del Valle J et al: Acid peptic disorders. In Yamada T, editor: *Textbook of gastroenterology,* ed 3, Philadelphia, 1999, Lippincott Williams & Wilkins.

Box 15-4　Epidemiology and Effects of *Helicobacter Pylori* Infection

■ *Helicobacter pylori* infection is very common and is generally acquired during childhood.
■ The infection rate is 90% in developing countries, 40% to 50% in developed countries.
■ About 15% to 20% of those infected develop peptic ulcer disease or gastric cancer.
■ *H. pylori* infection causes 90% to 95% of all duodenal ulcers.
■ *H. pylori* infection causes 50% to 70% of all gastric ulcers.
■ Infection is a significant risk factor for development of gastric cancer.
■ Infection carries little or no risk for development of GERD.

Adapted from Centers for Disease Control and Prevention: *Helicobacter pylori* and peptic ulcer disease, 2001, retrieved from *http://www.cdc.gov/ulcer/md.htm* on Nov 15, 2002; and Knigge KL: The role of *H. pylori* in gastrointestinal disease: a guide to identification and eradication, *Postgrad Med* 110(3):71-82, 2001.

Box 15-5   Use of Nonsteroidal Antiinflammatory Drugs (NSAIDs) and Peptic Ulcer Disease

■ An estimated 15 million to 25 million people in the United States use NSAIDs on a long-term basis.

■ Fifteen percent of those over age 65 use NSAIDs regularly.

■ Fifty percent of those taking NSAIDs will have mucosal erosions and 20% will have actual ulceration.

■ There is no correlation between NSAID-induced heartburn symptoms and the severity of erosion or ulceration.

■ Those with ulcerations may have no symptoms due to the analgesic effects of the NSAIDs.

■ The risk for ulceration increases dramatically with age, with history of prior gastrointestinal problems, and with diagnosis of severe rheumatoid arthritis.

■ Infection with *Helicobacter pylori* increases the risk of ulcer formation with NSAID use.

Adapted from Fennerty MB: NSAID-related gastrointestinal injury, *Postgrad Med* 110(3):87-94, 2001; and Laine L et al: Stratifying the risk of NSAID-related upper gastrointestinal clinical events: results of a double-blind outcomes study in patients with rheumatoid arthritis, *Gastroenterology* 123(4):1006-12, 2002.

---

substernal gnawing, burning pain. The pain may radiate to the back and typically occurs several hours after meals. It is generally relieved by the consumption of food or antacids, although spicy or acidic foods may exacerbate the discomfort. Anorexia, early satiety, nausea, belching, and abdominal bloating are additional symptoms that may occur. Some people with ulcers are awakened during the night by pain. It may be difficult to differentiate pain caused by an ulcer from pain of cardiac origin, because both may be experienced as substernal discomfort. One must remember that a significant portion of those with gastric inflammation experience no symptoms at all. Significant weight loss and vomiting are warning signs of potential complications and should be evaluated immediately. Vomiting may be due to the development of obstruction at the gastric outlet.

Diagnosis

Diagnosis of peptic ulcer disease begins with a complete history taking and physical examination. There are few external physical findings with ulcers, although some tenderness may be present in the epigastric area. Several diagnostic tests are available to detect infection with *H. pylori*. These should be used only when symptoms are present, because treatment is not indicated in asymptomatic cases. The most common test for *H. pylori* is the enzyme-linked immunosorbent assay. This antibody test indicates only exposure to the organism, not active infection, because

antibody levels remain elevated for years following infection and treatment. In the person with peptic ulcer symptoms but no history of treatment, positive results indicate the need for initiation of therapy, because *H. pylori* infection does not heal spontaneously. Urea breath testing is another means of determining the presence of *H. pylori* infection and is becoming the test of choice because of its ease and reliability (Cutler, 2001). In this test, the individual ingests radiolabeled urea. In the presence of *H. pylori*, the urea is converted into carbon dioxide and exhaled. Because this test gives positive results only when active infection is present, it is a useful tool to measure the success of treatment. Repeat testing is performed at least 4 weeks after therapy is completed and after PPI therapy has been stopped for at least 2 weeks. Urea testing may also be done by obtaining a venous blood sample after ingestion of the urea. A third test for *H. pylori* is the stool antigen test, which may also be used to determine the effectiveness of therapy (Cutler, 2001).

Diagnosis of peptic ulcer disease resulting from NSAID use generally relies solely on a history of symptoms and consideration of the type of NSAID being taken. Testing for *H. pylori* may also be performed, because its presence increases the risk of ulceration with NSAID therapy. Endoscopy with tissue biopsy is indicated if symptoms are severe or if gastric cancer is suspected.

Interdisciplinary Care

The focus of treatment for peptic ulcer disease is eradication of *H. pylori* infection and minimization of damage from NSAID use. Interdisciplinary team members include the primary care provider, the nurse, and in some cases a dietitian.

Drug Therapy

Pharmacologic therapy is the mainstay of management. Triple-agent therapy is indicated to eradicate *H. pylori*. This generally consists of a combination of a PPI plus two antibiotics, taken twice daily. The PPI reduces the amount of acid secretion, raises the pH, and inhibits the activity of *H. pylori* (Cutler, 2001). An alternate triple-agent therapy is the use of bismuth plus two antibiotics 4 times a day. This regimen was the original treatment for the infection but is more difficult to maintain because of the number of pills that must be taken each day and the sometimes unpleasant side effects of the bismuth. Table 15-5 outlines the medications used. Therapy is continued for 10 to 14 days and is 90% to 95% effective in preventing recurrence of the disease. In contrast, among those treated with traditional ulcer therapy (antacids, H_2 receptor blockers, and PPIs) without eradication of *H. pylori*, the disease recurs in 60% to 70% (Cutler, 2001). Long-term PPI therapy may be needed for those who had severe disease and for those for whom traditional therapy has not been effective.

The treatment of choice for NSAID-related peptic ulcer disease is to minimize or eliminate the use of NSAIDs. If

Table 15-5　Triple Therapy Regimens for Treatment of *Helicobacter Pylori* Infection

Category	Medication and Dosage	Patient Education
Regimen 1: Two Antibiotics Plus One Proton Pump Inhibitor Two antibiotics	Amoxicillin: 1 g PO BID for 10-14 days *or* Metronidazole (Flagyl): 500 mg PO BID for 10-14 days *and* Clarithromycin (Biaxin): 500 mg PO BID for 10-14 days	Report any unusual reactions (e.g., nausea and vomiting, diarrhea, rash). Amoxicillin may cause bone marrow depression, glomerulonephritis, vaginitis. Metronidazole may cause metallic taste in mouth; peripheral neuropathy, seizures, headache; may turn urine dark reddish brown; may cause Antabuse-type reaction if used with alcohol. Clarithromycin may cause Stevens-Johnson syndrome, hepatotoxicity, leukopenia, thrombocytopenia. Take all medication as prescribed; do not stop early if symptoms abate.
One proton pump inhibitor	Esomeprazole (Nexium): 40 mg PO QD *or* Lansoprazole (Prevacid): 30 mg PO BID *or* Omeprazole (Prilosec): 20 mg PO BID *or* Pantoprazole (Protonix): 40 mg PO BID *or* Rabeprazole (Aciphex): 20 mg PO BID *or* Ranitidine bismuth citrate (Tritec): 400 mg PO BID	Report any unusual reactions (e.g., nausea and vomiting, diarrhea, constipation, rash, headaches, dizziness, cough, epistaxis, taste changes, tinnitus, insomnia, dream abnormalities). Lansoprazole may cause chest pain, hematuria. Omeprazole may cause proteinuria, back pain, bone marrow suppression. Avoid use in pregnancy and lactation. Take before meals; do not chew/crush. Take all medication as prescribed; do not stop early if symptoms abate.
Regimen 2: Two Antibiotics Plus Bismuth Antibiotics	Tetracycline: 500 mg PO QID for 10-14 days	Report any unusual reactions (e.g., nausea and vomiting, diarrhea, rash). May cause bone marrow depression and hepatotoxicity. Take 1 hr before or 2 hr after dairy products or antacids. Take with a full glass of water. Avoid prolonged exposure to sunlight to minimize increased risk of sunburn. Take all medication as prescribed; do not stop early if symptoms abate.
	Metronidazole (Flagyl): 500 mg PO BID for 10-14 days	Report any unusual reactions (e.g., metallic taste in mouth; peripheral neuropathy, seizures, headache, dizziness). Urine may turn dark reddish brown. Avoid drinking alcohol, as Antabuse-type reaction may occur. Take all medication as prescribed; do not stop early if symptoms abate.

Continued

Table 15-5   Triple Therapy Regimens for Treatment of *Helicobacter Pylori* Infection—cont'd

Category	Medication and Dosage	Patient Education
Bismuth	Bismuth subsalicylate (Pepto-Bismol): 2 tablets PO QID for 10-14 days	Report any unusual reactions (e.g., confusion, increased bleeding time, tinnitus, metallic taste, black tongue [with chewable tablets], black stools). Chew tablets, do not swallow whole. Avoid concurrent use of other salicylates. Take all medication as prescribed; do not stop early if symptoms abate.

Adapted from Cutler AF: Eradicating *Helicobacter pylori* infection, *Patient Care* 35(7):91-100, 2001; and Skidmore-Roth L: *Mosby's 2003 nursing drug reference,* St Louis, 2002, Mosby.
BID, Twice a day; *PO,* by mouth; *QD,* every day; *QID,* four times a day.

NSAIDs must be continued, use of the lowest possible dosage is encouraged. This is especially the case when the NSAID is being taken for analgesia, not for its antiinflammatory effects. The dosage required for analgesia is much lower than that required to reduce inflammation. Substitution of acetaminophen or cyclooxygenase 2 (COX-2) inhibitor therapy for NSAID therapy is another option. Acetaminophen has no deleterious effects on the gastric mucosa, although large doses may adversely affect liver function. Examples of COX-2 inhibitor analgesics are celecoxib (Celebrex), valdecoxib (Bextra), and rofecoxib (Vioxx). Because COX-2 receptors are not found in the gastrointestinal system, these drugs do not produce the adverse reactions caused by the more traditional NSAIDs. For patients who must or wish to continue taking NSAIDs, PPIs appear to be the most effective means of reducing the incidence of ulcer. By decreasing the production of prostaglandins, they inhibit the formation of both duodenal and gastric ulcers and speed up the healing of any ulcers that already exist. The H_2 receptor antagonists are not as effective as the PPIs in healing ulcers from NSAID use (Wolfe, 2000). Anyone who has NSAID-induced peptic ulcer disease should also be tested for the presence of *H. pylori* infection and treated appropriately if it is found.

Nurse

As with GERD, the focus of nursing care for the individual with peptic ulcer disease is education. The individual with an ulcer needs to learn about disease etiology and long-term prognosis as well as to learn to recognize warning signs of complications. The treatment focus for ulcers has shifted dramatically over the past 15 years. Those with the disease may not be aware of the newer treatment philosophy and may have been self-treating for years with inappropriate therapy. This is an opportunity to convey to the patient that ulcers are curable and that living with chronic pain from ulcers is no longer the norm.

Because the mainstay of therapy is pharmacologic, the person with an ulcer must have a thorough understanding of the medications being used. Drug therapy is complex, and historically adherence to the drug regimen throughout the entire treatment period has been a problem for many individuals. Failure to complete the regimen will result in recurrence of the ulcer and the development of antibiotic-resistant *H. pylori*. Table 15-5 gives the specifics of education regarding peptic ulcer medications.

Peptic ulcer disease from chronic NSAID use is more complicated to manage, especially in the elderly population or in those with chronic arthritis, who may find it difficult to discontinue NSAID use. Collaboration between the physician, the person with the ulcer, and the nurse are important to identify the optimal type and dosage of NSAID to provide appropriate pain relief. In addition, the individual should be taught alternative therapies for relieving the pain from arthritis, with the goal of decreasing reliance on NSAIDs. Long-term prophylactic therapy with PPIs may be necessary to prevent recurrence of symptoms. If so, the individual will need education about the rationale for using the PPI and the importance of its continued use in the absence of symptoms.

The family should be included in any instruction about the disease process and medication management. Family members may not understand the importance of the complex medication regimen for disease management (see Table 15-3).

Primary Care Provider

Uncomplicated peptic ulcer disease may be managed by an internist or family practitioner. A gastroenterologist may be used in more complex cases. Once the diagnosis has been made, the ongoing care of peptic ulcer disease may be provided by an advanced practice nurse or a physician assistant.

Dietitian

Dietary changes are generally no longer recommended for those with an ulcer. In the past, the focus was on consuming a bland diet with frequent ingestion of milk and antacids. However, such a practice has been found actually to increase the production of gastric acid. Now the focus is on identifying those foods that tend to increase gastric distress and eliminating them from the diet. The registered dietitian may be called upon to provide counseling about appropriate food choices and to assist with weight loss if obesity is an issue. In addition, if symptoms appear when the stomach is empty, the addition of snacks or small meals during the day may help with pain control.

COMPLEMENTARY AND ALTERNATIVE THERAPIES

Several alternative therapies are available to relieve the distress of acid reflux and peptic ulcers. Those most commonly used are techniques to reduce pain and discomfort, such as relaxation methods, guided imagery, and behavioral techniques. Biofeedback may also be tried, although research into this methodology has shown mixed results (Agency for Healthcare Research and Quality, 2001). Acupuncture has been used to relieve nausea and heartburn. Research indicates that acupuncture does decrease acid production, although this effect does not continue long beyond the actual treatment (Sung, 2002). Herbal preparations are another alternative therapy used by some individuals (Box 15-6). Because of the potential for interaction of herbal preparations with other medications, the nurse must be careful to assess for their use and educate the individual about monitoring for adverse reactions.

Box 15-6   Herbs Used to Treat Upper Gastrointestinal Tract Disorders

- Allspice
- Butterbur
- Ginger
- Iceland moss
- Licorice
- Nutmeg

Adapted from Fetrow CW, Avila JR: *Professional's handbook of complementary and alternative medicines,* Springhouse, Pa, 1999, Springhouse Corp.

Think S for Success

Symptoms
- Manage gastric distress with appropriate medications.
- Teach about importance of completing therapy for *Helicobacter pylori* as ordered to prevent recurrence.
- Teach about minimizing use of nonsteroidal antiinflammatory drugs to prevent further symptoms.

Sequelae
- Instruct in signs of potential complications from peptic ulcers: hemorrhage, obstruction.

Safety
- Teach about appropriate drug therapy to prevent disease deterioration and complications.
- Teach recognition of potential adverse reactions.

Support/Services
- Provide support for patient and family in adhering to complex medication regimen and coping with chronic discomfort and pain.

Satisfaction
- Determine the degree to which peptic ulcer disease interferes with patient's ability to participate in daily activities.
- Discuss methods of adjusting lifestyle to achieve desired quality of life.

CASE STUDY

Patient Data

Mrs. B. is a 50-year-old government worker who lives at home with her husband and two teenaged sons. Work has been very busy lately, and her relationship with her sons has been tense at times because of "typical teenage antics." Mr. and Mrs. B. live in a small house in a neighborhood close to the city. While undergoing her annual physical examination with the nurse practitioner, Mrs. B. states that she has been under increased stress lately and is having a lot of heartburn, as well as a sour taste in her mouth much of the time. She states that she has experienced these symptoms off and on "for years" but sometimes goes for several years without any problems. Now she is taking an antacid when the heartburn is bothering her, and one ranitidine (Zantac) tablet in the morning "when she remembers." These measures have not appreciably helped her discomfort. She states that food consumption does not seem to make the heartburn any better or worse. The heartburn has been making her irritable throughout the day. Upon questioning by the nurse practitioner, she remembers that she was treated for "that ulcer bug" about 10 years ago and was told that her ulcer was gone when her medication was finished. In the intervening time she has had to take antacids and ranitidine occasionally. She supposes that the heartburn will get better again as it always does, but she is worried that her ulcer is coming back because of her increased stress.

Physical Examination

On physical examination, the nurse practitioner notes that Mrs. B. does not have abdominal tenderness and has normal bowel sounds. A stool test for occult blood gives negative results. Mrs. B. is noted to be 25 pounds overweight. The nurse practitioner also observes that Mrs. B. frequently needs to clear her throat and has a hoarse, gravelly voice. When questioned, Mrs. B. states that she sometimes has trouble sleeping because of a night cough from postnasal drip and frequently has to talk for a bit on awakening before her "voice gets going." The nurse practitioner suspects

Continued

CASE STUDY—cont'd

that Mrs. B. has GERD and prescribes esomeprazole (Nexium) 40 mg once a day to alleviate her symptoms. She also orders a urea breath test for Mrs. B., to be performed before she starts on the esomeprazole. The results of this test are negative. A referral is made to a local gastroenterologist for a complete workup.

Thinking It Through

- What is the significance of the negative urea breath test?
- What will be the most probable course of action in treating Mrs. B.?
- What are Mrs. B.'s concerns likely to be?
- What will be the focus of education for Mrs. B.?

Case Conference

After taking the esomeprazole for a week, Mrs. B. is evaluated by the gastroenterologist. Based on her history, as well as her previous history of treatment for *H. pylori* and her negative urea test result, he feels that she has GERD. Her cough and hoarseness are common symptoms of GERD, as is her heartburn. Although Mrs. B. has attributed her discomfort to increased stress, the physician explains that stress is no longer felt to be a major contributor to gastric inflammation and heartburn. He wants her to continue to take her medication for the next several months. He also schedules an endoscopy to evaluate the status of her esophagus and LES, and to look for evidence of Barrett's esophagus.

The office nurse meets with Mrs. B. to explain the medication regimen and lifestyle modifications to follow. She starts by explaining to Mrs. B. what GERD is and how her cough and hoarseness are probably caused by the reflux and not by postnasal drip. Mrs. B. is educated about the medication, with a focus on how important it is to take the drug on an empty stomach in the morning. Mrs. B. expresses dismay in response to this information, because she is in the habit of sleeping as late as possible and then eating on the run as she leaves the house, typically 30 minutes after she gets out of bed. The nurse suggests that perhaps she could leave a glass of water at the bedside, along with her medication, and take it in the early morning hours when she gets up to go to the bathroom or wakes when her husband gets up for the day. Mrs. B. agrees to try this. The physician has told Mrs. B. that she needs to sleep with the head of her bed elevated on wooden blocks and that she is not to lie down for 2 hours after eating. Although doubtful about how this will work, Mrs. B. says she will try it. The nurse also reviews with Mrs. B. which foods tend to exacerbate GERD and works with her to find alternatives to the sodas and chocolate that she

loves. In addition, the nurse makes a referral to a registered dietitian for weight loss counseling.

Mrs. B. returns to the office in 2 weeks, following her endoscopy. The physician reports that the examination showed no evidence of esophageal, gastric, or duodenal irritation or inflammation, nor of Barrett's esophagus. He wants Mrs. B. to continue taking esomeprazole and explains that tissue changes are not always present with GERD. The lack of findings does not mean that her symptoms are "all in her head," as Mrs. B. reports her husband's saying. Mrs. B. meets with the nurse again for additional education, as well as a check on how she is doing with her medication and her sleeping. Mrs. B. states that she had to lower the head of her bed because both she and her husband were ending up curled up at the bottom of the bed in the morning. Her husband was especially irritated with the elevation of the bed and repeatedly stated that he didn't think it was necessary. In addition, Mrs. B. found it very difficult to sleep soundly through the night because she could not find a comfortable position and was awaking feeling very groggy. Several days she forgot to take her medication. The nurse suggests to Mrs. B. that she try using a wedge for her bed, with several pillows on top of it. She also suggests having Mrs. B.'s husband remind her to take her medication when he gets up in the morning. They discuss her dietary changes and her success at losing weight. She has had three visits with the dietitian, and they have developed a workable diet plan. Mrs. B. will be making monthly visits to the dietitian for ongoing support and fine-tuning of her diet plan. Overall, Mrs. B. feels that her heartburn is beginning to get better. In addition, she is not coughing as frequently, especially at night.

At a follow-up visit at 3 months, Mrs. B. no longer complains of heartburn or cough and has found that sleeping with the wedge is working well for her. She has lost 15 of the 25 pounds she needs to lose, and states that she feels "great." The physician tells her to discontinue the esomeprazole. A final session with the nurse includes instructions to take ranitidine or an antacid as needed if the heartburn or cough returns. The nurse also explains that some people require ongoing maintenance therapy with a PPI to control their symptoms. Mrs. B. is instructed to return to the office if the symptoms do recur.

- How might the nurse have addressed some of Mr. B.'s concerns about his wife's treatment regimen?
- Discuss the complementary roles of the nurse and the dietitian in Mrs. B.'s care.
- How will the interdisciplinary team decide if surgical intervention is warranted in Mrs. B.'s case?

Internet and Other Resources

American College of Gastroenterology (ACG): *http://www.acg. gi.org;* telephone 703-820-7400; fax 703-931-4520; 4900-B South 31st St, Arlington, VA 22206-1656

American Gastroenterological Association (AGA): *http://www. gastro.org;* E-mail *info@gastro.org;* telephone 301-654-2055; Fax 301-654-5920; 4930 Del Ray Avenue, Bethesda, MD 20814

National Digestive Diseases Information Clearinghouse (NDDIC): *http://www.niddh.nih.gov/;* E-mail *nddic@info. niddk.nih.gov;* telephone 800-891-5389 or 301-654-3810; Fax 301-907-8906; 2 Information Way, Bethesda, MD 20892-3570

REFERENCES

Agency for Healthcare Research and Quality: Mind-body interventions for gastrointestinal conditions, Evidence Report/Technology Assessment No. 40, AHRQ Pub No. 01-E027, 2001, retrieved from *http://www.ahrq. gov/clinic/epcsums/mindsum.htm* on Nov 17, 2002.

American College of Gastroenterology: GI focus: the many faces of gastroesophageal reflux disease, 2002, retrieved from *www.acg.gi.org/ physicianforum/gifocus/gif_gerd.html* on Nov 13, 2002.

Chak A et al: Familial aggregation of Barrett's oesophagus, oesophageal adenocarcinoma, and oesophagogastric junctional adenocarcinoma in Caucasian adults, *Gut* 51(3):323-8, 2002.

Centers for Disease Control and Prevention: Economics of peptic ulcer disease and *H pylori* infection, 1998, retrieved from *http://www.cdc.gov/ulcer/economic.htm* on Nov 10, 2002.

Cutler AF: Eradicating *Helicobacter pylori* infection, *Patient Care* 35(7):91-100, 2001.

Del Valle J et al: Acid peptic disorders. In Yamada T, editor: *Textbook of gastroenterology,* ed 3, Philadelphia, 1999, Lippincott Williams & Wilkins.

DeVault KR, Castrell DO, the Practice Parameters Committee of the American College of Gastroenterology: Updated guidelines for the diagnosis and treatment of gastroesophageal reflux disease, *Am J Gastroenterol* 94(6):1434-42, 1999.

Enteric Medical Technologies: Enteryx procedure for the treatment of gastroesophageal reflux disease (GERD), patient information brochure, Foster City, Calif, 2003, Enteric Medical Technologies, retrieved from *http://www.fda.gov/ohrms/dockets/ac/03/briefing/3921b1_M3%20 patient% 20 booklet-FINAL 2.doc* on May 29, 2003.

Fennerty MB: Acid peptic disease, *Postgrad Med* 110(3):41, 2001a.

Fennerty MB: NSAID-related gastrointestinal injury, *Postgrad Med* 110(3):87-94, 2001b.

Fisher RS: Treatment of gastroesophageal reflux disease. In Wolfe M, editor: *Therapy of digestive disorder,* Philadelphia, 2000, WB Saunders.

Jackson Gastroenterology: Esophageal manometry, 2002, retrieved from *http://www.gicare.com/pated/epdgs31.htm* on May 29, 2003.

Kang JY, Ho KY: Different prevalences of reflux oesophagitis and hiatus hernia among dyspeptic patients in England and Singapore, *Eur J Gastroenterol Hepatol* 11:845-50, 1999.

Kaynard A, Flora K: Gastroesophageal reflux disease: control of symptoms, prevention of complications, *Postgrad Med* 110(3):42-53, 2001.

Khoury RM et al: Influence of spontaneous sleep positions on nighttime recumbent reflux in patients with gastroesophageal reflux disease, *Am J Gastroenterol* 94:2069-73, 1999.

Knigge KL: The role of H. pylori in gastrointestinal disease: a guide to identification and eradication, *Postgrad Med* 110(3):71-82, 2001.

Mullick T, Richter JE: Chronic GERD: strategies to relieve symptoms and manage complications, *Geriatrics* 55(11):28-44, 2000.

Murphy-Blake E: Management of clients with ingestive disorders. In Black J, Hawks J, Keene A, editors: *Medical-surgical nursing,* ed 6, Philadelphia, 2001, WB Saunders, pp 683-727.

Orlando RC: Reflux esophagitis. In Yamada T, editor: *Textbook of gastroenterology,* ed 3, Philadelphia, 1999, Lippincott Williams and Wilkins.

Sung JJ: Acupuncture for gastrointestinal disorders: myth or magic, *Gut* 51(5):617-9, 2002.

US Food and Drug Administration: FDA approves an implant for gastroesophageal reflux disease, 2003, retrieved from *http://www.fda.gov/bbs/topics/ANSWERS/2003/ANS01216.html* on May 29, 2003.

Wolfe MM: Therapy and prevention of NSAID-related gastrointestinal disorders. In Wolfe MM, editor: *Therapy of digestive disorders,* Philadelphia, 2000, WB Saunders, pp 96-112.

CHAPTER **16**

Disorders of the Intestines and Rectum

Loretta Normile, PhD, RN

OBJECTIVES

After reading this chapter, you should be able to do the following:

■ Summarize the prevention, screening, and detection methods used in inflammatory bowel disease, including Crohn's disease and ulcerative colitis, and in diverticular disease, irritable bowel syndrome, and malabsorption.

■ Explain the pathophysiology of inflammatory bowel disease, including Crohn's disease and ulcerative colitis, and of diverticular disease, irritable bowel syndrome, and malabsorption.

■ Describe the functional health patterns affected by inflammatory bowel disease, including Crohn's disease and ulcerative colitis, and by diverticular disease, irritable bowel syndrome, and malabsorption.

■ Explain the role of each member of the interdisciplinary team involved in the care of inflammatory bowel disease, including Crohn's disease and ulcerative colitis, and of diverticular disease, irritable bowel syndrome, and malabsorption.

■ Summarize the therapeutic approaches to the treatment of inflammatory bowel disease, including Crohn's disease and ulcerative colitis, and of diverticular disease, irritable bowel syndrome, and malabsorption.

ASSESSMENT OF THE LOWER GASTROINTESTINAL TRACT

Lower gastrointestinal tract signs and symptoms must be carefully assessed, because their causes range from normal responses to stress to severe life-threatening illness. A thorough medical history should be obtained and functional health patterns should be assessed (Box 16-1).

During the physical examination, the abdomen and lower gastrointestinal tract are evaluated using inspection, auscultation, palpation, and percussion.

DIAGNOSIS

Diagnosis is suggested by the symptoms present (Table 16-2) and is confirmed by stool analysis, radiography, and endoscopic examination (Box 16-2).

INFLAMMATORY BOWEL DISEASE

Inflammatory bowel disease (IBD) is a general term for the chronic bowel disorders characterized by profuse diarrhea and bloody stools. The exact cause of IBD is not known. These disorders are believed to result from a combination of genetic and environmental factors such as infections and irritants that interact with the body's immune system. Two potentially disabling inflammatory bowel conditions are Crohn's disease and ulcerative colitis. These inflammatory disorders affect millions, and costs of care are approximately $1.3 billion per year (Sandler et al, 2002).

Crohn's Disease

Crohn's disease, also referred to as regional enteritis or granulomatous colitis, is one of the most significant forms of inflammatory bowel disease and represents the most important cause of morbidity from inflammatory bowel disease (Krupnick and Morris, 2002). This disorder occurs most often in young adults or adolescents and quickly becomes a disease of long-lasting consequences. This chronic disease may affect employment, social activities, and overall life. Individuals with Crohn's disease are also at a greatly increased risk for intestinal adenosarcoma (McCance and Huether, 2002).

Estimates are that the associated direct costs of care for persons with digestive diseases total approximately $85.5 billion per year (Sandler et al, 2002). Chronic conditions of the lower gastrointestinal tract are associated with many problems, including chronic pain, altered elimination patterns, altered body image, fatigue, weakness, and debilitation. Chronic digestive disorders in the United States are related to a lifestyle of hurried eating, high-fat diets, stress, inactivity, and obesity. There are also demographic variations in the incidence of chronic lower gastrointestinal tract disorders (Table 16-1) This chapter discusses the chronic lower gastrointestinal tract conditions of inflammatory bowel disease, including Crohn's disease and ulcerative colitis, as well as diverticular disease, irritable bowel syndrome, and malabsorption.

Table 16-1 Demographic Differences in Incidence of Chronic Lower Gastrointestinal Tract Disorders

Disorder	Differences
Diverticulitis/diverticulosis	More common in aging and elderly in developed countries where consumption of refined foods is common.
Inflammatory bowel disease, Crohn's disease	Occur more frequently in whites than in African Americans or Asian Americans. Also occur more frequently in relatives of those with the disorders. More commonly seen in females than males and in upper middle class families.
Ulcerative colitis	More common in those with a family history of the disorder and in those of Jewish or Middle Eastern decent.
Irritable bowel syndrome	May show a familial tendency. More likely in those who are young and female.
Malabsorption	Most frequent cause in United States is cystic fibrosis, which is hereditary.

Box 16-1 Functional Health Pattern Assessment for Lower Gastrointestinal Tract Disorders

HEALTH PERCEPTION/HEALTH MANAGEMENT
- Does the patient have a history of smoking?
- What screening studies (e.g., stool occult blood) have been performed?
- Has the patient been exposed to known carcinogens?
- What is the patient's perception of his or her overall health?
- What medications, including over-the-counter drugs, does the patient take?
- What alternative therapies does the patient use?
- Does the patient use alcohol?
- Is there a family history of cancer or predisposing genetic conditions?

NUTRITION/METABOLISM
- What is the patient's current weight? Has there been a recent unexplained loss or gain in weight?
- Is the patient on a special diet?
- What is the condition of the skin and mucous membranes?
- What is the patient's typical dietary intake (daily)?
- Is there nausea and/or vomiting (if present, is it treatment related or anticipatory)?

ELIMINATION
- Have any changes occurred in bowel or bladder habits?
- What are the color, frequency, and caliber of stool? What triggers episodes of diarrhea?
- Is tenesmus present? Is there a history of irritable bowel disease?
- What are the color and character of the urine? Is dysuria or hematuria present?

ACTIVITY/EXERCISE
- Does the patient experience difficulty in walking or fatigue?
- Does the patient experience dyspnea on exertion? What dyspnea management strategies are used?
- What are the patient's regular exercise activities? In what recreational activities does the patient engage?

- Does the patient use mobility aids?
- Is the patient able to perform regular and instrumental activities of daily living?
- Does the patient use supplemental oxygen?

SLEEP/REST
- How many hours of uninterrupted sleep does the patient get at night?
- What sleep aids are used?
- Does the patient take naps or rest periods?

COGNITION/PERCEPTION
- What are the nature, location, and duration of pain? What factors aggravate and alleviate the pain?
- Does the patient experience paresthesias?
- How effective are current pain management strategies?

SELF-PERCEPTION/SELF-CONCEPT
- How does the patient describe himself or herself?
- How has the condition affected the patient's self-esteem?
- How has the condition changed the patient's body image?
- How has the condition affected the patient's sense of self?

ROLES/RELATIONSHIPS
- What kind of work does the patient perform?
- What role does the patient play in the home and family?
- What changes have occurred in the patient's ability to carry out role functions?
- How satisfied is the patient with his or her current roles and relationships?
- How has the condition affected the patient's family or significant others?
- What changes have occurred in family organization and function?

SEXUALITY/REPRODUCTION
- Is the patient sexually active?
- Is the patient satisfied with current sexual patterns?

Continued

Box 16-1   Functional Health Pattern Assessment for Lower Gastrointestinal Tract Disorders—cont'd

■ Has the patient experienced changes in sexual performance? Does the patient have concerns about potential changes in sexual performance or sexuality?

■ Have changes occurred in the menstrual cycle?

COPING/STRESS TOLERANCE

■ What are the patient's coping strategies?

■ What support systems are available to the patient?

■ Can the patient manage the condition in the current setting?

■ What level of hopefulness or despair has the patient exhibited?

■ What does the patient and/or family find helpful?

VALUES/BELIEFS

■ What constitutes good quality of life for the patient?

■ What is important to the patient?

■ What are the patient's spiritual beliefs?

■ What are the patient's health beliefs, including beliefs about the use of medications for pain control?

■ What are the patient's cultural beliefs and beliefs about locus of control? To what degree does the patient participate in cultural traditions and the cultural community?

Pathophysiology

The earliest lesions of Crohn's disease appear as tiny abscesses over nodules of lymphoid tissue. These abscesses lead to lymphedema and thickening of the bowel wall, and create an area with a cobblestone appearance that extends longitudinally and transversely to spread the disease into the lymphoid tissue. It is common for the lesions of Crohn's disease to occur in discontinuous segments of the bowel and in between healthy bowel segments (Swearingen, 2003). The terminal ileum and the colon are the areas most often affected (Beers and Berkow, 1999).

Crohn's disease affects each layer of the bowel: first the submucosa, then the mucosa, and finally the musculature.

Clinical Manifestations

Symptoms vary depending on the segment of intestine involved and the degree of inflammation. Common symptoms are cramps and diarrhea.

Diagnosis

Symptoms of inflammation or obstruction of the bowel in the absence of other gastrointestinal symptoms should trigger suspicion of Crohn's disease. Nonspecific diagnostic findings often include fever, arthritis, and anemia or erythema nodosum. Nonspecific laboratory test results such as leukocytosis, hyperalbuminemia, elevated levels of C-reactive protein, and an elevated erythrocyte sedimentation rate are commonly seen, but radiography is required to make a definitive diagnosis.

Barium enema testing shows a reflux of barium into the terminal ileum, which appears nodulous and stiff. In more

---

Box 16-2   Diagnostic Tests to Evaluate Gastrointestinal Function

■ Plain radiography

■ Air or barium contrast radiography

■ Endoscopy
  Esophagoscopy (esophagus)
  Gastroscopy (stomach)
  Duodenoscopy (small intestine)
  Colonoscopy (large intestine)
  Sigmoidoscopy (sigmoid colon)

■ Ultrasonography

■ Computed tomography

■ Magnetic resonance imaging

■ Stool studies

■ D-Xylose absorption studies

■ Gastric acid stimulation test

■ Manometry (use of water-filled catheters connected to pressure transducers passed into the esophagus, stomach, colon, or rectum to evaluate contractility)

■ Culture and sensitivity testing of duodenal contents

■ Breath tests
  Glucose breath test or D-xylose test
  Urea breath test

Table 16-2   Interpretation of Gastrointestinal Signs and Symptoms

Sign or Symptom	Possible Cause
Acute left lower quadrant pain	Diverticulitis
Abdominal tenderness	
Fever	
Mild nausea, usually without vomiting	
Constipation with onset of pain	
Cramping pain in right lower quadrant	
Nausea, usually without vomiting	Inflammatory bowel disease
Mild, urgent diarrhea	
Palpable mass in right lower quadrant	
Abdominal tenderness	
Flatulence	
Emotional stress	

advanced cases, marked ileal strictures and separation of bowel loops will be present. A small bowel radiographic series reveals the extent of the disease process. In very early cases, air double-contrast barium enema testing may be required for pathophysiologic changes to be seen.

Colonoscopy and biopsy are the confirming diagnostic tools. If Crohn's disease is present in the small bowel, differential diagnosis is required to rule out neoplasms and other inflammatory conditions.

Interdisciplinary Care

Primary Provider (Physician/Nurse Practitioner)

The goal of care in Crohn's disease is to reduce intestinal inflammation. Ultimately, this promotes the healing of tissues and relieves some of the associated symptoms. Drug therapy is the most common method for management of Crohn's disease, although surgery may be required.

The primary care provider orders routine blood tests and stool studies to rule out infection and other lower gastrointestinal tract problems. Some providers treat patients with mild Crohn's disease themselves and refer those with moderate or severe illness to a gastroenterologist.

Surgeon

Surgery may be required but is a treatment of last resort. If surgery does become necessary, there is a high likelihood that the colitis will not be cured. However, surgery can improve quality of life. Ileostomy and creation of an ileoanal anastomosis that preserves part of the anus are two of the surgical procedures that may be performed. In the latter, the surgeon attaches the ileum to the inside of the rectum and the anus, creating a pouch. Pouchitis is a possible complication of this procedure. The type of surgery performed depends on the severity of the disease and the patient's needs and lifestyle.

Drug Therapy

Several types of drugs are helpful in treating Crohn's disease. Abdominal cramps may be relieved by anticholinergics, loperamide, or codeine. Prednisone, often in dosages as high as 40 mg/day or more, is used to control inflammation (Beers and Berkow, 1999). Aminosalicylates or 5-aminosalicyclic acid (5-ASA) is also used to help reduce inflammation. Sulfasalazine (Azulfidine), a locally acting sulfonamide with antibacterial and antiinflammatory action, is used to produce and maintain remission. An immunosuppressant drug such as azathioprine (Imuran) may be prescribed. This drug may allow the dose of prednisone to be reduced to prevent some of the dangerous adverse effects of steroids (Lewis, Heitkemper, and Dirksen, 2000). Medications such as methotrexate (MTX) and infliximab (Remicade) may be given if the patient cannot tolerate other immunosuppressive drugs (Beers and Berkow, 1999). Metronidazole (Flagyl) may be used in patients with disease limited to the colon or confined to the perianal area (Lewis, Heitkemper, and Dirksen, 2000).

Nurse

The nurse monitors the patient with Crohn's disease for dehydration and maintains fluid and electrolyte balance. This begins with accurate recording of intake and output, including the amount of stool passed. Close attention must be paid to the patient's stools for signs of intestinal bleeding through inspection and stool testing for occult blood. Additional monitoring activities to detect bleeding and complications such as fistulas and infection include frequent checks of temperature, weight, hematocrit, hemoglobin level, and white blood count, especially if the patient is taking immunomodulators.

Dietitian

Surgical treatment, medications, and changes in the intestinal mucosa may result in malabsorption of nutrients and vitamins, especially vitamins D, E, K, and B_6 and folate, as well as malabsorption of some minerals such as iron, calcium, and potassium (Reinhard, 2002). Enteral feedings may be prescribed as part of nutritional therapy.

Ulcerative Colitis

Ulcerative colitis is characterized by long-term, intermittent inflammation and ulceration of the rectum and colon. Ulcerative colitis is probably as common in the elderly as in younger individuals and affects about 128 in 100,000 persons in the United States and Europe (Beers and Berkow, 1999). The incidence of this disease is increasing as the life span increases. It is distinguished from Crohn's disease on the basis of the mucosal pathology and the presence of bloody diarrhea.

The cause of this condition is unknown, although the disorder is seen more frequently in European and American Jews. The rate of occurrence is higher than average among white adult women. Risk factors identified in the literature include a family history of the disorder; a history of allergic reactions to food substances, which cause histamine release and an overproduction of enzymes; and the presence of an autoimmune disorder.

Pathophysiology

Ulcerative colitis ranges from a mild condition to a ravaging disease that culminates in perforation of the colon. Fatal peritonitis and toxic conditions are not uncommon in severe forms of the disease. Ulcerative colitis begins with degeneration of the reticulin fibers just under the mucosal epithelium of the rectum and sigmoid colon, and gradually moves upward to include the entire colon. Epithelial necrosis and mucosal ulceration eventually develop. The small intestine, except for the terminal ileum, is usually not affected.

Clinical Manifestations

The most frequently manifested symptoms of ulcerative colitis are abdominal pain or cramping and/or recurrent bloody diarrhea. Patients also may experience fatigue, nausea, anorexia, loss of body fluids and nutrients causing weight loss, and rectal bleeding. Most of the time, the symptoms are mild. Some persons suffer from other problems that initially seem unrelated, such as arthritis, liver disease (hepatitis, cirrhosis, and primary sclerosing cholangitis), osteoporosis, skin rashes, and anemia. It is believed that the immune system in individuals with ulcerative colitis triggers these conditions.

Diagnosis

A thorough history and physical examination are always required to diagnose ulcerative colitis and differentiate it from Crohn's disease or other intestinal conditions. Additional tests that aid in diagnosis include stool and blood analysis, radiography, and endoscopy to visualize the colon.

A colonoscopy or sigmoidoscopy provides direct visualization of inflammation, bleeding, or ulcers on the colon wall. During the examination, a biopsy may be taken. Barium enema testing, although not conclusive, provides a clear view of the colon, including ulcers, lesions, and other abnormalities.

Interdisciplinary Care

Primary Provider (Physician/Nurse Practitioner)

The goal of care in ulcerative colitis is control of intestinal inflammation, prevention of complications, and maintenance of nutrition and fluid volume. Supportive care is essential to ensure the patient's stability for possible surgery or medical recovery.

Surgeon

Most people with ulcerative colitis never require surgery. About 25% to 40% of ulcerative colitis patients undergo surgical intervention for hemorrhage, rupture of the colon, severe illness and debilitation, or risk of cancer. If a colectomy is necessary, the diseased segment of the bowel is removed and the two ends of healthy bowel are joined together. If anastomosis is not possible, the end of the remaining bowel is pulled through an opening in the abdomen to form a stoma.

Drug Therapy

Pharmacotherapy may induce and/or maintain remission. The sulfapyridine found in sulfasalazine poses the risk of uncomfortable side effects such as nausea, vomiting, diarrhea, dyspepsia, and headache. Other 5-ASA agents such as olsalazine (Dipentum), mesalamine (Pentasa), and balsalazide (Colazal), which have fewer side effects, may be used by people who cannot tolerate sulfasalazine.

In persons with moderate to severe ulcerative colitis or those who do not respond to 5-ASA drugs, corticosteroids can be given orally, intravenously, through an enema, or in a suppository, depending on the location of the inflammation. The corticosteroid drugs have great potential to cause side effects; therefore, they are not recommended for long-term therapy. The possible side effects include acne, hypertension, mood swings, weight gain, and an increased risk of infection.

Immunomodulators such as azathioprine (Imuran) and 6-mercaptopurine (Purinethol) reduce inflammation by acting on the immune system. These drugs are slow acting, and up to 3 to 6 months may be required before maximum benefit is seen. Their use is generally reserved for patients who have not responded to 5-ASA agents or to corticosteroids, or who have become dependent on corticosteroids. Individuals taking these immunomodulators must be monitored for complications, including pancreatitis and hepatitis as well as infection, for which they are at an increased risk. Cyclosporine A may also be used with 6-mercaptopurine (Purinethol) or azathioprine (Imuran) to treat active, severe ulcerative colitis in people who do not respond to intravenous corticosteroid therapy.

Analgesics, mild tranquilizers, sedatives, and other drugs such as selective serotonin reuptake inhibitors may be used very judiciously to relax the patient or to relieve pain during exacerbations.

Nurse

The role of the nurse in ulcerative colitis is one of careful monitoring. Accurate recording of intake and output, and monitoring of frequency and volume of stools are essential. Stool should be observed for blood. Careful attention must be paid to electrolyte levels and signs of dehydration such as poor skin turgor, decreased urine output, and rapid, irregular pulse.

The nurse promotes self-care, comfort, and effective nutrition. Strict observation for the effects of immunomodulator therapy is required, with attention to elevations in blood pressure. Edema and gastric irritation may signal an adverse reaction to prolonged therapy. The nurse must also observe for subtle signs of complications such as infection or perforation, because steroid therapy may mask signs of infection and inflammation.

If a stoma was created, the nurse and the wound, ostomy, and continence nurse work together to teach and support the patient and family. Stoma care varies slightly depending on the type of ostomy created (Figure 16-1). Regardless of the type of ostomy, however, the most important aspects of ostomy care are assessment of the stoma, care of the skin, selection of pouch and appliance, and support of the patient as he or she adapts to the change in body image and lifestyle (Box 16-3).

The patient and family and/or caregiver will need assistance and time to adjust to the changes in the appearance of the abdomen and to the odors that emanate from the ostomy site. Patients are frequently self-conscious about odors and fear that those around them can smell feces and can see the bulge of the appliance through the patient's clothing.

Physical closeness with others and sexuality are likely to be affected. In addition, depending on the ability of the patient to adjust to the changes associated with the ostomy,

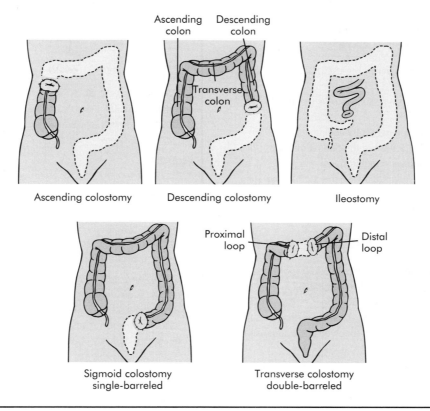

Figure 16-1 Types of ostomies. (From Lewis SM, Heitkemper MM, Dirksen SR: *Medical-surgical nursing: assessment and management of clinical problems,* ed 6, St Louis, 2004, Mosby.)

the patient may decline to leave home or to engage in activities that he or she once found meaningful or pleasurable. Patients and family members and/or caregivers may experience a period of grief as everyone adjusts.

The nurse and the interdisciplinary team allow the patient and family and/or caregivers to discuss fears and concerns in a safe environment (confidential and comfortable). The nurse may consult the medical social worker or a clinical psychologist or refer the patient to these professionals if the patient does not appear to be adjusting to the ostomy.

In addition to providing assistance with coping and with lifestyle changes, the nurse should be aware that the patient may not be taking in adequate or appropriate fluid or food. Excess fluid loss may occur with an ostomy, particularly an ileostomy. Certain foods may contribute to diarrhea, constipation, or flatulence. The nurse assesses the overall health status of the patient and plans and intervenes with the team to prevent and treat these problems. The nurse also teaches the patient and/or caregiver how to avoid fluid and electrolyte imbalance, infection, odor, and diarrhea and constipation. The nurse advises the patient and/or caregiver regarding the appropriate color and size of the stoma and the surrounding skin; the expected volume, color, and consistency of the drainage; the signs and symptoms indicating

possible infection; and the circumstances under which to call the nurse or physician for consultation. Some ostomies require irrigation, and the nurse and/or the wound, ostomy, and continence nurse teach the patient and/or caregiver how to perform this procedure in the inpatient facility and at home (Bliss and Sawchuk, 2000).

Medical Social Worker

In addition to the stress and strain of caregiving, families may experience stress due to the costs associated with this chronic disease. Outlays for equipment, drugs, and medical and other services, and lost wages for days taken off from work are some of the out-of-pocket expenses for families. A medical social worker may be called upon to help the family find financial assistance.

A sex therapist may be included on the team to offer strategies to help the couple to feel comfortable and satisfied with sexual activity. The occupational therapist can offer information about resources for clothes that may be more comfortable and may hide the ostomy better than the patient's usual clothing. Special cummerbunds and bathing suits are available, among other options.

The interdisciplinary team members should link the patient and caregiver with resources that can provide support

From McCloskey JC, Bulechek GM: *Nursing interventions classification (NIC),* St Louis, 2000, Mosby, p 483.

Box 16-3 Nursing Interventions for Ostomy Care

- Instruct the patient and caregiver in the use of ostomy equipment.
- Have the patient and caregiver demonstrate the use of the equipment.
- Assist the patient in obtaining necessary equipment.
- Provide support and assistance while the patient develops skill in caring for the stoma and surrounding tissue.
- Monitor the healing and adaptation of the stoma and surrounding tissue to ostomy equipment.
- Encourage the patient and caregiver to express feelings and concerns about changes in body image.
- Explain to the patient how ostomy care will affect his or her day-to-day routine.
- Teach the patient how to monitor for complications (e.g., mechanical breakdown, chemical breakdown, rash).
- Instruct the patient on methods to reduce odor.
- Teach the patient to chew thoroughly, avoid foods that caused digestive upset in the past, add new foods one at a time, and drink plenty of fluids.
- Discuss the patient's concerns about sexual functioning, as appropriate.
- Encourage participation in ostomy support groups.

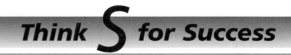

Think S for Success

Symptoms
- Manage periods of symptoms with corticosteroid therapy, immunomodulating drugs, and broad-spectrum antibiotics for infection. Severe episodes may require hospitalization and parental feedings.

Sequelae
- Prevent exacerbations by attention to triggers such as stress and to dietary factors.

Safety
- Teach individual and family about the importance of monitoring condition carefully and being alert for signs and symptoms of bleeding and/or infection. Steroids may mask signs of infection.

Support/Services
- Inflammatory bowel disease usually requires some type of long-term follow-up because exacerbations occur and the potential exists for medical crises. Direct patient to self-help groups such as United Ostomy Association and the Crohn's and Colitis Foundation of America, which can make the difference between adaptation and nonadaptation of patient and family to the many changes and needs.
- Provide resources to help patient and family cope with body changes and lifestyle changes. Those faced with decisions regarding surgery should obtain as much information as possible from doctors, enterostomal therapists, and other colon surgery patients. Patient advocacy organizations can help people locate support groups and other information resources.

Satisfaction
- Determine the degree to which patient's normal lifestyle and functional health patterns and quality of life are disrupted.

and information. The United Ostomy Association is an excellent resource.

Family and Caregiver Issues in Inflammatory Bowel Disease

Because IBD carries the potential for exacerbations and complications, care for the chronically ill person with IBD creates great challenges. The family and/or caregiver of a person with either Crohn's disease or ulcerative colitis may be very anxious and the learning curve may be steep, especially if the person has severe disease and/or undergoes surgery that results in creation of a stoma. The family must be fully educated about management and support of this debilitating disease with its exacerbations and complications. Much support will be necessary to assist the family in coping with the situation and caring for a person with an ostomy. Home health care providers and self-help groups can offer support, guidance, and instruction.

DIVERTICULAR DISEASES

Diverticulosis is a term for the presence of pouchlike formations (diverticula) anywhere in the digestive tract (Figure 16-2). Diverticular diseases are seen most frequently in developed or industrialized countries, particularly in the United States, where low-fiber diets are the norm, and are rarely encountered in Asian countries, where people eat diets rich in high-fiber vegetables.

Although diverticular disease is more likely to occur in persons younger than 40 years of age (Beers and Berkow, 1999), most people over the age of 60 have some diverticula. It is believed that *all* people over age 90 have diverticula. Today in the United States, millions of people are affected by diverticular disease. Because people are living longer and the population is aging, this chronic disease is likely to be seen in large numbers of people in years to come.

Pathophysiology

Diverticulosis begins with the development of small mucosal pouches in the wall of the colon. Although diverticulosis can be found anywhere in the gastrointestinal tract, it is usually

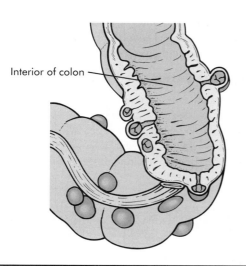

Interior of colon

Figure 16-2 Diverticula are outpouchings of the colon. When they become inflamed, the condition is diverticulitis. The inflammatory process can spread to the surrounding area in the intestine. (From Lewis SM, Heitkemper MM, Dirksen SR: *Medical-surgical nursing: assessment and management of clinical problems,* ed 6, St Louis, 2004, Mosby.)

seen in the sigmoid colon. Constipation leads to muscle straining to push hard stool through the colon. The excess pressure builds and causes weak spots in the colon, especially where arteries penetrate the tunica muscularis to nourish the mucosal layer of the colon (McCance and Heuther, 2002). Colonic pressure increases as the colon thickens and hypertrophies. Subsequently, the lumen of the colon decreases. Affected areas bulge out through the muscular layer of the colon and become diverticula. Diverticulitis occurs when the diverticula become infected or inflamed. The actual cause of the infection is unclear. It may begin when stool or bacteria are caught in the diverticula.

Clinical Manifestations

Most people with diverticulosis are asymptomatic. However, an attack of diverticulitis can develop suddenly when feces or bacertia become trapped in the diverticula causing inflammation and infection. The individual may experience pain, bloating, cramping, fever, nausea, vomiting, constipation, and tenderness in the left lower quadrant. The severity of the syptoms depends on the scope of the infection. A rare but life-threatening complication is blood vessel erosion, which could lead to bleeding and rupture.

Diagnosis

Diverticulosis or diverticulitis of the lower bowel can be either confirmed or ruled out by barium enema testing. Colonoscopic biopsy is contraindicated during acute diverticular disease.

Interdisciplinary Care
Primary Provider (Physician/Nurse Practitioner)

On the initial visit, the primary care provider may suspect diverticulitis if the patient complains of pain in the left lower abdomen and may order laboratory testing for leukocyte count and erythrocyte sedimentation rate. Treatment is based on the presenting symptoms. A lower gastrointestinal tract series or colonoscopy may be ordered to confirm the disease or rule out others.

Drug Therapy

For persons with mild to moderate pain but without any signs of perforation, a stool softener, a broad-spectrum antibiotic, an antispasmodic such as hyoscyamine, and an analgesic such as meperidine (Demerol) may be ordered. Meperidine will relieve discomfort as well as relax smooth muscles. Diverticulitis is typically treated with antibiotics.

Some people become dependent on the use of laxatives; therefore, the frequent use of laxatives should be discouraged. Long-term use of laxatives will result in a sluggish colon, and some stimulant laxatives may cause cramping. Consumption of a high-fiber diet and occasional use of a stool softener or a lubricant agent such as mineral oil can prevent progression of diverticulosis to diverticulitis.

Nurse

The role of the nurse in caring for persons with diverticular disease is mainly one of monitoring, managing pain, observing and educating. The stools of persons with diverticular disease should be monitored for color, consistency, and frequency. Explanation of diagnostic tests to be performed and thorough preparation for these tests is also a nursing role.

Monitoring for vasopressor-induced fluid retention requires more than observation of intake and output. Careful attention to symptoms such as abdominal cramps, oliguria, or anuria, and to other symptoms of shock such as hypotension, weak and rapid pulse, and clammy skin can result in rapid treatment to reverse this serious complication. A list of any instructions should be made and reviewed with the patient and family. If the patient requires a colostomy, colostomy care should be taught and a referral made to an enterostomal therapist. It may be necessary to teach stoma care to the entire family (Box 16-3).

Patients need a thorough explanation of what diverticulosis is and how diverticula form, and should be taught to avoid straining at stool and to prevent constipation by using bulk-forming laxatives and stool softeners.

Dietitian

Contrary to the common belief that individuals with diverticular disease should consume a low-fiber diet, the current teaching to patients is to include foods high in indigestible fiber in the daily diet to prevent the formation of diverticula.

Low-fiber, low-residue diets containing no milk products are ordered for acute flare-ups, followed by a gradual return to a diet high in roughage. Seeds, nuts, and skins of fruits and vegetables may be restricted. The merit of this restriction is still under investigation, but these foods should be avoided by those with severe disease. A liquid diet may be ordered for a short period to rest the colon. Total parenteral nutrition may be required in complicated cases. For many people with diverticulosis, adhering to a high-fiber diet may be the only treatment needed. Table 16-3 lists the fiber content of selected foods.

Counselor

Both patient and family may need help with coping skills, especially if surgical intervention and the creation of an ostomy is required. The change in body image may result in manifestations of depression, withdrawal, anger, and frus-

Table 16-3   Fiber Content of Selected Foods

Food	Amount of Fiber (g)
Fruits	
Apple (1 medium)	4
Peach (1 medium)	2
Pear (1 medium)	4
Tangerine (1 medium)	2
Vegetables	
Acorn squash, fresh, cooked (¾ cup)	7
Asparagus, fresh, cooked (½ cup)	1.5
Broccoli, fresh, cooked (½ cup)	2
Brussels sprouts, fresh, cooked (½ cup)	2
Cabbage, fresh, cooked (½ cup)	2
Carrot, fresh, cooked (1)	1.5
Cauliflower, fresh, cooked (½ cup)	2
Romaine lettuce (1 cup)	1
Spinach, fresh, cooked (½ cup)	2
Tomato, raw (1)	1
Zucchini, fresh, cooked (1 cup)	2.5
Starchy Vegetables	
Black-eyed peas, fresh, cooked (½ cup)	4
Lima beans, fresh, cooked (½ cup)	4.5
Kidney beans, fresh, cooked (½ cup)	6
Potato, fresh, cooked (1)	2
Grains	
Brown rice, cooked (¾ cup)	3.5
Cereal, bran flakes (¾ cup)	5
Oatmeal, plain, cooked (¾ cup)	3
White rice, cooked (1 cup)	1

From United States Department of Agriculture, Agricultural Research Service: Search the USDA national nutrient database for standard reference, retrieved from *http://www.nal.usda.gov/fnic/cgi-bin/nut_search.pl* on Jan 5, 2004.

tration as the patient avoids normal activities due to fear of odors, body changes, and disruption of normal bowel patterns. Counseling interventions include one-on-one counseling as well as participation in self-help groups.

Family and Caregiver Issues

Family members may be required to assist with care and must acquire the necessary knowledge and skill for that care. Assistance may be needed in dealing with child-bearing and ostomy issues. The use of self-help strategies may energize families and help them avoid feelings of frustration.

Think S for Success

Symptoms
■ Manage symptomatic periods by ensuring patient adherence to prescribed diet and medications.

Sequelae
■ Teach patient to prevent exacerbations by avoidance of foods that may cause cramping, such as nuts and seeds. A high-fiber diet and perhaps mild pain medications will help relieve symptoms in many cases. An attack of diverticulitis may be serious enough to require hospitalization and possible surgical intervention.

Safety
■ Teach individual and family about the importance of preventing constipation and straining.

Support/Services
■ Direct patient to resources that can provide support in coping with the disorder. This chronic disorder usually requires some type of long-term follow-up. Presence of a stoma creates alterations in body structure and function and causes drastic changes in lifestyle as a result of living with an ostomy. In addition, sexual dysfunctions may result from psychological or physiologic changes.

Satisfaction
■ Determine the degree to which diverticular disease affects normal day-to-day activities and quality of life.

IRRITABLE BOWEL SYNDROME

Irritable bowel syndrome (IBS), also referred to as spastic colon, spastic colitis, or nervous stomach, is relatively common, affecting approximately 20% of women and 10% of men (Drossman et al, 1997). IBS ranks second as a cause for loss of time on the job. For many years, IBS was considered to be a psychological problem with no physical basis. It is now recognized as a non–life-threatening, chronic condition causing much pain and discomfort and having the potential to significantly affect a person's quality of life.

Pathophysiology

IBS is an alteration of physiologic functioning rather than a change in structure or biochemistry. It appears to involve an interaction between the intestines, the brain, and the autonomic nervous system that results in a change in the regulation of motor and/or sensory function. The layers of muscle lining the walls of the intestine normally contract and relax at a coordinated pace as they move food from the stomach through the intestinal tract to the rectum. It is believed that, in IBS, various triggers cause the bowel to convert to weaker or stronger contractions that last longer than normal. If food passage through the intestines is slowed, stools become hard and dry. If food is forced through the intestines more quickly, the result is gas, bloating, and cramping with alternating periods of constipation and diarrhea. It is not unusual for a patient with IBS to experience several bouts of alternating diarrhea, cramping, bloating, and constipation over a period of days, weeks, or even months.

For reasons that still are not clear, individuals with IBS probably experience this disruption in the normal rhythm of colon contraction and relaxation in response to triggers that do not bother other people. Triggers for IBS can range from gas or pressure in the intestines to foods, medications, or powerful emotions. Alcohol, chocolate, and spices are some common foods that might cause constipation or diarrhea, for example. Any change in the daily routine may aggravate symptoms. A minor stressful episode such as a traffic backup at rush hour or a family disagreement at dinner might bring on colon spasm. Some researchers think IBS may have a hormonal trigger because women are two to three times more likely than men to have IBS. For many women, symptoms are worse during or around their menstrual periods.

Clinical Manifestations

IBS characteristically begins in adolescence or young adulthood. Individuals with IBS experience episodes of abdominal discomfort such as distension, bloating, and diarrhea alternating with normal stools or constipation. Diarrhea may be explosive and may be worse after eating a meal. Defecation is accompanied by straining and lower abdominal cramping. IBS episodes may be continuous, occurring every day of the year, with symptoms that range from mild to extreme or severe enough to disrupt daily activities.

Diagnosis

Diseases such as amebiasis, colon cancer, diverticulitis, and inflammatory bowel diseases may show symptoms similar to those of IBS. Therefore, diagnostic studies should be performed to rule out other more serious gastrointestinal disorders. IBS is a disorder that is not characterized by any inflammatory, infectious, or structural abnormality that can be identified using common examination methods, radiographs, or blood tests. Therefore diagnosis is made by ruling out other lower intestinal disorders.

Interdisciplinary Care
Primary Provider (Physician/Nurse Practitioner)

The goal of treatment for IBS is to relieve the symptoms caused by the disorder. No single treatment or therapy is completely effective for all who have IBS. Pharmacological, psychological, and nutritional interventions are often required.

Drug Therapy

Less than one third of those with IBS report satisfaction with the drugs and remedies used to treat their symptoms (International Foundation for Functional Gastrointestinal Disorders, 2003). Remedies used for IBS include aromatics such as peppermint oil to relieve cramping and anticholinergics given before meals or in conjunction with fiber agents (Beers and Berkow, 1999). Antispasmodics such as Donnatal (a belladonna-barbiturate combination) may be given, and tranquilizers such as alprazolam (Xanax) may be prescribed for short-term use. The chronic use of antidiarrheals and narcotic analgesics should be discouraged because tolerance and dependence may occur.

Nurse

It is essential for the nurse to develop a trusting relationship with the person who experiences IBS. The treatment plan should focus on support, counseling, and the eduction required for necessary lifestyle changes. The nurse must teach the importance of establishing regular bowel elimination patterns, especially during flare-ups. The person with IBS should know when to seek medical attention, for example, when fever, severe abdominal pain, and dehydration are present.

Dietitian

An individual with IBS may become reluctant to eat due to fear that a meal will trigger symptoms. Dietary treatment centers around establishment of regular eating patterns and avoidance of those food that provoke symptoms. One approach is for the patient to eat a bland diet and add only a few food items each day to identify which foods trigger symptoms. Some of the foods that may irritate the digestive tract are beverages containing caffeine, spices, lactose, and raw fruits and vegetables.

Counselor

Common life experiences such as changing jobs, eating out at a restaurant, traveling, and other aspects of social life have the potential to cause great anxiety for the person experiencing IBS. Counseling may be required to reassure the individual that the symptoms, which may be nearly incapacitating, are functional. Individuals may need help to deal with anxiety and stress, and to understand how stress affects their disorder. Some individuals may benefit from behavioral therapy.

Think **S** *for Success*

Symptoms
■ Teach patient to manage periods of diarrhea and constipation with normal diet and avoidance of foods and/or medications likely to cause symptom distress. Careful use of bulk-producing agents may help to alleviate constipation and also diarrhea by absorption of fluids.

Sequelae
■ Teach patient to prevent exacerbations by carefully watching stress, diet, and medications, which may cause recurrence and exacerbation.

Safety
■ Teach individual and family about importance of continual follow-up. Reinforce that there is no organic cause of the condition and that this is not a life-threatening disorder. Ensure that patient knows when to seek medical help.

Support/Services
■ This chronic disorder usually requires some type of long-term follow-up, especially reinforcement and guidance that no pathology is present. Provide information on opportunities to participate in clinical trials. New drugs are currently being tested and show some promise in alleviating the day-to-day struggles of those who live with irritable bowel syndrome.

Satisfaction
■ Determine degree to which irritable bowel syndrome is affecting patient's quality of life. Encourage person to continue with normal lifestyle and reestablishment of normal bowel routine.

Family and Caregiver Issues

IBS symptoms may affect the family because the quality of daily life is seriously altered for the person with IBS. Symptoms such as cramping and explosive diarrhea can interfere with daily comfort and may cause frequent absences at work or school as well as missed opportunities to participate in social activities with friends and/or family. One's professional career may also be hampered because occurrence and duration of symptoms are unpredictable. IBS can be incapacitating, and it is often difficult to ease the cramping and other symptoms, which may continue throughout the day. Symptoms of IBS occur infrequently at night.

MALABSORPTION SYNDROMES

Many diseases and conditions have been associated with malabsorption. Malabsorption syndrome is a chronic state manifested by impaired absorption of nutrients from the small intestine. Often, malabsorption occurs together with maldigestion, a malfunction of the biochemical processes of digestion. This makes diagnosis and treatment difficult.

Malabsorption may be brought on by surgical procedures such as gastric and intestinal resection, lesions, intestinal diseases, and vascular disorders (McCance and Huether, 2002).

Pathophysiology

Malabsorption can be the result of a broad spectrum of diseases and conditions (Box 16-4). Malabsorption can involve either the failure to absorb specific nutrients (including vitamins) or a general nonspecific malabsorption of food. Extended periods of malabsorption can lead to malnutrition and vitamin deficiencies.

Clinical Manifestations

Malabsorption generally manifests as weight loss, bruising and bleeding, flatulence, and abdominal discomfort such as bloating. However, different causes of malabsorption lead to distinct clinical manifestations. Malabsorption caused by lactose intolerance can produce explosive diarrhea and bloating after ingestion of milk. Malabsorption caused by pancreatic lipase deficiency is characterized by pale, soft, greasy stools containing undigested dietary fat (Beers and Berkow, 1999). Protein malabsorption may manifest with edema of the lower limbs.

Diagnosis

Signs and symptoms, especially steatorrhea, are suggestive of malabsorption, but laboratory studies are needed to confirm the diagnosis. The most reliable test for establishing a diagnosis of malabsorption syndrome is evaluation of fecal fat, which is measured for 3 to 4 days. Although steatorrhea is not always seen in malabsorption syndrome, its presence is absolute evidence of it. For an adult consuming the amount of fat typical in the American diet (approximately 50 to 150 g per day), a fecal fat level higher than 17 mEq/day or higher than 6% is considered abnormal. Stool inspections and microscopic examinations may reveal the presence of parasites or ova. Iron malabsorption may be inferred from low iron levels

---

Box 16-4 Causes of Malabsorption

■ Biliary atresia
■ Bovine lactalbumin intolerance (intolerance of cow's milk protein)
■ Celiac disease (gluten-induced enteropathy, sprue)
■ Cystic fibrosis
■ Infection with parasites such as *Giardia lamblia*, *Strongyloides stercoralis* (threadworm), *Necator americanus* (hookworm)
■ Lactose intolerance
■ Shwachman-Diamond syndrome
■ Soy milk protein intolerance
■ Vitamin B_{12} malabsorption
■ Zinc malabsorption

in the absence of chronic blood loss or accompanied by hypoalbuminemia.

Small-bowel endoscopic biopsies are frequently performed so that villi specimens can be examined for specific characteristics of conditions such as Whipple's disease and lymphosarcoma.

Other testing includes the 4C-triolein breath test and the D-xylose test. The D-Xylose test may give false-positive results in patients with chronic liver disease, diabetes mellitus, hyperlipidemia, obesity, thyroid disorders, or lung disease.

Interdisciplinary Care
Primary Provider (Physician/Nurse Practitioner)

Care varies depending on the cause of malabsorption syndrome. For example, antibiotics are used to treat Whipple's disease, whereas a gluten-free diet is prescribed to manage sprue.

Drug Therapy

The aim of pharmacotherapy is to correct deficiencies. Persons with iron deficiency are prescribed supplemental ferrous sulfate or ferrous gluconate tablets. Oral folic acid is administered to patients with folate deficiency, and intramuscular vitamin B_{12} injections are administered every month for a cobalamin deficiency. Patients with marked loss of fat will need supplementation of fat-soluble vitamins and calcium. Bacterial infections are treated with antibiotics.

Dietitian

Dietary management depends greatly on the cause of malabsorption syndrome. A low-residue diet will control diarrhea. A high-protein, low-fat, and high-calorie diet is given to those with severe weight loss. A low-fat diet will curb steatorrhea and bile salt excretion. Parenteral nutrition may be prescribed for persons with severe malnutrition who do not respond to oral feeding. Parenteral nutrition is given as the only source of nutrients for persons who must temporarily avoid enteral feedings. Only in rare situations is the long-term use of parenteral feeding required.

Nurse

The desired outcome in the care of the person with malabsorption syndrome is to keep the individual free of discomfort. Meticulous skin care and fluid replacement through either oral or parental means is required as well as assistance in overcoming activity intolerance during periods of weakness and fatigue.

Family and Caregiver Issues

The family may be responsible for continuing care for the patient with malabsorption. Family members may experience role strain as they attempt to care for the weakened and fatigued patient. The importance of follow-up visits with health professionals and adherence to the dietary aspects of the treatment plan should be reinforced.

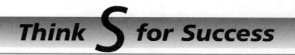

Think S for Success

Symptoms
■ Manage periods of discomfort throughout this chronic syndrome as well as during acute episodes.

Sequelae
■ Teach patient to prevent exacerbations by avoidance of triggers relating to malabsorption syndrome.

Safety
■ Teach individual and family about importance of adhering to medical and dietary regime. Ensure that emergency names and telephone numbers are known and accessible.

Support/Services
■ This chronic disorder usually requires long-term follow-up. Direct patient to organizations such as the National Digestive Diseases Information Clearinghouse *(http://www.niddk.nih. gov/index. htm)* that may have helpful information and the Celiac Disease Foundation, which may be able to provide resources. In addition, joining a support group in which members share common experiences and concerns helps patients and their families. More support resources are listed at the end of this chapter. Provide telephone follow-up and support.

Satisfaction
■ Determine the degree to which malabsorption syndrome affects the activities of daily living and quality of life of the patient and family and/or caregivers.

CASE STUDY
Patient Data

Ms. M. is a 35-year-old single mother of a 4-year-old son. She was born to a poor family in the South. She joined the armed forces at age 18 and is now a sergeant in the U.S. Army. Ms. M.'s 68-year-old mother, who had ulcerative colitis for many years, was recently diagnosed with colon cancer and underwent an abdominal-perineal resection. She currently resides with Ms. M. in military housing. Ms. M. has assumed most of the responsibility for her mother's care as her mother recovers from this surgery.

For several years now, Ms. M. has experienced bloating after meals, occasional periods of loose stools containing blood and mucus, and fleeting abdominal pain. Two years ago, she came to the military clinic with a weight loss of 15 pounds, weakness, and bloody stools. Since then, she has been taking prednisone, Lomotil (diphenoxylate and atropine) and "some sulfa drug." Today she returns to the emergency department. She appears weak and shaky. She reports having 10 to 20 stools a day with much mucus, blood, and abdominal cramping. Her temperature is 101.2° F, pulse rate is 122 beats per minute, and respiration

Continued

CASE STUDY—cont'd

rate is 24 breaths per minute. She says tearfully, "This illness is going to ruin my military career." She is admitted to the military hospital for the fourth time in the past year for an acute episode relating to her chronic ulcerative colitis.

Diagnostic Findings

■ Hematocrit: 25%
■ Hemoglobin level: 8.5 g/dl
■ Potassium level: 3.0 mEq/L
■ Sodium level: 129 mEq/L
■ Chloride level: 98 mEq/L
■ Serum albumin level: 2.4 g/dl (24 g/L)

Thinking It Through

■ How is Ms. M. similar to and/or different from the typical patient with ulcerative colitis?
■ To what medical complications is Ms. M. susceptible a result of her ulcerative colitis and what is the role of the nurse in preventing them?
■ Discuss Ms. M.'s laboratory results. What should you expect them to be after treatment?
■ Comment on the medications Ms. M. takes at home. What else does the nurse need to know? What education is necessary?
■ Based on the assessment data, identify one or more nursing diagnoses. What collaboration with other disciplines will be required?
■ Based on the information given, what is Ms. M.'s prognosis? What health teaching should be given?
■ How can the home health care nurse encourage self-care for Ms. M.'s 68-year-old mother?

Case Conference

The health care team meets with Ms. M. to determine how well she is coping at home and to identify any problems she may have in following her therapeutic plan. Ms. M. is aware that she needs help at home and is making arrangements to have her child attend a play group several times a week so that she can lower her stress level.

The nurse practitioner reviews the importance of hydration and explains the signs and symptoms of fluid and electrolyte imbalance. She also makes sure that Ms. M. knows how to check her stool for occult blood and reminds her to note any evidence of frank bleeding.

The dietitian compares Ms. M.'s diet diary with her record of exacerbations and notices that at this point Ms. M. is eating bland low-fiber foods. The dietitian explains that roughage is still needed in the diet and notes that foods high in residue should be limited, especially during exacerbations, but that some bulk in the diet is necessary for good bowel function.

The medical social worker discusses the resources available to assist Ms. M. in caring for her mother at home. Ms. M. does not want to discuss hospice at this time. They make an appointment for the social worker to visit Ms. M. at home and set up a family meeting to discuss care options.

■ Who else should be part of the case conference?
■ What role does the fact that Ms. M. is in the armed forces play in her illness and recovery?

Internet and Other Resources

Celiac Disease Foundation: *http://www.celiac.org*
Celiac Sprue Association/United States of America: *http://www.csaceliacs.org*
Crohn's and Colitis Foundation of America: *http://www.ccfa.org*
Gluten Intolerance Group: *http://www.gluten.net*
International Foundation for Functional Gastrointestinal Disorders (IFFGD): *http://www.iffgd.org;* E-mail *iffgd@iffgd.org*
MEDLINEplus Health Information: *http://www.nlm.nih.gov/medlineplus/encyclopedia.html*
National Institute of Diabetes and Digestive and Kidney Diseases: *http://www.niddk.nih.gov/*
Pediatric Crohn's and Colitis Association: *http://pcca.hypermart.net*
Reach Out for Youth with Ileitis and Colitis: *http://www.reachoutforyouth.org*
United Ostomy Association: *http://www.uoa.org*

REFERENCES

Beers MH, Berkow R: *The Merck manual of diagnosis and therapy*, ed 17, Whitehouse Station, NJ, 1999, Merck and Co.

Bliss DZ, Sawchuk L: Lower gastrointestinal problems. In Lewis SM, Heitkemper MM, Dirksen SR, editors: *Medical-surgical nursing,* ed 5, St Louis, 2000, Mosby, pp 1136-90.

Drossman DA et al: Irritable bowel syndrome: a technical review, *Gastroenterology* 112:2120-37, 1997.

International Foundation for Functional Gastrointestinal Disorders: Gastrointestinal functional and motility disorders, Nov 22, 2003, retrieved from *http://www.iffgd.org* on Jan 5, 2004.

Krupnick AS, Morris JB: The long-term results of resections and multiple resections in Crohn's disease, *Semin Gastrointest Dis* 11(1):41-51, 2000.

Lewis SM, Heitkemper MM, Dirksen SR, editors: *Medical-surgical nursing,* ed 5, St Louis, 2000, Mosby.

McCance KL, Heuther SE, editors: *Pathophysiology: the biologic basis for disease in adults and children,* ed 4, St Louis, 2002, Mosby.

Reinhard T: *Gastrointestinal disorders and nutrition,* Chicago, 2002, Contemporary Books.

Sandler RS et al: The burden of selected digestive diseases in the United States, *Gastroenterology* 122(5):1500-11, 2002.

Swearingen PL: *Manual of medical surgical nursing care: nursing interventions and collaborative management,* ed 5, St Louis, 2003, Mosby.

CHAPTER 17

Disorders of the Liver, Pancreas, and Gallbladder

Karen Rea, MSN, RN, BC

OBJECTIVES

After reading this chapter, you should be able to do the following:

- Describe the pathophysiology of chronic hepatitis C and cirrhosis, chronic cholelithiasis, and chronic pancreatitis
- Describe the clinical manifestations of chronic hepatitis C and cirrhosis, chronic cholelithiasis, and chronic pancreatitis
- Describe the functional health patterns affected by chronic hepatitis C and cirrhosis, chronic cholelithiasis, and chronic pancreatitis
- Describe the role of each member of the interdisciplinary care team involved in the care of persons with chronic hepatitis C, cirrhosis, chronic cholelithiasis, and chronic pancreatitis.
- Compare and contrast the progression and management of chronic hepatitis C and cirrhosis, chronic cholelithiasis, and chronic pancreatitis
- Describe the indications for use, side effects, and nursing considerations related to drugs commonly used to treat chronic hepatitis C and cirrhosis, chronic cholelithiasis, and chronic pancreatitis

Chronic diseases of the liver, gallbladder, and pancreas not only burden the health care system but also cause significant distress to those affected. Chronic hepatitis C is a major global health problem, with over 170 million cases in the world and over 4 million in the United States (LaBrecque et al, 2002). Although transmission has decreased due to the ability to screen blood for the causative virus, the sequelae of long-term infection will lead to a huge rise in the number of very ill persons within the next 10 years. Estimates predict a 61% increase in cirrhosis, a 68% increase in the need for liver transplants, and a 223% increase in deaths from liver-related disorders (LaBrecque et al, 2002). The affected individuals are those who are currently in their thirties and forties and who would be expected to be at the peaks of their careers when serious disease manifestations occur. Chronic

pancreatitis, although it does not affect as many individuals, is also most prevalent among those in their most productive adult years and thus places severe strain on these individuals and their families. The issue of alcohol abuse arises when cirrhosis and chronic pancreatitis develop, which complicates treatment success and affects family dynamics.

ASSESSMENT

Assessment varies somewhat according to the chronic disorder under consideration. However, it begins with a thorough history taking. Of particular importance are the presence of risk factors, a history of alcohol and/or drug use, and the pattern of specific symptoms. Table 17-1 present two commonly used tools to assess for alcohol usage, the CAGE (Cut Down, Annoyed, Guilty, Eye-opener) and AUDIT (Alcohol Use Disorders Identification Test) questionnaires (Desarathy and McCullough, 2003). Also important is information on the past occurrence and pattern of pain and discomfort; gastrointestinal upsets such as anorexia, nausea, and steatorrhea; and generalized feelings of malaise and fatigue. Physical examination focuses on abdominal assessment and general signs of malnutrition. The specialized diagnostic tests for chronic liver, gallbladder, and pancreatic disorders are discussed in the sections treating these specific diseases. Box 17-1 provides a framework for assessment encompassing common functional health patterns. Ethnic variations in the incidence of these disorders are outlined in Table 17-2.

CHRONIC DISORDERS OF THE LIVER

The two major chronic disorders of the liver are chronic hepatitis C and cirrhosis. Hepatitis is liver inflammation resulting from any of a variety of causes, including drugs, infection, and exposure to toxic chemicals. Cirrhosis is chronic degeneration of the liver, in which there is diffuse destruction and regeneration of the hepatic parenchymal cells. This chapter focuses on chronic hepatitis and cirrhosis caused by infection with the hepatitis C virus (HCV). After a discussion of the pathology and clinical recognition of each disorder, treatment and the roles of the

Table 17-1 Tools for Assessment of Alcohol Use

CAGE (Cut Down, Annoyed, Guilty, Eye-opener)	AUDIT (Alcohol Use Disorders Identification Test) Questionnaire
Assessment Questions	
1. Have you ever felt you should cut down on your drinking?	1. How often do you have a drink containing alcohol?
2. Have people annoyed you by criticizing your drinking?	2. How many drinks containing alcohol do you have on a typical day when you are drinking?
3. Have you ever felt bad or guilty about drinking?	3. How often do you have six or more drinks on one occasion?
4. Have you ever taken a drink the first thing in the morning (an eye-opener) to steady your nerves or get rid of a hangover?	4. How often during the last year have you found that you were not able to stop drinking once you had started?
	5. How often during the last year have you failed to do what was normally expected of you because of drinking?
	6. How often during the last year have you needed a first drink in the morning to get yourself going after a heavy drinking session?
	7. How often during the last year have you had a feeling of guilt or remorse after drinking?
	8. How often during the last year have you been unable to remember what happened the night before because you had been drinking?
	9. Have you or someone else been injured as a result of your drinking?
	10. Has a relative, friend, doctor, or other health worker been concerned about your drinking or suggested that you should cut down?
Interpretation	
There is a high likelihood of alcohol abuse if 2 or more of the questions are answered positively.	Score of 8 or more is indicative of alcohol abuse *Items 1-8 scoring*: 0 = never; 1 = monthly or less; 2 = 2-4 times/month; 3 = 2-3 times/week; 4 = 4 or more times/week *Items 9-10 scoring:* 0 = no; 2 = yes, but not in the last year; 4 = yes, during the last year

Adapted from Dasarathy S, McCullough A: Alcoholic liver disease. In Schiff E, Sorrell M, Maddrey W, editors: *Diseases of the liver,* ed 9, Philadelphia, 2003, Lippincott Williams and Wilkins.

interdisciplinary team member are described for both conditions together.

Chronic Viral Hepatitis
Pathophysiology

Viral hepatitis results from infection with one of several types of hepatitis virus. Hepatitis A and E are transmitted via the oral-fecal route. Hepatitis B, C, D, and G are transmitted by blood and bodily secretions. Hepatitis C is the most common cause of chronic viral hepatitis. HCV is a member of the Flaviviridae family of RNA viruses. It is able to mutate rapidly, which allows it to evade the defenses of the immune system. At least six genotypes of HCV exist. Genotypes 1a and 1b are the most common in the United States. Genotypes 2 and 3 are seen in approximately 20% of patients but have the best response to interferon treatment (National Institute of Diabetes and Digestive and Kidney Diseases [NIDDK], 2002). All genotypes are associated with about the same disease severity.

Of the various types of hepatitis, hepatitis C is the most serious and has the most devastating effects. It is the cause of most of the chronic liver disease today, affecting approximately 1.8% of the population in the United States, or 4 million people (Box 17-2). Three times as many individuals are infected with HCV than are infected with human immunodeficiency virus (Fathman, 2002). Hepatitis C is transmitted primarily by contact with blood and blood products. Prior to 1992, the main cause of transmission was transfusion of contaminated blood. Today, 60% of new cases occur in intravenous drug abusers (Reddy, 2002). Infection occurs early in drug abuse, and up to 80% of those infected develop chronic hepatitis C (Des Jarlais and Schuchat, 2001). Box 17-3 lists risk factors for contracting the disease. Figure 17-1 shows the epidemiologic trends associated with several risk factors. Chronic disease is more prevalent in African Americans, men, and those in their thirties and forties. Those with chronic disease who consume even moderate amounts of alcohol appear to be at increased risk of more rapid progression of liver disease and development of liver cancer (Centers for Disease Control and Prevention [CDC], 1998). Transmission via sexual activity is uncommon. When it does occur, it is seen more commonly in those with a his-

tory of multiple sexual partners (Hoofnagle and Heller, 2003).

The long-term consequences of hepatitis C are devastating. Approximately 15% to 25% of those with acute HCV infection recover without any long-term problems (CDC, 1998). The remainder develop chronic hepatitis, which may not cause any symptoms for years. Once it has developed, chronic hepatitis C rarely resolves spontaneously (Hoofnagle and Heller, 2003). Over 10 to 20 years, 20% of those with chronic disease progress to cirrhosis. The most common reason for liver transplantation in the United States is liver failure due to chronic hepatitis C. Superinfection

---

Box 17-1 Functional Health Pattern Assessment for Disorders of the Liver, Pancreas, and Gallbladder

HEALTH PERCEPTION/HEALTH MANAGEMENT
■ Is there a family history of liver, gallbladder, and/or pancreatic problems?
■ What is the patient's perception of the problem, including its severity and significance?
■ What over-the-counter medications does the patient take?
■ Does the patient use recreational drugs, especially intravenous drugs?
■ Does the patient use alcohol?
■ Is there a history of blood and/or blood product transfusion?

NUTRITION/METABOLISM
■ What is the patient's current height and weight? Have there been any recent unexplained changes in weight?
■ What are the patient's dietary habits and food tolerances? Is consumption of specific foods associated with pain or discomfort?
■ Is there anorexia, nausea, or vomiting?
■ Is hepatomegaly or splenomegaly present?

ELIMINATION
■ Does the patient experience diarrhea, abdominal cramping, or bloating?
■ Is the urine dark?

ACTIVITY/EXERCISE
■ Can the patient carry out normal activities without discomfort or undue fatigue?

SLEEP/REST
■ What are the patient's usual sleep and napping patterns?
■ How does the pain or discomfort affect sleeping?
■ Does the patient experience feelings of exhaustion, fatigue, and activity intolerance?

COGNITION/PERCEPTION
■ What are the location, duration, and characteristics of the pain, especially abdominal discomfort?
■ What makes the pain better or worse: positioning, medications, nonpharmacologic therapies?
■ Is there any evidence of neuropsychiatric changes, such as irritability, agitation, or mental status changes, especially if interferon is being used for treatment?

SELF-PERCEPTION/SELF-CONCEPT
■ What is the patient's response to having a chronic disorder that requires ongoing treatment?

■ How does the patient feel about the uncertainty in the success of treatment for chronic hepatitis C?
■ What are the patient's feeling about the long-term prognosis?
■ Does the patient feel guilty about events which occurred 10 to 20 years earlier that contributed to hepatitis C infection?
■ How has the disorder affected the patient's general self-image and feelings of worthiness?
■ What are the patient's feelings about past or present drug or alcohol abuse?
■ Does the patient show any signs of depression and suicidal ideation, especially if the patient is taking interferon?

ROLES/RELATIONSHIPS
■ How has the disorder affected family members and family dynamics?
■ What changes have occurred in the patient's role in the family?
■ What are family members' perceptions of the disorder?
■ Is the patient able to fulfill normal roles (in the family, workplace, religious group, etc.)?

SEXUALITY/REPRODUCTION
■ Does the patient have a history of multiple sexual partners?
■ How has the disorder affected sexual activity?
■ Does the patient with chronic hepatitis C use safe sex practices?
■ Is the patient using birth control, especially with ribavirin therapy?

COPING/STRESS TOLERANCE
■ Can the patient manage the condition in the current setting?
■ What support systems are available to the patient?
■ What are the patient's coping strategies?
■ Does the patient have financial concerns?

VALUES/BELIEFS
■ What are the patient's health beliefs regarding the chronic disease?
■ What are the patient's cultural beliefs about having the chronic disorder and its treatment?
■ What is the patient's attitude about locus of control (internal or external)?
■ What constitutes good quality of life for the patient?
■ What is important to the patient?
■ To what extent do the patient's cultural/spiritual beliefs influence decision making related to this condition?

Table 17-2 Demographic Differences in the Incidence of Chronic Liver, Gallbladder, and Pancreatic Disorders

Chronic Disorder	Demographic Differences
Hepatitis C	More prevalent in men in their thirties and forties, African Americans, and Mexican Americans.
Cirrhosis	Men more likely to have progressive disease. Slightly more common in white males than in females or African Americans.
Cholelithiasis	Women affected more than men. Highest incidence in Pima Indians of North America. Hispanics and those of Northern European descent have higher incidence than those of Asian or African American descent.
Pancreatitis	More prevalent in men in their thirties and forties. More common in cultures with high alcohol intake; no other cultural differences noted.

Adapted from Heitkemper M et al: Chronic hepatitis C: implications for health-related quality of life, *Gastroenterol Nurs* 24(4):169-75, 2001 (electronic version); Lee SF, Ko CW: Gallstones. In Yamada T, editor: *Textbook of gastroenterology*, ed 3, Philadelphia, 2000, Lippincott Williams and Wilkins; National Institute of Diabetes and Digestive and Kidney Diseases: Pancreatitis, NIH Pub No. 02-1596, Bethesda, Md, 2001, National Institutes of Health, retrieved from http://www.niddk.nih.gov/health/digest/pubs/pancreas/pancreas.htm on Nov 26, 2002; and Reddy KR: Public-health impact, natural history, diagnosis, and clinical management of hepatitis C: emerging clinical options with interferon-based therapies, retrieved from http://www.medscape.com/viewprogram/1809 on Nov 20, 2002.

Clinical Manifestations

Most of those with acute hepatitis C have no symptoms. If symptoms are present, they are very mild, and onset is less pronounced than with hepatitis A or B. Fatigue, mild upper right quadrant discomfort or tenderness, nausea and anorexia, muscle and joint pains, and mild flulike symptoms may be experienced 2 to 6 weeks after infection (NIDDK, 2002). Jaundice may occur in 20% to 30% of those infected, along with dark urine and clay-colored stools. Hepatomegaly and rarely splenomegaly may occur. Those who do experience symptoms with acute HCV are less likely to develop chronic infection (Reddy, 2002). With the development of cirrhosis from chronic hepatitis C, the individual experiences more severe symptoms. Extrahepatic manifesta-

with hepatitis A or B increases the risk of liver failure (Riley and Bhatti, 2001). After an additional 20 to 40 years, a small percentage of individuals develop liver cancer. Those who are heavy alcohol users, over age 40 at infection, and male are at increased risk for liver cancer. Approximately half the cases of primary liver cancer in the world are due to hepatitis C (NIDDK, 2002).

Box 17-2 Epidemiology of Hepatitis C

- Hepatitis C causes 50% to 60% of newly diagnosed cases of chronic liver disease.
- Seventy-five percent of those infected with hepatitis C virus develop chronic disease.
- Twenty percent of those with chronic hepatitis C develop cirrhosis within 20 years and liver cancer within 20 to 40 years.
- Only about 25% to 30% of those with chronic hepatitis C have been diagnosed.
- Worldwide, 170 million people, or 3% of the world's population, have hepatitis C.

Adapted from Hoofnagle J, Heller T: Hepatitis C. In Zakim D, Boyer T, editors: *Hepatology: a textbook of liver disease*, ed 4, Philadelphia, 2003, WB Saunders; Huber D: Does the "C" in hepatitis C stand for complex? *Gastroenterol Nurs* 24(3):120-6, 2001 (electronic version); National Institute of Diabetes and Digestive and Kidney Diseases: Chronic hepatitis C: current disease management, NIH Pub No. 02-4230, Bethesda, Md, 2002, National Institutes of Health, retrieved from http://www.niddk.nih.gov/health/digest/pubs/chrhepc/chrhepc.htm on Aug 27, 2002; and Reddy KR: Public-health impact, natural history, diagnosis, and clinical management of hepatitis C: emerging clinical options with interferon-based therapies, retrieved from http://www.medscape.com/viewprogram/1809 on Nov 20, 2002.

Box 17-3 Risk Factors for Hepatitis C

- Blood transfusion prior to 1992, when testing became available.
- Frequent exposure to blood products, as occurs in hemophilia, organ transplantation, chronic renal failure, cancer chemotherapy.
- Intravenous drug use (accounts for 60% of new cases today).
- High-risk sexual behavior (accounts for 20% of new cases).
- Intranasal cocaine use, especially with shared equipment.
- Health care occupation (transmission from needle-stick injuries).
- Infection of mother during pregnancy (5% of infants born to infected mothers contract the disease).
- In approximately 10% of cases, no cause or source is known.

From National Institute of Diabetes and Digestive and Kidney Diseases: Chronic hepatitis C: current disease management, NIH Pub No. 02-4230, Bethesda, Md, 2002, National Institutes of Health, retrieved from http://www.niddk.nih.gov/health/digest/pubs/chrhepc/chrhepc.htm on Aug 27, 2002.

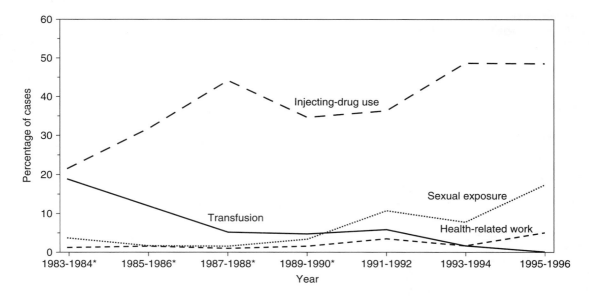

Figure 17-1 Reported cases of acute hepatitis C by selected risk factors. *Data presented for non-A, non-B hepatitis. (From Centers for Disease Control and Prevention: Recommendations for prevention and control of hepatitis C virus [HCV] infection and HCV-related chronic disease, *MMWR Morb Mortal Wkly Rep* 47[RR-19]:1-39, 1998 [electronic version], retrieved from *http://www.cdc.gov/mmwr/preview/mmwrhtml/00055154.htm* on Nov 24, 2002.)

tions may include cryoglobulinemia (Box 17-4), glomerulonephritis, porphyria cutanea tarda, nonspecific arthritis, and Sjögren's syndrome (Hoofnagle and Heller, 2003; NIDDK, 2002).

Diagnosis

In many cases the initial diagnosis of chronic hepatitis C is made during routine blood testing, and the diagnosis comes as a complete surprise to the individual being tested. Abnormal liver function test results, especially elevated serum levels of alanine aminotransferase, are generally the first indication of disease (NIDDK, 2002). The tests used to confirm the diagnosis are outlined in Table 17-3. A liver

---

Box 17-4 Manifestations of Cryoglobulinemia in Chronic Hepatitis C

■ Skin rashes: purpura, vasculitis, urticaria
■ Joint and muscle aches
■ Kidney disease
■ Neuropathy
■ Cryoglobulins, rheumatoid factor, and low complement levels in serum

From National Institute of Diabetes and Digestive and Kidney Diseases: Chronic hepatitis C: current disease management, NIH Pub No. 02-4230, Bethesda, Md, 2002, National Institutes of Health, retrieved from *http://www.niddk.nih.gov/health/digest/pubs/chrnhepc/chrnhepc.htm* on Aug 27, 2002.

---

biopsy is the most important tool for evaluating the degree of fibrosis present with hepatitis C. Those with severe fibrosis progress more rapidly to cirrhosis and end-stage liver disease (LaBrecque et al, 2002).

Cirrhosis and End-Stage Liver Disease

Over a 20-year period, chronic hepatitis C progresses to the development of cirrhosis in 20% of cases. Cirrhosis is a chronic degenerative process characterized by diffuse damage to and regeneration of hepatic parenchymal cells. Over a long period, this process of regeneration alters the normal vasculature and leads to impaired blood flow through the liver. The result is end-stage liver disease and eventual death from liver failure. Cirrhosis is the twelfth leading cause of death in the United States overall and was responsible for 26,000 deaths in 1999. It rises to become the fourth most common cause of death among both men and women in the sixth decade of life and is slightly more common in white males than in females or African Americans (CDC, 2001). Hepatitis C and alcohol abuse are the most common causes of cirrhosis in the United States (Table 17-4).

Pathophysiology

Damage from cirrhosis generally occurs over an extended period of time. Fibrosis and the formation of scar tissue gradually interfere with the normal functioning of the liver. Once significant liver damage occurs, multisystem problems begin to appear. Liver damage affects immune function, coagulation, bile metabolism, and the metabolism of proteins, fats,

Table 17-3   Diagnostic Tests for Chronic Hepatitis C

Test	Comments
Serum alanine aminotransferase level	May be elevated or normal. Not a good indicator of disease progression because levels fluctuate over time.
EIA for anti-HCV	95% sensitivity in high-risk populations. False positives common in low-risk populations.
Western blot: recombinant immunoblot assay	Used to confirm positive EIA result. If results are negative but EIA result was positive, the EIA result was most likely a false positive.
Polymerase chain reaction	Determines HCV viral RNA load. Viral RNA load does not correspond to disease severity. Indicates likelihood of positive response to therapy. Those with viral loads 1 million IU/ml are more likely to show positive response to therapy.
HCV genotype	Used to guide choice of treatments. Genotypes 2 and 3 respond more favorably to 24-week course of treatment. Genotype 1 requires a 48-week course of therapy.
Liver biopsy	Degree of fibrosis predicts the rate of HCV disease progression.

Adapted from National Institute of Diabetes and Digestive and Kidney Diseases: Chronic hepatitis C: current disease management, NIH Pub No. 02-4230, Bethesda, Md, 2002, National Institutes of Health, retrieved from *http://www.niddk.nih.gov/health/digest/pubs/chrnhepc/chrnhepc.htm* on Aug 27, 2002; and LaBrecque et al: Controversies in hepatitis C therapy, retrieved from *http://www.medscape.com/viewprogram/2053_pnt* on Nov 21, 2002.
EIA, Enzyme immunoassay; *HCV,* Hepatitis C virus.

and carbohydrates. Portal hypertension develops as a result of the fibrotic changes, and abdominal ascites, esophageal and gastric varices, and hepatorenal syndrome develop as blood backs up into the gastrointestinal and renal circulation. The inability to break down urea leads to hepatic encephalopathy from elevated serum ammonium levels (NIDDK, 2002). Metabolism of medications is also affected, with the potential for blood levels to increase beyond the therapeutic range. In most cases the long-term prognosis for those with cirrhosis is poor.

Clinical Manifestations

Cirrhosis has no symptoms in its early stages. The liver itself may be either enlarged or small and hard. As liver function fails, symptoms begin to appear. Early signs include anorexia, nausea, feelings of bloating, changes in bowel

Table 17-4   Causes of Cirrhosis and End-Stage Liver Disease

Cause	Comments
Viral hepatitis	Hepatitis C is the primary type of hepatitis leading to cirrhosis in the United States. Hepatitis B and D are more common causes worldwide. Chronic inflammation over many years creates fibrosis and scar tissue.
Alcohol abuse	Cirrhosis develops after many years of heavy drinking. Injury is due to blocking of normal metabolism of protein, fats, and carbohydrates.
Primary biliary cirrhosis	Of uncertain etiology; affects primarily women in middle age. Appears to be related to a problem with immunoregulation.
Autoimmune hepatitis	Caused by immune system dysfunction.
Nonalcoholic steatohepatitis	Caused by buildup of fat in the liver. Appears to be related to diabetes, protein malnutrition, obesity, coronary artery disease, and steroid treatment.
Biliary atresia	Seen in infants; damage results from blocked bile ducts.
Cystogenic cirrhosis	Etiology not known; up to 10% of cirrhosis falls into this category.
Wilson's disease	Copper builds up in liver tissue, causing tissue damage; hereditary disorder.
Other inherited diseases	Interfere in some way with liver function. Examples: α_1-antitrypsin deficiency, hemochromatosis, galactosemia, glycogen-storage disease.

Adapted from American Gastroenterological Association: Cirrhosis of the liver, retrieved from *http://www.gastro.org/clinicalRes/brochures/cirrhosis.html* on Nov 23, 2002; and National Institute of Diabetes and Digestive and Kidney Diseases: Cirrhosis of the liver, NIH Pub No. 04-1134, Bethesda, Md, 2004, National Institutes of Health, retrieved from *http://digestive.niddk.nih.gov/ddiseases/pubs/cirrhosis/* on Nov 23, 2002.

habits, and weight loss (NIDDK, 2000). Extreme fatigue is a major problem. There is generally tenderness over the upper right quadrant. As the disease progresses, multisystem manifestations begin to appear. These are identified in Figure 17-2.

Diagnosis

Cirrhosis is diagnosed by medical history taking to identify risk factors, by physical examination, and by liver function tests. Box 17-5 lists the laboratory tests commonly used to diagnose and monitor for liver damage. Liver computed tomography, ultrasonography, or magnetic resonance imaging may be performed to assess for liver size and density. Liver biopsy is the definitive means of determining the type and extent of liver damage. Esophagoscopy may be performed to visualize esophageal varices, and percutaneous transhepatic portography may be used to visualize the portal

venous system (American Gastroenterological Association, 2002).

Interdisciplinary Care

Chronic hepatitis C and cirrhosis exist along a continuum that ranges from disease with no outward manifestations to a severely compromised liver. The treatment goals are to minimize disease progression and development of complications, and to improve quality of life.

With chronic hepatitis C, an additional goal is to eliminate the disease. Up to 50% of those with HCV genotype 1 and 80% of those with genotypes 2 and 3 can be cured if appropriate treatment is given (LaBrecque et al, 2002). This means the disease will not progress to cirrhosis and liver cancer, and the individuals will no longer be a source of potential infection of others. Even in those who cannot be cured, disease progression may be slowed if appropriate

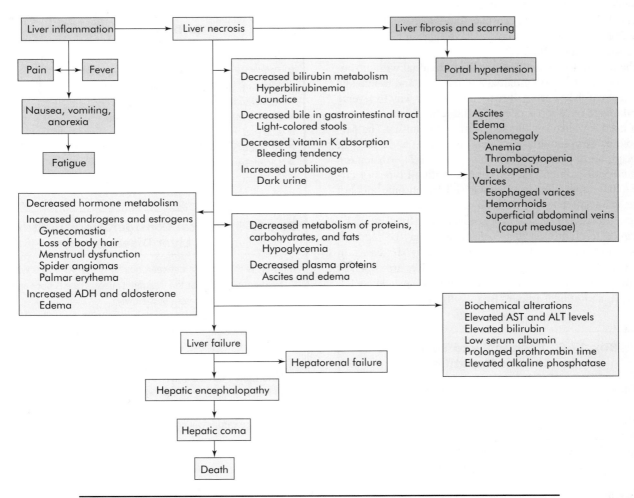

Figure 17-2 Clinical manifestations of cirrhosis. *ADH,* Antidiuretic hormone; *ALT,* alanine aminotransferase; *AST,* aspartate aminotransferase. (From McCance K, Huether S: *Pathophysiology: the biologic basis for disease in adults and children,* ed 4, St Louis, 2002, Mosby.)

Box 17-5 Laboratory Tests for Cirrhosis

■ Liver function indicators (alkaline phosphatase, alanine amino-transferase, lactic dehydrogenase, γ-glutamyl transferase levels): elevated
■ Serum bilirubin level: increased
■ Serum albumin level: decreased
■ Prothrombin time: prolonged
■ Complete blood count: decrease in red blood cells, white blood cells, and platelets
■ Glucose level: elevated
■ Serum ammonia level: elevated

Table 17-5 Treatment Focus for Cirrhosis of Varying Causes

Cause	Treatment
Hepatitis C	Peginterferon (PEG-intron, Pegasys) and ribavirin (Copegus, Rebetol) to eliminate virus from the body
Autoimmune cirrhosis	Steroid therapy to decrease inflammatory response
Wilson's disease	Chelation therapy to remove copper from the body
Primary biliary cirrhosis	Colchicine, ursodiol (Actigall), or methotrexate (Rheumatrex)
Alcohol abuse	Strict abstinence from alcohol

Adapted from Young-Mee L, Kaplan MM: Management of primary biliary cirrhosis. In Wolfe MM, editor: *Therapy of digestive disorders*, Philadelphia, 2000, WB Saunders.

interventions are carried out. However, determining who will respond to therapy and who will not is difficult. Box 17-6 describes the possible responses to therapy. Further treatment options are very limited for the individual who has not responded by the end of treatment. Generally, treatment is indicated for a person whose liver biopsy specimen shows some fibrosis but who does not yet have signs of liver decompensation (NIDDK, 2002).

The overall treatment goal for the individual with cirrhosis is to minimize further damage to the liver and to manage the effects of the existing fibrosis. There is no way to reverse liver damage once it has occurred. Table 17-5 lists the treatment used for cirrhosis due to a variety of causes. The person with symptomatic cirrhosis is given a variety of medications to control symptoms (Box 17-7). Abstention from alcohol is important for patients with all types of cirrhosis, but especially cirrhosis caused by chronic alcohol abuse. Paracentesis may be required to control abdominal ascites. In severe cases, a peritovenous shunt may be implanted to control ascites. Transfusions may be required for severe anemia and clotting deficiencies. In cases in which severe liver damage has occurred, liver transplantation may be indicated. This raises a host of psychosocial, financial, and ethical issues (Box 17-8). Social support for

Box 17-6 Responses to Treatment for Chronic Hepatitis C

■ *End-of-treatment response:* SVR sustained through posttreatment month 6.
■ *End-of-treatment response with relapse:* Initial SVR response, but evidence of hepatitis C virus (HCV) after cessation of treatment, usually within first 12 weeks.
■ *Nonresponse:* HCV present at end of treatment cycle.

Adapted from Bräu N: Pegylated interferons and advances in therapy for chronic hepatitis C, 2002, retrieved from *http://www.medscape.com/viewprogram/2035_pnt* on Nov 21, 2002.
SVR, Subviral response or undetectable HCV RNA 6 months after end of treatment.

Box 17-7 Medications Commonly Used to Treat Cirrhosis

■ *Diuretics:* to control ascites and fluid overload
■ *Pancreatic enzymes:* to assist with digestion
■ *Vitamins:* to ensure adequate intake to meet metabolic needs
■ *Antacids:* to treat gastric upset
■ *Stool softeners:* to relieve constipation
■ *Iron and folic acid:* to treat anemia
■ *Antibiotics:* as indicated to treat infections
■ *Lactulose:* to lower serum ammonia levels

Box 17-8 Ethical Considerations in Chronic Liver Disease

■ What is the balance between quality of life with and without treatment, given that the treatment success rate is poor and the disease often progresses very slowly?
■ What are the issues regarding treatment and allocation of resources in the presence of high-risk behaviors such as drug and substance abuse, chronic alcohol abuse, and sexual promiscuity?
■ Who should receive a liver transplant, given the limited supply of livers? What is the "fair" allocation of a scarce resource?
■ What are the issues involved when an individual's primary insurance carrier will not cover the cost of liver transplantation?

the individual with cirrhosis and his or her family is vital at all stages of the treatment process.

The interdisciplinary team generally consists of the physician, nurse, medical social worker, and perhaps therapists and home caregivers. Specialty nurses such as oncology specialists and psychiatric nurse specialists may be called on during treatment with peginterferon and ribavirin.

Drug Therapy

The mainstay of therapy for HCV infection is pharmacologic. Combination therapy with peginterferon and ribavirin for 24 to 48 weeks is the standard for individuals with newly diagnosed disease. However, this therapy is not effective for all individuals. Interferon alpha is a protein made by the body in response to viral infection. Recombinant forms of interferon alpha are used to decrease the viral load of HCV. Peginterferon is a chemically modified form of interferon alpha with a longer half-life. It is given subcutaneously weekly, instead of three times a week as with standard interferon alpha. In addition, peginterferon gives a more uniform blood level throughout the week and is more effective in inhibiting HCV than standard interferon (Bräu, 2002; NIDDK, 2002). Peginterferon alpha 2b (PEG-intron) is the current formulation approved for use within the United States. Peginterferon alpha 2a (Pegasys) is available only in clinical trials. Ribavirin is an oral antiviral agent taken twice a day along with peginterferon to increase the response rate and decrease the relapse rate. Both peginterferon and ribavirin cause significant side effects that require careful monitoring and management (Box 17-9). Laboratory tests (complete blood count and blood urea nitrogen, creatinine, and serum alanine aminotransferase levels) must be performed at regular intervals to monitor for treatment side effects and disease progression.

Box 17-9   Common Adverse Reactions to Medications Used to Treat Hepatitis C

PEGINTERFERON
- Influenza-like symptoms: fatigue, myalgia, arthralgia, anorexia, nausea and vomiting, fever
- Cytopenia: neutropenia, thrombocytopenia
- Neuropsychiatric effects: mood swings, depression, irritability, insomnia, suicidal tendency
- Autoimmune thyroiditis
- Alopecia

RIBAVIRIN
- Hemolytic anemia, especially between weeks 1 and 4 of therapy
- Skin rash
- Itching and nasal stuffiness
- Cough
- Hemolysis in those with renal disease
- Birth defects

Adapted from National Institute of Diabetes and Digestive and Kidney Diseases: Chronic hepatitis C: current disease management, NIH Pub No. 02-4230, Bethesda, Md, 2002, National Institutes of Health, retrieved from *http://www.niddk.nih.gov/health/digest/pubs/chrnhepc/chrnhepc.htm* on Aug 27, 2002.

The individual with cirrhosis and end-stage liver disease may be taking a multitude of medications (Box 17-7). Because these are chiefly for symptom management, the exact combination is highly individualized.

Nurses

The nursing needs of the individual with chronic liver disease are complex. Studies have shown that chronic HCV infection has a negative impact on health care quality of life, and patients perceive themselves as unwell even in the absence of disease-related complications. The impact of the disease is greater than that seen in persons with congestive heart failure and is similar to that of individuals with type 2 diabetes or chronic arthritis (Heitkemper et al, 2001). Education about the disease, its progression, and management of the expected effects of therapy is central for the affected person and his or her family (Tables 17-6 and 17-7). Many of those affected with chronic hepatitis C and cirrhosis are in their forties and fifties, a time when individuals are normally at their peak productivity as adults. Family members may have a difficult time understanding the severity of the disease and the need for treatment if the patient is asymptomatic. Therapy for HCV infection lasts an extended period of time (6 to 12 months); there is no guarantee of success and many unpleasant side effects occur. The exact course of chronic liver disease is difficult to predict. Some individuals do well for many years with appropriate support and interventions; others experience rapid liver decompensation and require intensive services.

Monitoring for disease progression is another focus of ongoing nursing care. This monitoring includes obtaining laboratory samples as indicated and assessing the effectiveness of medication. On each visit the nurse assesses for the presence of new symptoms. These findings must be discussed with the affected individual and related to any changes in the treatment plan. The nurse may need to "translate" information provided by the physician into understandable language. This is especially important if liver transplantation becomes a viable possibility.

The third focus of nursing care is the provision of ongoing psychosocial support. The individual with chronic liver disease may feel overwhelmed by the actual or potential severity of the disease. Treatment of hepatitis C with peginterferon may lead to irritability, mood swings, frank depression, and suicidal ideation (NIDDK, 2002). Those with preexisting psychiatric problems are particularly susceptible to development of these symptoms. Antidepressant therapy may be required to help control symptoms. The use of a depression scale with baseline measurements taken at the initiation of therapy is one means of monitoring mental status throughout treatment (Huber, 2001). If alcohol and/or drug use are present, ongoing substance abuse support services will be needed. As the disease progresses, those affected must be given an opportunity to talk about their feelings and fears. Providing assistance in locating ongoing

Table 17-6 Patient and Family Education Regarding Chronic Liver Disease

Topic	Teaching Points
Disease process	Definitions of hepatitis C and cirrhosis Transmission routes for hepatitis C virus Disease progression Treatment options
Lifestyle modifications	Complete avoidance of alcohol Cessation of high-risk activities such as intravenous drug abuse, intranasal cocaine use, and sexual relations with multiple partners Immunization against hepatitis A and B
Infection control precautions	Frequent hand washing Use of waterless hand gel when running water is not available Avoidance of crowds and those with known infections (colds, flu, etc.) Recognition of early signs of infection and need for treatment
Medication management	Name and purpose of all prescribed medications Dosage, administration times, and route Expected side effects and adverse reactions Possible interactions with other medications and/or foods
Appropriate use of over-the-counter medications	Need to check with physician before taking *any* over-the-counter medications Avoidance of nonsteroidal antiinflammatory drugs because they have unpredictable hepatotoxicity General safety of acetaminophen in dosages up to 2 g/day Need to avoid acetaminophen with alcohol use because it will cause liver damage Potential of vitamin A to cause liver damage in high doses Need to avoid multivitamins containing iron because iron accumulates in the liver
Careful use of prescription medications	Need to inform *all* physicians of diagnosis so that appropriate medication choices may be made Importance of taking prescribed medications exactly as ordered, notifying physician of any adverse reactions Prescription medications that may cause further liver damage: lipid-lowering drugs, antidiabetic medications, antifungal medications, anticonvulsants, hormones, and psychotropic medications
Nutritional guidelines	Consumption of small, frequent meals if nausea and anorexia are a problem Importance of focusing on foods with high nutritive value, following the daily Food Guide Pyramid Maintenance of adequate hydration Limitation of sodium intake to under 2000 mg/day if fluid retention and ascites are a problem Lack of need to eliminate any particular foods under normal circumstances Limitation of fat intake if steatorrhea is present Recommendation for protein intake of up to 1.5 g/kg of body weight per day, even if hepatic encephalopathy is present Recommended use of a multivitamin supplement to ensure adequate intake of folic acid and B vitamins
Liver transplantation	What is involved When it is appropriate

Adapted from American Dietetic Association: *Manual of clinical dietetics,* ed 6, Chicago, 2000, The Association; Huber D: Does the "C" in hepatitis C stand for complex? *Gastroenterol Nurs* 24(3):120-6, 2001 (electronic version); National Institute of Diabetes and Digestive and Kidney Diseases: Chronic hepatitis C: current disease management, NIH Pub No. 02-4230, Bethesda, Md, 2002, National Institutes of Health, retrieved from *http://www.niddk.nih.gov/health/digest/pubs/chrnhepc/chrnhepc.htm* on Aug 27, 2002; Reddy KR: Public-health impact, natural history, diagnosis, and clinical management of hepatitis C: emerging clinical options with interferon-based therapies, retrieved from *http://www.medscape.com/viewprogram/1809* on Nov 20, 2002; and Riley TR, Bhatti AM: Preventive strategies in chronic liver disease, Part I: alcohol, vaccines, toxic medications and supplements, diet and exercise, *Am Fam Physician* 64(9):1555-60, 2001.

support groups and sources of additional medical information is important. Part of this support is exploring with the individual his or her wishes for the future. This included thinking about quality-of-life issues, considering whether or not to seek a liver transplant, and making decisions about advance directives. Boxes 17-8 and 17-10 outline ethical and end-of-life considerations. The decision to seek a liver transplant and the transplantation process itself can be an emotional rollercoaster. Those involved in such decision making need continued psychosocial support throughout the process.

A psychiatric nurse specialist may join the team to provide counseling and ongoing support. An oncology nurse specialist may be called on to assist in managing the side effects of interferon therapy.

Table 17-7   Patient and Family Education Regarding Peginterferon and Ribavirin Therapy

Topic	Teaching Points
General medication management	Name, purpose, route, dose, frequency, and potential adverse reactions of drug
	Safe storage and preparation of peginterferon for injection
	Self-injection techniques for peginterferon
	Need for strict use of birth control methods (use of two different methods is recommended) while taking ribavirin and for at least 6 months following therapy because ribavirin causes birth defects
Management of flulike symptoms from peginterferon therapy	Generally self-limiting nature of symptoms and disappearance after a few weeks
	Use of acetaminophen prior to injection
	Administration of peginterferon at night so that symptoms occur during sleep instead of during the day
	Maintenance of adequate hydration
Management of neutropenia from peginterferon therapy	Use of appropriate infection control techniques
	Avoidance of crowds and those who are known to be ill
	Need to wash all raw fruits and vegetables well or avoid them completely in the case of severe neutropenia
	Avoidance of raw eggs and handling of raw poultry
	Avoidance of contact with animal waste products
	Avoidance of fresh-cut flowers because stagnant water harbors bacteria
Management of thrombocytopenia from peginterferon therapy	Use of soft toothbrush and avoidance of overly vigorous brushing and flossing
	Use of electric razor to minimize nicks and cuts
	Need to report any excessive bruising, nosebleeds, bleeding of gums, or other spontaneous bleeding
Management of anemia and severe fatigue from ribavirin therapy	Generally greater severity during the first month of therapy
	Benefit of keeping a fatigue log, using a rating scale of 1-10, to determine fatigue patterns
	Appropriate energy conservation techniques
	Need to pace activities
	Relaxation techniques
	Importance of maintaining a light exercise program

Box 17-10   End-of-Life Issues in Chronic Liver Disease

■ Progressive nature of the disease and frequently poor treatment outcomes

■ Issues surrounding the decision to seek a liver transplant and the possibility of failure of that transplant

■ Advance directive planning and decisions about how aggressive treatment should be

---

Primary Provider (Physician/Nurse Practitioner)

Medical care is generally directed by a physician, although an advanced practice nurse or physician assistant may be involved in ongoing monitoring and symptom management. The physician generally is a gastroenterologist or hepatologist. In some instances, an infectious disease specialist may play the primary role. For a person with advanced disease, a complex team of physicians may provide care: surgeon, cardiologist, rheumatologist, nephrologist, and internist. One physician should act as the coordinator for the medical care, ensuring that competing treatment protocols are not created. Even when many specialists are not involved, the primary physician must work closely with the patient's internist or family practitioner to coordinate care.

Medical Social Worker

The medical social worker is an invaluable member of the interdisciplinary team. The entire family should be the focus of intervention. The suddenness of the diagnosis, the possibility of severe side effects of treatment when the disease itself may have no symptoms, and the potentially poor long-term prognosis with life-threatening liver failure create much distress for the individual and family. The social worker can help them work through the various choices to be made and offer referral to appropriate support groups. Possible support groups include those for hepatitis, alcohol and/or drug abuse, and liver transplantation. Role changes in the family are not uncommon because of the side effects of treatment.

Finances may be an important issue for some individuals. With interferon treatment, the affected individual may not be able to work for prolonged periods. The cost of injectable medications is high, and many insurance companies require a copayment or do not cover the cost at all. The social worker must assist the family in identifying available financial resources.

Dietitian

The dietitian may be called on to provide nutritional counseling. Peginterferon therapy may cause anorexia and nausea. Appropriate food selections and methods of stimulating the appetite are discussed with the family. Although generally no specific diet is required for patients with hepatitis, healthy dietary habits should be encouraged to ensure availability of adequate nutrients for tissue regeneration. If the affected individual has a history of alcohol abuse, he or she may be malnourished and require dietary interventions to regain a proper nutritional balance. Some research has suggested that a low-fat diet, combined with exercise, may improve liver function test results (Riley and Bhatti, 2001). Additional dietary adjustments may be required in response to specific symptoms, such as fluid retention and protein wasting. Protein-restricted diets are no longer recommended for the individual experiencing hepatic encephalopathy (American Dietetic Association, 2000).

Physical and Occupational Therapists

Severe fatigue is a significant problem for many individuals undergoing treatment for hepatitis C and for those coping with cirrhosis. The physical therapist may be called on to teach energy conservation techniques. The therapist may also develop a plan for light exercise to maintain muscle tone and prevent deconditioning. An occupational therapist may assess the home environment for possible modifications to promote energy conservation. He or she may also assist in developing a work simplification plan (Duchene, 2002). Box 17-11 gives energy conservation tips.

Homemaker or Personal Care Aide

In cases in which fatigue is severe, a homemaker, companion, or personal care aide may perform household tasks or assist the individual with personal care. The family may need the help of the nurse or social worker in accessing the appropriate level of service and financing such care.

Complementary and Alternative Therapies

A significant portion of those diagnosed with HCV infection use alternative therapies (Fathman, 2002). These include modalities such as herbal therapies, antioxidant therapy, acupuncture, biofeedback, and relaxation techniques. Herbal therapies are the most commonly used (Table 17-8). Although there is little scientific research to support their effectiveness, there is frequent anecdotal support for their use. The most promising herb for combating hepatitis C is milk thistle, or *Silybum marianum* (Lawrence et al, 2000; National Center for Complementary and Alternative Medicine, 2000).

Think **S** for Success

SYMPTOMS
■ Manage symptoms from drug therapy, which can be quite significant and worse than the disease symptoms.
■ Manage discomfort, pruritus, maldigestion and malnutrition, and fatigue.

SEQUELAE
■ Prevent, monitor for, and manage long-term complications from disease and medications.
■ Educate patient on importance of ceasing alcohol and drug use.

SAFETY
■ Ensure safety through medication management, counseling of patient on safe sex practices, and infection control.
■ Prevent injury from complications of cirrhotic process and from malnutrition, fatigue, and drug and alcohol abuse.

SUPPORT/SERVICES
■ Assist patient in coping with anxiety, depression, frustration with treatment modalities, family issues, and decisions about liver transplantation.

SATISFACTION
■ Address quality-of-life issues, especially because the disease itself has few symptoms but the treatment produces serious symptoms. Quality-of-life issues include deteriorating physical condition with cirrhosis, lack of energy, inability to work, multiple physical symptoms, and stress associated with waiting for a liver transplant.

Box 17-11   Energy Conservation Tips

■ Pace activities, with alternating periods of rest and activity.
■ Adjust work habits to minimize energy expenditure: perform activities sitting down, rearrange counter heights if possible, organizing supplies to minimize the number of steps back and forth.
■ Do errands at nonpeak times of day.
■ Delegate activities to other members of the family.
■ Reprioritize "essential" activities: what will happen if they are not done? Eliminate nonessential activities.
■ Use good body mechanics when performing activities.
■ Use a grabber tool to minimize bending and reaching for items.

Adapted from Duchene P: Sleep, rest, and fatigue. In Hoeman S, editor: *Rehabilitation nursing: process and application*, ed 3, Philadelphia, 2002, WB Saunders.

CHRONIC CHOLELITHIASIS
Pathophysiology

Cholelithiasis is the presence of gallstones in the gallbladder (Box 17-12). Approximately 20 million Americans have cholelithiasis, of whom two thirds are asymptomatic (Lee

Table 17-8 Herbal Therapies for Hepatitis C

Herb	Mechanism of Action	Comments
Desmodium (*Desmodium ascendens*)	Regenerates and protects hepatic cells	Taken as a tea infusion of nonflowering parts
Ginger (*Zingiber officinale*)	Acts as antiinflammatory Thought to strengthen gastric mucosal resistance; also increases gastric emptying	Used primarily to treat nausea secondary to interferon therapy Taken as a tea
Huang qi (*Astragalus membranaceus*)	Increases function of immune system, works synergistically with interferon	Commonly used in Chinese medicine Extracted from the root Given as an injection
Licorice root (*Glycyrrhiza glabra*)	Has antiviral and antiinflammatory properties	Taken as a tea or pill Has been used for many years in Japan for chronic hepatitis Has toxic effects on heart and blood pressure with intake of >100 mg/day
Milk thistle (*Silybum marianum*)	Stabilizes hepatocyte cell membrane, improves cell regeneration, acts as antioxidant	Taken as a capsule; does not dissolve well in water to make a tea
St. John's wort (*Hypericum perforatum*)	Has antiviral properties: interferes with reproduction of viral particles Has antidepressant action	Taken as a pill or a tea May be used for direct antiviral effect or for reduction of anxiety, stress, headaches, and depression
Schisandra (*Schisandra chinensis*)	Improves protein synthesis, speeds up repair of liver function	Berries are used Taken as dried fruit, capsule, or extract

Adapted from Lawrence V et al: Milk thistle: effects on liver disease and cirrhosis and clinical adverse effects, Evidence Report/Technology Assessment No. 21, AHRQ Pub No. 01-E025, Rockville, Md, October 2000, Agency for Healthcare Research and Quality, retrieved from *http://www.ahrqu.gov/clinic/epcsums/milktsum.htm* on May 23, 2003.; National Center for Complementary and Alternative Medicine: Hepatitis C and complementary and alternative medicine: 2003 update, Pub No. D004, NCCAM Clearinghouse, Bethesda, Md, 2003, National Institutes of Health, retrieved from *http://nccam.nih.gov/health/hepatitisc/* on Jan 15, 2004; and Useful herbal medicines, retrieved from *http://www.hepatitis-c.de/useful.htm* on Aug 30, 2002.

NOTE: **Except for milk thistle, there is little scientific evidence that herbal therapy is effective in the treatment of chronic hepatitis C.**

Box 17-12 Types of Gallbladder Disorder

- Cholelithiasis: gallstones
- Cholecystitis: inflammation of the gallbladder, generally from gallstones
- Choledocholithiasis: gallstones in the common bile duct
- Cholangitis: inflammation of the common bile duct

and Ko, 2000). Women are affected more than men; nearly 25% of all women have gallstones by age 60 and 50% have gallstones by age 75 (Gallstones and gallbladder disease, 2001). The overall incidence of gallstones has increased during the twentieth century as underdeveloped countries adopt a more Western-style diet high in fats and processed foods (Lee and Ko, 2000).

Two main types of gallstone are seen: those composed of cholesterol, and those composed of pigment. Cholesterol stones are more common in developed countries, and pigment stones are more common in underdeveloped countries. Table

17-9 lists the risk factors for development of each type of stone. Long-term complications of gallstones include cholecystitis, cholangitis, pancreatitis, perforation of the gallbladder, and fistula formation. Chronic cholelithiasis leads to thickening and scarring of the gallbladder, which results in less efficient emptying. Gallbladder disease by itself is seldom fatal but may cause intermittent distress over many years.

Clinical Manifestations

Chronic cholelithiasis generally is asymptomatic, and in many people gallstones are diagnosed incidentally when tests are undergone for other reasons. Studies have indicated, however, that once the stones begin to cause symptoms, they will most likely continue to cause problems (Lee and Ko, 2000). Symptoms range from mild bloating and upper right quadrant discomfort to frank biliary colic. Biliary colic is episodic, severe right upper quadrant pain that may radiate to the back accompanied by nausea and vomiting and extreme restlessness. The pain develops over a short period of time and generally resolves gradually over a number of hours. The period of time between attacks is unpredictable. The attacks frequently have a diurnal pattern,

Table 17-9 Risk Factors for Development of Gallstones

Risk Factor	Comments
Obesity	Overproduction of cholesterol by liver leads to supersaturation of bile.
Sex	Females have higher incidence, probably due to effects of estrogen on mobilization of cholesterol from the bloodstream.
Age	Risk increases with age because of increased time for stones to develop and grow.
Use of hormonal therapy	Estrogen therapy leads to increase risk of cholesterol stones.
Rapid weight loss	Cholesterol production by liver increases; chance of symptomatic gallstones is increased.
Primary biliary cirrhosis	Risk of pigment gallstone formation increased.
Gemfibrozil (Lopid) therapy	Drug is used to lower cholesterol levels; it acts by increasing excretion of cholesterol in bile and thus increases risk of stone formation.

Adapted from Lee SP, Ko CW: Gallstones. In Yamada T, editor: *Textbook of gastroenterology,* ed 3, Philadelphia, 2000, Lippincott Williams and Wilkins.

peaking in the middle of the night (Lee and Ko, 2000). The development of jaundice, fever, or chills signifies a serious condition that requires immediate medical attention.

Diagnosis

Diagnosis is generally by history and presenting symptoms. Laboratory tests are usually not specific, although there may be some leukocytosis and elevated serum amylase levels. Ultrasonography of the gallbladder is the test of choice because it detects most gallstones. Cholecystography after oral administration of a contrast agent is seldom done today. Liver scans and abdominal computed tomographic scans may be performed to evaluate the bile ducts and assess for the presence of tumors. Magnetic resonance cholangiography is a new test that allows visualization of the biliary tree (Lee and Ko, 2000).

Interdisciplinary Care

Minimal treatment is required for asymptomatic gallstones. Prophylactic cholecystectomy to prevent the development of complications appears to offer no benefit (Lee and Ko, 2000). Surgery is an appropriate option when repeated episodes of pain and discomfort occur. Alternatively, medications may be used to attempt to dissolve the stones if they are made of cholesterol and the individual is not a candidate for surgery. During the acute stage of cholelithiasis, the chief treatment is symptom control for the pain, nausea, and vomiting.

Nurse

The major nursing role in asymptomatic cholelithiasis is education about the disease process and the recognition of symptoms that require medical attention. The patient may also be educated on how to lower risk factors by losing weight and avoiding the use of estrogen therapy.

Primary Provider (Physician/Nurse Practitioner)

The physician may be an internist or a gastroenterologist. He or she monitors the disease progression and evaluates whether specific interventions are needed. If the gallstones are causing frequent episodes of distress, a referral may be made to a surgeon to have them removed. In the case of

asymptomatic disease, an advanced practice nurse or physician assistant may provide ongoing monitoring.

Dietitian

The dietitian may be called on to establish an appropriate low-fat diet and to help with weight loss strategies. Obesity and consumption of a high-fat, highly processed diet are considered risk factors for gallstone formation, although the role of a high-fat diet in stimulation of a gallbladder attack is controversial (Lee and Ko, 2000). Research has not shown a direct correlation between consumption of high-fat diet and the development of symptoms. However, it is prudent to instruct the patient to follow a healthy low-fat diet to help with weight loss and improvement of health in general. A high-fiber diet has been associated with a lower risk of gallstones and can also help with weight loss (Gallstone and gallbladder disease, 2001).

Think S for Success

SYMPTOMS
- Manage discomfort and pain from gallstones and inflammatory process; manage nausea and vomiting.

SEQUELAE
- Prevent cholangitis, pancreatitis, perforation of the gallbladder, and fistula formation.

SAFETY
- Ensure safe use of medications for pain management.

SUPPORT/SERVICES
- Refer patient to weight loss support group and possibly to chronic pain support group if surgical removal of gallstones is not an option.

SATISFACTION
- Assess level of discomfort and ascertain satisfaction with any dietary modifications made to minimize discomfort.
- Develop a plan to optimize and maintain quality of life.

CHRONIC PANCREATITIS

Pathophysiology

Chronic pancreatitis is pancreatic inflammation that lasts for many years and eventually leads to progressive loss of exocrine and endocrine function. It is most commonly seen in those with a long history of alcohol abuse. The disorder is especially prevalent in men in their thirties and forties who have abused alcohol for over 10 years. There is some evidence that consumption of a high-fat, high-protein diet in conjunction with alcohol abuse may predispose to the development of pancreatitis (Owyang, 2000). In approximately 40% of cases the cause is unknown (Freedman, 2002). Hereditary pancreatitis is seen in a small number of cases and usually appears in childhood. New studies indicate a link between mutations in the cystic fibrosis gene and development of chronic pancreatitis in adults (Freedman, 2002). Those with the mutation do not have overt manifestations of cystic fibrosis. In underdeveloped countries, chronic pancreatitis may result from chronic malnutrition and is seen mainly in children and young adults (Bornman and Beckingham, 2001). Long-term complications of pancreatitis are listed in Box 17-13.

Clinical Manifestations

The most common manifestation of chronic pancreatitis is a constant or intermittent severe, dull pain in the epigastric area with radiation to the back. Sitting in a forward-leaning position may relieve the pain somewhat, whereas lying supine exacerbates it. The pain is generally exacerbated almost immediately by eating and is accompanied by nausea and vomiting. In about 15% of those with chronic pancreatitis, however, there is no pain at all (Owyang, 2000). Weight loss may occur from anorexia and avoidance of food to control the pain. There is some indication that being dehydrated also contributes to pain, probably because it helps contribute to the formation of pancreatic sludge (Sellers, 2002). Late symptoms include the development of steatorrhea and diabetes mellitus. Steatorrhea occurs when 90% of the exocrine function has been destroyed (Bornman and Beckingham, 2001). Diabetes mellitus secondary to destruction of islet cells develops in about a third of those

---

Box 17-13 Long-Term Complications of Chronic Pancreatitis

- Ascites
- Diabetes mellitus
- Malnutrition
- Pancreatic cancer
- Pleural effusion
- Pseudocyst

---

with chronic pancreatitis. The occurrence of hypoglycemia in patients with diabetes is a particular problem because of the lack of available glucagon to help moderate low blood glucose levels (Bornman and Beckingham, 2001).

Diagnosis

Diagnosis relies heavily on history of symptoms and etiologic factors. Few changes are seen in the results of pancreatic studies early in the disease. Levels of pancreatic enzymes (amylase, trypsin, and lipase) are generally elevated during an acute exacerbation but may be normal during asymptomatic periods. A subnormal level of pancreatic polypeptide in response to a high-protein meal is also an indicator of advanced chronic pancreatitis, although the level is generally normal in mild to moderate pancreatitis (Owyang, 2000). Abdominal radiography, pancreatic ultrasonography, and computerized tomography may be used to detect evidence of calcification and changes in the pancreatic ducts. None of these methods will detect evidence of early chronic pancreatitis. In advanced disease, endoscopic retrograde cholangiopancreatography will show changes in the size of the pancreatic ducts and evidence of cysts, strictures, and calcification (Bornman and Beckingham, 2001). Glucose tolerance testing, hemoglobin A_{IC} testing, and routine fasting blood glucose testing may be performed to assess for the development of diabetes mellitus.

Interdisciplinary Care

The focus of care in chronic pancreatitis is the control of symptoms and the prevention of complications. The interdisciplinary team consists of the primary care provider, nurse, medical social worker, dietitian, and perhaps a pharmacist.

Drug Therapy

Management of pain is of primary concern in chronic pancreatitis, because pain is the symptom creating the most distress to the affected individual and family. Absolute abstinence from alcohol is the first step in controlling pain, although some studies have indicated that abstinence may not relieve pain in all cases (Forsmark and Toskes, 2000). However, alcohol abuse does contribute significantly to disease progression and to a poorer prognosis. Therapy with nonsteroidal antiinflammatory drugs is the first line of treatment for pain, although it is seldom sufficient to control it. Opioid narcotics are generally needed to control the pain; the lowest effective dose should be used to minimize the development of adverse reactions. Tricyclic antidepressants, as well as the anticonvulsant gabapentin, may be used as adjuvant therapy. Both act synergistically with the narcotic agents to improve pain control (Forsmark and Toskes, 2000). In addition to pain medications, pancreatic enzymes (pancreatin or pancrelipase) are prescribed to decrease the secretion of enzymes by the pancreas and to help control steatorrhea. High doses of pancrelipase (up to eight tablets at a time) are taken at mealtime and bedtime. Adherence to this regimen may be an issue for some individuals because of the number of pills to be taken. The use of octreotide, a synthetic form of somatostatin, to inhibit pancreatic secretions is currently being investigated to improve pain control (Owyang, 2000).

Late complications of chronic pancreatitis are diabetes mellitus and steatorrhea or maldigestion. For the individual who develops diabetes mellitus, oral antidiabetic agents or insulin is prescribed. However, the goal of therapy is not tight glucose control. This approach is to prevent the development of treatment-induced hypoglycemia, which may prove fatal (Forsmark and Toskes, 2000). To control steatorrhea, pancreatic enzymes are prescribed in large doses. These are the same enzymes used to help control pain. In some individuals who do not obtain relief from steatorrhea, histamine 2 receptor blockers may be used to decrease gastric acid production, because acid inactivates pancreatic enzymes (Owyang, 2000).

Nurse

As in chronic liver disorders, the focus of nursing care in chronic pancreatitis is education of the affected individual and family (Table 17-10). This includes education regarding the disease process, medication management, nutritional issues, and the need for strict abstinence from alcohol. The nurse is also heavily involved in issues of pain control. The use of nonpharmacologic pain control techniques should be explored with the affected individual.

These include techniques such as massage for back pain and the use of heat, guided imagery, and distraction. During severe pain episodes, however, narcotics will be needed. Education about appropriate use and management of side effects is crucial. For example, the individual must be taught methods of preventing constipation if opioids are used on a regular basis and steatorrhea is not a problem. Keeping a pain diary is helpful in determining the patterns of pain, what precipitates it, and what is most effective in relieving it. The services of a pain management specialist should be used if the individual experiences pain that is difficult to control.

The management of chronic steatorrhea may be very distressing for the affected individual. The loose, bulky stools may be foul smelling and cause skin irritation. The nurse must provide education about appropriate skin care and about dietary modifications such as eating smaller, more frequent meals, and avoiding high-fat foods.

If diabetes mellitus develops, the nurse must educate the individual and family about its management.

Psychosocial support of the individual in coping with abstinence from alcohol, as well as referral to a local support group such as Alcoholics Anonymous, may be required. Family support is needed to deal with issues of alcohol abuse and possible dysfunctional family dynamics. Family support is also needed in cases in which the individual with pancreatitis is ill enough to miss work on a regular basis. Role reversals and loss of a steady income place a severe strain on other

Table 17-10   Patient and Family Education Regarding Chronic Pancreatitis

Topic	Teaching Points
Disease process	Cause specific to the individual
	Expected disease progression and long-term prognosis
Prevention of further pancreatic damage	Need for complete abstinence from alcohol
	Recognition of early signs of possible complications that should be reported to health care team
Medication management	Name and purpose of all prescribed medications
	Dosage, administration times, and route
	Expected side effects and adverse reactions
	Possible interactions with other medications and/or foods
Pain control measures	Appropriate use of medications for pain control
	Self-assessment and analysis of pain levels through use of a pain diary
	Nonpharmacologic methods of controlling pain: guided imagery, relaxation, use of heat, use of massage, positioning
Nutritional adaptations	Use of low-fat diet to control steatorrhea
	Benefit of diet rich in antioxidants
	Ingestion of multivitamin daily if dietary intake is poor
	Need for calorie- and carbohydrate-controlled diet if diabetes mellitus is present
Management of steatorrhea	Perineal care to minimize skin irritation and breakdown
	Importance of taking pancreatic enzymes exactly as ordered to control steatorrhea
Management of diabetes mellitus	Disease process and relationship to chronic pancreatitis
	Treatment regimen: medications and diet
	Recognition of hypoglycemia and hyperglycemia
	Recognition of long-term complications

family members. Family members may also blame the victim (especially if alcohol abuse is involved) and may not believe that the individual is in as much pain as he or she says. Referral to a psychiatric nurse specialist or social worker may be necessary to provide more extensive counseling services to the individual and family. Referral to a pancreatic support group offers a forum for ongoing education and sharing of experiences (Shepp, Chase, and Rawls, 1999).

Primary Provider (Physician/Nurse Practitioner)

The internist, gastroenterologist, or pancreatologist is responsible for the overall treatment plan and monitoring of disease progress. A surgeon may be called in if pseudocysts develop and require drainage. An endocrinologist becomes involved if insulin production is affected and diabetes develops. An advanced practice nurse or physician assistant may be involved in ongoing monitoring and symptom control.

Medical Social Worker

As in management of chronic liver diseases, the social worker is an important member of the team. He or she offers individual and family counseling. As noted earlier, family members may blame the victim if the pancreatitis is due to chronic alcohol abuse. There may also be dysfunctional family patterns that must be addressed so that appropriate care can be given. The individual with chronic pancreatitis may be unable to work because of the pain and steatorrhea. If so, financial issues will be of concern. The social worker can assist the family in accessing local resources. Referral to

a pancreatic support group is another role of the social worker.

Dietitian

Malnutrition caused by malabsorption and steatorrhea is a common finding in chronic pancreatitis. A low-fat, high-carbohydrate diet is recommended. Adequate hydration is also important, because dehydration contributes to pancreatic sludge and duct blockage (Sellers, 2002). The dietitian provides nutritional counseling and ongoing support as dietary adjustments are made to decrease pain, nausea, and vomiting. If malnutrition is severe, parenteral nutrition may be needed. In this case, the dietitian works with the physician and pharmacist to ensure that adequate nutrients and micronutrients are included in the parenteral therapy formulation.

Pharmacist

The pharmacist becomes a member of the interdisciplinary team when parenteral therapy is indicated. He or she is responsible for the actual mixing of the parenteral fluids and works with the dietitian and physician to facilitate supply of nutritional needs.

Complementary and Alternative Therapies

A promising alternative therapy was developed by the Manchester Royal Infirmary in the early 1990s (MRI Pancreatitis Support Group, 2002). This therapy uses antioxidants to neutralize free radicals in the body. Research

---

Table 17-11   Antioxidant-Rich Foods

Antioxidant	Characteristics	Food Sources
Vitamin A	Beta-carotene, found chiefly in red, yellow, and orange foods and dark-green leafy vegetables	Melon, apricots, mangoes, peaches Carrots, broccoli, cabbage, brussels sprouts, tomatoes, spinach, sweet potatoes, winter squash
Vitamin C	Found in brightly colored fruits and vegetables	Berries, citrus fruits, pineapple, kiwi, bananas, cherries, guava Root vegetables, brussels sprouts, broccoli, tomatoes, parsley
Vitamin E	Found in vegetable oils and nuts as well as fruits and vegetables	Apples, bananas, blackberries Asparagus, spinach, lettuce, parsley, carrots, tomatoes, broccoli, peas Rapeseed oil, sunflower oil, olive oil Whole-grain products, seeds, nuts
Selenium	Found in meats, nuts, seafood	Brazil nuts, tuna, beef, cod, turkey Enriched bread and rice
Methionine	Found in protein-rich foods	Fish and shellfish, milk, yogurt and cheese, beef, chicken

Adapted from American Dietetic Association: Antioxidant vitamins for optimal health, 2001, retrieved from *http://www.eatright.org/nfs/nfs84.html* on Nov 30, 2002; National Institutes of Health Clinical Center: Facts about dietary supplements: selenium, 2001, retrieved from *http://www.cc.nih.gov/ccc/supplements/selen.html* on Nov 30, 2002; and MRI Pancreatitis Support Group: A decade of research yields treatment for pancreatic disease, retrieved from *http://www.pancreaticdisease.com/info/info9.htm* on Aug 30, 2002.

at Manchester Royal Infirmary suggested that those who developed chronic pancreatitis had diets deficient in fresh fruits and vegetables. Supplementing the diet with foods and tablets containing vitamins C, A, and E plus selenium and methionine reduced the severity of the disease and is now a routine part of the therapy regimen at the Infirmary. Table 17-11 lists foods that are rich in antioxidants.

Think S for Success

SYMPTOMS
■ Manage chronic pain and steatorrhea.

SEQUELAE
■ Prevent, monitor for, and manage long-term complications such as cyst formation, diabetes mellitus, and malnutrition.

SAFETY
■ Ensure safe use of narcotic pain medications.
■ Prevent malnutrition.

SUPPORT/SERVICES
■ Assist patient in coping with frustration and depression caused by chronic pain, dealing with difficulties in abstaining from alcohol use, and resolving family issues associated with adjustment to the chronic disease.

SATISFACTION
■ Assess changes in quality of life caused by chronic pain and repeated hospitalizations. Determine the extent to which the illness has led to changes in family roles, perhaps including the inability to work.

FAMILY AND CAREGIVER ISSUES IN CHRONIC LIVER AND PANCREATIC DISEASES

With chronic liver and pancreatic diseases, many family and caregiver issues which must be addressed so that appropriate care can be given. Box 17-14 lists some common issues. Resources for family members and caregivers can be found at the end of this chapter.

Box 17-14 Family and Caregiver Issues in Chronic Liver and Pancreatic Diseases

■ Difficulty in believing that the disorder really exists, given the usual lack of symptoms (with liver disease) or variable nature of chronic pain (with chronic pancreatitis)
■ "Blame-the-victim" mentality, especially if drug abuse or alcohol abuse is present
■ Uncertainty about success of therapy and long-term prognosis
■ Role reversals when family member is undergoing therapy because of inability to work, fatigue, and other side effects of medications
■ Altered family dynamics if chronic alcohol abuse is present
■ Financial concerns because of treatment expenses and loss of work

---

CASE STUDY
Patient Data

Mr. B. is a 45-year-old white factory worker recently diagnosed with hepatitis C virus (HCV) infection. He lives with his family in a suburban row house close to a major industrial city. His wife is a homemaker and is active in the Catholic Church and local community affairs. Their two sons attend the local high school, where one is a sophomore and the other is a junior. Mr. B. was diagnosed 2 weeks earlier with HCV infection as a result of routine blood testing prior to changing his health insurance carrier. He was referred by his primary care physician to the liver clinic at the local teaching hospital for evaluation and follow-up.

During the first visit, Mr. and Mrs. B. meet with the clinic nurse case manager assigned to Mr. B. The nurse begins by taking a history, which reveals that Mr. B. has always considered himself healthy and is bewildered by his diagnosis. The nurse explains the cause of HCV infection and questions Mr. B. about risk factors in his past. He received two transfusions following an automobile accident as a teenager and had two tattoos while visiting the Far East when he was in the Navy. The nurse explains that the transfusions were probably the source of his HCV, although getting tattoos is also a risk factor. Unfortunately, there was no way to detect the presence of HCV 25 years ago. Physical assessment by the nurse reveals no significant findings except

mild hypertension, with a blood pressure of 154/92. Mr. B. takes no medications other than an occasional ibuprofen tablet for aches and pains. He had a drinking problem in the past but stopped drinking alcohol several years ago and now attends weekly meetings of Alcoholics Anonymous. A review of his laboratory test results reveals a normal complete blood count and levels of electrolytes, glucose, blood urea nitrogen, and creatinine. Liver function testing showed elevated levels of enzymes: alanine aminotransferase, γ-glutamyl transferase, alkaline phosphatase, leucine aminopeptidase, and lactic dehydrogenase. His enzyme immunoassay test was positive. Following her assessment, the nurse discusses with Mr. and Mrs. B. the disease process with HCV infection and the usual disease progression. At this point the physician joins the group to discuss further evaluation and possible treatment options for Mr. B. Plans are made to perform a liver biopsy to determine the amount of liver damage and to obtain a serum blood sample for viral RNA testing for HCV genotype.

The B.'s returned to the clinic 10 days later, following the liver biopsy and additional laboratory work. The biopsy revealed moderate liver fibrosis, and the viral RNA testing revealed the presence of genotype 1 hepatitis C. Based on these findings, the physician discusses the possibility of starting a 48-week course of peginterferon and ribavirin therapy. Mrs. B. expresses concerns

CASE STUDY—cont'd

about their ability to handle the weekly injections, as well as the possibility that her husband will be out of work for a prolonged period of time. Mr. B. is not convinced of the need for treatment because he has no symptoms. The nurse and physician suggest that Mr. and Mrs. B. think about the treatment plan at home before making a decision and give them information about a local hepatitis support group and on-line resources to help them make their decision.

Thinking It Through
- If you were the nurse case manager, how would you describe the disease process of hepatitis C to Mr. and Mrs. B., based on the information you have at hand?
- How will the results of the liver biopsy and viral RNA testing affect the treatment regimen for Mr. B.?
- What are likely to be the major concerns of Mr. and Mrs. B. regarding treatment and long-term prognosis?
- If Mr. B. decides to undergo treatment, what will be the teaching involved?
- What other team members will most likely be involved in Mr. B.'s care?

Case Conference
Three weeks later, the B.'s return to the clinic. Mr. B. has decided to undergo therapy. The nurse initiates detailed teaching about the therapy and its side effects, and administers the first dose of peginterferon. Over the next few weeks, Mr. and Mrs. B. return to the clinic for the weekly injections and gradually assume responsibility for the injections. By the end of 3 weeks, they have each demonstrated their ability to give the injections safely. In addition, during these visits the nurse assesses Mr. B. for development of expected side effects. He has experienced extreme fatigue and has been unable to go to work since he received the second injection. He is expressing feelings of depression and repeatedly says, "How did I get like this? I can't even play ball with my sons anymore." He and his wife are very concerned about finances and how long he will have to be out of work. Although they have some savings, they do not have enough to cover months with no income. The medical social worker meets with the B.'s to assess their financial needs. She helps them apply for Medicaid to assist with medical expenses and to apply for food stamps. Together they discuss the possibility of tapping into the leave-sharing program at his workplace and finding out if the union has any health-related emergency

benefits available. The social worker also offers biweekly counseling sessions to help the B.'s adjust to the major upheavals caused by the disease. The nurse and the social worker both encourage Mr. B. to focus on day-to-day short-term goals and to remember that this is a temporary condition that will get better as his treatment progresses.

Over the next 10 months Mr. and Mrs. B. are seen regularly in the liver clinic. During the first several months of treatment, the focus of care is on management of side effects from the medications. Mr. B. experiences signs of bone marrow depression, developing an infection at one of his injection sites as well as severe bruising and bleeding gums. The nurse focuses her teaching on how to cope with these side effects and how to prevent further complications from occurring. Mr. B. is cautioned to use only acetaminophen for discomfort and not to resume drinking alcohol. His depression worsens, however, even as his physical symptoms of fatigue improve. The physician starts Mr. B. on a low-dose antidepressant, explaining that depression is a not uncommon effect of the peginterferon therapy.

Over the course of his treatment, Mr. B. meets with the treatment team at monthly intervals to assess his progress. The physician is encouraged by the steady decrease in his viral RNA load. The nurse follows up on earlier education and continues to assess for development of complications. Fortunately, Mr. B. shows no signs of developing kidney disease, cryoglobulinemia, or liver decompensation. Mr. and Mrs. B. receive periodic counseling from the social worker as they learn to come to grips with the ramifications of his chronic disease. Mr. B. is able to return to work part time after 5 months of therapy. The antidepressant medication and the return to work significantly improve his mood. At the conclusion of his therapy, he has a subviral response and again feels well. He is still virus free at his 6-month checkup, which indicates that the treatment was successful in eliminating the hepatitis virus. At his yearly checkup, the nurse continues to assess for any signs of hepatic decompensation and reinforces the need for continued abstinence from alcohol.

- Discuss the ramifications if Mr. B. had started drinking alcohol again to cope with his depression.
- For what signs will the team be alert as Mr. B. returns for periodic follow-up after his treatment?
- If a liver transplant were deemed necessary in the future, how would the team assist Mr. and Mrs. B. through the decision-making process?

Internet and Other Resources

American Liver Foundation: *http://www.liverfoundation.org;* E-mail *webmail@liverfoundation.org;* telephone 800-GO-LIVER (800-465-4837); 75 Maiden Lane, Suite 603, New York, NY 10038

Centers for Disease Control and Prevention, National Center for Infectious Diseases: *http://www.cdc.gov/ncidod/;* Office of Health Communication, Mailstop C-14, 1600 Clifton Rd, Atlanta, GA 30333

Frontline Hepatitis: *http://frontline-hepatitis-awareness.com;* E-mail *ane@frontline-hepatitis-awareness.com;* telephone 866-HEP-GOGO (866-437-4646); fax 775-542-5143; 701 West Elizabeth #54, Monroe, WA 98272

Hepatitis C Association: *http://www.hepcassoc.org;* E-mail *info@hepcassoc.org;* telephone 866-437-4377; fax 908-561-4575; 1351 Cooper Rd, Scotch Plains, NJ 07076

Hepatitis Foundation International: *http://www.hepfi.org;* E-mail *mail@hepfi.org;* telephone 800-891-0707; fax 301-622-4702; 30 Sunrise Terrace, Cedar Grove, NJ 07009-1423

National Digestive Diseases Information Clearinghouse: *http://www.niddk.nih.gov/health/digest/digest.htm;* E-mail *nddic@info.niddk.nih.gov;* telephone 800-891-5489; fax 301-907-8906; 2 Information Way, Bethesda, MD 20892-3570

National Hepatitis C Coalition: *http://www.nationalhepatitis-c.org;* telephone 909-658-4414; PO Box 5058, Hemet, CA 92544

National Pancreas Foundation: *http://www.pancreasfoundation.org;* E-mail *info@pancreasfoundation.org;* telephone 866-726-2737; PO Box 15333, Boston, MA 02215

United Network for Organ Sharing (UNOS): *http://www.unos.org;* telephone 800-24-DONOR (800-243-6667); 1100 Boulders Pkwy, Suite 500, PO Box 13770, Richmond, VA 23225-8770

REFERENCES

American Dietetic Association: *Manual of clinical dietetics,* ed 6, Chicago, 2000, The Association.

American Gastroenterological Association: Cirrhosis of the liver, retrieved from *http://www.gastro.org/clinicalRes/brochures/cirrhosis.html* on Nov 23, 2002.

Bornman PC, Beckingham IJ: Chronic pancreatitis, *BJM* 322(7287):660-3, 2001.

Bräu N: Pegylated interferons and advances in therapy for chronic hepatitis C, Nov 1, 2002, retrieved from *http://www.medscape.com/view program/2035_pnt* on Nov 21, 2002.

Centers for Disease Control and Prevention: Recommendations for prevention and control of hepatitis C virus (HCV) infection and HCV-related chronic disease, *MMWR Morb Mortal Wkly Rep* 47(RR-19):1-39, 1998 (electronic version), retrieved from *http://www.cdc.gov/mmwr/preview/ mmwrhtml/00055154.htm* on Nov 24, 2002.

Centers for Disease Control and Prevention: Deaths, percent of total deaths, and death rates for the 15 leading causes of death: United States and each state—1999, Sep 21, 2001, retrieved from *http://www.cdc.gov/nchs/data/ statab/ lcwk9.pdf* on Nov 24, 2002.

Dasarathy S, McCullough A: Alcoholic liver disease. In Schiff E, Sorrell M, Maddrey W, editors: *Diseases of the liver,* ed 9, Philadelphia, 2003, Lippincott Williams and Wilkins.

Des Jarlais DC, Schuchat A: Hepatitis C among drug users: déjà vu all over again? *Am J Public Health* 91(1):21-2, 2001.

Duchene P: Sleep, rest, and fatigue. In Hoeman S, editor: *Rehabilitation nursing: process and application,* ed 3, Philadelphia, 2002, WB Saunders.

Fathman A: Alternative therapy and hepatitis C: a quantitative study, 2002, retrieved from *http://access.nku.edu/hepatitis/altettherapy.htm* on Aug 30, 2002.

Forsmark CE, Toskes PP: Treatment of chronic pancreatitis. In Wolfe MM, editor: *Therapy of digestive disorders*, Philadelphia, 2000, WB Saunders, pp 235-45.

Freedman S: Chronic pancreatitis [National Pancreas Foundation website], 2002, retrieved from *http://www.pancreasfoundation.org/chronicpancre-atitisarticle.html* on Nov 26, 2002.

Gallstones and gallbladder disease, 2001, retrieved from *http://www. healthandage.com/html/well_connected/pdf/ doc10.pdf* on Nov 24, 2002.

Giese L: Herbs and hepatobiliary disease, *Gastroenterol Nurs* 24(1):38-40, 2001 (electronic version).

Heitkemper M et al: Chronic hepatitis C: implications for health-related quality of life, *Gastroenterol Nurs* 24(4):169-75, 2001 (electronic version).

Hoofnagle J, Heller T: Hepatitis C. In Zakim D, Boyer T, editors: *Hepatology: a textbook of liver disease,* ed 4, Philadelphia, 2003, WB Saunders.

Huber D: Does the "C" in hepatitis C stand for complex? *Gastroenterol Nurs* 24(3):120-6, 2001 (electronic version).

LaBrecque DR et al: Controversies in hepatitis C therapy, 2002, retrieved from *http://www.medscape.com/viewprogram/2053_pnt* on Nov 21, 2002.

Lawrence V et al: Milk thistle: effects on liver disease and cirrhosis and clinical adverse effects, Evidence Report/ Technology Assessment No. 21, AHRQ Pub No. 01-E025, Rockville, Md, October 2000, Agency for Healthcare Research and Quality, retrieved from *http://www.ahrqu.gov/ clinic/epcsums/milktsum.htm* on May 23, 2003.

Lee SP, Ko CW: Gallstones. In Yamada T, editor: *Textbook of gastroenterology,* ed 3, Philadelphia, 2000, Lippincott Williams and Wilkins.

MRI Pancreatitis Support Group: A decade of research yields treatment for pancreatic disease, retrieved from *http://pancreaticdisease.com/info/ info9.htm* on Aug 30, 2002.

National Center for Complementary and Alternative Medicine: Hepatitis C and complementary and alternative medicine: 2003 update, Pub No. D004, NCCAM Clearinghouse, Bethesda, Md, 2003, National Institutes of Health, retrieved from *http://nccam.nih.gov/health/hepatitisc/* on Jan 15, 2004.

National Institute of Diabetes and Digestive and Kidney Diseases: Chronic hepatitis C: current disease management, NIH Pub No. 02-4230, Bethesda, Md, 2002, National Institutes of Health, retrieved from *http://www.niddk. nih.gov/health/digest/pubs/chrnhepc/chrnhepc.htm* on Aug 27, 2002.

Owyang C: Chronic pancreatitis. In Yamada T, editor: *Textbook of gastroenterology,* vol 2, ed 3, Philadelphia, 2000, Lippincott Williams and Wilkins, pp 2151-77.

Reddy KR: Public-health impact, natural history, diagnosis, and clinical management of hepatitis C: emerging clinical options with interferon-based therapies, retrieved from *http://www.medscape.com/viewprogram/ 1809* on Nov 20, 2002.

Riley TR, Bhatti AM: Preventive strategies in chronic liver disease, Part I: alcohol, vaccines, toxic medications and supplements, diet and exercise, *Am Fam Physician* 64(9):1555-60, 2001.

Sellers K: Hydration and chronic pancreatitis [National Pancreas Foundation website], 2002, retrieved from *http://www.pancreasfoundation.org/ hydration.html* on Nov 26, 2002.

Shepp PH, Chase P, Rawls E: Pancreatitis partners: a sharing and educational support group, *Gastroenterol Nurs* 22(4):155-7, 1999 (electronic version).

Useful herbal medicines, retrieved from *http://www.hepatitis-c.de/useful. htm* on Aug 30, 2002.

CHAPTER 18

Chronic Kidney Disease

Leslie Jean Neal, PhD, RN, FNP-C

OBJECTIVES

After reading this chapter, you should be able to do the following:

- Describe the pathophysiology of chronic kidney disease (CKD)
- Describe the clinical manifestations of CKD
- Describe the functional health patterns affected by CKD
- Describe the role of each member of the interdisciplinary team involved in the care of persons with CKD
- Describe the indications for use of some drugs commonly employed to treat CKD
- Describe the latest trends with regard to dialysis and transplantation

---

The term *chronic kidney disease (CKD)* is now used to encompass all of the chronic disease entities that contribute to the ultimate failure of the kidney. Experts say that CKD is at epidemic levels. The highest incidence of end-stage-renal disease (ESRD), the final outcome of CKD, is seen in older adults between the ages of 65 and 84 years. The incidence is rising, so that by the year 2030 more than 20% of the population in the United States aged 65 and older will have CKD. The incidence is increasing by 6% to 8% or 50,000 people each year. The cost of ESRD is estimated to be more than $20 billion (National Kidney Foundation, 2002)

Diabetes mellitus (DM) and hypertension account for 75% to 80% of all ESRD cases that result from cardiovascular disease. CKD (defined in some reports as a serum creatinine [SCr] level of 1.5 mg/dl or higher) currently affects 6.2 million people; 16 million people have DM, and 50 million have hypertension (National Kidney Foundation, 2002).

In the United States the prevalence of kidney damage (defined as a glomerular filtration rate [GFR] of less than 90 ml/min/1.73 m^2) is more than 10 million cases. Approximately 300,000 individuals have kidney failure (GFR is lower than 15 ml/min/1.73 m^2 or the patient is on dialysis). In total, 22 million to 24 million people in the United States have CKD if one uses the GFR value as the criterion for CKD (National Kidney Foundation, 2002). If one uses the laboratory-determined SCr level as the criterion, then 6.2 million people in the United States have CKD. (The reader is cautioned to note that cutoff laboratory values for chronic renal failure and ESRD may vary according to the source.

ASSESSMENT

CKD is underrecognized and therefore undertreated in the United States because of controversy regarding the classification of CKD (National Kidney Foundation, 2002). The current trend in diagnosing CKD is to use the GFR as the diagnostic criterion. SCr level has traditionally been used to identify the presence of kidney disease. However, studies have found that a great opportunity exists for inaccurate results when SCr level alone is used. Normal SCr level is considered to be 0.8 to 1.5 mg/dl. However, due to the renal reserve, plasma levels of blood urea nitrogen and SCr increase after GFR decreases by 50%, and therefore SCr levels of 1.5 mg/dl for males and 1.2 mg/dl for females may indicate significant impairment of kidney function (National Kidney Foundation, 2002). Ultimately, CKD produces systemic symptoms because of its effects on the heart and circulation. Box 18-1 lists functional health patterns that are potentially disrupted by CKD and provides a framework for assessing its effects.

According to the National Kidney Foundation's Disease Outcome Quality Initiative (K/DOQI) (National Kidney Foundation, 2002), persons with CKD should be evaluated to determine the following:

- Type of kidney disease
- Comorbid conditions
- Risk for loss of kidney function
- Risk for cardiovascular disease
- Severity of the disease
- Complications present
- Medications taken and dosage needed based on kidney function
- Adverse effects of medication on the kidney
- Drug interactions that could impair kidney function
- Self-management behaviors

Box 18-1   Functional Health Pattern Assessment for Chronic Kidney Disease

HEALTH PERCEPTION/HEALTH MANAGEMENT
- What is the patient's family and personal history of chronic kidney disease, diabetes mellitus, and hypertension?
- What is the patient's perception of his or her overall health?
- What medications does the patient take?
- What alternative therapies does the patient use?

NUTRITION/METABOLISM
- What is the patient's current weight? Has there been any recent unexplained weight loss or gain?
- Is the patient on a special diet?
- What is the condition of the skin and mucous membranes?
- Is the patient on dialysis?
- What is the serum albumin level?

ELIMINATION
- Have any changes occurred in bowel or bladder habits?
- Does the patient have urinary retention?
- Is the patient on dialysis?

ACTIVITY/EXERCISE
- Does the patient experience fatigue or malaise?
- Is the patient able to perform regular and instrumental activities of daily living?

SLEEP/REST
- How many hours of uninterrupted sleep does the patient get at night?
- How often does the patient take naps or rest periods?
- Is the patient undergoing nocturnal dialysis?

COGNITION/PERCEPTION
- Does the patient experience pain?

SELF-PERCEPTION/SELF-CONCEPT
- How has the condition affected the patient's self-esteem?
- How has the condition changed the patient's body image?

ROLES/RELATIONSHIPS
- What kind of work does the patient perform?
- How has the patient's role in the home and family changed?
- What changes have occurred in the patient's ability to carry out role functions?
- How satisfied is the patient with his or her current roles and relationships?
- How has the condition affected the patient's family?

SEXUALITY/REPRODUCTION
- Is the patient sexually active?
- Has the patient experienced changes in sexual performance?
- Is the patient satisfied with current sexual patterns?
- Has the patient experienced any changes in the menstrual cycle?

COPING/STRESS TOLERANCE
- What are the patient's coping strategies?
- What support systems are available to the patient?
- Can the patient manage the condition in the current setting?

VALUES/BELIEFS
- What constitutes good quality of life for the patient?
- What is important to the patient?
- What are the patient's beliefs about locus of control?
- What are the patient's beliefs related to this condition?
- What are the patient's beliefs about death and dying?
- What are the issues for the patient regarding transplantation?
- To what extent do the patient's cultural/spiritual beliefs influence decision making related to this condition?

Ethnic Variations

Risk factors for CKD include advancing age, male gender, and race. A person who has a primary relative with a history of kidney disease has an almost 10-fold increase in risk for developing CKD. Both males and females are affected by CRF. However, males are more likely to have ESRD. Native Americans have the highest incidence of DM, which increases their risk of CKD. African Americans have the second highest risk of DM; however, this group has the highest overall incidence of CKD (National Kidney Foundation, 2002). The white population has the lowest incidence of ESRD.

PATHOPHYSIOLOGY

According to the K/DOQI, CKD includes "conditions that affect the kidney, with the potential to cause either progressive loss of kidney function or complications resulting from decreased kidney function … the presence of kidney damage or decreased level of kidney function for three months or more, irrespective of diagnosis" (National Kidney Foundation, 2002, p. S18) (Box 18-2).

The GFR reflects the ability of the glomerulus, a network of capillaries that loop into Bowman's capsule, to filter plasma. The glomerulus and Bowman's capsule comprise the renal corpuscle. Phagocytic cells support the glomerular capillaries and secrete vasoactive substances that influence the GFR. The glomerular filtration membrane has three layers, each with unique properties that allow filtration of blood components, except blood cells and heavy plasma proteins. The glomerular filtrate passes through the layers and becomes urine (Huether, 2002).

The GFR is the rate of filtration of plasma per unit of time and is related to perfusion pressure in the kidneys and to renal blood flow. Autoregulation, neural regulation, and hormonal regulation influence the GFR. Decreased arterial pressure causes the arteriole to relax and renal blood flow to increase. Fluid loss or a decrease in blood pressure affects

Box 18-2 Definition of Chronic Kidney Disease

1. Kidney damage for ≥3 months, as defined by structural or functional abnormalities of the kidney, with or without decreased glomerular filtration rate (GFR), as manifested by either of the following:
   ■ Pathologic abnormalities
   ■ Markers of kidney damage, including abnormalities in the composition of the blood or urine, or abnormalities on imaging tests
2. GFR of <60 ml/min/1.73 m² for ≥3 months, with or without kidney damage

From National Kidney Foundation: K/DOQI clinical practice guidelines for chronic kidney disease: evaluation, classification, and stratification, *Am J Kidney Dis* 39(2 suppl 1):S1-S266, 2002.

the secretion of renin, which converts angiotensin I to angiotensin II. This ultimately causes the secretion of aldosterone and antidiuretic hormone, which leads to the retention of sodium and water in the kidney. In addition, when the systemic arterial pressure decreases, the sympathetic nervous system responds by stimulating vasoconstriction, which decreases renal blood flow and reduces the GFR. The retention of sodium and water by the kidney increases blood volume and thereby increases blood pressure. If blood pressure is high, afferent arterioles constrict and restrict glomerular blood flow and filtration pressure. These mechanisms are part of the body's means of compensating for physiologic changes (Huether, 2002).

Hypertension is strongly associated with CKD because high systemic blood pressure leads to restriction of renal blood flow. Interestingly, hypertension may either cause CKD or be a consequence of it. According to the K/DOQI, "high blood pressure is associated with faster progression of CKD, development of cardiovascular disease, and likely, higher mortality in patients with chronic kidney disease" (National Kidney Foundation, 2002, p. S115). Studies have shown that a high number of patients with a low GFR and patients beginning dialysis have left ventricular hypertrophy, a consequence of hypertension. In addition, a strong association is seen between blood pressure and increased speed of progression of diabetic kidney disease and between high blood pressure and a declining GFR rate in nondiabetic kidney disease (National Kidney Foundation, 2002).

As the GFR decreases, kidney function is progressively impaired. The K/DOQI defines progression as (1) decreased kidney function as measured by the GFR, creatinine clearance, or SCr level, or (2) the beginning of kidney failure defined by the need to begin dialysis or to perform a kidney transplant (National Kidney Foundation, 2002). For diabetic patients with kidney disease, proteinuria is also used as a criterion.

In addition to the nonmodifiable risk factors mentioned in the section on ethnic variations, there are modifiable risk factors that play a significant role. Proteinuria, low serum albumin level, high blood pressure (over 140/90), poor glycemic control in patients with DM, smoking, dyslipidemia, and anemia have each been associated with a faster rate of decline in GFR (National Kidney Foundation, 2002). Table 18-1 lists the estimated prevalences of CKD associated with modifiable and nonmodifiable risk factors.

Of those with insulin-dependent DM, 80% develop nephropathy within 15 years if they have had sustained microalbuminuria, and 50% of these progress to kidney failure. Among those with non–insulin-dependent DM, nephropathy develops in 20% to 40% and leads to kidney failure in 20% of cases (National Kidney Foundation, 2002).

Various types of kidney disease predispose to CKD. These susceptibilities are listed in Table 18-2. Several types of kidney disease have been grouped under the label CKD. Table 18-3 lists these diseases, outlines their causes, and gives the prevalence of these diseases among persons with ESRD.

CLINICAL MANIFESTATIONS

According to one nephrologist, creatinine clearance should be the fifth vital sign (Sethi, 2001). The reason is that renal

Table 18-1 Prevalence of Individuals at Increased Risk for Chronic Kidney Disease (CKD)

Risk Factor	Estimated % with Risk Factor Who Have CKD
Diabetes mellitus	Diagnosed: 5.1% of adults ≥20 years of age Undiagnosed: 2.7% of adults ≥20 years of age
Hypertension	24% of adults ≥18 years of age
Systemic lupus erythematosus	~0.05% definite or suspected
Functioning kidney graft	~0.03%
African American race	12.3%
Hispanic or Latino ethnicity (any race)	12.5%
American Indian and Alaska native race	0.9%
Age 60-70 years	7.3%
Age >70 years	9.2%
Acute kidney failure	0.14%
Daily use of nonsteroidal antiinflammatory drug	~5.2% with rheumatoid arthritis or osteoarthritis (daily use assumed)

From National Kidney Foundation: K/DOQI clinical practice guidelines for chronic kidney disease: evaluation, classification, and stratification, *Am J Kidney Dis* 39(2 suppl 1):S74, 2002.

Table 18-2 Relationship Between Types of Kidney Disease and Risk Factors for Initiation of and Susceptibility to Chronic Kidney Disease (CKD)

Type of Kidney Disease	Risk Factors for CKD
Diabetes mellitus (DM) types 1 and 2	DM, high blood pressure, family history of CKD, membership in U.S. ethnic minority group
Glomerular diseases	Autoimmune diseases, systemic infections, neoplasia, drug or chemical exposure, family history
Vascular diseases	High blood pressure, family history of CKD, membership in U.S. ethnic minority group (non-Asian)
Tubulointerstitial diseases	Urinary tract infections, stones, obstruction, toxic drugs
Cystic diseases	Family history of CKD
Disease in the kidney transplant	Prior acute rejection, greater HLA mismatches, cyclosporine or tacrolimus therapy, glomerular disease in native kidneys

Adapted from National Kidney Foundation: K/DOQI clinical practice guidelines for chronic kidney disease: evaluation, classification, and stratification, *Am J Kidney Dis* 39(2 suppl 1):S74, 2002.

Table 18-3 Classification of Chronic Kidney Disease

Pathologic Findings	Selected Causes	Prevalence Among Patients with ESRD
Diabetic glomerulosclerosis	Diabetes mellitus types 1 and 2	33%
Glomerular disease (primary or secondary)	Systemic lupus erythematosus, vasculitis, bacterial endocarditis, chronic hepatitis B or C, HIV infection	19%
Proliferative glomerulonephritis		
Noninflammatory glomerular diseases	Hodgkin's disease	
Hereditary nephritis (Alport's syndrome)	HIV infection, heroin toxicity, drug toxicity, solid tumors, amyloidosis, light chain disease	
Vascular diseases		21%
Diseases of large vessels	Renal artery stenosis	
Diseases of medium-size vessels	Hypertension	
Nephrosclerosis		
Diseases of small vessels	Sickle cell disease, hemolytic uremic syndrome	
Microangiopathy		
Tubulointerstitial diseases		4%
Tubulointerstitial nephritis		
Pyelonephritis	Infection, stones	
Analgesic nephropathy	NSAID use	
Allergic interstitial nephritis	Antibiotic use	
Granulomatous interstitial nephritis	Sarcoidosis	
Autoimmune interstitial nephritis	Uveitis	
Noninflammatory tubulointerstitial diseases		
Reflux nephropathy	Vesicoureteral reflux	
Obstructive nephropathy	Malignancy, prostatism, stones	
Myeloma kidney	Multiple myeloma	
Cystic diseases	Autosomal dominant or recessive disorder	6%
Diseases in the kidney transplant	Cyclosporin or tacrolimus therapy	Not recorded as a cause of ESRD in the U.S. renal data system
	Glomerular diseases	

From National Kidney Foundation: K/DOQI clinical practice guidelines for chronic kidney disease: evaluation, classification, and stratification, *Am J Kidney Dis* 39(2 suppl 1):S67, 2002.
ESRD, End-stage renal disease; *HIV,* human immunodeficiency virus; *NSAID,* nonsteroidal antiinflammatory drug.

involvement and damage often go undiagnosed until late in the disease process because some measures of kidney function can be misleading. For example, GFR can be maintained with compensatory hyperfiltration and hypertrophy. In addition, the majority of kidney diseases are asymptomatic (National Kidney Foundation, 2002).

Current guidelines advise that patients be evaluated for risk for CKD based on certain standard criteria and that similar evaluation strategies then be implemented to prevent the progression of CKD. Thus, clinical manifestations of CKD include both laboratory indicators and the symptoms associated with the diseases that contribute to CKD. For example, persons with DM who show the typical signs and symptoms of DM may already have renal impairment. Individuals with hypertension, which is typically asymptomatic, may also have renal impairment. However, the K/DOQI (National Kidney Foundation, 2002) states that, even when the presence or stage of kidney disease has been identified, the practitioner should make an accurate assessment of the cause, extent of damage, level of overall function, presence of comorbidities, complications of decreased renal function, risk for cardiovascular disease, and loss of kidney function for a particular individual. The staging of CKD is to be used to help the practitioner apply appropriate clinical interventions and management strategies and should be tailored to the individual. Therefore, the focus is on diagnosis rather than on clinical manifestations.

DIAGNOSIS

Kidney damage is defined by the K/DOQI as "pathologic abnormalities or markers of damage, including abnormalities in blood or urine tests or imaging studies" (National Kidney Foundation, 2002, p. S46). GFR estimates are considered the most reliable indicators of kidney function. Equations are used to estimate the GFR. For adults, the Cockroft-Gault creatinine clearance formula or the MDRD (Modification of Diet in Renal Disease) study creatinine clearance formula is used. These formulas take into account variables such as age, gender, race, and body size as well as the SCr concentration, because SCr level is not a reliable measure of kidney function when used alone. The use of timed creatinine clearance tests does not yield better estimates of GFR than the use of prediction formulas. However, these tests are useful for estimating GFR in patients on special diets, for assessing nutritional status, and for determining the need for dialysis (National Kidney Foundation, 2002). A normal level for SCr in young adults is approximately 1.0 mg/dl (National Kidney Foundation, 2002).

Individuals with an estimated GFR of less than 60 ml/min/1.73 m^2 are considered to have CKD, and it is recommended that they be educated about their diagnosis and about the consequences of limited kidney function. Few data are available on the lower limit of normal GFR in elderly persons. Therefore, for elderly individuals with a low GFR, it is recommended that other CKD markers such as proteinuria and hypertension be evaluated (National Kidney Foundation, 2002).

DM, hypertension, and glomerular disease cause increased excretion of albumin (albuminuria is a more sensitive marker for CKD than is total protein for these diseases) and tubulointerstitial disease is usually accompanied by increased levels of low-molecular-weight globulins in the urine; therefore, proteinuria is an important indicator of CKD. According to the K/DOQI, untimed urine samples (morning samples are preferred) should be used for detection and monitoring of proteinuria in adults. Dipstick testing is acceptable to evaluate both total urine protein and albuminuria. If the dipstick test registers +1 or higher, then a quantitative measurement should be undertaken within 3 months to confirm proteinuria. If a patient has abnormal results on three or more quantitative tests within 1 to 2 weeks, then the individuals should be considered to have persistent proteinuria and should be further evaluated and managed for CKD (National Kidney Foundation, 2002).

Abnormalities in urine sediment and on imaging studies are other helpful CKD indicators. Individuals who have CKD or who are at risk for developing CKD should undergo urine sediment examination or dipstick testing for red and white blood cells, and imaging studies should be performed on selected at-risk individuals (National Kidney Foundation, 2002).

COMPLICATIONS

Early detection and treatment can prevent complications of CKD. The most common complications are hypertension, progression of kidney disease, diseases in a transplanted kidney, cardiovascular disease, and mortality. Anemia, poor nutritional status and its subsequent complications, and bone diseases and disorders also can occur.

The progression of CKD can be slowed by the following interventions (Sethi, 2002):

- Normalization of blood pressure (to less than 130/85)
- Normalization of protein intake
- Achievement of glycemic control (hemoglobin A_{1c} [HbA_{1c}] level less than 7%)
- Smoking cessation
- Avoidance of nephrotoxic drugs
- Normalization of lipid levels (low-density lipoprotein level less than 100 mg/dl)

Some factors that can lead to an acute decline in GFR include volume depletion, urinary tract obstruction, and use of various medications such as some antimicrobial agents, nonsteroidal antiinflammatory drugs including cyclooxygenase 2 inhibitors, angiotensin-converting enzyme (ACE) inhibitors, angiotensin II receptor blockers (ARBs), intravenous radiologic contrast media, cyclosporine, and tacrolimus. Persons with CKD should undergo annual testing for SCr level and estimation of GFR. Those with the following should be evaluated more frequently:

- GFR less than 60 ml/min/1.73 m^2
- Risk factors for fast progression
- Risk factors for acute GFR decline
- Rapid GFR decline in the past (more than 4 ml/min/1.73 m^2 per year)
- Ongoing treatment to slow progression

INTERDISCIPLINARY CARE

The care provided depends on the stage of the disease and the specific effects of the disease on the patient. As with other diseases or illnesses, nurses monitor the patient's status, provide the appropriate education, and collaborate with the physician. Therapists and nurses may provide strengthening exercises for patients who have experienced bone loss and muscle weakness as a result of ESRD (Colangelo et al, 1997). Dietitians are closely involved because diet is particularly important in managing chronic renal failure.

Drug Therapy

Drug therapy for persons with CKD is related to the disease that has contributed to CKD. Blood pressure should be controlled with ACE inhibitors and/or ARBs, β-blockers, α-blockers, or calcium channel blockers. Diuretics should be used with prudence. ACE inhibitors and ARBs provide cardiac protection, produce regression of left ventricular hypertrophy, reduce proteinuria, lead to regression of nephropathy, and delay the progression of renal ischemia (Sethi, 2002).

Drug therapy for patients with DM should be aimed at achieving excellent glycemic control. Insulin and/or oral agents and ACE inhibitors and ARBs should be used as needed. Persons with cardiovascular disease should be monitored to prevent disease progression. Those with CKD are at high risk for developing coronary artery disease. Individuals with anemia, protein malnutrition, or bone disease related to CKD should be treated accordingly. Once the patient has reached end-stage renal disease, therapy also includes drugs needed for successful dialysis and transplantation.

Cyclosporine is the drug credited with making transplantation possible. Cyclosporine and tacrolimus prevent transplant rejection. After the patient takes cyclosporine for 10 years, the drug becomes nephrotoxic and can cause hypertension, gingival hyperplasia, and hirsutism. Tacrolimus can cause DM but is a better immunosuppressant than cyclosporine. A new drug, sirolimus, is not known to be nephrotoxic but may raise cholesterol levels (Jonsson, 2002).

Dietitian

According to the K/DOQI, individuals whose GFR is less than 60 ml/min/1.73 m^2 should be assessed for dietary protein, energy intake, and nutritional status. Those with mal-nutrition or decreased dietary intake should be counseled regarding modification of the diet or specialized nutrition therapy (National Kidney Foundation, 2002). Protein and phosphorus restriction reduce the demands on the kidney, so calories must be derived from fats and carbohydrates for energy. Although sodium replacement may be needed initially to correct losses due to polyuria, sodium and fluid are otherwise restricted. Potassium may have to be restricted or reduced through dialysis. Metabolic acidosis may develop due to decreased renal excretion of hydrogen. This may cause cardiac dysfunction or muscle wasting. Calcium is often provided as a supplement to prevent bone deterioration and to restore phosphorus and calcium homeostasis. Other dietary restrictions may be necessary due to comorbidities and dialysis requirements (Kear, 2002).

Primary Provider (Physician/Nurse Practitioner)

The recommendation is that patients be referred to a nephrologist when the SCr level is above 1.2 mg/dl in females and above 1.5 mg/dl in males, and the GFR is less than 60 to 75 ml/min/1.73 m^2; thus, patients may be monitored closely by physician specialists before they become symptomatic and require interdisciplinary care. In fact, it has been suggested that primary care providers treat at-risk patients with stage 1 or 2 disease but work with the nephrologist as the disease begins to enter stage 3. By the time stage 5 is reached, the nephrologist is managing the care of the patient (Sethi, 2002).

The management goals for CKD vary depending on the comorbid conditions present (Table 18-4).

The K/DOQI has recommended a clinical action plan for each stage of CKD (Table 18-5).

Nurse

Nurses are involved in teaching health promotion strategies to patients and their families and in managing the symptoms and sequelae of renal disease, many of which are listed in Box 18-3.

Nurses play an important role in caring for patients who are on dialysis or are preparing for or undergoing transplant surgery.

TRENDS IN DIALYSIS

Dialysis is a mechanical means by which the patient's blood is filtered of toxins and waste products and electrolyte and fluid balance are restored (Visovsky, 2002) (Figure 18-1). Traditionally, peritoneal dialysis and hemodialysis were delivered within the hospital or outpatient setting. Home hemodialysis has become more common, but the number of people using this method is still very small compared with the number who receive hemodialysis in an outpatient center. Two new options for dialysis, nocturnal dialysis and daily short dialysis, are beginning to make the process of dialysis easier and more effective for persons with ESRD.

Table 18-4   Management Goals for Chronic Kidney Disease (CKD) with Comorbid Conditions

Type of Comorbid Condition	Examples	Management Goals
Disease causing CKD	Diabetes mellitus Hypertension Urinary tract obstruction	Improve CKD Improve functioning and well-being Integrate care with management of CKD
Disease unrelated to CKD	Chronic obstructive pulmonary disease Gastroesophageal reflux disease Degenerative joint disease Alzheimer's disease Malignancies	Improve function and well-being Integrate care with management of CKD
Cardiovascular disease	Atherosclerosis Left ventricular hypertrophy Heart failure	Evaluate for and manage traditional CKD-related cardiovascular risk factors Possibly improve CKD Improve function and well-being Integrate care with management of CKD

From National Kidney Foundation: K/DOQI clinical practice guidelines for chronic kidney disease: evaluation, classification, and stratification, *Am J Kidney Dis* 39(2 suppl 1):S68, 2002.

Nocturnal Dialysis*

Nocturnal dialysis began to be used in 1994 but is still not widely practiced throughout the United States. Nocturnal dialysis more closely mimics the functioning of the human kidney because dialysis occurs over a 10- to 12-hour period (the normal kidney functions 24 hours a day). The patient sleeps so that a slower and gentler dialysate can be used than is used for daytime dialysis. Patients who will receive nocturnal dialysis undergo 6 weeks of training during which time they sleep at the dialysis unit or hospital. The cumulative solute removal is analyzed at the end of each week and has been found to be consistently higher than with other

*Adapted from Krishnan M: Treatment options: nocturnal dialysis et al, paper presented at the meeting Survivors: Women with CKD, Fairfax, Va, October 2002.

forms of dialysis. In addition, other benefits have been found:

- Blood pressure is frequently normal without medications.
- Anemia improves so that less erythropoietin is required.
- Diet and fluids are not restricted.
- Sleep patterns return to normal.
- The person's general sense of well-being increases, and the person experiences less weakness and fatigue.
- Phosphate removal is improved so that patients can stop taking calcium supplements.
- If the catheter becomes dislodged, a few days instead of minutes or hours are available to correct the fluid overload.
- Albumin levels are improved so that the risk of death is decreased.

Table 18-5   Clinical Action Plans for Various Stages of Chronic Kidney Disease

Stage	Description	GFR (ml/min/1.73 m^2)	Action*
1	Kidney damage with normal or high GFR	≥90	Diagnosis and treatment Treatment of comorbid conditions Slowing of disease progression Reduction of cardiovascular disease risk
2	Kidney damage with mildly decreased GFR	60-89	Estimation of progression
3	Moderately decreased GFR	30-59	Evaluation and treatment of complications
4	Severely decreased GFR	15-29	Preparation for kidney replacement therapy
5	Kidney failure	<15 (or dialysis)	Kidney replacement (if uremia is present)

From National Kidney Foundation: K/DOQI clinical practice guidelines for chronic kidney disease: evaluation, classification, and stratification, *Am J Kidney Dis* 39(2 suppl 1):S65, 2002.
GFR, Glomerular filtration rate.
*Actions at each stage also include all actions for preceding stages.

Box 18-3 Components of Kidney Disease Requiring Nursing Interventions

- Changes in urinary function (polyuria, oliguria)
- Lethargy, fatigue
- Headaches, confusion related to increased blood urea nitrogen level
- Altered carbohydrate metabolism
- Dyslipidemia
- Gastrointestinal changes (nausea, vomiting, ulcerations, stomatitis, constipation, diarrhea)
- Skin changes (yellowish coloration; pruritus; dry, brittle hair and nails)
- Reproductive changes (infertility, decreased libido)
- Imbalances in fluid and electrolytes (potassium, calcium, phosphate, magnesium, sodium)
- Cardiovascular changes (anemia, hypertension, congestive heart failure, clotting abnormalities, uremic pericarditis)
- Respiratory changes (Kussmaul's respirations, dyspnea, uremic lung)
- Neurologic changes related to increased levels of toxins in the blood
- Musculoskeletal changes (renal osteodystrophy, osteomalacia)
- Thyroid function impairment (hypothyroidism)
- Personality and behavioral changes (emotional lability, withdrawal, depression)

Adapted Brunier G, Bartucci M: Acute and chronic renal failure. In Lewis SM, Heitkemper MM, Dirksen SR, editors: *Medical-surgical nursing*, ed 5, St Louis, 2000, Mosby, pp 1299-1341.

- Hospitalizations are decreased (hospitalizations for ESRD are usually due to fluid overload, infection, or electrolyte imbalances).
- In individuals with coexisting congestive heart failure, ejection fraction improves, extracellular fluid volume decreases, and left ventricular mass indices decrease.

Daily Short Dialysis*

A method of dialysis consisting of daily short periods of dialysis at home was introduced in 1996. Dialysis is administered in a 2- to 2½-hour session each day. The following benefits have been found:

- The need for erythropoietin therapy is decreased.
- Blood pressure decreases.
- The average number of hospitalizations declines.
- Total monetary savings per patient is approximately $4000.
- Quality of life is improved and employment increases.
- The average number of medications taken and the use of phosphate binders are decreased.

TRANSPLANTATION

Indications for kidney transplantation include end-stage renal failure as well as individual social factors, financial circumstances, and reproductive considerations for the person with

---

*Adapted from Krishnan M: Treatment options: nocturnal dialysis et al, paper presented at the meeting Survivors: Women with CKD, Fairfax, Va, October 2002.

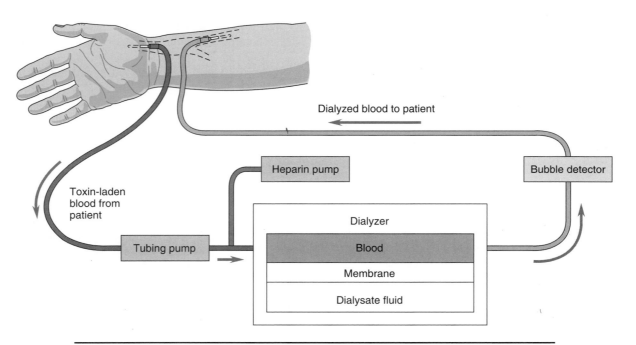

Figure 18-1 Hemodialysis. (From Copstead LC, Banasik JL: *Pathophysiology: biological and behavioral perspectives,* ed 2, Philadelphia, 2000, WB Saunders.)

CKD. For example, women are more likely to give birth successfully after transplantation, and some people cannot afford to continue dialysis for long periods (Jonsson, 2002).

The two most common types of transplant are cadaveric and living donor transplants. A living kidney donor may be related or unrelated to the patient. Surgery may be performed laparoscopically or abdominally as an open procedure. The use of transplants from living donors produces better long-term outcomes and may help some individuals avoid dialysis altogether. It is predicted that pig kidneys may be used for transplant in the future (Jonsson, 2002), and genetic or stem cell research might offer the prospect of a cure.

Think S for Success

SYMPTOMS
- Manage risk factors for chronic kidney disease (CKD); include creatinine clearance as a vital sign; monitor proteinuria.

SEQUELAE
- Prevent progression of CKD; consider new forms of dialysis; transplant early when possible.

SAFETY
- Teach patient and family the following:
  Definition and description of CKD
  Risk factors for developing CKD
  Ways of managing CKD
  Methods of preventing complications and progression of CKD
  Indications and contraindications of medications and treatments

SUPPORT/SERVICES
- Refer patient to financial and social support services and assistance when necessary. Patients and families waiting for a kidney for transplantation may need much encouragement and support.

SATISFACTION
- Determine the degree to which CKD is interfering with patient's lifestyle and develop a plan to help patient reach a desired quality of life.

END-OF-LIFE ISSUES

Persons with ESRD may face the same kind of end-of-life issues faced by others with a terminal disease. CKD is not curable, only manageable. Those with end-stage disease who are not candidates for transplantation require assistance to move through the stages of grief associated with a terminal illness. Families and caregivers also need support at this time. The patient can be in the end stage for a long period that varies according to the individual. Health care providers must recognize the signs of readiness in the patient and family to discuss and learn about end-of-life issues. Palliative care and pain control may play a role at varying times as the patient becomes less responsive to dialysis and other treatments. Pain is an issue during transplant recovery for both the donor and recipient. As always, it is vital that the nurse and other team members assess for pain and recognize the emotional issues that may arise.

FAMILY AND CAREGIVER ISSUES

Family members and caregivers may notice a significant alteration in lifestyle once a patient begins dialysis. Dialysis treatments are typically given from three to five times per week. Some patients need transportation to and from the dialysis facility. In addition, persons with CKD may require many medications and may need help in monitoring medication use. Persons on dialysis typically take 14 different medications.

Some family members and caregivers may resent the alteration in lifestyle, especially if they are angry with the patient for not taking care of himself or herself by controlling blood pressure or blood glucose levels over the years. They must be helped to recognize and manage these feelings so that they and the patient can maximize the quality of their remaining time together. Family members may be asked to donate a kidney for transplantation. The surgery is associated with a difficult recovery period and carries certain risks. Some family members experience guilt if they are uncomfortable considering kidney donation. Other family members expect something in return from the patient to whom they have donated a kidney. Referral to a medical social worker, psychologist, or psychiatrist may be helpful.

ETHICAL ISSUES

Various ethical dilemmas are likely to arise when dialysis and transplantation are being considered. Some issues concern the financial burden of providing dialysis or transplantation to a person who has several serious comorbidities and may have a small chance of surviving or enjoying an increased length or quality of remaining life. Other issues involve what the priority ranking of those on transplant lists should be and who is more entitled to receive a kidney than others on the list. Additional dilemmas are likely to arise as the technologies to manage and ultimately cure CKD (such as stem cell research) improve and expand.

CASE STUDY

Patient Data

Mrs. H. is a 60-year-old African American housewife. She has been newly diagnosed with DM type 2. She lives with her husband, two adult children, and three grandchildren in a small house near a major city. She is an active church member and spends a lot of her time helping friends and neighbors who are elderly and ill. She has been hypertensive for 10 years but does not always remember to take her medicine. A family history of hypertension and DM type 2 is noted. Mrs. H. is 5 ft 3 inches tall and weighs 200 lb. She was diagnosed with DM during a visit to her nurse practitioner, at which time she complained of polyuria, polyphagia, and polydipsia. A urine dipstick test in the office showed proteinuria and glucosuria. She also had her HbA_{1c} level measured that day and returned on another day to have her fasting blood glucose level tested.

Diagnostic Findings

HbA_{1c} level = 7%
Fasting blood glucose level = 130 mg/dl
Dipstick test for proteinuria: positive

Thinking It Through

■ What further testing, if any, should be done to satisfy the diagnosis of DM type 2?
■ Is there sufficient indication to place Mrs. H. on an oral antidiabetic agent?
■ Is there sufficient evidence to monitor Mrs. H. for CKD?
■ What are Mrs. H.'s concerns likely to be? How would you address them?
■ What might you do to increase the likelihood of adherence to a regimen to help slow the progression of CKD?

Case Conference

The interdisciplinary team that has gathered to discuss Mrs. H.'s case includes the nurse practitioner, the nephrologist, the endocrinologist, the dietitian, the registered nurse case manager, and Mr. and Mrs. H. The team has already reviewed the available data, which includes results of another fasting blood glucose measurement, a random measurement of blood glucose level, a blood chemistry panel, and a urinalysis.

The nephrologist presents his estimate of Mrs. H.'s GFR as well as her SCr level and albumin and total protein levels. He recommends that a urine sediment examination be conducted to further assist in predicting Mrs. H.'s risk for CKD. Mrs. H.'s estimated GFR is 90 ml/min/1.73 m². This value indicates that Mrs. H. is in stage 1 of CKD. The nephrologist suggests that she and the nurse practitioner work together with Mrs. H. to manage Mrs. H.'s care and slow the progression of CKD.

The endocrinologist reports that Mrs. H.'s HbA_{1c} level has remained at 7%, her fasting blood glucose level is 126 mg/dl, and her random blood glucose level is 200 mg/dl. He recommends that Mrs. H. be taught strict dietary management and glycemic control. He wants to give this approach a trial for 3 months before prescribing an oral antidiabetic agent.

The dietitian states that she has already begun to teach Mrs. H. about dietary and exercise management (exercise will be started once the patient receives clearance from a cardiologist after stress testing) and has provided her with oral and written instructions. She intends to meet with Mrs. H. in a month to monitor her progress. Mrs. H. comments that she is "feeling a bit overwhelmed by all of this" but will try very hard to watch her diet and follow everyone's instructions. Mr. H. laughs and says he'll be there by her side to "make sure she does!"

The nurse case manager remarks that she will reinforce the diet teaching and will obtain a glucometer and lancets for Mrs. H. and teach her how to use them and how to record her blood glucose levels. She makes sure that Mr. and Mrs. H. have her telephone numbers and understand that she will be the one to help them keep all of the regimens and health care providers straight.

Mr. H. speaks up and reluctantly admits that he is concerned about how to pay for all of this. The nurse case manager responds that she will be working with their health insurance representatives and with a medical social worker to help them to find ways of managing costs. She recommends that the physicians and the nurse practitioner prescribe generic medications when possible and provide samples of medication to the H.'s if they can.

Mr. H. is still concerned but states that he feels reassured that everyone will help them. He notes that their children and grandchildren are loving and supportive and comments that "that's a help." The team meeting concludes and the nurse case manager returns to her office to consider the results of the case conference.

■ What new information was gathered and how will it help the nurse design and monitor a plan of care?
■ What strengths do Mr. and Mrs. H. bring to the team?
■ What barriers must be overcome?
■ What are the potential positive and negative consequences of a collaboration between professionals in multiple specialists and disciplines in a complex case such as this case may become if Mrs.'s CKD progresses?

Internet and Other Resources

Kidney School: *http://www.kidneyschool.org*
National Guideline Clearinghouse (NGC): *http://www.guideline.gov*
National Institute of Diabetes and Digestive and Kidney Diseases (NIDDK): *http://www.niddk.nih.gov*
National Kidney Foundation (NKF): *http://www.kidney.org*

REFERENCES

Colangelo RM et al: The role of exercise in rehabilitation for patients with end-stage renal disease, *Rehabil Nurs* 22(6):288-92, 1997.
Huether SE: In McCance KL, Huether SE, editors: *Pathophysiology: the biologic basis for disease in adults and children*, ed 4, St Louis, 2002, Mosby, pp 1170-90.
Jonsson J: Transplant 2002, paper presented at the meeting Survivors: Women with CKD, Fairfax, Va, October 2002.
Kear TM: Nutritional management of renal failure, *Adv Nurses*, pp 23-4, April 15, 2002.
National Kidney Foundation: K/DOQI clinical practice guidelines for chronic kidney disease: evaluation, classification, and stratification, *Am J Kidney Dis* 39(2 suppl 1):S1-S266, 2002.
Sethi K: Evaluation of CKD care: what is CKD?, paper presented at the meeting Survivors: Women with CKD, Fairfax, Va, October 2002.
Visovsky C: Interventions for clients with acute and chronic renal failure. In Ignatavicius D, Workman M, editors: *Medical surgical nursing: critical thinking for collaborative care*, ed 4, Philadelphia, 2002, WB Saunders, pp 1664-1703.

CHAPTER 19

Disorders of the Urinary Bladder

Leslie Jean Neal, PhD, RN, FNP-C

OBJECTIVES

After reading this chapter, you should be able to do the following:

- Describe the pathophysiology of urinary incontinence and retention
- Describe the clinical manifestations of urinary incontinence and retention
- Describe the functional health patterns affected by urinary incontinence and retention
- Describe the role of each member of the interdisciplinary team involved in the care of persons with urinary incontinence or retention
- Describe the indications for use, side effects, and nursing considerations related to drugs commonly used to treat urinary incontinence or retention

OVERVIEW OF CHRONIC BLADDER DISORDERS

Over 13 million Americans have some type of voiding dysfunction (Dugan, Roberts, and Cohen, 2001). Voiding dysfunction, including urinary incontinence and retention, affects men and women, although urinary incontinence is more commonly seen in women and its incidence increases as women age (Newman and Giovannini, 2002). The care of people with voiding dysfunction costs more than $16 billion per year (Copstead and Banasik, 2000).

Urinary incontinence is defined as a voiding dysfunction in which the person is unable to control when urination occurs (Copstead and Banasik, 2000). Retention is the inability to empty the bladder fully (Gaynes, 2001).

ASSESSMENT

Individuals with chronic bladder impairment share common concerns that primarily center on social isolation and embarrassment. Those with chronic urinary incontinence may consider it a normal part of aging and may not describe their symptoms unless pressed (Dugan, Roberts, and Cohen, 2002). In a study sponsored by the Agency for Healthcare Research and Quality (AHRQ), those who did

not discuss their incontinence tended to be older and less bothered by leaking episodes than those who reported the problem. Even those who reported a fairly high frequency of incontinent episodes (average of 1.7 per day) did not consider incontinence to be either abnormal or a medical condition. The study found that the perception that incontinence is a normal part of getting older outweighed embarrassment or lack of awareness regarding treatment as a cause of underreporting of incontinence (Dugan, Roberts, and Cohen, 2001).

When people do inform health care providers about a problem with voiding dysfunction, the concerns they typically express are about the odor of urine or the interruption of daily activities by the need to void frequently. Limitations on activities outside the home, sexual dysfunction, reduced self-esteem, increased financial costs of managing incontinence, and skin breakdown and infection are all possible sequelae of incontinence.

Persons with urinary retention may be asymptomatic, because urinary retention tends to develop slowly. However, patients may experience pain and frequent urges to urinate. These symptoms may also cause the person to isolate himself or herself from others. In addition, urinary retention may lead to urinary incontinence.

Incontinence and retention may significantly alter functional health patterns (Box 19-1). Assessment specific to each condition of bladder impairment is discussed in detail in this chapter.

Ethnic Variations

The current literature does not indicate any ethnic variations in the incidence or prevalence of urinary incontinence or retention. However, urinary incontinence is associated with certain diseases, such as diabetes mellitus and multiple sclerosis, that do have associations with ethnicity.

PATHOPHYSIOLOGY

Micturition or the process of urination occurs because parasympathetic stimulation of the detrusor muscle causes the bladder to contract and sympathetic stimulation causes relaxation of the bladder sphincter so that urine is released from the bladder and urethra (Copstead and Banasik, 2000).

Box 19-1 Functional Health Pattern Assessment for Urinary Bladder Disorders

HEALTH PERCEPTION/HEALTH MANAGEMENT
- Does the patient view incontinence as normal?
- What medications, including over-the-counter drugs, does the patient take?
- What alternative therapies does the patient use?

ELIMINATION
- Does the patient have retention, as evidenced by pain, difficulty urinating, frequency, or urgency?
- Does the patient have incontinence, as evidence by frequency, urgency, or lack of bladder control?
- Does the patient lose urine and, if so, under what circumstances?

ACTIVITY/EXERCISE
- Does the condition affect the patient's ability to perform instrumental and other activities of daily living?
- Does the incontinence increase with movement?

SLEEP/REST
- Is sleep interrupted because of the need to urinate or change bed linens?

COGNITION/PERCEPTION
- Does the patient have pain due to retention?
- Does the patient experience burning due to bladder infection?

SELF-PERCEPTION/SELF-CONCEPT
- How has the condition changed the patient's body image?
- How has the condition affected the patient's self-esteem?

ROLES/RELATIONSHIPS
- What kind of work does the patient perform?
- Does the patient avoid social interaction?
- How satisfied is the patient with his or her current roles and relationships?

SEXUALITY/REPRODUCTION
- Is the patient sexually active?
- Has the condition affected the patient's sexual patterns?

COPING/STRESS TOLERANCE
- What coping strategies does the patient use?
- What support systems are available to the patient?
- Can the patient manage the condition in the current setting?

VALUES/BELIEFS
- What are the patient's beliefs about locus of control?
- What constitutes good quality of life for the patient?
- What is important to the patient?
- What are the patient's beliefs related to this condition?
- To what extent do the patient's cultural/spiritual beliefs influence decision making related to this condition?

Normal function of the urinary system depends on four basic factors (Rogers, Amador, and Bryan, 2000):
- Anatomic integrity
- Intact neurologic components for both voluntary control and synergistic emptying
- A predictable pattern of waste production
- Physical and mental ability and the psychological willingness to carry out toilet-related tasks

Any disruption in the process or in any of the aforementioned factors can cause voiding dysfunction. Immobility, confusion, or side effects of medications may contribute to urinary incontinence either by interfering with the person's ability to get to a toilet in time to void or by influencing the process of micturition (Copstead and Banasik, 2000).

Aging results in changes that contribute to the incidence of urinary incontinence and retention. Prostate enlargement increases urethral resistance, which leads to obstruction and causes the bladder to hypertrophy; the result is urinary retention. Menopause decreases estrogen levels and pelvic floor muscle tone. Thinning urethral mucosa and herniation of the urinary organs reduce urethral resistance. These factors contribute to urinary stress incontinence. A decreased bladder capacity associated with aging contributes to urgency and frequency, and increased detrusor contractions also contribute to urgency, frequency, and incontinence (Figure 19-1). Functional changes and medications may influence voiding dysfunction (Pires, 2002). Urinary incontinence is typically classified based on its symptomatology. Urinary incontinence and retention are discussed together because they often occur alternately and frequently have similar causes.

CLINICAL MANIFESTATIONS

Urge incontinence is urinary incontinence that is accompanied by a strong urge to void in response to overactivity of the detrusor muscle. The involuntary detrusor contractions may or may not be neurologic in orgin. If there is no neurologic abnormality, then the bladder is considered to be unstable; if a neurologic deficit is present, then the involuntary contraction is termed *detrusor hyperreflexia.* Detrusor hyperreflexia is frequently associated with stroke, multiple sclerosis, and suprasacral spinal cord lesions. When accompanied by external sphincter dyssynergia, as in the two latter conditions, urinary retention and renal damage may also occur (AHRQ, 1996).

Approximately 90% of cases of urge incontinence have no known cause. Back pain and cerebral vascular disease have been associated with urge incontinence, although the reason is unknown (Newman and Giovannini, 2002).

Stress incontinence is common in middle-aged women who have had children by vaginal delivery. Laxity of the

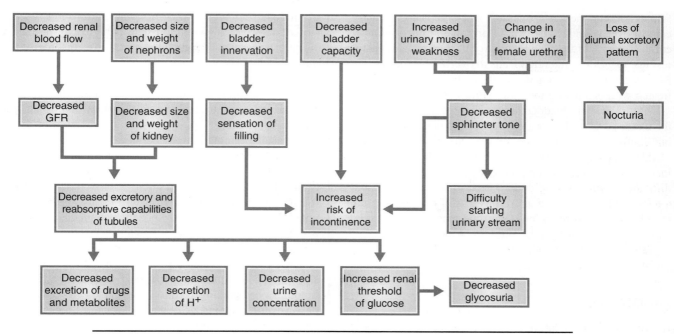

Figure 19-1 Changes in the renal system during the aging process. (From Copstead LC, Banasik JL: *Pathophysiology: biological and behavioral perspectives,* ed 2, Philadelphia, 2000, WB Saunders.)

pubococcygeus muscle, combined with increased intraabdominal pressure, contributes to leakage of urine, especially when the woman laughs, sneezes, or rises to a standing position. Men may experience stress incontinence following a prostatectomy. Mixed incontinence occurs when a person experiences both urge and stress incontinence.

Overflow incontinence refers to the dribbling that results when the bladder is overdistended. Urinary retention may also contribute to this type of incontinence. Overflow incontinence may be secondary to obstruction, detrusor underactivity, or a malfunction of the sphincter. Detrusor underactivity may be caused by medications, fecal impaction, radical pelvic surgery, low spinal cord lesion, diabetic neuropathy, vitamin B_{12} deficiency, or bladder weakness of unknown cause. Neurologic impairment or prostatic hyperplasia may cause overflow incontinence, and symptoms tend to resemble those of urge or stress incontinence (Copstead and Banasik, 2000). Women may also experience overflow incontinence as a result of pelvic prolapse into the vagina (AHRQ, 1996).

Functional incontinence is unrelated to internal or physiologic factors and occurs as a consequence of the inability to reach toilet facilities in time to void. Deficits in mobility, mental status, or physical ability contribute to functional incontinence. Other types of incontinence should always be ruled out before one decides on a diagnosis of functional incontinence (AHRQ, 1996).

Neurogenic causes of bladder dysfunction are related to neurologic injury. In uninhibited neurogenic bladder, the corticoregulatory tract or the supraspinal center is dysfunctional. Detrusor contractions are frequent and uninhibited, and the bladder empties completely. Because bladder capacity is decreased, urgency and involuntary voiding occur almost simultaneously. Urgency, frequency, and nocturia are common complaints (Pires, 2002).

Reflex neurogenic bladder (also called spastic or upper motor neuron bladder) occurs when motor and sensory tracts are unable to send messages to the bladder effectively. Involuntary and incomplete voiding occurs because of a lack of cerebral control. Detrusor muscle hypertrophy may eventually lead to renal damage. Reflex incontinence occurs because the individual does not sense that the bladder is full and cannot control voiding voluntarily. The bladder may contract while the external sphincter remains closed (detrusor sphincter dyssynergia), which causes resistance to outflow, high urine residuals, and incomplete emptying (Pires, 2002).

Autonomic neurogenic bladder (also called flaccid or lower motor neuron bladder) is caused by a disruption of sensory and motor impulses from the bladder to spinal cord to detrusor muscle to external sphincter. The individual experiences involuntary voiding when the bladder overflows. The person is unable to sense fullness and to start and stop voiding voluntarily. The external sphincter may have no motor activity or uncontrollable activity (Pires, 2002).

Sensory paralytic bladder results from damage to the sensory portion of the reflex arc. Persons with diabetic neuropathy may experience this type of incontinence. Bladder fullness or emptiness is not sensed, and there is no voluntary control over voiding. The overdistension and retention may cause atonicity of the bladder and result in large amounts of residual urine. The retention leads to overflow incontinence. Motor control is retained, so these individuals may be treated with behavioral measures (Pires, 2002).

Motor paralytic bladder occurs as a result of damage to the motor portion of the reflex arc. Sensation is experienced, but control of urination may or may not be voluntary. As bladder capacity is increased, residual urine volume is increased. Fullness and emptiness can be sensed. However, difficulty in initiating voiding, a need to strain to void, and a decreased urine stream as well as loss of detrusor muscle tone contribute to retention. Overflow incontinence results from decreased muscle tone and loss of motor function.

Table 19-1 lists conditions that contribute to urinary incontinence.

DIAGNOSIS

Diagnosis relies heavily on patient history. Elderly women, in particular, may be unaware that urinary incontinence is abnormal or may be uncomfortable discussing it. One must be sensitive when broaching the topic with men or women. A thorough health history helps focus the diagnosis of the type of incontinence the person is experiencing. In addition, a voiding diary (Box 19-2) in which the person records when the episode occurred and what happened may help narrow the possible types of incontinence if the record or diary is kept for several days. Determining whether the voiding dysfunction is a relatively new problem or a chronic one is important, because a change in health or functional status may have caused the problem to appear.

Persons with retention may complain of increasing dull lower abdominal pain and a strong urge to void despite being unable to void for several hours. Use of anticholinergic drugs or drugs with anticholinergic or α-adrenergic affects may initiate retention. Genital herpes, multiple sclerosis, and spinal cord lesions can cause retention, as can vigorous anal intercourse (Buttaravoli and Stair, n.d.).

The nurse should question the patient regarding the sensations of fullness or emptiness and their occurrence before or after voiding; changes in bowel habits; the presence of urgency, frequency, hesitancy, or straining; and alterations in mobility or the ability to remove clothing in time to void. The history should include information about any hematuria or dysuria, changes in sexual function, relevant surgeries, alterations in cognition, and the use of prescribed or over-the-counter medications (Pires, 2002). The environment should be assessed for hazards to mobility. Box 19-3 lists medications that may cause urinary incontinence.

Primary and secondary medical problems should be identified to determine their influence on voiding dysfunction.

Conditions such as spinal cord injury, Parkinson's disease, stroke, diabetes, dementia, prostate hypertrophy or cancer, chronic urinary tract infection, psychiatric disorders, and multiple sclerosis may contribute to urinary incontinence or retention. Previous surgery involving the pelvic or abdominal area, genitourinary system, or gastrointestinal system may be relevant to voiding dysfunction (Newman and Giovannini, 2002).

Physical examination includes evaluation of neurologic and psychosocial status, assessment of mobility and functional ability, abdominal and genital examination, rectal examination, and a stress test. In a stress test, the patient relaxes and then coughs vigorously, and any loss of urine is noted. The test is performed when the patient has a full bladder. Stress incontinence is suspected when the leakage of urine occurs spontaneously with coughing; urge incontinence is suspected when the loss of urine is delayed or persistent. The test may be performed with the patient in a lithotomy or standing position. During the test, the nurse observes for straining or hesitancy and notes the quality of the stream and the ability of the patient to control urinary flow voluntarily (Pires, 2002).

The person with retention may have a firm, distended bladder, and an enlarged or tender prostate or tumor may be palpated during the rectal examination. Tests may reveal stones lodged in the urethra or urethral strictures (possibly from gonorrhea), a tumor or clot in the bladder, prostatic cancer, benign prostatic hypertrophy, or prostatitis (Buttaravoli and Stair, n.d.). A magnetic resonance image or computed tomographic scan, white blood count, electrolyte count, and prostate specific antigen test as well as a renal ultrasonography and urethrography are helpful in ruling out these possible causes.

Specialized tests include a urinalysis to detect or rule out possible causes of incontinence such as infection, tumor, stones, or hyperglycemia. Blood urea nitrogen and creatinine levels may be assessed if an outlet obstruction, noncompliant bladder, or retention is suspected. Postvoid residual volume is measured to determine bladder emptying. Urodynamic testing to evaluate the function of the bladder, uroflowmetry to evaluate bladder emptying, and cystometry to determine detrusor function, including sensation, compliance, and capacity as well as the presence of voluntary or involuntary contractions, are other tests that may be ordered. Urethral pressure profilometry measures the pressures within the urethra and sphincter function. Electromyography may also be used to assess sphincter function (Pires, 2002).

In addition, cystourethroscopy may be performed to locate bladder and urethral lesions and identify sphincter deficiency if more than basic testing for incontinence is required. Intravenous pyelography and ultrasonography may be used to visualize the urinary system and the kidneys but are not routine (AHRQ, 1996; Pires, 2002). Table 19-2 gives the differential diagnosis for urinary retention.

Table 19-1   Identification and Management of Reversible Conditions That Cause or Contribute to Urinary Incontinence

Condition	Management
Conditions Affecting the Lower Urinary Tract	
Urinary tract infection (symptomatic with frequency, urgency, dysuria, etc.)	Antimicrobial therapy
Atrophic vaginitis and/or urethritis	Oral or topical estrogen.
Pregnancy, vaginal delivery, episiotomy	Behavioral intervention; avoid surgical therapy postpartum, because condition may be self-limiting.
Prostatectomy	Behavioral intervention; avoid surgical therapy until clear condition will not resolve.
Stool impaction	Disimpaction; appropriate use of stool softeners, bulk-forming agents, and laxatives if necessary; implementation of high fiber intake, adequate mobility, and fluid intake.
Increased Urine Production	
Metabolic (hyperglycemia, hypercalcemia)	Better control of diabetes mellitus. Therapy for hypercalcemia in accordance with underlying cause.
Excess fluid intake	Reduction in intake of diuretic fluids (e.g., caffeinated beverages).
Volume Overload	
Venous insufficiency with edema	Use of support stockings; leg elevation; sodium restriction; diuretic therapy.
Congestive heart failure	Medical therapy.
Impaired ability or willingness to reach a toilet; delirium	Diagnosis and treatment of underlying cause(s) of acute confusional state.
Chronic illness, injury, or restraint that interferes with mobility	Regular toileting; use of toilet substitutes; environmental alterations (e.g., bedside commode or urinal); removal of restraints if possible.
Psychological Disorders	Appropriate pharmacologic and/or nonpharmacologic treatment.
Drug Side Effects*	
Diuretics (polyuria, frequency, and urgency)	For all medications, discontinuance of or change in drug, as clinically possible.
Caffeine (aggravation or precipitation of incontinence)	Dosage reduction or modification (e.g., flexible scheduling of rapid-acting diuretics).
Anticholinergic agents (urinary retention; overflow incontinence; impaction)	
Antidepressants (anticholinergic actions; sedation)	
Antipsychotics (anticholinergic actions, sedation, rigidity, immobility)	
Sedatives, hypnotics, central nervous system depressants (sedation, delirium, immobility, muscle relaxation)	
Narcotic analgesics (urinary retention, fecal impaction, sedation, delirium)	
α-Adrenergic blockers (urethral relaxation)	
α-Adrenergic agonists (urinary retention; present in many cold remedies and over-the-counter preparations)	
β-Adrenergic agonists (urinary retention)	
Calcium channel blockers (urinary retention)	
Alcohol (polyuria, frequency, urgency, sedation, delirium, immobility)	

*Data from Fantl JA et al: Urinary incontinence in adults: acute and chronic management, AHCPR Pub No. 96-0682, Clinical Practice Guideline No. 2, March 1996, Rockville, Md, US Department of Health and Human Services, Public Health Service, Agency for Health Care Policy and Research.

INTERDISCIPLINARY CARE

Treatment of urinary incontinence may include behavioral techniques, drug therapy, surgery, or a combination of these.

Behavioral Therapist

Many different forms of behavioral therapy have been found to be effective for persons with urinary incontinence. There are three basic components to successful bladder retraining: education, scheduled voiding, and positive reinforcement (AHRQ, 1996). Education includes a description of what causes the incontinence and an explanation of how bladder retraining can be effective in treating it. The individual is

Box 19-3   Medications Associated with Urinary Incontinence

Calcium channel blockers	Metoclopramide
Clonazepam	Diuretics
Ethanol	Lithium
Misoprostol	Bromocriptine
Phenytoin	Antipsychotics and neuroleptics
Sedatives and hypnotics	Anticholinergics
Skeletal muscle relaxants	α-Adrenergic antagonists
Sympatholytics	α-Adrenergic agonists

From Martin CH: Urinary incontinence in the elderly [American Society of Consultant Pharmacists website], 1997, retrieved from *http://www.ascp.com/public/pubs/tcp/1997/aug/elderly.html* on August 28, 2002, p 3.

taught to void after progressively longer intervals. Consequently, involuntary urges to void or unscheduled voids are either integrated into the schedule and the next timed void is planned accordingly, or they are disregarded in favor of the schedule. For example, a patient may be taught to void every 2 hours initially. The urge to void more frequently is ignored. Kegel or pelvic floor muscle exercises may be used to help reduce the urge to void. If the person is unable to control urgency that occurs before the scheduled void time, then the unscheduled void may or may not be used to adjust the schedule. In other words, the person may start the 2-hour interval from the time of the involuntary void or may ignore it and maintain the schedule. The schedule is usually strictly maintained only during waking hours, and its use is augmented by adjustments in fluid intake and postponed voiding in an effort to increase bladder capacity. The caregiver is encouraged to offer frequent praise for successful timed voiding.

The health care provider communicates with the patient to determine when and how to increase scheduled intervals. This process usually occurs over several months. Prompted voiding is timed voiding that is used with persons who are confused or cognitively impaired. The caregiver prompts the patient to void on schedule. Stress and urge incontinence as well as incontinence related to detrusor instability, uninhibited neurogenic bladder, and sensory paralytic bladder may be resolved or improved by the use of timed or prompted voiding (AHRQ, 1996).

Scheduled voiding may be used by persons with neurogenic bladder. For example, the person with uninhibited neurogenic bladder may be able to prevent incontinence by voiding before the bladder is full enough to trigger a voiding reflex. If the individual can voluntarily start and stop the urine stream, bladder training may be successful (Pires, 2002).

Kegel or pelvic muscle exercises are very effective in strengthening the pubococcygeus muscle and thereby improving urethral resistance. The strengthened pubococcygeus muscle acts as a sling to support the urethra and bladder. The exercise is performed 30 to 80 times per day and each muscle contraction is sustained for 10 seconds. The exercise involves tightening the pubococcygeus muscle either by pulling in the

Table 19-2   Differential Diagnosis for Urinary Retention

Common	Occasional	Rare
Prostatic hypertrophy, benign or malignant	Constipation	Central nervous system disease
Anticholinergic drugs	"Holding on" (leads to prostatic congestion)	Pedunculated bladder tumor
Urethral calculus	Pelvic mass: pregnancy or fibroid uterus	Traumatic rupture of urethra
Bladder neck hypertrophy	Acute genital herpes	Foreign body inserted into anterior urethra
Prostatitis and prostatic abscess (also urinary tract infection)	Detrusor sphincter dyssynergia	Phimosis

From Urinary retention, retrieved from *http://www.doctorupdate.net/du_toolkit/s_sorters/s81.html* on Sept 2, 2002.

perivaginal muscles or by contracting the anal sphincter without contracting buttock, thigh or abdominal muscles. The exercise is performed as if the individual were trying to stop the flow of urine or prevent defecation. (One must avoid stopping the urine stream while actually voiding, however, to prevent urinary dysfunction or increase in the risk of infection). These exercises are particularly helpful to persons with stress incontinence, including men who have undergone prostatic surgery. In a study of older rural women with incontinence, researchers found that sequenced phases of intervention using self-monitoring, bladder training, and performance of Kegel exercises with biofeedback decreased the severity of incontinence by 61%. The control group who did not receive any intervention experienced an increase in severity of 184% (Urinary incontinence, 2002).

Vaginal cones may be used to assist the woman in performing Kegel exercises. The woman contracts vaginal muscles against increasingly heavier cones in an effort to retain the cone inside the vaginal vault. Biofeedback using electronic or mechanical devices may be provided to give individuals information about the effectiveness of pelvic floor exercises and physiologic mediation of detrusor control. In addition, electrical stimulation of the pelvic muscles and viscera can help some persons, especially those with neurologically impaired bladder or urethral dysfunction. These treatments may cause pain or discomfort, however (AHRQ, 1996).

Measures to reduce or eliminate functional incontinence include rearranging the person's environment for easier navigability and toilet access, evaluating and possibly changing medications that cause cognitive or mobility impairment, providing clothing that is easy to don and doff, ensuring sufficient lighting and privacy, installing grab bars, and providing color contrast to improve safety and visualization of toilet facilities. Supervision by or ready assistance from another person may also be needed to help the person with functional incontinence to reach the toilet in time to void.

Drug Therapy

Two main categories of drug are used to manage urinary incontinence: medications to treat urethral sphincter insufficiency and medications to treat detrusor overactivity (Table 19-3). Estrogen replacement and α-adrenergic agonists may be

Table 19-3   Medications Commonly Used to Treat Incontinence

Generic Name (Selected Trade Name)	Normal Adult Dosage	Therapeutic Uses	Major Adverse Effects/Cautions/ Interactions	Comments
Anticholinergic Agents Oxybutynin (Ditropan) Oxybutynin XL (Ditropan XL)	2.5-5 mg BID or QID 5-30 mg once daily	Overactive bladder	Dry mouth, blurred vision, constipation, confusion, tachycardia, orthostatic hypotension, dizziness, urine retention	Anticholinergics are the first-line drugs for therapy (oxybutynin or tolterodine are preferred).
Tolterodine (Detrol)	1-2 mg BID		Interactions: CYP 3A4 inhibitors; increased intraocular pressure with anticholinergics	
Tricyclic Antidepressants (TCAs)		Overactive bladder Stress or combined stress incontinence and overactive bladder (i.e., mixed incontinence)	Anticholinergic effects (as previously described), orthostatic hypotension, cardiac dysrhythmia	TCA use generally reserved for patients with an additional indication (e.g., depression, neuralgia) at an initial dose of 10-25 mg, 1-3 times/day.
Nortriptyline (Pamelor)	25-100 mg/day (with water or juice)			
Imipramine (Tofranil)	25-100 mg/day (with water or juice)			Do not use in patients with urinary obstruction.
Doxepin (Sinequan)	25-100 mg/day (with water or juice)		Interactions: monoamine oxidase inhibitors, sympatho-mimetic amines	

Continued

Table 19-3   Medications Commonly Used to Treat Incontinence—cont'd

Generic Name (Selected Trade Name)	Normal Adult Dosage	Therapeutic Uses	Major Adverse Effects/Cautions/Interactions	Comments
Estrogen Conjugated estrogen (Premarin)	0.5 g vaginal cream 3 times/wk, up to 8 mo; repeat course if symptom recurrence Or, estradiol vaginal insert/ring (2 mg [1 ring]), replaced after 90 days, if needed; If cream/insert ineffective, systemic therapy with conjugated estrogens, 0.3-0.625 mg/day orally immediately after food to decrease nausea Or, Estraderm or CombiPatch	Overactive bladder Stress or combined stress incontinence and overactive bladder (i.e., mixed incontinence)	Cream and vaginal insert: few adverse effects Systemic therapy: headache, vaginal spotting, edema, breast tenderness, possible depression Interactions: carbamazepine, phenobarbital, rifampin may decrease effect; may increase level or toxicity of cyclosporine; may decrease tamoxifen effect	Systemic therapy should not be used if there is suspected or confirmed breast or endometrial cancer, or active or past thromboembolism with previous use of oral contraceptive or estrogen, or pregnancy. Concurrent use of progestin (e.g., medroxyprogesterone 2.5-10 mg/day) necessary with intact uterus; progestin unnecessary without uterus or with short-term use of topical cream or vaginal insert. Pretreatment: periodic mammogram, gynecologic and breast examinations.
α-Adrenergic Agonists Pseudoephedrine (Sudafed)	15-60 TID (with food, water, or milk)	Stress incontinence	Anxiety, insomnia, agitation, palpitations, headache, angina, cardiac dysrhythmia, hypertension, tremor Should not be used in patients with obstructive syndromes and/or hypertension Interactions: methyldopa may increase pressor response	Pseudoephedrine is first-line therapy for women with no contraindications (notably hypertension).
α-Adrenergic Antagonists Terazosin (Hytrin)	1 mg at bedtime for first dose Increase by 1 mg every 4 days to 5 mg/day as needed	Overflow (because of benign prostate enlargement)	Postural hypotension, syncope in supine position, palpitations, edema, headache, dizziness, vertigo, drowsiness, weakness Interaction: antihypertensives may increase hypotension	Possible benefit in men with obstructive position of prostate, heart symptoms or benign prostatic hyperplasia. Monitor sitting and standing blood pressures with first dose and each dosage increase. May worsen female stress incontinence.

Table 19-3 Medications Commonly Used to Treat Incontinence—cont'd

Generic Name (Selected Trade Name)	Normal Adult Dosage	Therapeutic Uses	Major Adverse Effects/Cautions/Interactions	Comments
Doxazosin (Cardura)	1 mg at bedtime, with first dose in supine position Increase by 1 mg every 7-14 days to 5 mg/day, as needed		Same as for terazosin	Same as for terazosin
Tamsulosin (Flomax)	0.4 mg once daily Increase after 2-4 wk, if needed, to 0.8 mg/day		Same as for terazosin	Has benefit of lower incidence of orthostatic hypotension.
Antiandrogens Finasteride (Proscar)	5 mg/day Can be crushed but possibly pregnant woman should not handle	Overflow (because of benign prostate enlargement)	Erectile dysfunction, decreased libido, gynecomastia Interactions: falsely decreased prostate-specific antigen (PSA) concentration	Maximum therapeutic effect after 6-12 mo. Causes 50% decrease in PSA level.
Phytotherapeutic Agents Saw palmetto (*Serenoa repens*)	160 mg BID	Overflow (because of benign prostate enlargement)	Headache, gastrointestinal upset, hypertension, decreased libido, erectile dysfunction	Long-term efficacy and safety unknown.
Cholinergics Bethanechol (Urecholine)	1-30 mg QID	Overflow (because of atonic bladder)	Nausea, vomiting, abdominal cramps, diarrhea, bradycardia, bronchoconstriction, hypotension Interactions: effect decreased by anticholinergics	Avoid use in patients with asthma or heart disease Short-term use only.

Data from American Society of Health System Pharmacists: AHFS drug information, Bethesda, Md, 2000, The Society; and Lackner TE: Urinary health management in the long-term care setting, *Consultant Pharm* 14(suppl B):3-16, 1999.
BID, Twice a day; *QID,* four times a day; *TID,* three times a day.

prescribed to treat sphincter insufficiency that causes stress incontinence. Pseudoephedrine is initially used for stress incontinence if there are no contraindications, most notably hypertension (Pires, 2002). Estrogen may be administered orally or vaginally to postmenopausal women. The α-adrenergic blockers may increase stress incontinence and if used with estrogen may have a synergistic effect (Martin, 1997).

Overactivity of the detrusor muscle is treated with anticholinergic or antispasmodic agents to relax the detrusor muscle and increase the capacity of the bladder. These are typically used in patients with urge incontinence or uninhibited bladder.

New medications undergoing research include tolterodine, which treats urge incontinence by decreasing uncontrolled detrusor contractions, and duloxetine, which is used for stress and urge incontinence. Duloxetine is thought to increase bladder capacity (Martin, 1997). Darifenacin is an anticholinergic or muscarinic antagonist that affects the smooth muscle of the bladder. Transdermal oxybutynin is an anticholinergic drug delivered via skin patch to treat incontinence. Another anticholinergic, trospium chloride, may have fewer side effects (especially somnolence) than other anticholinergics. Desmopressin acetate, a synthetic form of vasopressin, reduces urine production to prevent nocturia (Newman and Giovannini, 2002).

Intermittent catheterization may be used in conjunction with anticholinergics in persons with reflex incontinence or may be used by itself in those with urinary retention, overflow incontinence, or neurogenic incontinence. Intermittent catheterization is generally performed using clean technique when the patient is residing outside of the hospital setting.

Surgeon

Surgery to treat bladder incontinence should be considered only after behavioral and pharmacologic treatments have failed or after a comprehensive clinical evaluation reveals that surgery is the best option. Table 19-4 describes surgical management of urinary incontinence.

Several surgical procedures are available for persons with neurogenic bladder impairment, including continent diversion, neurostimulation, neuromodulation, transurethral sphincterotomy, sphincter stent placement, enterocystoplasty, and augmentation (Pires, 2002). Surgery such as a prostatectomy or correction of a pelvic organ prolapse may be used to treat the cause of retention.

Nonsurgical Procedures

 Credé's method and Valsalva's maneuver may be used to help people with neurogenic urinary incontinence or retention. In Credé's method manual pressure is used to expel the urine from the bladder. This method should be used only with the permission of the physician and with the understanding that long-term use of the method has the potential to cause permanent renal damage or rectal or vaginal prolapse. Valsalva's maneuver is straining to expel urine from the bladder. Intermittent catheterization may be the most viable and least risk-laden method for preventing incontinence in patients with neurogenic urinary disorders (Pires, 2002).

Intermittent or indwelling catheterization may be used to treat people with chronic retention. Antispasmodic drugs may be given to reduce bladder contractions and relieve spasms. Use of medications that may contribute to retention should be reviewed and eliminated, if possible (Box 19-4).

Nurse

The nurse is frequently the first health care provider to detect that the individual has voiding dysfunction. When the health history is taken, the astute nurse will notice certain clues, such as hesitancy to leave the home environment and concerns about instrumental and other activities of daily living and odor. The nurse may observe the presence of diapers or excessive perfumes in the home or note that the individual is taking medications that have a strong likelihood of contributing to incontinence or retention.

The nurse recognizes that a problem exists and addresses it with sensitivity. Detailed and focused questioning will confirm the presence of voiding dysfunction. However, first the nurse must make the individual aware that voiding dysfunction is not normal and that treatments are available and are usually effective. Voiding dysfunction can have a significant impact on the individual's quality of life, and the knowledge that it can be diagnosed and treated may make a true difference in the individual's perspective on his or her lifestyle.

In addition to taking a thorough history, the nurse performs a physical examination and recommends laboratory tests and other diagnostic studies to the physician or advanced practice nurse (APN). If the nurse feels confident that the individual is experiencing stress incontinence, then the nurse might begin bladder retraining with the individual while awaiting the results of testing. If retraining is successful, then the individual may avoid pharmacologic and invasive treatments.

The nurse monitors behavioral therapy, refers the patient to a urologist as appropriate, instructs the individual regarding pharmacologic treatments, and provides care during the preoperative, perioperative, and postoperative periods should the individual require surgery. The nurse instructs the person to quit smoking because nicotine irritates the bladder

Table 19-4 Surgical Management of Urinary Incontinence

Type of Urinary Incontinence	Cause	Treatment
Stress	Hypermobility	Retropubic suspension, needle endoscopic suspension
Stress	Intrinsic sphincter deficiency	Sling (mostly in females), artificial sphincter, urethral bulking
Urge	Refractory detrusor instability	Augmentation cystoplasty
Overflow	Obstruction	Relieve obstruction (Intermittent catheterization, other therapy)
	Other than obstruction	

From Pires M: Bladder elimination and continence. In Hoeman S, *Rehabilitation nursing: process, application, and outcomes,* ed 3, St Louis, 2002, Mosby.

Box 19-4 Medications That Contribute to Retention

Some antidepressants
Chlorpheniramine
Diphenhydramine
Ephedrine
Pseudoephedrine

From Gaynes S: Urinary retention, April 6, 2001, retrieved from *http://www.emedicine.com/aaem/topic466.htm* on September 2, 2002.

Table 19-5 Specific Nursing Interventions for Incontinence or Retention

Bladder Dysfunction	Interventions
Stress incontinence	Bowel management
Urge incontinence	Kegel exercises
	Improvement of functional ability and/or environment
	Bladder retraining
	Toileting assistance
	Biofeedback
	Monitoring of electrical stimulation
	Monitoring of pharmacologic treatment
Overflow incontinence	Timed voiding
	Intermittent catheterization
	Care after prostatectomy or transurethral resection of the prostate
	Use of pessary or other device or medication to treat pelvic organ prolapse
Uninhibited neurogenic bladder	Timed voiding
	Catheterization, use of padding
	Monitoring of medications
Reflex neurogenic bladder	Intermittent catheterization
	Monitoring of medications
	Surgical care
Autonomic neurogenic bladder	Intermittent catheterization
	Valsalva's maneuver
	Credé's method if permitted
Motor paralytic bladder	Intermittent catheterization
	Valsalva's maneuver
	Credé's method if permitted
Sensory paralytic bladder	Timed voiding
	Intermittent catheterization

and to modify the diet by reducing caffeine, which increases detrusor pressure. In addition, alcohol, carbonated drinks, and aspartame may negatively affect bladder control. Weight reduction and the prevention of constipation may reduce pressure on the bladder (Newman and Giovannini, 2002).

The individual must understand that he or she is the leader of the team and that if he or she does not follow through with recommended behavioral therapies, then they will not be effective. Caregivers must be included as well, as appropriate. A cognitively intact, mobile individual may not want spouses or caregivers to participate in such intimate care. Other individuals, especially the cognitively impaired, will need other people to help them get to the bathroom; record the schedule and results; assist with hygiene, clothing manipulation, and prompting; and generally ensure that timed voiding occurs as scheduled. The nurse must maintain frequent contact with the individual and caregivers to ensure that timed voiding is progressing, Kegel exercises are being done properly, and medications are being taken appropriately, and must see that the rest of the health care team is apprised of the plan of care.

Nursing care that is specific to individuals with incontinence or retention is outlined in Table 19-5.

Primary Provider (Physician/Nurse Practitioner)

The physician, APN, or physician assistant (PA) is apprised by the nurse of the existence of voiding dysfunction. However, if pharmacologic or surgical interventions are not to be used to treat the problem, then the physician, APN, or PA may play only an ancillary role in the individual's treatment. The physician, APN, or PA should be made aware that bladder retraining and Kegel exercises are being implemented and should be kept current on their outcomes. The physician, APN, or PA is likely to agree to attempt behavioral therapies before other treatments if the patient is otherwise generally healthy.

If the individual has congestive heart failure or another health problem that may have initiated the voiding dysfunc-

tion, then the physician, APN, or PA may decide to treat that problem first or concurrently with bladder retraining. In addition, if laboratory tests, medications, use of vaginal cones, biofeedback, electrical stimulation, or surgery is necessary, the physician, APN, or PA must be more closely involved in the care of the patient.

Physical and Occupational Therapists

The therapist may be involved in identifying voiding dysfunction during the health history taking. Patient immobility may provide a clue to functional incontinence. In addition, the therapist may be involved in reinforcing bladder retraining and the use of Kegel exercises. Further, many therapists are involved in biofeedback and electrical stimulation interventions and may participate in the care of patients experiencing bladder dysfunction.

The therapist may prescribe a bedside commode to enable the patient to reach the toilet easily or an elevated toilet seat for persons who have undergone hip replacement.

COMPLEMENTARY AND ALTERNATIVE THERAPIES

The behavioral therapies discussed earlier in this chapter may be considered "alternative" therapies because they are alternatives to drug therapy or surgery. In addition, however, herbal remedies are used by some people to treat bladder problems. Parsley and nettle are examples of these (Fetrow and Avila, 2000). Cranberry juice has recently been validated as useful in treating urinary tract infection under certain circumstances. *Lactobacillus acidophilus* and *Bifidobacterium bifidus* may be taken along with antibiotics to prevent vaginal yeast infection (LaValle et al, 2000). Herbal and over-the-counter remedies may interact unfavorably with prescribed medications or treatments. It is important to make patients and families aware of this possibility and to advise them to consult their urologist before using herbal or over-the-counter alternative therapies.

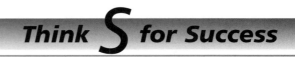
Think S for Success

Symptoms
■ Manage incontinence and retention with behavioral therapy, pharmacologic, or surgical interventions.

Sequelae
■ Prevent further loss of muscle tone with Kegel exercises. Prevent infection with interventions to prevent residual urine.

Safety
■ Identify and remove obstacles to reaching toileting facilities. Instruct patient and caregiver regarding medication use and adverse effects and contraindications.

Support/Services
■ Make appropriate referrals; locate financial assistance and adequate housing as needed.

Satisfaction
■ Determine the degree to which incontinence or retention is interfering with patient's quality of life or lifestyle and develop a plan to maintain or restore quality of life.

CASE STUDY

Patient Data

Mrs. Q. is a 55-year-old preschool teacher. She lives with her husband and has three grown children. She delivered all of her children vaginally and required an episiotomy during the first delivery. She started menopause at age 52 and takes no hormone replacement therapy. During the past several months, she has noticed that whenever she laughs, sneezes, or lifts one of the children at school, a little bit of urine leaks into her underwear. She has heard from some of her friends that this is a common occurrence and that it "just happens as we get older." She has seen many commercials on television about the problem and so assumes that it is normal. She finds herself bringing changes of underwear to work and being reluctant to wear close-fitting slacks or dressy clothes. She carries panty liners with her and changes them frequently but finds that the leakage is increasing and the pads are no longer enough. Wherever she goes, she feels that people are able to smell urine on her clothes, so she tries to avoid going out in groups of people. She has been reluctant to have sexual intercourse and has not explained the reason to her husband.

On a routine visit to the clinic for a physical, the nurse checks Mrs. Q.'s vital signs and height and weight. The nurse makes note of Mrs. Q.'s age and asks her if she has ever noticed any difficulty controlling her urine. Mrs. Q. is surprised to be asked and says, "Oh, sometimes, but doesn't everyone?"

The nurse takes a thorough health history and during the physical examination assists the nurse practitioner in performing abdominal, rectal, and genital assessments. Mrs. Q. undergoes a stress test, and the nurse notes an immediate leakage of urine when Mrs. Q. coughs. The nurse practitioner orders a urinalysis including culture and sensitivity testing to rule out infection as a cause of the incontinence. However, because Mrs. Q. reports experiencing no burning, dysuria, abdominal pain, fever, or chills, the nurse and nurse practitioner conclude that the most probable diagnosis is stress incontinence.

Thinking It Through
■ What nursing diagnoses might pertain to Mrs. Q.?
■ What should the nurse do next?
■ How should the nurse explain the importance of Mrs. Q.'s involvement in her treatment to its outcome?
■ Should Mr. Q. be involved in the discussion or treatment?

Case Conference

For a simple case of stress incontinence in an otherwise generally healthy patient, it is likely that only the patient, nurse, physician or APN, and possibly the pharmacist will be involved in the case. The nurse and/or nurse practitioner have assessed the patient, and the nurse practitioner has ordered laboratory tests to rule out other causes of the urinary incontinence.

The nurse and the nurse practitioner at the clinic discuss the likelihood of a diagnosis of stress urinary incontinence with Mrs. Q. They invite her to include her husband in the discussion because he drove her to the clinic. Mrs. Q. declines and states that she is embarrassed to involve him in their talk. The nurse and the nurse practitioner explain the causes of stress incontinence and suggest that Mrs. Q. begin a regimen of Kegel exercises and scheduled voiding. They recommend a padding system that masks odors and explain that the pads should be changed three or four times throughout the day when there is leakage.

The nurse practitioner explains that there are methods such as biofeedback, vaginal cones, and electrical stimulation that can be used if Mrs. Q. feels she is unable to perform Kegel exercises on her own 50 times each day for 10 seconds each. The nurse suggests that Mrs. Q. explain the cause of her avoidance of sexual activity to her husband and offers to help her explain by being present during their discussion or by providing pamphlets

CASE STUDY—cont'd

that Mrs. Q. can take home and share with him. The nurse also describes how to keep a voiding diary and asks Mrs. Q. to maintain the diary until the 6-week follow-up visit.

At the 6-week follow-up visit, Mrs. Q. states that she is having fewer episodes of leakage but that they are still occurring. She says that she is not always able to remember to perform the Kegel exercises and that, when she does remember, she usually does only about 10 to 20 repetitions of the exercise. She is keeping a voiding diary and does try to go to the toilet to void at regular 3-hour intervals during the day. Mrs. Q., the nurse, and the nurse practitioner confer and decide that Mrs. Q. should consider estrogen replacement therapy. Mrs. Q. states that she is less reluctant to have sexual intercourse but avoids it after she has drunk liquids. She says that her husband has been supportive.

The nurse practitioner confers with the pharmacist and Mrs. Q. is given an estrogen cream preparation. The nurse praises Mrs. Q. for her efforts at doing the Kegel exercises and bladder retraining and explains again the benefit of adhering to the plan of 50 Kegel exercises per day for 10 seconds each. The nurse arranges for Mrs. Q. to call for a follow-up visit in 3 months, or earlier if symptoms do not improve.

- What techniques or treatments might be recommended at the 3-month follow-up if the current therapies are unsuccessful?
- What strengths and weaknesses of Mrs. Q. and her situation affect the success of the plan of care?

Internet and Other Resources

American Foundation for Urologic disease: *http://www.afud.com*

National Association for Continence: *http://www.nafc.org*

Seek Wellness Today Incontinence Center: *http://www.Seekwellness.com*

U.S. Department of Health and Human Services Public Health Service: 2101 East Jefferson Street, Suite 501, Rockville, MD 20852; telephone 800-358-9295

REFERENCES

Agency for Healthcare Quality and Research: Clinical practice guideline: urinary incontinence in adults, Washington DC, 1996, Department of Health and Human Services.

Buttaravoli PM, Stair TO: Urinary retention. In *Common simple emergencies,* Washington DC, n.d., Longwood Information, retrieved from *http://www.ncemi.org/cse0709.htm* on Jan 8, 2003.

Copstead LC, Banasik JL: *Pathophysiology,* Philadelphia, 2000, WB Saunders.

Dugan E et al: Why older community-dwelling adults do not discuss urinary incontinence with their primary care physicians, *J Am Geriatr Soc* 49:462-5, 2001.

Gaynes S: Urinary retention, April 6, 2001, retrieved from *http://www.emedicine.com/aaem/topic466.htm* on Sep 2, 2002.

Fetrow CW, Avila JR: *The complete guide to herbal medicines,* Springhouse, Pa, 2000, Springhouse Corp.

LaValle JB et al: *Natural therapeutics pocket guide,* Hudson, Ohio, 2000, Lexi-Comp and Natural Health Resources.

Martin CH: Urinary incontinence in the elderly [American Society of Consultant Pharmacists website], 1997, retrieved from *http://www.ascp.com/public/pubs/tcp/1997/aug/elderly.html* on Aug 28, 2002.

Newman DK, Giovannini D: The overactive bladder: a nursing perspective, *Am J Nurs* 102(6):36-46, 2002.

Pires M: Bladder elimination and continence. In Hoeman SP, *Rehabilitation nursing,* St Louis, 2002, Mosby, pp 383-421.

Rogers ST, Amador MJ, Bryan TA: Physical and healthcare patterns and nursing interventions. In Edwards PA, editor: *The specialty practice of rehabilitation nursing,* Glenview, Ill, 2000, Association of Rehabilitation Nurses, pp 102-38.

Urinary incontinence in older rural women, *Am J Nurs* 102(5):21, 2002.

CHAPTER 20

Disorders of Hormone Regulation

Beth Cameron, ND, FNP, Mary C. Ewald, MS, RN,
Tracy L. Poelvoorde, MSN, BSN, BA, Dawn Rude, MS, BSN, and
Karen S. Wilson, MSN, RN

OBJECTIVES

After reading this chapter, you should be able to do the following:

- Describe the pathophysiology of insulin, thyroid hormone, cortisol, and growth hormone disorders.
- Describe the clinical manifestations of diabetes mellitus, hypothyroidism and hyperthyroidism, Cushing's syndrome, Addison's disease, and acromegaly.
- Describe the functional health patterns affected by insulin, thyroid, cortisol, and growth hormone disorders.
- Compare and contrast states of hormone excess and deficiency
- Describe the role of each member of the interdisciplinary team involved in the care of patients with diabetes mellitus, hypothyroidism and hyperthyroidism, Cushing's syndrome, Addison's disease, and acromegaly
- Describe the indications for use, side effects, and nursing considerations related to drugs commonly used to treat diabetes mellitus, hypothyroidism and hyperthyroidism, Cushing's syndrome, Addison's disease, and acromegaly

OVERVIEW OF HORMONES AND ENDOCRINE DYSFUNCTION

Hormones are chemicals naturally produced by the body that travel through the bloodstream to affect cells other than the glands in which they were produced. The major hormones and their target organs and regulatory effects are listed in Table 20-1.

Most hormones produce their effects on only one type of target cell, but some, such as insulin and thyroid hormone, act on many cells in the body. Hormones serve as regulators of many crucial body functions, including energy production, reproduction, fluid balance, growth and development, digestive tract activity, and mineral metabolism.

In a healthy person, feedback mechanisms control the level of circulating hormones in the blood. These feedback mechanisms often involve other hormones produced in the hypothalamus and pituitary glands. Significant pathology may result from the absence or overabundance of any hormone. In general, a decrease in the level of any hormone leads to a reduction in the expected effect and an increase in a hormone level leads to an exaggeration of the expected effect.

Because hormones are produced by glands, the most obvious cause of malfunctioning is a failure of the gland producing the hormone. However, disruption in other physiologic mechanisms also causes endocrine failure. This chapter reviews several major endocrine disorders associated with dysfunction in the production of or response to four important hormones: insulin (diabetes mellitus), thyroid hormone (hypothyroidism and hyperthyroidism), cortisol (Cushing's disease and Addison's disease), and growth hormone (acromegaly). These disorders are summarized in Table 20-2.

PATHOPHYSIOLOGY

The regulation of hormone production and the levels at which endocrine dysfunction can occur are outlined in Figure 20-1. Hormone regulation of body functions is compromised if the necessary chemicals are not available for hormone synthesis, the endocrine organ fails due to some pathophysiology of its own, the feedback pathway that stimulates production malfunctions, or the target organ fails to respond. In addition, mechanisms for transporting, metabolizing, and excreting the hormone affect the level of available hormone and may be compromised by protein malnutrition, cardiovascular dysfunction, kidney failure, and/or liver dysfunction.

The correct cause of the hormonal dysfunction must be identified if effective intervention and teaching plans are to be developed.

ASSESSMENT

Hormonal disorders may disrupt normal body functions in either subtle or catastrophic ways. Symptoms, which vary

Table 20-1 Major Hormones and Their Effects

Gland	Major Hormones	Target Organ/Cells	Major Regulation Effect
Hypothalamus	Corticotropin-releasing hormone	Pituitary	Pituitary release of adrenocorticotropic hormone
	Growth hormone–releasing hormone	Pituitary	Pituitary release of growth hormone
	Luteinizing hormone–releasing hormone	Pituitary	Pituitary release of luteinizing hormone
	Somatostatin	Pituitary	Inhibition of pituitary release of growth hormone
	Thyrotropin-releasing hormone	Pituitary	Pituitary release of thyroid-stimulating hormone
Pituitary	Adrenocorticotropic hormone	Adrenal cortex	Cortisol production
	Antidiuretic hormone		Fluid reabsorption in the renal tubule
			Gastrointestinal peristalsis
			Contraction of capillaries and small arterioles
	Follicle-stimulating hormone		Regulation of menstruation
			Sperm production
	Growth hormone	Bone and cartilage	Bone and cartilage growth
	Luteinizing hormone	Ovaries, testes	Ovulation
			Sperm development
			Testosterone production
	Oxytocin	Uterus	Uterine contraction
	Thyroid-stimulating hormone	Thyroid	Thyroid hormone production
Thyroid	Calcitonin	Bone	Bone formation
			Calcium regulation
	Triiodothyronine	Many cells and organs	Protein, carbohydrate, and lipid metabolism
			Protein synthesis
			Cell growth and differentiation
			Heart rate and stroke volume regulation
	Thyroxine	Many cells and organs	Converted to triiodothyronine in the body; see triiodothyronine effects above
Pancreas	Glucagon	Liver	Stimulation of gluconeogenesis
	Insulin	Many cells and organs	Uptake of glucose into cells
			Protein and lipid synthesis
			Inhibition of lipolysis and gluconeogenesis
Adrenal cortex	Androgens	Many cells and organs	Development of secondary sex characteristics
			Growth of muscle and bone
	Glucocorticoids (cortisol)		Carbohydrate and mineral metabolism
			Inflammatory and immune response
	Mineralocorticoids (aldosterone)		Regulation of extracellular volume
			Fluid and mineral regulation

widely based on the hormones involved, result in alterations in functional health patterns (Box 20-1). Careful assessment of these patterns is a primary focus for nursing interventions.

TREATMENT

Treatment of hormonal dysfunction depends on which hormone is involved and where and how the normal hormonal processes have been altered. Pharmacologic interventions include the use of synthetic or natural versions of hormones, drugs that suppress the production or disrupt the activity of hormones, drugs that alter target tissue response to hormones, and/or drugs that treat symptoms of hormonal imbalance. Frequently the entire health care team participates in helping the patient address the health management issues involved.

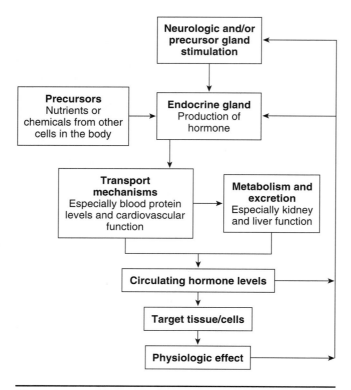

Figure 20-1 Hormonal regulation.

DIABETES MELLITUS

Approximately 17 million Americans (6.2% of the population) have diabetes mellitus, although one third of them do not know it (Centers for Disease Control and Prevention [CDC], 2003a). In the decade between 1990 and 2000, the prevalence of diagnosed diabetes in the United States increased from 6.7 million to 12 million Americans (CDC, 2003b). Diabetes mellitus is now the sixth leading cause of

Table 20-2 Major Endocrine Disorders

Condition	Hormone Pathology
Diabetes mellitus	Insulin underproduction or absence of production
	Insulin resistance
Hypothyroidism	Decreased production of thyroid hormone
Hyperthyroidism	Increased production of thyroid hormone
Cretinism	Decreased thyroid hormone in utero and/or first year of life
Cushing's syndrome	Increased cortisol levels
Addison's disease	Decreased cortisol levels
Acromegaly	Increased growth hormone levels in adulthood

death in the United States (CDC, 2003c), and 1 million new cases of diabetes are diagnosed each year (CDC, 2003a). Unfortunately, by the time of diagnosis, many patients have signs of diabetic complications such as neuropathy, nephropathy, cardiovascular changes, and/or retinopathy.

Ethnic Variations

Women are more likely than men to have the disease: 8.9% of women (9.1 million) and 8.3% of men (7.8 million) are affected (CDC, 2003a). The prevalence of diabetes increases with age. Although only 0.19% of Americans under 20 years of age have diabetes, 8.6% of those over 20 years of age have the disease, and 20.1% of all Americans over age 65 have it (CDC, 2003a). Race and ethnicity have a significant impact on risk for the disease: 7.8% of non-Hispanic whites have diabetes, 13% of non-Hispanic blacks, 10.2% of Hispanic or Latino Americans, and 15.1% of American Indians and Native Alaskans have the disease. Although the data for Native Hawaiians are limited, it appears that Native Hawaiians are 2.5 times more likely to have diabetes mellitus than white residents of Hawaii (CDC, 2003a).

Because age, familial customs, and societal cues strongly influence food choices and health care habits, each patient's cultural ways must be assessed individually. Patients must explore options, plan for the particular circumstances that occur within their own cultural and social systems, and weigh the consequences of their choices within their own belief systems. Health care providers tend to emphasize maintaining health to live longer, but some patients may feel that living longest is not living best.

Pathophysiology

Diabetes mellitus, primarily a disorder of glucose regulation, results from a failure in production of the hormone insulin and/or a lack of tissue response to naturally produced insulin. The two major types of diabetes mellitus are known as type 1 and type 2. Type 1 diabetes is characterized by a complete failure of the pancreatic cells that normally produce insulin. Type 2 diabetes is more complex and involves a resistance of the body's cells to naturally produced insulin in addition to a partial failure in the production of insulin. Possibly the insulin resistance of the cells occurs first, which causes an increased need for insulin, and the increased production of insulin over a long period of time eventually leads to exhaustion and failure of the pancreatic cells that are supposed to produce it.

Type 1 diabetes typically occurs in children and young adults, whereas type 2 diabetes is usually diagnosed in adults. The increase in childhood obesity in the United States over the last decade is associated with a recent increase in the diagnosis of type 2 diabetes in children and adolescents.

Normally, insulin acts to transport glucose into cells within the body, either for immediate use or for storage in the liver as glycogen. Without proper insulin functioning,

Box 20-1 Functional Health Pattern Assessment for Endocrine Disorders

HEALTH PERCEPTION/HEALTH MANAGEMENT
- Is there a family history of endocrine disorder?
- What is the patient's perception of his or her overall health?
- What medications, including over-the-counter drugs, does the patient take?
- What alternative therapies does the patient use?
- Is the patient at risk for injury and infection?

NUTRITION/METABOLISM
- What is the patient's current weight? Has there been any unexplained recent weight gain or loss?
- What is the patient's dietary history? Is the patient on any special diet? Has appetite changed?
- What is the condition of the skin and mucous membranes?
- Are fluid and electrolyte levels within normal limits?
- Is thermoregulation ineffective?

ELIMINATION
- Does the patient have constipation or diarrhea?
- What is the patient's fluid intake and output?

ACTIVITY/EXERCISE
- Does the patient experience fatigue, weakness, shortness of breath on exertion, or muscle or joint aches?
- Is the patient able to maintain normal routines?
- Is there a delay in growth and development?
- What are the patient's heart rate and blood pressure at rest and with exercise?

SLEEP/REST
- How many hours of uninterrupted sleep does the patient get at night? Does the patient take naps? What sleep aids does the patient use?
- Does the patient experience difficulty falling asleep or early awakening? Does the patient have the perception of being well rested?
- Does the patient display irritability, restlessness, or lethargy, have dark circles under the eyes, or yawn or change posture frequently?
- Does the patient show thick speech and use of incorrect words, distractibility, or memory deficits or problems?

COGNITION/PERCEPTION
- Have any changes been noted in mental function and problem-solving abilities? Does the patient experience memory difficulties?
- Have any alterations occurred in peripheral sensation or vision?

- Does the patient show loss of interest in usual activities, anxiety, apathy, irritability, altered communication patterns, or depressive thoughts?

SELF-PERCEPTION/SELF-CONCEPT
- How does the patient describe himself or herself?
- How has the condition affected the patient's self-esteem?
- How has the condition changed the patient's body image?
- Does the patient have worries or express feelings of helplessness or inadequacy? Does the patient avoid eye contact or withdraw from his or her social support system?
- Does the patient experience feelings of loneliness or rejection, or insecurity in public?

ROLES/RELATIONSHIPS
- What kind of work does the patient perform?
- What role does the patient play in the home and family?
- How has the condition changed the patient's self-perception of his or her roles and ability to perform role functions?
- How satisfied is the patient with his or her role performance?
- What are the effects of the condition on others?

SEXUALITY/REPRODUCTION
- Is the patient sexually active?
- Has the patient experienced any changes in sexual interest or in sexual behaviors and responses?
- Is the patient satisfied with current sexual patterns?
- Have any changes occurred in the menstrual cycle?

COPING/STRESS TOLERANCE
- What are the patient's coping strategies?
- What support systems are available to the patient?
- Can the patient manage the condition in the current setting?
- What family assistance is available?
- Does the patient experience depression?
- What community support and resources are available?

VALUES/BELIEFS
- What constitutes quality of life, for the patient?
- What is important to the patient?
- What would the patient like the provider to address and/or not to address based on his or her beliefs?
- What are the patient's spiritual beliefs and religious involvement? What is the patient's involvement in the community?
- What are the patient's health beliefs and cultural beliefs? To what degree do the patient's cultural and/or religious beliefs affect decision making?
- What are the patient's beliefs about locus of control?

glucose levels in the blood increase while cells in the body are starved of their principal source of energy. The cells signal their need for glucose to the brain, which sets in motion mechanisms to produce even more glucose, primarily the creation of symptoms of hunger and the breakdown of

glycogen and protein to extract glucose (gluconeogenesis). This further increases the blood glucose level but does not assist in getting energy to the cells that need it.

Gluconeogenesis releases glycerol and fatty acids into the bloodstream, which causes dyslipidemia, ketosis, and increased levels of antioxidants. As the body continues its attempts to increase glucose levels to feed starving cells, the high blood levels of glucose and the excretion of large amounts of ketones and glucose in the urine cause fluid and electrolyte imbalances that further destabilize body systems.

Long-term disruptions in blood levels of glucose, lipids, ketones, and antioxidants cause microvascular damage to the blood vessels and cells throughout the body, which lead to hypertension, retinopathy, nephropathy, and neuropathy (Cameron, 2002). Diabetes is the leading cause of blindness, renal failure, and nontraumatic lower extremity amputation in adults, and it is associated with an increased risk of cardiovascular disease, stroke, and death (CDC, 2003a).

Many additional types of diabetes mellitus have been identified by the American Diabetes Association (ADA) (Expert Committee, 2003). The constant factor in all types of diabetes mellitus is the deficient action of insulin. Researchers are investigating several hormones involved in the development of insulin resistance (Holst and Grimaldi, 2002; Kinney, 2002). Clinical trials are also being conducted on pancreatic islet cell transplantation, which has the potential to eliminate the need for exogenous insulin in type 1 diabetes mellitus (Robertson et al, 2000).

Clinical Manifestations

The classic symptoms of type 1 diabetes are polyuria, polydipsia, and unexplained weight loss. These same signs and symptoms may be seen in persons with type 2 diabetes when the blood glucose level rises rapidly, but the more common symptoms in type 2 diabetes are obesity, easy fatigability, lack of energy, shortness of breath, and blurring of vision. Other symptoms—such as frequent infections, increased healing time for cuts and infections, dry skin, pruritus, nausea, and continuous hunger—may also be indications of elevations in the blood glucose level.

Diagnosis

The ADA (2003b) has established standard criteria for diagnosis of diabetes mellitus (Box 20-2).

Box 20-2   Diagnostic Criteria for Diabetes Mellitus

1. A fasting plasma glucose level of 126 mg/ dl or higher (where "fasting" means no caloric intake for at least 8 hours), *or*
2. A 2-hour postload plasma glucose level of 200 mg/dl or higher during an oral glucose tolerance test, *or*
3. Symptoms of diabetes plus a casual plasma glucose level of 200 mg/dl or higher (where "casual" means measured at any time of the day without regard to time since last meal).

From American Diabetes Association: Screening for type 2 diabetes, *Diabetes Care* 26(suppl 1):S21-S24, 2003.

Treatment

Management of both types of diabetes centers on stabilizing blood glucose levels within a normal range through diet, weight control, exercise, and medication, as well as initiating health promotion measures to prevent complications from the disease. The course and severity of the disease in a given individual are determined by the success in maintaining good blood glucose control over many years. Medications, including insulin and oral antidiabetes drugs, are dose-adjusted to control the blood glucose level.

Persons newly diagnosed with diabetes usually receive extensive teaching about the disease and its management. A number of lifestyle adjustments are made at this time, including decisions to eat more meals at home and exercise more regularly. However, there are many cultural, societal, and media prompts for overconsumption of high-calorie, high-fat foods and sedentary lifestyles. Strong support is needed for patients to maintain their vigilance over the years.

The entire health care team must provide consistent and constant cues to action. Routine monitoring of blood glucose level and screening for complications should be considered critical and should be used to encourage continued adherence to the treatment regimen. Self-care activities reported by the patient must be encouraged and enthusiasm for self-management nurtured at every visit.

The ADA standards of care provide a comprehensive list of areas to be covered in the education of persons with diabetes (Mensing et al, 2003). These are listed in Box 20-3. In addition, the American Association of Diabetes Educators offers certification for health professionals who demonstrate competency in the education of persons with diabetes. Information regarding the scope of activity and standards of

---

Box 20-3   Diabetes Education Curriculum

- Description of the diabetes disease process and treatment options
- Nutritional management choices
- Physical activity recommendations
- Medication instruction
- Instructions for monitoring blood glucose level (and urine ketone levels when appropriate)
- Recommendations for preventing, detecting, and treating acute complications
- Behavior modification strategies to prevent, detect, and treat chronic complications
- Goal setting to promote health and problem solving for daily living
- Methods for psychosocial adjustment to the disease
- Need for preconception care and management during pregnancy

From Mensing et al: National standards for diabetes self-management education, *Diabetes Care* 26(suppl 1):S149-S156, 2003.

practice for these educators is available on-line at *http://www.aadenet.org*.

Monitoring

The presence of symptoms of hyperglycemia is a good indication that the blood glucose level is poorly controlled. Patients with type 2 diabetes may be symptom free and feel fine with significantly elevated glucose levels. All patients with diabetes must learn the importance of monitoring and controlling their glucose levels daily to maintain good control. Research has shown that even small improvements in blood glucose control over time have a major impact on the development of complications of diabetes (Diabetes Control and Complications Research Trial Group, 1993; United Kingdom Prospective Diabetes Study Group, 1998). For patients, this means that they must control their blood glucose level as tightly as possible, although an occasional slip from the regimen is not an overwhelming problem. The overall control achieved from month to month determines the sequelae of the disease.

Patients must have the information and equipment they need to self-monitor and self-regulate their blood glucose levels. Most patients with type 2 diabetes measure their blood glucose level once daily (usually before breakfast), whereas persons with type 1 diabetes may test their blood glucose levels four times a day or more. When patients are sick, are experiencing symptoms of hyperglycemia or hypoglycemia during the day, or have fluctuating morning blood glucose levels, it may be useful for them to test more frequently. Measuring preprandial and postprandial blood glucose levels and taking readings at bedtime and in the middle of the night give the patient and health care providers a more comprehensive view of the situation. All blood glucose readings should be recorded in a notebook that the patient shows to the health care team at every visit. Health care professionals should reinforce the importance of these records for adjustment of the management plan and attainment of the patient's goals.

Although patients should monitor blood glucose level daily at home, the most clinically significant measure of long-term glycemic control is the concentration of glycosylated hemoglobin (or hemoglobin A_{1c}). Hemoglobin becomes glycosylated—or attached to glucose molecules—when it is exposed to glucose in the blood; the higher the blood glucose level, the greater the percentage of hemoglobin molecules that attach to glucose (Pagana and Pagana, 2002). In healthy individuals, the hemoglobin A_{1c} concentration is less than 6%. In persons whose blood glucose level was elevated over the previous 3 months, the hemoglobin A_{1c} level may be two to three times the normal value. Table 20-3 compares average daily glucose values with the corresponding hemoglobin A_{1c} values.

The advantage of hemoglobin A_{1c} testing over routine blood glucose measurement is that it provides an estimate of the overall control of blood glucose over time. The blood

Table 20-3 Relation Between Hemoglobin A_{1c} Concentration and Average Blood Glucose Level

Hemoglobin A_{1c} Concentration (%)	Average Blood Glucose Level over Preceding 120 Days (mg/dl)
13	330
12	300
11	270
10	240
9	210
8	180
7	150
6	120
5	90
4	60

Adapted from Intermountain Health Care: Glycosylated hemoglobin, 2001, retrieved from *http://www.ihc.com/xp/ihc/documents/clinical/online/diabeteshemog.pdf* on Feb 5, 2004.

glucose level is a more direct measure that shows only the status at a given time and is affected by food intake during the previous 24 hours. Nurses and patients use blood glucose test results to assess immediate glucose status—to ascertain the effect of food and exercise on glucose level, to make adjustments in insulin dose, and to assess glucose response during sickness. The glycosylated hemoglobin level is used to assess long-term glucose control and provides both a measure of success in diabetes management and an estimate of the patient's risk for the development of diabetic complications.

Interdisciplinary Care

Depending on the severity and progression of the patient's diabetes, the interdisciplinary health care team for diabetes management may consist of nurses, doctors, podiatrists, health educators, pharmacists, social workers, and occupational and physical therapists. Every member of the team has the responsibility to do the following:

- Educate the patient that the treatment of diabetes requires a balance of dietary adjustment, weight control, exercise, and (frequently) medication
- Encourage and provide routine monitoring of the disease and its complications
- Stress that the patient's individual choices are the crux of management.

Primary Provider (Physician/Nurse Practitioner)

In addition to patient glucose monitoring at home, routine health care checks are recommended to evaluate long-term control of blood glucose level, to monitor for early signs of diabetic complications, and to institute early treatment for complications (ADA, 2003c). Primary care providers such as advanced practice nurses should educate patients that the recommended routine health promotion measures are part of a comprehensive plan to reach their goals for the control of this disease (Box 20-4).

Routine monitoring provides essential feedback to patients regarding their level of success in controlling diabetes and the need for alterations in the treatment program. Early treatment interventions for conditions such as nephropathy, retinopathy, hypertension, dyslipidemia, and neuropathy have been shown to have a significant impact in preventing serious sequelae. Pneumonia immunization and annual influenza immunization are recommended for all persons with diabetes, regardless of age, because those with diabetes are at higher risk of death due to these illnesses (CDC, 2003a).

Primary care providers should adopt procedures to cue routine monitoring activities through means such as flow sheets and signs posted in patient examination and waiting rooms. Office systems that automatically remind patients to come for testing at specified intervals may be useful in improving care and can be purchased commercially. The often slow progression of diabetes should not be used as an excuse for postponing monitoring activities. Missed appointments should be investigated and rescheduled as soon as possible. Designating one member of the care team to contact the patient on a regular basis about routine monitoring activities has been shown to result in better patient outcomes (Berg and Wadhwa, 2002). Nurse practitioners are ideally trained to educate, monitor, counsel, and intervene in this chronic disorder.

Drug Therapy

Pharmacologic interventions in type 1 diabetes include the use of various types of insulin to stabilize the blood glucose level and drugs to prevent or manage complications such as renal disease and hypertension (Table 20-4).

Short-acting insulins are given before meals and as needed to respond to surges in blood glucose level. Intermediate- and long-acting insulins are usually used in anticipation of rises in the blood glucose level and to maintain baseline blood glucose control. In either case, the administration of insulin requires continuing associated monitoring of the blood glucose level to determine if the appropriate dose is being administered.

Insulin needs are highly individualized. Persons with type 1 diabetes frequently take multiple doses of insulin each day. Rotation of injection sites can increase patient comfort, improve absorption, and prevent complications such as lipodystrophy. However, patients should be taught about the variation in absorption rates at different sites (e.g., absorption is fastest from the upper abdomen) and should be instructed to use a regular pattern of site rotation (upper arm, buttocks, upper abdomen, lower abdomen, thigh) as well as rotation within sites to give consistent glycemic response. Injections within sites should be given 1 inch apart, and specific injection points should be avoided for 2 to 4 weeks after an injection (Phipps et al, 2003). Progress has been reported in the use of insulin pumps to deliver basal and bolus doses of regular insulin 24 hours a day (Olohan and Zappitelli, 2003).

Many patients take two types of insulin at the same time. In general, two types of insulin can be mixed together in one syringe to minimize needle sticks. When insulin is mixed, the short-acting insulin should be drawn into the syringe first to avoid contamination of the short-acting insulin with insulin that might cause a slower response. Insulin glargine cannot be mixed with other insulins. Patients should be taught the times of onset and peak action of the types of insulin they are using so they can plan for adequate food intake at the appropriate times and adjust the insulin doses for changes in their daily routine.

Pharmacologic interventions in type 2 diabetes include the use of insulin and/or oral drugs to stimulate pancreatic

---

Box 20-4   Routine Health Promotion Measures for Persons with Diabetes

■ Blood for a glycosylated hemoglobin test should be drawn every 3 to 6 months. Every 1% decrease in the glycosylated hemoglobin concentration is associated with a 35% reduction in the risk of retinopathy, nephropathy, and possibly neuropathy (Diabetes Control and Complications Research Trial Group, 1993; United Kingdom Prospective Diabetes Study Group, 1998).

■ Blood pressure should be measured at every opportunity. Early detection and control of hypertension delays or prevents the development of nephropathy, stroke, and cardiovascular disease (United Kingdom Prospective Diabetes Study Group, 1998).

■ Blood lipid levels should be checked every 1 to 2 years beginning at the time of diagnosis. Early detection and control of dyslipidemia decreases the risks from atherosclerotic vascular disease.

■ Urine should be checked for microalbuminuria (the earliest indicator of renal disease) at least annually. Early detection and treatment of nephropathy (through means such as more strict glucose regulation, treatment of hypertension, and medications like angiotensin-converting enzyme inhibitors) may delay or prevent progression to end-stage renal disease.

■ Dilated-eye examinations should be performed annually. Early detection and treatment of retinopathy (using laser surgery and antidyslipidemia agents) may delay or prevent vision loss.

■ Foot examinations (checking for pressure sensitivity, vibration sensitivity, blood supply, skin integrity, structure, and ease of movement) should be performed at least annually. Use of protective footwear and increased attention to hygiene may prevent injuries to the feet and/or development of ulcers that might lead to amputation. Improved glycemic control through multiple methodologies may decrease neuropathy and vascular disease, which are associated with increased risk of amputation.

Table 20-4   Drug Treatment for Diabetes Mellitus

Drug	Side Effects	Nursing Considerations/Teaching Points
Rapid-Acting Insulins Insulin aspart (NovoLog) Insulin lispro (Humalog)	Hypoglycemia Pain at injection site	Onset 0.25-0.5 hr. Peak 0.5-3 hr. Take immediately before or after meals. Clear solutions.
Short-Acting Insulins Regular insulin	Hypoglycemia Pain at injection site	Onset 0.5-1.0 hr. Peak 1-5 hr. Take 30 min before meals. Change dose if altering food intake. Clear solutions.

Intermediate-Acting Insulins
NPH insulin (Humulin R, Iletin II R,
  Novolin R)
Lente insulin (Humulin L, Iletin
  II Lente, Novolin L)
	Hypoglycemia
	
	Pain at injection site
		Onset 1-4 hr.
		
		Peak 4-14 hr.
		Change dose if altering food intake.
		Cloudy white suspensions.

Long-Acting Insulins Insulin glargine (Lantus) Ultralente insulin (Humulin U)	Hypoglycemia Pain at injection site	Onset 1-10 hr. Glargine may have no pronounced peak; clear solution; given once a day; has >24-hr duration of action. Ultralente peaks at 8-20 hr; cloudy white suspension; duration of action 18-28 hr. Change dose if altering food intake.
α-Glucosidase Inhibitors Acarbose (Precose) Miglitol (Glyset)	Abdominal pain, diarrhea, flatulence	Delays carbohydrate digestion. Take at the beginning of meals. Monitor liver function.
Biguanides Metformin (Glucophage)	Megaloblastic anemia Lactic acidosis Gastrointestinal distress	Blocks release of glucose by the liver and absorption of glucose from the intestine. Decreases insulin resistance. Take with meals. Stop drug if dehydrated (due to risk of lactic acidosis). Monitor kidney function and blood counts.
Meglitinides Repaglinide (Prandin)	Hypoglycemia Headache	Stimulates release of insulin from pancreas. Take just 15-30 min before meals. Change dose if altering food intake. Skip dose if skipping meal.

Continued

Table 20-4   Drug Treatment for Diabetes Mellitus—cont'd

Drug	Side Effects	Nursing Considerations/ Teaching Points
Sulfonylureas Chlorpropamide (Diabinese) Glimepiride (Amaryl) Glipizide (Glucotrol) Glyburide (DiaBeta, Micronase) Tolazamide (Tolinase) Tolbutamide (Orinase)	Hypoglycemia Blood dyscrasias Weight gain	Stimulates release of insulin from pancreas. Monitor blood counts. Change dose if altering food intake. Contraindicated with sulfa allergy.
Thiazolidinediones Pioglitazone (Actos) Rosiglitazone (Avandia)	Hepatotoxicity Edema Anemia Weight gain	Sensitizes tissues to the action of insulin and increases glucose uptake. Monitor liver function.

cells to produce more insulin, make target cells more likely to respond to insulin, or alter gastrointestinal absorption of glucose. See Table 20-4 for an overview of oral antidiabetes drugs. Many persons with type 2 diabetes also use insulin to achieve their target levels of glucose. Oral antidiabetes drugs that stimulate the production of insulin or increase insulin sensitivity pose a significant risk for hypoglycemia.

In addition to using drugs that target blood glucose level, many persons with diabetes take medications for management of chronic complications of diabetes. Current guidelines for the treatment of hypertension, hyperlipidemia, retinopathy, nephropathy, and neuropathy are available in the ADA's Clinical Practice Recommendations (ADA, 2003a), which are published annually in *Diabetes Care* and can be obtained through the National Guideline Clearinghouse *(http:// www.guideline.gov).*

Dietitian

A registered dietitian may assist the patient in developing a diet plan that fits the patient's cultural and social needs. In the past, the ADA recommended an "exchange diet" that relied on lists of nutritionally equivalent foods within several food groups. Although the exchange diet is sound nutritionally, its complexity prevented many patients from using it successfully. For patients with diabetes, it is particularly important to have a plan for participating in family and other social gatherings involving food. Beliefs about physical fitness activities, attitudes toward use of health care services, and concepts of ideal weight also affect the success of diabetes mellitus treatment.

Since 1994, the ADA has recommended that persons with diabetes count carbohydrates in their food (Franz et al, 2003). Carbohydrates in food are converted directly to glucose in the body, and patients can learn to count the amount of carbohydrates in the foods they consume. Consistent adherence to targets for carbohydrate intake works together with the medications being used to provide an adequate blood glucose level without hyperglycemic or hypoglycemic episodes and to maintain control of blood glucose level. The patient is assessed for his or her individual glucose needs, response to the glucose in foods, and weight goals. The patient is then assigned a target number of 15-g servings of carbohydrate for each meal and snack, with carbohydrate intake spread across the day. Some 15-g carbohydrate choices are shown in Box 20-5.

A registered dietitian should assist the patient in identifying the target number of carbohydrates for each meal and snack. The target for the individual patient is based on a complex combination of body mass index, estimated activity level, and postprandial response to the carbohydrate load (Linekin, 2002). Once the target carbohydrate levels have been set, the patient may consume any combination of foods that provide that number of carbohydrates. Typically, patients consume three to five 15-g carbohydrate servings at each meal (Daly et al, 2003). This type of diet accommo-

---

Box 20-5   Foods Containing 15 Grams of Carbohydrates

½ cup fruit juice
½ cup regular soft drink
1 tbsp honey or sugar
½ cup ice cream
½ cup sweetened gelatin
1 slice bread
6 saltine crackers
1 small piece of fruit
1 cup milk
½ cup cooked pasta
⅓ cup cooked beans

dates most cultural needs. Food labels in the United States identify the amount of carbohydrates in each item sold, which can assist patients in determining appropriate serving sizes. Care should be taken that the patient understands the importance of maintaining a balanced diet (meat, starch, vegetables, fruit, milk, and fat) rather than simply counting carbohydrates.

The registered dietitian may also assist the person with diabetes in identifying a body weight target and appropriate intake target to reach this goal. A person with type 2 diabetes may benefit from information about weight loss programs in the community, whereas a person with type 1 diabetes usually must work to maintain the weight at an appropriate level. Because insulin contributes to the formation of body fat and weight gain, teenage girls with type 1 diabetes are at particular risk for taking insufficient insulin to keep their weight low, which may result in both immediate ketoacidosis and long-term diabetic complications.

Nurse

Nursing care of the person with diabetes centers on the provision of education, reinforcement of self-management behaviors, and coordination of health services. The key teaching points are strategies for safe day-to-day control of blood glucose level, monitoring for early identification of diabetic complications, and encouragement in routine health promotion activities.

The nurse helps the patient to assess current eating patterns and activity patterns, plan meals, identify acceptable physical activities to lower blood glucose level and control weight, learn blood-glucose monitoring activities, set realistic targets for lifestyle changes, and assess the effects of blood glucose control measures. Nursing interventions take place over a long period of time in a number of settings and reinforce the teaching of specialists in multiple other disciplines involved in the care of persons with diabetes.

For the patient to live safely with diabetes, the patient and the patient's family must be educated about the symptoms of hyperglycemia and hypoglycemia and the appropriate responses to prevent complications. Hyperglycemia may result from inadequate insulin, unexpected decreases in planned physical exertion, increased intake of carbohydrates, or the stress of illness. If untreated, hyperglycemia can lead to ketoacidosis and diabetic coma. The usually slow onset of hyperglycemia allows time for the patient to recognize the early symptoms of sweating, fatigue, and sluggishness and to respond by checking the blood glucose level, administering insulin or other medication, and/or decreasing carbohydrate intake.

The symptoms of hyperglycemia are sometimes missed when the patient is not feeling well because of another condition such as fever, infection, or gastrointestinal distress. The patient and family should be educated about the need to monitor blood glucose more frequently on sick days, because some of the symptoms attributed to the acute illness may actually be symptoms of hyperglycemia. Insulin needs increase when the body is under physical stress, even when the patient is too ill to eat. The patient should continue the usual medication and food intake as closely as possible when ill and should contact the primary care provider about illnesses that result in prolonged vomiting or diarrhea, prolonged hyperglycemia, or episodes of hypoglycemia. Many primary care providers also instruct patients (particularly those with type 1 diabetes) to monitor their urine for ketones on sick days to provide an early warning for the development of ketoacidosis.

In contrast to hyperglycemia, which often has a slow onset, hypoglycemia can develop rapidly in response to medication side effects, delays in food intake, or uncompensated exercise. Physical exertion causes an increased utilization of glucose by muscle and an associated fall in the available glucose for the brain, which results in dizziness and weakness. Untreated hypoglycemia from any cause can result in loss of consciousness and death. Patients taking insulin, or agents that stimulate the production of insulin or increase cell responsiveness to insulin, should know the importance of consistent food intake and exercise patterns in maintaining an adequate blood glucose level.

As mentioned earlier, the patient must know the times of onset and peak activity of the types of insulin taken so that food consumption can be planned accordingly and the insulin dose adjusted to changes in activity levels. The patient should also be able to recognize the symptoms of hypoglycemia (Box 20-6) and should always have a carbohydrate source such as a candy lozenge, juice, or pop immediately available for emergencies. Patients must know how to adjust their medications because most will want to vary their diets and activities to participate in social and community events that do not fit the normal daily routine. Hypoglycemia (usually defined as a blood glucose level of less than 50 mg/dl) can be either reactive or nonreactive.

Box 20-6   Signs and Symptoms of Hypoglycemia

REACTIVE HYPOGLYCEMIA
- Weakness
- Trembling
- Sweating
- Pallor
- Anxiety
- Irritability
- Rapid heart rate

NONREACTIVE HYPOGLYCEMIA
- Confusion
- Seizures
- Coma

Reactive hypoglycemia is a sudden drop in the blood glucose level that precipitates adrenergic symptoms. This may result from a sharp drop in the blood glucose level several hours after a meal, or it may be related to the use of insulin, oral antidiabetes agents, or alcohol. Exercise may also cause a sudden sharp drop in blood glucose levels. In nonreactive hypoglycemia, a slow decline in the availability of glucose to the brain results in neurologic symptoms. Both types of hypoglycemia respond to ingestion of carbohydrates. Some patients may be asymptomatic or only mildly symptomatic at a blood glucose of less than 50 mg/dl.

Another important safety concern for the patient with diabetes is foot care. People with diabetes have an increased risk for impaired peripheral circulation and neuropathy, both of which decrease sensory input from the feet (masking the symptoms of injury) and impair healing. The patient should be educated on the importance of daily foot hygiene and inspection of all aspects of the toes and feet. Small cuts or injuries should be cleaned and covered with a sterile dressing. Injuries that do not heal within 3 days should be reported to the primary care provider.

Drying the bottoms of the feet and between the toes is especially important because dampness increases the risk of bacterial and fungal growth. Toenails should be trimmed straight across and should be cut regularly. Some primary care providers recommend the use of lotion on the feet to keep the skin soft, although the nurse should caution the patient to avoid walking on feet slippery with lotion. Heating pads, hot water bottles, and harsh soaps should not be used. The use of garters or tight knee socks and sitting for prolonged periods reduce the blood flow to the feet and should be avoided. A person with diabetes should wear shoes that are neither too tight nor too loose (to prevent rubbing and the development of deformities) and that are sturdy enough to protect the feet from injury. The nurse should ask to inspect the feet of a patient with diabetes at every encounter with the health care system, both to identify problems and to reinforce the importance of daily foot inspection and care of the feet. The patient with advanced neuropathy, structural deformities of the feet, or vision limitation that might lead to self-injury during the use of trimming instruments may benefit from a podiatrist's care.

In reinforcing self-management behaviors of the person with diabetes, the nurse should concentrate on delivering positive messages specific to the patient's personal and cultural goals. Assessment of these goals and reinforcement of the connection between blood glucose control and the specific goals identified by the patient is central to effective treatment. To sell the patient on good health habits, the nurse must use a message that reaches the individual. Negative reminders that poor blood glucose control may result in blindness or amputations are ineffective. Indeed, some patients may even interpret the negative images as reminders to "have a good time while they can." Even when fear of disability is a strong motivating factor, reminders about the possible negative results lose their effectiveness when the patient does not see any immediate consequences of poor adherence to the management plan.

Nursing care of the person with diabetes is very complex. Numerous tools and lists have been developed to prompt the nurse to cover all the many important aspects of knowledge and skills that are needed for self-management.

Medical Social Worker

A social worker may be needed to assist the patient in locating resources to cover the cost of medications, treatments, and self-management activities. Many communities provide access to federally subsidized care through community health centers, which may help with eye examinations as well. Blood glucose meters are available at drugstores or through diabetes support groups. Often suppliers provide free glucose meters to those who request them, because the profit for the company comes from the glucose test strips that the meter uses. Medicare and some insurance companies provide assistance in paying for test strips. Health care providers may have to devise a less preferable but more affordable plan for monitoring blood glucose level less frequently if the patient has a limited income, does not have insurance to cover the cost of the test strips, and cannot locate financial assistance within the community.

The clinical social worker can help the patient and family adjust to the life changes and physical and emotional demands of the illness. One of the symptoms of hyperglycemia is increased irritability, which may negatively affect the patterns of interaction in the family. Often the entire family must change eating habits, become involved in the management of the disease, and cope with a change in roles and conflict over control of the patient's eating and activities. The social worker and registered dietitian may work together to help the family build new non–food-centered traditions for celebrations. A psychotherapist may be needed to assist in the management of depression, which is a common problem among persons with diabetes (Lloyd and Brown, 2002).

Physical and Occupational Therapists

A physical therapist may be called on to develop graded exercise programs, perform mechanical débridement of diabetic leg ulcers in whirlpool tubs and with pressurized water, and provide transfer education and gait training following amputation of a limb. An occupational therapist may identify and treat problems with activities of daily living that result from diabetic retinopathy and peripheral vascular disease.

Podiatrist

The podiatrist can assist in the management of diabetes by performing foot examinations, trimming toenails safely, and treating foot abnormalities with orthotics and surgical procedures.

Complementary and Alternative Therapy

Persons with diabetes use alternative therapies more often than persons who do not have diabetes. Egede et al (2002) found that persons with diabetes are 1.6 times more likely than other patients to use complementary and alternative medicine (CAM). For the most part, persons with diabetes seem to use CAM in conjunction with conventional diabetes care, and 57% reported discussing their use of CAM with their health care professional.

The types of CAM used included nutrition and diet therapy, spiritual healing, herbal remedies, massage, and meditation. Some of the nutritional therapies being used differed significantly from the ADA dietary recommendations. Herbal remedies have not been shown to be helpful in management of blood glucose level. Prayer and spiritual healing, however, have been shown to improve outcomes of therapy in other diseases.

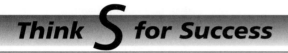

Think **S** for Success

Symptoms
- Manage symptoms of elevated blood glucose level with medication, diet, and exercise.

Sequelae
- Prevent complications by monitoring and controlling blood glucose level through medication, diet, and exercise; perform screening for early signs of complications.
- Seek early treatment for any developing complications.

Safety
- Teach symptoms of increased and decreased blood glucose levels and appropriate responses.

Support/Services
- Give encouragement for even small amounts of control.
- Help with obtaining medications and testing supplies.
- Use flowchart and automatic reminder system to ensure appropriate monitoring and testing.
- Make appropriate referrals for eye examinations, etc. Identify patient goals and motivating factors.
- Give patients self-management tools.

Satisfaction
- Determine the degree to which diabetes management is interfering with important aspects of patient's life and develop a plan to help patient reach or maintain desired quality of life.

ALTERED THYROID FUNCTION

Thyroid hormones perform several important functions in the body. They direct the rate of metabolism of proteins, carbohydrates, and lipids, effectively controlling the activity of body organs, the production of heat, and the consumption of oxygen. They also have a significant impact on heart rate and stroke volume and control protein synthesis, cell growth, and cell differentiation.

Euthyroidism is a state of normal thyroid secretion and functioning. Hyperthyroidism refers to increased secretion of thyroid hormone. Hypothyroidism is a state of decreased thyroid hormone secretion and function. Both hyperthyroidism and hypothyroidism can cause impaired cardiac function.

Gradations of thyroid hormone dysfunction exist that have many subtle symptoms not attributed to thyroid disorder until late in the course of the disease. It is therefore difficult to know the actual prevalence of thyroid hormone dysfunction. The American Association of Clinical Endocrinologists (AACE) (2003) estimates that 27 million Americans have thyroid disease and that it remains undiagnosed in half of them. Women are five times more likely than men to have hypothyroidism. By age 60, 17% of women and 9% of men will have thyroid disease. Hypothyroidism is more common than hyperthyroidism (Goldsmith, 1999; Li, 2002). Approximately 1% of American women will develop hyperthyroidism (Hormone Foundation, 2002).

Pathophysiology

The thyroid gland is responsible for secretion of the thyroid hormones thyroxine (T_4) and triiodothyronine (T_3). The gland is under the regulation of a negative feedback loop involving the hypothalamus, the anterior pituitary gland, and the thyroid gland. Low circulating levels of T_4 and T_3 stimulate the hypothalamus to secrete thyrotropin-releasing hormone (TRH), which in turn stimulates the anterior pituitary to secrete thyroid-stimulating hormone (TSH). TSH stimulates the thyroid gland to secrete both T_4 and T_3. High levels of T_4 and T_3 in the blood lower the hypothalamic secretion of TRH, which decreases the secretion of TSH; this reduction in TSH levels then causes less T_4 and T_3 to be secreted by the thyroid gland.

T_4 is converted to T_3 at the target tissues, and T_3 is the active thyroid hormone that produces the effects noted clinically. Adequate dietary iodine and protein are necessary for the synthesis and secretion of T_4 and T_3.

In hyperthyroidism, excessive amounts of T_3 and T_4 lead to a hypermetabolic state and an increase in sympathetic nervous system activity. The β-adrenergic receptors in cardiac tissue are stimulated, which results in tachycardia and increased cardiac output, stroke volume, and peripheral blood flow. The most common cause of hyperthyroidism is an autoimmune disorder known as Graves' disease. In Graves' disease, immunoglobulin G binds to TSH receptors on the surface of thyroid gland cells, which results in constant release of thyroid hormone. Because the feedback mechanism is subverted by the action of immunoglobulin G, increased thyroid hormone secretion continues in spite of hormonal signals from the hypothalamus and pituitary gland. Hyperthyroidism may also be caused by other dysfunctions of the thyroid gland or by toxic benign adenoma, thyroid carcinoma, toxic nodular goiter, or excessive ingestion of thyroid hormones. Many cases of hyperthyroidism eventually convert into hypothyroidism, either because of the destructive effects of medical therapies or "burn-out" of the thyroid gland.

In hypothyroidism, decreased levels of thyroid hormones cause physiologic effects opposite to those seen in hyperthyroidism (Figure 20-2).

Clinical Manifestations

Manifestations of thyroid disorders range from subclinical to severe (myxedema coma or thyroid storm) and are often first recognized by a health care professional (Table 20-5).

In hyperthyroidism, increased metabolic rate causes increased calorigenesis, lipid depletion, negative nitrogen balance, weight loss, and a state of nutritional deficit. Secretion and metabolism of hypothalamic, pituitary, and gonadal hormones are also altered in hyperthyroid states. In adult men, these alterations may result in diminished libido and erectile dysfunction. Affected women may experience oligomenorrhea or amenorrhea.

Conversely, in hypothyroidism the heart rate, cardiac output, stroke volume, and peripheral blood flow are all decreased, which results in peripheral edema, shortness of

breath, and easy fatigability. A decrease in the basal metabolic rate and alterations in lipid metabolism may cause constipation, weight gain, fatigue, sluggishness, depression, sensations of being cold, and decreased mental clarity. Skin may become dry, and hair may become brittle and fall out easily. Wound healing may be slowed. Medications are metabolized more slowly and remain active in the body longer. Menstrual periods may become heavier, and anovulation may lead to infertility. Men may experience decreased sperm production and diminished libido. Decreased absorption of nutrients from the gastrointestinal track may result in vitamin B_{12}, folate, iron, and protein deficiencies. Decreased protein synthesis may lead to abnormal red blood cell production with resulting anemias.

Myxedema, a medical emergency, is an altered level of consciousness that can occur when severe hypothyroidism is undiagnosed or undertreated. It is usually precipitated by a concurrent medical illness, infection, stress, or administration of sedatives or narcotics. It occurs almost exclusively in older adults with a history of longstanding untreated or undertreated primary hypothyroidism (Li, 2002). Patients with myxedema experience rapid development of stupor or coma, hypothermia without shivering, hypoglycemia, hypotension, hypoventilation, and signs of lactic acidosis. Treatment for myxedema consists of administration of levothyroxine, ventilatory support, slow adjustment of fluid balance, and rapid treatment of the precipitating illness.

Primary hypothyroidism typically develops as a primary autoimmune thyroid disorder known as Hashimoto's thyroiditis. However, it can be a manifestation of other forms of thyroiditis, some of which are transient illnesses (Table 20-6). Secondary hypothyroidism may occur as a result of insufficient thyroid gland stimulation due to failure of the TRH and TSH feedback mechanisms.

Diagnosis

The diagnosis of thyroid disorder is based on clinical presentation and evaluation of the levels of T_3, T_4, and TSH taken together. The T_3 and T_4 levels indicate the amount of hormone available to supply bodily needs, and the TSH level usually indicates the source of the disorder. Free T_4 level is more commonly measured than free T_3 level because of the cost, although free T_3 level is a more accurate reflection of the active thyroid stimulation of tissue. Low free T_3 levels accompanied by slightly elevated TSH levels are commonly found in patients who are severely ill; this situation is called *euthyroid sick syndrome,* and the patient should be evaluated by an endocrinologist before a condition of hypothyroidism is diagnosed (AACE, 2002).

In primary thyroid disorder, the thyroid gland malfunctions and does not respond to the TSH signals, continuing to produce either too much or too little hormone. In secondary thyroid disorders, the pituitary gland secretes inappropriate levels of TSH, to which the thyroid gland responds. In tertiary thyroid disorders, the hypothalamus secretes inappropriate levels of TRH to which both the pituitary and the thyroid

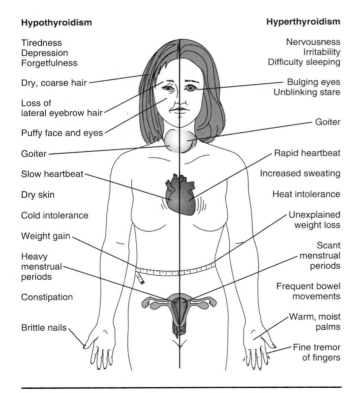

Hypothyroidism

Tiredness
Depression
Forgetfulness

Dry, coarse hair

Loss of
lateral eyebrow hair

Puffy face and eyes

Goiter

Slow heartbeat

Dry skin

Cold intolerance

Weight gain

Heavy
menstrual
periods

Constipation

Brittle nails

Hyperthyroidism

Nervousness
Irritability
Difficulty sleeping

Bulging eyes
Unblinking stare

Goiter

Rapid heartbeat

Increased sweating

Heat intolerance

Unexplained
weight loss

Scant
menstrual
periods

Frequent bowel
movements

Warm, moist
palms

Fine tremor
of fingers

Figure 20-2 Signs and symptoms of thyroid disease.

Table 20-5 Comparison of Hyperthyroidism and Hypothyroidism

Affected System	Hyperthyroidism	Hypothyroidism

Central nervous system	Agitation
	Nervousness
	Irritability
	Anxiety
	Insomnia
	Tremors
	Heat intolerance, increased sweating
	Fatigue
		Fatigue
		Cognitive impairments
		  Impaired attention
		  Decreased memory
		  Decreased motor speed
		Lethargy
		Slow speech
		Depression
		Dementia
		Cold intolerance

Cardiovascular system	Palpitations Atrial fibrillation Angina pectoris Hypertension	Bradycardia Low blood pressure Decreased cardiac output Increased risk of atherosclerosis Peripheral edema
Metabolism	Weight loss Increased frequency of bowel movements Increased appetite	Weight gain Constipation Anorexia Hyperlipidemia
Other	Thyroid enlargement Decreased menstrual flow	Thyroid enlargement Dry skin Slowed wound healing Heavy menstrual flow Joint stiffness and swelling Rheumatoid arthritis Weakness Muscle stiffness

gland respond. Table 20-7 shows the laboratory results for T_3, T_4, TSH, and TRH in each of these situations.

Other tests used in the diagnosis of thyroid disorders include ultrasonography, radioactive uptake scanning and stimulation testing. In a stimulation test, TRH is administered intravenously, followed by timed blood draws. The blood is analyzed for TSH level.

Interdisciplinary Care
Primary Provider (Physician/Nurse Practitioner)

The individual with a thyroid disorder may be cared for by a variety of providers, including the internist, family practice professional, and endocrinologist. Once the diagnosis has been made, the primary care provider monitors laboratory values of circulating hormones and compares this analysis to

Table 20-6 Types of Thyroiditis and Their Characteristics

Type	Characteristics
Chronic thyroiditis Hashimoto's thyroiditis	Autoimmune process characterized by inflammation and fibrosis.
Subacute thyroiditis Silent, painless thyroiditis/ lymphocytic thyroiditis	A form of thyroiditis increasing in frequency. Etiology unknown but possible autoimmune component. Symptoms include self-limiting form of hyperthyroidism and nontender, enlarged thyroid gland, which may be followed by hypothyroidism. Symptomatic treatment is provided during the hyperthyroid phase with β-adrenergic blockers but not antithyroid medications. Patients should be monitored annually for development of hypothyroidism.
Postpartum thyroiditis	Occurs within a few months after delivery in 1% to 5% of pregnant women. Clinical course is similar to that of silent, painless thyroiditis with transient toxic and hypothyroid phases that may be so mild that they go unnoticed in some patients. Permanent hypothyroidism occurs more frequently than after painless, silent thyroiditis.

From Phipps WJ et al: *Medical-surgical nursing: health and illness perspectives,* ed 7, Mosby, 2003, p 899.

Table 20-7   Diagnosis of Thyroid Disorders

Condition	T_3 and T_4	TSH	TRH
Hyperthyroidism			
Primary	↑	↓	↓
Secondary	↑	↑	↓
Tertiary	↑	↑	↑
Hypothyroidism			
Primary	↓	↑	↑
Secondary	↓	↓	↑
Tertiary	↓	↓	↓

↑, Increased; ↓, decreased; *T3*, triiodothyronine; *T4*, thyroxine; *TRH*, thyrotropin-releasing hormone; *TSH*, thyroid-stimulating hormone.

the symptoms reported. Responses to adjustments in medication are generally not manifested for 6 to 8 weeks, so careful follow-up and tracking of patient response to treatment are essential.

Treatment of hyperthyroidism is aimed at lowering thyroid hormone levels and returning the patient to a eumetabolic state. The three treatment modalities used to achieve normal thyroid functioning are antithyroid drug therapy, radioactive iodine (^{131}iodine) treatment, and thyroid surgery (AACE, 2002).

Surgeon

Thyroidectomy, is reserved for patients with thyroid carcinoma and toxic adenoma and is rarely used for individuals with Graves' disease, which is more commonly treated with antithyroid drugs or radioactive iodine). Indications for thyroidectomy include the presence of large goiters resistant to ^{131}iodine treatment, the presence of thyroid nodules, pregnancy, allergy to antithyroid drugs, and refusal of ^{131}iodine treatment (Singer et al, 1995). Following surgery, most patients will require thyroid hormone replacement for life; occasionally, a remaining fragment of thyroid gland tissue may begin secreting T_3 and T_4 months to years after surgery.

Drug Therapy

Hyperthyroidism

The most common treatment modality for hyperthyroidism in the United States is ^{131}iodine therapy (Table 20-8). The isotope, given as a pill, accumulates in the thyroid gland and selectively destroys gland tissue (McKenry and Salerno, 1998). Typically, one ^{131}iodine pill is given once, and a response is noted within 6 to 12 weeks (AACE, 2002). The patient should be taught precautions for disposal of excreta and the need to avoid close personal contact during the first 5 days after ingestion of the ^{131}iodine to protect the patient and others from the radioactive isotope (AACE, 2002). The most common side effect of treatment is the development of hypothyroidism, which usually requires thy-

roid hormone replacement therapy for life. Treatment with ^{131}iodine is contraindicated in pregnant and breast-feeding women.

Antithyroid drugs may be used as a primary treatment modality or they may be used to lower thyroid hormone levels prior to surgery or treatment with ^{131}iodine. Antithyroid drugs such as methimazole (Tapazole) and propylthiouracil (PTU) act by inhibiting biosynthesis of thyroid hormone, and 2 to 6 weeks may be required for their thyroid hormone–lowering effect to be demonstrated. As a primary modality, treatment with antithyroid drugs for 12 to 18 months may result in prolonged remission for 20% to 30% of those treated (American Thyroid Association, 2003). When the drugs are withdrawn, hyperthyroidism is likely to recur. Allergic reactions to antithyroid drugs manifest as skin rashes, hives, fever, and joint pain; the most serious side effect is a lowering of the white blood cell count. Patients receiving these drugs should know the symptoms of insufficient thyroid hormone (hypothyroidism) and should be monitored for them.

The β-blockers are used as adjunctive therapy to provide symptomatic relief from sympathetic nervous system effects until other modalities decrease the secretion of thyroid hormone. Commonly used β-blockers include propranolol (Inderol) and nadolol (Corgard). The calcium channel blocker diltiazem (Cardizem) is used in patients who cannot tolerate β-blocking agents (such as those with asthma).

Hypothyroidism

Drug therapy in the treatment of hypothyroidism focuses on replacement of thyroid hormones (see Table 20-8). Synthetic levothyroxine (Synthroid) is the treatment of choice for confirmed hypothyroidism. The levothyroxine dosage varies and is adjusted on an individual basis to attain a normal thyroid profile (normal T_3, T_4, and TSH levels). The required dosage is generally lower in the elderly because of decreased kidney clearance of T_4 (Li, 2002).

Because of the cardiovascular effects of thyroid hormone replacement, the initial dosage may be half or less of the anticipated final dosage (especially in the elderly), with the dosage gradually increased to the level that optimizes the thyroid profile and reduces the patient's symptoms. The thyroid profile should be reassessed 8 to 12 weeks after dosage changes, when it has achieved some degree of stabilization. Once the appropriate dosage is achieved, annual monitoring is usually sufficient.

For most persons with hypothyroidism, control of the disease is possible with one tablet of levothyroxine daily. A small percentage of those with hypothyroidism are unable to convert T_4 to T_3 efficiently (Guha, Krishnaswamy, and Peiris, 2002). These patients have symptoms of hypothyroidism even though T_4 and TSH levels indicate an adequate dose of replacement hormone. However, the T_3 level in these patients remains low with respect to the T_4 level unless they also receive direct replacement of the hormone T_3 as liothyronine (Cytomel). Liothyronine has a shorter half-life

Table 20-8 Drug Treatment for Thyroid Disorders

Drug	Side Effects	Nursing Considerations/Teaching Points
Hyperthyroidism *Antithyroid Drugs* Methimazole (Tapazole) Propylthiouracil	Rash, itching, arthralgia, jaundice, agranulocytosis	Contact physician if fever, rash, jaundice, arthralgia, or oropharyngitis develops. Use with caution in pregnancy.
Iodine 131	Early or late development of hypothyroidism	Contraindicated in pregnancy. For 5 days after treatment Avoid exchange of saliva and close contact with children Avoid close contact with pregnant women Flush toilet twice after use Wash hands thoroughly Avoid pregnancy for 6 months after discontinuing treatment.
Adjunctive Therapy Nadolol (Corgard) Propranolol (Inderal)	Fatigue, dizziness, bradycardia, rash, impotence, constipation, dry mouth	Use with caution if diabetes, renal impairment, severe congestive heart failure, or asthma is present.
Diltiazem (Cardizem)	Edema, headache, rash, nausea, dizziness, fatigue, hypotension, bradycardia	Use with caution if renal or hepatic impairment or pulmonary congestion is present.
Hypothyroidism Levothyroxine (Synthroid, Levothroid, Levoxyl)	Palpitations, increased appetite, tachycardia, nervousness, tremor, weight loss, diarrhea, abdominal cramps, insomnia.	Use with caution if cardiovascular disease or hypertension is present. Monitor thyroid levels annually and 6-12 wk after dosage adjustment.
Triiodothyronine (Cytomel)		

Adapted from American Association of Clinical Endocrinologists: Medical guidelines for clinical practice for evaluation and treatment of hyperthyroidism and hypothyroidism, *Endocr Pract* 8(6):457-67, 2002.

than thyroxine and must be administered in small doses several times a day. It is also the active form of the hormone, and cardiac side effects are more common. Some patients report feeling better when they take animal thyroid hormone, which contains both T_3 and T_4, rather than the synthetic levothyroxine (Guha, Krishnaswamy, and Peiris, 2002). Most patients who begin thyroid hormone replacement will need lifelong treatment.

Side effects of thyroid hormone replacement are primarily associated with the cardiovascular and musculoskeletal systems. Overdose of these hormones can cause rapid heart rate, angina, arrhythmia, and myocardial infarction. Long-term overdose of thyroid hormones is associated with symptoms of hyperthyroidism as well as with acceleration of osteoporosis, increased risk of fractures, and development of congestive heart failure. Undertreatment results in symptoms of hypothyroidism. A missed dose should not be taken the next day along with the regular dose because of the possible cardiovascular side effects.

The amount of available levothyroxine is sharply decreased when the pill is taken with food, especially products containing calcium and iron. The maximum dose of levothyroxine is obtained when the pill is taken on an empty stomach and the patient waits 1 to 2 hours before eating. However, the dose of the medication should be adjusted to correspond to the way that the patient takes it; if it is taken with food every day, the dose must be higher than if it is taken on an empty stomach. Patients should be instructed to take their thyroid hormone replacement medication every day at the same time with respect to their food intake, and they should know that if they are going to permanently alter their routine of food and medication intake, the dose must be reassessed. Occasional changes in routine do not affect the thyroid profile significantly, although patients may experience symptoms of excess thyroid stimulation or thyroid deficiency for a day or two if they alter their pattern.

Estrogen, whether in contraceptives or in hormone replacement therapy, may increase the protein binding of levothyroxine, so that the thyroid hormone replacement dose may have to be increased. Other drugs that interact significantly with thyroid replacement hormones are corticosteroids, tricyclic antidepressants, β-blockers, and phenytoin (Dilantin). Thyroid hormone replacement significantly increases the effectiveness of warfarin (Coumadin) and theophylline (Theo-Dur), and dose adjustments may be necessary. Some patients taking thyroid hormone replacement remain sensitive to stimulants such as caffeine and pseudoephedrine (in over-the-counter cold remedies) even when they are properly treated.

Nurse

When hyperthyroidism or hypothyroidism is properly treated, the patient lives a normal life except for the need for medication. The patient should be educated about the disease and its symptoms, about the need for lifelong monitoring of hormone levels, and about the side effects of the drugs taken. Annual measurement of the thyroid profile is usually sufficient for the patient receiving thyroid replacement hormones.

Many symptoms of worsening hyperthyroidism or hypothyroidism are subtle. In particular, symptoms of irritability, fatigue, and weight loss in hyperthyroid patients and decreased mental clarity, increased fatigue, frequent crying, and weight gain in hypothyroid patients are frequently mistaken for depression in women. Hoarseness, dry skin, deafness, constipation, cold sensitivity, and weakness in hypothyroidism may be mistaken for the aging process. The patient and health care providers should maintain a heightened alertness for the development of these symptoms in a person known to have thyroid disease.

An ophthalmic change called exophthalmos can occur in hyperthyroidism (Figure 20-3). The nurse should assess the ability of the individual to fully close the eyes. If the lids do not completely cover the eye, the patient should be instructed to use artificial tears to keep the corneas moist. The individual should also be instructed to gently tape the eyelids closed or to apply soft eye patches when going to bed to protect the eyes from abrasions and drying.

Dietitian

A registered dietitian should be consulted to ensure adequate nutrition for both hyperthyroid and hypothyroid patients. Hyperthyroid patients are at risk for malnourishment due to their rapid metabolic state and may need to follow a special diet to regain lost weight and replace body stores of nutrients. Hypothyroid patients may need a special diet to lose the weight gained prior to diagnosis of their illness and to address their anemia and hyperlipidemia, both of which should resolve rapidly with thyroid replacement.

Physical Therapist

Physical therapy may be indicated for gradual reconditioning of elderly patients with cardiovascular disease who have been diagnosed with thyroid disorders.

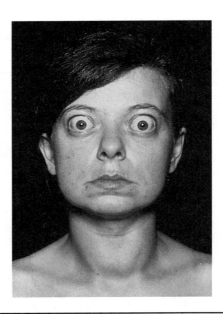

Figure 20-3 Ophthalmopathy caused by hyperthyroidism: exophthalmos. (From Seidel HM et al: *Mosby's guide to physical examination,* ed 5, St Louis, 2003, Mosby.)

Think S for Success

Symptoms
- Manage symptoms with appropriate medications.
- Teach patient the symptoms of hypothyroidism that may result from antithyroid therapies.

Sequelae
- Prevent complications by assessing treatment effectiveness and providing continued health assessment.
- Protect corneas.

Safety
- Monitor thyroid profile annually or 4-8 weeks after medication dosage adjustments. Teach safety measures for radioactive iodide 131.

Support/Services
- Educate patient about disease and management modalities.

Satisfaction
- Determine the degree to which thyroid disease management is interfering with important aspects of patient's life and develop a plan to help patient reach or maintain desired quality of life.

ADRENAL GLAND DYSFUNCTION

The adrenal cortex secretes glucocorticoids (cortisol), mineralocorticoids (aldosterone), and sex hormones. The adrenal cortex hormones affect mobilization of energy stores, inflammatory and immune response, fluid and electrolyte balance, growth and development, and secondary sex characteristics. A change in the level of any of the adrenal cortex hormones causes dysfunction in many organs and tissues of the body.

Of the many disorders caused by excesses and deficiencies of adrenocortical hormones, this chapter addresses only two, Cushing's syndrome and Addison's disease.

Pathophysiology

The adrenal glands secrete cortisol under the regulation of a negative feedback loop involving the hypothalamus, the anterior pituitary gland, and the adrenal cortex. Low circulating levels of cortisol stimulate the hypothalamus to secrete corticotropin-releasing hormone, which in turn stimulates the anterior pituitary to secrete adrenocorticotropic hormone (ACTH). ACTH stimulates the adrenal cortex to secrete cortisol. High levels of cortisol in the blood lower the hypothalamic secretion of corticotropin-releasing hormone, which decreases the secretion of ACTH and thus causes less cortisol to be secreted by the adrenal gland.

Cushing's Syndrome

Cushing's syndrome is a spectrum of clinical abnormalities caused by excess adrenocortical activity. The most common form of Cushing's syndrome, known as Cushing's disease, is caused by a pituitary adenoma that secretes excessive amounts of ACTH. Other potential causes of Cushing's syndrome are ACTH-secreting tumors outside of the pituitary (as in some lung cancers), and exogenous administration of corticosteroids.

Cushing's syndrome is relatively rare, affecting about 10 people per 1 million population; most cases occur in people between 20 and 50 years of age (National Institute of Diabetes and Digestive and Kidney Diseases [NIDDK], 2002). Cushing's disease accounts for 70% of the cases of Cushing's syndrome; women are five times more likely than men to have Cushing's disease (Cushing's Support and Research Foundation, 2002).

Clinical Manifestations

The clinical manifestations of Cushing's syndrome can be grouped according to the effects of the various hormones of the adrenal cortex. Figure 20-4 shows the effects of cortisol excess and Table 20-9 lists the manifestations of adrenocortical hormone dysfunction.

Symptoms of excess glucocorticoids are profound and affect most body systems. One of the most common effects of glucocorticoid excess is weight gain resulting from the accumulation of adipose tissue in the trunk, face, and cervical area. This can be accentuated by weight gain from sodium and water retention induced by excess mineralocorticoids. Because of protein and muscle wasting caused by the catabolic effects of cortisol on the peripheral tissues, the patient has thin extremities and loss of strength. Cardiac myopathy may develop rapidly as a result of muscle wasting.

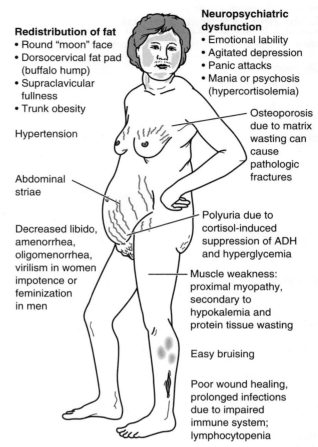

Redistribution of fat
- Round "moon" face
- Dorsocervical fat pad (buffalo hump)
- Supraclavicular fullness
- Trunk obesity

Hypertension

Abdominal striae

Decreased libido, amenorrhea, oligomenorrhea, virilism in women impotence or feminization in men

Neuropsychiatric dysfunction
- Emotional lability
- Agitated depression
- Panic attacks
- Mania or psychosis (hypercortisolemia)

Osteoporosis due to matrix wasting can cause pathologic fractures

Polyuria due to cortisol-induced suppression of ADH and hyperglycemia

Muscle weakness: proximal myopathy, secondary to hypokalemia and protein tissue wasting

Easy bruising

Poor wound healing, prolonged infections due to impaired immune system; lymphocytopenia

Complications
Cardiovascular complications are the major causes of morbidity and mortality. Other complications:
- Congestive heart failure
- Hypertension
- Dependent edema
- Left ventricular hypertrophy
- Pathologic fractures
- Masked infections

Figure 20-4 Clinical manifestations of Cushing's syndrome. *ADH,* Antidiuretic hormone. (From Luckmann J: *Saunders manual of nursing care,* Philadelphia, 1997, WB Saunders.)

High levels of cortisol antagonize insulin and vitamin D, which leads to inhibition of glucose uptake and bone formation. Hyperglycemia and the symptoms of diabetes are a common result. Increased risk for atherosclerosis with subsequent effects on the heart is a serious consequence of the altered fat metabolism. Loss of protein bone matrix may lead to osteoporosis and pathologic fractures. Thin skin and capillary fragility occur because collagen synthesis is inhibited. Bluish red stretch marks often appear on the abdomen, thighs, buttocks, arms, and breasts as a result of weakened connective tissue. Wound healing is delayed. Excess cortisol inhibits many functions of the immune system, which results in an increased risk of infection.

Table 20-9   Clinical Manifestations of Adrenocortical Hormone Dysfunction

Affected System	Hypofunction (Addison's Disease)	Hyperfunction (Cushing's Syndrome)
Glucocorticoids		
General appearance	Weight loss	Truncal (centripetal) obesity, thin extremities, rounding of face (moon face), fat deposits on back of neck and on shoulders (buffalo hump)
Integumentary system	Bronzed or smoky hyperpigmentation of face, neck, hands (especially creases), buccal membranes, nipples, genitalia, and scars (if pituitary function normal); vitiligo, alopecia	Thin, fragile skin; purplish red striae; petechial hemorrhages; bruises; florid cheeks (plethora); acne; poor wound healing
Cardiovascular system	Hypotension, tendency to develop refractory shock, vasodilation	Hypervolemia, hypertension, edema of lower extremities
Gastrointestinal system	Anorexia, nausea and vomiting, cramping abdominal pain, diarrhea	Increase in secretion of pepsin and hydrochloric acid, anorexia
Urinary system		Glycosuria, hypercalciuria, kidney stones
Musculoskeletal system	Fatigability	Muscle wasting in extremities, proximal muscle weakness, fatigue, osteoporosis, awkward gait, back and joint pain, weakness
Immune system	Propensity toward coexisting autoimmune diseases	Inhibition of immune response, suppression of allergic response, inhibition of inflammation
Hematologic system	Anemia, lymphocytosis	Leukocytosis, lymphopenia, polycythemia, increased coagulability
Fluids and electrolytes	Hyponatremia, hypovolemia, dehydration, hyperkalemia	Sodium and water retention, edema, hypokalemia
Metabolic system	Hypoglycemia, insulin sensitivity, fever	Hyperglycemia, negative nitrogen balance, dyslipidemia
Emotional/psychological status	Neurasthenia, depression, exhaustion or irritability, confusion, delusions	Psychic stimulation, euphoria, irritability, hypomania to depression, emotional lability
Mineralocorticoids		
Fluid and electrolytes	Sodium loss, decreased volume of extracellular fluid, hyperkalemia, salt craving	Marked sodium and water retention, tendency toward edema, marked hypokalemia
Cardiovascular system	Hypovolemia, tendency toward shock, decreased cardiac output, decreased heart size	Hypertension, hypervolemia
Androgens		
Integumentary system	Decreased axillary and pubic hair (in women)	Hirsutism, acne
Reproductive system	No effect in men, decreased libido in women	Menstrual irregularities and enlargement of clitoris (in females); gynecomastia and testicular atrophy (in males)
Musculoskeletal system	Decrease in muscle size and tone	Muscle wasting and weakness

When increased cortisol level is accompanied by increased levels of mineralocorticoids (also produced in the adrenal glands), the patient may also exhibit changes in sodium and potassium regulation, fluid balance (excess volume), and acid-base balance as well as hypertension. Adrenal androgen excesses may cause virilization in women and feminization in men. In women, menstrual disorders are common, as is hirsutism. Mood disturbances, insomnia, irrationality, and occasionally psy-chosis alter the mental health of the patient and affect the family.

Diagnosis

Patients with Cushing's syndrome frequently report the following symptoms during the initial nursing history taking: a recent onset of weakness, increase in weight or abdominal girth, more frequent infections and poor wound healing, roundness of face, increasing acne, depression, and mood alterations.

A complete physical examination reveals evidence of some of the other clinical manifestations noted in Table 20-9.

Laboratory tests are used to confirm the diagnosis. Plasma cortisol levels may be elevated and show a loss of diurnal (daytime) variation. Plasma ACTH levels may be normal, increased, or decreased depending on the underlying cause. ACTH level is normal or increased with pituitary or hypothalamic causes of Cushing's syndrome; it is decreased with adrenal causes. The most specific test for diagnosing Cushing's syndrome is the 24-hour urine free cortisol level (NIDDK, 2002). The patient's urine is collected over a 24-hour period and tested for the amount of cortisol. Levels higher than 100 μg/day for an adult suggest Cushing's syndrome (NIDDK).

Once Cushing's syndrome is diagnosed, the cause must be determined. The dexamethasone suppression test helps to distinguish Cushing's syndrome caused by excess production of ACTH by pituitary adenomas from Cushing's syndrome caused by ectopic ACTH-producing tumors (NIDDK, 2002). Patients are given dexamethasone, a synthetic glucocorticoid, by mouth over a period of days, and serum and urinary cortisol levels are measured over the same period. In persons with normal response or a pituitary source of excess ACTH, the exogenous glucocorticoid will cause a decrease in ACTH secretion and a drop in the level of cortisol measured in the urine. In patients with ACTH-secreting tumors elsewhere in the body, ACTH and cortisol secretion will not be suppressed. The dexamethasone suppression test can give false-positive results in the presence of stress, depression, alcohol abuse, acute illness, and high estrogen levels (Cushing's Support and Research Foundation, 2002). Several other tests are used to distinguish less common causes of Cushing's syndrome (NIDDK, 2002).

Identification of the cause of Cushing's syndrome is imperative for the successful therapeutic management of the condition. Surgical intervention is indicated for pituitary tumors and for some ACTH-secreting neoplastic tumors.

Interdisciplinary Care

Drug Therapy

Drugs used in the treatment of Cushing's syndrome are listed in Table 20-10. Patients receiving these drugs are at risk for adrenal insufficiency (see following section on Addison's disease). Adrenal enzyme inhibitors such as mitotane (Lysodren) may be used to destroy adrenocortical cells when surgical removal of the adrenal gland is not recommended. When adrenocortical cells are destroyed, the patient will require life-long corticosteroid replacement.

Dietitian

The patient with Cushing's syndrome experiences weight gain from increased glucose metabolism, increased appetite, and sodium and water retention. Diet therapy focuses on providing a low-calorie, high-nutrient diet that includes protein, vitamin C, and calcium. Oral calcium and vitamin D are recommended to minimize loss of bone density. Sodium is restricted in the diet to decrease fluid volume excess. A registered dietitian can provide guidelines for meal planning and sources of sodium in food.

Nurse

The patient with Cushing's syndrome is at risk of developing infections due to immunologic suppression. In addition, increased cortisol levels can mask common signs of infection. Infection protection, such as use of a meticulous sterile technique when performing invasive procedures, is a priority. Prevention of cross contamination through effective hand washing is important for the entire interdisciplinary team. The patient and family should be taught to look for subtle signs of infection, such as fatigue and general feelings of discomfort, and to seek evaluation by a health professional when these occur. The patient should also be cautioned to avoid situations carrying a high likelihood of exposure to persons with infections, such as crowds.

The patient's risk for injury is a priority for nurses when counseling a patient with Cushing's syndrome. Altered skin integrity due to greater skin friability and changes in capillary permeability increases the risk of infection and injury. Because the bone matrix is weakened, pathologic fractures can result from vigorous movements or minor accidents. Vertebral fractures and back pain may cause significant discomfort. Fatigue and dizziness from the cardiovascular effects of the disease can lead to an unsteady gait, which increases the likelihood of injury. The patient's home should be assessed for safety, and potential dangers, such as loose throw rugs and missing handrails on stairs, should be remedied when possible. Teaching the family and patient to be alert for safety risks is an important nursing function.

Fluid and electrolyte imbalances due to fluid and sodium retention can increase the risk of circulatory problems, so the patient should learn to monitor fluid balance through daily measurement of weight and general observation of intake and output.

Chronic changes in the body—a round "moon" face, dorsocervical fat pad or "buffalo hump," trunk obesity, abdominal striae, and easy bruising—may significantly affect the patient's self-image. Active listening, measures to enhance self-esteem, and reinforcement of the support systems are important.

Physical Therapist

The patient with Cushing's syndrome experiences loss of protein matrix in the bone when the normal cycle of bone resorption and bone formation is disrupted. Weight-bearing exercise stimulates bone formation and maintenance. The physical therapist should be consulted when the patient has

Table 20-10 Drug Treatment for Cortisol Excess or Deficiency

Drug	Side Effects	Nursing Considerations/Teaching Points
Adrenal Cytotoxic Drugs Mitotane (Lysodren)	Adrenal insufficiency Depression Sedation Dizziness Nausea Skin rash	Use caution in operating vehicles. Take drug with food. Keep taking drug even if skin rash occurs—contact health care provider.
Corticosteroids *Glucocorticoids* Cortisone (Cortone) Dexamethasone (Decadron) Hydrocortisone (Cortef) Methylprednisolone (Medrol)	Suppression of immune response Behavioral changes Mood swings Euphoria Depression Psychotic behavior Insomnia Hypertension Heart failure Cardiac arrhythmias Thromboembolism Gastrointestinal irritation and/or peptic ulcer Pancreatitis Cushingoid symptoms: moon face, buffalo hump, central obesity Muscle weakness and wasting, thin extremities Osteoporosis Vertebral compression fractures Hyperglycemia Menstrual cycle changes Bruising Acne Frequent infections Poor wound healing	Assess for signs of adrenal insufficiency periodically during therapy. Teach about side effects with long-term use. Monitor potassium, glucose, and plasma cortisol levels. Weigh daily. Monitor for edema and decreased urine output. Take with food in morning. Take missed doses when remembered, but do not double doses. Supplemental doses may be needed during stress. Avoid alcohol. Carry Medic Alert identification indicating steroid use. Use is contraindicated in patients with systemic fungal infections. Medication must not be discontinued except on physician's order. Diet high in protein, calcium, and potassium, and low in sodium and carbohydrates is recommended. After long-term use, acute adrenal insufficiency may result after withdrawal of drug (especially with stress).
Mineralocorticoids Fludrocortisone (Florinef)	Sodium and water retention Hypertension Heart failure Hypernatremia Hypokalemia Bruising	Usually given with glucocorticoid medication Monitor blood pressure Monitor fluid and electrolyte balance Teach signs of electrolyte imbalance: muscle weakness, numbness, fatigue, anorexia, nausea, arrhythmia Teach about need to discontinue medication slowly under provider's care Instruct to carry medical alert information about condition and medications Instruct to contact provider at first sign of infection

difficulty beginning an exercise program because of overall poor conditioning and muscle wasting. Physical therapy is also recommended for muscle strengthening. Walking can be suggested as an initial approach to combat bone de-

mineralization. Stretching exercises, strength training, and other weight-bearing exercises will also improve muscle strength. For the patient who is better conditioned, aerobic exercise for 30 to 60 minutes every other day should be

encouraged. The patient should be taught to avoid high-impact or rotational-type exercises of the spine to avoid the risk of pathologic fractures. If pathologic fractures occur, the physical therapist can provide guidance and support to the patient. Splinting devices to provide alignment and instruction in transferring techniques to support spinal integrity may be needed.

Occupational Therapist and Medical Social Worker

A patient with Cushing's syndrome caused by an inoperable tumor or chronic reliance on adrenocortical medications may deal with the complications of the syndrome for years. In addition to fatigue, altered mobility, and potential for pathologic fractures the patient may also experience cardiovascular effects. Congestive heart failure, hypertension, edema, and left ventricular hypertrophy can severely restrict the patient's ability to perform activities of daily living. The ability to carry out job responsibilities may be limited. The occupational therapist can assist the patient in adapting the home and work environment and teach the patient to perform tasks in a way that optimizes waning strength. The licensed clinical social worker may assist with evaluation of financial circumstances and identification of resources and appropriate living arrangements to maximize independence and support the patient's emotional and physical needs.

Think S for Success

Symptoms
- Identify and manage symptoms of excess adrenal hormones with drug therapy.

Sequelae
- Emphasize to patient that treatment will be lifelong.
- Educate patient that inadequate treatment may lead to death from cardiovascular complications.

Safety
- Educate patient and family on ways to avoid infections and to prevent accidental injuries, especially pathologic fractures.
- Teach patient about the importance of adhering to medication regime.

Support/Services
- If necessary, help patient obtain financial assistance and emotional support for alteration in appearance.

Satisfaction
- Determine the degree to which symptoms and disease treatment are interfering with important aspects of patient's life. Develop a plan to help patient reach and maintain desired quality of life.

Addison's Disease

Addison's disease, also called chronic adrenocortical insufficiency, occurs either as a result of a primary defect or disease of the adrenal gland or secondarily as a result of ACTH deficiency. Addison's disease is rare, occurring in only 1 in 100,000 people. It affects men and women equally with 95% of the cases occurring before the age of 60 (O'Sullivan, 1998).

Autoimmune or idiopathic atrophy of the adrenal gland accounts for 80% of cases of primary Addison's disease (Sabol, 2001). Other causes include systemic infection, histoplasmosis, metastatic tumors, surgical removal of the adrenal gland, and tuberculosis (Dresh, 2000). Tuberculosis was once the primary cause of Addison's disease, and the resurgence of tuberculosis in the United States has raised concerns about a potential increase in cases of Addison's disease.

Secondary failure of adrenal cortex hormone production can occur because of hypothalamic or pituitary disease, infarctions, or tumors, which result in release of insufficient amounts of ACTH. Another cause of adrenal insufficiency is the suppression of the hypothalamic-pituitary axis by long-term treatment with exogenous steroids (Sabol, 2001).

Lower levels of circulating glucocorticoids lead to decreased gluconeogenesis in the liver, which may cause hypoglycemia. Laboratory tests show low glucose and sodium levels and elevated levels of potassium. When circulating ACTH is not used by the adrenal cortex, it combines with melanocyte-stimulating hormone, which produces hyperpigmentation of the skin (O'Sullivan, 1998). When the adrenal cortex produces inadequate amounts of mineralocorticoids, the decrease in aldosterone production causes sodium and water loss and an increase in resorption of potassium in the kidneys.

Clinical Manifestations

Symptoms related to primary Addison's disease do not appear until 90% of the adrenal glands is destroyed (Sabol, 2001) (see Table 20-9). Many symptoms of Addison's disease are nonspecific, which makes diagnosis difficult. Muscular weakness, fatigue, and weight loss begin gradually and progress slowly. Abdominal complaints may include pain, nausea, vomiting, diarrhea or constipation, and anorexia. Hyperpigmentation occurs in primary Addison's disease, especially at pressure areas (knees, elbows, knuckles), in skin creases, on exposed skin, and on the buccal mucosa. Personality changes are seen in 60% to 70% of people with Addison's disease and include depression, restlessness, apathy, confusion, and irritability (Dresh, 2000). Chronic dehydration results in low blood pressure, postural hypotension, and dizziness or near-syncopal episodes.

A thorough health history may indicate recent exposure to stresses and changes in energy and activity levels, easy fatigability, profound muscle weakness, difficulty concentrating, depression, nausea, abdominal pain, anorexia, weight loss, and darkening of the skin in the skin folds and areas of pressure. The physical examination should include assessment of the activity level, emotional and mental status, skin pigmentation and turgor, weight, orthostatic blood pressure and pulses, abdominal tenderness, and muscle strength.

About 25% of patients have an addisonian crisis as the first manifestation of Addison's disease. The symptoms of severe adrenal insufficiency include electrolyte imbalances, hypotension, increased heart rate, increased respiration rate, fever, change in level of consciousness, and vascular collapse. Addisonian crisis is a medical emergency, and immediate action is required to sustain life. The primary goal of management initially is to reverse the shock by administering fluids and corticosteroids to restore blood volume. Addisonian crisis can also occur if a patient with chronic Addison's disease stops taking glucocorticoids abruptly or fails to increase the medication dose in response to major stressors such as infection, surgery, and trauma.

Diagnosis

If adrenal insufficiency is suspected, cortisol levels are tested initially by measuring a random early morning serum cortisol level. If the cortisol level is low, the diagnosis is clear (Sabol, 2001). Results of diagnostic tests may be normal if the adrenal insufficiency is mild. When a low-normal value is found in an unstressed patient, one must consider whether the patient has sufficient stored cortisol to respond to stress. Conversely, a stressed patient may have "normal" cortisol levels when the amount of stress should result in significantly higher levels of circulating cortisol. Either situation requires further testing for correct diagnosis.

The ACTH stimulation test is the most specific test for diagnosing Addison's disease. In a rapid ACTH stimulation test, ACTH is administered and cortisol levels are measured after an appropriate interval (30 minutes if the ACTH was administered intravenously and 60 minutes if given intramuscularly). A normal response of increased cortisol levels excludes adrenal insufficiency (Pagana and Pagana, 2002). When the response to a rapid test is abnormal, a longer ACTH stimulation test is performed, with ACTH injected over 24 to 72 hours. Patients with primary adrenal insufficiency do not respond to ACTH stimulation because the adrenal cortex is not functioning. Patients with secondary adrenal insufficiency (pituitary failure to produce ACTH) demonstrate a gradual increase in cortisol production as the adrenal cortex responds to the ACTH.

Interdisciplinary Care

Drug Therapy

All individuals with adrenal insufficiency need lifelong replacement of glucocorticoids. Several different types of corticosteroid medication may be used (Table 20-10), but all patients must take them every day. The dose and frequency

of medication is adjusted to keep the patient symptom free and maintain normal electrolyte levels.

During times of stress, the amount of glucocorticoids must be increased to meet the body's increased demand. Stresses that may require a dosage increase include vomiting and diarrhea, temperature over 100° F, major trauma, and surgery. Glucocorticoid dosages are generally doubled for minor stress such as vomiting, diarrhea, and fever. If the patient is unable to take oral medications, intramuscular injections must be administered. The patient or caregiver can be taught to administer the injection. The major stress of trauma and/or surgery requires parenteral hydrocortisone, which is usually given in a medical setting. As the patient's condition improves, the glucocorticoid should be tapered to the maintenance dose.

Patients receiving long-term glucocorticoid drug therapy, such as those with rheumatoid arthritis, Crohn's disease, ulcerative colitis, and asthma, are at risk of developing exogenous Cushing's syndrome as a complication of the drug therapy. Patients taking medications such as prednisone (Deltasone), prednisolone (Delta-Cortef), methylprednisolone (Solu-Medrol), and dexamethasone (Decadron) require monitoring for cushingoid effects. See Table 20-10 for the side effects of glucocorticoid therapy. Some possible medication regimens to limit the probability of developing Cushing's syndrome include alternate-day dosing, reduction in total dosage, and/or gradual discontinuation of the medication altogether. When an alternate-day regimen is used, the patient takes twice the daily dosage of a shorter-acting corticosteroid (such as Cortef or Solu-Cortef) every other morning. This approach allows the hypothalamic-pituitary-adrenal axis to recover on the day when the drug is not administered (Olin et al, 1993).

Dietitian

An individual with Addison's disease must maintain hydration and electrolyte balance. Ingestion of fluids and foods high in sodium and low in potassium is encouraged. Nausea, vomiting, and diarrhea should be controlled. In hot weather, a patient going outside should increase intake of fluids and salt to maintain fluid and electrolyte balance. Daily weight measurement assists in the monitoring of fluid and nutritional balance. A registered dietitian may be consulted to help the patient develop appropriate food plans.

Nurse

A person with Addison's disease can lead a normal, symptom-free life if adequate corticosteroid therapy is maintained during times of health, stress, and illness. The patient and his or her family or significant others need knowledge about Addison's disease and addisonian crisis to deal with the disease on a daily basis. The patient must take the prescribed medicine regularly every day (for the rest of his or her life) and must know how to respond to stress, when to increase the medication dose, and how to assess and correct fluid balance. The patient must know the signs of both excess corticosteroid therapy and inadequate replacement. With education, the patient may be able to make adjustments in medications and dietary intake to compensate for routine changes in life stress. Activities that could result in dehydration or stress due to increased physical or mental demands must be identified. The nurse should assist the patient in developing clear guidelines for when to self-manage and when to seek medical help. Indicators of inadequate replacement include decreased energy level, decreased muscle strength, mental status changes, low blood pressure with orthostatic changes, decreased weight, and poor skin turgor. Regular appointments with the primary care provider are important for routine monitoring of electrolyte and glucose levels and adjustment of dosage. Stress management and other coping skills should be explored and enhanced.

The patient should wear a Medic Alert bracelet or necklace and carry an identification card indicating that he or she has Addison's disease and noting the medications used.

Other Specialists

The physical therapist can assist the patient in regaining strength and increasing activity once the disease is managed. The medical social worker can help the patient and the family deal with the disease and identify stressors that may interfere with maintaining good health.

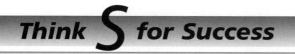

Think S for Success

Symptoms
- Identify and manage symptoms of deficient adrenal hormones with replacement therapy.

Sequelae
- Emphasize to patient that treatment will be lifelong.
- Educate patient that inadequate treatment may lead to death.

Safety
- Provide education about need to take medication every day.
- Educate patient and family regarding ways to manage stress, identify symptoms of overreplacement and underreplacement of hormones, self-adjust replacement hormones, maintain hydration status, and monitor weight.

Support/Services
- Help patient obtain assistance with finances if necessary.
- Educate patient that regular alterations in lifestyle may be significant.

Satisfaction
- Determine the degree to which symptoms and disease treatment are interfering with important aspects of patient's life. Develop a plan to help patient reach and maintain desired quality of life.

ACROMEGALY

Deficiency or excess of growth hormone (GH) produces chronic conditions including dwarfism, gigantism, and acromegaly. Dwarfism occurs when there is a deficiency of GH during infancy or childhood (although there are many other causes as well). Gigantism is seen when there is an excess of GH during infancy or childhood. Acromegaly occurs as a result of excess GH during adulthood.

Acromegaly is a relatively uncommon (3 cases per 1 million population per year) chronic hormonal disorder of middle-aged persons in which excess GH causes slow thickening of the bones of the skull, hands, and feet (Henry, Alexander, and Eng, 1996). This disorder occurs more frequently in women than in men and is diagnosed most often in adults in their forties and fifties (McCance and Huether, 2002). Scientists estimate that 40 to 60 of every 1 million people have the disease at any given time (National Institutes of Health [NIH], 2002). Because the clinical diagnosis of acromegaly is often missed, however, these figures probably underestimate the frequency of the disease (NIH, 2002).

Typically, the disease is present for many years before it is diagnosed. Untreated, acromegaly can result in serious illness, and it is associated with a decreased life expectancy (McCance and Huether, 2002). Once acromegaly is recognized, it is treatable in most patients, but because of its insidious onset the disease has often caused serious and disfiguring changes by the time of diagnosis (NIH, 2002) (Figure 20-5).

Pathophysiology

The hypothalamus produces GH–releasing hormone, which stimulates the pituitary gland to produce GH. Secretion of GH by the pituitary causes the production of yet another hormone, insulin-like growth factor I (IGF-I), in the liver. IGF-I directly stimulates the growth of bones (causing linear increase) and other tissues of the body. GH also promotes growth of soft tissues, maintains a normal rate of protein synthesis, promotes fat mobilization, is essential for proliferation of cartilage cells at the epiphyseal plates, and has an antiinsulin (hyperglycemic) effect. Elevated IGF-I levels signal the hypothalamus to release somatostatin, a hormone that inhibits the pituitary release of GH.

When the pituitary continues to make GH independent of the normal regulatory mechanisms during adulthood, the level of IGF-I continues to rise, which leads to bone growth, organ enlargement, and changes in glucose and lipid metabolism (NIH, 2002). Elevated levels of GH cause connective tissue proliferation and an increase in the cytoplasmic matrix, as well as bony proliferation that results in the characteristic appearance of acromegaly (McCance and Huether, 2002). The severity of the acromegaly depends on the degree of the overproduction of GH and the age at which the condition begins.

Hyperglycemia may be seen as a result of GH inhibition of peripheral glucose uptake and increased hepatic glucose production, followed by compensatory hyperinsulinism and

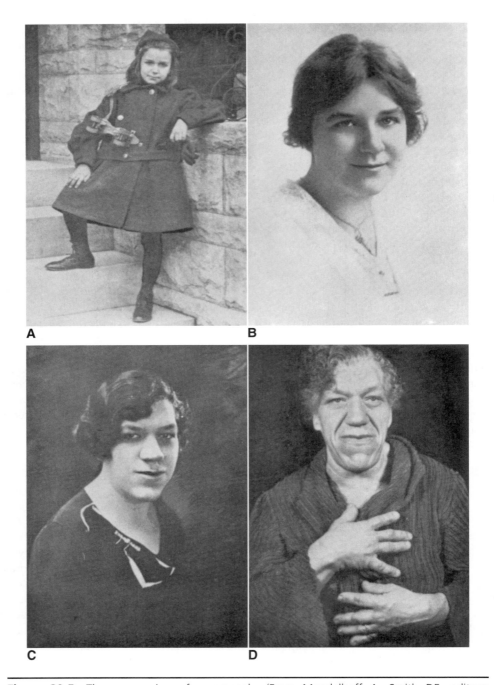

Figure 20-5 The progression of acromegaly. (From Mendelhoff A, Smith DE, editors: Acromegaly, diabetes, hypermetabolism, proteinuria, and heart failure, Clinical Pathological Conference, *Am J Med* 20:133, 1956.)

subsequent insulin resistance. Diabetes mellitus occurs when the pancreas is unable to secrete enough insulin to off-set the effects of GH. Approximately one third of individuals who are affected by acromegaly develop glucose intolerance before diagnosis, and they continue to be at higher risk for developing diabetes even during treatment (McCance and Huether, 2002).

In those with normally functioning pituitary glands, GH is secreted episodically in brief surges followed by long periods of inactivity. These surges are affected by sleep, exercise, stress, food intake, and blood glucose levels. Secretion occurs more frequently and at higher levels during youth. With age, the surges decrease (Sachse, 2001).

Over 90% of patients with acromegaly have a benign tumor of the pituitary gland, somatotropic adenoma, which is the cause of the overproduction of GH (Damjanov, 2000). Occasionally acromegaly is not caused by a pituitary tumor but by a tumor in the pancreas, lungs, or adrenal glands. These tumors can also lead to an excess of GH, either because they produce GH themselves or because they produce GH-releasing hormone.

Clinical Manifestations

The many possible manifestations of the disease are reviewed in Table 20-11.

Patients receiving treatment may experience a regression of many of these symptoms, but the bony enlargement of the face and hands is usually permanent.

The most serious chronic health consequences of acromegaly are diabetes mellitus, hypertension, and cardiovascular disease. Hypertension and left-sided heart failure are seen in one third to one half of individuals with this disease (McCance and Huether, 2002). Patients with acromegaly are also at increased risk for precancerous polyps of the colon and are therefore at risk for developing colon cancer.

Diagnosis

Patients with acromegaly do not show the usual GH baseline secretory pattern with sleep-related peaks. A totally unpredictable secretory pattern is seen (McCance and Huether, 2002). Thus, a single measurement showing an elevated blood GH or IGF-I level is not enough to diagnose acromegaly. Demonstration of elevated GH levels both at baseline and after a glucose challenge is the most reliable method of confirming a diagnosis of acromegaly (NIH,

Table 20-11 Clinical Manifestations of Acromegaly

Cause	Clinical Effect
Connective tissue proliferation	Enlarged lips and nose Interstitial edema Deepening of voice (due to enlarged sinuses and vocal cords) Snoring (due to upper airway obstruction) Increased size and function of sebaceous glands and sweat glands (which causes increased odor) Skin tags Thick, coarse skin and body hair Elongation of ribs at bone-cartilage junction Barrel-chested appearance Increased cartilage in joints
Soft tissue swelling	Swelling of hands and feet (often an early feature); patients may notice a change in ring, glove, or shoe size
Bony proliferation	Changes in facial features: protrusion of brow and jaw Nasal bone enlargement Increase in spacing of teeth Periosteal vertebral growth Enlargement of bones in hands and feet
Bone overgrowth and soft tissue thickening impeding peripheral nerves	Carpal tunnel syndrome Muscle weakness Muscular atrophy Foot drop
Enlargement of body organs	Liver enlargement Spleen enlargement Kidney enlargement Heart enlargement
Overgrowth of bone and cartilage	Arthritis Arthralgia Backache
Other	Headache (occurs in 50% to 87% of individuals with acromegaly and does not seem to be related to level of growth hormone, size or extension of the associated pituitary tumor, or hypertension) Muscle pains

2002). Magnetic resonance imaging and computerized tomography assist in evaluation of the pituitary for abnormal structure and tumors.

Interdisciplinary Care
Primary Provider (Physician/Nurse Practitioner)

The goals of treatment are to reduce GH production to normal levels, to relieve the pressure caused by the growing pituitary tumor on the surrounding brain areas, to preserve normal pituitary function, and to reverse or ameliorate the symptoms of acromegaly. Currently, treatment options include surgical removal of the tumor, drug therapy, and radiation treatment of the pituitary. Surgery is a rapid and effective treatment and is therefore the treatment of choice. Surgical success is indicated by normalization of GH and IGF-I levels.

Even when surgery is successful and hormone levels return to normal, the patient must be carefully monitored for years for possible recurrence. If hormone levels do not return to normal after surgery, the patient may require additional treatment with radiation and/or medications (NIH, 2002). Radiation to the pituitary gland delivered in divided doses over 4 to 6 weeks will lower GH levels by about 50% over 2 to 5 years. However, radiation therapy may result in a gradual decrease in the production of other pituitary hormones as well (NIH, 2002).

The patient diagnosed with acromegaly usually has sustained significant alterations in appearance, and he or she may need assistance in adjusting to the permanent disfigurement. Providers should offer support through active listening, and the patient should be referred for psychotherapy if indicated.

Drug Therapy

Bromocriptine (Parlodel), a dopamine agonist, and octreotide (Sandostatin), a synthetic form of somatostatin, both reduce GH secretion and tumor size (Table 20-12). Bromocriptine may be taken orally; its major side effect is gastrointestinal distress. Octreotide must be injected subcutaneously every 8 hours; it also causes gastrointestinal side effects, including the development of gallstones in 25% of patients. Withdrawal of either of these drugs can lead to recurrence of the high levels of GH secretion.

Table 20-12 Drug Treatment for Acromegaly

Drug	Side Effects	Nursing Considerations/Teaching Points
Dopamine Agonists Bromocriptine (Parlodel)	Dizziness Headaches Dry mouth Seizures Confusion, hallucinations Hypotension Stroke Acute myocardial infarction Insomnia Gastrointestinal disturbances Peptic ulcer	First dose should be taken where and when patient can lie down. Start with low dose. Take with food. Teach about orthostatic changes and monitor blood pressure. Avoid alcohol. May impair ability to perform tasks that require alertness and coordination. Do not double up doses if missed. Women should use nonhormonal method of birth control Contact physician immediately if symptoms of enlarging pituitary tumor (headache, blurred vision, severe nausea) are present.
Somatostatin Analogs Octreotide (Sandostatin)	Hypoglycemia Hyperglycemia Cholelithiasis Dizziness, drowsiness, visual disturbances Gastrointestinal disturbances: diarrhea, abdominal pain, distention Hypothyroidism	Inject subcutaneously every 8 hr. Teach correct injection technique and rotation of sites. Administer between meals and at bedtime. Do not double up doses. Avoid driving or other tasks that require concentration. Should not be used, or used with caution, when oral antidiabetes drugs are taken. Watch for symptoms of hypoglycemia.

Think S for Success

Symptoms
- Enlargement and distortion of the bones of the face, hands, and feet; headache; visual changes; hyperglycemia.

Sequelae
- Distorted appearance; vision changes or blindness; colon cancer; diabetes mellitus; hypertension.

Safety
- Ensure that patient obtains routine eye examinations.
- Screen for colon cancer.
- Screen for diabetes mellitus and provide treatment as indicated.
- Treat hypertension and cardiovascular disease.

Support/Services
- Listen to concerns about altered appearance.
- Help with planning for health-monitoring activities. Use flowchart to assist with appropriate monitoring and testing.
- Educate patient about medications or other treatments.
- Make appropriate referrals. Support groups or counseling may help patient meet emotional needs related to acceptance of change in body image.

Satisfaction
- Determine the degree to which management of acromegaly and related complications is interfering with important aspects of patient's life and develop a plan to help patient reach or maintain desired quality of life.

Nurse

Patient education should focus on the need for annual (or more frequent) monitoring for recurrence of the GH disorder and for diabetes, cardiac disease, hypertension, and colon polyps or colon cancer. The patient must know the symptoms of these disorders and the importance of consistent contact with the health care provider. Some patients may need counseling to deal with body image disturbances and poor-quality social interactions related to ridicule or self-consciousness about changes in appearance.

FAMILY AND CAREGIVER ISSUES

Family and caregiver issues related to chronic disorders of hormone regulation include the following:
- Hormone disorders are frequently invisible to others, which decreases the sympathy and assistance offered.
- Others may view diet and activity measures as optional.
- Awareness of stress and its effects on health may be lacking.
- Normal life stresses can cause exacerbations in spite of all the sacrifices made to control the condition.
- Fatigue may require lifestyle and medication management.
- Chronic fear may be present.

CASE STUDY

Patient Data

Mrs. W. is a 62-year-old widow who works as a bookkeeper at a small garden supply store in a Midwestern city. She lives alone in a neighborhood in which one of her two children, two of her three sisters, and her mother also live. She is active in her women's group at church and is renowned for her contribution of apple strudel at potluck dinners. She must be frugal with her resources but has a large social group of family and friends. She is not physically active and has hired neighborhood youths to do her outside house and yard work since her husband died 5 years ago. She has been feeling "tired" for the last 2 or 3 years and becomes fatigued easily with exertion. She has had monthly (or more frequent) episodes of diaphoresis and weakness, which she says usually occur 1 to 2 hours after eating. She comes to the clinic for treatment of a sore on her toe that will not heal. She has not seen a medical practitioner in 5 years. The nurse notes that Mrs. W. is 50 lb overweight, with a body mass index of 32; her blood pressure is 160/95. An examination reveals a draining 1-cm ulcer on the right great metatarsal-phalangeal joint and a loss of vibratory and touch sensation below the ankle bilaterally. The nurse practitioner orders a random blood glucose test, and results come back at 325 mg/dl. The patient is then given an appointment at which blood pressure is again taken; blood is drawn for a complete blood count and measurement of levels of fasting blood glucose, hemoglobin A_{1c}, lipids, and electrolytes; and an electrocardiogram is taken.

Diagnostic Findings

Hemoglobin A_{1c}: 12%
Fasting blood glucose level: 200 mg/dl
Hematocrit: 39%
Blood pressure: 140/90
Lipid level: normal
Electrocardiogram: normal

Thinking It Through
- What nursing diagnoses pertain to Mrs. W.?
- Does the care of a person with type 1 diabetes mellitus differ from that of a person with type 2 diabetes mellitus? If so, in what way?
- How can the health care team contribute to Mrs. W.'s quality of life?
- What are Mrs. W.'s concerns likely to be? How would you as the nurse address them?

Case Conference

The interdisciplinary team that has gathered to discuss and plan Mrs. W.'s care includes the nurse practitioner, internist, nurse, registered dietitian, diabetes educator, physical therapist, Mrs. W., and her daughter.

The nurse practitioner has already reviewed the findings with Mrs. W., explained to her that she has type 2 diabetes, and outlined the lifestyle modifications that are recommended for controlling the disease. She has further explained that Mrs. W.'s

Continued

CASE STUDY—cont'd

blood pressure is elevated, that it must be assessed several more times before hypertension may be diagnosed, but that lifestyle modifications are indicated to control the condition. She asked the patient's permission to initiate standard diabetes teaching protocols and checked with the insurance company about payment before arranging for the diabetes educator and the registered dietitian to attend the conference. The internist has not yet met Mrs. W. but has already arranged an appointment to see her later in the week. He asked the physical therapist to attend the conference to initiate a reconditioning program so that Mrs. W. can begin exercising regularly. The nurse has already explained to Mrs. W. that she will act as case manager to arrange appointments, record routine care, and serve as a central contact point for the patient.

The nurse practitioner introduces all the members of the health care team and explains their roles. Mrs. W. tells everyone that she hopes to avoid having a leg amputation as did her mother; she also states that she wants to try to control her diabetes with dietary changes. Her daughter interjects that Mrs. W. will have to make significant alterations in her consumption of chocolate candy and ice cream. The registered dietitian intervenes in this mother-daughter interaction to say that she will work with Mrs. W. to identify an acceptable diet plan and teach her to adjust her food intake for weight loss. She explains the basics of carbohydrate counting and the nutrition pyramid. Mrs. W. encourages her daughter to join her in trying the dietary changes and the internist agrees, stressing the genetic predisposition to diabetes that runs in the family. The diabetes educator explains that she will see Mrs. W. at least twice privately and offers her a series of six classes geared to persons with newly diagnosed diabetes. Mrs. W. and her daughter both decide to attend. The diabetes educator approves this choice, explaining that support from others is very important in adhering to lifestyle changes.

Mrs. W. asks if she should continue the dressing changes on her toe that were prescribed by the nurse practitioner. The internist says that he will assess the effectiveness of the current treatment at the visit later in the week. When Mrs. W. says that the ulcer on her toe began as a cut from her toe-trimming clippers, the internist recommends that Mrs. W. see a podiatrist on a regular basis, both for toenail trimming and regular evaluation of her feet. Mrs. W. is amenable to this but says that she will check her health insurance coverage before deciding on podiatric care.

The nurse asks Mrs. W. about her mother's experience with diabetes and Mrs. W. expresses her concerns about her mother's loss of vision, confinement to a wheelchair, and inability to pick up small objects because of loss of feeling in her hands. The nurse practitioner explains that recent research reports indicate that better glycemic control may prevent or delay such complications of diabetes. Mrs. W. states that she will do whatever she must to control her blood glucose level and lose weight.

The physical therapist says he will assess her physical abilities and help her get ready to begin a program of regular exercise. Mrs. W. says that she would like to walk around her neighborhood and to the local grocery store. Since talking to the nurse practitioner, she has inquired about joining the local YMCA and feels that she can spare the money for a single senior membership. Her daughter expresses surprise that her mother is considering using the weight room at the YMCA and says that her family already has a membership but only the kids go—maybe she will go too. The physical therapist supports these plans, only cautioning Mrs. W. to receive her physical therapy evaluation before undertaking sudden increases in activity.

The nurse asks if Mrs. W. and her daughter have more questions. Mrs. W. reiterates her determination to control her diabetes and says that she is looking forward to learning more in the classes. Appointments are made with the physical therapist, registered dietitian, and diabetes educator. The internist tells Mrs. W. that he will arrange a referral to a podiatrist when she comes for her visit later in the week. The nurse practitioner makes an appointment with Mrs. W. for a complete baseline physical examination in 2 weeks.

Once the team meeting is over, the nurse returns to her office and thinks about the meeting as she develops a plan of care for Mrs. W.

■ What new information was gathered that would assist the nurse in developing the plan of care?
■ What strengths does Mrs. W. bring to the team?
■ What barriers to therapy must be overcome?
■ Identify two collaborative problems that the plan of care should address.

Internet and Other Resources

General

Endocrine Society: *http://www.endo-society.org;* telephone 301-941-0200; 8401 Connecticut Avenue, Suite 900, Chevy Chase, MD 20815-5817

National Guideline Clearinghouse: *http://www.guideline.gov*

National Institute of Diabetes and Digestive and Kidney Disease: *http://www.niddk.nih.gov;* Office of Communications and Public Liaison, NIDDK, NIH, Building 31, Room 9A04, Center Drive, MSC 2560, Bethesda, MD 20892-2560

Pituitary Network Association: *http://www.pituitary.com;* telephone 805-499-9973, 800-642-9211; 16350 Ventura Blvd, Suite 231, Encino, CA 91436

Diabetes

American Association of Diabetes Educators: *http://www.aadenet.org;* telephone 800-338-3633; 100 West Monroe Street, Suite 400, Chicago, IL 60603

American Diabetes Association: *http://www.diabetes.org;* telephone 800-DIABETES, 800-342-2383; Attn: National Call Center, 1701 North Beauregard Street, Alexandria, VA 22311

National Diabetes Information Clearinghouse: *http://www.niddk.nih.gov/health/ diabetes/diabetes.htm;* telephone 301-654-3327, 800-860-8747; 1 Information Way, Bethesda, MD 20892-3560

Thyroid disorders

American Association of Clinical Endocrinologists: *http://www.aace.com;* telephone 904-353-7878; 1000 Riverside Avenue, Suite 205, Jacksonville, FL 32204

American Foundation of Thyroid Patients: *http://www.thyroidfoundation.org;* telephone 432-694-9966; 4322 Douglas Avenue, Midland, TX 79703

American Thyroid Association: *http://www.thyroid.org;* telephone 703 998-8890; 6066 Leesburg Pike, Suite 650, Falls Church, VA 22041

Adrenal disorders

Cushing's Support and Research Foundation: *http://csrf.net;* telephone 617-723-3824, 617-723-3674; 65 East India Row, Suite 22B, Boston, MA 02110

National Adrenal Diseases Foundation: *http://www.medhelp.org/nadf;* telephone 516-487-4992; 505 Northern Blvd, Suite 200, Great Neck, NY 11021

REFERENCES

American Association of Clinical Endocrinologists: Medical guidelines for clinical practice for evaluation and treatment of hyperthyroidism and hypothyroidism, *Endocr Pract* 8(6):457-67, 2002.

American Association of Clinical Endocrinologists: Facts about thyroid disease, 2003, retrieved from *http://www.aace.com/pub/tam2003/facts. php* on March 2, 2003.

American Diabetes Association: Clinical practice recommendations, *Diabetes Care* 26(suppl 1):1-156, 2003a.

American Diabetes Association: Screening for diabetes, *Diabetes Care* 26(suppl 1):S21-S24, 2003b.

American Diabetes Association: Standards of medical care for patients with diabetes mellitus, *Diabetes Care* 26(suppl 1):S33-S50, 2003c.

American Thyroid Association: Hyperthyroidism, 2003, retrieved from *http://www.thyroid.org/patients/brochures/Hyper_brochure.pdf* on Feb 9, 2004.

Berg GD, Wadhwa S: Diabetes disease management in a community-based setting, *Manag Care* 11(6):45-50, 2002.

Cameron BL: Making diabetes management routine, *Am J Nurs* 102(2): 26-33, 2002.

Centers for Disease Control and Prevention: National diabetes fact sheet, Dec 11, 2003a, retrieved from *http://www.cdc.gov/diabetes/pubs/ factsheet.htm* on May 25, 2003.

Centers for Disease Control and Prevention: Prevalence of diabetes: number of persons with diagnosed diabetes, United States, 1980-2000, March 17, 2003b, retrieved from *http://www.cdc.gov/diabetes/statistics/ prev/national/fig1.htm* on May 25, 2003.

Centers for Disease Control and Prevention: Diabetes: disabling, deadly, and on the rise: at a glance, 2003c, retrieved from *http://www.cdc.gov/ nccdphp/aag/aag_ddt.htm* on Feb 9, 2004.

Cushing's Support and Research Foundation: Cushing's support and research fact sheet, 2002, retrieved from *http://world.std.com/~csrf/ factsheet.html* on Nov 15, 2002.

Daly A et al: Diabetes mellitus nutrition therapy: practical tips improve outcomes, *J Am Acad Nurse Pract* 15(5):206-11, 2003.

Damjanov I: *Pathology for the health-related professions,* Philadelphia, 2000, WB Saunders.

Diabetes Control and Complications Research Trial Group: The effect of intensive treatment of diabetes in the development and progression of long-term complications in insulin-dependent diabetes mellitus, *N Engl J Med* 329(14):977-86, 1993.

Dresh JW: Assessment and management of patients with endocrine disorders. In Smeltzer SC, Bare BG, editors: *Textbook of medical-surgical nursing,* ed 9, Philadelphia, 2000, JB Lippincott, pp 1026-80.

Egede LE et al: The prevalence and pattern of complementary and alternative medicine use in individuals with diabetes, *Diabetes Care* 25(2): 324-9, 2002.

Expert Committee on the Diagnosis and Classification of Diabetes Mellitus: Report of the Expert Committee on the Diagnosis and Classification of Diabetes Mellitus, *Diabetes Care* 26(suppl 1):S4-S20, 2003.

Franz MJ et al: Evidence-based nutrition principles and recommendations for the treatment and prevention of diabetes and related complications, *Diabetes Care* 26(suppl 1):S51-S61, 2003.

Goldsmith C: Hypothyroidism, *Am J Nurs* 96(6):42-3, 1999.

Guha B, Krishnaswamy G, Peiris A: The diagnosis and management of hypothyroidism, *South Med J* 95(5):475-80, 2002.

Henry JB, Alexander DR, Eng CD: Evaluation of endocrine function. In Henry JB, editor: *Clinical diagnosis and management by laboratory methods,* ed 19, Philadelphia, 1996, WB Saunders, pp 322-73.

Holst D, Grimaldi PA: New factors in the regulation of adipose differentiation and metabolism, *Curr Opin Lipidol* 13(3):241-5, 2002.

Hormone Foundation: Thyroid: overview, 2002, retrieved from *http://www. hormone.org/learn/thyroid_1.html* on Nov 23, 2002.

Kinney JM: Insulin resistance in the elderly—the focus enlarges, *Curr Opin Clin Nutr Metab Care* 5(1):11-17, 2002.

Li TM: Hypothyroidism in elderly people, *Geriatr Nurs* 23(2):88-93, 2002.

Linekin PL: Diabetes pattern management, *Home Healthc Nurse* 20(3): 169-78, 2002.

Lloyd CE, Brown FJ: Depression and diabetes, *Curr Womens Health Rep* 2(3):188-93, 2002.

McCance KL, Huether SE, editors: *Pathophysiology: the biologic basis for disease in adults and children,* ed 4, St Louis, 2002, Mosby.

McKenry LM, Salerno E: *Mosby's pharmacology in nursing,* ed 20, St Louis, 1998, Mosby.

Mensing C et al: National standards for diabetes self-management education, *Diabetes Care* 26(suppl 1):S149-S156, 2003.

National Institute of Diabetes and Digestive and Kidney Diseases: Cushing's syndrome, NIH Pub No. 02-3007, June 2002, retrieved from *http://www.niddk.nih.gov/health/endo/pubs/cushings/cushings.htm* on July 18, 2002.

National Institutes of Health: Acromegaly, NIH Pub No. 02-3924, June 2002, retrieved from *http://www.niddk.nih.gov/health/endo/pubs/acro/acro.htm* on Aug 23, 2002.

Olin B et al: *Drug facts and comparisons,* St Louis, 1993, Facts and Comparisons.

Olohan K, Zappitelli D: The insulin pump: making life with diabetes easier, *Am J Nurs* 103(4):48-57, 2003.

O'Sullivan S: Nursing management of adults with hypothalamus, pituitary, or adrenal disorders. In Beare PG, Myers JL, editors: *Adult health nursing,* ed 3, St Louis, 1998, Mosby, pp 1350-81.

Pagana KD, Pagana TJ: *Mosby's manual of diagnostic and laboratory tests,* ed 2, St Louis, 2002, Mosby.

Phipps WJ et al: *Medical-surgical nursing: health and illness perspectives,* ed 7, St Louis, 2003, Mosby.

Robertson RP et al: Pancreas and islet cell transplantation for patients with diabetes, *Diabetes Care* 23(1):112-6, 2000 (technical review).

Sabol VK: Addisonian crisis, *Am J Nurs* 101(7):24AAA-24DDD, 2001.

Sachse D: Acromegaly: early recognition of this rare multisystem disorder results in considerable benefits to patients, *Am J Nurs* 101(11):69-74, 2001.

Singer PA et al: Treatment guidelines for patients with hyperthyroidism and hypothyroidism, *JAMA* 273(10):808-12, 1995.

United Kingdom Prospective Diabetes Study Group (UKPDS): Intensive blood-glucose control with sulphonylureas or insulin compared with conventional treatment and risk of complications in patients with type 2 diabetes, *Lancet* 352(9131):837-953, 1998.

CHAPTER 21

Disorders of the Brain

Jennifer H. Matthews, PhD, APRN,BC

OBJECTIVES

After reading this chapter, you should be able to do the following:

■ Describe the pathophysiology of chronic disorders of the brain, including headache, migraine, cerebrovascular accident (CVA), traumatic brain injury (TBI), and epilepsy
■ Describe the clinical manifestations of chronic disorders of the brain, including headache, migraine, CVA, TBI, and epilepsy
■ Describe the functional health patterns affected by chronic headache, migraine, CVA, TBI, and epilepsy
■ Describe the role of each member of the interdisciplinary team involved in the care of patients with chronic headache, migraine, CVA, TBI, and epilepsy
■ Describe the indications for use, adverse events, and nursing considerations related to drugs commonly used to treat chronic headache, migraine, CVA, TBI, and epilepsy.

This chapter focuses on the care of individuals who have chronic brain disorders ranging from episodic conditions that are temporarily disabling to conditions that permanently affect the individual's life. The disorders covered include headaches and migraines, epilepsy, stroke, and traumatic brain injury.

ASSESSMENT

Similar assessment techniques are used regardless of the nature of the brain disorder. Taking a thorough history and performing a complete physical examination including a neurologic examination are standard practice. Other diagnostic aids include neuroimaging of the brain by angiography, computed tomography (CT), magnetic resonance imaging (MRI), and positron emission tomography. Box 21-1 lists some of the common diagnostic tests and functional assessment instruments used and Box 21-2 provides a framework for functional health pattern assessment.

HEADACHE AND MIGRAINE
Headache

Headache is one of the most common neurologic symptoms or conditions that humans experience. Headache may be a symptom of an underlying neurologic condition or disease, or the result of a neurologic insult that interferes with the individual's ability to function.

Chronic headaches are seen in individuals who suffered traumatic brain injuries and stroke and are experienced by individuals with epilepsy.

Assessment

In addition to performing a complete functional health assessment (Box 21-2), the health care provider should develop a headache symptom profile for any individual who complains of persistent or severe headache (Box 21-3). Evaluation should also include the degree of disability that an individual experiences related to the headaches. The Migraine Disability Assessment Scale (MIDAS) can be used to gather information about the level of disability and to track progress (Stewart et al, 1992). Sample questions from the MIDAS instrument are listed in Box 21-4.

Pathophysiology

Headache, as a symptom, can be associated with serious disorders such as systemic diseases, intracranial immune responses, or space-occupying lesions. Benign headaches may stem from irritation in networks of nerves, muscles, or blood vessels. The brain itself is not the origin of headache pain because brain tissues are insensate.

Six major causes of headache have been identified. These are listed in Box 21-5. However, headaches can also originate from spasms (myodystonia) in the muscles of the scalp, cervical area, or upper shoulders. Causes of such headaches are whiplash, rotational injuries, direct trauma to the muscles, or regular strain and tension in the muscles.

Tension-Type Headache

Tension-type headaches (TTHs) are the most prevalent type of headache. Women are more likely to experience TTH, with the peak prevalence between 30 and 39 years of age (Schwartz et al, 1998). TTH has episodic and chronic forms,

---

Box 21-1 Diagnostic Tests and Functional Assessment Tools

DIAGNOSTIC TESTS
- Cerebral angiography
- Computed axial tomography
- Electroencephalography
- Lumbar puncture and cerebrospinal fluid analysis
- Magnetic resonance imaging
- Nerve function tests
- Neurologic assessment with focal signs
- Positron emission tomography

FUNCTIONAL ASSESSMENT TOOLS
- Barthel Index
- Beck Depression Inventory (BDI)
- Chronic Illness Resources Survey (CIRS)
- Functional Disability Inventory (FDI)
- Functional Independence Measure (FIM)
- Functional Status Index (FSI)
- Functional Status Questionnaire (FSQ)
- Short Form 12 (SF-12) Health Survey
- Short Form 36 (SF-36) Health Survey
- Sickness Impact Profile (SIP)

---

both of which may interfere with the individual's ability to work.

Cluster Headache

Cluster headaches are attacks of severe unilateral pain in the forehead and temporal regions that last from 15 to 180 minutes and may occur up to eight times a day. The onset is likely to be sudden and often occurs during the dreaming (rapid eye movement) phase of sleep. These headaches occur more frequently in men than in women.

Migraine

Migraine is a complex neurologic condition characterized by recurring acute events with neurologic, vascular, hormonal, and neurotransmitter components. An individual may experience his or her first migraine during childhood, but most often the disorder begins during adolescence. Migraine episodes continue at the same intensity through middle age and then subside in frequency and severity.

Migraine headaches affect 28 million Americans or about 11% of the population. Peak prevalence is between the ages of 30 and 50 years, and 75% of those with migraine are women (Lipton et al, 2002; National Institute of Neurological Disorders and Stroke, 2001).

Median attack frequency is about 1.5 per month with a duration of about 24 hours. However, about 10% of migraineurs have weekly episodes and 20% have attacks lasting 2 to 3 days (Lipton et al, 2002; Stewart et al, 1992).

Individuals experiencing migraines are frequently disabled by the attack. Thirty-eight percent report missing days of work or school due to the headaches; 57% of those who continue with activities report working at 50% capacity (Lipton et al, 2001).

The International Headache Society (IHS) (1998) has classified migraines into seven categories (Box 21-6).

Pathophysiology

TTH is most likely the result of two interacting mechanisms: the hypersensitivity of pain fibers of the trigeminal nerve and the contraction of the muscles of the jaw and neck. This causes pain and tenderness in the pericranial muscles, which evolve into TTH.

Cluster headaches appear to involve primarily trigeminal nerve mechanisms. They are not life threatening and do not seem to cause permanent structural damage. The pain can be so severe, however, that it may cause the individual to have suicidal ideations.

The migraine center is located in the aminergic nuclei of the brainstem. This center is responsible for processing or modulating sensory and nociceptive (pain) input. The migraine is initiated as a neural event that causes dilation of cranial blood vessels. In migraines without aura, ion channels in the neurons dysfunction and alter impulse conduction (Goadsby, Lipton, and Ferrari, 2002). The occurrence of migraines with aura has a familial component with inherited abnormalities in the cells of nuclei in the brainstem (NIH, 2001). Abnormal cells trigger a reduction in cortical activity and reduced blood flow (oligemia). These changes in blood flow stimulate the release of vasoactive neuropeptides, serotonin (5-hydroxytryptamine, or 5-HT), and inflammatory products, which excite the trigeminal nerve (cranial nerve V, or CN-V). The CN-V ophthalmic division becomes inflamed and causes the visual symptoms of aura and migraine, and the CN-V parasympathetic outflow branch affects nerve roots of cranial nerve II, producing pain over the frontal, temporal, parietal, occipital, and high cervical regions (Goadsby, Lipton, and Ferrari, 2002). Inflammatory products also disturb the blood-brain barrier at the postrema and cause nausea and vomiting (McCance and Huether, 2002).

A migraine may be triggered by external or internal factors: stress, fatigue, lack of sleep, or jet lag; weather changes, spring, winter, or exposure to light or sunlight; foods such as red wine, cheese, or chocolate; and hormonal variations related to menstruation, ovulation, or oral contraceptive use.

Clinical Manifestations
Tension-Type Headache

Individuals with TTH experience headaches with the following characteristics:
- Mild to moderate pain
- Bilaterality

Box 21-2 Functional Health Pattern Assessment for Brain Disorders

HEALTH PERCEPTION/HEALTH MANAGEMENT
- Is there a family history of headaches, epilepsy, hypertension, stroke, or depression?
- What are the individual's and family's perception of the patient's overall health?
- Does the patient accept and adhere to the therapeutic regimens, including use of prescribed and over-the-counter medications and complementary and alternative therapies?

NUTRITION/METABOLISM
- What is the patient's current weight? Has there been any unexplained recent weight gain or loss?
- What are the patient's cultural beliefs about food and eating?
- What are the patient's dietary habits and choices? Is the patient on a special or prescribed diet? What is the condition of the skin and mucous membranes?
- Does the patient have a history of peptic ulcer or gastrointestinal bleeding?
- Is the patient able to swallow?
- Is the patient fed by percutaneous endogastric tube with instillation of prescribed formula? What are the ethical considerations with regard to nutrition and hydration?

ELIMINATION
- Have any changes occurred in bowel or bladder habits?
- Does the patient have any deficits in elimination sensations? What are the patterns of continence? Does the patient experience pain on or difficulty in urinating?
- Does the patient use adult undergarments? Does the patient require bowel and bladder training?
- Does the patient show decreased discrimination of environmental cues to appropriate facilities? Does the patient use an elevated toilet seat, assistive devices, and/or grab bars?

ACTIVITY/EXERCISE
- Does the patient experience difficulty in walking, fatigue, or malaise?
- What are the patient's regular exercise activities? In what recreational activities does the patient engage?
- What mobility aids does the patient use?
- Have patterns of cooperation been established to allow performance of instrumental and other activities of daily living?
- Does the patient participate in passive and active range of motion and restorative activities?

SLEEP/REST
- How many hours of uninterrupted sleep do the patient and caregiver obtain at night? Does the individual or caregiver take naps or rest periods?
- What complementary-alternative and prescribed sleep aids are used?

COGNITION/PERCEPTION
- What is the nature of the pain? Describe using the mnemonic COLDER: Character, Onset, Location, Duration, Exacerbation, Relief.
- What is the patient's cognitive awareness of self, family, others, environment, time, and place?
- Is the patient able to recognize and appropriately respond to sensory messages from the body?
- Can the patient communicate his or her ideas or needs and manipulate items in the environment?
- Does the patient show symmetrical involvement, paresthesias, paralysis, or neglect syndrome?

SELF-PERCEPTION/SELF-CONCEPT
- How does the patient describe himself or herself?
- How has the condition affected the patient's self-esteem?
- How has the condition changed the patient's body image?
- What are the effects of the condition on the patient's sense of self?
- Can the patient communicate and interact with the family and environment?

ROLES/RELATIONSHIPS
- Is the patient employed or does the patient play a dependent role in the home or family?
- What changes have occurred in the patient's ability to carry out role functions?
- How satisfied is the patient with his or her current roles and relationships?
- How has the condition affected the patient's family and/or significant others?

SEXUALITY/REPRODUCTION
- Is the patient sexually active?
- Has the condition led to changes in sexual performance?
- Is the patient satisfied with current sexual patterns?
- Have any changes occurred in the menstrual cycle?
- Do hormonal changes play a role in triggering neurologic events?

COPING/STRESS TOLERANCE
- What are the patient's coping strategies?
- What support systems are available to the patient?
- Can the individual and family manage the condition in the current setting?
- Do the patient and family recognize the impact of the changes that have occurred and plan for the future?
- How hardy and resilient are the individual and family?
- What is the caregiver burden?

VALUES/BELIEFS
- What constitutes quality of life for the patient?
- How are individual and family values upheld?
- What are the patient's spiritual beliefs, health beliefs, and cultural beliefs?
- How involved is the patient in cultural practices? How does the patient's cultural community influence health practices?
- What are the patient's views on locus of control?

Box 21-3   Headache Symptom Profile

■ What is the headache history for the individual, that is, are the current headaches similar to headaches experienced prior to injury or disease?

■ Is there a family history of headaches? Are these headaches similar to those experienced by other family members?

■ Do neurologic symptoms occur with the headache? These might include an aura that precedes the headache, numbness or tingling in another body part, nausea or vomiting, or an altered mental status.

■ What is the degree of functional disability associated with the headache? Does it interfere with work or school, hamper activities of daily living, or cause a change in lifestyle during the episode?

Box 21-4   Sample Questions from the Migraine Disability Assessment Scale

1. On how many days in the last 3 months did you miss work or school because of your headaches?

2. On how many days in the last 3 months did you not do household work because of your headaches?

3. On how many days in the last 3 months did you miss family, social, or leisure activities because of your headaches?

Adapted from Stewart et al: Development and testing of the Migraine Disability Assessment (MIDAS) Questionnaire to assess headache-related disability, *Neurology* 56:S20-S28, 2001.

Box 21-5   Major Causes of Headache

■ Displacement of structures within the skull, such as from space-occupying lesions (solid tumors or hematomas)
■ Inflammation from intracranial, extracranial, or cervical sources
■ Changes in vascular dynamics and/or metabolic changes
■ Increased muscle tone or spasm in the head or neck
■ Inflammation or irritation of the meningeal membranes
■ Increased pressure within the skull
■ Musculoskeletal disorders
Cervical sympathetic nerve syndromes (involving C1 to C3 autonomic nerves damaged in excessive flexion and extension injury)
Temporomandibular joint dysfunction
Hypersensitivity of pain fibers of the trigeminal nerve and the contraction of the muscles of the jaw and neck
Neuritic and neuralgic pain syndromes (entrapment of large scalp nerves by muscles in spasms)

Box 21-6   Classification of Migraine

■ Migraine without aura
■ Migraine with aura
■ Ophthalmoplegic migraine
■ Retinal migraine
■ Childhood periodic syndromes that are precursors to migraine
■ Complications of migraine (status migrainosus)
■ Migraine disorders that do not fall into any of the above categories

■ Gradual onset of the pain
■ Nonpulsatile nature
■ Pain likened to a tight band, pressure, or tightening feeling and not aggravated by activity

Chronic TTH is differentiated from episodic TTH by the frequency of the attacks. Individuals with chronic TTH experience more than 15 episodes per month and may have additional symptoms such as nausea, photophobia, and phonophobia (IHS, 1998).

Cluster Headache

Cluster headaches have autonomic symptoms that involve the nose and eye areas, such as conjunctival and eyelid swelling, lacrimation, nasal congestion and rhinorrhea, miosis and ptosis, and forehead and facial sweating from vasodilation (IHS, 1998). The headaches occur in series during a cluster period that may last for weeks, months, or a year before the individual has a remission (episodic cluster headaches). A remission is defined as a 14-day period without headache. Headaches that occur for 1 year without a remission lasting more than 14 days are considered chronic phase cluster headaches. Ten percent of individuals with cluster headaches experience chronic phase attacks (IHS, 1998).

Migraine

Migraineurs who experience no aura have pain for 4 to 72 hours if the migraine is untreated. The pain is unilateral, is moderate to severe, is described as throbbing, and is aggravated by movement. The migraineur may also have nausea, vomiting, photophobia, or phonophobia.

Migraines accompanied by an aura have different associated features than those that are not accompanied by an aura. Often, the aura causes reversible focal neurologic symptoms such as visual scotomas, scintillations or temporary blindness, aphasia, sensory deficits such as tingling or numbness, clumsiness, or weakness. The aura may last 5 to 20 minutes but rarely longer than 60 minutes. The migraine may last up to 72 hours or may be absent after the aura (IHS, 1998).

Interdisciplinary Care

Primary Provider (Physician/Nurse Practitioner)

Many individuals with episodic TTH do not seek medical care but treat mild headaches with ice packs, rest, and stress reduction. More severe TTHs are treated with aspirin or nonsteroidal antiinflammatory drugs (NSAIDs). The primary provider is the first person to whom an individual goes for help when self-management is inadequate. Individuals with chronic TTH often seek medical care for the treatment of their headaches. The provider makes a diagnosis on the basis of the history and physical assessment. Closer evaluation of these individuals reveals that many also experience migraines.

The goals of treatment for the individual with cluster headache are to prevent the headache from occurring and to relieve symptoms. Triggers are identified through the use of a headache diary. The individual should record as much about the headache as possible: foods consumed and activities performed for 24 hours prior to the headache, current level of stress, the time the headache began, duration of the headache, and activities or medications that relieved the pain. The provider and the individual review the diary over time to help establish probable triggers and means of relief.

Management of migraine is more complex, and the primary provider may refer the patient to a neurologist or physician specializing in treatment of individuals with migraine. The goals of long-term migraine treatment are to prevent headache, reduce attack frequency and severity, avoid the need to increase headache medication, reduce disability, improve quality of life and ultimately educate the individuals to enable the person to manage his or her condition (Silberstein and the US Headache Consortium, 2000).

Drug Therapy

Medications prescribed for the individual with TTH are analgesics and antiinflammatories such as aspirin or other NSAIDs (Table 21-1). Chronic TTH is also treated with tricyclic antidepressants, and a trial of migraine medications may be considered. Long-term use of analgesics, opiates and muscle relaxants, tranquilizers, and antihistamines is avoided.

Use of analgesics is ineffective and is not recommended in the treatment of cluster headache, and may lead to rebound or worsening of symptoms. The inhalation of 100% oxygen for several minutes has been shown to be effective for some individuals who suffer with cluster headaches at night. Generally, a combination of medications is needed to control the symptoms (see Table 21-1). New medications are released yearly, and the health care provider should try combinations of medications to control the symptoms. With cluster headaches, the response of the individual to a medication may change over time, and the medications must be alternated and recombined to achieve adequate relief.

Newer antiepileptic medications, such as divalproex, reduce cluster headache frequency and pain during an attack (Cutrer, 2001; Rozen, 2001). Ergot preparations (containing ergotamine alone or in combination with other medications) and methysergide are effective for some individuals and may be preventive; unfortunately, the side effects may be severe. Other medications that may be used to treat or prevent symptoms include antihistamines, lithium, calcium channel blockers, propranolol, amitriptyline, verapamil, and cyproheptadine. All preventive medications should be tapered off slowly during periods of remission (no headache). Corticosteroid medications such as prednisone have provided short-term relief in cluster headache episodes, but their long-term use is not advised because of side effects.

Injection of chemicals and surgery on trigeminal nerve ganglion cells near the brain have shown initial success in highly selected cases when drug therapy is ineffective.

When medications are used to treat migraine, 2 to 3 months of monitoring and adjusting of dosages may be required to achieve the desired effects. The most effective medications are listed in Table 21-1 and include tricyclic antidepressants, antiepileptics, β-blockers, calcium channel blockers, and serotonin agonists.

As soon as the individual detects that a migraine is imminent, he or she should take adequate doses of an analgesic and antiinflammatory medication to aid in minimizing pain during the period before other medication becomes bioavailable, followed by medication that will prevent the migraine from developing (Goadsby, Lipton, and Ferrari, 2002). The triptans are the most effective group of drugs that directly interfere with migraine development.

The triptans ($5\text{-HT}_{1B/1D}$ receptor agonists) activate the serotonin receptors, causing constriction of cranial vessels, inhibition of peripheral neurons, and inhibition of impulses in the neurons of the trigeminal-cervical nerve complexes. Several triptans available are sumatriptan (oral, subcutaneous, nasal spray), naratriptan (oral), rizatriptan (oral), and zolmitriptan (oral).

The ergot alkaloids, long the mainstay of migraine therapy, are less favored today because of their erratic pharmacokinetics, potent sustained generalized vasoconstrictor effects, and ability to cause overuse syndromes and rebound headaches (Goadsby, Lipton, and Ferrari, 2002).

Antiemetics such as ondansetron HCl and trimethobenzamide HCl and chlorpromazine are also prescribed for the associated symptoms of nausea and vomiting.

Medications that are given when migraine treatment has failed are called rescue medications. These include opiate analgesics such as butorphanol nasal spray, meperidine (intramuscular or intravenous), and methadone (intramuscular); barbiturates such as butalbital-containing analgesics; and corticosteroids (for status migrainosus) (Matchar et al, 2000).

Nurse

One of the primary roles of the nurse is support of the individual with migraine and his or her family in learning to

Text continues on p. 323.

Table 21-1 Medications Commonly Used to Treat Brain Disorders

Medications	Indications/Uses	Side Effects	Nursing Considerations/Teaching Points
NSAIDs Aspirin Celecoxib (Celebrex) Diclofenac (Voltaren) Diflunisal (Dolobid) Fenoprofen (Nalfon) Ibuprofen (Advil, Motrin) Indomethacin (Indocin) Meclofenamate (Meclomen) Naproxen (Aleve, Naprosyn) Piroxicam (Feldene) Rofecoxib (Vioxx) Sulindac (Clinoril) Tolmetin (Tolectin)	Analgesic and antiinflammatory Tension-type headache, migraine headache, chronic daily headache, cluster headache, TBI	GI irritation, peptic ulcer, GI bleeding, nausea, vomiting, dizziness, rash, headache, tinnitus, nephrotoxicity, exacerbation of asthma Aspirin and diflunisal: salicylate toxicity	Before giving drug assess for bleeding disorders, peptic ulcer disease, gastritis, liver disease, kidney disease, or asthma. Administer drug with food, milk, or antacids if prescribed. Do not crush if enteric coated. Do not give aspirin and other NSAIDs together. Use caution with anticoagulants. Educate *patient to avoid alcohol*. Instruct patient to report signs of bleeding, edema, weight gain of more than 5 lb in 1 week, rashes, persistent headaches. Monitor BP, blood glucose.
Antiepileptic Drugs (AEDs) *Hydantoins* Mephenytoin (Mesantoin) Ethotoin (Peganone) Phenytoin (Dilantin) Fosphenytoin (Cerebyx)	Partial and generalized tonic-clonic seizures	CNS: fatigue, clumsiness, confusion, mood alterations, low attention span, reduced ability to problem solve. Other: hirsutism, gingival hyperplasia and sensitivity, nausea, vomiting, constipation, blood dyscrasias, hepatotoxicity	Observe for reduction of seizure activity. Assess for side effects; monitor for therapeutic levels, perform blood and liver function tests. Educate patient to avoid alcohol because it reduces medication adequacy. Educate patient on proper tooth-brushing technique.
Barbiturates Phenobarbital (Luminal) Pentobarbital sodium (Nembutal)	Adjunct therapy to AEDs, especially phenytoin Migraine headache	CNS: depression, mental or physical dependence, dizziness, ataxia, headache, slurred speech, drowsiness and somnolence, fatigue, insomnia in the elderly Other: skin rashes, Stevens-Johnson syndrome, bronchospasm	Observe for reduction of seizure activity. Observe for sleep pattern disturbances and daytime sedation, hangover. Monitor for blood dyscrasias, serum levels. Encourage increased folic acid intake, safety measures for coordination changes.
Succinimides Ethosuximide (Zarontin)	Absence seizure		Monitor for reduction in seizure activity. Evaluate results of liver, renal, and hematologic studies. Educate patient to take with food, milk, or antacid as ordered.
Benzodiazepines Clonazepam (Klonopin)	Adjunct therapy to AED Absence and myoclonic	CNS: headache, drowsiness, personality changes	Observe for tolerance and dependency.

Continued

Table 21-1 Medications Commonly Used to Treat Brain Disorders—cont'd

Medications	Indications/Uses	Side Effects	Nursing Considerations/Teaching Points
Benzodiazepines—cont'd			
Diazepam (Valium) Clorazepate (Tranxene)	seizures	Other: epigastric pain, nausea, anorexia, vomiting, rash, pruritus, Stevens-Johnson syndrome, hepatic and renal dysfunction	Use tapered dosage to discontinue. Monitor results of liver function tests and periodic CBC. Educate patient to avoid alcohol.
Miscellaneous			
Valproate (Depakote, Depakene)	Absence and myoclonic seizures; dementia behavior modification		Patient must be free of hepatic dysfunction. Observe for reduction of seizure activity.
Topiramate (Topamax)	Tonic-clonic seizure; adjunct therapy for partial seizure; migraine headache	CNS: drowsiness, lassitude, loss of dexterity, dizziness, blurred vision, hallucination, unsteadiness Other: pruritus, skin rash, hiccups, dry mouth, nausea, vomiting	Observe for reduction of seizure activity. Must maintain adequate fluid intake; monitor food intake to avoid weight loss.
Carbamazepine (Tegretol; related in structure to tricyclics; effects like those of phenytoin)	Partial and tonic-clonic seizure, mixed seizure patterns, chronic nerve pain, dementia behavior modification	Same as for Topiramate	Contraindicated in absence, atonic, or myoclonic seizures. Can exacerbate AV heart block, blood disorders, and bone marrow depression. Observe for fluid retention. Do not administer with antacids.
Oxcarbazepine (Trileptal) Gabapentin (Neurontin)	Partial seizures, chronic nerve pain	Tremors, weight gain, irregular menses, hepatotoxicity	Observe skin for rashes. Note changes in seizure activity.
Lamotrigine (Lamictal)	Partial seizures Used as adjunct therapy	Drowsiness, ataxia, dizziness, tremor, nervousness, anxiety, depression, confusion	Dosage is gradually increased.
Triptans (5-HT$_{1D}$ receptor agonists)			
Sumatriptan (Imitrex; oral, SC, nasal spray) Naratriptan (Amerge; oral) Rizatriptan (Maxalt; oral) Zolmitriptan (Zomig; oral)	Treatment of prodroma, aura, or acute-onset migraine headache	CNS: drowsiness, confusion, ataxia, muscle aches Other: Stevens-Johnson and SLE-type syndromes, SIADH	Onset of action is rapid. Contraindicated in individuals with a history of ischemic heart disease, uncontrolled hypertension, or CVA. Do not give with other vasoconstrictors. Do not use within 24 hours of ergotamine administration. Tablet can taste unpleasant.
Ergot Alkaloids **Serotonin agonist** Methysergide (Sansert)	Prevention of migraine	Drowsiness, dizziness, tiredness, ataxia, peripheral edema, fibrotic thickening in some tissues	Do not administer for longer than 6 mo. Contraindicated with other vasoconstrictors and in hypertension, angina, TIA-CVA
α-Adrenergic blocker Dihydroergotamine (DHE, Migranal, injectable, nasal spray)	Acute-onset migraine		
Antihypertensives **β-blockers** Propranolol (Inderal) Timolol (Blocadren)	Adjunct therapy in migraine control CVA: HTN TBI: lower impulsivity	Drowsiness, weakness, nasal congestion, difficulty sleeping, bradycardia, bronchospasms, depression, cold hands and feet	Contraindicated in individuals with heart failure, heart block, or bradycardia Monitor BP and heart rate; hold dosage if heart rate <60 beats/min—notify prescriber. Taper dose slowly.

Table 21-1 Medications Commonly Used to Treat Brain Disorders—cont'd

Medications	Indications/Uses	Side Effects	Nursing Considerations/Teaching Points
α₂-Agonists Clonidine (Catapres) Tizanidine (Zanaflex)	CVA: HTN TBI: lower impulsivity Tension and daily headache	Nausea, vomiting, constipation, weakness, hypotension, decreased sexual drive	Avoid use in individuals with coronary insufficiency, MI, CVA. Monitor BP frequently. Monitor for signs of anticholinergic effects—urinary retention.
Calcium Channel Blockers Nimodipine (Nimotop) Verapamil (Calan)	Adjunct therapy for migraine CVA: HTN	Headache, nausea, hypotension, dizziness, skin rash or flushing, ankle edema, dry mouth, tachycardia	Monitor BP, cardiac rhythms for slow AV conduction; report heart rates <60 beats/min Monitor renal and liver function test results. Educate patient to avoid alcohol and grapefruit juice.
Angiotensin-Converting Enzyme Inhibitors Captopril (Capoten) Enalapril (Vasotec) Lisinopril (Prinivil, Zestril)	CVA: HTN	Dry cough and dyspnea, headaches, insomnia, diarrhea, loss or impairment of taste, nausea, dizziness, hypotension, rash, fever, joint pain, angioedema (rare)	Dosing is dependent on brand. May be given in combination with diuretics; monitor for hypotension. Monitor CBC regularly; monitor sodium and potassium levels, and renal function test results, especially for proteinuria
Anticoagulants and Antiplatelet Drugs Warfarin (Coumadin) Aspirin Dipyridamole (Persantine) Clopidogrel (Plavix)	CVA	Alopecia, anorexia, abdominal cramps or distress, leukopenia, nausea, vomiting, diarrhea, fatal uncontrolled bleeding	Monitor PT or INR frequently (target INR: 2.0-3.0). Monitor CBC, renal and liver function test results. Be aware of early signs of infection. Educate individual to be aware of ease of bruising after small trauma and to carry card containing information on anticoagulant/antiplatelet drug therapy. Observe for occult bleeding. Advise patient not to use salicylates or alcohol if taking warfarin.
Antilipidemics, Statins Pravastatin (Pravachol) Torvastatin (Lipitor) Simvastin (Zocor)	CVA with hyperlipidemia; suspected protective action in dementia	GI: gas, stomach cramps and pain, constipation or diarrhea, nausea Other: rash, headaches, myalgia, myositis	Monitor liver function test results for elevated transaminase and creatine levels; test serum CK level if muscle tenderness occurs. Observe for urinary retention.
Antidepressants **Tricyclic** Amitriptyline (Elavil)	Adjunct treatment for migraine, tension-type headache, epilepsy, TBI, dementia	Anticholinergic effects of dry mouth, urinary hesitancy, constipation, drowsiness; orthostatic hypotension, cardiac dysrhythmias, weight gain, impotence, insomnia	Avoid giving to individuals with active alcoholism, GI disorders with risk of paralytic ileus, cardiovascular disorders such as dysrhythmias, heart failure, and heart block. Encourage intake of fluids for dry mouth. Monitor for suicidal ideation.

Continued

Table 21-1 Medications Commonly Used to Treat Brain Disorders—cont'd

Medications	Indications/Uses	Side Effects	Nursing Considerations/Teaching Points
Selective Serotonin Reuptake Inhibitors			
Fluoxetine (Prozac) Sertraline (Zoloft)	Epilepsy, CVA, TBI, dementia	Insomnia, agitation, anxiety, GI distress, dry mouth, hepatic dysfunction	Monitor liver function test results. Monitor for positive effects. Observe for suicidal ideation. Few cardiac side effects occur. Do not affect the seizure threshold.
Anxiolytics			
Diazepam (Valium) Lorazepam (Ativan)	TBI, dementia	Drowsiness, lassitude, loss of dexterity Extrapyramidal side effects of dystonia, akathisia, tardive dyskinesia; sleepiness, dizziness, dry mouth, constipation, nasal congestion	Monitor use of drug over time; caution patient regarding dependency on drug. Monitor liver function test results and CBC periodically.
Antiemetics			
Ondansetron (Zofran) Granisetron (Kytril) Trimethobenzamide (Tigan)	Migraine secondary effects of nausea and vomiting	CNS: headache, drowsiness, dizziness, fatigue CV: bradycardia, hypotension GI: constipation, diarrhea	If used long term, observe for adverse reactions, monitor renal and liver function tests. Monitor for relief of nausea and vomiting, electrolytes, fluid balance.
Psychostimulants			
Methylphenidate (Ritalin)	TBI	Anorexia, nausea, abdominal pain, increased nervousness, insomnia, headache, drowsiness, dizziness, hypertension, tachycardia, chest pain and trembling, easy bruising	Monitor for appetite suppression and weight loss. Can cause dependency. Taper periodically and reassess for continued need of medication.
Corticosteroids			
Dexamethasone (Decadron)	Migraine rescue Antiinflammatory, potentiates vasoconstrictor effects	Short-term use: insomnia, headache, restlessness, hypotension, visual disturbances	Monitor for side effects and desired effects in treating migraine. IV dosing in emergency; if oral administration used, may need schedule to taper dosage.
Opiate Analgesics			
Meperidine (Demerol)	Migraine rescue	Vertigo, lightheadedness, fatigue, sleepiness, nausea and vomiting, nervousness, increased anxiety, mental confusion, pruritus and skin rash	Monitor vital signs closely; report tachycardia and respiratory depression. Monitor pain relief, encourage individual to use pain scale to rate pain.

$5\text{-}HT_{1D}$, 5-Hydroxytryptamine (serotonin) 1D; *AV*, atrioventricular; *BP*, blood pressure; *CBC*, complete blood count; *CK*, creatinine kinase; *CNS*, central nervous system; *CVA*, cerebrovascular accident; *GI*, gastrointestinal; *HTN*, hypertension; *INR*, international normalized ratio; *IV*, intravenous; *NSAID*, nonsteroidal antiinflammatory drug; *MI*, myocardial infarction; *PT*, prothrombin time; *SC*, subcutaneous; *SIADH*, syndrome of inappropriate secretion of antidiuretic hormone; *SLE*, systemic lupus erythematosus; *TBI*, traumatic brain injury; *TIA*, transient ischemic attack.

prevent and manage migraine attacks and improve quality of life. Goals of behavioral and physical treatments for migraine include the following (Campbell, 2000):

- Reduce the frequency and severity of headache
- Reduce headache-related disability
- Reduce reliance on poorly tolerated or unwanted pharmacotherapies
- Enhance personal control of migraine
- Reduce headache-related distress and psychological symptoms

The emphasis is on assisting the individual in discovering the trigger events and supporting the person in creating lifestyle changes that will accommodate work and life responsibilities, yet avoid the stress and trigger events that lead to migraine.

The nurse teaches the individual about the prescribed medication regimen, including the effects and adverse effects of the drugs. In addition, the individual (and support person) must learn to administer medications by several routes:

- Injection for medications to treat the acute attack and possibly for rescue medication
- Nasal spray
- Rectal suppository

Complementary and Alternative Therapies

Massage therapy may be beneficial to individuals with headaches after trauma or with TTH to relieve the muscle spasms. There are a variety of forms of massage therapy. The individual should be treated by a licensed massage therapist and monitored by health professionals for improvement in quality of life as noted by a decrease in the frequency and severity of headache.

Cognitive and behavioral treatments that control muscle tension and mental relaxation have proven effective in preventing migraines. These encompass techniques such as visual imagery, meditation, and passive relaxation. Some individuals benefit from combining relaxation techniques with preventive migraine medication such as β-blockers or tricyclic antidepressants. Those who pursue these methods should be guided by a trained therapist who supports, teaches, and monitors progress in achieving therapeutic goals.

Cognitive-behavioral therapy includes psychotherapeutic interventions to identify stress and minimize the effects of stress. As much as a 50% improvement in headache activity can be achieved through such therapy (Campbell, 2000).

Physical treatments such as acupuncture, transcutaneous electrical nerve stimulation, cervical manipulation, and hyperbaric oxygen therapy have not been proven effective in evidence-based research.

EPILEPSY

A seizure is the result of sudden uncontrolled neuronal discharges and subsequently altered brain function. It may be a symptom of metabolic or neurologic disorders. When

---

Think *S* for Success

Symptoms
- Help patient manage lifestyle to avoid headache triggers.
- Instruct patient to begin therapeutic regimen at initial symptom to abort headache or decrease its severity.
- Monitor development of secondary symptoms and medicate as necessary.
- Educate patient to seek medical attention if no relief is obtained.

Sequelae
- Prevent chronic cycles of headache events that lead to depression and despair.

Safety
- Teach individual and family the importance of the following:
  Adhering to therapeutic regimen
  Checking for signs of gastrointestinal bleeding if taking nonsteroidal antiinflammatory drug for headache pain
  Maintaining preventive medication administration regimen during periods when headaches do not occur
- Teach individual and family technique for administering medications intramuscularly and via suppository.
- Caution patient to avoid operating machinery and driving during and directly after an event.

Support/Services
- Arrange for assistance with finances or community reintegration if needed.
- Make appropriate referrals for evaluation, treatment, and monitoring of headaches.
- Ascertain financial need if individual has frequent absences from work.
- Recommend community support groups for headache or chronic pain.

Satisfaction
- Determine degree to which the headache interferes with important aspects of patient's life.
- Develop a plan to maintain or restore quality of life.

---

no underlying correctable cause of seizures can be discovered, the term *epilepsy,* a Greek word meaning "to be seized upon or taken," is applied. Epilepsy is a chronic primary disorder that can cause disability and restrict an individual's activities. Epilepsy has been diagnosed in approximately 2 million Americans, with the highest prevalence among the elderly (Browne and Holmes, 2001; McCance and Huether, 2002). Epilepsy is distinctive among chronic brain disorders in that enacted legislation regulates or denies driving privileges to many individuals who have it out of concern for public safety (Berg and Engel, 1999).

Pathophysiology

Twenty percent of individuals with epilepsy have a genetic mutation on chromosome 21. These individuals will most likely show evidence of the disorder before age 20 years. Some persons whose disease does not have a familial component have cellular-level defects. One primary defect appears to be depolarization shifts in the resting potentials of the cell plasma membranes in groups of neurons. Alterations in the interstitial environment precipitated by trigger events cause instability, which changes potassium and calcium ion diffusion. Other persons have defects in the neurohormonal inhibitory system or excitatory transmission systems (Dudek, 2001; McCance and Huether, 2002; McDonald, 2001, National Institute of Neurologic Disorders and Stroke, 2000).

About 30% of seizures are secondary to another disorder and are halted when the underlying cause is treated. Examples of these disorders include infection, fever higher than 106° F (41° C), diabetic crisis, primary neurologic diseases, and head trauma. Epilepsy is medically irreversible, however, and produces recurrent seizures in approximately 60% of cases, A seizure is often precipitated by trigger events (Box 21-7).

Assessment and Diagnosis

Seizures are characterized by clinical manifestations (e.g., tonic-clonic, absence), site of origin (e.g., primary motor area, frontal lobe), electroencephalographic (EEG) characteristics (e.g., slow, focal, 3-Hz spike), and response to therapy (e.g., refractory, intractable). Most health care professionals use the international classification guidelines and criteria for epileptic seizures provided by the International League Against Epilepsy (Devinsky, 1999; McCance and Huether, 2002) (Table 21-2).

Seizures are classified broadly as either partial or generalized. In generalized seizures consciousness is always lost as the discharge begins subcortically, bilaterally, and symmetrically and flows downward into the brainstem. The activity in partial seizures begins in the cortical neurons and is superficial and unilateral within one hemisphere. The individual remains conscious if the neuronal activity remains in one hemisphere. If the activity spreads to the other hemisphere, the individual loses consciousness and the seizure becomes generalized secondarily.

A thorough history taking and physical examination is essential. The seizure may be secondary to treatable disorders, and some chronic conditions mimic epilepsy and must be considered in the differential diagnosis. Examples of these disorders include migraine, headaches, transient ischemic attacks, stroke, syncope of cardiovascular origin, and psychogenic seizures (Browne and Holmes, 2001; Leppik, 2001).

Diagnostic tests include serial EEGs, neuroimaging by CT and MRI, general blood chemistry studies, and hepatic function examinations. When the disorder is managed by long-term drug therapy, blood assays are required to ensure that therapeutic levels have been achieved and to monitor the effects of the antiepileptic medications on organ function.

Clinical Manifestations

Some seizures are highly dramatic unforgettable events whereas others go unnoticed. Furthermore, seizures are but one manifestation of epilepsy. Other phenomena may occur both before and after the actual seizure activity. Phenomena that occur before a seizure are referred to as prodroma and aura. Phenomena occurring after a seizure are called postictal events.

Prodroma, a set of events that occurs from a few days to hours before a seizure, may take the form of headache, malaise, or depression. Individuals come to learn these signs and take measures to remain safe or to abort the seizure. Aura, sensations that occur minutes to moments before the seizure, are simple partial seizures that precede the generalized seizure. These sensations may be auditory, gustatory, or visual, and a sense of dizziness or numbness may be present (Devinsky, 1999).

Postictal phenomena may last a few minutes or several hours. Some individuals experience momentary fatigue, headache, disorientation, and hallucination. Others require from 24 hours to 2 weeks to feel fully recovered.

The manifestations of a seizure relate directly to the brain area that is the epileptogenic center. Generalized seizures of multifocal origin begin with collapse and flexion of the extremities, with both tonic and clonic activity noted. Shortly thereafter the person extends the arms and legs and stiffens the back. The jaw clamps shut and a cry is emitted from forceful air expulsion. The tonic phase lasts 10 to 60 seconds, during this time the individual is apneic and may become cyanotic, the pupils dilate, and incontinence occurs. The clonic phase begins as inhibitory signals in the brain try to cancel the rapid impulses of the tonus. Muscular relaxation alternates with the tonic muscular jerking. At this point, there is excess saliva, the eyes may roll, and increased sweating and tachycardia are present. The tonic-clonic com-

---

Box 21-7   Events That Trigger Some Types of Seizure

- Hypoglycemia
- Hyperthermia
- Fatigue and lack of sleep
- Stress (emotional and physical)
- Concurrent disease
- Hyperventilation
- Stimulant drugs or caffeine
- Alcohol
- Withdrawal from chemicals or alcohol
- Intrusive environmental stimuli such as loud noise, blinking and bright lights

Table 21-2   Classification of Epileptic Seizures by Clinical Type (International League Against Epilepsy)

Type of Seizure	Clinical Features or Symptoms
Partial (seizure begins locally)	
Simple (without impairment of consciousness)	Motor signs (twitch, tingling)
	Sensory or somatosensory symptoms (simple hallucinations, tingling, light flashes, buzzing)
	Autonomic symptoms (epigastric sensation, sweating, flushing, pupil dilation)
	Psychic symptoms from higher cerebral functions (déjà vu, fear, perception of time distortion)
Complex (with impairment of consciousness)	May begin as simple seizure with motor, sensory, autonomic, and psychic symptoms then impaired consciousness—awake but unable to respond appropriately
	Onset has impaired consciousness (with or without automatisms—automatic acts which the person does not recall)
Secondarily generalized partial seizures	Begins as simple partial seizure (as above) and evolves into generalized tonic-clonic seizure; person is comatose after the seizure and recovers slowly; may bite tongue, may be incontinent
Generalized (seizure onset is bilaterally symmetric and without a local onset)	
Tonic, clonic, or tonic-clonic	Consciousness is lost; loss of consciousness may be preceded by tonic increase in muscle tone, subsequent rhythmic clonic jerks that subside slowly; person is comatose after the seizure and recovers slowly; may bite tongue, may be incontinent
Absence seizures, simple and complex types	Simple: seizure begins rapidly with brief period of unresponsiveness of approximately 10 sec; increased or decreased muscle tone
	Complex: loss of consciousness with brief tonic, clonic, or automatic movements

Others:
  Lennox-Gastaut syndrome
  Juvenile myoclonic epilepsy
  Infantile spasms
  Atonic seizures	

Specialized Epileptic Syndromes	
Myoclonus and myoclonic seizure Reflex epilepsy Acquired aphasia with convulsive disorder Febrile and other seizures of infancy and childhood Hysterical seizure Seizure caused by metabolic/toxic factors—eclampsia, alcohol, drugs, nonketotic hyperglycemia	

ponent lasts 2 to 5 minutes (Figure 21-1). When the muscular activity is over, breathing quiets and the postictal period begins. The person may be in a stupor or may not respond appropriately. The individual has no recall of the seizure and may complain of headache, confusion, muscle aching, and fatigue.

Brain damage with gradual loss of mental capacity can occur from anoxic periods during seizures (Brodie and Kwan, 2002; Engel, 2001; Meador, 2002), especially when seizures are frequent, severe, and long lasting.

Death can occur in two epileptic events: status epilepticus and sudden unexpected death in epilepsy (SUDEP) (Browne and Holmes, 2001; Walczak et al, 2001). Status epilepticus is unremitting seizure activity that results in brain anoxia and accumulation of lactic acid, which destroys neurons and other cells. Although there is no other life-threatening illness associated with SUDEP and the results of autopsy reveal no explanation for the death, Walczak and colleagues (2001) suggest that postictal central apnea causing anoxia and positional asphyxia are the causes of death.

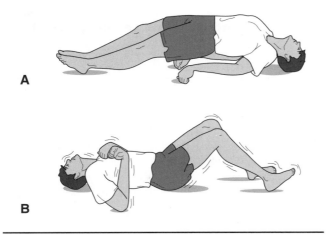

Figure 21-1 **A,** Tonic and **B,** clonic phases of a seizure.

Partial seizures may be accompanied by jerking or twitching of a single extremity or changes in sensation in the face. Other sensations can be tingling, a pins-and-needles feeling, or numbness in the muscles.

Absence seizures are characterized by an abrupt cessation of activity with an arrest of consciousness. The individual does not collapse but has a vacant stare and may respond to conversation. The seizure passes in 10 to 30 seconds and the individual resumes his preseizure activity.

Depression is a significant clinical manifestation of epilepsy and is most likely to occur in individuals with partial seizures that originate in the temporal or frontal lobes and in individuals with poor suppression of seizures (Kanner and Balabanov, 2002).

Interdisciplinary Care

Because of the irreversible, chronic nature of epilepsy, the individual with this disorder needs an extensive support system to assist in managing the disease: these include the primary care provider, neurologist, nurse, psychologist, and social worker, as well as the family and a network of significant others.

Primary Provider (Physician/Nurse Practitioner)

Management of epilepsy requires long-term therapy, constant monitoring, and reevaluation as new treatments evolve, new pharmaceuticals emerge, and technology improves. The treatment goals are the following:

- Suppression of seizures without adverse effects of treatment
- Positive management by the individual and family
- Maintenance of cognitive function and mental health
- Achievement of optimal quality of life

The view of epilepsy as an incurable disease is being challenged, because some individuals are cured through surgery. However, a universal cure has not been achieved. Therefore epilepsy must be broadly approached as a chronic

disorder affecting multiple facets of the individual's life and support network. The treatment plan focuses on enabling the individual to carry out the prescribed treatment, create a lifestyle conducive to managing the seizures, and manage his or her life (Buelow, 2001).

Specialists

Neurologist

The neurologist helps determine the diagnosis of primary epilepsy or epilepsy secondary to other disorders and establishes the primary treatment plan. The neurologist also evaluates the appropriateness of the treatment plan as new therapies evolve, new pharmaceuticals emerge, and technology improves. The primary provider assists in executing the treatment plan.

Neurosurgeon

The neurologist consults the neurosurgeon when the individual does not respond to pharmacotherapy. Workup for surgery should be considered after failure to suppress seizures has occurred in two pharmacotherapy trials in which the individual did not achieve desired effects. The earlier in the course of epilepsy that the disorder is identified as refractory to treatment with antiepileptic drugs and the patient is considered a candidate for surgery, the better the therapeutic outcomes in terms of cure of the seizures, good quality of life, and maintenance of cognitive function and mental health (Engel, 2001). In well-screened candidates, successful surgery can "cure" the epilepsy in over 50% of cases and significantly reduce the frequency and severity of seizures in the remaining individuals (Engel et al, 2003; Wiebe et al, 2001). Advances in technology allow for precise surgical access to epileptogenic areas, most notably in the temporal lobe.

Another treatment executed by the neurosurgeon, in collaboration with the neurologist, is vagal nerve stimulation (VNS). VNS has shown safety and efficacy in the treatment of individuals with refractory partial seizures and secondary generalized seizures (Fisher and Handforth, 1999). VNS produces significant seizure reduction (by as much as 75%) but does not result in complete seizure remission. This treatment requires electrode implantation and a period during which current pulse stimulation of the left vagus nerve is increased to achieve optimal seizure suppression. Individuals who are unable to tolerate or benefit from antiepileptic drugs (AEDs) are candidates for this therapy (Fisher and Handforth, 1999). The benefits are attributed to increased blood flow to the thalamic areas of the brain and activation of synaptic sites in the brainstem and cerebral hemispheres. Adverse effects from this therapy are voice hoarseness and occasional shortness of breath. SUDEP occurs at the same rate in those undergoing VNS as in those treated with AEDs.

Drug Therapy

The mainstay of treatment is pharmacologic through the administration of AEDs in monotherapy or combination therapy. Individual AEDs have specific actions on different neuron centers and types of seizure syndrome (Box 21-8). In general, AEDs have considerable adverse effects and cause neurotoxicity (see Table 21-1).

The outcome of the first use of an AED is a powerful predictor of treatment success for an individual in long-term therapy. Seizure suppression is achieved with the first or second drug selected in 60% of patients (Brodie and Kwan, 2002). Among individuals in whom monotherapy does not successfully prevent seizures, 10% experience suppression with combination therapy and another 40% experience improvement in seizure suppression with combination therapy (Devinsky, 1999). If an individual has not had a seizure after 2 or more years of treatment with AEDs, discontinuation of therapy with drug tapering can be attempted in combination with close monitoring and restrictions on dangerous activities for 1 year (Browne and Holmes, 2001).

In more than 30% of individuals, epilepsy is refractory to AED treatment and the drugs produce inadequate or no suppression of seizures (Brodie and Kwan, 2002; Devinsky, 1999; Engel, 2001; Sisodiya et al, 2002). For these individuals, other treatment methods should be sought as soon as possible.

Nurse

The nurse assists the patient in making lifestyle accommodations and adhering to prescribed therapy to help maintain and enhance quality of life. To do this, the nurse must have a thorough understanding of how the individual perceives himself or herself, the disorder, and its impact on the person's life. Buelow (2001) developed guidelines for interviewing to help professionals gain this understanding (Box 21-9).

A major symptom the nurse must address is the depression frequently associated with seizures. Kanner and Balabanov (2002) postulate that a bidirectional relationship exists between depression and epilepsy and suggest that

---

Box 21-8   Selected Antiepileptic Drugs Used for Specific Types of Seizure

PARTIAL SEIZURES
■ Carbamazepine (Tegretol)
■ Divalproex (Depakote)
■ Oxcarbazepine (Trileptal)
■ Phenytoin (Dilantin)

ABSENCE SEIZURES
■ Ethosuximide (Zarontin)
■ Divalproex sodium (Depakote)

GENERALIZED TONIC-CLONIC SEIZURES
■ Divalproex sodium (Depakote)
■ Phenytoin (Dilantin)
■ Fosphenytoin (Cerebyx)

Box 21-9   Guide for Interviewing a Person with Epilepsy

■ Tell me how you feel about your life right now.
■ Tell me how epilepsy affects your life.
■ Tell me about situations you have encountered in your life that have been affected by epilepsy.
■ Tell me about what you do to manage those situations.
■ Tell me about things that you do to manage seizures that were not prescribed by your physician.
■ Tell me about how you learned what strategies work.
■ Tell me about how important these strategies are for managing seizures.
■ Tell me about what your doctor asks you to do to manage your seizures.
■ Tell me about how easy or difficult it is to carry out these instructions.
■ Tell me about how you feel about carrying out the treatment regimen that is prescribed for you.
■ Tell me what others can do to help you maintain your ability to care for yourself.
■ Tell me what self-management means to you.
■ Is there anything else that you would like me to know about your epilepsy?

From Buelow JM: Epilepsy management issues and techniques, *J Neurosci Nurs* 33(5):260-6, 2001.

---

neurotransmitter dysfunction is the common link between the two. The transmitters implicated in both disorders are serotonin, noradrenalin (norepinephrine), dopamine, and γ-aminobutyric acid.

The symptoms of depression may be atypical, such as dysphoria, anxiety, fear, an inability to experience pleasure in anything, guilt, suicidal ideation, and change in body patterns (sleep, eating, libido). Because the adverse effects of AEDs can cause symptoms that mimic those of depression, it is important to ascertain when the symptoms of depression began and the timing of any changes in these symptoms (i.e., before or after introduction of AED therapy).

Individuals with epilepsy and depression can be treated successfully with selective serotonin reuptake inhibitors, other antidepressants, and, if necessary, tricyclic antidepressants in conjunction with their AEDs (Kanner and Balabonov, 2002).

The adverse effects of AEDs cause some individuals such discomfort that they forego the medication and endure increased seizure activity. The nurse must teach and support the patient in making choices consistent with the treatment plan. In addition, family and friends should be included in education regarding what to do in the event of a seizure (Box 21-10) and how to support the treatment regimen and create a safe environment.

Box 21-10 Topics for Teaching Related to Safety

- Adherence to antiepileptic drug regimen to achieve seizure control
- Need to learn prodromal symptoms and respond with prescribed measures to abort impending seizure
- Need to learn aura symptoms (if present) and to take immediate actions to alert others that assistance is required and to put self in safest position possible—ease individual to the floor or ground
- Appropriate family interventions during the seizure
  - If individual is standing, ease individual to the floor and protect the head if possible.
  - Loosen clothing around the neck.
  - Guide individual onto his or her side so that secretions can drain out.
  - Do not force anything into the mouth or try to restrict arm or leg movement.
  - Clear the area of any objects that may cause injury to the individual during the seizure.

- Appropriate family interventions after the seizure
  - Seek medical attention for the individual if the seizure was different in pattern or longer than prior seizures
  - Remain with the individual during postictal period and provide reassurance, because person may have disorganized thoughts, impaired judgment, and inability to process information
  - Maintain the individual's self-esteem by assisting in hygiene if the individual experienced incontinence
  - Check for physical injury.
- Information about the seizure to be entered in the individual's treatment diary by the family member or nurse
  - Prodroma, aura, trigger event
  - Onset time and duration of seizure
  - Sounds emitted at onset of seizure
  - Movements of arms, legs, and head
  - Incontinence patterns
  - Patterns in resumption of breathing
  - Postictal behavior patterns

Medical Social Worker

The social worker helps the individual with epilepsy and his or her family to understand government regulations regarding driving motor vehicles and participating in certain types of employment and recreational activities. In addition, the social worker assesses the household financial situation and determines eligibility for government assistance.

The social worker recommends community-based social support groups for the individual and family based on their needs and unique stressors. As the individual with epilepsy undergoes successful pharmacologic or surgical treatment of epilepsy and the societal restrictions are lifted, the social worker figures prominently in the adjustment of the person from a state of dependency to a psychosocial state of "normality" in the aspects of life in which this was formerly not the case (Wilson, Bladin, and Saling, 2001). Without adequate guidance, structure, and rehabilitation, the individual's new role may cause anxiety as the individual enters situations for which he or she is not prepared. The areas most strongly affected are vocational functioning, social and role redefinition, and the sense of well-being and ability to discard the sick role.

Ethical Considerations

In certain segments of society, misconceptions of lay people about individuals with epilepsy result in social stigmatization, isolation, and exclusion of the individual with epilepsy from the mainstream. These misconceptions, combined with legislative restrictions, may limit an individual's ability to interact freely and engage in a variety of normal activities.

The nurse educates individuals, groups, and communities about epilepsy and its causes and treatments.

STROKE

Stroke, or cerebrovascular accident (CVA), is the third leading cause of death in the United States (Centers for Disease Control and Prevention [CDC], 1999; Minino and Smith, 2001). Although age-adjusted stroke death rates have declined by 70% since 1950 (CDC, 1999), 167,000 persons die from stroke each year.

Approximately 590,000 individuals in the United States survive stroke annually, so that there are more than 4 million living stroke survivors (American Heart Association [AHA], 2001; National Stroke Association [NSA], 2002a) (Table 21-3). Among the survivors, approximately one third have mild impairments or disabilities, another third are moderately impaired, and the remainder are severely impaired, which makes stroke the leading cause of adult disability in the United States (AHA, 2001; Habel, 2001; NSA, 2002a). Between 30% and 40% of stroke survivors will experience another stroke within 5 years. Health professionals are challenged to expand efforts to prevent first and subsequent strokes.

Ethnic Variations

African Americans have a higher incidence of stroke and experience more extensive physical disabilities from stroke than any other racial group. Mortality rates follow a similar trend.

Think S for Success

Symptoms
- Help patient manage lifestyle to avoid epilepsy triggers.
- Instruct patient to begin therapeutic regimen at the first prodromal or aura symptoms to abort the seizure or to decrease its severity.

Sequelae
- Prevent cognitive decline by seeking medical means to decrease the frequency and duration of seizure activity.
- Evaluate seizure activity and effectiveness of recommended treatment regimen.

Safety
- In postictal state, evaluate patient for injury, fatigue, mental acuity, and judgment.
- Teach individual and family the importance of the following:
  Adhering to therapeutic regimen
  Monitoring for adverse effects of medications; ensure that individual adheres to schedule for recommended laboratory blood tests
- Teach patient and family techniques to protect patient during and after seizure.

Support/Services
- Support individual in maintaining normalcy in life within treatment regimen.
- Plan alternative transportation means.
- Arrange for assistance with finances or community reintegration if necessary.
- Ascertain financial need if individual is unable to work or is frequently absent from work.

Satisfaction
- Determine degree to which epilepsy and seizures interfere with important aspects of patient's life.
- Develop plan to help individual reach or maintain desired quality of life.

Table 21-3   Mortality from Stroke

Age Group (Years)	Percentage of Strokes Resulting in Death
>85	40.1
75-84	34.3
65-74	14.4
<65	11.2

From Centers for Disease Control and Prevention: State-specific mortality from stroke and distribution of place of death—United States, 1999, *MMWR Morb Mortal Wkly Rep* 51(20):429-33, May 24, 2002.

In addition, regional differences exist in the incidence of stroke related to demographics and habits such as dietary choices. The region with the highest stroke mortality rate is comprised of 12 contiguous states (Virginia, North Carolina, South Carolina, Georgia, Florida, Alabama, Mississippi, Louisiana, Arkansas, Tennessee, Kentucky, and Indiana) and the District of Columbia. Stroke death rates in these states and in Washington, D., are consistently 10% higher than in the rest of the country. This area is often referred to as the "stroke belt" (CDC, 1999, 2002; NSA, 2002a).

Pathophysiology

Stroke is the result of neuronal death of brain tissue. Although stroke has a variety of causes, including global hypoperfusion secondary to shock, the two primary categories of stroke are ischemic stroke and hemorrhagic stroke. The region of the brain affected by the ischemia determines the sequelae and deficits that the individual will experience. The area most commonly affected is the region supplied by the middle cerebral artery, which perfuses cortical motor, sensory, and speech areas as well as the temporal lobe optic segment. Only rarely does an atraumatic stroke occur without one or more risk factors present. Common risk factors are listed in Table 21-4.

Ischemic strokes, also known as ischemic infarcts, pale infarcts, or white strokes, result from occlusions in the arterial vasculature. They are classified as either thrombotic or embolic and account for 61% of all strokes (AHA, 2001). Thrombi form as platelets and fibrin are activated while passing over rough atherosclerotic plaques in the intracranial vessels supplying the brain. Other conditions that lead to increased coagulation and thrombi include hemoconcentration such as in dehydration and polycythemia and blood stasis during hypotension or during prolonged vasoconstriction. Embolic strokes occur when fragments break from a stationary thrombus or when an embolus forms as a result of plaque, atrial fibrillation, myocardial infarction, or disorders of the aorta, carotids, or vertebral-basilar circulation.

Ischemic strokes usually involve the cerebral hemispheres. As the blood flow stops, the central zone of cells loses function and the neurons die. A zone of surrounding cells (the penumbra) is injured from the hypoxemia, and without reperfusion some cells may die in an hour. Six hours is the upper limit to reverse this process and regain some function. After 6 hours cellular membranes lose their integrity, which allows extracellular ions to enter; the mitochondria cease production of adenosine triphosphate; lactic acid forms and damages intracellular and extracellular structures causing necrosis; edema occurs; and macrophages appear to remove the debris. If reperfusion does take place, then because the integrity of vessel walls has been compromised, a bleeding or red stroke may result as circulation resumes, causing further tissue damage.

Hemorrhagic stroke is the third most common type of stroke after thrombotic and embolic strokes and results from hypertensive insults that lead to leakage from or rupture of vessels, aneurysms, vascular malformations, bleeding within a tumor, or anticoagulation conditions. Hypertension is the most common initiating factor. Vascular wall defects

Table 21-4   Common Risk Factors Associated with Cerebrovascular Accidents

Risk Factor	Comments
Ethnicity	Incidence is 2.5 times higher in the African American population than in the white population; African American survivors suffer greater physical disability from stroke and higher rate of mortality.
Hypertension with elevations in systolic and/or diastolic pressure	Systolic and diastolic pressures are independent risk factors. Isolated systolic hypertension in the elderly is a significant risk factor.
Coronary heart disease	Risk for ischemic stroke after myocardial infarction is 31% in first month and 1% to 2% each year after myocardial infarction.
Atrial fibrillation	Ischemic stroke risk is 5 times higher in those with this risk factor.
Diabetes mellitus (DM)	DM with macrovascular and microvascular changes increases the risk of ischemic stroke by 2.5 to 3.5 times.
Insulin resistance	Insulin resistance is an independent risk factor for ischemic stroke.
High blood lipid levels and high dietary intake of cholesterol	Independent risk factor for ischemic stroke.
Cigarette smoking, including exposure to second-hand smoke	Increases risk of stroke by 50%.
Heavy alcohol consumption	Carries increased risk for hemorrhagic stroke that is dose dependent.
Carotid artery occlusion	Risk increases as degree of stenosis increases.
Physical inactivity	Increases risk because it contributes to obesity, hypertension, and DM.
Obesity	Increases risk of stroke because it contributes to hypertension and DM.
Hyperhomocysteinemia	Increases risk and is an independent risk factor in ischemic stroke.

occur in aneurysms (Figure 21-2), vessel bifurcations, and vascular malformations, as well as from plaque erosion. These defects begin to leak or rupture under increased blood pressure. As the mass of blood forms, it displaces and compresses brain tissue and vessels and impedes blood flow, which causes ischemia and a reactionary vasodilation and edema. This series of events increases intracranial pressure, and seepage into ventricular spaces may occur.

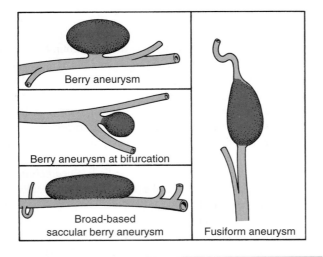

Figure 21-2   Types of aneurysm. (From McCance KL, Huether SE, editors: *Pathophysiology: the biologic basis for disease in adults and children,* ed 4, St Louis, 2002, Mosby.)

A hemorrhage several centimeters in diameter is considered massive and a hemorrhage 1 to 2 cm in diameter is referred to as small. Hypertensive hemorrhages occur in the putamen of the basal ganglia, the thalamus, the cortex and subcortex, the pons, and the cerebellum (McCance and Huether, 2002). Other causes of hemorrhage are bleeding and coagulation disorders, head trauma, and illicit drug use.

Clinical Manifestations

Ischemic stroke can have one of several presentations. In 50,000 Americans, it begins as a transient ischemic attack (TIA) in which there is intermittent blockage of blood flow. The signs and symptoms most frequently experienced include loss of speech, visual disturbances, headache, tingling or twitching in facial muscles, numbness or loss of function of a body part, confusion, and loss of immediate memory. None of these signs and symptoms or any residual defect remains at the end of 24 hours. Without treatment, however, TIAs occur more frequently over time, and a subsequent attack becomes an irreversible stroke. If the effects of a TIA last longer than 24 hours and the signs and symptoms reverse, the attack is known as reversible ischemic neurologic defect (RIND). A stroke in evolution is a thrombotic stroke evolving in a step-by-step progression over minutes to hours. A completed stroke is one that has reached its maximum destructiveness and full neurologic damage (McCance and Huether, 2002).

Development and resolution of cerebral edema is a significant factor in the final outcome of stroke; the more the edema and the longer the resolution phase, the greater the chance of extended neurologic deficit. Most individuals survive the first ischemic stroke of the hemispheres. Infarcts of the vital brainstem are generally fatal.

The manifestations of hemorrhagic stroke depend on the area and size of the hemorrhage. Focal neurologic deficits and loss of consciousness occur. The onset is usually sudden, although some individuals experience a momentary severe headache before losing consciousness. If coma with unresponsiveness develops, the prognosis is poor.

Manifestations of stroke include motor hemiplegia, hemiparesis, flaccidity, spasticity, and rigidity; loss of sensation in areas affected by motor problems; communication deficits with problems in expression (agnosia and aphasia) and comprehension; perceptual alteration and sensory neglect (unilateral neglect); visual impairments; weakness and paralysis of facial muscles, ocular muscles, and tongue and difficulty with mastication; ataxia, alterations in balance and coordination; incontinence; and altered level of consciousness. The deficits manifested are determined by the brain hemisphere affected. For example, deficits caused by right hemisphere damage include cognitive and behavioral changes that lead to emotional lability and poor judgment, whereas a stroke in the left hemisphere often causes loss of speech comprehension and the motor ability to form words. Table 21-5 lists common deficits associated with damage to each brain hemisphere.

Depression is frequently noted in individuals with stroke. Initially, the depression was considered a reaction to the stroke and adjustment to altered roles and disability. More research has shown that it may be due to primary effects on key cortical and subcortical structures that mediate cognition, emotion, and interpersonal capabilities, which affect an individual's perception, thinking, emotional processing, social cognition, empathy, and interpersonal abilities (Eslinger, Parkinson, and Shamay, 2002).

Two pain syndromes are experienced by individuals with stroke. The first is referred to as central poststroke pain. The mechanism is not fully known, but the thalamus is thought to be involved, causing a hyperexcitable response to incoming sensory stimulation (Vestergaard et al, 2001). The pain may follow the distribution of numbness the individual experiences. It may be severe and may limit the ability of the individual to recover fully or to care for himself or herself. Lamotrigine, an AED that has shown success in treating other nerve pain (trigeminal neuritis), decreases the pain in individuals with central poststroke pain (Vestergaard et al, 2001).

The second pain syndrome, shoulder pain, affects between 16% and 80% of individuals with stroke (Snels et al, 2002). The first of the two primary origins is referred pain from the neck, visceral regions, or thalamus. The second origin is local pain from damage to the rotator cuff, spasticity, subluxation of the joint, or tendonitis or from disuse atrophy syndrome (Snels et al, 2002). There is little agreement on how to relieve the pain. Exercise and strengthening of arm, shoulder, and accessory muscles are the therapies of choice. Prevention of a "frozen" shoulder joint is

Table 21-5 Stroke-Related Deficits by Site of Blockage

Site of Circulation Blockage	Deficit
Middle cerebral artery, right or left	Contralateral impairment of motor and sensory functions, i.e., right blockage affects left-side
	Motor: varying degrees of weakness in face, arm, or leg; hemiparesis or hemiplegia
	Sensory: follows motor pattern
	Transient to permanent visual neglect on contralateral side
	Some short-term memory loss and short attention span; long-term memory intact
Left middle cerebral artery	Loss of function in spoken or written language comprehension (Wernicke's aphasia)
	Expressive: loss of ability to speak or form words due to loss of Broca's motor area (Broca's aphasia, nonfluent aphasia, dysarthria)
	Possible loss of ability to read or write
	Behavioral change to slow, cautious style, requires information to be repeated with feedback and reassurances
Right middle cerebral artery	Spatial and perceptual deficits; misjudgment of distances (leading to falls) and lack of eye-hand coordination
	Behavioral changes: impulsive style and lack of awareness of impairments and inability to perform the same tasks as before the stroke
	Visual impairment, which leads to neglect of objects and body parts on the left side
Posterior circulation to hindbrain and midbrain	Deficits from interferences in nerve conduction between major pathways between brain and spinal cord causing total incapacitating sensory and motor abnormalities; paralysis
	Deficits in many areas, lack of coordination and balance; dizziness and nausea

imperative. NSAIDs and occasionally muscle relaxants are used for short-term treatment; pain medications are avoided, however, because long-term use can be detrimental.

Assessment and Diagnosis

As long as 2 weeks may be required before the individual with stroke can be accurately assessed. The individual can be more precisely evaluated during the recovery period in rehabilitation as risk factors are stabilized and the healing process moves forward. The health care team assesses the individual in the rehabilitation unit using one of a variety of scales developed for this purpose. In the rehabilitation setting the instrument may be the Functional Independence Measures (FIM) tool. In the home setting it may be the Outcome Assessment Information System (OASIS) tool. FIM contains 18 areas designed to assess an individual's physical and behavioral functioning with regard to self-care, cognition, elimination, and control of eating. A companion complementary assessment tool, the Functional Assessment Measure (FAM), was developed to assess the individual's ability outside of the home. Its scale and rating process are the same as those of the FIM instrument. Each item is assigned a score ranging from 1, which indicates that total assistance is needed, to 7, which indicates complete independence (Cavanaugh et al, 2000). Individuals with a score of 6 or 7 can safely perform the given activity and can live independently if they choose. Areas assessed by FAM are listed in Box 21-11.

In addition, the ability of the caregiver to provide care to the individual with stroke should be assessed. Physical ability, endurance, and hardiness of the caregiver, as well as the existence of support systems for the caregiver, are vital aspects of providing care. An average of 8.6 hours a week is needed to care for an individual with a stroke if there are no stroke-related health problems. An additional 10 hours is required if stroke-related health problems are present (Hickenbottom et al, 2002).

Box 21-11   Areas Evaluated by the Functional Assessment Measure

- Swallowing ability
- Community access
- Writing ability
- Emotional status
- Employability
- Attention level
- Ability to execute car transfers
- Reading ability
- Speech intelligibility
- Adjustment to limitations
- Orientation ability
- Safety awareness/judgment

Interdisciplinary Care

The residual physical, social, and psychological impairments of stroke affect every aspect of the individual's life. Key members of the interdisciplinary team include the primary care health care provider; physician specialist, that is, neurologist or physiatrist; nurse; dietitian; social worker; physical therapist; occupational therapist; speech therapist; psychologist; and vocational rehabilitation counselor. The goals of care are the following:

- Management of risk factors that contributed to the stroke
- Avoidance of the toxic effects of therapy
- Management of poststroke disabilities
- Maintenance of functional status
- Maximization of quality of life

Primary Provider (Physician/Nurse Practitioner)

In the community setting, after the individual who experienced a stroke is discharged from the hospital or rehabilitation center, the person's care is managed by a primary provider. Through close management, the provider seeks to lower or eliminate the risk factors that influenced the occurrence of the first CVA (see Table 21-4), such as diabetes mellitus, obesity, hypertension, hyperlipidemia, and hyperhomocysteinemia. The primary provider collaborates frequently with the family and the nurse involved in caring for the individual.

Specialists

The neurologist who cared for the individual during the acute care phase generally remains part of the poststroke treatment team and provides expert consultation to the team members as needed. The neurologist may see the individual on a periodic basis. If the individual develops a pain syndrome, the neurologist may be the physician who treats this condition or refers the individual to a clinic specializing in pain management.

The physiatrist, in collaboration with the individual, the family, and the rehabilitation team, creates a management plan to optimize the individual's integrative functioning when the stroke has resulted in motor, sensory, and cognitive deficits. The physiatrist assesses the individual and develops the goals for the team in keeping with the functional abilities and potential of the individual. Based on this assessment, the course of treatment and therapeutic regimen are prescribed. The emphasis is on physical functioning to assist the patient in maintaining independence through mobility and transfer ability.

Drug Therapy

In the poststroke period, the medications most frequently ordered depend on the cause of the stroke and the risk factors associated with the stroke event. Anticoagulants and antiplatelet drugs are used to prevent thrombus formation, antilipidemics are used to control hyperlipidemia, and antihypertensives are used to control blood pressure. (see Table 21-1).

Dietitian

The nonpharmacologic approach of diet management is the treatment of choice for the individual with stroke and should be used in conjunction with pharmacologic agents. The dietitian, together with the individual and primary health care provider, can devise a diet to meet the needs of the individual. Adherence to diet therapy is a central factor in the prevention of a second stroke, and every attempt must be made to create a diet acceptable to the individual (National Cholesterol Education Program, 2001). Some lifestyle considerations in dietary therapy are the following:

- What coexisting illnesses and conditions can benefit from dietary adjustments?
- What is the dietary history of the individual: likes and dislikes; weight loss or gain?
- What foods can be selected that are within the patient's budget?
- Has stroke changed the individual's eating pattern?

The desired outcomes of diet therapy are for the individual to achieve a healthy diet in accordance with recommended government guidelines by maintaining the following:

- Glycemic control with the hemoglobin A_{IC} concentration consistently lower than 7.0% and plasma glucose levels 125 mg/dl or lower (American Diabetes Association, 2002).
- Weight and body mass index within guidelines for age and height; male waistline size of 40 inches or less; female waistline size of 35 inches or less (AHA, 2002)
- Reduction of sodium sufficient to prevent fluid retention
- Low-density lipoprotein cholesterol levels consistent with the recommendations of the National Cholesterol Education Program (2001) (Table 21-6)

Nurse

The nurse is the central figure for the individual with stroke and his or her family. The nurse establishes a trusting relationship by providing physical care and emotional support to the individual and to the family. Because of this trust, the nurse learns more about the individual and his or her coping ability and inner strengths, and applies this knowledge in the healing, restorative, and rehabilitative processes. The nurse uses the same processes in caring for the family and preparing the caregiver(s) for the responsibilities of caring for the individual in the home. Eaves (2000) identified themes in the adaptation process; two of these are discovering the impact of stroke and reconstructing life. It is a slow process for the individual and the family to understand the extent of the changes in the patient's independence, roles, and expectations.

The degree of impact depends on the FIM score, the level of pain (or discomfort), the resilience of the individual, and the level of depression. The experiences of nurses and other professionals demonstrate the importance of the support of the family and/or significant others and their attitudes toward assisting in recovery to restructure lifestyles and "make things work." For the caregivers the task can seem overwhelming and fatigue can be constant as they attend to the needs of the individual. It is critical that the nurse be available to listen, accept emotional outpourings, give counsel, provide anticipatory guidance, teach, and monitor the environment and the individual. By listening and by asking "How is this or that for you?" the nurse provides the opportunities for the individual or caregiver to express frustrations, anger, and other emotions. The nurse keeps communication open with the caregiver to prevent the development of isolation, frustration or feelings of futility, and burnout. In addition to physical changes, an individual with stroke can experience mood swings, emotional lability, behavior changes, and changes in personality that greatly alter the individual's being and persona . It can be difficult for the caregiver to remain caring, emotionally involved, and connected to an individual who bears little resemblance to his or her former self—to a loved one the caregiver no longer knows.

Maintaining focus on quality-of-life issues and ways to overcome physical and emotional barriers maximizes abilities, minimizes disabilities, and encourages engagement in life. Social isolation may become a problem if the individual has low self-esteem and perceives himself or herself as unacceptable to society, has communication problems, or experiences depression. Strategies the nurse can teach the family and caregivers to enhance communication are listed in Box 21-12.

The nurse must take advantage of opportunities to teach the individual and family to understand their resources and rights under the provisions of the Americans with Disabilities Act, which prevents discrimination in employment and reduces barriers to accessing buildings and facilities in public areas. The nurse teaches the individual and family to select and incorporate new technology and devices that meet their needs, such as the following:

- To enhance communication: computers, electronic devices for voice enhancement
- To aid in accomplishing physical tasks: kitchen and cooking modifications; motorized wheelchairs and transport devices
- To assist with continence issues: continence products

Table 21-6 Recommended Levels of Low-Density Lipoprotein (LDL) Cholesterol Based on Risk

Risk Level	LDL Cholesterol Goal
Patient has cardiovascular disease, coronary heart disease, or history of stroke.	Reduce to <100 mg/dl.
Patient has two risk factors (e.g., obesity, diabetes).	Reduce to <130 mg/dl.
Patient has no risk factors.	Keep below 160 mg/dl.

From National Cholesterol Education Program: The third report of the expert panel on detection, evaluation, and treatment of high blood cholesterol in adults, National Heart, Lung, and Blood Institute, 2001, Bethesda, Md, National Institutes of Health.

Box 21-12 Strategies to Enhance Communication after Stroke

■ Base the communication on respect.
■ Approach and treat the individual as an adult; avoid child or baby talk.
■ Face the individual and speak clearly and slowly.
■ Use short, simple statements and questions.
■ Do not assume that the individual who does not respond verbally cannot hear or has not heard the speaker; do not raise the voice to repeat.
■ Allow adequate time for the individual to respond.
■ When the individual responds and the speech is not understood, be honest and say so.
■ Acknowledge the individual's frustration at his or her inability to communicate.
■ Use alternate methods to communicate, such as statements that can be answered with a single word or a yes or no response; flash cards or a picture board; writing tablets; computerized talking boards; or other electronic devices.

■ To provide greater ease in grooming and dressing: use of hand rails and safety devices, one-handed clothing closures

If the individual has not regained sufficient upper body control or cannot maintain posture and balance, the nurse must ensure that the family understands the physical safety needs. In conjunction with the physical therapist, the nurse teaches the individual and caregiver to use special devices or equipment prescribed to assist the individual in maintaining body position and control while sitting. Caregivers must remain alert to shifts in body position or slumping, especially while the individual is eating foods or drinking fluids. A further complication often seen as part of upper body control deficit is unilateral neglect syndrome, in which the individual no longer senses, detects, or recognizes part of the body. The nurse teaches the family to protect that body part—for example, to protect the arm so that it does not become entrapped between the body and a chair or dangle unsupported when the patient sits or stands. In positioning the individual in bed, care must again be taken to maintain proper alignment and prevent entrapment. The individual remains important to the management of his or her body and should be encouraged to use the dominant side to care for the affected or neglected side. The strategy may be gentle reminders from the caregivers to care for the neglected side and to use the dominant side to perform self-care and activities of daily living.

The nurse may need to develop a time schedule or checklist for the caregivers and the individual so that the individual is moved regularly with a goal of maintaining adequate circulatory and tissue perfusion to prevent decubitus ulcers or damage to sensory-deprived areas. The nurse will teach and reinforce positioning techniques that maintain anatomic alignment, enhance respiratory effort, enhance circulatory

dynamics and unrestricted venous and lymphatic return flows, and consider any motor or sensory deficits the individual has.

Medical Social Worker

The medical social worker assesses the home, caregiver, and individual for areas of need related to community reintegration. The social worker collaborates with a variety of the health professionals to ensure that the individual with stroke and his or her family have access to community resources. For example, the social worker may arrange for a weekly in-house caregiver to care for the individual a half-day while the family caregiver is away running errands, shopping, and engaging in community activities. The social worker may arrange for special telephone services if the individual has hearing or visual impairment or needs the services of an emergency alerting system through a local health care facility.

The social worker also assesses financial resources and determines eligibility for medical programs that provide financial payment, specialized services, or home care medical equipment. The social worker may also play the role of counselor and provide emotional support to the individual, the family, or the caregiver. Because the social worker is not physically involved in the personal care of the individual, it may be easier for the family or individual to discuss personal issues with the social worker.

Physical Therapist

The physical therapist focuses primarily on control of the larger muscle groups, that is, the muscles of posture, ambulation, and gross movement. The greater the muscle abilities of the individual, the greater the level of independence. The physical therapist carefully evaluates the individual for muscle strength and body control required to sit, change positions, transfer, and ambulate, and determines the need for devices that will maintain proper body alignment and function. The therapist creates arm slings to prevent subluxation of the shoulder joint if the individual has no shoulder strength or has neglect syndrome. The individual's physical therapy needs will change over time, and adjustments must be made in the treatment plan and communicated to other team members. The therapist develops an individualized exercise program to accomplish the following:

■ Promote flexibility and relaxation of the muscles on the affected side
■ Help the patient return to more normal movement
■ Improve balance and coordination
■ Decrease pain and stiffness
■ Maintain range of motion in the affected arm and leg

After learning the exercises, the individual and his or her caregiver perform the exercises at home daily. Examples of exercises to increase muscle strength and independence in individuals moderately affected by stroke can be found on the NSA website (*http://www.stroke.org;* NSA, 2002a, 2002b).

Occupational Therapist

The occupational therapist assists the individual with control of smaller muscle groups, eye-hand coordination, and adaptations to accommodate the activities of daily living. Part of this therapy may be the use of molded hand splints and arm cradles to maintain alignment during sleep and relaxation periods. Often the focus is on regaining arm and hand movement and control, and the ability to manipulate small objects. The goal of this therapy is to develop the means whereby the individual can provide as much of his or her own personal care as possible. Other goals relate to activities in the home such as food and meal preparation.

Speech Therapist

Two major goals of speech therapy are to enhance the communication abilities of the individual and to determine the ability of the individual to swallow. One of the greatest frustrations for the individual with a stroke is the inability to communicate freely. The speech therapist determines what program and exercises are needed for vocalization.

Estimates are that 43% to 54% of individuals with stroke who have difficulty swallowing (dysphagia) experience aspiration. Without proper assessment, diagnosis, and treatment, approximately 37% of these individuals will develop pneumonia, and 3.8% will die of that pneumonia (Agency for Health Care Policy and Research, 1999). The speech therapist teaches the individual with swallowing difficulties techniques to improve swallowing, exercises that strengthen muscles, and modifications in diet to avoid aspiration. Interventions for preventing aspiration are listed in Box 21-13.

The eating environment should be pleasant and free of distractions. If the individual is distracted by nearby activity, the likelihood of aspiration increases. Small bites of food should be placed behind the front teeth on the unaffected side of the mouth. As the individual takes the food, she or he should tilt the head backward and concentrate on swallowing. The caregiver can assist the individual by giving step-by-step instructions in eating. The mouth should be checked to ensure that food has not become pocketed in the affected cheek.

Rehabilitation Specialist

The goal of rehabilitation is self-care and an optimal quality of life for the individual with stroke and for the caregivers. Vocational rehabilitation specialists work to return the individual with stroke to the workplace, allow the individual to participate in a beneficial pastime, and provide the person with skills to live independently in the community. The vocational counselor builds on the success of the individual in overcoming challenges and physical disability. Through the work of the counselor, self-esteem, self-pride, and a sense of accomplishment are rebuilt in the individual.

Box 21-13   Interventions to Prevent Aspiration

- Assess for gag reflex and swallowing ability.
- Have patient eat in upright position.
- Feed in small amounts.
- Avoid liquids or thicken liquids before feeding.
- Provide soft or pureed foods.
- Cut food into small pieces.
- Crush medications or obtain in liquid form.
- Have patient maintain upright position for 30 to 45 minutes after eating.
- Consider placement of feeding tube.

Think S for Success

Symptoms
- Manage poststroke health problems.

Sequelae
- Prevent disability, loss of function, and recurrence of stroke.
- Maintain skin integrity.
- Maintain joint mobility; prevent contractures and disuse syndrome.
- Observe for signs of lack of self-care and initiative due to depression.
- Observe for new onset of TIA/stroke.

Safety
- Teach patient and family importance of adhering to therapeutic regimen in medication, diet, and physical therapy.
- Monitor risk factors.
- Monitor for changes or difficulty in swallowing.
- Create and maintain a safe, clutter-free environment.

Support/Services
- Arrange for assistance with finances.
- Obtain devices and technology to assist in performance of activities of daily living.
- Prevent caregiver burden and burnout with community reintegration.
- Make appropriate referrals, including referral for counseling for depression.
- Assist patient and/or family in accessing resources such as nutritional services, Meals on Wheels, community-based support groups, adult day care and home care services, community-based rehabilitation services, and hospice care.
- Educate patient and family about resources such as the American Heart Association, American Stroke Association, and National Stroke Association.

Satisfaction
- Determine degree to which patient's disabilities interfere with important aspects of his or her life.
- Develop plan to assist patient and family in reaching and maintaining desired life quality.
- If applicable, help patient obtain vocational rehabilitation to allow independent living or retraining or assistive devices to reenter the workplace.

Family and Caregiver Issues and Concerns

Family members who are caregivers frequently become overwhelmed and stressed and are unable to recognize their situation. The nurse can provide supportive care for the caregiver by listening and helping the caregiver to express concerns, needs, and emotions. Using anticipatory guidance, the nurse can help the family recognize the point at which further assistance is needed.

End-of Life Issues

Up to 14% of stroke survivors experience a second stroke within the first year after stroke, and 47% of those who survive this second stroke die within the first year (AHA, 2001). Individuals surviving the first or second stroke may be critically ill with uncertain outcomes, and family members or significant others may have to make decisions about continuing treatment, placing the individual in an extended care facility, withdrawing life support, and so on, at a time when such decision making is difficult. It is helpful to discuss the advantages and disadvantages of all the options with the family and allow them time to reach a decision. (Advance directives are discussed in Chapter 27.) Encouraging family members to discuss end-of-life options in all cases, even those in which the outlook is good, helps prepare the family for future decisions. If the individual appears unlikely to survive beyond a 6-month period, hospice services should be explored.

TRAUMATIC BRAIN INJURY

A traumatic brain injury (TBI) is an insult to the brain that is not degenerative or congenital but is caused by an external physical force that may produce a diminished or altered state of consciousness and results in an impairment of cognitive abilities or physical functioning. It can also result in the disturbance of behavioral or emotional functioning (Brain Injury Association, 2002).

About 5.3 million Americans are currently living with disabilities resulting from TBI (National Centers for Injury Prevention and Control [NCIPC], 2001). One in four adults with TBI is unable to return to work 1 year after the injury (NCIPC, 2001).

Motor vehicle crashes are the leading cause of TBI and account for 50% of TBIs. Falls and violence (from firearms) account for the remaining 50%. The most frequent cause of TBI varies by age group. Among persons older than 65 years, falls are primary; motor vehicle crashes and transportation-related accidents predominate among persons aged 5 to 64 years (NCIPC, 2001). After the first brain injury, the risk for a second injury is three times higher; after a second injury, the risk for a third injury is eight times higher.

The costs associated with TBI in the United States are estimated to total $48.3 *billion* annually. Hospitalization accounts for $31.7 billion. Fatal brain injuries cost the nation $16.6 billion each year (NCIPC, 2001). Technologic

advances, aggressive treatment at the scene of an injury, specialized care units staffed by highly specialized health care personnel, aggressive surgical techniques, and fluid and pressure management along with the use of pharmacologic agents have significantly increased the number of survivors.

Pathophysiology

A variety of insults can injure the brain. The trauma can be blunt force in which the cranium remains intact or an open penetrating injury in which the dura is pierced or the brain contents are exposed to elements of the environment. The trauma is rated as mild, moderate, or severe. Three types of injury can result from the trauma, producing cumulative damage (McCance and Huether, 2002):

■ Primary injury: from the direct impact; causes neuronal and support cell damage; vascular permeability occurs.

■ Secondary injury: occurs due to cerebral edema, brain swelling, hemorrhage, infection, and intracranial pressure; this leads to tissue hypoxia from ischemia and increased cell permeability and cell death.

■ Tertiary injury: caused by apnea, hypotension, change in pulmonary resistance, and arrhythmias

Two broad categories of injury may occur—focal injury and diffuse axonal injury—and both may occur in the same traumatic event. A focal injury is a specific observable brain lesion such as a contusion or hematoma from a force-of-impact trauma or a penetrating trauma from compound fractures and missiles (knives, rocks, bullets). The damage remains localized to the impact area and may include swelling. It does not become a whole-brain injury. The classic double injury from acceleration-deceleration trauma is the "coup and contrecoup" brain injury in which there are strike and rebound focal points (Figure 21-3). This type of injury frequently leads to diffuse brain injury.

Penetrating injuries can result in more bleeding, infection, and entrance and exit wounds with a track wound in between that becomes ischemic and collapses.

Diffuse brain injury (diffuse axonal injury, or DAI) results from a shaking effect (e.g., from whiplash or rotational force, coup-contrecoup) that causes strains and distortions within the brain tissue. DAIs cause mild, moderate, or severe concussions. The force leads to shearing, tearing, and stretching of nerve fibers that damage the axons. Long axons from the frontal and temporal tracts are vulnerable to injury from motor vehicle crashes; such axonal injury contributes to significant cognitive and affective deficits after these traumas.

At the cellular level, injury causes the influx of calcium across plasma membranes; this damages intracellular cytoplasmic structures, interferes with production of adenosine triphosphate (ATP), and leads to the formation of lactic acid, which accelerates cell damage and death. Wide variations occur in release of the body's "fight or flight" hormones. This, coupled with fluctuations in the levels of neurochemi-

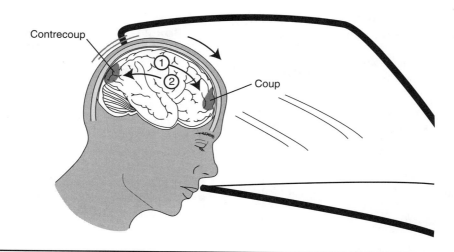

Figure 21-3 Coup and contrecoup brain injury. A double injury from acceleration-deceleration trauma in which there are strike (1) and rebound (2) focal points.

cals and neurotransmitters, has a significant effect on communication pathways in the brain and in behavior. The most notable hormones and transmitters involved are cortisol, norepinephrine, epinephrine, serotonin, dopamine, acetylcholine, and glutamate.

Clinical Manifestations

The clinical manifestations vary greatly depending on the extent of actual injury to the body and the head, concurrent medical conditions, age and hardiness of the individual, presence of behavioral or psychiatric problems prior to the injury, and expertise of those providing prehospital and in-hospital treatment.

In focal injury, level of consciousness, length of loss of consciousness, and reflex responses are indicators of injury and predictors of recovery. If contusions, hematoma, or local swelling expands, manifestations may include increasing headache, vomiting, seizures, hemiparesis-hemiplegia, confusion, and altered level of consciousness. Recovery may take hours to days, and some individuals may never regain functioning level of consciousness.

Similarly, in open penetrating wounds, the effects and sequelae depend on the location and extent of injury, depth of coma, length of unresponsiveness, and secondary injuries.

Individuals with diffuse brain injury experience disruptions in physical, cognitive, psychological, behavioral, and social processes. Sequelae include spastic paralysis, peripheral nerve injury, swallowing disorders, dysarthria, visual and hearing impairments, and taste and smell deficits. The cognitive impact manifests as disorientation and confusion, short attention span, memory deficits, learning difficulties, dysphasia, poor judgment, and perceptual deficits. Behavior changes include agitation, impulsiveness, flat affect, social withdrawal, and depression (McCance and Huether, 2002). The three levels of DAI are mild, moderate, and severe.

Moderate and severe DAI may be associated with long periods of coma, decorticate or decerebrate posturing, memory loss, emotional lability, and other cognitive deficits.

Decorticate posturing is a result of lesions of the corticospinal tracts. Decerebrate posturing occurs with lesions in the lower brain structures of the midbrain, pons, or diencephalon and has a poorer prognosis (Figure 21-4).

The most severe DAIs involve the neural connections between the cerebral hemispheres and between the diencephalon and the brainstem, and lead to autonomic dysfunction, respiratory compromise, and severe sensorimotor and cognitive deficits. The Glasgow Coma Scale, a neurophysiologic rating scale (lowest score 3, highest score 15), is used to rate basic reflex responses in an individual (Table 21-7). Scores of 13 to 15 indicate mild TBI; 9 to 12, moderate TBI; and 3 to 8, severe TBI.

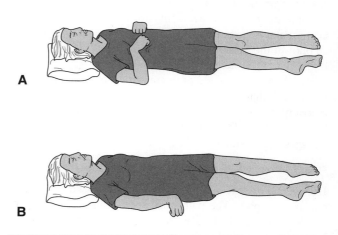

Figure 21-4 A, Decorticate posturing. **B,** Decerebrate posturing.

Table 21-7 Glasgow Coma Scale

Eye Opening

Spontaneous	4 points
To speech	3 points
To pain	2 points
None	1 point
Unable to assess: closed—dressing or swelling	

Verbal Response

Answers appropriately	5 points
Conversation is confused	4 points
Uses inappropriate words	3 points
Makes incomprehensible sound	2 points
No verbal response	1 point
Unable to assess: endotracheal or tracheal tube	

Motor Response

Obeys commands	6 points
Localizes pain	5 points
Withdraws to pain	4 points
Shows decorticate flexion	3 points
Shows decerebrate extension	2 points
Flaccid	1 point
Total score	_____

Box 21-14 Typical Characteristics of Individuals with Traumatic Brain Injury

BEHAVIORAL AND PSYCHOLOGICAL
- Apathy
- Lack of initiative
- Lack of social skills and/or interaction
- Depression
- Inability to concentrate
- Social withdrawal
- Lack of ability to enjoy pleasures
- Ineffectual communication: receptive or expressive
- Agitation and restlessness
- Aggression outburst
- Mood swings

COGNITIVE
- Deficits in attention and information processing
- Deficits in reasoning
- Difficulty in planning
- Deficits in writing and reading comprehension
- Difficulties in problem solving and decision making
- Inability to meet vocational needs
- Deficiencies in judgment
- Memory problems

Behavioral and Psychological Consequences

Motor and sensory deficits can affect any part of the body. Nevertheless, with time and technology, the individual can often compensate and function despite the deficits. It is the behavioral and psychological consequences of TBI that can be the most limiting and devastating (Bogner et al, 2001; Jean-Bay, 2000; Yasuda et al, 2001). Psychiatric problems such as depression may be present prior to the injury, as suggested by the fact that 66% of TBIs due to firearms injury were the result of a suicide attempt. Impulsivity may be a factor in motor vehicle accidents involving young adults and alcohol abuse, because 41% of TBI victims test positive for alcohol in the blood at the time of injury (Traumatic Brain Injury Model Systems, 2001).

The longer the period of unconsciousness, the greater the likelihood that behavior problems will be present after recovery from the wound. Cognitive changes also affect behavior. Box 21-14 lists typical behavioral and cognitive changes in individuals with TBI.

Pain

During and after rehabilitation the individual with TBI often experiences pain. The pain is persistent although it may be episodic and may be headache, neck and shoulder pain, lower back pain, or general diffuse pain. Any pain can interfere with the ability of the individual with TBI to implement the treatment plan, eat, sleep, or interact socially, and can alter other behaviors as well. The individual may not be able to express that pain exists, although change in the person's attention and behavior may signal its presence. The treatment currently recommended avoids reliance on pain medication and instead uses alternative, positive measures such as attention diversion by increasing physical and social activity, counseling for emotional distress and stress relief, biofeedback, and comfort measures such as ice or hot packs and massages.

Diagnosis

The report of the causative event and description and assessment of the injury provide significant information. Serial neuroimaging by CT and MRI is critical in determining points of primary injury and the development (and subsequent resolution) of secondary injury such as an increase in hematoma, development of edema, brain tissue shifts, and herniations from increased intracranial pressure. Additional diagnostic tools are cerebral angiography, EEG, and measurement of intracranial pressure.

Assessment

Assessment focuses on physical, cognitive, and psychological-behavioral status and the degree of social interaction. It may take weeks from the time of discharge from the acute care facility to a rehabilitation unit to determine the extent of recovery. Preinjury conditions such as age of the individual, presence of coexisting illness, tobacco or alcohol abuse, and presence of depression and psychiatric disorders influence the outcomes. These conditions must be assessed and managed as well. Various scales and indicators have been developed to aid in the prediction of functional outcomes (Box 21-15). No consensus exists regarding which is the best to use (Bogner et al, 2001; Yasuda, et al, 2001).

The Functional Independence Measure is the most widely accepted functional assessment tool in use in the rehabilitation community. Another instrument frequently used by the rehabilitation team, the Satisfaction with Life Scale, is designed to identify quality-of-life issues and concerns of the individual and caregivers. The Neurobehavioral Functioning Inventory is specifically designed to assess the neurobehavioral adaptation of the TBI survivor and family. The information that is learned through this instrument allows the health care team to devise—and revise—the treatment plan. The instrument is a 76-item self-report inventory divided into six subscales: depression, somatic complaints, memory and attention, communication, aggression, and motor problems (Jean-Bay, 2000; Kreutzer, Seel, and Marwitz, 1999).

Interdisciplinary Care

The interdisciplinary team that cares for the individual with TBI is large and includes the individual and his family and/or significant others. The team is composed of a primary health care provider, physician specialists such as a neurologist or neuropsychiatrist and physiatrist, nurse, pain management specialist, physical therapist, occupational therapist, speech therapist, behaviorist, and social worker. Good communication among the team members is essential.

Primary Provider (Physician/Nurse Practitioner)

When the individual makes the transition from the rehabilitation center to the home setting, the primary care provider takes responsibility for managing the day-to-day, month-to-month care of this individual. It is important that a strong relationship be developed between the provider and the individual. Through frequent interactions and wellness assessments, the individual with TBI and the provider can develop familiarity and trust, so that when an acute event arises, the provider, aware of the norms for the individual, can more readily focus on diagnosing the illness and prescribing a treatment.

Specialists

Neurologist

The neurologist participates primarily in the acute care and early rehabilitation settings for the individual recovering from TBI. As the individual's condition stabilizes, the neurologist has fewer and fewer interactions with the individual and family, until finally he or she performs only an annual examination and evaluation of the individual. The neurologist may be the specialist handling pain management or may refer the individual to a specialty clinic.

Neuropsychiatrist, Neuropsychologist, and Behaviorist

Because the behavior of the individual after TBI may be unpredictable and aggressive, a thorough evaluation is helpful to distinguish problems arising from neurologic factors from those arising from environmental factors. The general practice is to administer a series of tests to aid in identifying problems with functioning related to specific areas of the brain as well as strengths and weaknesses in mental performance. With this information, the practitioner can devise strategies that create consistency in the interactions of various people with the individual and address environmental issues, the individual's needs, the behavior, or the mental functional ability. Examples of strategies include controlling the environment, being honest and respectful at every interaction, and using praise, rewards, and positive approaches to encourage positive behavior and to create gentle deterrents in response to unacceptable behavior. The psychiatrist can prescribe medications to control behavior as part of the treatment plan (see Table 21-1). One member of this team may be a behaviorist who is at the rehabilitation center (or the day care center) and who interacts daily with the staff and the individual one on one.

Physiatrist

The physiatrist in the rehabilitation setting has much the same responsibilities as outlined in the section on stroke. The physiatrist collaborates with the therapists to determine the functional abilities of the individual and then devises a plan of treatment to achieve the optimal outcome.

Drug Therapy

After hospitalization, there are only a few specific medications that may be prescribed. The drug therapy is for treatment of

---

Box 21-15 Assessment Scales Used in Traumatic Brain Injury

- Glasgow Coma Scale (GCS)
- Glasgow Outcome Scale (GOS)
- Extended Glasgow Outcome Scale (GOSE): provides a measure of overall functional outcome but does not address the specifics of functional limitations
- Functional Independence Measure (FIM)
- Functional Assessment Measure (FAM): used in conjunction with FIM
- Functional Status Examination (FSE): in addition to identifying functional limitations, provides insight into factors contributing to them
- Beck's Depression Inventory (BDI)
- Satisfaction with Life Scale (SWLS)
- Neurobehavioral Functioning Inventory (NFI)

symptoms (Glenn, 2002; O'Shanick, 2001) (see Table 21-1). The medication categories and their indications for use in TBI are listed in Table 21-8.

Dietitian

The diet that is prescribed addresses any coexisting conditions and attempts to achieve proper body mass while conforming to the individual's cultural preferences. If the individual is unable to swallow easily and a risk for aspiration exists, food consistency must be adjusted. If more severe problems exist, the individual may have a percutaneous endogastric (PEG) tube for direct instillation of food, formula, fluids, and medications into the stomach. If a PEG tube is required, the dietitian selects the type of feeding that is most consistent with nutritional goals.

Nurse

The primary role of the nurse is that of care coordinator in the rehabilitation center and community or home setting. The amount of time required and level of professional care needed depends on the individual's level of functioning. Individuals with mild or moderate TBI may need bimonthly or monthly visits. Those with severe TBI or low-level brain function (Hauber and Testani-Dufour, 2000) may require weekly assessments and supervision; these individuals may be in a minimally conscious state or a persistent vegetative state (PVS). The individual in a minimally conscious state

Table 21-8 Medications Used to Treat Individuals with Traumatic Brain Injury

Drug Category	Indications/Comments
Anticonvulsants	For seizure control
Antidepressants, including SSRIs	SSRIs do not affect seizure threshold
Antianxiety agents	For short-term use
Neuroleptics	Should rarely be used with agitation and aggressive behavior because these agents lower seizure threshold, decrease memory, and cause dystonias and tardive dyskinesia
Anti-Parkinson agents	To increase dopamine activity; improve deficits in motivation and initiative
Psychostimulants	To decrease drowsiness, increase attention and concentration; for short-term use
Anticholinergics meclizine (Antivert)	To treat dizziness and insomnia; can lower seizure threshold and cause dry mouth, confusion
Antihypertensives	β-Blockers: to treat headaches and aggressiveness and impulsivity; α-blockers (clonidine [Catapres]): to decrease impulsivity and reduce blood pressure

SSRIs, Selective serotonin reuptake inhibitors.

or PVS requires an intense level of nursing care, initially by a licensed professional and later by family members as they begin to assume more of the care. While the nurse is in the setting, the nurse uses his or her skills to assess the physical and emotional environments of the individual and the family and the interaction and interpersonal environment in the living space.

The nurse can provide direct care as well as coach the individual and family as they learn skills and problem-solving approaches to meet new challenges. The nurse observes and assesses for any change in the individual's condition. Such changes could be indicators of skin pressure areas; changes in the skin integrity of wounds (e.g., PEG tube site); changes in weight, nutrition, or hydration status; changes in communication patterns; or changes in bowel and bladder habits that indicate infection or constipation. The nurse teaches and reinforces positive behaviors and adherence to the treatment plan.

The nurse assesses the individual's and caregiver's burden, resilience, and ability to continue to care for the individual. The individual with TBI may become frustrated at his or her own limitations and develop destructive responses such as depression, emotional outbursts, impulsivity, and harmful actions toward himself or herself and others. Early awareness of changes and prompt intervention can prevent a situation from spiraling out of control.

Physical and Occupational Therapists

See Interdisciplinary Care in the section on stroke.

Speech Therapist

See Interdisciplinary Care in the section on stroke. Most individuals with TBI regain the ability to produce speech and sound. A speech therapist is needed when motor problems are present, as evidenced by the following (Blosser and DePompei, 2001):

■ Slurred production of words
■ Drooling
■ Difficulty swallowing
■ Hoarse or nasal voice quality
■ Slowed rate of speech
■ Absence of verbal speech due to paralysis of the vocal mechanisms

Rehabilitation

The interdisciplinary team supports the individual with TBI and his or her family and/or significant others during rehabilitation and lifestyle adjustment. In the United States, tremendous gains have been realized in the survival rate of individuals with TBI, and successes have been achieved by individuals in overcoming disabilities. Among the behaviors that interfere with the learning of new skills and maintenance of independence are restlessness and posttraumatic agitation (Bogner et al, 2001). It is critical that the interdisciplinary team address these issues and be aware of underlying problems. A goal of the team is to engage the individual in meaningful work. Employment opportunities for the individual with TBI may be found in a sheltered situation, specialty workshop, or in independent employment.

Family and Caregiver Issues and Concerns

The success of the individual with TBI in achieving recovery goals is tied to the support of the family. The strength of the preinjury home environment is a strong predictor of the long-term outcomes in recovery (Hauber and Testani-Dufour, 2000). Each member of the family is distressed, and each member must have an opportunity to verbalize feelings and emotions during the stressful acute care period as well as in the long term. Family issues include the following:

- Commitment of time
- Reversal of roles in dependence and independence
- Restructuring of the lifestyle to accommodate the individual with TBI
- Long-term financial commitment
- Emotional strain: guilt, anger, horror, sadness, depression, anxiety, stress, uncertainty, sorrow
- Stress of caring for an individual who may not recognize them or who is apathetic and unemotional or ungrateful for their efforts
- Need to perform care regarding functions they find embarrassing or are uncomfortable with: toileting, cleansing, bathing, and clothing the family member
- Decisions about life support

PERSISTENT VEGETATIVE STATE

The vegetative state is a clinical condition of complete unawareness of the self and the environment, accompanied by sleep-wake cycles with either complete or partial preservation of hypothalamic and brainstem autonomic functions. The condition may be transient, marking a stage in the recovery from severe acute or chronic brain damage, or permanent, as a consequence of the failure to recover from such injuries. PVS cannot be declared until there has been no recovery or activity for 1 year (Adams, Graham, and Jennett, 2000). Box 21-16 lists the criteria that must be met for the determination of a vegetative state.

PVS is a state of total dependency of one human being on another or on a system of network support. All functions of the body and the environment in which the individual exists must be monitored and controlled to ensure safety (Multi-Society Task Force on PVS, 1994a, 1994b) (Box 21-17).

Family and Caregiver Issues and Concerns

According to the findings of the Multi-Society Task Force for PVS (1994b), the mean survival time of an adult in PVS is 3 to 5 years, although cases of long-term survival

---

Think S for Success

Symptoms
- Maximize physical abilities to ensure continued competence.
- Manage persistent pain: headache, muscle spasms.
- Manage behavioral and psychological factors.

Sequelae
- Prevent disability by monitoring for immobility, impaired body awareness, or impaired deficit awareness.
- Address behavioral and psychological problems to prevent destructive actions.

Safety
- Teach individual and family the importance of the following:
  Adherence to treatment plan and therapeutic regimen
  Periodic examinations and diagnostic tests to monitor therapy and progress
  Understanding of eating patterns and positioning to prevent aspiration
  If patient is taking medications, adverse effects and restrictions while on medications
  Understanding and avoidance of triggers that lead to stress, upset, and mood swings

Support/Services
- Provide continual contact with social worker if necessary to obtain financial assistance.
- Make appropriate referrals within the community.

Satisfaction
- Determine factors that interfere with patient's quality of life and focus on eliminating or minimizing these factors.
- Help patient to engage in meaningful employment.
- Assist patient in arranging the least restrictive living environment possible given patient's capabilities.

Box 21-16   Criteria for Vegetative State

1. No evidence of awareness of self or environment and an inability to interact with others
2. No evidence of sustained, reproducible, purposeful, or voluntary behavioral responses to visual, auditory, tactile, or noxious stimuli
3. No evidence of language comprehension or expression
4. Intermittent wakefulness manifested by the presence of sleep-wake cycles
5. Sufficiently preserved hypothalamic and brainstem autonomic functions to permit survival with medical and nursing care
6. Bowel and bladder incontinence
7. Variably preserved cranial nerve reflexes (pupillary, oculo-cephalic, corneal, vestibulo-ocular, and gag) and spinal reflexes

Adapted from Multi-Society Task Force on PVS: Medical aspects of persistent vegetative state (part 1), *N Engl J Med* 330(21):1499-1507, 1994.

Box 21-17   Systems to Be Monitored in Individuals in a Persistent Vegetative State

RESPIRATORY
- Ineffective airway clearance
- Aspiration of saliva or gastric tube feedings from lack of protective mechanisms
- Ineffective breathing pattern

CARDIAC
- Hypovolemia from dehydration
- Nutritional anemia, which decreases hemoglobin level and hematocrit
- Cardiac pump depression

GASTROINTESTINAL/NUTRITIONAL
- Inadequate oral hygiene, which may lead to the following:
  Dental caries
  Sialolithiasis
  Gingival disease and hyperplasia from antiepileptic drugs
  Periodontal disease
  Possible tooth damage from gritting and grinding of teeth during facial muscle spasms
- Malnutrition caused by inadequate nutrient intake in enteral formula or effects of the gastric feeding
- Bowel incontinence due to neuromuscular impairment

MUSCULOSKELETAL (DISUSE SYNDROME)
- Loss of muscle mass and strength secondary to passive condition

- Constipation from lax pelvic muscles and inability to evacuate bowel
- Possible contractures, immobilized joints
- Osteoporosis from lack of weight bearing

INTEGUMENTARY (TISSUE INTEGRITY)
- Possible development of decubitus (pressure) ulcers
- Macerations and infection caused by moisture on skin

GENITOURINARY
- Urinary incontinence
- Possible decubitus ulcers caused by skin moisture from incontinence
- Urinary retention
- Possible renal stones
- Males: improper scrotal positioning, which can lead to edema or torque
- Females: irregularities, hormonal fluctuations, and menses

IMMUNE
- Possible infection

HOMEOSTATIC
- Impaired thermal regulation
- Impaired fluid and electrolyte balance

---

beyond 10 years have been recorded. Long-term planning and home assessment are vital parts of the preparation to send home the individual in PVS (Hauber and Testani-Dufour, 2000). The caregiver must have hardiness, compassion, and understanding to care tenderly for the individual who requires total care. The compassionate attitude of the caregiver provides an environment of comfort, nurturing, and acceptance.

The interdisciplinary team must provide many opportunities for the family to learn the skills and techniques needed to care for the individual. The nurse is generally responsible for coordinating the long-term care of the individual with PVS and ensuring that the appropriate disciplines are involved in managing and monitoring the patient's progress and the family's ability to continue in the caregiving role. Areas included in the ongoing assessment are listed in Box 21-18.

Box 21-18   Areas of Ongoing Assessment for the Individual in a Persistent Vegetative State

FAMILY CAREGIVERS
- Family commitment and understanding of responsibilities
- Family hardiness, including physical health and stamina of family members, strength and spiritual resolve, stress management, role strain, caregiver fatigue, and coping abilities and techniques
- Family constellation and support network for the family members themselves as well as for the individual in a persistent vegetative state (PVS); includes an understanding of the dynamics of family process alteration
- Development of a routine and schedule of care management to assure care throughout the 24-hour day over the period of time the individual is at home

RESOURCES AND FINANCES
- Family member(s) responsible for resources management
- Ability of the family to manage the day-to-day living expenses of the household
- Planning for unexpected and emergency expenses
- Need for assistance in managing the family debt and resources: eligibility for assistance programs, medical debt from hospitalizations, ability to meet current and ongoing medical and supply expenses

Box 21-18 Areas of Ongoing Assessment for the Individual in a Persistent Vegetative State—cont'd

HOUSING SITUATION

■ Availability of adequate and acceptable space to provide care to the individual in PVS (access to water, storage for supplies, and facilities for cleaning soiled linens; adequate ventilation, heating and cooling, lighting)

■ Ability to get the individual in and out of the house easily

■ Availability of adequate and acceptable space for family life so that the family can have comfortable routines

INDIVIDUAL'S PERSONAL HYGIENE AND HEALTH CARE

■ Family members' levels of abilities and skills as caregivers (teaching should be continued as learning opportunities occur)

■ Teaching and support for family management of therapeutic regime

■ Education of family members to discriminate changes in the condition of the individual

■ Monitoring by health care professional(s) regarding care and their astuteness in assessing changes in condition

---

CASE STUDY

Patient Data

Mrs. M. is a 78-year-old African American who is a central person in her community. She is widowed. Mrs. M. is known for her great spirituality, her warmth and generosity, her pleasant manner, and her laughter. She is also known for her talents in the kitchen and seems to cook nonstop for her family, extended family, neighbors, and many community fund-raising activities. She has three adult daughters and two adult sons; each of them has several children. Most folks are amazed that she never seems to age and she never rests; she prides herself on her stamina.

Recently, at times, her right hand and arm feel tingly and numb for a few minutes and she loses her train of thought at the same time. She has avoided seeing her physician for over a year since he told her to lose some weight (she currently weighs about 280 lb) and to watch her blood pressure and blood glucose level, both of which were elevated at her last two visits. Mrs. M.'s head throbs at times and her vision blurs, but she tells herself these symptoms are part of aging. More family is coming to visit and she scurries about the kitchen carrying heavy pots back and forth to get her cooking finished as she mentally goes through the list of what must be done.

Mrs. M.'s next memory is of sounds and voices she does not recognize and she is in bed—but it is not as comfortable as her bed at home. Someone is asking her to lift her arm, squeeze her hand, push her foot against the footboard, answer a question—she opens her eyes and mouth but she speaks only garbled words. Mrs. M. has suffered a CVA (stroke) involving the left middle cerebral artery; it was a thrombotic-ischemic event. She was found moments after she collapsed to the floor and was rushed to a regional medical center. For an hour after arriving at the hospital, she remained unresponsive and she received a protocol stroke treatment of thrombolytics. She now finds herself in the intensive care unit for recovery. Her family and community of faith have been supportive and unwavering in their prayers and in providing for each other in her absence.

Diagnostic Findings

Blood pressure: 178/90 mm Hg at admission; 138/74 mm Hg now

Plasma glucose level: 310 mg/dl at admission; 150 mg/dl fasting now

Cholesterol level: 286 mg/dl (low level of high-density lipoproteins and high level of low-density lipoproteins)

Triglyceride level: 500 mg/dl

Glasgow Coma Scale score: 9

MRI scan: left middle cerebral artery involvement

Weight: 285 lb

Height: 62 inches

Mrs. M.'s medical condition steadily improves, and therapies for neuroprotection and for management of her plasma glucose level, cholesterol level, and weight are initiated. She is moved to a rehabilitation center where her functional abilities are evaluated and a treatment plan is devised. She has worked very hard to accomplish the goals she set for herself and now wants to go home. Mrs. M. requests that the team convene a care conference to discuss her progress and the possibility of her going home.

Thinking It Through

■ What nursing diagnoses pertain to Mrs. M?

■ What risk factors did she have that may have contributed to the stroke?

■ What types of deficits are typical of individuals with left middle cerebral artery CVAs?

■ If Mrs. M. seeks discharge from the rehabilitation facility, what questions and concerns will the team members have?

■ What challenges does Mrs. M. face?

■ What types of accommodations will have to be made at home for her?

■ What challenges do her family and caregivers face?

■ What are the nurse's concerns in her transition to home?

Case Conference

The team conference includes Mrs. M.; two adult daughters, Suzan and Jackie; and the physiatrist, nurse, speech therapist, physical therapist, registered dietitian, and medical social worker. Each team member reports on Mrs. M.'s progress and current functional abilities.

The physiatrist reviews the circumstances leading to Mrs. M.'s stroke, notes her risk factors, and summarizes her course of hospitalization. Mrs. M. has a visual deficit that affects her right field of vision. She is alert and appears to comprehend and engage in the activities around her. Her current therapeutic regime includes ticlopidine (Ticlid) 250 mg BID; glipizide (Glucotrol) 5 mg daily; lisinopril (Prinivil) 10 mg daily; gemfibrozil (Lopid) 600 mg BID; and propoxyphene (Darvon) 65 mg for occasional moderate pain; and a healthy diet for weight control. Overall, the physiatrist is pleased with Mrs. M.'s determination, attitude, and progress.

The nurse reports that Mrs. M. has established a daily routine and strives for self-management in personal hygiene; she showers seated on a shower stool and requires help in bathing her left side and perineal area. She uses the self-medication packets provided by the pharmacy and thus far each day since her arrival has

Continued

appropriately administered her own medication. She requires assistance in performing the finger stick for self-monitoring of plasma glucose level morning and evening. Her glucose levels are in the 130s in the morning and 150s in the evening. Her vital signs are normal with blood pressure generally in the 130s/70s. Mrs. M. has skin care difficulties in the perineal and rectal areas as well as in deep folds of the skin. Although she appears to be continent, there is constant perianal moisture and some stress incontinence may be present. The nurse is concerned that the area will become macerated and a yeast infection will begin. Thus far, Mrs. M. has not been constipated but has a diminished sense of rectal fullness. The nurse also reports that Mrs. M. has been very emotional and tearful at times; she allows Mrs. M. to cry and stays with her and accepts the emotions even when the words are not clear.

The speech therapist reports that there is some improvement in Mrs. M.'s expressive aphasia. She has progressed from guttural sounds to slow enunciation of single and two-word phrases to communicate. Mrs. M. becomes frustrated when she is unable to make herself understood and has cried at times. The therapist has created a word board for Mrs. M. to point to when she wants to communicate faster than she is able to speak. She has difficulty chewing food and swallowing completely. Food has a tendency to become pocketed in the right cheek, and Mrs. M. does not completely chew the food on the right side.

The physical therapist reports continued work to strengthen muscles in Mrs. M.'s arms and legs. There is significant right-sided weakness (hemiparesis) and right-side neglect. The therapist is adapting a walker for Mrs. M. so that she can use her strong left hand and employ a cradle and handle for her right arm to move the walker forward. The therapist is concerned that, if Mrs. M. is not watching her right arm, it will dangle at her side and the weight of it will cause shoulder joint problems. Mrs. M. is adapting to her right leg brace, which aids in stability and support of the leg. Her skin is moist, and the therapist is concerned that maceration may develop due to the brace straps. Mrs. M.'s weight is a hindrance to progress in walking and stairstep maneuvers. Mrs. M. has not learned to transfer independently and becomes confused as to whether she should pivot to the right or left as she transfers. She is not stable in transferring to the wheelchair. Because of her weight, the therapist is concerned that the attendant or caregiver could suffer injury in an attempt to assist or support Mrs. M.

The registered dietitian reports that Mrs. M.'s current weight is 265 lb and that her fasting plasma glucose level is 135 mg/dl; there has been a slight lowering of the cholesterol level. The dietitian has developed a meal plan for Mrs. M. that is based on many of the foods consumed in her culture; however, preparation of these foods will have to change to reduce salt, lower reliance on animal fats, and reduce concentrated carbohydrates, and greater emphasis must be given to fresh soft vegetables and fruits. The dietitian reports that she met with Mrs. M.'s daughter Suzan, who will be the primary caregiver providing food for Mrs. M. Suzan also wants to benefit from a healthier diet and agrees to adhere to the new plan and recipes. The dietitian has been with Mrs. M. at meals and concurs with other team members that Mrs. M. neglects the right side, not chewing fully, not swallowing fully, and not eating foods from the right side of the plate. There is also some drooling out of the right edge of the mouth.

The social worker gives high praise to Mrs. M. and to her daughters and family for the emotional and physical support they have provided. The family members are eager to learn to care for Mrs. M. and have begun searching for support groups in their community. Mrs. M. is eligible for Medicare and will receive her medications through a medication grant program; she is eligible to receive medical equipment such as a hospital bed and wheelchair and glucose testing machine. On Mrs. M.'s return

home she is eligible for home health care and teaching by registered nurses and for weekly visits by a home health aide.

The sons have revamped the entrance of Mrs. M.'s house to accommodate a walker or wheelchair and have provided a long, shallow-sloped ramp. There is a fully equipped bathroom on the first floor. The sons are renovating it by removing the bathtub and installing an open shower with grab bars; the toilet will have a raised seat and will also have grab bars. The dining room is being screened off to become Mrs. M.'s bedroom. The family decided not to renovate the kitchen to accommodate Mrs. M. It was felt that Suzan would be the cook and it should not be made too easy for Mrs. M. to feel that she could become involved at the level she was before her stroke. The sons are also renovating Suzan's home, changing the entrance and the downstairs bathroom to accommodate Mrs. M. if she visits or needs to stay at Suzan's house. Church and community members are reviewing issues of access to community buildings to ensure ease of access by Mrs. M. as well as all community members.

Suzan and Jackie report that they are committed to caring for their mother. The three daughters and two sons all live within 15 miles of Mrs. M. Suzan lives 50 feet from her house. Suzan's children are grown and gone, and she feels that she can manage two households. There will always be a responsible person with Mrs. M. at night; during the day, as she continues to improve, she may be left alone for short periods of time. Jackie is an elementary school teacher and lives close by. She is not able to be there daily but can visit frequently to relieve Suzan. She can do the household shopping and would like the challenge of coaching her mother to improve her communication skills. Both daughters have assisted the nurse in daily hygiene for Mrs. M. and have been able to demonstrate the required techniques. Both feel comfortable in giving personal care, can perform the finger stick to obtain a blood sample and operate the glucose monitoring machine, and have learned the exercises that Mrs. M. must perform daily to maintain her strength. Both are learning the mobility and transfer techniques needed to help Mrs. M.

Mrs. M. indicates that she is no longer self-sufficient but is determined to go home and find her optimal level of functioning there and enjoy her community and family.

The team members discuss the newly shared information and decide when Mrs. M. can make the transition to home. There is some discussion about whether she should first go to a skilled care unit in a long-term care setting. The physical therapist recommends that Mrs. M. remain for another week at the rehabilitation center and that a physical therapist from a home health care agency evaluate Mrs. M. at home and continue supervised therapy for another 2 weeks. The speech therapist agrees and feels that this would allow time for Jackie to participate in several coaching sessions to learn the goals and techniques of therapy. The social worker agrees to the time period because this provides the time to order and install the necessary home medical equipment and visit the home for an assessment. The nurse also agrees to the time frame; it allows her to provide several more teaching sessions to Suzan, and she can meet with the home health nurse. In addition, the nurse wants to focus on Mrs. M.'s skin care and determine the source of the perineal moisture and address it.

Once the team meeting is over, the nurse returns to her office and thinks about the meeting as she develops a plan of care for Mrs. M.

■ What new information was gathered that can assist the nurse in developing the plan of care?
■ What strengths do Mrs. M.'s daughters and family bring to the team?
■ What barriers to therapy must be overcome?
■ Identify two collaborative problems that the plan of care should address.

Internet and Other Resources

General

Centers for Disease Control and Prevention: *http://www.cdc. gov;* telephone 800-311-3435

Family Caregiver Alliance: *http://www.caregiver.org;* E-mail *info@caregiver.org;* telephone 415-434-3388, 800-445-8106; fax 415-434-3508; 690 Market Street, Suite 600, San Francisco, CA 94104

National Center for Injury Prevention and Control: *http://www. cdc.gov/ncipc/default.htm;* telephone 770-488-1506; Mail stop K65, 4770 Buford Highway NE, Atlanta, GA 30341-3724

National Council on Patient Information and Education: *http://www.talkaboutrx.org;* E-mail *ncpie@ncpie.info;* telephone 301-656-8565; fax 301-656-4464; 4915 St. Elmo Avenue, Suite 505, Bethesda, MD 20814-6053

National Family Caregivers Association: *http://www.nfcacares. org;* E-mail *info@nfcacares.org;* telephone 301-942-6430, 800-896-3650; fax 301-942-2302; 10400 Connecticut Avenue, Suite 500, Kensington, MD 20895-3944

National Institute of Neurological Disorders and Stroke (NINDS): *http://www.ninds.nih.gov/;* telephone 800-352-9424; National Institutes of Health, Neurological Institute, PO Box 5801, Bethesda, MD 20894

National Organization for Rare Disorders (NORD): *http:// www.rarediseases.org;* E-mail *orphan@rarediseases.org;* telephone 203-744-0100; voice mail 800-999-NORD (800-999-6673); fax 203-798-2291; PO Box 1968, 55 Kenosia Avenue, Danbury, CT 06813-1968

National Rehabilitation Information Center (NARIC): *http:// www.naric.com;* E-mail *naricinfo@heitechservices.com;* telephone 301-459-5900; 4200 Forbes Boulevard, Suite 202, Lanham, MD 20706

Uniform Data System for Medical Rehabilitation: *http://www. udsmr.org;* E-mail *info@udsmr.org;* telephone 716-817-7800; fax 716-568-0037; 270 Northpointe Parkway, Suite 300, Amherst, NJ 14228

United States Department of Education, National Institute on Disability and Rehabilitation Research (NIDRR): *http:// www.ed.gov/about/offices/list/osers/nidrr/index.html;* telephone 202-205-8134; 400 Maryland Avenue SW, Washington, DC 20202-2572

Epilepsy

American Epilepsy Society: *http://www.aesnet.org/;* E-mail *Info@aesnet.org;* telephone 860-586-7505; fax 860-586-7550; 342 North Main Street, West Hartford, CT 06117-2507

Citizens United for Research in Epilepsy (CURE): *http://www. CUREepilepsy.org;* E-mail *CUREepi@aol.com;* telephone 312-923-9117; fax 312-923-9118; 505 North Lake Shore Drive, #4605, Chicago, IL 60611

Epilepsy Foundation: *http://www.efa.org;* E-mail *postmaster@ efa.org;* telephone 800-332-1000; 4351 Garden City Drive, Landover, MD 20785-7223

Epilepsy Institute: *http://www.epilepsyinstitute.org;* E-mail *website@epilepsyinstitute.org;* telephone 212-677-8550; fax 212-677-5825; 257 Park Avenue South, Suite 302, New York, NY 10010

International League Against Epilepsy: *http://www.ilae epilepsy.org/;* telephone 011-32-(0)-2-774-9547; fax 011-32-(0)-2-774-9690; Avenue Marcel Thiry 204, B-1200 Brussels, Belgium

National Institute of Neurological Disorders and Stroke (NINDS): *http://www.ninds.nih.gov/health_and_medical/ disorders/epilepsy.htm;* National Institutes of Health, Neurological Institute, PO Box 5801, Bethesda, MD 20894; helpful publications include Seizures and Epilepsy: Hope Through Research; information booklet on seizures, seizure disorders, and epilepsy; Headache and Migraine

National Society for Epilepsy: *http://www.epilepsynse.org.uk;* telephone 01494-601300; fax 01494-871927; Chesham Lane, Chalfont St. Peter, Bucks SL9 0RJ United Kingdom

Headache

American Headache Society: *http://www.ahsnet.org;* telephone 856-423-0043; fax 856-423-0082; 19 Mantua Road, Mount Royal, NJ 08061

International Headache Society: *http://www.i-h-s.org*

National Institute of Neurological Disorders and Stroke (NINDS): *http://www.ninds.nih.gov/;* National Institutes of Health, Neurological Institute, PO Box 5801, Bethesda, MD 20894; helpful publication is Headache and Migraine

Stroke

American Stroke Association (division of American Heart Association): *http:// www.americanheart.org;* telephone 888-4-STROKE (478-7653); 7272 Greenville Avenue, Dallas, TX 75231-4596

National Stroke Association: *http://www.stroke.org;* E-mail *info@stroke.org;* telephone 303-649-9299, 800-STROKES (800-787-6537); fax 303-649-1328; 9707 East Easter Lane, Englewood, CO 80112-3747

Traumatic Brain Injury

Brain Injury Association: *http://www.biausa.org;* E-mail *public relations@biausa.org;* telephone 703-761-0750, helpline 800-444-6443; 8201 Greensboro Drive, Suite 611, McLean, VA 22102

Brain Trauma Foundation: *http://www.braintrauma.org;* E-mail *info@braintrauma.org;* telephone 212-772-0608; fax 212-772-0357; 523 East 72nd Street, 8th Floor, New York, NY 10021

Traumatic Brain Injury Model Systems (TBIMS) National Database (funded by National Institute on Disability and Rehabilitation Research): *http://www.tbindc.org;* Traumatic Brain Injury National Data Center, c/o Kessler Medical Rehabilitation Research and Education Corporation, 1199 Pleasant Valley Way, West Orange, NJ 07052

Traumatic Brain Injury National Data Center (TBINDC) (funded by National Institute on Disability and Rehabilitation Research): *http://www.tbindc.org/registry/about_registry.php/;* E-mail *tbindc@kmrrec.org;* Traumatic Brain Injury National Data Center, c/o Kessler Medical Rehabilitation Research and Education Corporation, 1199 Pleasant Valley Way, West Orange, NJ 07052

Assessment Tools

FIM (Functional Independence Measures) System: trademark of the Uniform Data System for Medical Rehabilitation, a division of UB Foundation Activities, Inc., *http://www.udsmr.org;* E-mail *info@udsmr.org;* telephone 716-817-7800; fax 716-568-0037; 270 Northpointe Parkway, Suite 300, Amherst, NY 14228

Neurobehavioral Functioning Inventory (NFI): proprietary, copyright owned by Psychological Corporation, *http://www. psychcorp.com;* E-mail *HBINTL@HARCOURTBRACE.COM;* telephone 800-211-8378; fax 800-232-1223; TDD 800-723-1318; Psychological Corporation, Order Service Center, PO Box 839954, San Antonio, TX 78283-3954

REFERENCES

Adams JH, Graham DI, Jennett B: The neuropathology of the vegetative state after acute brain injury, *Brain* 123:1327-38, 2000.

Agency for Health Care Policy and Research: Diagnosis and treatment of swallowing disorders (dysphagia) in acute-care stroke patients, Evidence Report/Technology Assessment No. 8, March 1999, Rockville, Md, Agency for Health Care Policy and Research, retrieved from *http://www.ahrq.gov/clinic/epcsums/dysphsum.htm* on Jan 19, 2004.

American Diabetes Association: ADA clinical practice recommendations, *Diabetes Care* 25:S1-S2, 2002.

American Heart Association: *2002 Heart and stroke statistical update*, Dallas, 2001, American Heart Association.

American Heart Association: AHA guidelines for primary prevention of cardiovascular disease and stroke: 2002 update: consensus panel guide to comprehensive risk reduction for adult patients without coronary or other atherosclerotic vascular diseases, *Circulation* 106(3):388-91, 2002.

Berg AT, Engel J: Restricted driving for people with epilepsy, *Neurology* 52(7):1306-7, 1999.

Blosser JL, DePompei R: Crossing the communication bridge—speech, language, and brain injury, The Road to Rehabilitation Series, Alexandria, Va, 2001, Brain Injury Association.

Bogner JA et al: Role of agitation in prediction of outcomes in traumatic brain injury, *Am J Phys Med Rehabil* 80:636-44, 2001.

Brain Injury Association: The costs and causes of traumatic brain injury [BIA Information and Support web page], 2002, retrieved from *http://www.biausa.org* on accessed July, 2002.

Brodie MJ, Kwan P: Staged approach to epilepsy management, *Neurology* 58(suppl 5):S2-S8, 2002.

Browne TR, Holmes GL: Epilepsy: primary care, *N Engl J Med* 344(15):1145-51, 2001.

Buelow JM: Epilepsy management issues and techniques, *J Neurosci Nurs* 33(5):260-6, 2001.

Campbell JK, Penzien DB, Wall EM: Evidence-based guidelines for migraine headaches: behavioral and physical treatments, St Paul, April 2000, US Headache Consortium and American Academy of Neurology.

Cavanaugh SJ et al: Stroke-specific FIM models in an urban population, *J Neurosci Nurs* 32(1):17, 2000.

Centers for Disease Control and Prevention: Decline in deaths from heart disease and stroke—U.S. 1900-1999, *MMWR Morb Mortal Wkly Rep* 48(30):649-56, Aug 6, 1999.

Centers for Disease Control and Prevention: State-specific mortality from stroke and distribution of place of death—United States, 1999, *MMWR Morb Mortal Wkly Rep* 51(20):429-33, May 24, 2002.

Cutrer FM: Antiepileptic drugs: how they work in headache, *Headache J Head Face Pain* 41(s1):3-11, 2001

Devinsky O: Patients with refractory seizures, *N Engl J Med* 340(20):1565-70, 1999.

Dudek FE: Zinc and epilepsy, *Epilepsy Curr* 1(2):66-70, 2001.

Eaves YD: "What happened to me": rural African American elders' experiences of stroke, *J Neurosci Nurs* 32(1):37, 2000.

Engel J: Finally, a randomized, controlled trial of surgery for epilepsy: an editorial, *N Engl J Med* 345(5):365-6, 2001.

Engel J et al: Practice parameter: temporal lobe and local neocortical resections for epilepsy: a report of the Quality Standards Subcommittee of the American Academy of Neurology, *Neurology* 60(3):538-47, 2003.

Eslinger PJ, Parkinson K, Shamay SG: Empathy and social-emotional factors in recovery from stroke, *Neurology* 15(1):91-7, 2002.

Fisher RS, Handforth A: Reassessment: vagus nerve stimulation for epilepsy: a report of the Therapeutics and Technology Assessment Subcommittee for the American Academy of Neurology, *Neurology* 53:666-9, 1999.

Glenn MB: A differential diagnostic approach to the pharmacological treatment of cognitive, behavioral, and affective disorders after traumatic brain injury, *J Head Trauma Rehabil* 17(4):273-83, 2002.

Goadsby PJ, Lipton RB, Ferrari MD: Migraine—current understanding and treatment, *N Engl J Med* 346(4):257-70., 2002.

Habel M: Brain attack: raising awareness about the leading cause of adult disability, *NurseWeek* May 12, 2001.

Hauber RP, Testani-Dufour L, Coleman K: Living in limbo: the low-level brain injured patient and the patient's family, *J Neurosci Nurs* 32(1):22-6, 2000.

Hickenbottom SL et al: A national study of the quantity and cost of informal caregiving for the elderly with stroke, *Neurology* 58:1754-9, 2002.

International Headache Society: The international classification of headache disorders, ed 2, *Cephalgia* 24(suppl 1), 2004.

Jean-Bay E: The biobehavioral correlates of post-traumatic brain injury depression, *J Neurosci Nurs* 32(3):169-76, 2000.

Kanner AM, Balabanov A: Depression and epilepsy: how closely related are they? *Neurology* 58(suppl 5):S27-S39, 2002.

Kreutzer JS, Seel RT, Marwitz JH: Neurobehavioral functioning inventory, Resources for occupational therapists and physiotherapists, 1999, retrieved from *http://www.tpc-international.com/resources/title.cfm?ID=95* in July 2002.

Leppik IE: Treatment of epilepsy in the elderly, *Epilepsy Curr* 1(2):46-7, 2001.

Lipton RB et al: Migraine diagnosis and treatment: results from the American migraine study II, *Headache* 41(7):638-45, 2001.

Lipton RB et al: Migraine in the United States: epidemiology and patterns of health care use, *Neurology* 58(6):885-94, 2001.

Matchar DB et al: Evidence-based guidelines for migraine headache in the primary care setting: pharmacological management of acute attacks, St Paul, April 2000, US Headache Consortium and American Academy of Neurology.

McCance KL, Huether SE, editors: *Pathophysiology: the biologic basis for disease in adults and children,* ed 4, St Louis, 2002, Mosby.

McDonald RL: GABA$_A$ receptor defects can cause epilepsy, *Epilepsy Curr* 1(2):74-5, 2001.

Meador KJ: Cognitive outcomes and predictive factors in epilepsy, *Neurology* 58(suppl 5):S21-S26, 2002.

Minino AM, Smith BL: Death: preliminary data for 2000, *National Vital Statistics Reports* 49(12), 2001.

Multi-Society Task Force on PVS: Medical aspects of persistent vegetative state (part 1), *N Engl J Med* 330(21):1499-1507, 1994a.

Multi-Society Task Force on PVS: Medical aspects of persistent vegetative state (part 2), *N Engl J Med* 330(22):1572-79, 1994b.

National Centers for Injury Prevention and Control: Injury fact book 2001-2002, Atlanta, 2001, Centers for Disease Control and Prevention.

National Cholesterol Education Program: The third report of the Expert Panel on Detection, Evaluation, and Treatment of High Blood Cholesterol in Adults, National Heart, Lung, and Blood Institute, Bethesda, Md, 2001, National Institutes of Health.

National Institute of Neurologic Disorders and Stroke: Epilepsy benchmarks: curing epilepsy: focus on the future, a NINDS/NIH research agenda for epilepsy, Bethesda, Md, 2000, National Institutes of Health, retrieved from *http://www.ninds.nih.gov* and *http://www.epilepsy benchmarks@ninds.nih.gov* on Jan 19, 2004.

National Institute of Neurological Disorders and Stroke: Migraine update, 2001, retrieved from *http://www.ninds.nih.gov* on June 24, 2002.

National Stroke Association: United States stroke statistics, Stroke is a brain attack, 2002a, retrieved from *http://www.stroke.org/brain_stat.cfm* on July 14, 2002.

National Stroke Association: HOPE: the stroke recovery guide—exercises and recommendations, 2002b, retrieved from *http://www.stroke.org* on July 14, 2002.

O'Shanick G: Mapping the way—drug therapy and brain injury, The Road to Rehabilitation Series, Alexandria, Va, 2001, Brain Injury Association.

Rozen TD: Antiepileptic drugs in the management of cluster headache and trigeminal neuralgia, *Headache J Head Face Pain* 41(1):25-33, 2001.

Schwartz BS et al: Epidemiology of tension-type headaches, *JAMA* 279(5):381-3, 1998.

Silberstein SD, the US Headache Consortium: Practice parameter: evidence-based guidelines for migraine headache (an evidence-based review): report of the Quality Standards Subcommittee of the American Academy of Neurology, *Neurology* 55:754-63, 2000.

Sisodiya SM et al: Drug resistance in epilepsy: expression of drug resistance proteins in common causes of refractory epilepsy, *Brain* 25(1):22-31, 2002.

Snels IA et al: Treating patients with hemiplegic shoulder pain, *Am J Phys Med Rehabil* 81(2):150-60, 2002.

Stewart WF et al: Prevalence of migraine headache in the United States: relation to age, income, race, and other sociodemographic factors, *JAMA* 267:64-9, 1992.

Traumatic Brain Injury Model Systems (TBIMS): Data update: facts and figures from the TBIMS National Database—2001, *Traumatic brain injury: facts and figures* 7(1), 2001.

Vestergaard K et al: Lamotrigine for central poststroke pain: a randomized trial, *Neurology* 56:184-90, 2001.

Walczak TS et al: Incidence and risk factors in sudden unexpected death in epilepsy: a prospective cohort study, *Neurology* 56:519-25, 2001.

Wiebe S et al: A randomized, controlled trial of surgery for temporal lobe epilepsy, *N Engl J Med* 345(5):311-8, 2001.

Wilson S, Bladin P, Saling M: The "burden of normality": concepts of adjustment after surgery for seizures, *J Neurol Neurosurg Psychiatry* 70(5):649-55, 2001.

Yasuda S et al: Return to work for persons with traumatic brain injury, *Am J Phys Med Rehabil* 80:852-64, 2001.

CHAPTER 22

Dementias

Lin E. Noyes, PhD, RN

OBJECTIVES

After reading this chapter, you should be able to do the following:

- Describe the pathophysiology of Alzheimer's disease, vascular dementia, frontal lobe dementias, and dementias with Lewy bodies
- Describe the clinical manifestations of dementia
- Describe the functional health patterns affected by dementia
- Describe the role of each member of the interdisciplinary team involved in the care of patients with dementia
- Describe the indications for use, adverse events, and nursing considerations related to drugs commonly used to treat people with dementia

This chapter focuses on the care of individuals with Alzheimer's disease and other irreversible dementias. Irreversible dementias are life-changing illnesses that generally start with subtle changes in memory and/or the executive functioning of the brain and progress until the affected person is so impaired that someone else must provide totally for the person. The caregiver, often called "the second victim of dementia," is both a partner in the illness and a member of the care team.

The term *dementia* means a lack of mental abilities. The word has been used since the time of Cicero to mean "senseless," "out of one's mind," or "insane." Contemporary medicine uses the term to describe a neurodegenerative syndrome with the following characteristics:

- Global loss of intelligence is noted.
- Deficits are seen in at least two brain functions, memory and one other function.
- Symptoms occur in a state of clear consciousness.
- Symptoms represent a change from previous behavior.

If these symptoms are present, the person exhibiting them is said to have dementia. Dementia affects 20% of older adults.

There are approximately 140 causes of dementia, including reactions to medication, physical illnesses, emotional illnesses, and neurologic conditions. Twenty percent of dementias are caused by conditions that may be treatable (thyroid irregularities, vitamin B_{12} and folate deficiencies, heavy metal intoxication, and normal-pressure hydrocephalus). The most common cause of irreversible dementia is Alzheimer's disease (50% to 70% of cases), followed by vascular or multiinfarct disease (20%). Individuals may also have a mixed dementia (Alzheimer's disease and vascular dementia).

Other neurologic illnesses that cause dementia include Pick's disease, diffuse Lewy body disease, Creutzfeldt-Jakob disease, and Parkinson's disease (30% of cases). Research on dementing illnesses is relatively new, and discoveries regarding diseases and conditions that cause dementia are unfolding. A variety of terms are used to describe the condition of dementia (Box 22-1). In this chapter, "person with dementia" refers to individuals with irreversible dementia.

PATHOPHYSIOLOGY

A common irregularity in many neurodegenerative dementias is the presence of abnormal aggregations of proteins in the brain. Alzheimer's disease is recognized microscopically by the presence of amyloid plaques and neurofibrillary tangles on brain autopsy (Figure 22-1). Simultaneous changes in brain chemistry result in a decrease in neurotransmitters and a loss of nerve cells. As various brain cells become affected, corresponding function is diminished. These changes occur first in the hippocampus, then proceed to the cortex, and eventually involve the entire brain. As the disease progresses brain atrophy occurs and electrical activity in the brain is diminished.

Unlike Alzheimer's disease, vascular dementia results from brain cell damage due to disruption of blood flow to brain tissue. Blood vessels may break or become clogged and disrupt the flow of blood to brain tissue, which results in necrosis (infarct) and a lack of function of those cells. The occurrence of small infarcts throughout the brain over time results in dementia. Multiinfarct dementia is considered "treatable" in some cases because reducing the occurrence of infarcts will reduce future damage to brain cells.

Pick's disease (associated with frontotemporal dementia) is an accumulation of abnormal protein that begins in the frontal lobes of the brain and progresses to involve the whole brain. Dementia with Lewy bodies is a disease microscopically similar to Alzheimer's disease except that Lewy bodies (another abnormal aggregation of proteins) are present in the brain. Creutzfeldt-Jakob disease is a rare prion disease caused by an abnormal folding of a prion protein and resulting in rapidly progressive dementia (National Institute on Aging, 2003).

The similarities between Parkinson's disease and Alzheimer's disease are being investigated, because people with Parkinson's disease may develop Alzheimer's disease–type memory loss and people who have Alzheimer's disease may develop some of the physical symptoms of Parkinson's disease. Some other dementias are considered to be genetically linked, but these account for relatively few cases of dementia.

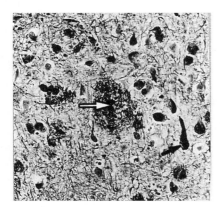

Figure 22-1 Pathologic changes in Alzheimer's disease. Senile plaque with central amyloid core *(white arrow)* next to a neurofibrillary tangle *(black arrow)* in the histologic specimen from a brain autopsy. (From Damjanov I, Linder J: *Pathology: a color atlas,* St Louis, 2000, Mosby.)

ASSESSMENT

Assessment of a person with dementia begins with an interview and physical examination. Due to memory loss and possible lack of insight into the illness, the person coming for assessment should be accompanied by his or her care partner so that an accurate medical history can be obtained. Hospitalized patients and others with no history of dementia who have sudden changes in cognitive status and/or level of consciousness should be evaluated for delirium and treated for underlying causes, including medical conditions, intoxication by substances, or withdrawal from substances (Insel and Badger, 2002). Depression must also be considered as a cause of the presenting symptoms, because a high rate of depression occurs in older adults (Bagulho, 2002) and the presence of depression is often masked by (or mistaken for) the presenting symptoms of early dementia. Older adults without a previous history of depression may be experiencing the onset of dementia (Insel and Badger, 2002).

Neuropsychological and cognitive status assessment tools administered in the earlier stages of dementia as well as depression scales rely heavily on verbal and writing skills and thus become less useful tools as the disease progresses. Most tools that depend on self-report are also of little value. Ongoing assessment of health status and changes in functional health patterns requires astute observational skills (Box 22-2). Periodic evaluation of the person's abilities and the care partner's assessment of changes are essential to document the progression of symptoms and reactions to treatment interventions. Box 22-3 lists tools that may be useful for clinical assessment during the course of a dementing illness. Although the Mini-Mental State Examination is widely used, people in early stages of Alzheimer's disease can perform quite well on this test. Another tool that is useful for screening is to ask the individual to draw the face of a clock with the hands at a specific position. The person with Alzheimer's disease most likely will not be able to complete this task (Figure 22-2).

DIAGNOSIS

The *Diagnostic and Statistical Manual of Mental Disorders*, fourth edition, identifies the essential features of dementia as follows:

Impairment in short- and long-term memory, associated with impairment in abstract thinking, impaired judgment, other disturbances of higher cortical function, or personality change. The disturbances are severe enough to interfere significantly with work or usual social activities or relationships with others (American Psychiatric Association, 1994).

The diagnosis of dementia is made when all other possible causes of cognitive symptoms have been excluded. After the history taking and physical and neurologic evaluation, the following tests are performed to rule out other causes of the symptoms: computed tomography or magnetic resonance imaging, tests for vitamin B_{12} deficiency, thyroid function tests to detect hypothyroidism, and assessment for depression

Box 22-2   Functional Health Pattern Assessment for Dementia

HEALTH PERCEPTION/HEALTH MANAGEMENT

- Is there a family history of stroke, Alzheimer's disease, or other dementia disorder?
- What are the individual's and family's perceptions of the patient's overall health?
- Do the patient and family accept and adhere to the therapeutic regimens and practices, including using prescribed medications?
- Does the patient use alternative therapies?
- Does the patient engage in measures to promote brain health such as physical exercise and challenging mental activities?
- Are the patient and family amenable to education and support?

NUTRITION/METABOLISM

- What is the patient's current weight? Has there been any unexplained recent weight gain or loss?
- Does the patient consume a diet consistent with healthy brain functioning?
- What are the patient's cultural beliefs about food and eating?
- What are the patient's dietary habits and choices? Is the patient on a special or prescribed diet?
- Have there been alterations in independent eating behaviors? Is the patient able to swallow?
- What are the ethical considerations in nutrition and hydration?

ELIMINATION

- Have any changes occurred in bowel or bladder habits?
- Does the patient experience pain or difficulty in urinating?
- Does the patient have deficits in elimination sensations? What are the patterns of continence?
- Does the patient use adult undergarments? Does the patient require bowel and bladder training?
- Does the patient show decreased discrimination of environmental cues to appropriate facilities?
- Does the patient use an elevated toilet seat, assistive devices, and/or grab bars?
- Does the patient accept assistance from a caregiver?

ACTIVITY/EXERCISE

- Does the patient experience difficulty walking, apathy, or depression?
- What are the patient's regular exercise activities? In what recreational activities does the patient engage?
- What mobility aids does the patient use?
- Have patterns of cooperation been established to allow performance of instrumental and other activities of daily living?
- Does the patient perform range of motion and restorative functions daily?

SLEEP/REST

- How many hours of uninterrupted sleep do the patient and caregiver obtain at night? Does the individual or caregiver take naps or rest periods?
- What complementary-alternative and prescribed sleep aids are used?

COGNITION/PERCEPTION

- What is the patient's cognitive awareness of self, family, others, environment, time, and place?
- Can the patient recognize and appropriately respond to sensory messages from the body?
- Can the patient communicate his or her ideas or needs and manipulate items in the environment?
- Does the patient show symmetrical involvement, paresthesias, paralysis, or neglect syndrome?

SELF-PERCEPTION/SELF-CONCEPT

- How does the patient describe himself or herself?
- How has the condition affected the patient's self-esteem?
- Has the patient experienced changes in recognizing self? How has the condition affected the sense of self?
- Can the patient communicate and interact with the family and environment?

ROLES/RELATIONSHIPS

- Is the patient employed or does the patient play a dependent role in the home or family?
- What changes have occurred in the patient's ability to carry out role functions?
- How satisfied is the patient with his or her current roles and relationships?
- How has the condition affected the patient's family and/or significant others?

SEXUALITY/REPRODUCTION

- Has the condition led to changes in sexual performance?
- Does the patient recognize his or her partner?
- Have there been occurrences of inappropriate sexual behavior?

COPING/STRESS TOLERANCE

- What are the patient's coping strategies?
- What support systems are available to the patient?
- Can the individual and family manage the condition in the current setting?
- Do the patient and family recognize the impact of the changes that have occurred and plan for the future?
- How hardy and resilient are the individual and family?
- What is the caregiver burden?

VALUES/BELIEFS

- What constitutes quality of life for the patient?
- What is important to the patient and family?
- What are the patient's beliefs relating to this condition?
- How are individual and family values upheld?
- What are the patient's spiritual beliefs, health beliefs, and cultural beliefs? To what extent do these beliefs influence decision making?
- What are the patient's views on locus of control?
- Has the patient engaged in end-of-life decision making?

(Knopman et al, 2001). Confirmation of the diagnosis is possible only at autopsy, but a thorough diagnostic workup yields a correct diagnosis in about 90% of cases.

CLINICAL MANIFESTATIONS

Alzheimer's disease is progressive and irreversible, has an insidious onset, and manifests itself in numerous ways. *Early-, middle-,* and *late-stage Alzheimer's disease* are terms used loosely to describe the progression of the disease. Table 22-1 compares the manifestations of the disorder in each stage.

Staging Alzheimer's disease is unlike staging cancer because changes in brain tissue and function vary greatly. The length and progression of illness varies and, in the end, leaves the individual completely dependent on others for nutrition, hydration, and total care.

Vascular dementia shows a stepwise progression of symptoms with some loss of function after each ischemic episode. Individuals may temporarily regain the lost skill (cognitive, sensory, or neuromuscular) until the next episode occurs.

Repeated ischemic episodes leave the person with cumulative and progressive losses similar to those found in Alzheimer's disease. The later stages of vascular dementia are almost indistinguishable from dementia caused by

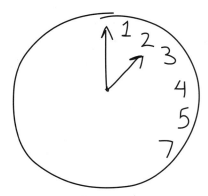

Figure 22-2 A method of screening for Alzheimer's disease. When asked to draw the face of a clock with the clock hands at a specific position, the patient with Alzheimer's will not be able to complete the task.

Alzheimer's disease. Pick's disease initially manifests as memory problems, disinhibitions, and an increase in childlike behaviors that progress to the generalized losses of dementia.

INTERDISCIPLINARY CARE

The goal of care for individuals with dementia is to keep the person functioning as independently as possible for as long as possible and to decrease the period of dependency.

Primary Provider (Physician/Nurse Practitioner)

The family physician may diagnose and rule out physical and physiologic causes of dementing symptoms, help chart the progress of the illness, refer the family to community services as needed, and treat concurrent illnesses such as high blood pressure and infections. Treatment of hypertension is known to reduce the incidence of stroke activity.

Specialists

The neurologist determines the cause of dementia, charts the progress of neurologic decline, treats untoward behaviors when they occur, and treats seizures, which may occur in the later stages of dementia.

The neuropsychologist identifies the specific areas of brain function affected and compares changes over time in individuals with very mild symptoms or with questionable dementia. Knowing the areas of the brain that are particularly affected helps team members plan effective interventions. A psychiatrist may become involved if the individual has depression or other concurrent psychiatric manifestations.

A psychologist or counselor can help the individual in the early stages of dementia deal with anger and feelings of loss and help caregivers adjust to the changes caused by the illness and cope with their own reactions to their caregiving role.

Drug Therapy

No drugs can cure Alzheimer's disease. Drugs that treat the cognitive symptoms of dementia began to appear in the 1990s and are aimed at preventing the breakdown of the neurotransmitter acetylcholine in the brain. Other drugs used in Alzheimer's disease include behavior-modifying drugs and drugs thought to prevent or delay the onset of Alzheimer's disease.

Drugs used to treat the symptoms of cognitive decline in Alzheimer's disease include galantamine (Reminyl), rivastigmine (Exelon), and donepezil (Aricept). These drugs may slow the symptoms of the disease but will not stop it from progressing. All of these drugs are most effective in the initial stages of Alzheimer's disease and at best slow down the progressive decline for a while. Vascular dementias may be treated with antistroke drugs. Drug adherence must be monitored closely, because forgetfulness is the main feature of dementia.

Nonsteroidal antiinflammatory drugs, estrogen, vitamin E, and nerve growth factor are under investigation as agents that may delay or diminish the effects of Alzheimer's disease.

Table 22-1   Manifestations of Alzheimer's Disease in Early, Middle, and Late Stages

Manifestations	Early Stage	Middle Stage	Late Stage
Functional			
Eating	Loses ability to cook and shop appropriately. May need reminders about when to eat or limits on how much food is consumed.	May not eat without supervision or cueing, even when food is in front of the person.	Gradually becomes unable to feed self enough to satisfy nutritional needs. Requires full assistance with eating. Choking and coughing may occur and swallowing becomes impaired.
Dressing	Can dress self but may wear same clothes over and over again. May need to have clothes laid out in order of dressing and other clothes locked up.	Unable to dress without supervision and cueing.	Must be dressed by another.
Toileting	May not be able to find the bathroom when needed but can toilet self if directed to bathroom.	Has difficulty in manipulating clothing, finding the commode, and cleaning self. Can maintain continence with bathroom schedule and supervision. May require assistance with wiping.	Gradually becomes incontinent of urine and feces, requiring full assistance and use of adult undergarments.
Bathing	May lose ability to bathe/shower and groom self. May bathe less and not notice body odor (change from premorbid behavior).	May refuse to accept help needed to bathe or groom self, especially when help comes from close relative.	May be afraid of bathing and become verbally and physically aggressive during bathing.
Cognitive			
Amnesia	Memory loss begins gradually, often observed by others; newer memories more easily forgotten than memories from the past.	Memory loss increases. May confabulate (make up things) to hide memory loss. Unable to recall significant people's names or relationship. Orientation to time and place may be diminished.	Profound short-term and long-term memory loss evidenced in lack of recognition of people and/or familiar surroundings. May remember words to familiar songs and sing along. Orientation to time and place absent.
Aphasia	Loss of spoken language and comprehension of spoken language occurs. Word finding impaired. Hesitations and pauses exhibited in conversation.	Conversations may become very concrete and limited. May repeat what speaker says or use all-purpose pat phrases. May revert to use of childhood language.	Communication severely limited in regard to number of words spoken and comprehension of the meaning of words spoken or heard. May repeat same word over and over with little attachment to its meaning (chanting).
Apraxia	Ability to do complex tasks requiring coordination and multiple steps diminishes.	Coordination of purposeful movement to complete everyday tasks begins to deteriorate. Can follow step-by-step directions.	Unable to coordinate actions to perform activities of daily living. May continue a repetitive task started or guided by someone else. Becomes unable to stand, walk, or transfer by self.
Agnosia	Brain's ability to recognize what the eye sees begins to diminish. Moving objects may be misinterpreted.	Brain's ability to recognize what the eye sees in stationary situations diminishes.	May be unable to make sense of objects seen by the eye and appear functionally blind.
Executive function	Ability to work diminishes; unable to initiate, plan, or organize complex activity.	Unable to plan or initiate any meaningful activity.	Complete inability to perform executive functions.

Table 22-1   Manifestations of Alzheimer's Disease in Early, Middle, and Late Stages—cont'd

Manifestations	Early Stage	Middle Stage	Late Stage
Cognitive—cont'd			
Decision-making capacity	Able to make decisions for self and plan for the future in the initial stages of the illness. May or may not have insight into the changes occurring. Judgment regarding self or others may be impaired.	Able to make decisions for self regarding some everyday issues but unable to weigh risks, benefits, or consequences of major decisions. Judgment regarding personal safety, belongings, and appropriate actions may be impaired	Unable to make or express decisions regarding self.
Psychological	May exhibit apathy, depression, loss of regard for self and others, frustration, anger, agitation, suspiciousness, disinhibition. May blame others or defer to care partner for all information and guidance. May hide things in unusual places.	May become blissfully unaware of cognitive difficulties or become angrier and frustrated in performing everyday tasks. May use pejorative terms and foul language. May feel useless, restless, and bored. May be aware of new losses and become saddened by them.	Paucity of thought may be reflected in blank expression on the person's face. May appear frightened when approached. May be uncooperative and resistive to care.
Behavioral	May take notes or attempt to use reminders excessively. May engage in repetitive tasks such as buying objects that are useless or unnecessary. May complete an activity when given a specific command. May have accidents driving or cooking. May shadow care partner and wait for all directions. May become lost when driving or walking. May hide important objects (money, keys) for safety and be unable to retrieve them when needed	May make comments that are not socially appropriate. May mistake household products for food substances. Sleep-wake cycle may be disturbed, may sleep excessively or stay awake for days before sleeping. May lose the ability to use simple household tools like utensils and brushes. May exhibit restlessness and hyperactivity. Restlessness or wandering behaviors may signify unmet physical needs.	May cry out to keep contact with the environment. May pick at clothing or bed covers. May sleep most of the time but can be engaged in the environment and relate to others for short periods of time with encouragement. Agitation and increased body movements or facial grimaces may indicate physical pain or discomfort.
Social	May dress in layers or dress inappropriately for the occasion. May shy away from routine social engagements.	Unable to use telephone or recognize voices in telephone conversations. Manners deteriorate. Enjoyment of nonroutine events lessens.	Returns smiles and uses friendly tone of voice even though words may not make sense.
Performance	Unable to carry out routine work functions, pay bills, or use complicated machinery.	May be able to do parts of tasks and complete tasks if presented one step at a time.	May sit doing nothing unless prompted by others.
Physical	Weight loss or gain, otherwise no changes.	Countenance may appear vacant or watchful; as coordination deteriorates, may have more accidents and/or injuries.	More susceptible to infections and pressure ulcers. Focal neurologic signs may appear. General body wasting occurs.

There are no dementia-specific behavior-modifying drugs. Antidepressants, antipsychotics, and sedatives are given to manage behavioral symptoms, generally in much smaller dosages than are otherwise typically used. Pharmaceutical management of untoward behaviors is used as a last resort; however, when the right drug is found by trial and error, it is usually mildly effective. The risk of side effects for all drugs is weighed against the benefits of the medication. Individuals taking behavior-modifying drugs may quickly lose already fragile self-care abilities (see Table 21-1).

Nurse

The nurse focuses on the needs and well-being of both the individual with dementia and his or her caregivers. Interventions vary as the illness progresses, as illustrated in Table 22-2 for eating strategies. These strategies can be adapted to fit other areas of assistance.

In the early stages the nurse advocates for a thorough diagnostic workup and supports both the individual and family through any denial of what is happening. For the individual with dementia who is aware of the illness, the nurse can provide support either individually or in a group setting. Individuals in the early stages of their illness may be eager to do whatever they can to make themselves as healthy as they can be. They may want to participate in drug trials, perform cognitive remediation exercises, and adopt healthy lifestyle changes. They want to know what they can expect and if what they are experiencing is "normal" given their illness.

The nurse as health educator helps the person gain knowledge about the illness, and because dementia takes a unique course in each individual, the information should be future oriented. The nurse can also help the individual focus on issues that he or she can take control of while the person is still able to do so. For instance, an individual in the early stages of dementia can make decisions about whom to appoint as his or her health care and business power of attorney.

Choices about future health care interventions including end-of-life care and do-not-resuscitate orders should be discussed. Doing so gives the individual a sense of control about the future and also helps the family or designated representative make future decisions confidently. Elder law attorneys can often assist the individual with dementia and the family in creating documents specifying the wishes of the person for future use. Box 22-4 lists special issues in decision making for people with dementia.

The nurse assists family members in understanding the illness, finding respite (temporary breaks in caregiving), and receiving support. All caregivers must preserve their own health during long-term caregiving. The nurse may lead a support group in which families have the opportunity to compare experiences, share helpful solutions, and vent unpleasant emotions. The nurse often helps family members learn caregiving skills and communication techniques that lessen the burden of day-to-day caregiving.

In addition to memory loss, people with dementia have difficulty using and understanding words (aphasia) because of changes in the brain. Fortunately, communication is more than words. Only 3% of communication is verbal (words and their meanings); 38% is voice (pitch, tone, tempo, volume) and 55% is body language (expression, eyes, breathing, posture, movements, gestures, and tenseness). At times the caregiver sends one message with words and a different message with body language. When words and body language do not match, the person with dementia will most likely believe the body language. Box 22-5 offers guidelines for communicating with people with dementia.

As the disease progresses, the nurse manages problem behaviors that arise. Knowing the person's usual routine, using good communication techniques, and keeping the environment calm are steps for managing behavioral outbursts (Box 22-6). After a problem behavior occurs, what was going on in the environment, what the demands of the interaction were, and what role the caregiver played in the behavior should be reviewed to determine what can be changed so that the behavior does not occur again.

Caregivers

Caregivers provide the day-to-day, hands-on care for the person with dementia. The specific interventions depend on the clinical manifestations of the illness, beginning with supervision to ensure safety and progressing to the provision of total care. (See Table 22-2 for examples of caregiver interventions for eating.) Family members are often the primary caregivers. They know the person's past lifestyle, likes and dislikes, and normal routines and should be encouraged to share this information with other members of the health team.

Paid caregivers such as certified nursing assistants or others with less formal training step in intermittently or on a full-time basis, or when family is not available. Most care is given in a home setting, but as the disease progresses and when the family decides, the person with dementia may be placed in an assisted living facility or a nursing home. The advantage of residential care is the potential availability of a team of hands-on caregivers.

Dietitian

The registered dietitian assesses the individual's nutritional status and identifies and suggests foods and ways of eating that can help the individual maintain adequate nutritional status as eating skills diminish. Nutrients thought to be healthy for the brain are listed in Box 22-7, and although there is no research documenting the benefits of eating these foods, including foods high in antioxidants and omega-3 fatty acids as part of a well-balanced diet is recommended.

Physical Therapist

The physical therapist's interventions are aimed at maintaining independence in walking and transferring, and bolstering the individual against the apraxia that accompanies brain deterioration. Ensuring that the individual in the earlier stages of the illness performs exercises aimed at maintaining full range of motion, flexibility, and muscle

Text continued on p. 359.

Table 22-2 Comparison of Eating Strategies for People in Early, Middle, and Late Stages of Dementia

Early Stages		Middle Stages		Late Stages	
Intervention	Rationale	Intervention	Rationale	Intervention	Rationale
1. Encourage safe meal preparation for as long as possible.	1. Preserving daily habits promotes feelings of self-esteem and mastery.	1. Bring the individual to the table and place food in front of the person.	1. Sitting with other people who are eating cues the expected behavior.	1. If the individual loses the ability to chew food or chews but does not swallow, serve foods with a pudding-like consistency.	1. The process of chewing and swallowing effectively can deteriorate. Individuals lose the ability to sequence the task of eating. Foods that must be chewed and swallowed are much more difficult to eat. One-step eating (as with pudding) is safer (decreases chance of choking and aspirating during meals).
2. Make and adhere to a regular routine for meal preparation; do not vary from it.	2. Routine enhances procedural memory.	2. Tell the individual that the food is in front of him or her and that it is time to eat. (May need to repeat this frequently until all the food is consumed.)	2. The individual may not recognize things visually and may need auditory cues to help attend to the task at hand.	2. Inspect the mouth for "pocketing" of food along the gum line and remove any residual food after eating before leaving the individual alone after a meal.	2. Food that is left in the mouth may never be swallowed and can cause choking and aspiration.
3. Monitor the individual and the environment.	3. Bit by bit the individual loses abilities to do routine procedures. Monitoring allows one to observe whether or not the individual uses utensils and appliances safely.	3. Remove all items from the table except the plate of food; use a place mat and plate of contrasting colors.	3. Removing visual distractions helps the individual focus on the task at hand. Contrast helps heighten visual cues.	3. The individual may be able to feed self part of the food but then become tired. If you must assist the individual with the meal by feeding the person, sit down next to the individual to help him or her. Sometimes if you use two spoons, one for you and one for the individual, the person will accept the help more easily.	3. Allowing the individual to participate as fully as possible enhances feelings of mastery and self-control. Helping the individual when he or she becomes tired allows a good balance between fostering independence and ensuring adequate nutrition. Sitting beside the individual instead of standing provides a more natural setting to assist the individual in eating and decreases appearances and feelings of dependency.

Continued

Early Stages		Middle Stages		Late Stages	
Intervention	Rationale	Intervention	Rationale	Intervention	Rationale
4. Modify the environment for safety if needed. Put away electric appliances, knives, poisonous substances that may be mistaken for food products. Disarm the stove by removing the fuse on an electric stove and knobs on a gas stove. Set items needed where the individual can see them, label drawers and cabinets so the individual can find necessary items.	4. The individual's ability to manipulate appliances and kitchen utensils safely diminishes with progression of the disease. In addition, judgment, recognition of items and their use, and motor skills also diminish.	4. Cue the individual, "Pick up your fork and take a bite."	4. Cueing reminds the individual how to begin the task.	4. If the individual has trouble swallowing or keeping the food in the mouth, start the meal with ice cream or something else cold.	4. Cold substances stimulate the muscles and nerves and enhance the person's ability to take food into the mouth and then swallow.
5. Simplify food preparation or prepare the food for the individual.	5. The balancing of safety with feelings of independence and self-worth changes for each individual in each situation. If the risk of harm is high (fire, injury) then safety should be valued more; if the risk of harm is low (the person can do the task but makes a mess), then independence should be valued more.	5. If the individual still does not eat, hand the person the fork and say, "Here is your fork, it's time to eat."	5. Help the individual initiate the task by involving him or her in the first step of the process of eating.	5. If eating a large meal at one time is difficult, offer shorter, more frequent meals.	5. As the disease progresses, the individual may tire easily; frequent small meals may be more tolerable.

6. Encourage the individual's participation in meal preparation as much as ability allows; work co-operatively with the individual. Allow the person to do all tasks he or she can still do, then do the rest.	6. Coaching step by step promotes a sense of mastery and inclusion. Sequencing promotes involvement that memory loss disrupts.	6. Put the fork in the individual's hand and guide it to the food and then to the mouth.	6. Hand-over-hand technique may prompt motor memory so the person can continue the task on his or her own.	6. Use a thickening agent in liquids if drinking liquids causes choking.	6. Liquids that are nectar consistency are more easily swallowed and therefore safer when swallowing is problematic.
7. Prepare the food for the individual, place it in front of the person at the table when it is time to eat, and tell the person, "Here is your food."	7. Environment (table, presence of food) and word cue the person to begin eating.	7. If the individual cannot manipulate the utensils, provide finger food. Almost everything can be turned into a sandwich.	7. Using utensils is a higher-level cognitive task than using hands to eat and will be lost earlier. Being able to feed oneself is a quality-of-life issue and is valued over being fed.	7. Don't serve combination foods that have more than one consistency (e.g., chicken noodle soup has things that must be chewed in a liquid broth).	7. Multiconsistency foods confuse the person about whether to chew or swallow and induce choking.
8. If the individual eats more than he or she should or focuses on eating sweets in abundance, remove these items from accessibility and put low-calorie alternatives in clear sight. Keep eating times as routine as possible and make sure the individual has "tasks" or "chores" to do in between meals.	8. The individual's recognition of satiation or hunger becomes undependable. The person may forget having eaten. Gorging may occur, resulting in weight gain. The individuals may eat out of boredom.	8. Allow the individual sufficient time and supervision to complete the meal.	8. The individual may be slower due to decreased abilities but can finish the task if given repeated cues and the time to complete the task.	8. If the individual is only able to take in very small amounts, give small spoonfuls frequently and give calorie-dense foods.	8. As the disease progresses, the individual may tire easily, and frequent small meals may be more tolerable. Eating calorie-dense foods provides more nutrition with less work for the individual.

Continued

Table 22-2 Comparison of Eating Strategies for People in Early, Middle, and Late Stages of Dementia—cont'd

Early Stages		Middle Stages		Late Stages	
Intervention	Rationale	Intervention	Rationale	Intervention	Rationale
9. Make sure that food is wrapped in plastic or that containers are labeled so that the food can be seen.	9. The individual may not recognize that milk is in the container or that the dinner plate is under the warming cover so will not eat.	9. If the individual mixes foods and liquids or stacks the dishes without finishing eating, place only one item in front of the person at a time.	9. As the individual loses knowledge of the purpose of things, he or she may manipulate plates and utensils in a meaning-less way and/or become overwhelmed with the choices.	9. Hold the individual's head erect and/or position the individual in a sitting position to prevent choking; keep the individual sitting for half an hour after a meal.	9. Weakened muscles in the esophagus no longer propel food into stomach. Sitting erect enhances the effects of gravity and lessens the chances of vomiting and aspirating.
		10. If the individual says, "This is too much, I can't eat it," then put very small portions on the plate and add more only when the platen is empty.	10. Limiting choices helps to focus attention. Proportion and size lose meaning; seeing a full plate may overwhelm the individual.	10. Discussions of feeding tubes should include the latest research on the benefits and risks of feeding tubes. Although the family is the decision maker, health care professionals inform the decision by giving all the facts to the family.	10. Family members make decisions based on facts presented to them about the normal course of disease and the risks and benefits of using feeding tubes versus continuing natural feeding techniques.
		11. If the individual eats but is untidy, assess whether or not the mess is upsetting to the individual; if it is not, allow the individual to continue to feed self. Protect clothing with an apron (adult word—do not say bib) and cover the furniture.	11. Eating independently is valued more highly than eating neatly and adds to the individual's self-esteem.		

Box 22-4 Special Issues in Decision Making for the Individual with Dementia

- Who will make legal, financial, health, and day-to-day decisions?
- Where does the individual want to live and be cared for when he or she can no longer live at home?
- What medical procedures and care interventions does the individual want in the final stages of life?
- What are the patient's choices related to participating in research studies?

Box 22-6 Guidelines for Managing Difficult Behaviors

1. Intervene early, never say no, and ask for help and cooperation.
2. Change the interaction, environment, or caregiver.
3. Use a nonchallenging stance:
   - Stand outside the individual's personal space; 3 ft is a comfortable distance for people not engaged in an aggressive action.
   - Increase the distance if the person's behavior is escalating.
   - Do not block the exit.
   - Stand at an angle to the person, not face to face.
   - Keep your hands in full view, with palms up, not in pockets or behind you.
4. Use the following safety techniques to reduce occurrences of injury:
   - Never turn your back on a person who is acting out.
   - Make sure you have an exit route.
   - Protect yourself from injury.
   - Know your limits.
   - Call 911 if you need to do so.

strength helps the individual keep fit and healthy. Exercise has also been shown to be an antidote for restless and agitated behaviors. The physical therapist can also help teach family caregivers how to assist with transferring, lifting, and moving the individual in the later stages of the illness.

Occupational Therapist

The loss of a skill required to perform the activities of daily living is usually caused by deterioration in the ability to organize and sequence the steps in a task; that is, the knowledge that step A comes before step B. The more advanced the dementia is, the more the caregiver must simplify each task. The occupational therapist teaches the caregiver how to use cueing, task breakdown, and hand-over-hand techniques to help the individual complete a task (Box 22-8). This helps the individual maintain as much independence as possible because the caregiver provides appropriate assistance rather than performing the full task for the individual.

Box 22-5 Guidelines for Communicating with People with Dementia

- Make every effort to match verbal and nonverbal messages.
- Remember to convey a positive attitude with a smile, a warm and friendly tone, and an open, noncontrolling stance or posture.
- Give one message at a time.
- Use adult language in word choice and tone of voice.
- Use e-x-p-a-n-d-e-d speech. Practice speaking slowly, which allows the person with dementia to process information and respond.
- Never say, "No, don't do that."
- Watch the person's body language, facial expressions, and tone of voice and use these to help you formulate a response.
- Agree with some part of the individual's message; limit later.
- Change the subject instead of arguing facts.
- Ask for the person's help to distract the person from an undesirable activity.
- Redirect the individual to a more desirable location or activity.
- Try to be proactive instead of reactive.

From Noyes LE: Loss and Alzheimer's disease. In Doka KJ, editor: *Living with grief: loss in later life*, Washington, DC, 2002, Hospice Foundation of America, pp 59-70.

Medical Social Worker

The medical social worker helps the family locate community resources and services to ease the burden of caregiving, and promotes the highest quality of care possible for the individual who has been diagnosed with dementia. Because most of the long-term care of individuals with Alzheimer's disease is not paid for by Medicare or other insurance programs, the social worker may assist the family in finding coverage for needed services through Medicaid or veteran's programs if appropriate.

Only half of the individuals with dementia have family members available to help them. If the individual is living alone or with other unrelated people and has no family members, then local social services agencies must step in and provide the services to protect the person from the effects of his or her own disease. Adult protective service workers may be needed to get an unwilling person to the doctor for diagnosis and/or treatment.

Elder Law Attorneys

Lawyers who specialize in helping older adults can help the individual with dementia and the family with legal and

Box 22-7 Nutrients for a Healthy Brain

- Antioxidants found in brightly and darkly colored fruits and vegetables, including spinach, kale, Swiss chard, and blueberries
- Omega-3 fatty acids found in salmon and other fish, safflower oil
- Endorphin boosters found in chocolate
- Adequate water

Box 22-8   Task Organization Aids for Persons with Dementia

EARLY AND EARLY MIDDLE STAGE

■ Write reminders.

■ Give visual cues.

■ Help structure activities.

■ Provide companionship.

■ Encourage and praise for participating in a task.

MIDDLE STAGE

■ Give verbal cues and prompts: Say, "It's time to brush your teeth."

■ Break the task into segments: Say, "Turn on the water"; when completed, say "Wet your toothbrush," then say, "Put toothpaste on the toothbrush," then "Now brush your teeth," then "Rinse your mouth" and continue these step-by step directions until the task is completed.

■ Help the person get started in the activity: hand the person the wash cloth and soap.

LATE STAGE

■ Give hand-over-hand guidance: guide the person's hand with your own hand each step of the way. Often, once the task is started, the person with dementia will be able to continue independently with verbal cues and praise.

---

financial issues related to diminishing capacity and decision making for the future.

Speech Therapist

When swallowing becomes a problem, a speech therapist may assess the individual's swallowing abilities and teach family members strategies to promote swallowing and avoid aspiration pneumonia.

ALTERNATIVE THERAPIES

Ginkgo biloba has been widely touted as a treatment for dementia because it is thought to have antioxidant, antiinflammatory, and anticoagulant properties. Research results have not demonstrated positive effects from taking *Ginkgo biloba*. Individuals considering taking this herb should consult with their primary care providers, because it may have an additive anticoagulant effect with other medications and cause harm.

Tai chi, an exercise program, is being investigated as a means of preserving complex motor skills and balance to lengthen the time individuals can perform complex tasks such as getting in and out of a car and transferring from sitting to standing or sitting down at a table.

Acupuncture treatments have been tried in the early stages of Alzheimer's disease to prevent deterioration with marginal success.

Individuals in the earlier stages of dementia benefit from cognitive remediation. Mental exercises aimed at promoting word fluency, problem solving, and recall help the individual in day-to-day life. Eventually the individual will get worse, but in the early stages doing something to ward off the illness has both psychological and cognitive benefits. Physical exercise, because it promotes feelings of overall well-being, should also be strongly encouraged.

Think *S* for Success

Symptoms

■ Monitor and identify changes in symptoms of dementia and monitor progress of illness.

■ Manage symptoms as decline progresses.

■ Keep daily activities in a routine to promote feelings of well-being and control for individual with dementia.

■ Provide support, education, and respite for caregivers.

Sequelae

■ Prevent unnecessary and premature losses of function by encouraging independence and participation in routine activities.

■ Assess individual's ability for self-care at regular intervals.

■ Teach family and caregivers to watch for early warning signs of untoward behaviors and intervene early.

■ Monitor family and/or caregivers for signs of distress and caregiver burnout. Help family find respite resources, education, and support.

■ Keep family members informed about the changes in individual's functioning noted by nurse and help them develop an alternate plan if they are unable to continue caregiving.

Safety

■ Modify individual's environment to ensure physical and psychological safety.

■ Teach family and/or caregiver how to prepare and manage behavioral outbursts if they occur.

■ As the disease progresses, teach family good body mechanics and methods of transferring and physically helping individual complete activities of daily living.

Support/Services

■ Acknowledge and recognize individual's humanity by treating individual with respect and talking to individual as an adult.

■ Encourage family members to join support groups.

■ Teach family about the changes to expect in the illness, acknowledging that each individual is different and may not experience every change in a predictable way.

Satisfaction

■ Help person to function at highest level possible.

■ Ensure that person is free to move about in a safe environment.

■ Ensure that family members have energy and resources to continue caregiving.

■ Determine the degree to which dementia is interfering with relationships, employment, independence, and other important aspects of the patient's and family's lives.

■ Develop a plan to help the patient and family reach or maintain the desired quality of life.

CASE STUDY
Patient Data

Mrs. T. is a 70-year-old retired music teacher who was diagnosed with dementia of the Alzheimer's type 6 years earlier. Mrs. T.'s daughter is not well and cannot physically care for her mother. Adult protective services was called to place Mrs. T. in a foster home, where she has been living for the last 5 years. Mrs. T. attends a dementia-specific adult day center located in the back of a church on weekdays while the foster family provides child care during the day.

Mrs. T. is brought to the day center by a transportation service for people with disabilities and does not have a consistent driver. She arrives between 7:30 AM (when the center opens) and 8:30 AM depending on traffic and whether the van shows up on time. The van provides only door-to-door service and the driver does not accompany Mrs. T. into the church to the day center area.

When Mrs. T. is at the center she takes part in the various activities and enjoys the routine of day care and being with other people. Recently she has become more disinhibited and has been kissing other participants and hugging them to show her affection. Many of the participants do not like this, and staff members have to intervene frequently to redirect her activity. Her attention span has shortened and she frequently walks in the halls when she can no longer attend to an activity. She wants to walk outside more frequently than staff are able to accompany her.

The foster family is having increasing difficulty with Mrs. T.'s restlessness on the weekends and holidays and her declining self-care skills. It is becoming increasingly difficult for the foster family to help Mrs. T. get up and get dressed and out the door to the van as children arrive in the mornings.

Twice in the past month, the high school located next to the adult day center has called early in the morning to say that the van dropped Mrs. T. there by mistake, and a day center staff member has had to go to the school and bring her to the center.

Thinking It Through

- What are possible reasons for the changes in Mrs. T.'s behavior and who in the care team can help assess the changes?
- What issues must be addressed immediately?
- What are the long-term issues that must be addressed?
- What are the roles of the day center, adult protective services, Mrs. T.'s daughter, and her foster family in this situation?
- What is Mrs. T.'s role in this process?

Case Conference

The foster family, adult protective services worker, and adult day center nurse and program assistant most familiar with Mrs. T.'s care attend the case conference to discuss what steps are necessary to keep Mrs. T. safe in transit and to talk about whether the current combination of services is sufficient to meet her present needs.

The daughter was invited but could not attend and reported to the day center staff before the meeting. She had taken her mother to a physician, who found no urinary tract infection or other signs of infection and said that no changes in medications were necessary.

The adult protective services social worker states her concern that Mrs. T. may end up truly lost if the school is not open or if she starts walking away. She fears that Mrs. T. may be a victim of the elements or may fall and hurt herself if she wanders away.

The foster family does not want to change the time Mrs. T. goes to the center because Mrs. T. resists leaving the foster home once the children have arrived for care.

The day center nurse asks the daughter to contact the Alzheimer's Association and register Mrs. T. with the "Safe Return" program. Mrs. T. will then wear a bracelet with contact information, and if someone finds her wandering, her caregivers can be contacted.

In addition, the center staff compose and copy notes for Mrs. T.'s foster family to give to the driver in the morning so that each driver is reminded of the correct destination and knows that Mrs. T. cannot be counted on for reliable directions. The center staff also ask the foster family to call the center when Mrs. T. gets into the van so they know when to expect her at the center.

The foster family agree to try to do these things but states that mornings are very hectic and it will be an additional burden on them to comply. They also express the concern that Mrs. T.'s care is becoming more and more demanding, and they do not know how much longer she will be able to stay with them.

The protective services social worker says he will follow up on the three safety recommendations and will begin to work with the family to find other living arrangements, because it seems unlikely that the current combination of services will be adequate much longer.

- What are the benefits and disadvantages of changing Mrs. T.'s living arrangements at this point?
- What are some interventions that could be tried to manage the restlessness and overly affectionate behaviors that Mrs. T. is exhibiting?
- What are some of the factors that must be considered in choosing alternate residential care for Mrs. T.?
- What are some interventions that will make the transition to residential care easier for Mrs. T. and her daughter?

Internet and Other Resources

Alzheimer's Association: *http://www.alz.org;* telephone 800-272-3900

Alzheimer's Disease Education and Referral Center (ADEAR): *http://www.alzheimers.org;* telephone 800-438-4380

REFERENCES

American Psychiatric Association: *Diagnostic and statistical manual of mental disorders,* ed 4, Washington, DC, 1994, American Psychiatric Association.

Bagulho F: Depression in older people, *Curr Opin Psychiatry* 15:417-22, 2002.

Folstein MF, Folstein SE, McHugh PR: Mini-Mental State: a practical method for grading the state of patients for the clinician, *J Psychiatr Res* 12:189-98, 1975.

Insel KC, Badger TA: Deciphering the 4 D's: cognitive decline, delirium, depression and dementia—a review, *J Adv Nurs* 38(4):360-8, 2002.

Knopman DS et al: Practice parameter: diagnosis of dementia (an evidence-based review): report of the Quality Standards Subcommittee of the American Academy of Neurology, *Neurology* 59(9):1143-53, 2001.

National Institute on Aging: Alzheimer's disease: unraveling the mystery, NIH Pub No. 02-3782, Bethesda, Md, 2003, National Institutes of Health.

Reisberg B et al: The Global Deterioration Scale for assessment of primary degenerative dementia, *Am J Psychiatry* 139(9):1136-9, 1982.

Yesavage JA et al: Development and validation of a geriatric depression screening scale: preliminary report, *J Psychiatr Res* 17:37-49, 1983.

Zarit SH, Todd PA, Zarit JM: Subjective burden of husbands and wives as caregivers: a longitudinal study, *Gerontologist* 26(3):260-6, 1982.

CHAPTER **23**

Disorders of the Spinal Cord

Sharon Mailey, PhD, RN, and Sheila Sparks, DNSc, RN

OBJECTIVES

After reading this chapter, you should be able to do the following:

- Describe the pathophysiology of spinal cord impairment, tetraplegia, and paraplegia
- Describe types of spinal cord injury using the American Spinal Cord Injury Association Impairment Scale
- Describe the role of each member of the interdisciplinary team involved in the care of patients with a chronic disorder of the spinal cord
- Describe the indications for use, side effects, and nursing considerations related to drugs commonly used to treat chronic disorders of the spinal cord
- Describe nursing care measures to prevent secondary disabilities
- Discuss nursing care management of secondary disabilities

Each year approximately 11,000 Americans sustain spinal cord injury (SCI) from car accidents (41%), gunshot wounds or other violence (22%), falls (22%), or sports (7%), primarily diving. Because of modern treatment methods, only 20% die before reaching a hospital and 85% of those who live 24 hours are still alive 10 years later. SCI primarily affects younger people who are employed (63%), single (53%), and between the ages of 16 and 30 years (53%). The average age at injury is 32 years. It is estimated that approximately 243,000 Americans are living with disabilities resulting from SCI. Some 88% are living in a private, non-institutional residence (in most cases their homes before injury). The great majority, more than 81%, are men (44% of them aged 16 to 30 years). Among those injured since 1990, the majority are Caucasian (59%); 28% are African American and about 8% are Hispanic. These facts and figures are from the database maintained by the National Spinal Cord Injury Statistical Center (NSCISC), which had its inception in 1973 and currently is the hub of 16 federally funded regional Model Spinal Cord Injury Care Systems (NSCISC, 2003).

Accounting for a little less than one half of all spinal cord injuries, paraplegia results from injury to the thoracic, lum-

bar, or sacral regions of the spinal cord. There may be complete or incomplete loss of motor and/or sensory function (Figure 23-1). Persons with tetraplegia (formerly called *quadriplegia*) (52%), have sustained injuries to one of the eight cervical segments of the spinal cord. More than 90% of these injuries are caused by sports trauma. The trends over time indicate an increase in the number of persons with incomplete paraplegia and a decrease in the number of persons with tetraplegia (NSCISC, 2003).

The NSCISC (2003) reports that the average yearly health care and living expenses (Table 23-1) and estimated lifetime costs (Table 23-2) that are directly attributable to SCI vary greatly according to the severity of the injury.

The life expectancies for persons with SCI continue to increase but are still below normal life expectancies for those with no SCI (Tables 23-3 and 23-4) (NSCISC, 2003). Mortality rates are significantly higher during the first year after injury (NSCISC, 2003). Due to medical advances, renal failure is no longer the leading cause of death for SCI patients. Among those individuals enrolled in the National Spinal Cord Injury Database of NSCISC since its inception in 1973, the cause of death has shifted to pneumonia, pulmonary emboli, and septicemia.

Acute and long-term survival rates for persons with SCI have improved in the last 50 years. The occurrence of secondary disabilities reduces survival, and the most significant prognostic factors related to survival are age and measures of injury severity such as neurologic level of injury, degree of injury completeness, and ventilator dependency. Pulmonary and cardiovascular conditions such as deep vein thrombosis, pulmonary embolus, and autonomic dysreflexia are also major causes of morbidity and mortality. Metabolic dysfunctions in SCI are associated with altered endocrine function, sedentary lifestyle, and impaired neurogenic influence. These include heterotopic ossification, osteoporosis, pathologic bone fractures, and immobilization hypercalcemia. Pressure ulcers are a frequent complication of SCI. Urinary tract infections are the most common secondary complication of SCI, and upper tract urologic complications are more threatening to long-term health and survival. Secondary neuromusculoskeletal disabilities include spasticity, contracture, pain, posttraumatic syringomyelia, osteoporosis with limb fracture, and heterotopic ossification. All SCI patients with

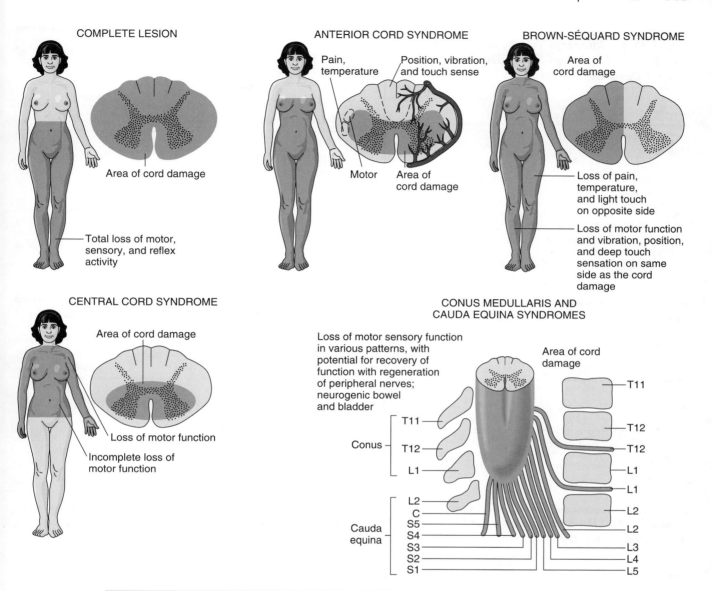

COMPLETE LESION

Area of cord damage

Total loss of motor, sensory, and reflex activity

ANTERIOR CORD SYNDROME

Pain, temperature

Position, vibration, and touch sense

Motor

Area of cord damage

BROWN-SÉQUARD SYNDROME

Area of cord damage

Loss of pain, temperature, and light touch on opposite side

Loss of motor function and vibration, position, and deep touch sensation on same side as the cord damage

CENTRAL CORD SYNDROME

Area of cord damage

Loss of motor function

Incomplete loss of motor function

CONUS MEDULLARIS AND CAUDA EQUINA SYNDROMES

Loss of motor sensory function in various patterns, with potential for recovery of function with regeneration of peripheral nerves; neurogenic bowel and bladder

Area of cord damage

Conus — T11, T12, L1

Cauda equina — L2, C, S5, S4, S3, S2, S1

T11, T12, T12, L1, L1, L2, L2, L3, L4, L5

Figure 23-1 Common spinal cord syndromes. (From Ignatavicius DD, Workman ML: *Medical-surgical nursing: critical thinking for collaborative care,* ed 4, Philadelphia, 2002, WB Saunders.)

neurologic deficit experience some change in sexual function and/or sexual health. Individual differences in the experience of disability make it difficult to generalize about psychological changes after SCI. Society generally devalues individuals with disabilities, however, and therefore they have a greater probability of experiencing depression and negative self-concept, body image, and self-esteem requiring resocialization. These secondary disabilities are major factors in the patient's quality of life, relationship to his or her family, and adaptation to a lifelong disability.

Current demographic data indicate that the proportion of Americans older than age 65 has increased to approxi-

mately 13%, and the age group 85 years of age and older is the fastest growing segment of this aging population. A trend in SCI is the increase in the proportion of those who were at least 61 years of age at injury. In the 1970s, 4.7% of persons in the NSCISC database were older than 60 years of age at injury, compared with 10% in the 1990s, and since 2000, this has increased to 11.4% of new injuries. Also, data for the 1990s revealed that approximately 25% of all individuals with SCI had survived for more than 20 years after the initial injury and were entering their fifth and sixth decades of life (Grudinskas and Nee, 2002).

Table 23-1 Average Yearly Health Care and Living Expenses for Individuals with Spinal Cord Injury (in 2000 Dollars)

Severity of Injury	First Year	Each Subsequent Year
High tetraplegia (C1-C4)	$626,588	$112,237
Low tetraplegia (C5-C8)	$404,653	$45,975
Paraplegia	$228,955	$23,297
Incomplete motor function at any level	$184,662	$12,941

From National Spinal Cord Injury Statistical Center, Spinal Cord Injury Information Network: *Spinal cord injury facts and figures at a glance*, Dec 2003, retrieved from *http://spinalcord.uab.edu/show.asp?durki= 21446* on Feb 8, 2004.

Table 23-2 Estimated Lifetime Costs of Spinal Cord Injury by Age at Injury (Discounted at 2%)

Severity of Injury	Age at Injury	
	25 Years	50 Years
High tetraplegia (C1-C4)	$2,393,507	$1,409,070
Low tetraplegia (C5-C8)	$1,353,360	$857,050
Paraplegia	$799,721	$545,460
Incomplete motor function at any level	$533,474	$386,619

From National Spinal Cord Injury Statistical Center, Spinal Cord Injury Information Network: *Spinal cord injury facts and figures at a glance*, Dec 2003, retrieved from *http://spinalcord.uab.edu/show.asp?durki= 21446* on Feb 8, 2004

Table 23-3 Life Expectancy for Persons with Spinal Cord (SCI) Injury Who Survive the First 24 Hours after Injury

Age at Injury	No SCI	Motor Functional at Any Level	Paraplegia	Low Tetraplegia (C5-C8)	High Tetraplegia (C1-C4)	Ventilator Dependent at Any Level
20 yr	57.8	52.9	45.3	40.5	36.0	16.3
40 yr	38.9	34.4	27.7	23.7	20.1	7.0
60 yr	21.6	17.8	12.7	10.0	7.7	1.3

From National Spinal Cord Injury Statistical Center, Spinal Cord Injury Information Network: *Spinal cord injury facts and figures at a glance*, Dec 2003, retrieved from *http://spinalcord.uab.edu/show.asp?durki=21446* on Feb 8, 2004.
NOTE: Figures are average remaining years of life.

Table 23-4 Life Expectancy for Persons with Spinal Cord Injury (SCI) Who Survive at Least 1 Year after Injury

Age at Injury	No SCI	Motor Functional at Any Level	Paraplegia	Low Tetraplegia (C5-C8)	High Tetraplegia (C1-C4)	Ventilator Dependent at Any Level
20 yr	57.8	53.4	46.0	41.8	38.2	23.3
40 yr	38.9	34.9	28.3	24.7	21.8	11.1
60 yr	21.6	18.2	13.2	10.7	8.8	2.9

From National Spinal Cord Injury Statistical Center, Spinal Cord Injury Information Network: *Spinal cord injury facts and figures at a glance*, Dec 2003, retrieved from *http://spinalcord.uab.edu/show.asp?durki=21446* on Feb 8, 2004.
NOTE: Figures are average remaining years of life.

ASSESSMENT

In addition to a physical examination of the spine, a comprehensive neurologic assessment is essential to establish baseline neurologic impairment and to determine rehabilitation goals for the individual with SCI. The neurologic assessment involves the examination of motor function, sensation, and reflex activity and is a shared responsibility of the health care team members, with the nurse integrating the findings into the nursing process (Evans and Love, 2001). The American Spinal Injury Association (ASIA) has

developed a classification system for grading muscle strength after SCI that makes possible standardized testing and reproducible examinations for research purposes, outcomes assessment, evaluation of progress, and classification of injures. The ASIA neurologic classification of motor and sensory status is presented in Figures 23-2 and 23-3. The ASIA's standardization of testing allows for competence in neurologic assessment, which ensures appropriate communication to patient and family by health care providers. The ASIA assessment should be performed on

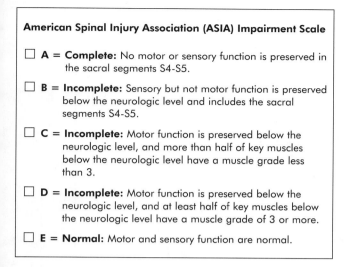

American Spinal Injury Association (ASIA) Impairment Scale

☐ **A = Complete:** No motor or sensory function is preserved in the sacral segments S4-S5.

☐ **B = Incomplete:** Sensory but not motor function is preserved below the neurologic level and includes the sacral segments S4-S5.

☐ **C = Incomplete:** Motor function is preserved below the neurologic level, and more than half of key muscles below the neurologic level have a muscle grade less than 3.

☐ **D = Incomplete:** Motor function is preserved below the neurologic level, and at least half of key muscles below the neurologic level have a muscle grade of 3 or more.

☐ **E = Normal:** Motor and sensory function are normal.

Figure 23-2 American Spinal Injury Association Impairment Scale. (From American Spinal Injury Association, *International standards for neurological functional classification of spinal cord injury patients [revised],* Chicago, 2002, American Spinal Injury Association.)

admission and postoperatively, and should be used to reassess for changes in condition (especially in cervical lesions) at least annually.

The ASIA Impairment Scale identifies SCI as complete or incomplete. Complete SCI is total disruption of the spinal cord with complete loss of motor and sensory function below the level of injury and is irreversible; tetraplegia results from lesions in the cervical region and paraplegia from lesions in the thoracic, lumbar, or sacral region. In incomplete SCI, motor and sensory functions below the level of the lesion are preserved. Consequences of traumatic SCI may be manifested as the ASIA-defined clinical syndromes or as vertebral fractures, as follows (Barker, 2001a, 2001b, 2002):

Anterior cord injury (see Figure 23-1)—Nursing assessment and considerations should focus on signs and symptoms of immediate motor loss below the level of injury, loss of pain and temperature sensation below the level of injury, and sensations of touch, proprioception, and vibration that remain intact.

Brown-Séquard syndrome (see Figure 23-1)—Nursing assessment and considerations should focus on motor and sensory deficits below the level of injury; bowel, bladder, and sexual functions; and ambulation and functional recovery potential.

Central cord syndrome (see Figure 23-1)—Nursing assessment and considerations should focus on motor and sensory changes including sacral sparing; degree of spinal tract damage and/or recovery; bowel, bladder, and

sexual functions; resolution of edema during recovery with progressive return of function; supportive care in recognition of loss of hand and arm function; and safety factors and prevention of injury during ambulation due to spasticity and inability to guard with upper extremities in a fall.

Cauda equina syndrome (see Figure 23-1)—Nursing assessment and considerations should focus on the subjective complaints of pain and tingling of the legs; changes in bowel, bladder, and sexual functions; sacral paresthesia; hematoma at site of lumbar surgery; sudden loss of function at the level of a herniated disc; absent or diminished reflexes; and peripheral nerve regeneration, which makes some recovery possible under ideal situations.

Conus (sacral cord) medullaris syndrome (see Figure 23-1)—Nursing assessment and considerations should focus on the areflexic bladder, bowel, lower limbs, and sexual function.

Vertebral injuries—Nursing assessment and considerations should focus on vulnerability to fracture and damage from trauma and the aging process as well as the combination of the two.

The neurologic assessment should begin with the determination of level of consciousness, along with consideration of factors that may influence the data, such as cognitive impairment, head injury, chemical impairment, or hypothermia. A mental status examination should be performed and the responses quantified using the Glasgow Coma Scale. The cranial nerve assessment and the neurologic level of injury or impairment based on the motor and sensory response of the ASIA should be evaluated. Determining the awareness of reflex activity below the level of injury, particularly of the perianal reflexes, helps in formulating diagnosis, prognosis, and the treatment plan; management of bladder, bowel, and sexual dysfunction are specifically influenced by these findings (Evans and Love, 2001). In addition to this assessment, common diagnostic tests to evaluate level and/or type of SCI may be performed (Box 23-1).

Because of the demographic shift to an increase in the number of people over age 65 and an increase in the proportion of people over age 60 sustaining an SCI, it is essential to use comprehensive tools and methods to collect assessment data and to develop appropriate plans of care. To facilitate a comprehensive assessment of individuals with an SCI who are aging, a geriatric functional health pattern tool was developed by the Veterans Administration Boston Healthcare System, West Roxbury Campus, for collecting pertinent data and establishing an appropriate plan of care. With the trends in health care and aging, and the escalating costs associated with living with a chronic and debilitating injury, an understanding of the trajectory of aging and its impact on structure and function is of paramount importance (Grudinskas and Nee, 2002).

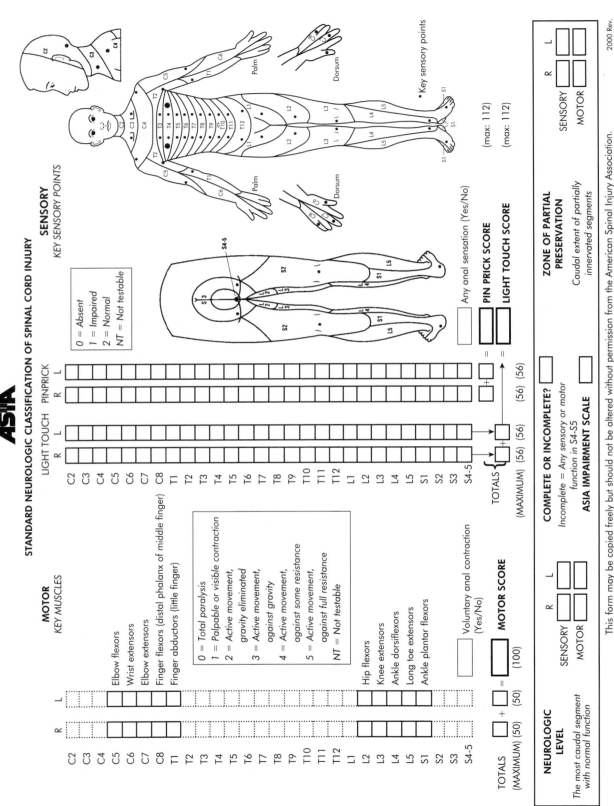

Figure 23-3 Standard neurologic classification of spinal cord injury. (From American Spinal Injury Association, *International standards for neurological functional classification of spinal*

PATHOPHYSIOLOGY

The spinal cord begins where nerve tissue exits the skull at the foramen magnum. It tapers along the cervical, thoracic, lumbar, and sacral regions and ends in the conus medullaris at the level between the first and second lumbar vertebrae. The spinal cord has 31 segments, and each has a pair of spinal nerves. The spinal cord also serves as a center for spinal reflexes, knee-jerk reflex, and withdrawal reflex.

The spinal cord conducts nerve impulses between the brain and parts of the body outside the central nervous system through two types of nerve tract (Figure 23-4). Ascending tracts transmit motor impulses and sensory information from the body parts to the brain. Descending tracts transmit motor impulses from the brain to the muscles and glands. The nerve tracts are further delineated in terms of function.

Ascending Tracts

The fasciculus gracilis and fasciculus cuneatus conduct sensory impulses from skin, muscles, tendons, and joints to the brain. Sensations of touch, pressure, and body movement are interpreted. These nerve fibers decussate (cross over) at the medulla oblongata; therefore, impulses originating on the left side of the body are interpreted by the right side of the brain.

The lateral and ventral spinothalamic tracts conduct impulses to the brain that are interpreted as sensations of pain and temperature. These nerve fibers decussate.

The fibers of the dorsal spinocerebellar tract do not decussate; those of the ventral spinocerebellar tract do cross over. These tracts transmit impulses from the legs and trunk and allow for coordination of muscular movement.

Descending Tracts

The lateral and ventral corticospinal tracts conduct motor impulses from the brain to spinal nerves and then to skeletal muscles. They are also called pyramidal tracts and function to control voluntary movement.

The lateral, anterior, and medial reticulospinal tracts transmit motor impulses from the brain and control muscle

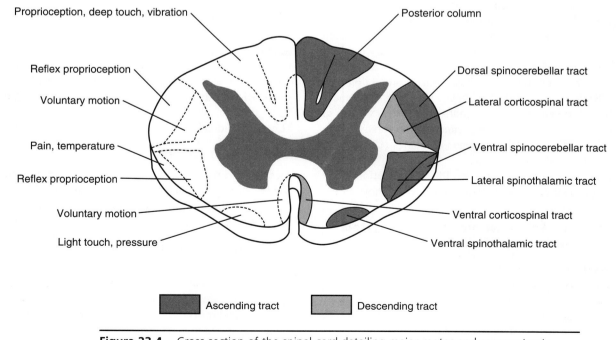

Proprioception, deep touch, vibration

Reflex proprioception

Voluntary motion

Pain, temperature

Reflex proprioception

Voluntary motion

Light touch, pressure

Posterior column

Dorsal spinocerebellar tract

Lateral corticospinal tract

Ventral spinocerebellar tract

Lateral spinothalamic tract

Ventral corticospinal tract

Ventral spinothalamic tract

■ Ascending tract   ■ Descending tract

Figure 23-4   Cross section of the spinal cord detailing major motor and sensory tracts.

tone and the sweat glands. They are also called extrapyramidal tracts.

The rubrospinal tract carries motor impulses from the brain to skeletal muscles and assists with muscular coordination and posture control.

Spinal Nerves

Thirty-one pairs of spinal nerves emerge from the spinal cord (Box 23-2 and Figure 23-5). In early childhood the spinal cord extends the length of the vertebral column, but as the individual ages the column grows and the spinal cord ends at the space between the first and second lumbar vertebrae. A spinal nerve injury may occur during birth, as a result of an accident, or from pressure caused by a tumor in a surrounding area. Injuries that occur in the cervical plexus result in headache and pain in the neck; injury to the brachial plexus may lead to thoracic outlet syndrome, which causes constant pain in the neck, shoulder, or arm. Thoracic outlet syndrome may also be caused by congenital malformations and may limit or restrict shoulder and arm movement. Each spinal nerve has two roots: motor and sensory (see Figure 23-4). The anterior root carries nerve impulses away from the central nervous system in motor (efferent) fibers that cause skeletal muscles to contract. The posterior root carries nerve impulses to the central nervous system in sensory (afferent) fibers that communicate pain, touch, vibration, and temperature.

CLINICAL MANIFESTATIONS OF SECONDARY DISABILITIES

Once the person with an SCI has undergone acute treatment and rehabilitation, the effects of the SCI may result in secondary disabilities or the occurrence of autonomic dysreflexia (Consortium for Spinal Cord Medicine, 2001). Public health officials are supporting efforts to prevent secondary disabilities (Wilber et al, 2002). Prevention of secondary disabilities is also the focus of community-based health promotion programs (Rimmer and Braddock, 2002). However, differences in patient characteristics, in the course of medical events, in psychological, social, and environmental supports, and in cognitive abilities strongly influence outcomes (Consortium for Spinal Cord Medicine, 1999).

Secondary disabilities are health complications that cause additional functional difficulties beyond those of the

original injury (Sparks, 2001). Secondary disabilities are related to the effects of aging with an SCI and to the physiologic changes that accompany paralysis, including losses in sensation, movement, bone density, and bowel and bladder function (Menter and Hudson, 1995). Some secondary disabilities increase with age; these include pneumonia, contractures, pressure ulcers, acquired scoliosis, pain, and dependence in self-care activities. Other secondary disabilities, such as spasticity, fevers, and urinary tract infections, decrease with age (Menter and Hudson, 1995). In addition, persons with SCI may experience physical barriers in accessing preventive health care such as screening mammograms or gynecologic care (Welner, Simon, and Welner, 2002). In the discussion that follows, secondary disabil-ities are grouped into five areas—cardiovascular and cardiopulmonary, genitourinary and gastrointestinal, neuromusculoskeletal, psychosocial, and skin—and the essential elements necessary for the prevention and management of secondary disabilities in the SCI population are described.

Cardiovascular and Cardiopulmonary Secondary Disabilities

Cardiovascular secondary disabilities include pulmonary embolus, autonomic dysreflexia, reflex sympathetic dystrophy, and deep vein thrombosis. Persons with SCI are at greater risk of heart disease due to autonomic nervous system changes and hazards of immobility. If there was preexisting cardiac disease, an aggressive cardiac prevention program must be implemented. Cardiopulmonary secondary disabilities include pneumonia, aspiration, atelectasis, and ventilatory failure.

Pulmonary Embolus

Pulmonary embolus is the sudden occlusion of a pulmonary artery, which decreases blood supply to the lung. A frequent cause is a thromboembolus from the right side of the heart. Pulmonary embolus is common with deep vein thrombosis. Risk factors include blood stasis, immobility, trauma, heart disease, obesity, age, and use of oral contraceptives (LeMone and Burke, 1999).

Deep Vein Thrombosis

Deep vein thrombosis is the formation of a clot in the deep veins causing complete or partial occlusion of blood flow. The primary cause is venous stasis; trauma and increased blood coagulation may also cause deep vein thrombosis.

Reflex Sympathetic Dystrophy

Reflex sympathetic dystrophy is pain and autonomic dysfunction in the shoulder, hand, and arm of the affected side. Clinical manifestations include edema, pain, and altered sweating and skin color; later there is atrophy of the skin and bone and a contracture forms. The condition is also called shoulder-hand syndrome.

Box 23-2   Spinal Nerves and Associated Groups of Vertebrae

■ Cervical nerves: 8 pairs, C1 to C8
■ Thoracic nerves: 12 pairs, T1 to T12
■ Lumbar nerves: 5 pairs, L1 to L5
■ Sacral nerves: 5 pairs, S1 to S5
■ Coccygeal nerves: 1 pair

Spinal Cord Injury Functional Activity Chart

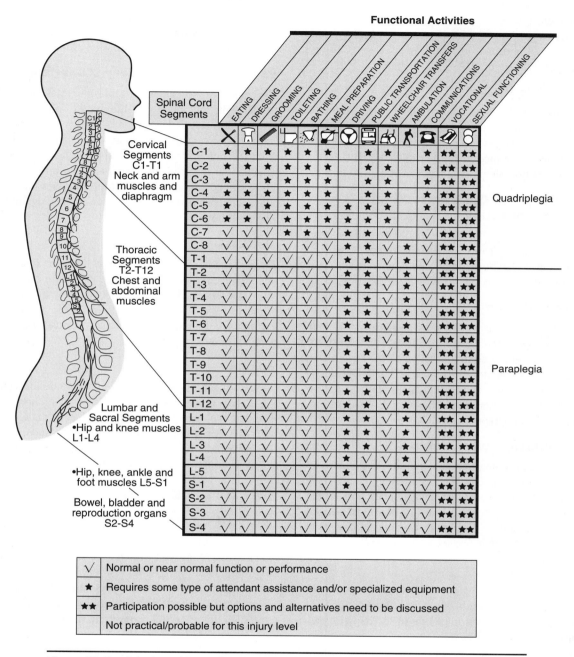

Figure 23-5 Spinal cord injury functional activity chart. (From Murphy M: Traumatic spinal cord injury: an acute care rehabilitation perspective, *Crit Care Nurs Q* 22[2]:51, 1999.)

Pneumonia

Pneumonia is infection of the lung parenchyma by bacteria, viruses, fungi, or protozoa (infectious pneumonia) or aspiration or inhalation of toxic gases (noninfectious pneumonia) (LeMone and Burke, 1999). Its frequency depends on the level of injury; the incidence is lowest in incomplete paraplegia. Patients with nontraumatic SCI have an incidence of 2.6%; those with traumatic SCI have an incidence of 26.6% (McKinley, Tewksbury, and Godbout, 2002). Identification and treatment of respiratory complications may reduce morbidity and mortality (Lanig and Peterson, 2000).

Atelectasis

Atelectasis is incomplete expansion or collapse of lung tissue. The incidence increases as the level of injury increases. With complete tetraplegia the incidence averages 2.6%; the incidence does not appear to increase as years since injury increase (Ragnarsson et al, 1995).

Ventilator Failure

Ventilator failure is the need for partial or total ventilator support for longer than 7 days. Ventilator failure is associated with the level of injury. The incidence is lowest in paraplegia, less than 1% in incomplete tetraplegia, and 0.5% to 2.3% in complete tetraplegia (Ragnarsson et al, 1995).

Genitourinary and Gastrointestinal Secondary Disabilities

Genitourinary secondary disabilities include urinary tract infections and upper tract urologic complications. Gastrointestinal secondary disabilities include gallstone disease, esophageal dysfunction, and altered bowel elimination.

Urinary Tract Infection

Urinary tract infection is defined as bacteriuria (colony count of 1 to 100,000 colonies or more than 100,000 colonies). It is the most common secondary complication after discharge from acute care. Trautner and Darouiche (2002) report that "antiinfective catheter materials, antibiotics, and antiseptic agents are not beneficial for long-term prevention of UTI in persons with SCI" (p. 283).

Upper Tract Urinary Complications

Upper tract urinary complications include vesicoureteral reflux, hydronephrosis, pyelocaliectasis, renal calculi, renal and perirenal infection, and renal insufficiency and failure (Cardenas et al, 1995). Renal calculi are the most serious complication. Incidence is higher in individuals with indwelling catheters and increases with an increase in the years since SCI.

Gallstone Disease

Gallstone disease, or cholelithiasis (formation of stones or calculi), can lead to obstruction of bile in the hepatic, cystic, or common bile duct. Cholecystitis is inflammation of the gallbladder. Clinical manifestations include abdominal pain or cramping (which may be referred to the subscapular area), nausea, vomiting, bile reflux and jaundice, pancreatitis, intolerance of fatty foods, fever, and changes in laboratory test results (high white blood count and elevated levels of serum bilirubin, alkaline phosphatase, and serum amylase).

Esophageal Dysfunction

Esophageal dysfunction includes esophagitis, heartburn, and dysphagia.

Altered Bowel Elimination

Altered bowel elimination may be related to poor dietary management, chronic constipation or bowel incontinence, or impaired transit time (Cardenas et al, 1995; Consortium for Spinal Cord Medicine, 1998b).

Psychosocial Secondary Disabilities

Psychosocial secondary disabilities relate to adaptation, adjustment, and quality-of-life issues following SCI. Psychosocial rehabilitation models of care address behavioral and psychological adaptation to disability (Antai-Otong, 2003). Employment, marital status, living arrangements, and educational level all influence, and are influenced by, psychosocial adjustment. This section discusses three psychosocial secondary disabilities: depression, suicide, and impaired coping following SCI.

Depression

Depression has been identified as the most frequent postinjury diagnosis and usually appears within the first month. The depression has been associated with the profound impact of the SCI on the individual's life and the period of enforced helplessness after injury (Consortium for Spinal Cord Medicine, 1998a).

Suicide

Suicide is taking one's own life. For some individuals with SCI, the suicide attempt may be obvious (substance abuse, accidents) or may be related to self-neglect (failure to maintain the skin or to maintain nutritional balance) or refusal of necessary care (such as operations or rehabilitation). Suicide is more common during the first few years after injury; rates are similar to those in the rest of the population after 5 to 10 years (Dijkers et al, 1995).

Impaired Coping

Impaired coping is difficulty in learning to adapt and adjust to changes. Quality of life and life satisfaction generally are high in persons with SCI. Preinjury personality, availability of social support systems, and quality of rehabilitation are related to the patient's coping abilities and level of satisfaction with life after SCI. Long-term management and follow-up are needed to enhance coping, socialization, and adjustment. A recent study indicates that 41% of persons with SCI may have lower life satisfaction scores than those without SCI (Kemp and Krause, 1999).

Skin Secondary Disabilities

Skin secondary disabilities include pressure ulcers, skin tears, and abrasions. Up to 85% of persons with SCI develop a pressure ulcer during their lifetimes (Mahoney, 2001). An evaluation instrument developed specifically for persons with SCI is the Pressure Ulcer Risk Assessment Scale (Salzberg et al, 1998). In addition to pressure, other major risk factors for pressure ulcer include serum albumin level of less than 3.5 dl and the presence of friction, and shearing forces.

Neuromusculoskeletal Secondary Disabilities

Neurologic secondary disabilities include autonomic dysreflexia, spasticity, syringomyelia, and pain. Musculoskeletal secondary disabilities include contractures, heterotopic ossification, osteoporosis, and fractures. Shoulder pain due to overuse is common in persons with SCI.

Autonomic Dysreflexia

Autonomic dysreflexia (Figure 23-6), a medical emergency, can lead to stroke or seizures due to severe hypertension. This emergency can be fatal. Persons with SCI above the T6 level are susceptible to this condition, which is caused by high-level sympathetic discharge in response to a stimulus below the level of the SCI. Signs and symptoms include any or all of the following: pounding headache; flushing and sweating of the skin, especially the head and neck area; sys-

tolic blood pressure above 140 mm Hg; chills; goose bumps; nasal congestion; irritability or feeling of apprehension; and slowing of heart rate. Some of the common causes are distended bladder or bowel (constipation), pressure ulcer, fracture, burns, urinary tract infection, ingrown toenail, or any procedure causing pain or discomfort below the level of the person's injury.

Spasticity

Spasticity is hyperactivity of deep tendon reflexes and increased muscle tone, and is expected because of the pathophysiology of injury to the spinal cord above the conus medullaris (Maynard et al, 1995). Spasticity has some benefit for health and functioning. It becomes problematic when it is severe enough to require medication or surgical treatment. Spasticity occurs before discharge from initial hospitalization in 32.2% of persons listed in the National Spinal Cord Injury Database of NSCISC, increases to 42.7% by the end of the first year after injury, and decreases to 35% by 10 years after injury (Maynard et al, 1995).

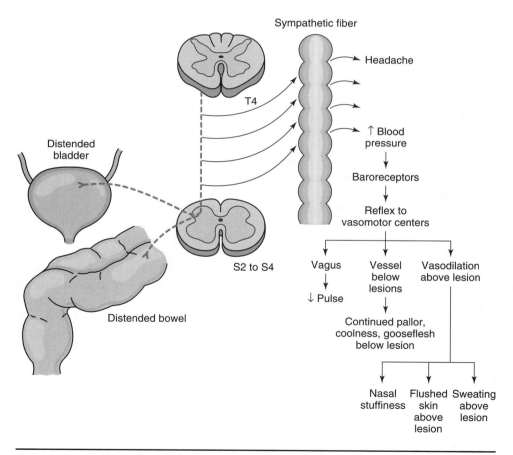

Figure 23-6   Causes and results of autonomic dysreflexia. (From Phipps W et al: *Medical-surgical nursing: health and illness perspectives,* ed 7, St Louis, 2003, Mosby, p 1426.)

Syringomyelia

Syringomyelia is the presence of a fluid-filled cystic cavity in the central intramedullary gray matter. Syringomyelia causes pain, motor weakness and loss of sensation, and spasticity. The condition may be treated with surgical drainage and/or placement of permanent shunts. Incidence of symptomatic syringomyelia varies from 1% to 3%; incidence may be as high as 67% for cysts with no symptoms (Maynard et al, 1995). More research is needed to determine the natural course of these cysts and their development into symptomatic cysts.

Pain

Pain may be neurogenic or musculoskeletal. The symptoms of neurogenic pain (central pain, phantom pain, deafferentation pain, dysesthetic pain, central dysesthetic syndrome, spinal cord pain) include burning, tingling, or aching diffuse pain below the level of injury (Maynard et al, 1995). Pain impulses ascend within the lateral spinothalamic tract to the thalamus and cerebral cortex, where the perception of pain is mediated. The presence of neurogenic pain lowers quality of life. Musculoskeletal pain is more common in the shoulder and hand than in the wrist. Pain management options include nonpharmacologic measures such as guided imagery, diversional activities, relaxation techniques, hypnosis, acupuncture, and meditation.

Contracture

Contracture is permanent shortening of connective tissue. After contracture develops, the inelasticity limits body movement. Preventive measures include proper positioning and repositioning, splinting, and regular range-of-motion and stretching exercises. Contracture is considered a preventable complication of SCI, and rates are lower in patients treated in Model Spinal Cord Injury Systems. Incidence increases with time since injury, with higher rates seen in tetraplegia and in those with spasticity and heterotopic ossification (Maynard et al, 1995).

Heterotopic Ossification

Heterotopic ossification is an accumulation of calcium, especially in joints distal to the level of injury such as the hips and knees. It restricts joint range of motion, limits functional abilities, and may lead to pressure ulcers. Treatment is with disodium etidronate, early initiation of stretching exercises, joint range-of-motion exercises, and avoidance of flexion positions. Antiinflammatory agents may be of some benefit. Incidence is 16% to 53% of persons with SCI (Mahoney, 2001).

Osteoporosis

Osteoporosis is a metabolic bone disorder in which bone resorption proceeds at a higher rate than bone formation. Bone mass is reduced, risk for bone fracture increases, and other degenerative changes take place. Cases of osteoporosis resulting in fractures are coded in the National Spinal Cord Injury Database of NSCISC; estimated incidence is approximately 1%, which is probably a low figure. Rapid bone loss occurs early after injury; bone loss increases over time and with aging.

Immobilization Hypercalcemia

Immobilization hypercalcemia is increased reabsorption of calcium from bones that leads to muscle weakness, fatigue, altered mental status, ataxia, personality changes, decrease in level of consciousness, abdominal pain, nausea and vomiting, constipation, weight loss, and dysrhythmias. The condition is treated with a low-calcium diet and administration of calcitonin; acute therapy is with intravenous sodium phosphate or potassium phosphate.

Acquired Scoliosis

Acquired scoliosis is a lateral curvature of the spine that occurs after an injury. It may lead to pain, shortness of breath, and gastrointestinal disturbances. Scoliosis is treated with braces, electrical stimulation, and traction in young patients and with weight reduction, active and passive exercises, and braces in adults. Metal straightening rods may be inserted surgically to reduce the curvature and provide rotational stability.

Fracture

Fracture is a break in the continuity of a bone that results from trauma or disease (such as cancer or osteoporosis). Fracture is classified as open or closed, complete or incomplete, and stable or unstable. The most common site of fracture in a person with SCI is the femur.

DIAGNOSIS

Diagnosis is based on patient history, assessment data, and results of diagnostic tests to evaluate level and/or type of SCI (see Box 23-1). Other diagnostic studies include chest radiography, electrocardiography, lung scanning (perfusion and ventilation), pulmonary angiography, pulse oximetry, arterial blood gas levels, and blood coagulation studies (activated partial thromboplastin time and prothrombin time). Based on the assessment of presenting signs and symptoms, appropriate diagnostic studies are included. Trauma to the spinal cord is classified as closed or direct (open) trauma. Automobile accidents, falls, and injuries sustained in sports such as diving, skiing, football, and soccer result in closed injuries; gunshot wounds and stab wounds are examples of direct trauma.

INTERDISCIPLINARY CARE

Because of the complexity and severity of SCI, appropriate care is best provided through the interdisciplinary team. The overwhelming majority of individuals with SCI are discharged to private residences within the community (96% of those treated at Model Spinal Cord Injury Systems and 90% of individuals treated at facilities subscribing to the Uniform Data System) (Consortium for Spinal Cord Medicine, 1999). To foster discharge and maintain these individuals in the community, an interdisciplinary approach is imperative. Under optimal circumstances, the management goals reflect expected functional outcomes in the areas of mobility, performance of instrumental and other activities of daily living, and communication skills (see Table 23-5). To optimize achievement of the goals, an interdisciplinary approach to care must be achieved. Immobility contributes to many of the secondary disabilities experienced by individuals with SCI. The short-term goal of the team is to minimize the effects of immobility and the long-term goal is to prevent or treat complications of immobility.

Drug Therapy

The medical provider may prescribe corticosteroids such as dexamethasone (Decadron) for their antiinflammatory and edema-reducing effects, although corticosteroids may interfere with health. Atropine is used to treat bradycardia if the pulse falls below 50 beats per minute. For patients with severe muscle spasticity (usually those with upper motor neuron injuries), medications are given to help control spasticity. During the chronic phase of SCI, many patients experience pain, and a drug therapy program must be tailored to the individual. Pharmacologic agents are used to treat specific autonomic dysfunction such as gastrointestinal hyperactivity, bleeding, bradycardia, orthostatic hypotension, inadequate emptying of the bladder, and autonomic dysreflexia. Other drugs to prevent or treat complications of immobility may be needed, such as bowel and bladder maintenance therapies.

Diet Therapy

The dietitian provides a comprehensive assessment of nutritional needs and prescribes a program that helps the patient to maintain an ideal body weight and promotes bowel and bladder elimination. The dietitian addresses any possible complications, such as outlining procedures to follow if problems such as diarrhea or infection develop.

Nursing

As leader of the health care team, the nurse must perform a comprehensive assessment of the patient's functional disability, environment, and family and support system. The nurse helps the patient learn self-care, mobility skills, bladder management (intermittent catheterization), and bowel retraining. The nurse, in collaboration with the therapists, instructs the caregiver in procedures for accomplishing the activities of daily living, such as transfer, feeding, bathing,

dressing, positioning, and skin care, as appropriate. In addition, the nurse consults with the dietitian regarding nutritional education at the time of discharge, teaches the patient about his or her drug therapy, and addresses issues of sexuality and self-image.

Medical Management

The medical management of the patient with SCI depends on the type of injury and the presence of any other associated injuries. Treatment may be surgical, nonsurgical, or a combination of both. In chronic disease management, the physician's role is to minimize or prevent secondary disabilities and provide drug therapy and referrals as needed.

Physical Therapy

The physical therapist, in collaboration with the nurse and occupational therapist, determines the most appropriate positioning and exercise techniques, assesses the need for hand and wrist splints, and develops a plan to prevent foot drop. To maintain and improve physical mobility and activity skills, the physical therapist performs isometric and isotonic exercises and instructs the caregiver in their use as appropriate. The physical and occupational therapists collaborate in developing an exercise program and defining adaptive equipment needs. The use of lower limb functional electric stimulation can improve lower limb strength and outcomes (Phillips et al, 1998). The physical therapist encourages activity to the patient's tolerance level to facilitate optimal independence.

Occupational Therapy

In the chronic stage of SCI, the occupational therapist tries to establish a balance among self-care, leisure, and productivity. Specht et al (2002) report that involvement in leisure activity provides mental and physical health benefits, enjoyment, opportunity to develop a self-concept and increase self-esteem, and opportunities to build and enhance social relationships. Recent advances in neuroprosthetics include Food and Drug Administration approval of the NeuroControl Freehand System, a surgically implanted device for people with tetraplegia that restores the ability to grasp, hold, and release objects of various sizes. For individuals who retain the ability to use the shoulder, upper arm, and elbow, have adequate range of motion and hand muscles that respond to electrical impulses, and have mature skeletons, this device provides a functional hand grasp. In addition to complex treatments, the occupational therapist provides orienting materials (clock, radio, and calendar) and encourages contact with staff, family, and friends.

Medical Social Work

The medical social worker assesses the patient, family, and caregiver to determine their ability to meet the patient's psychosocial and financial needs. The medical social worker is a key player in obtaining adaptive devices and assessing the home environment to ensure that it is free from hazards and can accommodate the patient's special needs (e.g., a wheelchair). Because of the escalating costs of care, the medical social worker assists the patient in obtaining the resources to support high-quality care and achieve outcomes that promote health. Providing the patient's family with counseling on how to avoid promoting dependency is an essential role. The medical social worker provides referrals for vocational rehabilitation and assists with placement in adapted work settings.

COMPLEMENTARY AND ALTERNATIVE THERAPY

Massage therapy is a treatment modality that assists the patient and caregivers in the management of muscle spasms and provides stimulation to improve circulation. Many massage techniques exist, such as moving the hands or fingers over the skin slowly or briskly with long strokes or in circles (superficial massage) and applying firm pressure to the skin to maintain contact while massaging the underlying tissues (deep massage).

Think S for Success

Symptoms
■ Manage symptoms with appropriate medications and treatment modalities.

Sequelae
■ Prevent secondary disabilities and promote independence.

Safety
■ Teach patient, family, and caregiver the importance of intervention for signs and symptoms of autonomic dysreflexia.

Support/Services
■ Assist patient with finances or community reintegration if needed.
■ Assist patient in coping with body changes if needed.
■ Arrange for patient to receive counseling and vocational retraining if needed. Encourage frank discussion about fears and concerns.
■ Make appropriate referrals.

Satisfaction
■ Determine degree to which spinal cord injury is interfering with important aspects of patient's life and develop a plan to help patient reach or maintain desired quality of life.

FAMILY AND CAREGIVER ISSUES

A chronic illness or disability such as SCI causes a profound life change for the injured person, the family, and the designated caregiver and may place the patient in a dependent relationship with family and caregivers (Canave-Jimenez, 2001). Role change and immobility issues are physically and mentally stressful and require new coping skills and strategies. The recommendation is that the patient avoid using family members as caregivers if possible. Spouses, parents, or siblings can offer emotional support, but their role may get blurred or confused if they are also the caregivers (Parsa, 1999). Being a caregiver can be stressful.

Because of the nature of the dependence in SCI, the patient may need to hire a caregiver. This patient population is vulnerable to abusive relationships, and a thorough background check of prospective caregivers must be performed. The patient must be sensitive to the risk for becoming a victim of physical, verbal, emotional, sexual, and/or financial abuse.

Parsa (1999) has identified elements of domestic abuse and provided guidelines for avoiding relationships that may lead to abusive behaviors. Patients with spinal cord impairment may be at higher risk of becoming a victim of abuse because of the following:

■ Decreased strength and mobility
■ Dependence on others for personal care
■ Decreased or increased financial resources
■ Increased alcohol or drug misuse
■ Loss of control over the environment
■ Depression
■ Low self-esteem
■ Limited availability of in-home services
■ Lack of housing options

Caring for a patient with SCI requires much time and effort; it can be physically and emotionally draining. This can cause caregivers to experience considerable stress, especially when they must also cope with problems involving the family, finances, personal health, and so on. Increasing levels of stress can lead to caregiver burnout. At its extreme, this can lead to neglect or emotional or physical abuse. An intervention plan to reduce stress can include the following (Ward and Parsons, 2000):

■ Engaging in cognitive restructuring—finding a benefit in a stressful event
■ Increasing knowledge of SCI issues, which can reduce feelings of inadequacy and powerlessness
■ Identifying the things that cannot be changed and setting them aside as uncontrollable
■ Taking time for leisure to relax and energize
■ Finding quiet time
■ Interacting with others—talking it out and getting it off one's chest

Those who care for other people can do a better job of caregiving if time and attention are also given to their own personal needs.

ETHICAL CONSIDERATIONS

The quality-of-life changes that confront an SCI patient present the health care team, family, and patient with many ethical issues. Recognition of the patient's autonomy in determining treatment and extent of care has become part of the patient's rights in the decision making regarding his or her care. Bioethical dilemmas and uncertainties occur with this shift of autonomy to the patient through the "reaffirmation of informed consent and decisional capacity of the patient defined in legal documents such as durable power of attorney for health care and living wills" (Lemke, 2001, p. 68). The dilemma becomes even more apparent when there is a difference of opinion between the patient and the health care provider.

The nurse is in a unique position to provide for the patient's physical needs as well for the emotional needs of the patient and family. In this bonding process, it is important for "nurses to be aware of their own bias and to realize that rehabilitation is a voluntary choice and that the individual cannot be forced to complete the program" (Lemke, 2001, p. 72). "The request to discontinue care for a patient who is cognitively intact, nonterminal, and disabled is related to his/her perception of benefits versus burdens, placing his/her death as a better option" (Lemke, 2001, p. 69). Most patients choose life with disability and survive, but a few choose not to live with the disability, and the nurse must respect the patient's decision and be an advocate for the patient's decision making. Legal and ethical standards must be followed in the patient's, family's, and institution's decision processes.

Ventilator care and the issue of "removing a ventilator is possibly responsible for more right to die cases than any other treatment" (Rundquist, 2002, p. 7). The ethical principles of autonomy (the patient's right to determine the course of action), beneficence (protection from harm), nonmaleficence (the responsibility to do no harm), and veracity (telling the truth) are all involved and may be in conflict with each other in the determination of such cases. Ethics committees and the legal system are important resources available to assist in resolving the conflict for the patient, family, and health care provider.

CASE STUDY

Patient Data

Mr. G. is a 45-year-old Mexican American who had a motorcycle accident 10 years previously that resulted in complete paraplegia at the T10 level. He is independent in all activities, has been married for 24 years, and has three children (boys 13 and 14 years of age, a girl 17 years of age). He is employed as a computer programmer, uses an electric wheelchair, and drives an adapted personal vehicle. His Functional Independence Measure score has recently decreased from his baseline level of 106 to 99. The decrease is especially significant in the area of motor function, and he has become more dependent in the areas of self-care, sphincter control, mobility, and locomotion; his scores have remained stable in the cognitive areas. On examination, he is noted to have urinary retention, jaundice, and spasticity. He also complains of nausea and intolerance of fatty foods. His wife is concerned because he has stopped participating in his weekly poker game with friends and no longer accompanies her to school activities related to their children or to church.

Diagnostic Findings

- Hemoglobin level: 11 g/dl
- Hematocrit: 34%
- White blood count: 20,000/mm³
- Alkaline phosphatase level: 120 U/L
- Serum bilirubin level (total): 1.8 mg/dl

Thinking It Through

- As the primary nurse for this patient, what other assessment data will you need to assist Mr. G. in maintaining and restoring his health?
- What secondary disabilities may be present? Provide a rationale for your choices.
- How can the health care team contribute to Mr. G.'s quality of life?
- What nursing diagnoses pertain to Mr. G.?

Case Conference

The interdisciplinary team that has gathered to discuss and plan Mr. G.'s care includes the medical internist, neurologist, nurse, physical therapist, occupational therapist, medical social worker, psychologist, Mr. G., and his wife.

The medical internist and neurologist have discussed the need to admit Mr. G. to the hospital for further evaluation. Mr. G. expresses concern about the family's finances and the cost of the hospitalization because of his insurance coverage. Mrs. G. begins to cry.

The nurse, who has been working with this family for the last 5 years, leads the discussion to obtain more diagnostic information. Mr. G. speaks of his increase in alcohol consumption to cope with the stress at work and his fear of losing his job. He discusses the increasing cost of maintaining his household with three teenagers and his inability to increase his income. He is very

Internet and Other Resources

American Association of Spinal Cord Injury Nurses (AASCIN): *http://www.aascin.org*

American Association of Spinal Cord Injury Psychologist and Social Workers (AASCIPSW): *http://www.aascipsw.org*

American Paraplegia Society (APS): *http://www.apssci.org*

American Physical Therapy Association (APTA): *http://www.apta.org*

American Spinal Injury Association (ASIA): *http://www.asiaspinalinjury.org*

Christopher Reeve Paralysis Foundation: *http://www.ChristopherReeve.org*

International Spinal Cord Society (ISCoS): *http://www.iscos.org.uk*

MEDLINEplus: *http://www.nlm.nih.gov/medlineplus*

Model Spinal Cord Care Systems (MSCIS): *http://www.spinalcord.uab.edu/*

National Rehabilitation Information Center: *http://www.naric.com*

National Spinal Cord Injury Association (NSCIA): *http://www.spinalcord.org*

Paralyzed Veterans of America (PVA): *http://www.pva.org*

United Spinal Association (formerly Eastern Paralyzed Veterans Association): *http://www.unitedspinal.org*

REFERENCES

Antai-Otong D: Psychosocial rehabilitation, *Nurs Clin North Am* 38(1):151-60, 2003.

Barker E: Anatomy and physiology of the spine and spinal cord. In Nelson A, editor: Nursing practice related to spinal cord injury and disorders: a core curriculum, New York, 2001a, Eastern Paralyzed Veterans Association, pp 65-80.

Barker E: Consequences of traumatic spinal cord injury. In Nelson A, editor: *Nursing practice related to spinal cord injury and disorders: a core curriculum,* New York, 2001b, Eastern Paralyzed Veterans Association, pp 81-8.

Barker E: *Neuroscience nursing: a spectrum of care,* ed 2, St Louis, 2002, Mosby.

Canave-Jimenez F: Caregivers: training and support. In Nelson A, editor: *Nursing practice related to spinal cord injury and disorders: a core curriculum,* New York, 2001, Eastern Paralyzed Veterans Association, pp 423-40.

Cardenas D et al: Management of gastrointestinal, genitourinary, and sexual function. In Lanig IS et al, editors: *A practical guide to health promotion after spinal cord injury,* Gaithersburg, Md, 1995, Aspen, pp 120-44.

Consortium for Spinal Cord Medicine: *Depression following spinal cord injury: a clinical practice guideline for primary care physicians,* Washington, DC, 1998a, Paralyzed Veterans of America.

Consortium for Spinal Cord Medicine: *Neurogenic bowel management in adults with spinal cord injury,* Washington, DC, 1998b, Paralyzed Veterans of America.

Consortium for Spinal Cord Medicine: *Outcomes following traumatic spinal cord injury: clinical practice guidelines for health-care professionals,* Washington, DC, 1999, Paralyzed Veterans of America.

Consortium for Spinal Cord Medicine: *Acute management of autonomic dysreflexia: clinical practice guidelines,* ed 2, Washington, DC, 2001, Paralyzed Veterans of America.

Dijkers M et al: The aftermath of spinal cord injury. In Stover SL, DeLisa JA, Whiteneck GG, editors: *Spinal cord injury: clinical outcomes from the model systems,* Gaithersburg, Md, 1995, Aspen, pp 185-212.

Evans H, Love L: Neurological assessment related to spinal cord injury. In Nelson A, editor: *Nursing practice related to spinal cord injury and disorders: a core curriculum,* New York, 2001, Eastern Paralyzed Veterans Association, pp 105-10.

Fuhrer M: The subjective well-being of people with spinal cord injury: relationships to impairment, disability, and handicap, *Topics Spinal Cord Injury Rehabil* 1:56-71, 1996.

Grudinskas L, Nee M: An assessment tool for the older person with spinal cord injury, *SCI Nurs* 19(2):61-6, 2002.

Kemp BJ, Krause JS: Depression and life satisfaction among people aging with post-polio and spinal cord injury, *Disabil Rehabil* 21(5-6):241-9, 1999.

Lanig IS, Peterson WP: The respiratory system in spinal cord injury, *Phys Med Rehabil Clin North Am* 11(1):29-43, 2000.

Lemke D: Patient requested removal of ventilatory support in high-level tetraplegia: guidelines for the health care provider, *SCI Nurs* 18(2):67-73, 2001.

LeMone P, Burke K, editors: *Medical-surgical nursing: critical thinking in client care,* ed 2, Menlo Park, Calif, 1999, Addison-Wesley.

Mahoney D: Nursing management of the patient with spinal cord injury. In Derstine JB, Hargrove SD, editors: *Comprehensive rehabilitation nursing,* Philadelphia, 2001, WB Saunders, pp 368-423.

Maynard F et al: Management of the neuromusculoskeletal systems. In Stover SL, DeLisa JA, Whiteneck GG, editors: *Spinal cord injury: clinical outcomes from the model systems,* Gaithersburg, Md, 1995, Aspen, pp 145-69.

McKinley W, Tewksbury M, Godbout C: Comparison of medical complications following nontraumatic and traumatic spinal cord injury, *J Spinal Cord Med* 25(2):88-93, 2002.

Menter R, Hudson L: Effects of age at injury and the aging process. In Stover SL, DeLisa JA, Whiteneck GG, editors: *Spinal cord injury: clinical outcomes from the model systems,* Gaithersburg, Md, 1995, Aspen, pp 272-88.

National Spinal Cord Injury Statistical Center, Spinal Cord Injury Information Network: Spinal cord injury facts and figures at a glance, Dec 2001, retrieved from *http://spinalcord.uab.edu* on Feb 8, 2003.

Parsa C: *Gary's story: what you should know about domestic abuse and spinal cord injury,* Bellflower, Calif, 1999, Nelson Healthcare Staff Development.

Phillips WT et al: Effect of spinal cord injury on the heart and cardiovascular fitness, *Curr Probl Cardiol* 23(11):641-716, 1998.

Ragnarsson K et al: Management of pulmonary, cardiovascular, and metabolic conditions after spinal cord injury. In Lanig IS et al, editors: *A practical guide to health promotion after spinal cord injury,* Gaithersburg, Md, 1995, Aspen, pp 79-99.

Rimmer J, Braddock D: Health promotion for people with physical, cognitive, and sensory disabilities: an emerging national priority, *Am J Health Promot* 16(4):ii, 2002.

Rundquist J: The right to die—ethical dilemmas in persons with spinal cord injury, *SCI Nurs* 19(1):7-10, 2002.

Salzberg C et al: Predicting and preventing pressure ulcers in adults with paralysis, *Adv Wound Care* 11(5):237-46, 1998.

Sparks SM: Prevention and management of secondary disability in persons with spinal cord injury. In Nelson A, editor: *Nursing practice related to spinal cord injury and disorders: a core curriculum,* New York, 2001, Eastern Paralyzed Veterans Association, pp 449-68.

Specht J et al: The importance of leisure in the lives of persons with congenital physical disabilities, *Am J Occup Ther* 56(4):436-45, 2002.

Trautner B, Darouiche R: Prevention of urinary tract infection in patients with spinal cord injury, *J Spinal Cord Med* 25(4):277-83, 2002.

Ward K, Parsons L: Managing work-related stress in times of uncertainty: a care plan for the caregiver, *SCI Nurs* 17(2):59-63, 2000.

Welner S, Simon J, Welner B: Maximizing health in menopausal women with disabilities, *Menopause* 9(3):208-19, 2002.

Wilber N et al: Disability as a public health issue: findings and reflections from the Massachusetts survey of secondary conditions, *Milbank Q* 80(2):393-421, 2002.

CHAPTER **24**

Neuromuscular Disorders

Leslie Jean Neal, PhD, RN, FNP-C, and Julie Ries, MA, PT, GCS

OBJECTIVES

After reading this chapter, you should be able to do the following:

- Describe the pathophysiology of multiple sclerosis, Guillain-Barré syndrome, Parkinson's disease, Huntington's disease, amyotrophic lateral sclerosis, and myasthenia gravis
- Describe the clinical manifestations of these diseases
- Describe the functional health patterns affected by these diseases
- Describe the role of each member of the interdisciplinary team involved in the care of persons with these diseases
- Describe the indications for use, side effects, and nursing considerations related to drugs commonly used to treat these diseases

Persons with a family history of neurologic disorders such as stroke, epilepsy, multiple sclerosis, amyotrophic lateral sclerosis, or brain or spinal tumors may be at increased risk for neurologic disease. In addition, increased age, hypertension, cigarette smoking, heredity, diabetes mellitus, carotid artery disease, polycythemia, and heart disease place people at high risk for neurologic conditions. Drug and alcohol use also increase risk. Many chronic diseases affect the communication between the nerves and muscles. This chapter discusses several of these: multiple sclerosis, Guillain-Barré syndrome, Parkinson's disease, Huntington's disease, amyotrophic lateral sclerosis, and myasthenia gravis. However, Charcot-Marie-Tooth disease (CMT), Duchenne's muscular dystrophy (DMD), and Becker's muscular dystrophy (BMD) are mentioned briefly because the reader may encounter patients with these diseases. These disorders are not discussed in detail because CMT is not a common focus of the interdisciplinary team and muscular dystrophy occurs in childhood, with patients living only into young or middle adulthood.

Both CMT and muscular dystrophy are inherited. CMT is the most commonly encountered inherited neurologic disease, and 1 in 2500 people has some form of the disorder. The neuropathy of CMT affects sensory and motor nerves. The disease is characterized by weakness and atrophy of the distal muscles, decreased sensation, and impaired deep tendon reflexes. There are two types of CMT, CMT-1 and CMT-2, which are differentiated by genetic testing. Signs and symptoms begin in the lower extremities and progress to the upper extremities. A high-stepped gait with frequent tripping or falling and foot deformity such as high arches are common elements in the medical history. The disease typically appears in the first or second decade or in middle age. Clinical manifestations are highly variable. Physical therapy, orthotics, and sometimes surgery are methods of treatment. However, no therapy is available to prevent disease onset or to halt the progression of disability (Chance and Bird, 2001).

DMD is the most frequently encountered neuromuscular disease of children. Death typically occurs by the third decade of life. BMD is less common but has a later onset and slower progression, with most persons surviving until the fourth or fifth decade of life. DMD and BMD primarily affect the heart and skeletal muscles. Dystrophin, a protein that stabilizes the cell plasma membrane during muscle contractions, is missing in persons with DMD and is reduced in persons with BMD. As a result muscle fibers deteriorate and regenerate until the muscles can no longer repair themselves as necessary. Irreversible degradation of the muscle fibers occurs, and muscle is replaced by connective tissue and fat. Extreme muscle weakness and muscle wasting characterize both diseases (Altman and Gilchrist, 2003).

ASSESSMENT

Persons with neuromuscular diseases share common lifestyle changes and similar assessment findings. Primary areas of concern are pain, mobility, the ability to perform the activities of daily living (ADL) and instrumental activities of daily living (IADL), and bowel and bladder function. Some of these diseases predispose to mental status changes, whereas others do not. Box 24-1 lists the functional health patterns that may be affected by this group of neuromuscular diseases. Because disease signs and symptoms, diagnostic testing, and interdisciplinary care are similar for persons with the conditions discussed in this chapter, these topics are discussed together early in the chapter. Details for specific neuromuscular conditions are highlighted separately.

Box 24-1 Functional Health Pattern Assessment for Neuromuscular Disorders

HEALTH PERCEPTION/HEALTH MANAGEMENT
- Is there a family history of neuromuscular disease?
- What is the patient's perception of his or her overall health?
- What medications, including over-the-counter drugs, does the patient take? Does the patient use recreational drugs?
- What alternative therapies does the patient use?
- Is there a history of previous hospitalizations?
- What are the patient's safety practices? For example, has the patient been exposed to lead?

NUTRITION/METABOLISM
- What is the patient's current weight? Has there been any unexplained recent weight gain or loss?
- Is the patient on a special diet?
- What is the condition of the skin and mucous membranes?
- Does the patient have difficulty swallowing or chewing?
- Is there a history of vitamin deficiencies (especially of B vitamins)?
- Does the patient use alcohol?

ELIMINATION
- Have any changes occurred in bowel or bladder habits (incontinence, constipation)?
- Does the patient use an elevated toilet seat?
- Does the patient have pain or difficulty urinating?
- What prescription and/or over-the-counter medications does the patient use to control elimination?

ACTIVITY/EXERCISE
- Does the patient have difficulty walking or transferring?
- Does the patient experience weakness, fatigue, or malaise?
- Is paresthesia or paralysis present?
- Does the patient have poor balance or coordination?
- What are the patient's regular exercise activities?
- What mobility aids does the patient use?
- In what recreational activities does the patient participate?
- Is the patient able to perform regular and instrumental activities of daily living?

SLEEP/REST
- How many hours of uninterrupted sleep does the patient get at night?
- Does the patient take naps or rest periods?
- What sleep aids are used?

COGNITION/PERCEPTION
- What are the nature, character, location, and duration of the pain?

- What factors alleviate and aggravate the pain? What treatments has the patient tried?
- Is involvement symmetrical?
- Are paresthesias present?
- Have changes in memory occurred?
- Does the patient have numbness, tingling, vertigo, aphasia, or changes in vision (especially diplopia)?

SELF-PERCEPTION/SELF-CONCEPT
- How does the patient describe himself or herself?
- How has the condition affected the patient's self-esteem?
- How has the condition changed the patient's body image?
- What are the effects of the condition on the patient's sense of self?

ROLES/RELATIONSHIPS
- What kind of work does the patient perform?
- What role does the patient play in the home and family?
- What changes have occurred in the patient's ability to carry out role functions?
- How satisfied is the patient with his or her current roles and relationships?
- How has the condition affected the patient's family and/or or significant others?

SEXUALITY/REPRODUCTION
- Is the patient sexually active?
- Have changes occurred in sexual performance?
- Is the patient satisfied with current sexual patterns?
- Have changes occurred in the menstrual cycle?
- Does the patient have concerns about the genetic-familial aspects of the condition?

COPING/STRESS TOLERANCE
- What are the patient's coping strategies?
- What support systems are available to the patient?
- Can the patient manage the condition in the current setting?

VALUES/BELIEFS
- What constitutes quality of life for the patient?
- What is important to the patient?
- What are the patient's spiritual beliefs, health beliefs, and cultural beliefs?
- What is the patient's attitude toward locus of control?
- How important to the patient are his or her beliefs and how can health care providers best support those beliefs while the patient receives health care?

The health history, review of systems, physical examination, results of specific tests, and assessment of the person's environment together form a comprehensive picture of the individual's past and current health status. This allows the clinician, in conjunction with the individual and caregivers, to formulate logical and scientific nursing diagnoses to serve as the basis for interventions.

It is important for the clinician to evaluate the mental status of the patient before proceeding to gather other data. If the patient is not likely to be a reliable source of information, then information should be solicited from a family member or friend.

The medication history is important, particularly with regard to the use of ephedrine (implicated in brain attacks), which is often found in Chinese medicines, and dietary supplements, tranquilizers, sedatives, and mood elevators, which can cause drowsiness and dizziness. Use of antispasmodic and antiepileptic medications may indicate that the patient has a neurologic condition. Exposure to toxic substances in utero or in the newborn period may have altered neurologic development.

Persons with confirmed or suspected neurologic disease should be given a complete and thorough physical examination, because neurologic conditions are likely to affect the entire body. The person's mental status should also be assessed (Neal, 1997). The simple mnemonic tool "Is Anybody Home?" designed to help the clinician remember the many parts of the neurologic assessment is included in Box 24-2. Observation of the person with neurologic disease is especially important because changes in alertness, mood, affect, appearance, and appropriateness of behavior are often clues to changes in neurologic status (Neal, 2002).

Assessment of the person's environment is vital to assisting the individual in integrating the neuromuscular condition into his or her lifestyle. Arranging both the tangible and intangible aspects of the environment is integral to an adaptive lifestyle. Tangible aspects include the location of furniture, the width of doorways, the availability and suitability of equipment and adaptive devices, the financial ability to afford food, medicine, and treatment, the ability to obtain and use transportation, and other similar factors. Intangible aspects include the person's support system, spiritual and religious comfort, psychosocial satisfaction and pleasure, and self-esteem and self-actualization. Careful assessment of both tangible and intangible aspects of the environment is the responsibility of the treating team. Suggestions for modifications to tangible factors can help ease the transition of the individual with neuromuscular

disease and his or her family and/or significant others in learning to live with the disease. Making suggestions for improving intangible aspects of the environment is also within the scope of activity of the treating team.

Caregivers of chronically ill persons frequently become worn down by the demands of caring for the individual, and although they endeavor to provide tangible and intangible support they may unintentionally lose patience with the individual. An important and often overlooked part of adapting the environment is ensuring that both the patient and caregiver have changes in scenery and in persons with whom they have contact. Assisting the caregiver to arrange periods of relief or respite is an important part of the care provided by the interdisciplinary team.

DIAGNOSIS

For all of the diseases discussed in this chapter, the past medical history, family medical history, clinical presentation, and results of a complete neurologic examination are integral to making an accurate diagnosis. These data and the findings of specific tests and procedures assist in ruling in or ruling out various neuromuscular pathologies. Several tests and procedures are used to diagnose neuromuscular conditions. Table 24-1 describes the most common of these.

INTERDISCIPLINARY CARE

The goals of interdisciplinary care are generally the same for persons with all of the neuromuscular diseases discussed in this chapter. According to *Healthy People 2010* (Department of Health and Human Services, 2000) the primary goals for the care of persons with neuromuscular diseases are the following:

- To increase quality and years of life
- To eliminate health disparities

The health care team members strive to support the patient, family, and caregivers in meeting these goals. In addition to the patient, family, and caregivers, the primary members of the health care team include the physician, nurse practitioner, clinical nurse specialist, and/or physician assistant; the nurse; the physical therapist; the occupational therapist; the dietitian; and the certified nurse's aide. A housekeeper or companion may also be involved so that caregivers can obtain respite. In addition, a medical social worker may be called in to help the patient obtain sufficient funds for treatment or locate an appropriate place to live. The medical social worker or psychologist may also provide counseling to the patient and caregivers. A respiratory therapist may be needed once ventilatory support is required, and when speech or swallowing is affected, a speech and language pathologist is frequently added to the team.

All of the team members work together with the patient and family to provide rehabilitative care. Interdisciplinary care in all settings is patient specific and focuses on the alterations experienced by the person with neuromuscular

---

Box 24-2   Is Anybody Home?

I: Intellect, including thought processes and reasoning, judgment, and simple calculations

S: Sensation, including touch, pain, temperature

A: Appearance, appropriateness, affect

N: Nerves, cranial

Y: Yak, yak; communication and use of language

B: Balance

O: Orientation

D: Deep tendon reflexes

Y: Yesterday; short- and long-term memory

H: Health history

O: Observe for alterations between assessments

M: Muscle strength and motor ability

E: Energy level and emotional state

From Neal LJ: Is anybody home? *Home Healthc Nurse* 15(3):158-67, 1997.

Table 24-1   Studies and Procedures Used in Diagnosis of Neuromuscular Conditions

Study or Procedure	Description and Purpose
Computed tomography	X-ray beam scanning of head in cross-sectional slices to provide images of the brain; distinguishes differences in densities
Positron emission tomography	Computer-assisted imaging of organ function; allows measurement of blood flow, brain metabolism, and tissue composition
Magnetic resonance imaging	Use of a magnetic field to generate images; gives information about intracellular chemical changes
Single photon emission computed tomography	Three-dimensional imaging; contrasts normal and abnormal tissue
Cerebral angiography	Radiographic imaging of cerebral circulation using contrast dye
Electromyography	Measurement of changes in electrical potentials in skeletal muscles using needle electrodes
Nerve conduction studies	Stimulation of a peripheral nerve to record muscle action potential or sensory action potential
Lumbar puncture and cerebrospinal fluid examination	Spinal tap to remove cerebrospinal fluid for analysis

From Smeltzer SC, Barre BG: *Medical-surgical nursing,* Philadelphia, 2000, JB Lippincott.

disease and maintenance of hope and quality of life. Nursing diagnoses that characterize these include (Neal, 2002):

- Impaired breathing: increased risk for aspiration and respiratory failure
- Pain: paresthesias and neuropathy that tend to be chronic and intermittent
- Injury: risk for injury related to alterations in balance, mobility, and cognition
- Altered nutrition: increased risk for dysphagia and aspiration
- Activity intolerance: fatigability
- Impaired communication: due to muscular weakness
- Altered thought processes: possible cognitive changes and depression or anxiety
- Altered elimination: bowel or bladder incontinence, urinary retention, constipation
- Altered mobility: weakness, paralysis, paresthesias, paresis
- Altered skin integrity: caused by altered mobility and altered nutrition
- Changes in psychosocial status: social isolation, depression, hopelessness, helplessness, sexual dysfunction, concerns about pregnancy and passing on the disease to offspring
- Self-care deficit: loss of personal control
- Sexual dysfunction: may be an early sign of disease
- Caregiver role strain: related to progressive debility of disease, changes in patient's cognition and physical ability

Primary Provider (Physician/Nurse Practitioner)

Several physicians may be involved in the care of the person with a neuromuscular condition. The primary care physi-

cian, nurse practitioner, clinical nurse specialist, or physician assistant may be the first provider to suspect and possibly diagnose the neurologic condition. However, it is likely that the patient will be referred to a neurologist to determine the causes of the neuromuscular changes. Both the neurologist and the primary care provider monitor the patient's condition as it progresses. However, the physiatrist, a physical medicine and rehabilitation physician, may direct and monitor care while the patient receives rehabilitation.

Nurse

In the inpatient setting, the nurse cares for the patient during the diagnostic period and during exacerbations and complications, and provides end-of-life care. Rehabilitation nurses in inpatient or outpatient facilities teach patients and families about the condition and how to integrate the changes brought on by the condition into the patient's lifestyle. Nurses employed in long-term care facilities strive to prevent exacerbations and complications and care for patients who cannot be managed or manage themselves at home. In the outpatient setting, the nurse provides intermittent or private duty skilled care depending on the needs of the homebound patient.

The nurse instructs the patient and family regarding medications and their indications and use. The nurse monitors medication use and alerts the physician, physician assistant, or advanced nurse practitioner of any adverse effects or contraindications. In addition, the nurse monitors the patient's pain and recommends pain management protocols to the prescribing provider. Wounds that may develop as a result of immobility or decreased mobility may be assessed initially by the nurse, who may suggest treatment strategies. The nurse confers with the other members of the team regarding the patient's nutrition and exercise to maintain health and maximize energy and self-care ability.

The nurse teaches the patient and/or caregiver to perform intermittent catheterization using a mirror to see the genitalia. Some patients and caregivers are reluctant to perform the procedure but when informed that it can reduce wetting episodes, the need for an indwelling catheter, and the risk of urinary tract infection, many patients and caregivers are willing to learn. If intermittent catheterization is not yet needed to control urine, the patient may be taught timed voiding. With this method, the patient attempts to urinate in the toilet at specific intervals and thus "train" the brain to signal the bladder at specific times. Prompted voiding consists of caregiver reminders to void if the patient is cognitively impaired. Finally, if indwelling catheterization is called for, the nurse performs the catheterizations and monitors the catheter to prevent infection.

The nurse works with the physical and occupational therapists to design and implement a plan of care to address safety, mobility, strengthening, and vocational issues. The nurse reinforces instruction from the speech pathologist and respiratory therapist regarding independent and safe eating or feeding and optimal respiratory status.

Therapists

The physical therapist and occupational therapist work with the individual with neuromuscular diseases to maximize independence in functional activities. Therapeutic interventions might include stretching, strengthening, motor control training, balance training, functional mobility training, gait training, self-care and ADL training, and instruction in energy conservation techniques. Both types of therapist also advise and instruct regarding durable medical equipment (wheelchairs, walkers, canes, hospital beds, bedside commodes) and adaptive equipment (eating utensils, dressing aids), as well as high-technology equipment such as computerized equipment control units for patients with significant physical impairment (Figure 24-1). The therapist works with the nurse to teach the patient how to maintain functional mobility skills and the ability to perform ADL and IADL for as long as possible. As the patient loses the ability to function independently, the therapist can instruct the family and caregiver on how to safely and effectively assist the patient.

The speech language pathologist (SLP) or therapist assesses and treats cognitive and communicative disorders, as well as oral-motor and swallowing deficits. The SLP is instrumental in assisting the patient to maximize communication and in educating family and/or significant others in how to communicate most effectively with the patient. Through swallowing studies, the SLP assesses the risk of aspiration and may recommend the use of gastrostomy or other feeding tubes if swallowing becomes severely impaired.

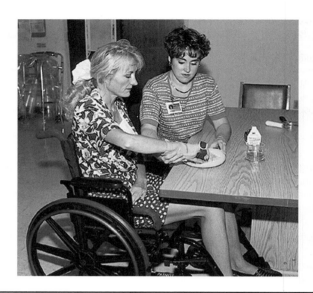

Figure 24-1 Patient participating in occupational therapy using mobile arm supports and upper extremity orthotics. (From Lewis SM et al: *Medical-surgical nursing: assessment and management of clinical problems,* ed 5, St Louis, Mosby, 2000.)

Dietitian

The dietitian ideally works with the patient throughout the course of the disease. Fatigue discourages patients from eating and drinking in necessary quantities. Dysphagia and feeding tubes present many nutritional challenges. Wound prevention and wound healing related to changes in mobility require a diet rich in protein (unless coexisting renal disease limits protein intake) and in other nutrients, especially vitamin C for healing. Hyperalimentation may be needed to maintain adequate nutrition.

Certified Nurse's Aide

Once the individual with a neuromuscular disease or his or her caregiver is unable to perform ADL safely and capably, the role of the certified nurse's aide becomes vital to retaining the person in the community and providing long-term care. The certified nurse's aide also provides assistance with ADL and personal care when the patient is hospitalized. Assistance with bathing, grooming, dressing, eating, transferring, and ambulation is especially helpful.

Drug Therapy

Many of the drugs used to treat persons with neuromuscular disease are the same for all such disorders. Pharmacologic agents used to treat the diseases discussed in this chapter are listed in Tables 24-2 and 24-3. These tables should be referred to for drug treatment of all of the neuromuscular diseases discussed in this chapter.

Table 24-2 Drugs Commonly Used to Manage Neuromuscular Diseases

Medication	Use	Disease
Corticosteroids	Treat exacerbations	MS, MG, GBS
Immunomodulators	Treat exacerbations	MS, MG
Cholinergics	Treat urinary retention	MS
Anticholinergics	Treat urinary frequency	MS
	Reduce tremor	PD
Muscle relaxants	Reduce spasticity	MS, SCI
Antispasmodics	Treat urinary retention	MS, SCI
Dopaminergic agents	Treat bradykinesia, tremor, rigidity	PD, SCI
	Maintain mean arterial pressure	
Antihistamines	Treat tremor, rigidity	PD
MAO inhibitors	Treat bradykinesia, tremor, rigidity	PD
Anticholinesterase agents	Prolong action of acetylcholine	MG
Antipsychotics, antichorea agents	Reduce psychosis, chorea	HD
Antidepressants	Reduce depression	All
Methylprednisolone	Improve blood flow, reduce edema	SCI
COMT inhibitors	Inhibit breakdown of levodopa	PD
Antioxidants	Slow disease progression	PD
Methotrexate	Provide immunosuppression	MS
T-cell receptor peptides	Inhibit immune system attack	MS
Monoclonal antibodies	Suppress abnormal immune response	MS
Stool softeners	Prevent constipation	All
β-Agonist/GABA antagonists	Treat spasticity	MS
Riluzole (Rilutek)	Reduce release of glutamate from cells	ALS
G_{M1} ganglioside	Increase functional recovery	SCI

ALS, Amyotrophic lateral sclerosis; *COMT,* catechol-O-methyltransferase; *GABA,* γ-aminobutyric acid; *GBS,* Guillain-Barré syndrome; *HD,* Huntington's disease; *MAO,* monoamine oxidase; *MG,* myasthenia gravis; *MS,* Multiple sclerosis; *PD,* Parkinson's disease; *SCI,* spinal cord injury.

Table 24-3 Drug Therapy for Neuromuscular Diseases

Medication	Use	Side Effects	Nursing Considerations	Disease
Corticosteroids: prednisone	Treat exacerbations	Cushing's syndrome, GI irritation, osteoporosis, HTN, steroid psychosis, acne hirsutism, increased risk of infection	Teach patient to titrate doses.	MS, MG, GBS
Immunomodulators: Copaxone	Treat exacerbations	Mild flulike symptoms, injection site reactions	Copaxone: rare reaction of chest tightness, dyspnea, flushing, anxiety	MS, MG
Cholinergics: Bethanechol	Treat urinary retention	Sweating, salivation, GI distress and cramps	Advise patient of side effects.	MS
Anticholinergics: Ditropan	Treat urinary incontinence	Dry mouth, reduced GI motility, increased heart rate, urinary retention	Advise patient of side effects; suggest sucking on candy to avoid dry mouth.	MS
Muscle relaxants: Flexeril	Treat spasticity	Dizziness, drowsiness, fatigue, weakness	Instruct patient to avoid abrupt withdrawal.	MS
Antispasmodics: Atropine	Treat urinary retention	Dry mouth, blurred vision, tachycardia, constipation	Do not use in patients with narrow angle glaucoma. Use with care in elderly because of possibility of glaucoma.	MS
Methotrexate	Provide immuno-suppression	Dizziness, drowsiness, headache	Be aware that NSAIDs, salicylates, sulfonylureas, tetracyclines may increase toxicity.	MS

Continued

Table 24-3   Drug Therapy for Neuromuscular Diseases—cont'd

Medication	Use	Side Effects	Nursing Considerations	Disease
T-cell receptor peptides	Inhibit immune system attack			MS
Monoclonal antibodies	Suppress abnormal immune response			MS
Stool softeners: Colace	Prevent constipation	Throat irritation, mild cramps	Administer with full glass of water or juice.	All
β-Agonists/GABA antagonists	Treat spasticity			MS
Antidepressants: SSRIs	Reduce depression, fatigue	Anxiety, drowsiness, headache, insomnia, nervousness	Discontinue MAO inhibitors for 14 days before therapy.	All
Levodopa Carbidopa	Enhance, substitute for dopamine	Nausea, vomiting, cardiac arrhythmias, hypotension	Advise patient of "on-off" effect. Instruct patient to take on empty stomach. Advise patient that withdrawal from drug must be gradual.	PD
Cholinesterase inhibitors: Pyridostigmine	Provide first-line MG management	Cholinergic crisis	Expect day-to-day variations in dosing depending on symptoms. Give with food. Treat cholinergic crisis with atropine.	MG

GABA, γ-Aminobutyric acid; *GBS,* Guillain-Barré syndrome; *GI,* gastrointestinal; *HTN,* hypertension; *MAO,* monoamine oxidase; *MG,* myasthenia gravis; *MS,* multiple sclerosis; *NSAIDs,* nonsteroidal antiinflammatory drugs; *PD,* Parkinson's disease; *SSRIs,* selective serotonin reuptake inhibitors.

COMPLEMENTARY AND ALTERNATIVE THERAPIES

Fatigue can be partially managed by maintaining adequate fluid intake; eliminating caffeine, sugars, refined carbohydrates, and excess fat from the diet; and adding fresh fruits, vegetables, and fiber. Also eliminating chocolate, alcohol, and gluten-containing products may be useful. Stress management classes, group therapy, and avoidance of exposure to temperature extremes, pesticides, insecticides, heavy metals, and other immune irritants may alleviate symptoms. Various herbs such as astragalus, cat's claw, evening primrose, grape seed, and olive leaf have been suggested as potentially useful for patients with neuromuscular diseases. Vitamin, mineral, and other nutritional supplements that may be helpful include magnesium, N-acetyl cysteine, *Lactobacillus acidophilus,* fish or flaxseed oils, vitamin B$_{12}$, vitamins C and E, and phosphorus (Lavalle et al, 2001).

Other alternative therapies that have been studied for use in multiple sclerosis include homeopathy, biofeedback, yoga (Schwartz et al, 1999), guided imagery, massage (Whitmore and Leake, 1996), acupuncture, chiropractic, vitamin C therapy (Berkman et al, 1999), administration of other vitamins, and magnet therapy (Huntley and Ernst, 2000).

There are many contraindications to these remedies, and they may interact with prescribed medications or may include ingredients that are not listed on the product's labels. Patients and families must be educated regarding the safety concerns associated with the use of any over-the-counter remedy.

MULTIPLE SCLEROSIS

Multiple sclerosis (MS) is twice as common in women as in men and tends to appear between the ages of 20 and 50 years. However, MS may also affect adolescents or the elderly (Halper, 2002). The disease is more prevalent in whites and in people living furthest from the equator. Fifteen percent of people with MS have a relative who has or had the disease. Currently, 350,000 people living in the United States have MS, 200,000 of whom are women (National Multiple Sclerosis Society, 2003a).

Pathophysiology

MS is a disease of the central nervous system (CNS) in which the myelin sheath covering the axon of the nerve fiber is destroyed. Infection with a slow-growing virus that triggers a hypersensitivity reaction and subsequent repeated inflammation is one possible cause. Another is an autoimmune response of the body to myelin. Inflammation eventually destroys the myelin. The site of myelin destruction is reflected in the symptoms. Most frequently, patients seek treatment for ocular changes that reflect demyelination of the optic and oculomotor cranial nerves.

Changes in coordination, balance, motor ability, gait, and sensation are caused by demyelination of the cerebellar, corticospinal, and posterior column systems. Extreme fatigue is an often-cited symptom, as are dysphagia and dysarthria. Some individuals develop cognitive changes.

The National Multiple Sclerosis Society (2003b) has developed new diagnostic categories for persons with MS:

- Relapsing-remitting: shows periods of worsening of symptoms without disease progression between exacerbations
- Primary-progressive: continuous worsening without interruption
- Secondary-progressive: relapsing-remitting initially, then becomes progressive
- Progressive-relapsing: progressive from onset with acute relapses

Relapsing-remitting is the type most commonly identified in patients newly diagnosed with MS. The term refers to the tendency of the disease at this initial stage to be characterized by relapses or exacerbations followed by full or partial recovery. The disease course is stable, without progression, between these exacerbations. Pseudoexacerbations may occur during which existing MS symptoms flare without new inflammation or demyelination (Halper, 2002). Research has demonstrated that motor ability, brainstem function, and elimination change as the disease progresses over time. The ability to perform ADL, communicate, socialize, and engage in intimate acts declines (Gulick, 1998).

Diagnosis

The diagnosis is primarily clinical (Halper, 2002). In addition to the diagnostic procedures mentioned earlier, a thorough history taking and assessment of the patient, urodynamic studies in cases of urinary incontinence or retention, and evoked potential studies to evaluate the transmission of nerve impulses to the CNS should be performed. Imaging studies and electrophoretic analysis of cerebrospinal fluid may confirm suspicions of MS. Of the diagnostic tests listed in Table 24-1, the most useful for confirming a diagnosis of MS are magnetic resonance imaging, which reveals plaques of demyelination in most patients (Halper, 2002); cerebrospinal fluid analysis, the results of which can reveal an inflammatory process in the CNS; and measurement of evoked potentials, which may show slowing of nerve conduction velocities.

Clinical Manifestations

Clinical manifestations of MS depend on the location of plaques in the brain and/or spinal cord. Persons with MS often seek treatment for ocular changes, fatigue, and ataxia. Extreme fatigue is an often-cited and disabling symptom. Heat sensitivity is another important complaint: an increase in core temperature seems to have a negative effect on motor status. Other changes, such as alterations in coordination, balance, gait, and sensation, are individualized and relate to the site of demyelination. Cognitive changes tend to occur later in the disease, and these often precipitate psychosocial problems with family and caregivers. Changes in skin integrity and contractures occur if caregivers are not careful to reposition and exercise the patient frequently.

Changes in motor ability as the disease progresses tend to include weakness in the extremities, difficulties in balance, falling, spasms, tremors, and knee locking. Brainstem changes include diplopia, dysphagia, forgetfulness, and blurred vision. Urinary frequency and incontinence or urinary retention and constipation usually develop. Neuropathic pain is related to demyelination and may be acute, chronic, paroxysmal, or subacute (Halper, 2002).

Acute exacerbations are typically preceded by bacterial or viral infection and are usually managed with corticosteroids. It is important to treat infections early. Relapsing MS may be treated with interferon immunomodulators (Table 24-3) as well as with glatiramer, a nonsteroidal, noninterferon agent self-administered by injection that does not have the side effects of interferon immunomodulators. Mitoxantrone is used for MS that is worsening but is not primary-progressive. It has been shown to lower relapse rates and reduce neurologic deficits but, as a chemotherapeutic drug, can produce heart, liver, or blood toxicity over time (Halper, 2002).

Think S for Success

Symptoms
- Manage individual symptoms with rest periods and drug treatment. Drug therapy for multiple sclerosis is aimed at treating the symptoms and controlling disease progression.

Sequelae
- Change position frequently.
- Provide care to avoid infections and pressure ulcers and other wounds.

Safety
- Teach patient and caregivers about medications.
- Teach patient and caregivers to do the following:
  Allow patient to participate in self-care as much as possible.
  Use equipment safely because patients are at risk for falls related to fatigue and difficulties with balance.
  Avoid activities and environments that will exacerbate symptoms (strenuous exercise, heat).
  Combat fatigue with energy conservation and pacing of activities.

Support/Services
- Refer patient to community resources.
- Provide assistance with finances and community reintegration.
- Work with family to handle patient role changes related to extreme fatigue.

Satisfaction
- Determine degree to which multiple sclerosis is interfering with quality of life and develop a plan to accomplish short- and long-term goals toward an acceptable quality of life.

GUILLAIN-BARRÉ SYNDROME

Guillain-Barré syndrome (GBS) occurs slightly more frequently in men than in women and affects approximately 1 in 100,000 people in the United States (Worsham, 2000). Whites are more likely to get GBS than African Americans, and people over the age of 45 years are most susceptible. GBS occurs throughout the world, although climactic and seasonal variations are noted.(Copstead and Banasik, 2000). Persons with chronic diseases such as systemic lupus erythematosus, Hodgkin's disease, and human immunodeficiency virus infection have an increased risk for developing GBS (Smeltzer and Barre, 2003).

Pathophysiology

Whereas MS affects the myelin sheath of neurons in the CNS, GBS affects the myelin sheath of neurons in the peripheral nervous system (Table 24-4). GBS is also known as acute infectious polyradiculoneuritis and is characterized by acute inflammation, paralysis, and motor weakness. Segmental demyelination slows nerve conduction and disperses nerve impulses. Cranial and motor nerves are more commonly affected than less heavily myelinated nerves, which results in tingling, pain, or the sensation of crawling skin. The cause of GBS is unknown. However, the onset of symptoms typically occurs 1 to 8 weeks after an infection, which suggests a cell-mediated immune response. Yet, the humoral immune system is thought also to be involved. Other risk factors include trauma, surgery, upper respiratory tract infection, immunization, gastrointestinal illness, and the presence of antibodies to Epstein-Barr virus or cytomegalovirus. These conditions may cause sensitization of the T cells to the person's myelin (Ignatavicius and Workman, 2002; Smeltzer, and Barre, 2003).

Diagnosis

Along with the diagnostic studies described earlier in the chapter, analysis of cerebrospinal fluid for protein and nerve conduction studies should be performed. The protein content of the cerebrospinal fluid is elevated, and nerve conduction velocity (NCV) testing shows slowed impulse transmission. Interestingly, the slowed conduction on NCV studies may not be apparent during the first few weeks of illness, and abnormal NCV findings persist after the patient has made a full clinical recovery. It is important to gather a through history to rule out other possible causes of the symptoms.

Clinical Manifestations

The classic form of GBS takes 2 to 4 weeks to progress from symptom onset to nadir. The initial primary symptom is symmetrical ascending weakness. Numbness, tingling, and weakness typically begin in the lower extremities. Later, muscles of the chest, trunk, upper extremities, and neck and those innervated by the cranial nerves are affected. In up to 30% of cases, mechanical ventilation is required during this acute period. Pain and paresthesia often develop. However, vibratory and proprioceptive changes in sensation are more common. Because both the sympathetic and parasympathetic nervous systems are affected, the patient may experience high blood pressure or orthostatic hypotension, bowel or bladder dysfunction, diaphoresis, and bradycardia (Lewis et al, 2000).

Recovery because of remyelination is usually spontaneous and tends to occur in a descending fashion. Typically, recovery extends over a period of months to years. Prognosis is generally good with eventual full recovery or only mild residual problems, such as diminished or absent deep tendon reflexes. A small number of individuals do experience permanent disability, however, and complete flaccid paralysis requiring chronic mechanical ventilation may occur (Bullock and Henze, 2000).

Think S for Success

Symptoms
- Manage symptoms as they appear. Some persons will need ventilatory support temporarily.

Sequelae
- Prevent permanent disability by treatment of symptoms, proper positioning, and physical and occupational therapy.

Safety
- Make patient and caregivers aware of potential safety hazards related to motor weakness, paresthesias, and postural hypotension; strenuous exercise during acute period is contraindicated.

Support/Services
- Ensure that patient obtains assistance with instrumental and other activities of daily living and emotional support as necessary until recovery is complete.
- Assess coping strategies and available resources.

Satisfaction
- Determine degree to which Guillain-Barré syndrome interferes with lifestyle and help patient maintain quality of life.
- Help caregivers and family members provide support to patient and each other.

Table 24-4 Comparison of Multiple Sclerosis and Guillain-Barré Syndrome

Multiple Sclerosis	Guillain-Barré Syndrome
Affects central nervous system	Affects peripheral nervous system
Demyelinating	Demyelinating
Symptoms are variable	Ascending weakness is primary symptom
Progressive	Most people recover, 7-22% left with disability
Death occurs from complications	Death may occur from symptoms

PARKINSON'S DISEASE

Parkinson's disease (PD) most commonly appears in persons between 58 and 62 years of age and occurs more frequently in men than in women. Approximately 30 to 300 people in 100,000 get PD, and estimates are that 500,000 people living in the United States have the disease (McCance and Huether, 2002).

Pathophysiology

PD is a disease of the basal ganglia characterized by a deficiency of the neurotransmitter dopamine. Primary or idiopathic PD accounts for the majority of cases of parkinsonism. In primary PD, there is a loss of neurons in the substantia nigra. In secondary parkinsonism, disorders other than PD cause a PD-like movement disorder. Atherosclerosis, neoplasm, trauma, toxins, infection, and drug intoxication are examples of causes of secondary parkinsonism. Among the drugs that can induce parkinsonism are antihypertensives, antiemetics, and neuroleptics as well as some recreational drugs. The parkinsonian effects are usually reversible with discontinuation of the drug (McCance and Huether, 2002).

Although the etiology of PD is unknown, there is support for genetic, toxin-induced, and viral causes. Symptoms of PD occur because of an imbalance between levels of dopamine and acetylcholine in the substantia nigra. Typically these neurotransmitters balance one another, with dopamine causing inhibition of neural stimulation and acetylcholine contributing to excitation of neuronal activity. This balance allows motor function to continue normally. The relative excess of acetylcholine results in the classic triad of PD: tremor, rigidity, and bradykinesia. The severity of the disease appears to be directly proportional to the amount of neuronal loss in the substantia nigra (McCance and Huether, 2002). A fourth symptom recently added to this triad is postural abnormalities.

Diagnosis

The presence of two of the three symptoms in the classic triad, including either resting tremor or bradykinesia, is diagnostic of PD. Positron emission tomography may be used to demonstrate reduced uptake of dopamine.

Clinical Manifestations

In addition to the classic triad and postural abnormalities, persons with PD exhibit decreased arm swing, dysarthria, dysphagia, flat affect, foot drag, and hoarseness. Although symptoms may begin unilaterally, they typically become bilateral. The Hoehn-Yale scale is used to stage symptoms: 0—no visible disease; 1—unilateral involvement; 2—bilateral involvement with minimal gait difficulty; 3—bilateral involvement with postural instability; 4—bilateral involvement with inability to walk (Lieberman, 1995).

Disease onset is insidious. However, for some individuals micrographia is an early sign (Imke, 2000). Tremor at rest, particularly of the upper extremities, is the most common

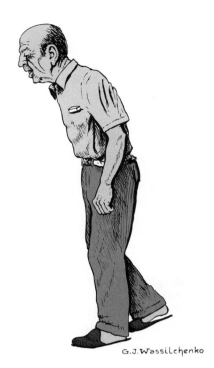

G.J.Wassilchenko

Figure 24-2 Characteristic shuffling gait of a patient with Parkinson's disease. (Modified from Rudy EB: *Advanced neurological and neurosurgical nursing,* St Louis, 1984, Mosby.)

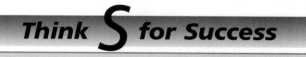

Think **S** for Success

Symptoms
- Manage symptoms with medication, rest, and reduced levels of stress.
- Consider thalamotomy, pallidotomy, and thalamic stimulation as surgical alternatives.

Sequelae
- Prevent pneumonia, a leading cause of death in persons with Parkinson's disease.

Safety
- Teach patient and family how to make environment safe for movement; how to choose, obtain, and use assistive and adaptive devices; and how to use medications appropriately.

Support/Services
- If necessary, help patient obtain assistance with finances, community integration, and occupational and vocational rehabilitation or maintenance. Seek appropriate referrals.

Satisfaction
- Determine degree to which Parkinson's disease is interfering with patient's and caregiver's lives and mutually develop a plan to minimize disruption caused by symptoms.

sign. Rigidity may first appear as muscle cramping in the hands or toes and is revealed by resistance during passive range-of-motion movements. Cogwheel rigidity, manifested by brief jerking movements, is characteristic.

Bradykinesia is responsible for fatigue, lack of fluidity of movement, flat affect, dysarthria, dysphagia, and micrographia. The person with PD may also freeze when initiating certain types of movement.

Postural abnormalities develop, and the person with PD assumes a posture characterized by a bent head and neck and stooped shoulders. Shuffling replaces smooth movements during ambulation and a loss of equilibrium occurs. Gait and balance impairment in PD is due to a multitude of factors, including the loss of postural control, range-of-motion and strength limitations, visuospatial deficits, start hesitation, and freezing. Orthostatic hypotension and vertigo may be complicating factors. Falls are a significant problem in the patient with PD. Typical parkinsonian gait is a stooped postured, narrow-based, festinating gait (short, shuffling steps with diminished stopping ability) with minimal or no arm swing (Figure 24-2).

In addition to these manifestations, persons with PD may display diaphoresis, postural hypotension, constipation, urinary retention, gastric retention, and seborrhea. Clinical as well as situational depression may develop, and dementia may or may not evolve. Dementia is most common in persons over age 70 and is related to a loss of cholinergic cells and the presence of neurofibrillary tangles, which are also characteristic of Alzheimer's disease. Bradyphrenia, sleep disturbances, and cognitive changes, including confusion and difficulty with calculations and abstract thought, may develop (McCance and Huether, 2002).

MYASTHENIA GRAVIS

Myasthenia gravis (MG) is a chronic autoimmune disease that affects 5 to 10 persons in 100,000 in the United States. Among young adults, more women than men are affected, but among those over age 50, more men get the disease. Thymic tumors are present in up to one quarter of persons with the disease, and up to 80% have abnormal changes in the thymus. The disease is associated with other autoimmune diseases, such as systemic lupus erythematosus and rheumatoid arthritis (McCance and Huether, 2002).

Pathophysiology

Whereas PD is a disorder of dopamine activity at the neuromuscular junction, MG is a disorder of acetylcholine activity. Receptor sites for acetylcholine are destroyed, which results in diminished neural transmission. This destruction occurs because acetylcholine receptors are recognized as foreign and the body initiates an immune response that prevents the binding of acetylcholine at the receptor. Acetylcholine is a neural transmitter responsible for excitatory activity. When acetylcholine transmission is reduced, muscle weakness and fatigue result.

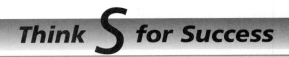

Think S for Success

Symptoms
- Manage muscle weakness with anticholinesterase drugs, steroids, immunosuppressants, and thymectomy when appropriate.

Sequelae
- Prevent myasthenic crisis by encouraging compliance with medication regimen and ensuring adequate dosing.
- Prevent cholinergic crisis by avoiding overdosing of anticholinesterase medications.

Safety
- Teach patient and family how to arrange the environment to prevent injury related to muscle weakness.
- Assist patient and family in obtaining assistive and adaptive devices and teach their use.
- Discourage driving and other dangerous activities during times of muscle weakness.
- Keep medication handy in several locations.

Support/Services
- If necessary, help patient obtain assistance with finances or community integration and occupational and vocational assistance.

Satisfaction
- Determine degree to which muscle weakness is interfering with patient's lifestyle and normal activities and work with patient and family to design a plan to enhance quality of life.

Three main types of MG are seen in adults: ocular MG in which muscle weakness occurs only in the eyes; generalized MG, which involves proximal muscles and is characterized by remissions and exacerbations; and bulbar MG, which involves muscles innervated by cranial nerves IX, X, XI, and XII. Generalized MG may be slowly progressive or may progress rapidly; bulbar MG is typically rapidly progressive and fulminating (Neal, 2002).

Diagnosis

The Tensilon test is used to diagnose MG. Tensilon (edrophonium) is administered intravenously. If immediate improvement in muscle strength occurs, then MG is diagnosed. Tests to detect the presence of anti–striated muscle antibodies may also assist diagnosis. Electromyographic testing is also used to assess muscle weakness. Computed tomography and magnetic resonance imaging of the thymus are performed to search for a thymoma, because 75% of individuals with MG have thymus gland abnormalities.

Clinical Manifestations

The most common presenting symptom is fatigue, and the history reveals frequent upper respiratory tract infections. Onset is slow and insidious, with repetition of activity causing exacerbation of signs and symptoms and rest therapeutically diminishing signs and symptoms. Muscle weakness is manifested by ptosis, diplopia, dysarthria, facial drooping, and dysphagia. Patients tend to spontaneously compensate for facial muscle weakness (e.g., by using posterior head tilt to facilitate eye contact when lids are drooping or using hand placement to facilitate jaw closure). The muscles of the neck, shoulder, and hip may be weak initially, followed by involvement of all muscle groups and the need for mechanical ventilation.

Progression is highly variable, and the disease course ranges from mild with spontaneous remissions to more rapid progression and death. Ocular MG has an excellent prognosis (McCance and Huether, 2002).

An emergency condition caused by myasthenic crisis or profound muscle weakness may occur if the dosage of medication is inadequate. Intravenous administration of anticholinesterase drugs (to block the enzyme cholinesterase, which breaks down acetylcholine) results in immediate improvement in strength. Anticholinesterase therapy may cause a cholinergic crisis, however. Weakness, ptosis, dyspnea, diarrhea, nausea, abdominal cramping, sweating, and vomiting may occur within an hour of dosing.

HUNTINGTON'S DISEASE

Huntington's disease (HD) occurs in 5 of every 100,000 persons regardless of gender or race. The disease is inherited. Children have a 50% chance of acquiring the disease if they have one affected parent. Onset is between the ages of 30 and 50 years.

Pathophysiology

HD is another degenerative neuromuscular disease characterized by psychiatric, cognitive, and movement disorders. The genetic defect causing HD has been localized to a long repeated trinucleotide (CAG) on chromosome 4. The more repeats beyond the normal number of 9 to 34, the earlier in life the disease will appear (McCance and Huether, 2002). By the time individuals know they have the disease, in middle age, they have typically passed on the abnormal autosomal dominant gene to their progeny.

In HD, abnormal levels of glutamine in the brain destroy brain cells, which causes degeneration and atrophy of the basal ganglia, the cerebral cortex, and the cerebellum. The neurotransmitters acetylcholine and γ-aminobutyric acid are lost, and there is a relative excess of dopamine. A buildup of lactic acid occurs because production of fuel for energy within the neurons is impaired (McCance and Huether, 2002; Neal, 2002).

Diagnosis

In addition to the tests listed in Table 24-1, studies are performed to identify the genetic marker: 28 or fewer CAG repeats is diagnostic of HD. Some family members of persons with HD have chosen to be tested for the genetic marker so they can begin to plan for a future of likely institutionalization and make a decision regarding whether or not to have children.

Clinical Manifestations

Clinical manifestations of HD are directly correlated with the pathophysiology of HD. Because the basal ganglia control movement; the cerebral cortex is involved in thought processes, judgment, memory, and perception; and the cerebellum modulates coordination and balance, movement, cognition, and coordination are most affected.

The relative excess of dopamine and deficiency of γ-aminobutyric acid and acetylcholine are manifested by chorea-like symptoms: hypotonia and hyperkinesia (fragmented, involuntary movements). Incoordination, balance and gait disturbances, impaired eye movements, dysarthria, and dysphagia are other motor impairments associated with HD. As the disease progresses, persons with HD experience dementia, sometimes manifested by violence, irritability, impaired judgment, paranoia, and hallucinations. Emotional changes also occur and can range from depression to euphoria and anger, and suicidal tendencies may decrease as the disease progresses. Affected individuals generally live 10 to 15 years after diagnosis and typically die from complications of choking, pneumonia, infection, falling, or heart failure (Smeltzer and Barre, 2000).

Think S for Success

Symptoms
■ Manage symptoms. Individual may have to be institutionalized when symptoms become unmanageable at home.

Sequelae
■ Prevent suicide if suicidal ideation or depression is present.
■ Prevent infection, choking, falls, heart failure, and pneumonia by treating symptoms.

Safety
■ Assist family and caregivers in creating a safe environment when patient develops balance and gait instability.

Support/Services
■ Ensure that patient obtains the necessary emotional support to deal with anticipation of getting the disease if family members have it or if individual chooses to be tested for the genetic marker.
■ Ensure that family obtains the necessary emotional support once patient becomes difficult to manage.

Satisfaction
■ Assist patient and family in getting the most out of life despite anticipation of developing the disease.
■ Help patient and family to manage symptoms so patient can enjoy good quality of life for as long as possible.

AMYOTROPHIC LATERAL SCLEROSIS

Amyotrophic lateral sclerosis (ALS) is more prevalent in men than in women until the age of menopause, then prevalence is equal. The disorder affects approximately 6 in 100,000 persons. Five thousand people are newly diagnosed with ALS each year in the United States. The disease occurs worldwide, and incidence does not appear to vary based on race, socioeconomic status, or ethnicity (McCance and Huether, 2002). Onset may occur in the fourth decade of life but peak incidence is in the fifth decade. There appears to be a familial component to ALS among approximately 10% of those who acquire the disease.

Pathophysiology

The majority of ALS cases are of unknown cause. A familial form of ALS (responsible for approximately 10% of all cases) has been linked to chromosome 21, and a defective gene appears to be responsible for one quarter of the cases that are familial. ALS affects the upper and lower motor neurons and leads to profound muscle weakness, respiratory failure, and death. Individuals usually die 3 to 5 years following the onset of symptoms. The gene normally codes for an enzyme that destroys free radicals.

A sporadically occurring genetic abnormality seems to be the best current explanation for ALS. However, the pathogenesis is unknown. Glutamate and hydrogen peroxide production may be abnormal (McCance and Huether, 2002). Upper and lower motor neuron degeneration occurs without inflammation but with subsequent axonal degeneration, demyelination, and glial scarring. Unaffected lower motor neurons attempt to compensate for those that have degenerated.

Diagnosis

Medical history and physical examination as well as electromyographic testing aid in the diagnosis of ALS. Abnormal electromyographic findings include muscle fibrillations and fasciculations and giant motoneuron spikes.

Clinical Manifestations

The initial site of weakness is variable and individual. However, some common characteristics are seen in muscle weakness in persons with ALS. Weakness generally begins with one muscle group and is asymmetrically distributed. Muscles of the eye and the myocardium are usually affected in the end stage of the disease. Paresis may be spastic or flaccid and eventually progresses to paralysis. Persons with ALS usually retain bowel and bladder control, and cognition and autonomic nerve functions are unimpaired until death occurs (McCance and Huether, 2002).

The lower motor neuron flaccidity of ALS causes muscle atrophy as a result of weakness. Range of motion against resistance decreases, as do deep tendon and other reflexes. Muscle wasting, fibrillations, and fasciculations with corresponding changes in the skin are characteristic. The hair may thin whereas the nails thicken, and perspiration and body hair decrease. Upper motor neuron spasticity includes weakness that progresses to paralysis and atrophy related to lack of use of muscle groups. Deep tendon reflexes may become hyperactive, and the patient may have clonus and a positive Babinski's sign.

As a result of muscle weakness, individuals are gradually less able to perform ADL and IADL. Muscle atrophy and wasting progress to immobility with its associated complications. Communication becomes difficult because of dysarthria and dysphagia and excessive or inadequate salivation. Diaphragmatic and intercostal muscle weakness leads to dyspnea and respiratory failure.

Think S for Success

Symptoms
- Manage symptoms.

Sequelae
- Maintain optimum function and mobility for as long as possible. Provide ventilatory support as needed. Provide assistance with feeding to prevent aspiration.

Safety
- Teach patient and family to modify environment at work and at home to prevent injury related to muscle weakness. Assist with acquisition and use of assistive and adaptive devices to maximize remaining strength and ability to engage in self-care.

Support/Services
- Assist in locating resources for financial and community assistance.

Satisfaction
- Assist family and caregivers in understanding importance of including patient in self-care as much and for as long as possible. Patient will remain intact cognitively, so teach importance of including patient in decision making and home life.
- Assist with equipment to maximize strength and maintain involvement in instrumental and other activities of daily living for as long as possible.
- Help patient to find alternative ways of enhancing quality of life if customary activities are limited because of muscle weakness.

REHABILITATION FOCUS

All of the neuromuscular diseases addressed in this chapter with the exception of GBS are degenerative. In rehabilitation the focus is on the physical, psychological, and social well-being of the patient. The hallmark of neurodegenerative disease is diminishing functional ability of the patient. This may be relentless in its progression, as in ALS, or much more gradual and subtle, as in many cases of MS. This anticipated decline in status necessitates a unique rehabilitation paradigm in which the goals of intervention may shift in focus during the transition from early stages of the disease to later stages. In early stages, patients and their families may be dealing with the impact of the diagnosis and may face many uncertainties. During middle stages of the disease, patients and families are beginning to deal with losses of function and perhaps beginning to make decisions about changes regarding their roles in life. Finally, during late stages of disease, patients and families are dealing with end-of-life issues. The rehabilitation focus shifts from restorative and preventative during early stages of the disease to more compensatory and palliative during later stages.

END-OF-LIFE ISSUES

Each of the diseases discussed in this chapter has associated end-of-life issues. Individuals with GBS may fully recover and, even if they do not, are still likely to have an average life span despite having had the disease. Persons with any of the other diseases, however, are likely to die of complications of the disease. The interdisciplinary team can make a very significant contribution toward assisting the individual and family or caregivers to prepare for the end of life. Helping the patient draft a living will and a power of attorney so that the patient's wishes will be observed is an important function of the team. Provision of support as needed to enhance quality of life for the patient and those involved in her or his life and to enhance quality of death when the time comes should be considered throughout planning and intervention in patient care. Hospice professionals and ancillary personnel can help prepare patients and families for the end of life and can offer chaplain and counseling services whenever needed, including during the year following the patient's death.

FAMILY AND CAREGIVER ISSUES

The diseases discussed in this chapter are all degenerative with the exception of GBS. Families and caregivers as well as patients are continually expected to adjust their lifestyles as the disease progresses. It is optimal for the interdisciplinary team members to work together to minimize drastic alterations in lifestyle by offering strategies and assistive and adaptive devices that can help patients and their families integrate the disease and its symptoms into their way of life.

Families and caregivers find themselves grieving for the patient long before the patient reaches the end of life because so much of the patient's previous functional ability is progressively lost. Families and caregivers need support and encouragement to seek respite care, to take time off, to join support groups, and to have fun. It is important to help them not to feel guilty for engaging in some activities away from the patient's bedside and to find activities that rejuvenate their energy and spirit. Local newspapers often list local support group information.

ETHICAL CONSIDERATIONS

Several ethical considerations may potentially arise with regard to the diseases discussed in this chapter. Box 24-3 lists some of these.

Box 24-3   Ethical Considerations

- The pursuit of measures to prolong life
- The decision to withhold or withdraw treatments
- The right to die
- Euthanasia and physician-assisted suicide
- The pursuit of genetic testing to determine propensity for the disease
- The decision to institutionalize the patient
- The decision about whether to have children
- The decision about whether to try experimental treatments

CASE STUDY
Patient Data
Mrs. N. is a 38-year-old white woman with relapsing-remitting MS. She was diagnosed with the disease 2 years ago. She has three children ranging in age from 6 to 17 years. She has been married to an Army officer for 18 years. The home health nurse notes in the history that the husband attempted suicide twice since the diagnosis and that Mrs. N. has become very controlling with unpredictable moods and frequent episodes of depression. Mrs. N. states that she has difficulty controlling her bladder. During the home visit, she complains to the nurse that she is overwhelmed with fatigue but discusses several outings she took the previous week to shop and lunch with friends. The nurse notes that Mrs. N. does not use any assistive devices and seems to be unsteady when moving about the house.

Thinking It Through
- What nursing diagnoses pertain or potentially pertain to Mrs. N. and her family?
- What kinds of medications might help Mrs. N.?
- What help might you offer her regarding her bladder problems?
- Prioritize Mrs. N.'s health needs.

Case Conference
The interdisciplinary team gathers in the home health agency conference room to discuss Mrs. N.'s case. The patient has chosen not to participate but her husband is in attendance as are the nurse, neurologist, medical social worker, husband's psychologist, occupational therapist, and physical therapist. The therapists are new to the case and have conducted only preliminary assessments of Mrs. N.

Continued

CASE STUDY—cont'd

The nurse suggests that Mr. N. express his concerns to the group. He states that life has been very difficult for him and his family since his wife was diagnosed with MS. He has felt helpless to handle the situation and that is why he attempted suicide. He states that the psychologist has assisted him in learning coping strategies that have helped, but his children appear to be suffering as well. He states that his wife's behavior and moods are unpredictable and that he and the children feel like they are living in a volatile environment.

The social worker confirms that during her counseling sessions with Mrs. N. she has ascertained that Mrs. N. suffers from intermittent manic and depressive episodes. The social worker suggests that a referral to a psychiatrist be initiated so that Mrs. N. can be started on appropriate medications. The psychologist states that he will be happy to see the husband and children in family counseling.

The occupational therapist comments that she has begun to teach Mrs. N. how to use some assistive devices to conserve her strength. The physical therapist mentions that she believes Mrs. N. could benefit from the use of a quad cane to increase her stability and that therapeutic interventions will focus on strengthening, energy conservation, and prevention of falls. The nurse and social worker agree that they will reinforce these instructions during their visits.

The nurse also asks the neurologist about medications to enhance Mrs. N.'s bladder control and suggests that Mrs. N. begin learning timed voiding techniques. The neurologist agrees and asks the nurse to teach Mrs. N. about the techniques and the medication and to keep him informed if catheterization becomes necessary.

The neurologist agrees to confer with and update Mrs. N.'s primary physician, who could not attend the meeting. He asks Mr. N. to encourage Mrs. N. to make an appointment with him soon so that he can reassess her. The nurse reminds him that she gives Mrs. N. weekly injections of interferon beta a1 (Avonex) and that Mrs. N. may be due for a check on her hemoglobin level and hematocrit because mild anemia is sometime a side effect of the drug.

The nurse also suggests that Mrs. N.'s diet be supplemented with calcium and vitamin D and that she moderate caffeine, alcohol, and phosphate intake to reduce the risk of osteoporosis, because women with MS are at increased risk for this disorder (Sharts-Hopko and Sullivan, 2002).

Mr. N. expresses gratitude for the conference and states that he will help in any way he can and will try to convince his wife to become a more active member of her health care team. The team disperses after agreeing to meet in 3 months to reassess the case.

Internet and Other Resources

Healthlink USA: *http://www.healthlinkusa.com*

Information Resource Center and Library, National Multiple Sclerosis Society: *http://www.nmss.org;* 733 Third Avenue, New York, NY 10017

MS Toll-Free Information Hotline: 800-FIGHT MS (800-344-4867)

National Multiple Sclerosis Society: *http://www.nmss.org;* 733 Third Avenue, New York, NY 10017

REFERENCES

Altman DJ, Gilchrist JM: Dystrophinopathies, Nov 12, 2003, retrieved from *http://www.emedicine.com/neuro/topic670.htm* on Jan 31, 2004.

Berkman CS et al: Use of alternative treatments by people with multiple sclerosis, *Neurorehabil Neural Repair* 13(4):243-54, 1999.

Bullock BL, Henze RL: *Focus on pathophysiology,* Philadelphia, 2000, Lippincott Williams and Wilkins.

Chance PF, Bird TD: Charcot-Marie-Tooth disease and other inherited neuropathies. In Braunwald E et al, editors: *Harrison's principles of internal medicine,* ed 15, New York, 2001, McGraw-Hill, pp 2512-5.

Copstead LC, Banasik JL, editors: *Pathophysiology,* ed 2, Philadelphia, 2000, WB Saunders.

Department of Health and Human Services: Healthy people 2010, ed 2, Washington, DC, November 2000, US Government Printing Office, retrieved from *http://www.healthypeople.gov* on July 20, 2003.

Gulick EE: Symptom and activities of daily living trajectory in multiple sclerosis: a 10-year study, *Nurs Res* 47(3):137-46, 1998.

Halper J: Multiple sclerosis care, *Clin Rev* 12(5):66-71, 2002.

Holland N, Halper J: Primary care management of multiple sclerosis, *Adv Nurse Pract* 7(3):27-32, 1999.

Huntley A, Ernst E: Complementary and alternative therapies for treating multiple sclerosis symptoms: a systematic review, *Complement Ther Med* 8:97-105, 2000.

Ignatavicius DD, Workman ML, editors: *Medical surgical nursing: critical thinking for collaborative care,* ed 4, Philadelphia, 2002, WB Saunders.

Imke S: Parkinson's: a medical management update, *Parkinson Rep* 19(30):1-7, 2000.

Lavalle JB et al: *Natural therapeutics guide,* Hudson, Ohio, 2001, Lexi-Comp and Natural Health Resources.

Lewis SM et al: *Medical-surgical nursing: assessment and management of clinical problems,* ed 5, St Louis, 2000, Mosby.

Lieberman AS: Hitler, Parkinson's disease and history, *Barrow Neurol Inst Q* 11(3):4-1, 1995.

McCance KL, Huether SE, editors: *Pathophysiology: the biologic basis for disease in adults and children,* ed 4, St Louis, 2002, Mosby.

National Multiple Sclerosis Society: Library and literature: epidemiology, March 2003a, retrieved from *http://www.nationalmssociety.org/Sourcebook-Epidemiology.asp* on Jan 26, 2004.

National Multiple Sclerosis Society: What is multiple sclerosis? August 12, 2003b, retrieved from *http://www.nationalmssociety.org/What%20is%20MS.asp* on Jan 26, 2003.

Neal LJ: Basic neurological assessment of the home health client, *Home Healthc Nurse* 15(3):156-69, 1997.

Neal LJ: Neuromuscular disorders. In Hoeman SP: *Rehabilitation nursing,* ed 3, St Louis, 2002, Mosby, pp 484-506.

Sharts-Hopko NC, Sullivan MP: Beliefs, perceptions, and practices related to osteoporosis risk reduction among women with multiple sclerosis, *Rehabil Nurs* 27(6):232-6, 2002.

Schwartz CE et al: Utilization of unconventional treatments by persons with MS: is it alternative or complementary? *Neurology* 52:626-9, 1999.

Smeltzer SC, Barre BG: *Brunner and Suddarth's medical-surgical nursing,* Philadelphia, 2003, Lippincott.

Whitmore SM, Leake MB: Complementary therapies: an adjunct to traditional therapies, *Nurse Pract* 21(8):10, 12, 13, 1996.

Worsham TL: Easing the course of Guillain-Barré syndrome, *RN* 63(3):46-50, 2000.

CHAPTER **25**

Disorders of the Joints and Connective Tissues

Sharron Guillett, PhD, RN, and Lee A. Bazzarone, DC, CCSP

OBJECTIVES

After reading this chapter, you should be able to do the following:

- Describe the pathophysiology of osteoarthritis, rheumatoid arthritis, gout, systemic sclerosis, and systemic lupus erythematosus
- Describe the clinical manifestations of osteoarthritis, rheumatoid arthritis, gout, systemic sclerosis, and systemic lupus erythematosus
- Describe the functional health patterns affected by osteoarthritis, rheumatoid arthritis, gout, systemic sclerosis, and systemic lupus erythematosus
- Describe the role of each member of the interdisciplinary team involved in the care of patients with osteoarthritis, rheumatoid arthritis, gout, systemic sclerosis, and systemic lupus erythematosus
- Compare and contrast the progression and management of osteoarthritis and rheumatoid arthritis
- Describe the indications for use, side effects, and nursing considerations related to drugs commonly used to treat osteoarthritis, rheumatoid arthritis, gout, systemic sclerosis, and systemic lupus erythematosus

According to the National Academy on an Aging Society (2000) 66% of the United States population reports having some form of arthritis. Current predictions are that by 2020 the number of people with arthritis will reach 60 million (Zarlinden, 2000).

Stated simply, arthritis is joint (*arthr-*) inflammation (*-itis*). It is part of a broader group of conditions termed *rheumatic disorders*. Rheumatic disorders are conditions characterized by inflammation, degeneration, and displacement of joints and related tissues. These disorders are associated with significant disability and expense, straining personal and financial resources.

The American Rheumatism Association classifies rheumatic disorders based on their nature and associated characteristics (Box 25-1). This chapter discusses chronic disorders in the categories of degenerative joint diseases (osteoarthritis), metabolic diseases (gout), and diffuse connective tissue diseases (rheumatoid arthritis, systemic lupus erythematosus, and systemic sclerosis).

ASSESSMENT

Individuals with chronic conditions affecting the joints and connective tissues experience many of the same symptoms and encounter similar difficulties regardless of the specific disorder. Therefore, the focus of overall assessment of these individuals does not differ markedly. The areas of primary concern are pain and mobility. These two areas greatly affect other functional health patterns and overall quality of life. A general guide for assessing functional health patterns is shown in Box 25-2. Ethnic differences in the incidence of these disorders are presented in Box 25-3. A list of instruments that have been developed to assist nurses in the assessment of functional health patterns is provided in Box 25-4. Concerns specific to a particular condition are addressed in the discussion of nursing care for patients with the given condition.

DEGENERATIVE JOINT DISEASE
Osteoarthritis

Osteoarthritis (OA), a degenerative disorder of the articulating joints, is the most common arthritic disease. It affects nearly 16 million Americans over the age of 60 and is the leading cause of disability in the aged (Summer, O'Neill, and Shirey, 2000). Weight-bearing joints are most often affected by this degenerative process, and it is more common in men than in women. OA may be primary (idiopathic) or secondary to trauma, infection, congenital defects, metabolic disorders, or overuse.

Degeneration of articular cartilage progresses slowly, affecting range of motion in the involved joint and producing varying degrees of pain and stiffness. Symptoms range from occasional or mild discomfort to painful disability. Although the incidence of OA increases with age, painful joints and/or alterations in functional mobility are not normal findings in any population and should be investigated.

<table>
<tr><td>

Box 25-1 American Rheumatism Association Classification of Rheumatic Diseases

Class 1: Diffuse connective tissue diseases
Class 2: Arthritis associated with spondylitis
Class 3: Degenerative joint disease
Class 4: Arthritis associated with infection
Class 5: Arthritis associated with metabolic and endocrine disorders
Class 6: Neoplasms
Class 7: Neuropathic disorders
Class 8: Bone and cartilage disorders with associated arthritis
Class 9: Nonarticular rheumatism
Class 10: Miscellaneous

</td></tr>
</table>

Pathophysiology

The body's joints are surrounded by a synovial membrane that secretes a liquid containing hyaluronic acid and glucoproteins, which help the fluid stick to the articular cartilage surface. Secretion of synovial fluid is achieved by mechanical stretch of the surrounding soft tissues and compression of the cartilage, which is normally smooth and translucent. Synovial fluid carries nutrients to cartilage, carries away debris, lubricates joints, and acts as a shock absorber when joint pressure is increased.

When there is too much stress on a joint over time, the articular components begin to break down. As the cartilage degenerates it begins to soften and becomes opaque with rough surfaces. The spaces between bones become narrower, and cartilage may crack and break loose, which

---

Box 25-2 Functional Health Pattern Assessment for Joint and Connective Tissue Disorders

HEALTH PERCEPTION/HEALTH MANAGEMENT
- Is there a family history of arthritis?
- What is the patient's perception of his or her overall health?
- What medications, including over-the-counter drugs, does the patient take?
- What alternative therapies does the patient use?

NUTRITION/METABOLISM
- What is the patient's current weight? Has there been any unexplained recent weight gain or loss?
- Is the patient on a special diet?
- What is the condition of the skin and mucous membranes?
- Is there a history of peptic ulcer or gastrointestinal bleeding?

ELIMINATION
- Have any changes occurred in bowel or bladder habits?
- Does the patient use an elevated toilet seat?
- Does the patient experience pain or difficulty in urinating?
- Is there a history of renal calculi?

ACTIVITY/EXERCISE
- Does the patient experience difficulty in walking, fatigue, or malaise?
- Does the patient have joint stiffness in the morning or after sitting for prolonged periods?
- What are the patient's regular exercise activities and recreational activities?
- What mobility aids does the patient use?
- Is the patient able to perform regular and instrumental activities of daily living?

SLEEP/REST
- How many hours of uninterrupted sleep does the patient get at night?
- Does the patient take naps or rest periods?
- What sleep aids are used?

COGNITION/PERCEPTION
- What are the nature, character, location, and duration of the pain?

- What factors aggravate and alleviate the pain?
- Is involvement symmetrical?
- Are paresthesias present?

SELF-PERCEPTION/SELF-CONCEPT
- How does the patient describe himself or herself?
- How has the condition affected the patient's self-esteem?
- How has the condition changed the patient's body image?
- What are the effects of the condition on the patient's sense of self?

ROLES/RELATIONSHIPS
- What kind of work does the patient perform?
- What role does the patient play in the home and family?
- What changes have occurred in the patient's ability to carry out role functions?
- How satisfied is the patient with his or her current roles and relationships?
- How has the condition affected the patient's family and/or significant others?

SEXUALITY/REPRODUCTION
- Is the patient sexually active?
- Have changes occurred in sexual performance?
- Is the patient satisfied with current sexual patterns?
- Have changes occurred in the menstrual cycle?

COPING/STRESS TOLERANCE
- What are the patient's coping strategies?
- What support systems are available to the patient?
- Can the patient manage the condition in the current setting?

VALUES/BELIEFS
- What constitutes quality of life for the patient?
- What is important to the patient?
- What are the patient's spiritual beliefs, health beliefs, and cultural beliefs?
- What is the patient's view about locus of control?

causes the synovium to become inflamed. The synovial membranes hypertrophy and synovial fluid becomes abnormally viscous. In areas where the cartilage has been totally destroyed, subchondral bones become dense and hard, and bony overgrowths develop. The reason cartilage begins to break down is not well understood. There is some evidence that inadequate nutrition plays a role, and genetic factors are known to influence the development of bony outgrowths (Heberden's nodes) (Bush, 2000).

Clinical Manifestations

Symptoms depend on the joints involved and the degree of degeneration present. The most common symptoms are stiffness and pain on movement. The stiffness associated with OA is not long lasting and generally improves with minimal activity. The pain associated with OA, described as deep aching, is localized and improved by rest. It is usually related to swelling, displacement, and inflammation of the

tissues surrounding the joint rather than to the joint itself. On palpation the affected joints feel hard and cool. As the pain increases, joint mobility and function decrease, which can affect posture, gait, and coordination. Symmetrical joint involvement is unusual, and wrists, elbows, and ankles are rarely affected unless they are injured. The joints most often affected are those of the fingers, thumb, lumbar vertebrae, and cervical vertebrae. Knees and hips are also frequently affected; arthritis of the knees is more commonly found in older women (especially in the presence of obesity) and arthritis of the hip occurs more often in men. Hip involvement is particularly debilitating. As pain increases and mobility decreases, it becomes difficult for the patient to bear weight, sit, and get up out of chairs, which results in significant disability.

Another common manifestation of OA is the development of bony overgrowths called nodes or nodules. Heberden's nodes are bony overgrowths that develop in the distal interphalangeal joints. They are associated with an autosomal gene that is dominant in women and therefore tends to appear in families. Bouchard's nodes involve the proximal interphalangeal joints and are less common than Heberden's nodes. Although the nodes themselves generally do not interfere with function, they are disfiguring and therefore distressing to patients (Figure 25-1).

A serious complication of degenerative changes in the spinal cartilage is a herniated nucleus pulposus (herniated disk). The herniated disk compresses the nerve root, creating pain and muscle spasm. A herniated disk requires immediate attention (see Chapter 26).

Diagnosis

Diagnosis is based on patient history and radiographic findings. Radiographs show a narrowing of the joint space, sclerosis, and bony overgrowths. There are no laboratory tests specific to OA. The erythrocyte sedimentation rate, usually elevated in inflammatory disorders, is generally within normal limits. Synovial fluid aspirate is normal in appearance and character.

Interdisciplinary Care

The goals of care include management of pain, maintenance of function, avoidance of the toxic effects of therapy, and maximization of quality of life. The team approach is the most effective way to accomplish these goals. Members of the team include the patient and patient's family, physicians, nurses, and physical and occupational therapists. Referrals to medical social workers can be made if warranted by the patient's need for additional resources.

Primary Provider (Physician/Nurse Practitioner)

Individuals with OA self-manage their symptoms until pain or discomfort interferes with function. At that point they may turn to the primary provider for help. It is essential that the provider attend to these complaints of pain and provide appropriate pain relief. In the past providers have tended to

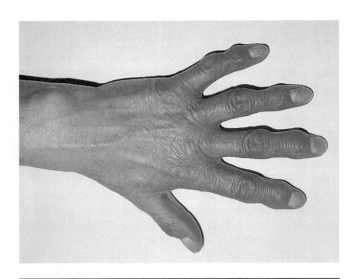

Figure 25-1 Heberden's nodes. (From Stevens A, Lowe J: *Pathology: illustrated review in color,* ed 2, London, 2000, Mosby-Wolfe.)

dismiss complaints of aches and pains as part of the aging process and have encouraged patients to take over-the-counter analgesics, rest, and apply heat to aching joints. This practice leads people to stop voicing complaints of pain, which contributes to undertreatment. There is also the potential of over-medication, especially with nonsteroidal antiinflammatory drugs (NSAIDs), which can lead to gastric complications. Providers should encourage people to stay active within limits of tolerance, recommend weight loss programs if appropriate, and advise patients about the types of medications that will be most effective. Information regarding the combining of drugs, safe dosage levels, and side effects should be discussed and reviewed at every visit. If medication is ineffective, surgery should be recommended before the onset of deformity (American Pain Society, 2002).

Drug Therapy

Pharmacologic treatment of OA is aimed at pain control. For many patients with mild to moderate joint pain, relief can be obtained from simple analgesics such as acetaminophen. For patients unable to control their pain with acetaminophen, NSAIDs and cyclooxygenase 2 (COX-2) inhibitors have been found to be effective (American College of Rheumatology, 2000). Caution must be used when patients taking warfarin are given high doses of acetaminophen, because acetaminophen can prolong the half-life of the warfarin. Prothrombin times must be watched carefully. Caution must also be used when giving NSAIDs to persons over 65 years of age because of the increased risk of adverse events such as gastrointestinal bleeding. Studies have shown that, in people over the age of 65 years, between 20% and 30% of hospitalizations and deaths involving peptic ulcer disease were related to NSAID therapy (Smalley and

Griffin, 1996). Risk factors that should be considered before encouraging patients to take NSAIDs are age older than 65 years, history of peptic ulcer disease, history of gastrointestinal bleeding, use of anticoagulants, and use of oral glucocorticoids. Topical analgesics may be used in combination with acetaminophen or alone by patients for whom acetaminophen is not effective and NSAIDs or COX-2 inhibitors are not an option. Table 25-1 provides a description of the drugs commonly used in the treatment of joint and connective tissue disorders. Recommendations for managing arthritis pain developed by the American Pain Society are shown in Box 25-5. The effectiveness of drug therapy is enhanced when it is combined with the nonpharmacologic measures described elsewhere in this chapter.

Nurse

As leader of the health care team, the nurse must assess the patient's functional ability, satisfaction with pain management, knowledge of the illness and therapeutic regimen, environment, support systems, and resources (see Box 25-2). Based on this information, the nurse develops the plan of care and makes the appropriate referrals. Patient education is critical to the successful management of OA and is the area on which nursing care should be focused. Studies have shown that patients who participate in self-management programs have less joint pain, make fewer visits to the doctor, and report improvement in quality of life (Subcommittee on Osteoarthritis, 2000). When self-management is not a realistic goal, the family and/or significant others should be taught how to carry out the therapeutic regime. The Arthritis Foundation offers self-management programs as well as other educational materials that help the patient and family gain confidence that the disease is manageable.

The plan of care includes teaching the patient and family how to do the following:
- Strengthen muscles and maintain or improve range of motion
- Develop strategies for protecting joints and conserving energy (Box 25-6)
- Maintain appropriate weight through diet and exercise
- Select appropriate clothing and footwear
- Use mobility aids and assistive devices safely
- Maintain a safe home and work environment (Box 25-7)
- Manage pain using drugs and nonpharmacologic methods

Social support has also been found to have a positive affect on functional status and adherence to therapy. The nurse can work with the health care team to establish a system of periodic telephone calls or visits from friends, family, and trained volunteers.

If the patient or family is unable to implement the plan of care adequately, the nurse should seek a referral to a medical social worker, who can explore home care services for which the patient may be eligible or pursue placement outside of the home.

Table 25-1   Drugs Used in the Treatment of Joint and Connective Tissue Disorders

Drug	Side Effects	Nursing Considerations/Teaching Points
NSAIDs Aspirin Choline salicylate (Arthropan) Celecoxib (Celebrex) Diclofenac (Voltaren) Diflunisal (Dolobid) Fenoprofen (Nalfon) Ibuprofen (Advil, Motrin) Indomethacin (Indocin) Meclofenamate (Meclomen) Naproxen (Aleve, Naprosyn) Piroxicam (Feldene) Rofecoxib (Vioxx) Sulindac (Clinoril) Tolmetin (Tolectin)	GI irritation, peptic ulcer, GI bleeding, nausea, vomiting, dizziness, rash, headache, tinnitus, nephrotoxicity, exacerbation of asthma Aspirin, choline salicylate, and diflunisal: salicylate toxicity	Before giving drug assess for bleeding disorders, peptic ulcer disease, gastritis, liver disease, kidney disease, and asthma. Administer drug with food, milk, or antacids if prescribed. *Do not* crush if enteric coated. *Do not* give aspirin and other NSAIDs together. *Use caution with anticoagulants.* *Do not use alcohol.* Report signs of bleeding, edema, weight gain more than 5 lb in 1 week, rashes, persistent headaches. Monitor BP, blood glucose level.
DMARDs **Gold salts** Gold sodium thiomalate (Myochrysine) Aurothioglucose (Solganal) Auranofin (Ridaura)	Parenteral: dermatitis, stomatitis, metal taste in mouth, blood dyscrasias, nephrotoxicity, diarrhea Oral (less toxic): GI irritation, renal complications	Give deep IM in buttocks. Check urine for blood and protein before each dose and *do not give if results are positive.* Check CBC. Do not taper. Caution women not to become pregnant while taking drug.
Antimalarials Chloroquine (Aralen) Hydroxychloroquine (Plaquenil)	Nausea, rash, headache, dizziness, blood dyscrasia, corneal opacity, retinopathy	Administer with food, milk, or antacid as ordered. Perform ophthalmologic examination each 6-12 mo. Avoid sun exposure. Report rashes and visual changes. Monitor CBC and liver enzyme levels.
Immunosuppressants Azathioprine (Imuran) Cyclophosphamide (Cytoxan) Cyclosporin (Sandimmune) Leflunomide (Arava) Methotrexate (Rheumatrex) Penicillamine (Cuprimine, Depen) Sulfasalazine (Azulfidine)	GI irritation and ulceration, alopecia, stomatitis, dermatitis, blood dyscrasia, bone marrow depression Same as above plus hemorrhagic cystitis, sterility Hypertension, hyperkalemia, hepatic and renal toxicity GI irritation, nausea, hair loss, diarrhea GI irritation, stomatitis, infertility, photosensitivity, blood dyscrasia, hepatotoxicity GI irritation, diarrhea, rash, pruritus, myasthenia gravis, blood dyscrasias, glomerulonephropathy, anorexia, nausea, vomiting, rash, yellow-orange skin, headache, thrombocytopenia, neutropenia, infertility, hepatic, renal, CNS toxicity	Warn about teratogenic effects. Monitor CBC, platelet levels, and urinalysis results. Use with caution in patients with liver or kidney disease. Same as above. Same as above plus give with meals. Avoid alcohol, report jaundice. Teratogenic; use birth control until at least 3 mo after discontinuing drug. Check CBC and liver enzyme levels. Give on empty stomach. Contraindicated with gold therapy. Monitor CBC, urinalysis results, liver enzyme levels. Avoid sun exposure. Check CBC and liver enzyme levels.

Continued

Table 25-1 Drugs Used in the Treatment of Joint and Connective Tissue Disorders—cont'd

Drug	Side Effects	Nursing Considerations/Teaching Points
Corticosteroids Dexamethasone (Decadron) Hydrocortisone (Solu-Cortef) Methyl prednisolone (Solu-Medrol) Prednisone (Deltasone) Triamcinolone (Aristocort)	Cushing's syndrome, GI irritation, osteoporosis, hypertension, steroid psychosis, acne, hirsutism, increased risk for infection	Use only as last resort and for short periods of time. Taper dose slowly. Monitor BP, weight, CBC, blood glucose level.
Biologic Response Modifiers Etanercept (Enbrel)	Injection site reactions, headache, sinusitis, rhinitis, URI, diarrhea	Use only in patients who have not responded to other DMARDs. Patient should not receive live vaccines. Notify physician immediately if urticaria, difficulty breathing, or new infection develops.
Analgesics *Nonnarcotic* Acetaminophen (Tylenol) Capsaicin cream	Rash, hives, leukopenia, hepatotoxicity Local burning sensation, redness	Avoid alcohol use. Do not exceed recommended dosage. Must be used regularly to maintain effect.
Narcotic Propoxyphene with acetaminophen or aspirin (Darvocet, Darvon) Codeine with acetaminophen or aspirin (Tylenol No. 3, No. 4, Empirin No. 3, No. 4) Oxycodone with acetaminophen or aspirin (Percodan, Percocet, Tylox) Hydrocodone with acetaminophen or aspirin (Lorcet Vicodin)	Arrhythmias, constipation, nausea, vomiting, sedation, headache, respiratory depression	Monitor CBC and liver enzyme levels. Caution about sedation. Take measures to prevent constipation. Report respiratory distress.
Drugs for Gout Colchicine (Novocolchine) Allopurinol (Zyloprim)	Nausea, vomiting, diarrhea, abdominal cramping, bleeding GI distress, bone marrow depression, rash; prolongs half-life of warfarin	Avoid use of alcohol. Drink 3 L of fluid per day. Report easy bruising or bleeding. Report nausea, vomiting, diarrhea. Give with meals. Drink 3 L fluid per day. Monitor BUN and creatinine levels. Check CBC, prothrombin time.
Uricosurics Probenecid (Benemid) Sulfinpyrazone (Anturane)	Headache, dizziness, nausea, vomiting, renal colic, fever, hives, anaphylaxis GI distress, GI bleeding, hypoglycemia	Do not take aspirin products. Drink 3 L fluid per day. Give after meals or with milk. Give with meals. Do not take aspirin products. Check for bleeding, monitor CBC. Drink 3 L fluid per day.

BP, Blood pressure; *BUN,* blood urea nitrogen; *CBC,* complete blood count; *CNS,* central nervous system; *DMARDs,* disease-modifying antirheumatic drugs; *GI,* gastrointestinal; *IM,* intramuscularly; *NSAIDs,* nonsteroidal antiinflammatory drugs; *URI,* upper respiratory tract infection.

Box 25-5   Recommendations for Managing Arthritis Pain

- All treatment should begin with a thorough assessment of pain and function.
- Acetaminophen is the drug of choice for mild to moderate arthritis pain.
- Cyclooxygenase 2 (COX-2) inhibitors such as Vioxx and Celebrex are the drugs of choice for moderate to severe pain.
- Nonselective nonsteroidal antiinflammatory drugs should not be taken unless patients are not responsive to COX-2 drugs because of the potential for gastrointestinal side effects.
- Opioids are recommended for severe pain unrelieved by other drugs.

Adapted from American Pain Society: Guideline for the management of pain in osteoarthritis, rheumatoid arthritis and juvenile chronic arthritis, 2002, retrieved from *http://www.ampainsoc.org/pub/arthritis.htm* on July 30, 2003.

Box 25-6   Tips for Protecting Joints and Conserving Energy

- Press water out of wash cloths instead of squeezing or wringing.
- Use padded pens and pencils and kitchen utensils, and loosen grip often.
- Use arms rather than fingers to carry baskets.
- Slide objects instead of lifting them.
- Use palms rather than fingers to push up from sitting position.
- Use elevated toilet seats.
- Use chairs with firm seats and arm rests.
- Do not sit in chairs with hips lower than knees.
- Use a firm mattress or add bed boards.
- Use carts to transport items from room to room.
- Pace activities to balance rest and work.
- Spread household chores out over the week.
- Sit on stool rather than stand when possible, for example, at sink, kitchen counter, stove.
- Use grooming aids like button hooks, shoe horns, and long-handled brushes.
- Use light-weight dishes and eating and cooking utensils.
- Modify clothing to use Velcro closures instead of buttons, zippers, or ties.
- Maintain normal weight and good posture.
- Avoid repetitive motions, painful activities, and heavy tasks.

Box 25-7   Home and Work Environment Safety Checklist

- Remove scatter rugs.
- Make certain that hallways, walkways, and work areas are well lighted.
- Use night lights.
- Add grab bars to bathroom tubs and toilets.
- Add hand rails to stairs and ramps.
- Modify work environment to allow for joint-protective adaptations.*

*The Americans with Disabilities Act requires employers to make reasonable accommodations and prevents job discrimination against people requiring them.

Physical Therapist

The physical therapist plays a central role in the care of the patient with a functional disability. On the initial visit the therapist measures range of motion and assesses muscle strength and joint mobility. The therapist is also concerned about pain management because pain interferes with the ability to participate actively in the therapy program. The therapist and the nurse work closely to design an exercise program that is both safe and effective. The therapist may also recommend the use of heat or mobility aids.

Chiropractor

The chiropractor has been specifically trained to diagnose abnormal joint motion and its associated signs of joint stiffness and muscle tightness at an early stage. He or she makes specific adjustments of the facet joints where adhesions are most likely to form (Cramer, 2000). These adjustments free the joints and restore normal joint mobility, which is paramount in stopping the progression of OA and preventing joint pathology.

The chiropractor also provides nutritional counseling and prescribes specific exercises to promote a healthy lifestyle.

In advanced stages of chronic OA, chiropractic treatment is mainly palliative and focuses on lessening or relieving pain by the use of heat, transdermal electrical stimulation, and low-impact adjustments.

Occupational Therapist

The occupational therapist is particularly helpful to the patient with OA because the therapist works on the small joints that are primarily affected by OA. The occupational therapist, too, assesses joint mobility and alignment and recommends devices such as splints that protect the joints as well as assistive devices to improve joint function (Figure 25-2).

Complementary and Alternative Therapies

The use of alternative therapies for treating OA is quite high, especially among older patients (Cherniak, Senzel, and, Pan, 2001; Ramsey et al, 2001). Therefore it is important to ask patients if they are using any of these therapies before recommending traditional therapies. Some herbal remedies such as St. John's wort are known to interfere with a number of other drugs, and careful exploration of the patient's use of herbs and supplements is important for patient safety.

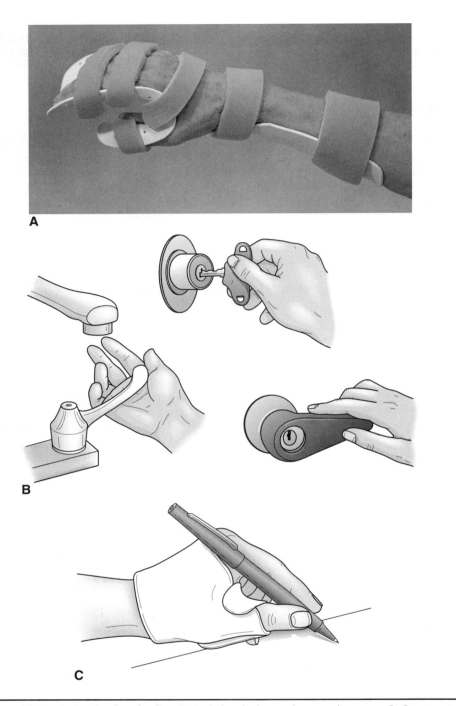

Figure 25-2 **A,** Resting hand splint. **B,** Assistive devices to increase leverage. **C,** Carpometa-carpal splint to decrease pain during activity.

Alternative therapies commonly used in the treatment of joint and connective tissue disorders are listed in Box 25-8. A number of research studies have been conducted to test the effectiveness of these methods. Early studies have demonstrated that several complementary and alternative therapies have positive benefits. However, the National Institutes of Health has released a statement that not enough conclusive evidence exists at present to make a decision either in favor of or against their use. The largest clinical trial to date of the use of glucosamine and osteochondroitin has recently been funded by the National Institutes of Health to determine if the claims that they improve arthritic symptoms can be supported.

Box 25-8   Alternative Therapies

- Acupuncture
- Diet modifications
  Consumption of avocado and soybean preparations
  Avoidance of nightshade vegetables (e.g., tomatoes)
  Consumption of pineapple (antiinflammatory)
  Consumption of fish oil supplements
- Chiropractic treatments
- Feng shui
- Herbal remedies
  Glucosamine
  Chondroitin
  St. John's wort (for depression)
  Chinese herbs (especially for gout)
- Massage
- Meditation
- Copper jewelry
- Yoga

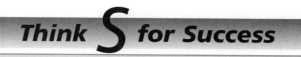

Think S for Success

Symptoms
- Manage painful inflamed joints with medication, joint rest, and protection.

Sequelae
- Prevent disability by instructing patient to protect affected joints and follow exercise regimen outlined by physical therapy.

Safety
- Teach patient and family the importance of the following:
  - Adhering to therapeutic regimen
  - Checking for signs of bleeding if patient is taking non-steroidal antiinflammatory drugs (NSAIDs)
  - Avoiding aspirin while taking other NSAIDs
  - Avoiding anticoagulants while taking NSAIDs
  - Using mobility aids safely

Support/Services
- Help patient obtain assistance with finances or community reintegration if needed.
- Make appropriate referrals.

Satisfaction
- Determine degree to which osteoarthritis is interfering with important aspects of patient's life and develop a plan to help patient reach or maintain desired quality of life.

DIFFUSE CONNECTIVE TISSUE DISEASES
Rheumatoid Arthritis

Approximately 1% of adults in the United States have rheumatoid arthritis (RA), a chronic progressive, debilitating, systemic disease characterized by symmetrical inflammation of the joints and related structures. Unlike OA, RA affects both large and small joints, including the shoulders, elbows, wrists, and hands. Other differences between the two include the higher proportion of women among those

with RA (3:1) and the systemic manifestations that accompany it. Table 25-2 compares the two disorders.

RA usually appears in the third decade of life and clinical complications occur most often in the fourth and fifth

Table 25-2   Comparison of Rheumatoid Arthritis and Osteoarthritis

	Rheumatoid Arthritis	Osteoarthritis
Incidence	1% of population	66% of population
Age at onset (years)	20-50	>40
Gender predilection	More common in women	No difference
Onset	May develop suddenly over weeks or months	Develops slowly over a number of years
Joints affected	Small and large joints Symmetrical involvement	Small joints, hips, knees, cervical and lumbar vertebrae Wrists, elbows, ankles and shoulders usually not affected
Nodules	Present	Heberden's
Signs and symptoms	Redness, swelling, warmth, prolonged morning stiffness Fatigue, fever, weight loss, malaise, depression Joints spongy and warm on palpation	Morning stiffness that improves with activity Painful joints with minimal redness and swelling No systemic symptoms Joints hard and cool on palpation
Radiographs	Narrowing, erosions, osteoporosis	Sclerosis, bony overgrowth
Laboratory results	Positive for rheumatoid factor, elevated erythrocyte sedimentation rate (ESR), anemia common	Negative for rheumatoid factor, normal ESR, anemia uncommon

decades. If left untreated, the disease leads to disability and premature death. Even with treatment, 7% of those affected will experience some degree of disability within 5 years of being diagnosed, and 50% will be unable to work after 10 years (Chen, 2000). The financial burden is also considerable; the annual individual direct costs for medical care are about $5000, and total U.S. expenditures related to the disease reach almost $9 billion per year (Ramsburg, 2000).

Pathophysiology

The cause of RA is unclear. Something triggers the release of massive amounts of macrophages and T lymphocytes into the synovial fluid. These cells release cytokines, small proteins that not only induce the inflammatory response but also interfere with bone formation, stimulate bone resorption, and erode cartilage. The four stages of disease progression are described in Box 25-9. Several triggers have been suggested, including infections, autoimmunity, genetic factors, environment, nutrition, and metabolic disorders.

Diagnosis

The American College of Rheumatology has identified criteria for the diagnosis of RA and defined a functional status classification of patients diagnosed with RA. These are presented in Box 25-10. The patient is said to have RA when four of the seven criteria are present and criteria 1 through 4 have been present for at least 6 weeks (Arnett et al, 1988).

Clinical Manifestations

RA has both systemic and articular manifestations and is characterized by periods of remission and exacerbation. The onset of RA may be abrupt or insidious, with patients complaining of nonspecific stiffness and aching accompanied by fatigue, malaise, and weight loss. Joints are red, swollen, stiff, and painful. On palpation, involved joints feel spongy

---

Box 25-9   Stages of Disease Progression in Rheumatoid Arthritis

- Stage 1: Inflammation of synovial membrane and fluid
- Stage 2: Development of granulation tissue (pannus) that covers the surface of the joint cartilage and eventually invades the joint capsule
- Stage 3: Replacement of pannus with fibrous tissue that blocks the joint space and interferes with motion and alignment
- Stage 4: Calcification of fibrous tissue, which may lead to complete immobility of the joint

Adapted from Lewis SM, Heitkemper MM, Dirksen SR: *Medical-surgical nursing: assessment and management of clinical problems,* ed 6, St Louis, 2004, Mosby.

Box 25-10   American College of Rheumatology Classification of Rheumatoid Arthritis

DIAGNOSTIC CRITERIA*
1. Morning stiffness lasting at least 1 hour
2. At least three joints with hot, soft tissue swelling or fluid simultaneously
3. At least one of the swollen areas present in a wrist, metacarpophalangeal joints, or proximal interphalangeal joints
4. Simultaneous bilateral involvement of joints
5. Presence of subcutaneous nodules
6. Elevated levels of serum rheumatoid factor
7. Radiographic changes (erosions or bony decalcifications must be present)

FUNCTIONAL CLASSIFICATION
Class I: Completely able to perform self-care, vocational and recreational activities
Class II: Able to perform self-care and vocational activities but limited in recreational activities
Class III: Able to perform self-care but limited in vocational and recreational activities
Class IV: Limited ability to perform any activities

*A patient is said to have rheumatoid arthritis if he or she has satisfied at least four of the seven criteria. Criteria 1 through 4 must have been present for at least 6 weeks.

---

and warm. Joint involvement is symmetric. The stiffness of RA is prolonged, lasting an hour or more.

As RA progresses the joint is destroyed and the supporting structures are weakened, which leads to deformity. Deformities of the hands include ulnar deviation of the fingers and subluxation of the metacarpophalangeal joints. Swan-neck deformity (hyperextension of proximal interphalangeal joints and flexion of distal interphalangeal joints) and boutonnière deformity (flexion of proximal interphalangeal joints and hyperextension of distal interphalangeal joints) are common. Deformities of the feet include subluxation and hallux valgus (deviation of the great toe toward the other toes) (Figure 25-3).

As stated earlier, patients also have a number of extraarticular symptoms. When the disease is active, patients are likely to experience fatigue, weakness, fever, weight loss, and anemia. As many as one half of all patients with RA also develop rheumatoid nodules as a result of vasculitis.

Interdisciplinary Care

Primary Provider (Physician/Nurse Practitioner)

The goals of care for the patient with RA are to control disease activity, slow the rate of joint damage, manage pain, maintain function for instrumental and other activities of daily living, and maximize quality of life.

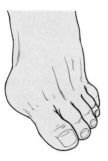

Figure 25-3 Hallux valgus. (From Lewis SM, Heitkemper MM, Dirksen SR: *Medical-surgical nursing: assessment and management of clinical problems,* ed 6, St Louis, 2004, Mosby.)

Patients with progressive systemic disorders experience disruptions in all functional health patterns and therefore have many health care needs. The care of individuals with RA is very complex, and once the diagnosis has been made, most individuals are referred to a rheumatologist, who then becomes the primary provider.

Drug Therapy

Drug therapy in RA is important not only to manage the symptoms but also to slow the disease progression. Drugs used include NSAIDs, corticosteroids, disease-modifying antirheumatic drugs (DMARDs), and biologic response modifiers (see Table 25-1).

All NSAIDs are similar in their efficacy. Factors to be considered when selecting the appropriate NSAID include cost, duration of action, patient preference, and incidence of side effects. NSAIDs should be taken with food to decrease gastrointestinal complications. Combining NSAIDs should be avoided because this practice does not increase effectiveness and adverse reactions may be additive.

Corticosteroids are used intraarticularly to treat flare-ups in one or two joints. Steroids may be given intramuscularly if several joints are affected. Because of their serious side effects, oral steroids are generally used only as bridge therapy until one of the longer acting drugs can take effect. Burst therapy may be initiated for an acute flare-up. In burst therapy oral steroids are given in high dosages that are tapered quickly over 1 to 2 weeks.

DMARDs have become the cornerstone of treatment because they have been shown to slow disease progression, retard the advancement of disability, and lower costs associated with the disease. Administration of DMARDs, which include gold salts, antimalarial agents, immunosuppressants, sulfasalazine, and penicillamine, is started early in treatment because these drugs take weeks to months to take effect. Methotrexate (Rheumatrex) is the most widely used DMARD because it shows long-term effectiveness, and in spite of its significant side effects most people manage to continue taking the drug for at least 3 years (Ramsburg, 2000).

Biologic response modifiers are a new group of drugs that attempt to balance the inflammatory process by using exogenously created tumor necrosis factor receptor molecules. The first drug in this category, etanercept (Enbrel), was approved by the Food and Drug Administration in 1998. Etanercept is administered via injection, and the most common side effect is a mild to moderate reaction at the injection site during the first few weeks of treatment.

Nurse

Education, pain management, and support are the priorities of care for the patient with RA. It is essential that both patient and family be aware of the systemic nature of the disease and the importance of adhering to the therapeutic regime. Family members should recognize that, even when the patient appears well, the patient may not be able to engage in normal activities or perform usual roles. The patient and family should be actively involved in discussing ways that they can work together with the health care team to manage the patient's condition and maintain family functioning. The patient should be given assistance in developing a realistic plan to balance rest and exercise and should be able to recognize symptoms indicating that the plan should be modified.

Pain can be managed by taking NSAIDs, applying heat or cold, and using other nonpharmacologic strategies referred to earlier. It is extremely important for the nurse to assess the character and level of pain at each visit. Pain signals disease activity, and a change in the nature or intensity of pain and/or stiffness may warrant a change in the plan of care. It is also important for the patient to have a thorough understanding of the way to use pain medications and the need for careful monitoring to prevent adverse events.

Because of the progressive nature of this disease, many patients become depressed. Supporting the patient and family as they work through the changes in functional status, body image, and roles is vital to helping the patient achieve the important possibilities of his or her life. Listening actively, identifying strengths, and validating the patient's concerns are useful strategies. Referring the patient to a social worker or counselor is sometimes necessary. A number of support groups exist to assist patients and families as they struggle with this disease. The Arthritis Foundation is an excellent resource.

The nurse also collaborates with physical and occupational therapists to determine what equipment or devices may be of benefit. The nurse reinforces the therapists' teaching in the use of assistive devices and encourages their use.

Physical Therapist

The physical therapist provides therapeutic exercises to improve joint mobility and maintain function. The physical therapist also makes recommendations regarding the use of mobility aids and devices to maintain body alignment. Splinting or casting may be necessary to prevent internal rotation of the hip or flexion contractures of the knees and elbows.

The physical therapist also applies heat using paraffin baths, whirlpool baths, heating pads, and moist heat packs. Applying ice to relieve pain may also be recommended. The modality used depends on the location and severity of the pain, as well as the ease and cost of the application. The patient can be shown how to use ordinary household items such as bags of frozen vegetables, wash cloths moistened and warmed in the microwave, and so on. It is very important that the patient limit applications of heat to 20 minutes and applications of ice to 10 minutes to avoid injury.

Occupational Therapist

The occupational therapist contributes significantly to the overall well-being of the patient because he or she provides strategies that promote independence. The occupational therapist observes the patient in the patient's environments to determine methods for simplifying work and reducing the stress on small joints. Something as simple as the weight of the dishes used by the patient may unduly stress the joints of the hands and wrists. Devices that allow the patient to continue self-care provide a sense of control and contribute greatly to self-esteem. The therapist can recommend grooming aids and suggest ways to adapt clothing for ease, comfort, and independence.

Medical Social Worker

The medical social worker assesses the psychosocial and financial needs of the patient and family. The social worker provides resources to help the patient and family manage the financial burden associated with RA. The social worker is very knowledgeable about services covered by Medicare and Medicaid and by any other programs provided by state or federal governments. The social worker also provides referrals for vocational rehabilitation and assists with placement in an adapted work setting if necessary.

Systemic Lupus Erythematosus

Systemic lupus erythematosus (SLE) is a multisystem inflammatory disease that gets its name from the common manifestation of facial rash, which gives the face a lupine (wolflike) appearance. SLE is an autoimmune disorder. Although the exact cause is unknown, genetic, environmental, and hormonal factors contribute to development of the disease. Because SLE is underdiagnosed and underreported, the true incidence of the disease is hard to determine (Bush, 2000). About 1 in 2000 individuals in the United States is known to have the disease. The disorder is much more prevalent in women, with a female/male ratio of 9:1 (Porth, 1998). The course of SLE is variable and unpredictable, with periods of remission and exacerbation. Although SLE was once thought to be fatal, the survival rate is now 70% 10 years after diagnosis.

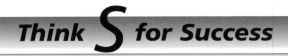

Think S for Success

Symptoms
■ Manage painful inflamed joints with medication, pacing, joint rest and protection, and careful applications of heat and cold.

Sequelae
■ Prevent disability by instructing patient to maintain proper positioning, reduce stress on joints, use good body mechanics, and follow physical therapy regimen.

Safety
■ Teach patient and family the importance of the following:
  Managing pain adequately
  Adhering to therapeutic regimen
  Reporting any side effects related to drug therapy
  Maintaining a safe home and work environment
  Not using over-the-counter drugs before checking with health care team

Support/Services
■ Help patient obtain assistance with finances, counseling, work, or community reintegration if needed.
■ If necessary, assist patient in managing depression, which is common.
■ Make appropriate referrals.

Satisfaction
■ Determine degree to which rheumatoid arthritis is interfering with daily, vocational, and recreational activities, roles and relationships, and important aspects of patient's life and develop a plan to help patient reach or maintain desired quality of life.

Pathophysiology

SLE is characterized by an overaggressive response of antibodies against normal body constituents related to impaired T-cell function and subsequent B-cell hyperactivity. SLE antibodies form immune complexes that trigger inflammatory responses in the connective tissues of the kidneys, heart, brain, lung, spleen, gastrointestinal tract, musculoskeletal system, peritoneum, blood vessels, and lymph vessels. The inflammatory response to the immune complexes causes localized tissue damage.

Clinical Manifestations

The early symptoms of SLE are similar to those of RA, including both systemic and musculoskeletal symptoms. Ninety percent of patients with SLE report joint symptoms, but the arthritis associated with SLE, unlike that in RA, does not generally result in deformity.

One of the most common manifestations of SLE is disturbance in blood cells. Some people have a tendency to bleed, whereas others have a tendency to form clots, but virtually all patients have anemia, three fourths have leukopenia, and about one third have thrombocytopenia.

The majority of people with SLE also have skin disturbances. The characteristic rash is a red butterfly-shaped rash across the cheeks and bridge of the nose (Figure 25-4). Other skin manifestations include hives, alopecia, discoid lesions, ulcerations of the oral and nasal mucosa, and a maculopapular rash that appears on surfaces exposed to the sun.

A large proportion of patients have cardiopulmonary manifestations at some point during the illness. Pleurisy and pleural effusions are common. Pericarditis, atherosclerosis, and vasospastic disorders are less common (about 20% of patients) and indicate advanced disease.

Almost one half of individuals with SLE have renal involvement and up to 10% develop renal failure. Lupus nephritis is the leading cause of death in SLE.

Central nervous system (CNS) disturbances include seizures, organic brain syndrome, and stroke. Organic brain syndrome is characterized by intellectual decline, disorientation, memory loss, psychosis, and depression. CNS involvement ranks second as a cause of death among patients with SLE. Patients also develop conjunctivitis and may be photophobic. Retinal vasculitis may cause transient blindness. Gastrointestinal symptoms include anorexia, nausea, and diarrhea.

Patients with SLE should be cautioned that pregnancy carries risks for both mother and fetus. Women should seek advice before becoming pregnant and plan the pregnancy during a time when disease activity is low. Women with advanced renal, cardiac, or CNS involvement should not become pregnant. Pregnancy can produce eclampsia-like symptoms that may result in fetal death. Other risks to the fetus include prematurity and stillbirth. Exacerbations of SLE are more likely in the postpartum period.

Diagnosis

The American College of Rheumatology criteria for a diagnosis of SLE are presented in Box 25-11. The presence of four of the criteria is indicative of SLE. It is important to consider history, clinical manifestations, and laboratory results together, because any single finding may be present in other conditions. Even a positive result on the lupus erythematosus preparation test is nonspecific because it may occur in other rheumatologic diseases.

Interdisciplinary Care

Primary Provider (Physician/Nurse Practitioner)

Care of the individual with SLE is similar to that of the individual with RA. The patient is usually cared for at home. However, close follow-up is warranted because of the powerful drugs used for treatment and the unpredictable nature of the disease. A flare-up can result in admission to a critical care unit. The patient is instructed to monitor temperature daily because fever is often the first sign of an exacerbation (Ignatavicius, 2002).

Drug Therapy

The drugs used to treat SLE are similar to those used to treat other rheumatic disorders. Patients with mild disease may manage symptoms effectively with aspirin or other NSAIDs. Patients with skin disruptions or arthritis may be given antimalarials. If so, an eye examination must be performed every 6 to 12 months. Steroids may be used topically for skin lesions and may also be administered to suppress acute exacerbations or treat life-threatening involvement in vital organs. Steroid dosage is gradually

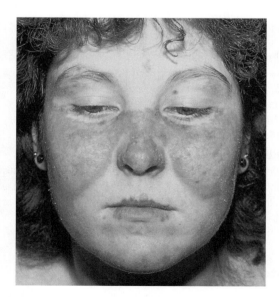

Figure 25-4 Butterfly rash of systemic lupus erythematosus. (From Habif TP: *Clinical dermatology: a color guide to diagnosis and therapy,* ed 4, St Louis, 2004, Mosby.)

Box 25-11   American College of Rheumatology Criteria for Diagnosis of Systemic Lupus Erythematosus

Presence of four or more of the following is indicative of systemic lupus erythematosus:
- Malar rash
- Discoid rash
- Photosensitivity
- Oral ulcers
- Nonerosive arthritis
- Pleuritis or pericarditis
- Renal disorder
- Seizures or psychosis
- Hematologic disorder
- Immunologic disorder
- Antinuclear antibodies

tapered as the exacerbation resolves. If conservative treatment is not effective, immunosuppressants may be ordered.

Nurse

The goals of care for the patient with SLE are to prevent exacerbations, manage pain, and maintain self-esteem. As is often the case, the chronic care nurse concentrates on health care teaching to promote self-care management and adherence to the plan of care. Health teaching should focus on skin care, medication management, avoidance of precipitating factors and infections, careful monitoring, and follow-up.

Skin care is important. The patient should be instructed to avoid prolonged sun exposure, excessive drying of the skin, and irritating soaps, shampoos, hair dyes, permanent waves, and so on and encouraged to use sunscreen products and hypoallergenic soaps and cosmetics. If hair loss is distressing, wigs, scarves, or other accessories can be worn until the hair grows back.

The patient should be instructed not to use over-the-counter drugs without checking with the health care team. The patient taking steroids must be cautioned not to abruptly discontinue the drugs for any reason. The patient should also be cautioned against taking aspirin and NSAIDs together. The patient taking antimalarials must be told to report any changes in vision and must undergo regular eye examinations.

Factors that precipitate an exacerbation of SLE include physical and emotional stress, infection, prolonged exposure to the sun, and some drugs and foods. The patient should be encouraged to balance rest and activity to avoid becoming fatigued. Drugs known to aggravate SLE are the sulfonamides and the antihypertensives procainamide and hydralazine. Oral contraceptives should be used with caution because they may also aggravate the disease.

Foods that may trigger a flare-up include sprouts, celery, parsley, and shiitake mushrooms. Relaxation techniques can be used to relieve emotional stress, and the patient should be encouraged to share fears and concerns with the nurse. The patient and family should be actively involved in the plan of care and participate in decision making to decrease feelings of helplessness and increase self-esteem.

Patients with SLE are susceptible to infection. Measures to limit exposure to infection include avoiding large crowds, staying way from friends or relatives who are ill, and using good hand-washing technique. Measures to increase resistance include ensuring sufficient rest and good nutrition. If anorexia is a problem the nurse can suggest dietary supplements.

The patient should also be taught to monitor himself or herself for signs and symptoms of a flare-up or worsening of the disease, including fever, chills, chest pain, malaise, oliguria, dysuria, increased fatigue, or changes in mental status, and to notify the physician if any such signs and symptoms are present. The patient should also watch for signs of medication side effects such as bleeding, swelling, nausea, or vomiting. The nurse should also encourage the patient to wear a Medic Alert bracelet.

Medical Social Worker

The medical social worker helps the patient and family adjust to the chronic yet unpredictable nature of the illness by helping them obtain the necessary financial resources and community supports. The patient may have difficulties with work or school that the social worker can help resolve.

The social worker also provides referrals to support groups, assists with family planning, and smoothes transitions from acute to chronic settings.

Think S for Success

Symptoms
- Manage symptoms with appropriate medication.
- Encourage frequent rest periods. Pain and fatigue are most frequently cited as interfering with quality of life.

Sequelae
- Prevent exacerbations by instructing patient to avoid known triggers such as the following:
  Infection
  Stress
  Sun exposure
  Certain drugs and foods

Safety
- Teach patient and family the importance of the following:
  Good skin care
  Appropriate use of steroids
  Monitoring for flare-ups or worsening of disease
  Conservation of energy
  Planning of pregnancies

Support/Services
- Assist patient in coping with body changes if necessary.
- Assist patient in obtaining counseling and financial support if necessary.
- Encourage frank discussion about fears and concerns.
- Teach family about patient's limitations.
- Promote positive outlook.
- Make appropriate referrals.

Satisfaction
- Determine degree to which systemic lupus erythematosus is interfering with relationships, employment, independence, and other important aspects of patient's life and develop a plan to help patient reach or maintain desired quality of life.

Systemic Sclerosis

Systemic sclerosis is more commonly referred to as scleroderma because the initial and most obvious manifestation of the disease is diffuse thickening and tautness of the skin. Scleroderma can be localized just to the skin or can be generalized, involving visceral organs.

The disease is relatively uncommon, affecting about 250,000 people in the United States (Scleroderma Foundation, 2004). Women are affected more frequently than men, especially during the child-bearing years, when the ratio of women to men increases from 3:1 to 15:1. The age of onset is generally between 20 and 50 years.

Pathophysiology

The cause of scleroderma is unknown, but genetic, environmental, and immune factors are thought to contribute to its development. Collagen is overproduced in skin, blood vessels, lungs, kidneys, and gastrointestinal tract. Eighty percent of persons with generalized systemic sclerosis have limited involvement; the remainder develop a severe form of the disease with diffuse visceral organ effects that progresses rapidly and is ultimately fatal.

Clinical Manifestations

Localized scleroderma produces changes in the skin that give it a taut, shiny appearance. The skin predominantly affected is that of the face and fingers. As the skin tightens, facial lines disappear and the mouth takes on a pursed-lip appearance. The fingers are pulled into a semiflexed position. As the skin over the bony prominences tightens, the skin may crack and split, which increases the susceptibility to infection.

Generalized scleroderma is frequently manifested by CREST syndrome:

Calcium deposits in the tissues
Raynaud's phenomenon
Esophageal hypomotility
Sclerodactyly
Telangiectasia (flat, reddened areas on the face and hands and in the mouth)

Arthralgias and morning stiffness are common early symptoms, as is Raynaud's phenomenon. Dysphagia is also common due to the inability to open the mouth wide enough for food to enter and the loss of esophageal motility. Pulmonary involvement leads to exertional dyspnea and eventually to right-sided heart failure. Cardiac involvement is manifested by dysrhythmias and episodes of pericarditis. Many patients also suffer from frequent bouts of diarrhea, which lead to malnutrition, dehydration, and in some cases social isolation as patients become reluctant to leave home for fear of not reaching a bathroom in time.

Diagnosis

No specific test exists for systemic sclerosis, and diagnosis is usually made on the basis of clinical manifestations. Skin biopsy and analysis may be performed to confirm the diagnosis. Laboratory studies usually reveal an elevated erythrocyte sedimentation rate and the presence of antinuclear antibodies.

Interdisciplinary Care

Primary Provider (Physician/Nurse Practitioner)

The primary provider attempts to keep the disease in remission through the use of immunosuppressants and high doses of steroids. Continuing care is aimed at managing symptoms, and referrals may be made to specialists based on individual needs. For example patients who develop esophageal strictures are referred to gastroenterologists for dilation procedures, whereas those who have skin conditions see a dermatologist.

Drug Therapy

No cure exists for systemic sclerosis; therefore, the drugs used are targeted to the symptoms present. Immunosuppressants and corticosteroids are useful in slowing the progression of pulmonary fibrosis in severe cases. Esophageal problems are treated with histamine 2 receptor blockers such as cimetidine (Tagamet) or ranitidine (Zantac). Patients with kidney disease are given angiotensin-converting enzyme inhibitors such as lisinopril (Prinivil) and captopril (Capoten). Calcium channel blockers like nifedipine (Procardia) may be prescribed for patients with Raynaud's disease.

Dietitian

The dietitian helps the patient identify nutritious foods that are easy to swallow. Consumption of fluids should be encouraged. If diarrhea is a problem, low-residue diets should be explained and their use encouraged. Vitamin supplements may be suggested to keep skin healthy and intact.

Nurse

Nursing care of the patient with systemic sclerosis depends on the symptoms present. The goals of care are to manage symptoms and maintain adequate nutrition, independence, and self-esteem. Health teaching is the primary mechanism for accomplishing these goals.

The patient and family should be taught strategies to conserve energy and protect hands and fingers. A patient with Raynaud's phenomenon should be encouraged to wear gloves to protect the fingers from heat and cold, even when lifting iced or hot drinks. Patients should be encouraged to stop smoking and instructed to avoid blood draws using the finger-stick method.

The patient with dysphagia should be taught to eat six small meals per day, chew food completely, and sit erect while eating. If reflux is a problem, the patient should sleep with the head elevated on pillows. Oral hygiene is very important and poses a problem because the mouth does not open wide. The patient should find a dentist who is familiar with the disease and can work with smaller oral openings.

Emotional support is another area on which the nurse must focus. The patient and family need information about the nature of the disease and an opportunity to discuss their fears and concerns. The changes in physical appearance, eating habits, and elimination pose threats to self-esteem and may generate feelings of helplessness or hopelessness. Sexual activity may be painful or the patient may avoid intimacy because of feeling undesirable. The patient may withdraw from social contact, creating disturbances in family and other relationships. Employment in the chosen career field may no longer be possible. The nurse should listen actively to patient and family concerns and make referrals to a social worker, counselor, or vocational rehabilitation specialist as needed.

Physical and Occupational Therapists

The physical therapist teaches and helps the patient to perform gentle range-of-motion exercises and keep muscle groups strong to maintain mobility.

The occupational therapist uses the same techniques to help the patient with scleroderma that are used to help the patient with RA.

Think S for Success

Symptoms
■ Manage symptoms with appropriate medication.

Sequelae
■ Prevent disability by ensuring that patient follows physical therapy regimen.

Safety
■ Teach patient and family the importance of the following:
Taking good care of the skin
Protecting feet and hands from heat, cold, and injury
Eating small, frequent meals of food that is easy to swallow
Conserving energy and protecting joints

Support/Services
■ Assist patient in coping with body changes if necessary.
■ Assist patient in obtaining counseling and vocational retraining if necessary.
■ Encourage frank discussion about fears and concerns.
■ Make appropriate referrals.

Satisfaction
■ Determine degree to which scleroderma is interfering with relationships, employment, independence, and other important aspects of patient's life and develop a plan to help patient reach or maintain desired quality of life.

METABOLIC DISEASE ASSOCIATED WITH ARTHRITIS

Gout

Gout is arthritis that occurs in the presence of increased levels of serum uric acid (hyperuricemia). This increased uric acid level may be the result of a hereditary inability to properly metabolize purines (primary gout) or the result of other conditions or medications that alter uric acid secretion (secondary gout).

Primary gout occurs predominantly among men between the ages of 30 and 50. Gout is rare among women, who tend to have lower uric acid levels than do men until after menopause. Women who do develop gout generally experience their first attack between the ages of 50 and 70.

Secondary gout is associated with conditions that either increase the amount of uric acid the body produces or interfere with the ability of the kidneys to excrete it. These conditions include alcoholism, arteriosclerosis, diabetes, hyperlipidemia, hypertension, obesity, renal disease, prolonged bed rest, prolonged fasting, and sudden or severe illness or injury. Drugs such as those used for cancer chemotherapy, immunosuppressants, thiazide diuretics, and low-dose aspirin can also cause increased serum uric acid levels.

Clinical Manifestations

Untreated gout develops in four stages. The first stage is characterized by an asymptomatic rise in uric acid levels to 9 to 10 mg/dl. If uric acid levels do not rise beyond that point, the risk of disease progression is slight. Only 5% to 20% of people with hyperuricemia progress to the second stage of the disease, acute gouty arthritis.

Acute gouty arthritis is usually precipitated by a specific event such as surgery, trauma, infection, or ingestion of alcohol (especially beer). Acute attacks may involve more than one joint but usually not more than four. The joint most commonly affected is the great toe. Other joints affected include the wrists, olecranons, knees, ankles, and midtarsals. These joints may appear cyanotic or reddened and inflamed and are very tender.

Once the initial attack subsides the patient enters the third stage, which is called the intercritical period. During this time there are no symptoms. This stage can last up to 10 years, but most people experience another attack within the first year.

The final stage, chronic gout, is characterized by involvement of multiple joints and the presence of urate crystals called tophi in the synovia, subchondral bone, vertebrae, cartilage, and tendons. The diagnosis of gout is made only when these urate crystals are found in joint fluid. Tophi generally take years to develop and can become so large that they deform joints and tear overlying skin.

Gout is experienced differently by different individuals. Some people have infrequent attacks that are mild, whereas others have frequent attacks that are severe and progressively disabling. The severity of the attacks and the progression of the disease are related to the levels of uric acid in the blood. Even though uricemia by itself is not diagnostic of gout, high uric acid levels appear to be associated with increased severity and the early development of tophi.

Complications of gout include OA, pyelonephritis, renal calculi, and infection related to disruption of skin over large tophi.

Diagnosis

Elevated serum uric acid levels are associated with a number of drugs and conditions other than gout. Therefore, although serum uric acid levels are almost always elevated in gout, serum uric acid levels are not diagnostic of gout. The diagnosis is made on finding urate crystals in the synovial fluid of an inflamed joint. To compensate for fluctuations in serum uric acid levels, urine may be collected over 24 hours to determine whether there is overproduction of uric acid.

Interdisciplinary Care

Primary Provider (Physician/Nurse Practitioner)

The primary provider prescribes maintenance medications and follows patient progress.

Drug Therapy

The purpose of drug therapy is to stop an acute episode and prevent future episodes. Antiinflammatory drugs are used to halt an attack. Colchicine (Novocolchine) usually stops the pain of an acute attack within 24 to 48 hours and is the drug of choice. Colchicine is so effective in treating gout that a positive response aids in establishing the diagnosis. NSAIDs are also used for pain management but contribute nothing diagnostically. Corticosteroids are used only when administration of colchicine and NSAIDs is contraindicated.

The drugs used to prevent future episodes are those that act either to increase uric acid excretion (uricosurics) or to decrease uric acid production. The drug most commonly used to increase uric acid excretion is probenecid (Benemid), and that most commonly used to decrease production is allopurinol. Colchicine has also been used as a maintenance drug because it reduces the frequency of acute episodes. It has no effect on uric acid levels, however.

The patient receiving drug therapy should be instructed to have serum uric acid levels checked at regular intervals. A patient taking a uricosuric drug must be cautioned not to use aspirin because aspirin blocks the drug's effect. Acetaminophen may be used for mild pain relief if needed.

Dietitian

The patient with gout may be placed on a weight reduction diet if obesity contributes to the condition. Some dietitians recommend restricting alcohol and foods high in purine such as sardines, anchovies, liver, kidneys, goose, and sweetbreads. Others place no dietary restrictions on the patient.

Nurse

Nursing care is directed at maintaining quality of life by managing symptoms, preventing disability, and assisting the patient in obtaining needed services and equipment. Inflamed joints must be supported and rested and may need to be immobilized. A foot board or cradle may be needed to keep the weight of bed coverings off of affected extremities. Open sores should be cleansed and an appropriate dressing applied if drainage is present. The patient and family should be instructed in the use of clean dressing and wound care techniques to prevent secondary infection. The patient and family should also be educated about gout and its management. The nurse should stress that gout is a chronic condition that can be controlled through careful attention to drug management and avoidance of factors known to bring on an attack.

Referrals should be made to physical and occupational therapists for assessment of joint function and recommendation of appropriate aids to promote independence in activities of daily living. Depending on the degree of joint deformity, the patient may need adapted eating utensils, dressing and grooming aids, mobility aids, and so on. A social worker is rarely involved in the care or disposition of the patient with gout. However, if the gout has resulted in a level of disability that interferes with the patient's ability to work or carry out expected roles, the social worker can assist the patient in finding the resources and support needed.

Think **S** for Success

Symptoms
- Manage painful inflamed joints with medication, joint rest, and protection.

Sequelae
- Prevent disability by monitoring and controlling uric acid levels.

Safety
- Teach patient and family the importance of the following:
  Adhering to therapeutic regimen
  Having serum uric acid levels checked regularly
  Avoiding aspirin while taking uricosuric drugs
  Understanding factors that lead to an attack

Support/Services
- Help patient obtain assistance with finances or community reintegration if needed.
- Make appropriate referrals.

Satisfaction
- Determine degree to which gout is interfering with important aspects of patient's life and develop a plan to help patient reach or maintain desired quality of life.

FAMILY AND CAREGIVER ISSUES

A number of family and caregiver issues arise in disorders of the joints and connective tissues. Family members or caregivers may tire of the complaints of the person with arthritis or joint pain, or minimize or disbelieve the patient's symptoms. There may also be a lack of understanding of the need to permit the patient to perform maximal self-care by modifying the environment to fit the patient's new lifestyle.

ETHICAL CONSIDERATIONS

SLE is a disease in which ethical dilemmas may arise. For example, Ms. Jones is 25 years old and has not experienced a remission of her SLE symptoms or disease since diagnosis at age 19. During one of her routine visits to the rheumatologist, she excitedly states that she and her husband are eager for her to get pregnant and have a beautiful healthy baby. What is the ethical obligation of the nurse (or other health care provider) on hearing this information? The nurse may choose to support Ms. Jones' decision because it is the patient's decision whether or not to attempt to become pregnant. However, the nurse may feel that she has an ethical duty to share information with Ms. Jones and her husband regarding the significant risks related to pregnancy, delivery, and the health of the newborn for a patient with SLE. What if the patient refuses to hear this information when the nurse offers to share it with her?

CASE STUDY

Patient Data

Mrs. T. is a 70-year-old retired piano teacher. She lives with her husband, also retired, in a three-bedroom brick home in the suburbs. She has a large back yard and since her retirement spends a lot of time gardening. Her two children are grown and live in other states. She has six grandchildren who take turns staying with her over the summer when school is not in session.

She is active in her church as well as in a number of civic organizations. Over the past several weeks she has been feeling "achy" and tired but states that "at my age you begin to expect good days and bad days." She started taking ibuprofen (Motrin) but the recommended dosage did not seem to help much. When the aching and fatigue kept her from her gardening and volunteer work, her husband began to worry and suggested that she go to the clinic. The nurse noted that the knuckles on both hands were red and swollen and warm to the touch. Range of motion was limited in the hands and fingers and grip was weak bilaterally. Mrs. T. was unable to make a fist. The physician ordered radiographs, a complete blood count with differential, erythrocyte sedimentation rate, and test for rheumatoid factor.

Diagnostic Findings

■ Hemoglobin level: 11 g/dl
■ Hematocrit: 33%
■ White blood count: 5000/mm^3
■ Erythrocyte sedimentation rate: 55 mm/hour
■ Rheumatoid factor: positive
■ Radiographs: within normal limits

Thinking It Through

■ What nursing diagnoses pertain to Mrs. T.?
■ Does the care of an older patient with RA differ from that of a younger patient? In what way?
■ How can the health care team contribute to Mrs. T.'s quality of life?
■ What are Mrs. T.'s concerns likely to be? How would you as the nurse address them?
■ What are Mr. T.'s concerns likely to be? How would you as the nurse address them?

Case Conference

The interdisciplinary team that has gathered to discuss and plan Mrs. T.'s care includes the rheumatologist, nurse, physical therapist, occupational therapist, and Mrs. T. and her husband.

The rheumatologist has already reviewed her findings with Mrs. T., explaining that Mrs. T. has early signs of RA. At this meeting the physician will provide the prescriptions necessary for Mrs. T. to receive the drugs and therapies the team feels are warranted.

The nurse, who also has already spent some time talking with Mrs. T. and her husband about the impact that the diagnosis is likely to have on their every day life and future plans, will act as case manager and coordinate the activities of the therapists. The nurse teaches Mrs. T. about the DMARDs she will be taking and any potential side effects, stressing those that should be reported to either her or the physician. Mrs. T. expresses concern about the cost of the drugs because the family is on a fixed income and she does not have prescription drug coverage through Medicare. The nurse suggests that the doctor write a referral to social services to explore other sources of financial support. The nurse also recommends that Mrs. T. call the local Area Agency on Aging to learn what resources are available. Mrs. T. does not own a computer but her grandchildren are quite computer literate, so the nurse suggests that Mrs. T. and her grandchildren go on-line to get information about "Medigap" insurance as well as support groups for people with RA.

Discussion about the computer prompts the occupational therapist to address the issue of protecting small joints. She warns Mrs. T. about the dangers of activities that use repetitive motions or place hands, fingers, and wrists in unnatural positions. If Mrs. T. uses a keyboard she should have built-up wrist pads and should rest frequently. Mrs. T. laughs and indicates that she probably will not spend much time at the keyboard but that she wonders if she can continue gardening. The occupational therapist suggests that she make a home visit to see what the garden looks like and observe how Mrs. T. works there. Then she can suggest some modifications that may allow Mrs. T. to engage in those activities she most enjoys.

At this point Mr. T. speaks up and tells his wife that he doesn't want her to do anything that will hurt her. He says that she should just rest and get better and let him worry about the garden. The nurse recognizes Mr. T.'s anxiety and encourages him to talk about that. Once he has voiced his concerns the nurse reassures him that, although balancing rest and activity is important, in people of Mrs. T.'s age it is important to keep moving. There is more danger of developing complications from disuse than from exercise. If working in the garden becomes painful, then other hobbies can be explored.

The physical therapist asks Mrs. T. if she has a heating pad at home and explains the correct way to apply heat for comfort. She also gives Mrs. T. a pamphlet on body mechanics and ways to avoid injuries to both small and large weight-bearing joints. The physical therapist, too, would like to make a home visit to look at chairs, beds, stairs, and so on to determine if any mobility aids are likely to be needed. She encourages Mrs. T. to let Mr. T. carry groceries and other packages for her. She also suggests that they get a little pushcart so that Mrs. T. can push rather carry items from room to room as well as a kitchen stool so that Mrs. T. can sit rather than stand at the sink and stove.

The nurse notices that Mrs. T. has been rubbing her hands throughout the discussion and asks her if she is in pain. Mrs. T. replies, "Oh, it's nothing I can't handle." The nurse talks to Mrs. T. about the importance of pain management and suggests that she begin taking aspirin for the pain. If that is not effective, the

CASE STUDY—cont'd

doctor can prescribe a different pain medication for her, such as ibuprofen. The nurse explains that it will take a few weeks for the DMARD to take effect and that it is important to treat the pain and inflammation until this happens so that the damage to her joints can be minimized. The nurse cautions Mrs. T. not to take any medicines other than those prescribed and to check with her or the physician before taking cough syrups or cold remedies because they may increase the likelihood of adverse reactions.

Mrs. T. asks if she should be on any special diet. The physician states that as long as Mrs. T. maintains her weight she should be fine and adds that, if the medicine or illness causes a loss of appetite or weight, she should supplement her diet with Ensure or something similar. Mr. T. assures the doctor that he will make certain Mrs. T. eats right.

The nurse asks Mr. and Mrs. T. if they have any questions. At this point they are fairly overwhelmed and cannot think of any-thing to ask. The nurse gives them her card and tells them to call her if they think of anything once they are home. The physical therapist and occupational therapist schedule a time for a home visit, and the nurse states that she will call in about a week to see how Mrs. T. is feeling. Mrs. T. is given a prescription for methotrexate, and a return appointment is scheduled for the next month.

Once the team meeting is over, the nurse returns to her office and thinks about the meeting as she develops a plan of care for Mrs. T.

■ What new information was gathered that would assist the nurse in developing the plan of care?
■ What strengths do Mr. and Mrs. T. bring to the team?
■ What barriers to therapy must be overcome?
■ Identify two collaborative problems that the plan of care should address.

Internet and Other Resources

American Pain Society: *http://www.ampainsoc.org*
Arthritis Foundation: *http://www.arthritis.org*
Lupus Foundation of America: *http://www.lupus.org*
National Institute of Arthritis and Musculoskeletal and Skin Diseases: *http://www.niams.nih.gov*
Scleroderma Foundation: *http://www.scleroderma.org*

REFERENCES

American College of Rheumatology, Subcommittee on Guidelines: Recommendations for the medical management of osteoarthritis of the hip and knee, *Arthritis Rheum* 43(9):1909-15, 2000.

American Pain Society: Guideline for the management of pain in osteoarthritis, rheumatoid arthritis and juvenile chronic arthritis, 2002, retrieved from *http://www.ampainsoc.org/pub/arthritis.htm* on Feb 6, 2003.

Arnett FC et al: The revised criteria for the classification of rheumatoid arthritis, *Arthritis Rheum* 31:315-24, 1988.

Bush M: Arthritis and connective tissue diseases. In Lewis SM, Heitkemper MM, Dirksen SR, editors: *Medical-surgical nursing: assessment and management of clinical problems*, ed 5, St Louis, 2000, Mosby.

Chen S: Pain and rheumatoid arthritis: an update, *Drug topics* 144(17):47, 2000.

Cherniak EP, Senzel RS, Pan CX: Correlates of use of alternative medicine by the elderly in an urban population, *J Altern Complement Med* 7(3):277-80, 2001.

Cramer G: Effects of side-posture positioning and side-posture adjusting on the lumbar zygapophysial joints as evaluated by magnetic resonance imaging; a before and after study with randomization, *J Manipulative Physiol Ther* 23(6):380-94, 2000.

Ignatavicius D: Interventions for the client with connective tissue disease. In Ignatavicius D, Workman M, editors: *Medical surgical nursing: critical thinking for collaborative care,* ed 4, Philadelphia, 2002, WB Saunders, pp 328-63.

National Academy on an Aging Society: Arthritis: a leading cause of disability in the United States, 2000, retrieved from *http://www.agingsociety. org/agingsociety/pdf/arthritis.pdf* on March 4, 2004.

Porth CM: *Pathophysiology: concepts of altered health states,* ed 5, Philadelphia, 1998, Lippincott.

Ramsburg K: Rheumatoid arthritis, *Am J Nurs* 100(11):40-3, 2000.

Ramsey SD et al: Use of alternative therapies by older adults with osteoarthritis, *Arthritis Rheum* 45(3):222-7, 2001.

Scleroderma Foundation: What is scleroderma?, retrieved from *http://www. scleroderma.org/medical/overview.htm* on Feb 9, 2004.

Smalley WE, Griffin MR: The risks and costs of upper gastrointestinal complications attributable to NSAIDs, *Gastroenterol Clin North Am* 25:373-96, 1996.

Summer K, O'Neill G, Shirey L: Arthritis: a leading cause of disability in the United States, Washington, DC, March 2000, National Academy on an Aging Society.

Zarlinden J: New pain relief for arthritis, *Nurs Spectrum* 10:14-6, March 6, 2000.

CHAPTER 26

Musculoskeletal Disorders

Dottie Roberts, MSN, MACI, CMSRN, RN, BC, ONC

Chronic musculoskeletal disorders are a common cause of impairments and disability. They affect an individual's ability to participate in society and maintain an acceptable quality of life. This chapter explores the incidence, pathogenesis, and treatment of such common musculoskeletal disorders as osteoporosis, fibromyalgia, Paget's disease, osteomyelitis, and low back pain.

ASSESSMENT

Although chronic musculoskeletal disorders have unique causes and treatments, the affected individuals share many symptoms such as pain and immobility. Problems in these two areas affect other health patterns and overall quality of life. A general framework for assessing functional health patterns is provided in Box 25-2. For the patterns identified in the box, those issues related to self-perception/self-concept and roles/relationships may be of most significance because the physical changes that mark most of these diseases can greatly affect an individual's self-confidence and role performance. Additional assessment instruments are listed in Box 26-1.

Ethnic Variations

Of the musculoskeletal conditions discussed in this chapter, osteoporosis is the only one with recognized ethnic differences in incidence. Whites, Hispanics, and Asians are at higher risk of developing osteoporosis than any other ethnic groups. However, approximately 300,000 African American women also have the disease (Agency for Healthcare Research and Quality, 2001; Sedlak and Doheny, 2002).

OSTEOPOROSIS

Osteoporosis is a systemic skeletal disease characterized by low bone mass (or bone mineral density [BMD]) and deterioration of bony tissue, with increased bone fragility and susceptibility to fracture. According to the National Osteoporosis Foundation (2002a), almost 44 million men and women 50 years of age or older have osteoporosis or low bone density. If the diagnostic categories of the World Health Organization (1999) are used, then as many as 70% of women over 80 years of age have osteoporosis (Table 26-1).

Pathophysiology

Bone is a dynamic tissue that undergoes a continuous process known as remodeling, in which old bone is replaced by new bone. Remodeling begins with activation of osteoclasts, cells that resorb a small portion of bone over approximately 7 to 10 days. Osteoblasts then form an organic matrix that mineralizes new bone. In osteoporosis, a disturbance occurs in the normal balance of osteoblastic and osteoclastic activity. Mineral and protein components are diminished in the bony matrix, and BMD decreases (Geier, 2001).

Peak bone mass is reached by about 30 years of age in both men and women. Bone mass is enhanced by adequate calcium intake and weight-bearing exercise. Between the age of 30 and menopause in women, BMD may plateau or decrease slightly. A perimenopausal woman begins to experience a marked decrease in BMD because of decreases in the amount of natural estrogen (Roberts and Lappe, 2001). Bone loss accelerates in the 2 years before a woman's last menstrual period, and rapid loss continues for another 2 years after the end of menses. Rapid bone loss can also occur following surgical menopause, a result of the removal of the ovaries.

Box 26-1 Functional Assessment Instruments

- Barthel Index
- Beck Depression Inventory (BDI)
- Chronic Illness Resources Survey (CIRS)
- Functional Disability Inventory (FDI)
- Functional Independence Measure (FIM)
- Functional Status Index (FSI)
- Functional Status Questionnaire (FSQ)
- Index of Extended Activities of Daily Living
- Katz Index of Independence in Activities of Daily Living (Katz ADL)
- Minnesota Multiphasic Personality Inventory-2–based Personality Psychopathology Five (PSY-5) scales
- Owestry Disability Questionnaire
- Physical Performance Test (PPT)
- Quebec Back Pain Disability Scale
- Roland-Morris Disability Questionnaire
- Short Form 12 (SF-12) Health Survey
- Short Form 36 (SF-36) Health Survey
- Sickness Impact Profile (SIP)

Box 26-2 Risk Factors for Osteoporosis

- Female gender
- Increasing age
- Family history of osteoporosis*
- Personal history of fractures as an adult
- Small-boned, thin body build
- White or Asian ethnicity
- Menopausal status, history of loss of menses before menopause
- Lifestyle choices
  Inadequate calcium intake
  Nutritional disorders (e.g., anorexia nervosa)
  Lack of weight-bearing exercise
  Smoking*
  Alcohol use
- Other factors
  Hypogonadism*
  Use of certain medications (glucocorticoids are especially damaging)*
  Hypercalciuria*
  Hyperthyroidism
  Hyperparathyroidism
  Multiple myeloma
  Transplantation
  Chronic disease

Adapted from Burgess E, Nanes MS: Osteoporosis in men: pathophysiology, evaluation, and therapy, *Curr Opin Rheumatol* 1(4):421-8, 2002c; and National Osteoporosis Foundation: Prevention: who's at risk? 2002, retrieved from *http://www.nof.org/prevention/risk.htm* on April 27, 2003.
*Significant for men.

Although many studies have evaluated osteoporosis in women, less is known about loss of bone density in men. According to Burgess and Nanes (2002), men present unique challenges with regard to osteoporosis screening, differential diagnosis, and treatment. Risk factors for osteoporosis are identified in Box 26-2. Those that are significant for men are indicated with an asterisk. Men have a higher peak bone mass than women. Therefore, the loss of 1 standard deviation unit in BMD leaves men with a higher resid-

ual bone mass than women. The true relationship between male T scores (a measure of BMD) and fracture risk must be determined to allow osteoporosis to be defined accurately and treated appropriately in men.

Clinical Manifestations

The patient with osteoporotic vertebrae usually shows progressive spinal deformity and shortened stature. As kyphosis (dowager's hump) increases, the lower ribs eventually come to rest on the iliac crests. Downward pressure on the internal organs causes abdominal distention and bloating, and breathing can be impaired by restricted lung expansion (Figure 26-1). The patient may complain of difficulty in finding clothing that fits well.

In many individuals, the diagnosis of osteoporosis is made after a fracture. Patients with osteoporosis are especially prone to *fragility fractures* caused by low-trauma events, such as sneezing or bending to pick up a newspaper, that would not cause fractures in healthy individuals. If an osteoporotic vertebral body collapses on itself (compression or crush fracture), the patient may complain of a sudden onset of severe back pain that worsens with movement and

Table 26-1 World Health Organization Definitions of Osteopenia and Osteoporosis

Term	Definition
Normal	Bone mineral density (BMD) or bone mineral content (BMC) no more than 1 standard deviation (SD) below the young adult mean
Low bone mass (osteopenia)	BMD or BMC between 1.0 and 2.5 SDs below the young adult mean
Osteoporosis	BMD or BMC more than 2.5 SDs below the young adult mean
Severe (established) osteoporosis	BMD or BMC more than 2.5 SDs below the young adult mean *and* the presence of one or more fragility fractures

Adapted from Roberts D, Lappe J: Management of clients with musculoskeletal disorders. In Black JM, Hawks JH, Keene AM, editors: *Medical-surgical nursing: clinical management for positive outcomes,* ed 6, Philadelphia, 2001, WB Saunders, pp 551-85.

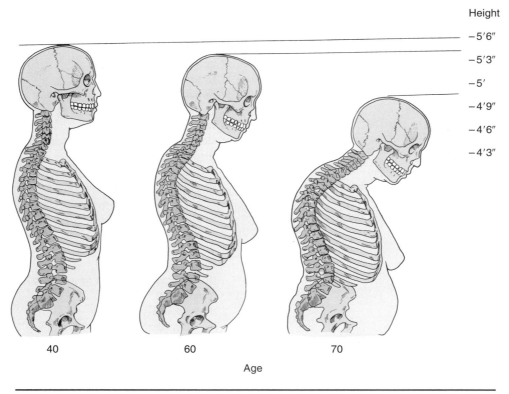

Height
— 5'6"
— 5'3"
— 5'
— 4'9"
— 4'6"
— 4'3"

40   60   70

Age

Figure 26-1   Osteoporotic changes. A normal spine at age 40 years and osteoporotic changes at ages 60 and 70 years. These changes may result in dorsal kyphosis and loss of height. (From Roberts D, Lappe J: Management of clients with musculoskeletal disorders. In Black JM, Hawks JH, Keene AM, editors: *Medical-surgical nursing: clinical management for positive outcomes,* ed 6, Philadelphia, 2001, WB Saunders.)

is relieved by rest. However, many fractures are discovered accidentally either on routine radiographs or during radiologic evaluation of suspected pneumonia.

Hip fractures often occur in patients with osteoporosis when an unstable gait leads to a fall. Hip fractures continue to be associated with high rates of mortality and loss of independence. About 24% of patients aged 50 and older who sustain a hip fracture die within 1 year following their injuries. A year after hip fracture, 40% of patients are unable to walk without assistance, and only one third of patients fully regain their preinjury level of independence (National Osteoporosis Foundation, 2001). Because men generally experience decreased BMD later than women, they account for only about 20% of hip fractures. Approximately 17% of men have had a hip fracture by the age of 90, compared with 32% of women (Ott, 1999).

Fractures of the wrist may also occur with a fall. Osteoporosis can also affect the mandible. Decreased BMD in the jaw can lead to loss of teeth or to poor fitting of dentures, and can also cause changes in the appearance of the face.

The impact of osteoporosis is not limited to the skeleton. The patient with osteoporosis must also cope with associ-

ated functional problems, low self-esteem, and psychological distress (Roberto and Reynolds, 2001). The patient often describes decreasing involvement with family and friends, acknowledging that the ability to participate in valued social activities has been influenced by the pain caused by osteoporotic changes.

Diagnosis

Standard radiographic examination does not reveal the presence of osteoporotic changes until approximately 30% of bone mass has been lost (Sedlak and Doheny, 2002). Among bone studies used to diagnose osteoporosis, dual-energy x-ray absorptiometry (DEXA) is the gold standard. This test carries low risk and takes relatively little time to perform. The spine and the hip are the sites most commonly measured during a DEXA scan. Results are reported as a T score representing the difference between the patient's BMD and that of a normal young adult of the same gender. This difference is expressed as the number of standard deviations above or below the normal result. For example, a patient with a T score of −2.0 has a BMD that is two standard deviations below the normal for a young adult of the same gender.

Diagnostic evaluation of osteoporosis may also include analysis of serum and urinary markers of bone remodeling. Serum calcium and phosphorus levels are usually normal in the presence of osteoporosis, but urinary calcium level may be elevated. Osteocalcin, which is synthesized by the osteoblasts and is therefore a biochemical marker of bone formation, is increased in conditions of rapid bone turnover. Biochemical markers of bone resorption include urinary alkaline phosphatase. The levels of these markers may offer some perspective on changes in bone remodeling within a relatively short time after they occur and before changes in BMD can be detected. However, marker levels do not indicate bone mass and cannot predict fracture risk (Osteoporosis Prevention, 2000).

Interdisciplinary Care

Primary Provider (Physician/Nurse Practitioner)

Goals for the care of the patient with osteoporosis include pain management, optimization of function and quality of life, and minimization of any adverse effects of therapy. In addition, the progress of confirmed osteoporosis must be slowed.

The primary provider measures the patient's height at every visit and orders appropriate screening tests based on the patient's age and history. Current screening and educational efforts are directed at younger women to prevent osteoporosis or detect it early enough to successfully intervene. The provider should stress that no single step is sufficient to prevent the disease and should encourage a combination of interventions that may be effective (Box 26-3). Once osteoporosis is confirmed, the patient needs information that will help him or her live successfully with the disease.

Surgeon

Painful vertebral compression fractures are initially treated conservatively with rest, analgesics, and occasional bracing. Discomfort can last for weeks to months, however, and analgesics may not always effectively manage the pain of compression fractures. As one surgical treatment option, vertebroplasty can be performed in indicated patients to correct partially collapsed and painful vertebrae. Percutaneous vertebroplasty involves injection of an acrylic polymer into the vertebral body. Kyphoplasty is a more advanced, minimally invasive alternative to vertebroplasty. In this procedure a catheter is introduced into the vertebral body and a balloon

---

Box 26-3   Interventions to Prevent and Manage Osteoporosis

- A balanced diet rich in calcium and vitamin D
- Weight-bearing exercise
- A healthy lifestyle with no smoking or excessive alcohol use
- Bone density testing and use of medications when appropriate

---

is inflated. The inflated balloon helps to restore vertebral height. The space created by the balloon is injected with an acrylic, polymethylmethacrylate (PMMA), under much lower pressure than in traditional vertebroplasty, which makes kyphoplasty a safer procedure. Both vertebroplasty and kyphoplasty are conducted under fluoroscopic guidance. The goals of these procedures are to decrease pain and to achieve fracture stability. Multiple case studies have demonstrated positive outcomes following these procedures, although no controlled studies have compared them with conservative treatment of osteoporotic compression fractures.

Drug Therapy

Pharmacologic interventions can be used to prevent osteoporosis if they are initiated before bone loss occurs. They can also be used to decrease fracture risk in the patient with confirmed osteoporosis (see Table 26-2 for specific medications).

Estrogen is commonly prescribed in postmenopausal women for the prevention of osteoporosis. Although the exact mechanism of action is unclear, estrogens do appear to inhibit bone resorption by attaching to specific receptors in the bone cells. They also promote the synthesis of calcitonin, affect the intestinal absorption of calcium, and improve the availability of the active metabolite of vitamin D that decreases bone resorption. Evidence suggests that osteoporotic fractures can be prevented in women receiving estrogen (Osteoporosis Prevention, 2000).

Estrogen replacement therapy continues to be controversial. Estrogen has been shown to exacerbate some preexisting conditions, including gallbladder and hepatic disease, coagulopathy, and hypertension. These adverse effects have been reduced through use of the transdermal patch delivery system, which bypasses the gastrointestinal tract to deliver estrogen directly through the skin into the vascular system. Debate continues, however, regarding the use of estrogen in women with a history of or familial risk for breast cancer. Because estrogen taken alone can also increase the risk of endometrial cancer, it is typically prescribed together with progestin for women with an intact uterus.

Androgen replacement therapy is important for hypogonadal men. Long-term testosterone replacement in men with primary or secondary hypogonadism has been found to increase spine BMD (Burgess and Nanes, 2002). However, no large randomized trials of testosterone treatment have targeted fracture risk as the primary end point. Recent trials have been conducted on the use of parathyroid hormone in men to stimulate new bone formation.

Bisphosphonates such as alendronate (Fosamax) and risedronate (Actonel) are approved for both the prevention and treatment of osteoporosis. They act specifically to inhibit osteoclast-mediated bone resorption. Alendronate has been shown in multiple long-term studies to increase BMD in the spine (Sedlak and Doheny, 2002). Because alendronate is poorly absorbed from the gastrointestinal tract, it should be taken with 6 to 8 oz of plain water at least

Table 26-2 Medications Used to Treat Musculoskeletal Disorders

Medication	Side Effects	Nursing Considerations
Hormones Estrogen (Vivelle, Premarin, Prempro, Premphase) Testosterone (Testoderm TTS, Androderm) Methyltestosterone (Android, Testred, AndroGel)	Increased risk for endometrial cancer Possible breast enlargement and increased risk for prostate cancer in older men with prolonged usage of any form	Adverse effects can be reduced by use of transdermal patch delivery system. Because of rapid liver breakdown of pill and capsule forms, blood levels high enough to be useful cannot be attained unless large doses (40-50 mg/day) are given. Site of gel application should be covered or direct contact with women and children should be avoided.
Bisphosphonates Alendronate (Fosamax) Risedronate (Actonel) Etidronate (Didronel) Tiludronate (Skelid) Pamidronate (Aredia)	Esophagitis, esophageal ulcers	Once-weekly administration is as effective as daily dosing. Instruct patient to take alendronate with 6-8 oz plain water at least 30 min before first food, drink, or medication of day; remain upright for 30 min after AM dose. Warning: Concomitant use of bisphosphonates and estrogen is not recommended because of uncertain interaction potential. Different dosing schedule is followed for Paget's disease. Treatment typically given for 2 to 6 mo only. Repeat course of etidronate can be given after rest period of 3-6 mo.
Selective Estrogen Receptor Modulators Raloxifene (Evista)	Possible exacerbation of thromboembolic conditions	Warning: Raloxifene has not been evaluated in combination with any form of estrogen that comes in a pill, patch, or injection, and should not be taken with any of these forms of estrogen.
Calcitonin Injectable (Calcimar) Nasal spray (Miacalcin)	Rhinitis (when used as a nasal spray)	Insufficient evidence exists to support use in men. Drug should be administered with adequate calcium and vitamin D. Teach injection technique if parenteral form prescribed. Refrigerate nasal spray if in use for more than 14 days. May need to discontinue drug for 6-12 mo before resuming therapy because some people develop resistance to salmon calcitonin. Only injectable form approved by FDA for treatment of Paget's disease.

Table 26-2   Medications Used to Treat Musculoskeletal Disorders—cont'd

Medication	Side Effects	Nursing Considerations
Tricyclic Antidepressants Amitriptyline (Elavil) Doxepin (Sinequan)	Drowsiness	Many patients cannot tolerate the sedative side effects of the tricyclic medications. Caution patient not to operate machinery or drive while taking drug.
Selective Serotonin Reuptake Inhibitors Fluoxetine (Prozac) Sertraline (Zoloft) Paroxetine (Paxil)	Insomnia	May be taken with sedating tricyclic.
Muscle Relaxants Cyclobenzaprine (Flexeril)	Drowsiness	Most often taken at night, although some patients can also tolerate in the morning. Caution patient not to drive a motor vehicle while taking this medication.
Antineoplastic Agents Plicamycin (Mithracin, Mithramycin)	Nephrotoxicity, hepatotoxicity, thrombocytopenia, anemia	Used for treatment of hypercalcemia (not specifically approved by FDA for use in Paget's disease). May be repeated as needed; check laboratory test results for renal and liver function, assess for bleeding.

FDA, Food and Drug Administration.

30 minutes before the first food, drink, or medication of the day. The patient must be instructed to remain in an upright position for 30 minutes after taking the morning dose. A once-weekly form of alendronate is also available, and this therapy has been shown to be as effective as daily dosing. Concomitant use of alendronate and estrogen is not currently recommended because of a lack of clinical data regarding the interaction of these two drugs.

Although calcitonin (Calcimar) has been used for many years to treat osteoporosis in women, insufficient evidence exists to recommend its use in men (Burgess and Nanes, 2002). Calcitonin is available in either a parenteral or nasal spray preparation. It is a peptide hormone that is destroyed in the gastrointestinal tract and therefore cannot be administered orally. Some patients develop resistance to salmon-derived calcitonin after about 2 years, which makes the drug ineffective for long-term treatment. Discontinuing the drug for 6 to 12 months before resuming therapy usually eliminates the resistance. Patient education regarding route of administration is critical.

Selective estrogen receptor modulators (SERMs) maximize the effect of estrogen on the bone while minimizing its potentially negative effects on the breast and endometrium. Raloxifene (Evista) is one drug in this class that has been shown to reduce fracture risk and increase BMD in the spine and femoral neck. Unlike the bisphosphonates, raloxifene can be taken once a day at any time. This medication can be taken with or without food and can also be taken with calcium or vitamin D supplements. A major concern with raloxifene is the risk of thromboembolism and superficial thrombophlebitis.

Calcium supplements are available in numerous forms. To prescribe the most appropriate form for the individual patient, the provider must evaluate the patient's resources and commitment to treatment. Calcium citrate is often recommended because it is easily absorbed. Because each tablet contains only 21% elemental calcium, however, more tablets are needed to obtain the recommended allowance and cost is therefore higher. Calcium citrate can also cause stomach upset and diarrhea. Calcium carbonate is widely used because it contains 40% elemental calcium. Calcium lactate and calcium gluconate are less concentrated forms (15% elemental calcium); although they are as absorbable as calcium citrate, they are much more expensive. Calcium carbonate can cause constipation and bloating. Supplements made of bone meal and dolomite are high in elemental calcium but may contain lead and other toxic metals. Calcium-based antacids (e.g., Tums) contain about 40% elemental calcium and are one of the cheapest supplements available. However, an antacid that also contains aluminum must be avoided because it will leach the calcium from the body (Petras, 2002).

For back pain that accompanies vertebral compression fractures, analgesics may be needed for 1 to 2 weeks.

Nurse

As the pivotal member of the health care team, the nurse must assess the patient's functional ability, attainment of pain management goals, knowledge of illness and prescribed therapies, sociocultural environment and support systems, and financial and personal resources. Using this information, the nurse develops a plan of care and makes appropriate referrals.

Patient education is central to the plan of care. Information about osteoporosis prevention is important to adolescents and young adults who are still forming bone. It is also critical to perimenopausal women, who, without intervention, may begin to experience a rapid and dramatic decrease in bone density. According to the National Osteoporosis Foundation (2002b and 2002c), four elements are involved in osteoporosis prevention, as shown in Box 26-3. The nurse should stress that no single element is sufficient to prevent the disease, but the combination of these interventions may be effective.

Once osteoporosis is confirmed, the patient needs information that will help him or her live successfully with the disease. The National Osteoporosis Foundation offers a variety of educational brochures for patients, with information on varied topics such as disease treatment, fall risk, and fashion tips for dressing comfortably with osteoporosis. Using educational materials, the nurse develops and refines a plan of care that will support the patient's efforts at disease management (Box 26-4).

Because the patient's social support systems affect his or her functional status and ability to adhere to the therapeutic regimen, assessment of family and community support is extremely important. The nurse must determine the role that the patient's partner or caregiver can play in successful disease management. If the patient's spouse or significant other is in poor health, the nurse must find community resources that can support the patient in independent living. A religious group or community organization may become involved, or the patient may need skilled home care services. Referral to a medical social worker can help in determining the appropriate resources for the patient.

In addition, the nurse should assess the patient's psychological well-being and make referrals as needed for evaluation of depression. Women with osteoporosis may be forced to accept help from others, losing the traditional female role

---

Box 26-4 Teaching Points Related to Management of Osteoporosis

■ Exercise appropriately to maintain optimal bone quality and minimize risk for injury.

■ Assess the home environment and institute fall prevention strategies.

■ Use mobility aids and assistive devices as needed.

■ Adequately manage pain using pharmacologic and nonpharmacologic methods.

■ Make dietary choices that support bone health.

■ Select comfortable clothing and footwear that promote a positive self-image as well as physical safety.

■ Use positive coping strategies to address the psychological impact of living with a chronic disabling disease.

---

of caregiver that they may have filled throughout their lives. Fear of becoming a burden is also very real to many women, and they worry that their increasing frailty will affect their ability to live independently. The patient's response to illness must be fully assessed to ensure that appropriate resources are available.

If the nurse provides home care, he or she must understand surgical procedures for the repair of hip fractures and the subsequent precautions the patient may need to observe. Weight bearing may be restricted for the individual who has had a fracture repaired by open reduction and/or internal fixation. Additional precautions may be required if a total hip arthroplasty was performed. Interventions vary based on the surgical approach (posterior versus anterior) and whether a cemented or noncemented prosthesis was used. The nurse should consult with the surgeon and physical therapist to ensure that appropriate precautions are implemented.

Dietitian

In developing the plan of care for the patient with osteoporosis, the dietitian encourages intake of dietary sources of calcium. Although calcium is not a treatment for osteoporosis, daily mineral intake is necessary to promote optimal bone health. If the patient's diet contains the recommended age-related daily allowance of calcium, no supplementation is necessary. However, most individuals do not have adequate dietary calcium intake. Recommended allowances of elemental calcium are presented in Table 26-3. Supplementation with vitamin D may also be necessary to maximize calcium absorption if the individual does not get adequate sun exposure (e.g., during the winter months, and in cases of institutionalization).

Physical Therapist

The physical therapist and nurse work closely in developing an exercise program that is both safe and effective for the patient with osteoporosis. Both weight-bearing exercise and

Table 26-3 Recommended Daily Allowance (RDA) for Calcium

Age	RDA (mg)
Children	
9-18 years	1300
Adults	
19-50 years	1000
51 years and older	1200
Pregnant/Lactating Women	
14-18 years	1300
19-50 years	1000

Adapted from Sedlak CA, Doheny MO: Metabolic conditions. In Maher AB, Salmond SW, Pellino TA, editors: *Orthopaedic nursing*, ed 3, Philadelphia, 2002, WB Saunders, pp 423-67.

strength training are recommended. Mall walking is a safe indoor activity that provides the added benefit of social support. For strength training, the patient should begin with light weights and gradually increase to tolerance. A mobility aid may be prescribed to facilitate safe ambulation. The patient who has had surgical repair of a hip fracture may also need equipment such as an elevated toilet seat. Because unrelieved pain can interfere with the patient's ability to participate in an exercise program, the therapist is also concerned with pain management and may recommend the use of other modalities such as heat or cold to assist in pain treatment.

Fall prevention education is an important intervention for the physical therapist. Assessment of the home may be needed to ensure elimination of environmental hazards. The therapist also instructs the patient in the use of nonskid shoes. Exercises to improve balance are helpful for the patient who is at risk for falls.

Occupational Therapist

The occupational therapist focuses on the patient's ability to perform activities of daily living (ADL) and assesses independence in self-care skills. If the patient needs assistive devices such as long-handled reaching devices or dressing aids, the occupational therapist prescribes them and instructs the patient in their use.

Medical Social Worker

If the patient is unable to manage the plan of care adequately, the medical social worker may identify home services for which the patient is eligible or consider placement outside of the home.

Complementary and Alternative Therapies

Many patients with decreased BMD are reluctant to use allopathic therapies prescribed by their health care providers. They avoid estrogen replacement, in particular, because of its link to cancer and its potentially unpleasant effects. Soy isoflavones may offer a more natural alternative. Soy isoflavones are non-

steroidal molecules with a chemical structure similar to that of SERMs like raloxifene (Evista). Health food stores sell soy powders that can be mixed with a variety of foods or beverages. Calcium supplements are also sold with soy additives, which can satisfy patients who wish to avoid prescribed estrogen replacement.

Researchers have recently learned that menopausal loss of progesterone also has an effect on BMD (Kessenich, 2002). Progesterone is known to temper the adverse effects of estrogen withdrawal, including hot flashes, irritability, and insomnia. To combat these symptoms, some women choose natural or bioidentical progesterones in a transdermal cream preparation. Natural progesterones, which have no known adverse effects, have been marketed in Europe for decades. They should not be confused with the wild yam creams that are currently sold in health food stores. The yam creams contain two precursors of progesterone that cannot be used by humans because humans lack the necessary enzymes to produce progesterone from those substances.

As an alternative to conventional exercise, the patient with osteoporosis may prefer to practice movement therapies such as yoga or t'ai chi. T'ai chi, an ancient form of Chinese exercise, has been proven to enhance flexibility, improve balance, and reduce the risk of falls in the elderly (Kessenich, 2002). The meditative aspects of t'ai chi may also be beneficial to patients with a chronic disease such as osteoporosis.

Think S for Success

Symptoms
- Manage pain with activity modification and medication.
- Advise patient to choose comfortable clothing to minimize appearance of skeletal deformity.

Sequelae
- Decrease disability by teaching patient to protect against skeletal injury and follow exercise plan developed by physical therapist.

Safety
- Teach patient and family the importance of the following:
  Taking medications and supplements as prescribed
  Using mobility aids correctly
  Using assistive devices as needed for safe performance of activities of daily living
  Modifying environmental conditions that increase fall risk

Support/Services
- Assist with referrals for financial aid or community support.

Satisfaction
- Assess degree to which osteoporosis interferes with aspects of life patient considers important (e.g., role responsibilities, relationships, employment) and assist patient in developing a plan to reach or maintain optimal quality of life.

FIBROMYALGIA

Fibromyalgia syndrome (FS) is the second most commonly diagnosed musculoskeletal disorder and a recognized cause of disability (Roberts, 2001). However, varied symptoms among patients and misinformation or lack of current information among health care providers often lead to misdiagnosis. An estimated 3 million to 6 million people in the United States have been diagnosed with FS (National Institute of Arthritis and Musculoskeletal and Skin Diseases, 1999).

Fibromyalgia is a syndrome of widespread nonarticular musculoskeletal pain and fatigue with multiple tender points. Although the former name of *fibrositis* implies generalized inflammation of muscles and other soft tissue, fibromyalgia is in fact noninflammatory, nondegenerative, and nonprogressive. The disease occurs primarily in women of child-bearing age. However, it also appears in children and men, and incidence has increased in the geriatric population. It frequently occurs with rheumatic diseases such as rheumatoid arthritis or systemic lupus erythematous, or with myofascial pain syndrome.

Pathophysiology

Because of the multiple features of fibromyalgia, its etiology is elusive. Abnormalities of musculature have been suggested, but none has been reproduced or confirmed. Light microscopy has not shown evidence of inflammation in the muscles or tendons of affected patients. However, severe damage to myofilaments has been revealed by electron microscopy and supports the veracity of patients' complaints.

Preliminary research has suggested a role for autoimmunity in disease development. Recent findings also indicate that disturbances of the neuroendocrine axis may be central to the development of fibromyalgia, particularly disturbances related to the patient's sleep patterns. Loss of stage 4 non-REM (rapid eye movement) sleep is common in approximately 75% of FS patients (Lindberg and Iwarsson, 2002). Hormones are released during the various stages of sleep. Growth hormone, for example, is released primarily during stage 3 and stage 4 of non-REM sleep. Up to one third of FS patients have low levels of insulin-like growth factor, an indication of low growth hormone secretion. Disturbances in non-REM sleep can also lead to ineffective tissue restoration and pain modulation.

Other endocrinologic and neurologic findings in FS reflect disturbances in the autonomic and endocrine stress response systems. Up to three times the normal levels of substance P (a neurotransmitter associated with enhanced pain perception) have been measured in the cerebrospinal fluid of FS patients.

An alteration in the hypopituitary-adrenal axis also creates low overall production of cortisol in individuals with fibromyalgia. In addition, an abnormality in serotonin metabolism can alter patients' perception of pain in involved tissues.

Clinical Manifestations

Individuals with FS typically describe diffuse, burning pain that alternately increases and decreases during the day. They generally find it difficult to localize pain to particular muscles, joints, or soft tissues. Sleep deprivation with resulting fatigue and weakness is common. Fatigue followed by pain is often reported to cause limitations in daily activity and negatively affect quality of life. Stress is frequently related to decreased functional level in FS patients and to exacerbations of the disease. Individuals with FS commonly have one or more comorbid conditions (Box 26-5).

Physical examination reveals soft tissue tenderness, especially in skin folds, and point tenderness at areas not generally known by the patient. Not all areas may be involved simultaneously, but pain may occur in the occiput, neck, shoulders, thoracic and lumbar spine, paraspinous regions, buttocks, hips, elbows, and knees. Reactive hyperemia (localized redness) may remain after point palpation, but the classic inflammatory signs of redness, swelling, and heat are absent. The health care provider may note that the patient has a weary look with a flat or anxious affect.

Diagnosis

Fibromyalgia should be considered in any patient who presents with musculoskeletal pain unrelated to a clearly defined anatomic cause. Diagnosis is made on the basis of history and physical examination because routine laboratory studies reveal little or nothing about the symptoms and course of fibromyalgia. Occasionally a low antinuclear antibody titer is seen but is not considered to be diagnostic. A muscle biopsy specimen may reveal a nonspecific moth-eaten appearance in some fibers and atrophy in others, but this is not a common finding.

The American College of Rheumatology (1990) has developed diagnostic criteria for fibromyalgia based on the patient's clinical presentation (Box 26-6). Failure to meet these criteria, however, does not absolutely exclude the possibility of fibromyalgia.

Box 26-5 Comorbid Conditions Associated with Fibromyalgia

- Migraine headache
- Chronic fatigue
- Irritable bowel syndrome
- Depression
- Restless legs syndrome
- Temporomandibular joint syndrome
- Myofascial pain syndrome

Adapted from Millea PJ, Holloway RL: Treating fibromyalgia, *Am Fam Physician* 62(7):1575-82, 2000.

Box 26-6   American College of Rheumatology Criteria for Classification of Fibromyalgia

1. History of widespread pain for at least 3 months
   - Pain is considered widespread when all of the following are present: pain on both left and right sides of the body; pain both above and below the waist; axial skeleton pain (cervical spine, anterior chest, thoracic spine, or low back). Shoulder and buttock pain is considered to be pain for each involved side; low back pain is considered lower segment pain.
2. Pain in 11 of 18 tender points on digital palpation
   - *Occiput:* bilateral, at the suboccipital muscle insertions.
   - *Low cervical:* bilateral, at the anterior aspects of the intertransverse spaces at C5-C7.
   - *Trapezius:* bilateral, at the midpoint of the upper border.
   - *Supraspinatus:* bilateral, at origins, above the scapular spine near the medial border.
   - *Second rib:* bilateral, at the second costochondral junctions, just lateral to the junctions on the upper surfaces.
   - *Lateral epicondyle:* bilateral, 2 cm distal to the epicondyles.
   - *Gluteal:* bilateral, in upper outer quadrants of buttocks in anterior fold of muscle.
   - *Greater trochanter:* bilateral, posterior to the trochanteric prominence.
   - *Knee:* bilateral, at the medial fat pad proximal to the joint line.

   Digital palpation should be performed with an approximate force of 4 kg. For a tender point to be considered "positive," the patient must state that the palpation was painful. "Tender" is not considered "painful."

   The patient is said to have fibromyalgia if both criteria are satisfied. The presence of a different clinical disorder does not exclude the diagnosis of fibromyalgia.

Adapted from American College of Rheumatology: 1990 Criteria for the classification of fibromyalgia, *Arthritis Rheum* 33(2):160-72, 1990.

Interdisciplinary Care
Primary Provider (Physician/Nurse Practitioner)

Underdiagnosis or late diagnosis of fibromyalgia because of the belief that the symptoms are "all in the patient's head" is a very real concern. The patient's complaints of chronic pain may be met with cynicism when laboratory data or radiologic studies fail to pinpoint the cause of symptoms. Health care providers with a poor understanding of fibromyalgia may consider the pain to be related to the patient's mental well-being and attempt to diagnose depression or anxiety, rather than believing that the patient experiences the level of pain described. The prevalence of depression and anxiety is high in FS patients, but the complications and problems associated with fibromyalgia in fact most often lead to the psychiatric disorders. Health care providers need an increased understanding of the symptoms of fibromyalgia, a greater willingness to take patients' complaints seriously, and an interest in initiating prompt treatment to minimize the impact of the disease.

Managing chronic pain of any kind requires that the provider not only listen carefully to complaints of pain but inquire about pain and encourage patients to describe their experiences with pain. Knowledge gained in the field of chronic pain management indicates that combined therapies are more likely to be successful than drug therapy or behavioral therapy alone. The primary provider works with the patient to develop individualized strategies and identify resources.

Drug Therapy

Fibromyalgia is not generally responsive to corticosteroid therapy, and symptoms are likely to be only minimally affected by nonsteroidal antiinflammatory drugs (NSAIDs). Adjunctive medications are often prescribed for use at bedtime to decrease pain and improve sleep. Low-dose tricyclic antidepressants, selective serotonin reuptake inhibitors, or a combination of the two types of drug may result in mild to moderate improvement in symptoms. Dosage should be individualized and can be gradually increased if necessary as long as the recommended maximum is not exceeded. Some patients do find that their symptoms worsen when they are taking antidepressants, so use of these medications must be carefully monitored. Benzodiazepines or muscle relaxants can also be included in the therapeutic regimen. Localized pain can be treated with topical agents such as EMLA (lidocaine with prilocaine) or capsaicin creams, or with corticosteroid injection at tender points.

Chronic opioid therapy should be reserved for FS patients with moderate to severe pain or significant functional impairment, or for those for whom other therapies are ineffective or contraindicated. For intermittent pain relief, an oral opioid combined with acetaminophen may be prescribed.

Treatment with recombinant growth hormone offers some promise in reducing symptoms and improving quality of life for FS patients who have low levels of insulin-like growth factor. The cost of growth hormone therapy is unfortunately prohibitive for most patients and is often not covered by health insurance.

Nurse

Because medical treatment options for fibromyalgia are limited, the nurse may have more opportunities to discuss self-management strategies and alternative therapies with the patient. Both the patient and the family may need assistance in managing stress, coping with the psychosocial effects of chronic disease, and maintaining as normal a life as possible given the patient's functional limitations. The nurse can suggest that the patient become involved in an exercise program to decrease pain and improve sleep. Maintenance of exercise regimens may be poor in FS patients, so the nurse can encourage participation with a companion to improve adherence and allow the patient to receive optimal benefit.

Patient education is important, and pain management is a critical topic. Besides providing the patient with information about any medications prescribed for the pain of FS, the nurse may be able to discuss alternative therapies at this point.

Dietitian

Clinical research continues to evaluate the possible use of dietary supplements or specific nutrients to manage FS symptoms. A dietitian can review available supplements and nutrients and develop an individual plan of care for the patient with FS. S-adenosylmethionine (SAM-e) may be one source of relief for the affected individual. SAM-e (pronounced "sammy") occurs naturally in all living cells, but levels do decrease with age and in the presence of depression or deficiencies of B vitamins or methionine. Supplements have been used to treat mild osteoarthritis and depression. B vitamins (800 mg of folic acid, 1000 mg of vitamin B_{12}) should be taken to help the body utilize SAM-e.

The anthocyanidins are a group of food supplements sometimes recommended for treatment of FS. Anthocyanidins are members of the flavonoid group of plant-derived chemicals, nonnutritive compounds that have been intensively investigated in recent years for their possible protective effects against chronic disease. In a study that was small but demonstrated statistically significant results (Edwards, Blackburn, and David, 2000), anthocyanidins were shown to have benefits when administered at a dosage of 80 mg/day. Possible food triggers for symptom exacerbation should also be discussed with the FS patient. Foods frequently identified as triggers include cereals made of wheat or corn, dairy products, caffeine, yeast, and citrus.

Physical Therapist

The physical therapist provides instruction in both aerobic and strength training activities to help improve disease symptoms. Because adherence to the program is a considerable problem, the patient with FS should be made aware that pain and stiffness will occur immediately after exercise and do not indicate that the condition has worsened. With adherence to an exercise regimen, the patient will eventually experience decreased pain and improved sleep. The therapist may also recommend the use of other modalities such as heat or cold to assist in pain management.

Occupational Therapist

The occupational therapist focuses on the patient's ability to perform ADL and assesses independence in self-care skills. If the patient needs assistive devices such as long-handled reaching devices or dressing aids, the occupational therapist will prescribe them and instruct the patient in their use. Energy conservation measures are listed in Box 25-6.

Medical Social Worker

If the patient is unable to manage the plan of care adequately, the medical social worker may explore home services for which the patient is eligible. If the patient has severe disability, placement outside of the home may be considered.

Complementary and Alternative Therapies

Nutrients that may be helpful for sleep disturbances include melatonin and Calms Forte, a mixture of herbs, calcium, and magnesium phosphates. The amino acid L-threonine has been used to alleviate restless legs syndrome, which is frequently experienced by FS patients, and peppermint oil may help with irritable bowel syndrome.

Behavioral therapies such as relaxation response training or meditation may be helpful. Massage and reflexology may also be suggested to alleviate the pain of FS, and acupuncture has proven helpful for some individuals. The patient who is interested in alternative therapies should be assisted in selecting a reputable practitioner who is certified by a professional organization for the given discipline (e.g., the American Association of Medical Acupuncture).

Anecdotal evidence suggests that reiki may be an effective treatment modality for fibromyalgia (see Chapter 3). The National Center for Complementary and Alternative Medicine (2003) is currently recruiting patients for a clinical trial that will evaluate the ability of reiki to relieve pain and improve psychological well-being in patients with fibromyalgia.

Think **S** for Success

Symptoms
- Listen to and believe patient's complaint.
- Manage pain with activity modification, medication, and alternative therapies.
- Teach patient to develop personal habits that facilitate sleep (e.g., bedtime routines).

Sequelae
- Instruct patient to decrease pain and improve sleep by following exercise plan developed by physical therapist.

Safety
- Teach patient and family the importance of the following:
  Taking medications and supplements as prescribed
  Making dietary changes that may help with symptom management
  Using mobility aids correctly
  Using assistive devices as needed for safe performance of activities of daily living

Support/Services
- Assist with referrals for financial aid or community support.

Satisfaction
- Assess degree to which fibromyalgia interferes with aspects of life patient considers important (e.g., role responsibilities, relationships, employment) and assist patient in developing a plan to reach or maintain optimal quality of life.

OSTEOMYELITIS

Osteomyelitis is a severe infection of the bone and surrounding tissues. In adults the infection is usually subacute or chronic, developing in response to an open injury to bone and the adjacent soft tissue. Adult men are more frequently affected than women because of the increased incidence of blunt trauma in men. Osteomyelitis may be more difficult to treat in the presence of other disorders that affect the body's ability to fight infection, including malnutrition, alcoholism, acquired immunodeficiency syndrome, and kidney or liver failure. Patients with diabetes mellitus or severe atherosclerosis are also at greater risk of developing chronic infection because of vascular insufficiency. Patients with sickle cell disease are particularly susceptible to osteomyelitis because they have both a compromised immune status and poor circulation. Osteomyelitis can also develop as a complication of pressure ulcers. Because osteomyelitis is a complex disease state and prognosis is affected by the patient's general health status, various classification systems have been developed to guide diagnosis (Box 26-7).

Box 26-7   Cierny-Mader Staging System for Osteomyelitis

ANATOMIC TYPE
- Stage 1: medullary osteomyelitis
- Stage 2: superficial osteomyelitis (outer surface of bone); soft tissue compromise common
- Stage 3: diffuse osteomyelitis; well-marginated sequestration of cortical bone
- Stage 4: permeative destructive lesion causing instability

PHYSIOLOGIC CLASS
- A host: normal immune status
- B host
- Bs—systemic compromise
- Bl—local compromise
- Bls—local and systemic compromise
- C host: significant immunocompromise; treatment worse than the disease

FACTORS AFFECTING IMMUNE SURVEILLANCE, METABOLISM, LOCAL VASCULARITY
- Systemic factors (Bs): malnutrition, renal or hepatic failure, diabetes mellitus, chronic hypoxia, immune disease/immune deficiency/immunosuppression, extremes of age
- Local factors (Bl): chronic lymphedema, venous stasis, major vessel compromise, arteritis, extensive scarring, radiation fibrosis, small-vessel disease, neuropathy, tobacco abuse

Adapted from Carek PJ, Dickerson LM, Sack JL: Diagnosis and management of osteomyelitis, *Am Fam Physician* 63(12):2413-20, 2001; and Wheeless CR: Cierny classification of osteomyelitis. In *Wheeless' textbook of orthopaedics*, 1996, retrieved from *http://www.ortho-u.net/ortho1/500.htm* on April 27, 2003.

Pathophysiology

Infecting organisms reach the bone by one of three routes: through the bloodstream from another site of infection (hematogenous infection), by extension from adjacent soft tissue infection (contiguous focus), or by direct introduction into the bone through trauma or recent surgery. Hematogenous osteomyelitis, the most common type of infection, occurs primarily in children before the age of epiphyseal closure. However, it also has a peak incidence in advanced middle age and older adulthood. A single organism is usually the infecting agent, entering the bone via the bloodstream from a distant site of infection. Common sources of infection in adults include urinary tract infection and upper respiratory tract infection. Even a relatively trivial trauma such as an ordinary cut can allow entrance of bacteria into the bloodstream. Osteomyelitis secondary to a contiguous infection (e.g., skin and soft tissue infections such as pressure sores or burns) is primarily a disease of adults.

Bacteria generally seed the more vascular bones, becoming trapped in the metaphyses. *Staphylococcus aureus* is the most common causative organism in both acute and chronic infection. Chronic osteomyelitis can also be caused by *Staphylococcus epidermidis, Pseudomonas aeruginosa, Serratia marcescens,* and *Escherichia coli.*

The body's inflammatory and immunologic responses to the bacterial invasion lead to pus formation, edema, and vascular congestion. Without treatment, pus continues to collect. Increasing pressure within the rigid bone causes vascular occlusion and ischemia. The Volkmann and haversian canals within the infected bone also support bone necrosis by allowing the pus to spread to other areas of the bone, which creates even more pressure and further compromises the vascular supply.

If initial treatment is either delayed or inadequate, the necrotic bone separates from the living bone to form segments (sequestra) that serve as a medium for additional growth of microorganisms. During this chronic infectious process, the sequestra continue to enlarge and may extrude through the bone into the surrounding soft tissue. In an attempt to heal the infected bone, osteoblasts isolate the dead fragments and form an involucrum (layer of new bone surrounding necrotic bone). The involucrum interferes with the normal process of phagocytosis and decreases the ability of antibiotics to reach the infective site, which further contributes to development of chronic osteomyelitis. Once the infection reaches the outer surface of the bone (periosteum), soft tissue abscesses and cutaneous sinus tracts can develop. The sinus tracts provide a route for chronic wound drainage as well as a port for entry of new organisms (Figure 26-2). The infection can also become walled off by fibrotic tissue and remain localized in a formation known as Brodie's abscess. Areas of severe cortical bone destruction are prone to pathologic fracture.

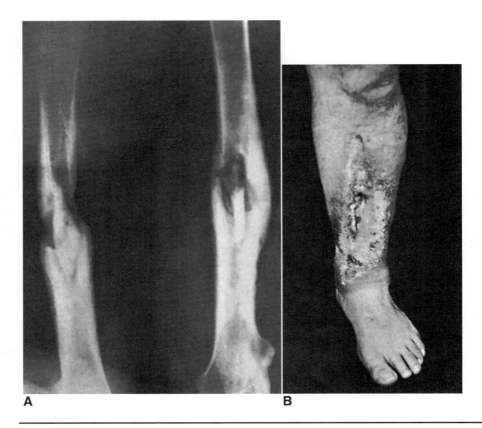

A   B

Figure 26-2 A, Chronic osteomyelitis of the femur with large retained sequestrum. **B,** Chronic osteomyelitis of the tibia with marked scarring and draining sinuses. (From Salmond SW, Fine C: Infections of the musculoskeletal system. In Maher AB, Salmond SW, Pellino TA, editors: *Orthopaedic nursing,* ed 3, Philadelphia, 2002, WB Saunders.)

Clinical Manifestations

If treatment of acute osteomyelitis is only partially successful, the resulting chronic infection will be marked by persistent bone pain, tenderness, and sinus drainage. Infection may also lead to disabling consequences such as a pathologic fracture or a malignant transformation to squamous cell carcinoma in a draining tract. Vertebral osteomyelitis also produces localized back pain with associated paravertebral muscle spasm, and painful involvement of the foot results in mobility impairment.

Diagnosis

Laboratory tests and radiologic studies are important tools to confirm the health care provider's suspicion of osteomyelitis. Definitive diagnosis requires isolation of the infecting organism. Both aerobic and anaerobic blood cultures should be performed before the initiation of antibiotic therapy. Gram's staining can provide some basic information about the organism's identity and aid in the selection of optimal antibiotic therapy. Cultures of superficial specimens from open wounds, skin ulcers, or cutaneous tracts do not always reveal the cause of deep-seated bone infections.

Instead, needle aspiration or open bone biopsy is used to obtain a specimen for culture and sensitivity testing. In the patient with suspected chronic infection, bone specimens should be obtained during surgery. Accuracy of biopsy can be limited by poor specimen collection technique and the patient's previous antibiotic use.

Even with large pus collections in a bone's medullary cavity, radiographic proof of infection lags behind the patient's clinical presentation by at least 7 to 10 days. In fact, in most cases changes are not seen for 3 to 4 weeks, because 30% to 50% of the bone matrix must be lost for a lytic lesion to be apparent on plain radiographs (Salmond and Fine, 2002). Early radiography is performed primarily to rule out fracture. Radioisotope bone scans show abnormalities earlier than plain films, but infection, fractures, and tumors cannot be distinguished based on the areas of uptake. Perhaps the most reliable diagnostic tool is magnetic resonance imaging (MRI), which is able to differentiate bone and soft tissue infection.

Interdisciplinary Care

The chronicity of osteomyelitis is due to both the avascular nature of the sequestra and the porosity of bone. In spite of advances in antibiotic therapy, a cure for chronic osteomyelitis remains elusive. Chronic osteomyelitis is characterized by variable periods of quiescence and flare-ups that may continue throughout a patient's lifetime. The long-term recurrence rate remains approximately 20% to 30% (Wirganowicz, 1999). A multifocal interdisciplinary approach is needed to treat the disease effectively and to minimize the risk for disability.

Primary Provider (Physician/Nurse Practitioner)

The primary provider confirms the diagnosis and begins treatment with aggressive antibiotic therapy. If the infection is not responsive to antibiotics, surgical débridement may be necessary.

Surgeon

The goals in the treatment of chronic osteomyelitis are to eradicate the infection and maintain optimal function for the affected area. Antibiotic therapy alone is frequently unable to provide long-term arrest of chronic osteomyelitis. Surgery often becomes necessary to remove all infected material and the surrounding scar tissue and to restore adequate blood flow to the area. The dead space created by the removal of the sequestra and scar tissue, however, is at risk for reinfection. To decrease the risk for recurrence, surgical dissection should be fairly aggressive—similar to the method used in treatment of a benign, aggressive bone tumor such as a giant cell tumor. In cases in which the structural integrity of the bone appears compromised, autologous bone grafting can later be done using grafts from the posterior iliac crest. Allograft may also be mixed with the autologous graft if the size of the bony defects exceeds the amount of bone that can be obtained from the patient. Appropriate antibiotic therapy should continue concomitantly with surgical treatment.

Drug Therapy

Acute osteomyelitis can be managed effectively with careful isolation of the causative microorganism and a 4- to 6-week course of appropriate parenteral and oral antibiotics. After cultures have been obtained, a regimen of nafcillin (Unipen) plus either cefotaxime (Claforan) or ceftriaxone (Rocephin) is often initiated (Carek, Dickerson, and Sack, 2001). The antibiotic regimen may be revised when the organisms are positively identified. If antibiotic therapy fails to eradicate the infection, surgical débridement may be necessary and another course of parenteral antibiotics becomes essential. Without adequate débridement, chronic osteomyelitis does not respond to most antibiotic regimens no matter how long the course of treatment.

As an alternative to parenteral administration, a high concentration of medication can be delivered directly to the site of infection through the use of antibiotic-impregnated implants. The most widely used implants have traditionally been beads of PMMA, which both offer localized treatment and provide some stability for the infected area. However, the beads have low biocompatibility and a low release ratio (as low as 5% for several antibiotics), and thermal damage to the antibiotic may occur because of the heat used to load it into the beads (Laeseke, 2000). In addition, a second operation is required to remove the beads.

To alleviate some of the problems with PMMA, hydroxyapatite blocks are being used to treat patients with chronic osteomyelitis. Hydroxyapatite has excellent biocompatibility and is effective in filling defects in bone. Any antibiotic can be used with hydroxyapatite because centrifugation rather than heat is used to mix the antibiotic with the block. Additional surgery is unnecessary because hydroxyapatite blocks are incorporated into the bone over time. Although use of the blocks has been successful clinically, additional research is needed to determine how long the release of antibiotic can be sustained (Laeseke, 2000).

Nurse

In addition to the nursing care already described for patients with chronic musculoskeletal conditions, the nurse must provide thorough teaching about the long-term use of antibiotics and infection control measures such as hand washing and proper handling of wound drainage or dressings. Monitoring of the patient's adherence to the antibiotic regimen is critical. The patient and family must understand the consequences of inadequate treatment of osteomyelitis and the need to continue antibiotic therapy for the prescribed period of time.

Mild to severe local pain or joint pain is expected with osteomyelitis, and the patient and family need instruction on the use of prescribed analgesics. The patient should be encouraged to take medications around the clock rather than on an as-needed basis.

The presence of a painful condition with long-term health implications can be frightening for the patient and family. Family disruption and role changes can create considerable stress and anxiety. The nurse can help reduce the feelings of powerlessness that contribute to this response by providing consistent communication about tests, treatments, and expected progress. The nurse can also introduce relaxation and guided imagery techniques as useful strategies for the anxious patient.

In some cases, the presence of resistant infection may necessitate amputation. The nurse must be prepared to help the patient and the family cope with the impact of amputation on both role function and personal relationships (Box 26-8).

Physical Therapist

The physical therapist implements range-of-motion and other exercises to mobilize unaffected joints. If approved by the physician, passive range-of-motion exercises can be performed on the affected joints to decrease the risk of contracture. Progressive ambulation will allow active range of

---

Box 26-8   Nursing Interventions to Help Patients Cope with Amputation

■ Assist individual and family with grieving:
  Identify the loss and encourage verbalization of feelings about the loss.
  Explain stages of grieving likely to be experienced.
  Identify strengths and sources of support.
■ Explore patient's feelings about body image.
■ Encourage patient's socialization with peers and others.
■ Identify resources for physical, financial, and emotional support.
■ Help patient set realistic goals for return to previous roles.
■ Manage chronic pain and/or phantom limb pain.
■ Teach patient to care for residual limb:
  Prevent contractures.
  Assess for skin breakdown.
  Assess for proper fit of appliance or prosthesis.

Table 26-4   Alternative Therapies for Osteomyelitis

Therapy	Benefit
Maggots	Feeding maggots are introduced into a wound to eliminate necrotic tissue.
Electrical stimulation	Necrotic tissue is solubilized for débridement.
Magnets	Local circulation is increased, which reduces swelling and inflammation.
Copper bracelets	Electrical charges generated on the skin from the bracelet travel along acupuncture meridians to relieve pain at distant sites.
Hyperbaric oxygen	Directly kills or inhibits growth of strict anaerobes

---

motion for an involved lower extremity. However, activity is based on the patient's ability to tolerate joint stress and the need to avoid pathologic fracture or other musculoskeletal problems. The affected area may also be immobilized with braces or casts to facilitate movement. Instruction in the use of a walker or crutches may be indicated. For the amputee, instruction on wrapping the residual limb and preparing for and caring for a prosthesis is included.

Medical Social Worker

If the patient lacks the financial resources for treatment of osteomyelitis, the medical social worker may need to arrange assistance in the purchase of medication and possibly home care services. Chronic or recurrent infection may affect the patient's ability to hold a job, and the medical social worker may need to assist the patient in accessing additional aid programs or obtaining alternate vocational training. In addition, social support may be especially needed by the patient whose progressive, resistant infection has necessitated amputation or additional treatment in a long-term care facility.

Complementary and Alternative Therapies

The high incidence of recurrence of osteomyelitis has led patients to consider multiple alternative treatment methods (Wirganowicz, 1999). Table 26-4 lists these therapies and their believed benefits.

The results of these experimental procedures are often inconclusive. As an adjunctive therapy, however, hyperbaric oxygenation has offered some benefit in soft tissue healing following surgical débridement for refractory osteomyelitis. Hyperbaric oxygen directly kills or inhibits the growth of organisms that prefer a low-oxygen environment (strict anaerobes) and may be a useful adjunct to antibiotic therapy (Undersea and Hyperbaric Medicine Society, 2003).

Think S for Success

Symptoms
■ Manage pain with activity modification, medication, and joint stabilization.

Sequelae
■ Maintain optimal function by instructing patient to follow exercise plan developed by physical therapist.
■ Use bracing as prescribed to maintain normal joint alignment.
■ Prevent amputation by following therapy with antibiotics.
■ Encourage patient's attention to diseases such as diabetes that increase risk for recurrent infection.

Safety
■ Teach patient and family the importance of the following:
  Completing antibiotic regimen as prescribed, even if symptoms appear to resolve
  Using appropriate infection control and wound care strategies
  Using mobility aids correctly
  Using assistive devices as needed for safe performance of activities of daily living
  Caring for the residual limb and prosthesis following amputation

Support/Services
■ Assist with referrals for financial aid or community support.
■ Explore vocational alternatives for patient who is unable to continue in previous employment.

Satisfaction
■ Assess degree to which osteomyelitis interferes with aspects of life patient considers important (e.g., role responsibilities, relationships, employment) and assist patient in developing a plan to reach or maintain optimal quality of life.

Ethical Considerations

Treatment for chronic osteomyelitis is at best an extended process that can control the lives and consume the resources of its victims. If affected individuals also happen to be uninsured or underinsured, their limited access to health care makes the likelihood of a cure even lower. Uninsured persons with traumatic injuries are less likely to be admitted to the hospital, receive fewer services if they are, and are more likely to die than are insured victims. When uninsured individuals with diseases such as diabetes receive inadequate or infrequent treatment, they also increase their risk of related vascular insufficiency and osteomyelitis. Until the disparity in health insurance is adequately addressed, individuals with chronic disease or infection will continue to run the risk of undertreatment, with resulting increases in morbidity and mortality.

PAGET'S DISEASE (OSTEITIS DEFORMANS)

Paget's disease is a common metabolic bone disorder, second only to osteoporosis in prevalence and impact on the geriatric population. The disease is equally prevalent in men and women, but incidence is increased in those over the age of 50 years. Approximately 3% of the population in the United States is affected, and as many as 10% of those over 80 years of age have Paget's disease (Schneider and Hofmann, 2002).

Pathophysiology

The cause of Paget's disease is unknown, but there is evidence of a familial tendency. Up to 40% of those with Paget's disease have at least one relative with the disorder (Sedlak and Doheny, 2002). Researchers suggest that Paget's disease may be caused by infection by certain blood-borne viruses that stimulate proliferation of osteoclasts. In the United States, the measles viral antigen is the antigen most commonly detected in patients with Paget's disease. However, a great deal of attention has been focused recently on a susceptibility locus on chromosome arm 18q, and a genetic cause for the disorder is now proposed (Schneider and Hofmann, 2002).

Paget's disease results from excessive osteoclastic activity, which in turn stimulates increased bone formation and accelerated bone remodeling. The resulting bone, which is highly vascular and structurally weak, is susceptible to deformity and fracture. The disease occurs in three phases. The initial phase includes intense osteoclastic activity and bone resorption. Resulting bone turnover is as high as 20 times the normal rate. An osteolytic-osteoblastic phase follows, during which osteoblasts begin to produce an abundance of woven bone but with ineffective mineralization. During the final phase of the disease, dense cortical and trabecular bone deposition occurs, but it is sclerotic, disorganized, and weaker than normal bone. The disease most often affects the axial skeleton, but any area can be involved (Table 26-5). In one third of patients with Paget's disease,

Table 26-5   Bones Affected by Paget's Disease

Bone	Percentage of Patients with Paget's Disease
Pelvis	72
Lumbar spine	58
Femur	55
Thoracic spine	45
Skull	42
Tibia	35
Humerus	31
Cervical spine	14

Adapted from Schneider D, Hofmann MT: Diagnosis and treatment of Paget's disease of bone, *Am Fam Physician* 65(10):2069-72, 2002.

only one bone is affected. In most patients, however, the disorder affects at least two bones.

Clinical Manifestations

Approximately 70% of patients with Paget's disease are asymptomatic (Schneider and Hofmann, 2002). In others, symptoms may be vague and difficult to distinguish from those of other diseases. Pain is the most common complaint, described as continuous discomfort that increases with rest, on weight bearing, when limbs are warmed, and at night. Paget's disease can cause osteoarthritis if the affected section of bone is near a joint, which makes diagnosis more difficult and adds to the difficulties in managing the patient's pain.

Bone deformity, often accompanied by mobility impairment, is also a common finding. The variety of deformities includes kyphosis, shortened or bowed limbs, and dental abnormalities. The kyphotic deformities can lead to vertebral compression fractures. Bowing of the tibia is common, often leading to a pathologic fracture that may be the first indication of Paget's disease (Figure 26-3, *A*). Fractures heal slowly and often incompletely. Progressive deformity of the skull can also occur over many years, leading to a soft, thick, enlarged cranium that may actually be difficult for the patient to hold erect in severe cases (Figure 26-3, *B*). Because of the increased vascularity of the bone, affected areas are warm to the touch; local temperature may be as much as 5° F higher than the remainder of the body's surface (Sedlak and Doheny, 2002).

The patient with Paget's disease may also complain of neurologic symptoms, which arise from nerve compression caused by bony growth. One possible complication is hearing loss, which results from enlargement of the temporal bone in the skull. Other deficits may include impairments in vision, swallowing, speech, and balance.

The most alarming complication of Paget's disease is development of a malignant bone tumor in a preexisting pagetic lesion. Incidence of malignant degeneration ranges from less than 1% to 10%, depending on the severity of the

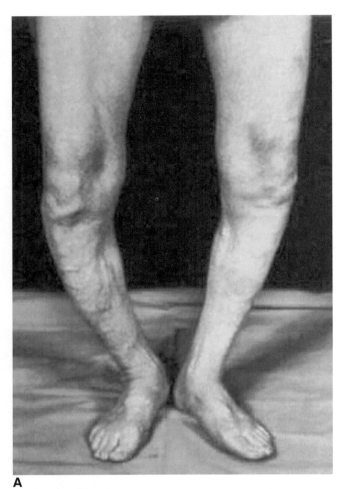

A

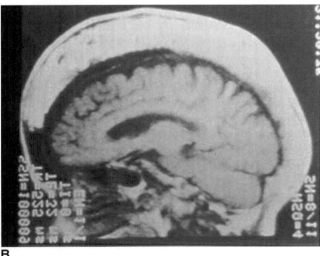

B

Figure 26-3   A, Tibial bowing caused by Paget's disease. **B,** Magnetic resonance image of skull showing enlarged cranium. (Courtesy the Paget Foundation, New York, NY.)

disease (Schneider and Hofmann, 2002). Tumors are usually highly malignant. A marked increased in pain or deformity may signal this complication. Any acute increase in symptom severity indicates the need for further assessment and possible bone biopsy.

Heart failure is a relatively rare complication among elderly patients affected by Paget's disease and results from the heart's attempts to pump blood through the vessels in active pagetic bone. This complication is more likely when at least one third of the skeleton is affected. Other cardiovascular abnormalities associated with Paget's disease include hypertension, atherosclerosis, systolic murmurs, and calcification of the aortic valve.

Diagnosis

In asymptomatic persons, the disease is often found incidentally on radiographs and laboratory studies. In the early stages of the disease, characteristic osteolytic lesions are noted in the long bones and skull. As the disease progresses, an adjoining overgrowth of bone gives the radiographic image a coarse, irregular appearance. Enlargement of the bone contours is also evident. After the patient becomes symptomatic, the weakened bone usually shows a characteristic mosaic pattern. Annual radiographs are recommended for patients with active osteolytic lesions.

Radioactive bone scanning may be performed to evaluate the metabolic activity of pagetic lesions. The radioactive isotopes are deposited at sites of high bone turnover, which makes them useful in determining the number, extent, and activity of lesions. MRI of the skull can also be performed.

The high serum levels of alkaline phosphatase (ALP) found in patients with Paget's disease indicate excessive osteoblastic activity. Normal serum ALP level is 30 to 115 IU/L. The patient with Paget's disease may have a level from high normal to more than 1000 IU/L. Serum ALP level is a commonly used biochemical marker, and a good correlation exists between the results and the extent of the disease. However, the ALP value is diminished in the presence of hepatic disease and pregnancy. Patients with end-stage Paget's disease typically have low ALP levels. Expert health care providers recommend assessment of serum ALP levels three or four times annually for patients receiving pharmacologic treatment for Paget's disease. In addition, asymptomatic patients who have a first-degree relative also affected by the disease should be screened with an ALP test every 2 to 3 years. Many health care providers recommend initiating treatment when the serum ALP level rises to 125% to 150% of normal values.

Tests of other biochemical substances that serve as markers of bone resorption and disease activity may also support the diagnosis. These include urinary hydroxyproline, pyridinoline and deoxypyridinoline, N-telopeptide, and C-telopeptide.

Assessment of calcium levels is indicated for the patient who has had an acute episode of immobility related to the disease. The patient with impaired mobility is particularly at risk for hypercalciuria, hypercalcemia, and renal calculi.

History, physical examination, and laboratory and radiologic examinations are usually enough to confirm a diagnosis of Paget's disease. In a few cases, however, the health care provider must perform a bone biopsy to clarify an unusual clinical or radiologic finding. Bone biopsy is also indicated if the health care provider has a high suspicion of malignancy because of the patient's increased pain or deformity. Because Paget's disease can cause severe hearing loss, a patient older than 50 years of age should also have audiograms measured regularly for early detection of deficits.

Interdisciplinary Care

Primary Provider (Physician/Nurse Practitioner)

The primary provider usually discovers the changes associated with Paget's disease incidentally. Asymptomatic patients with Paget's disease require no treatment, and those with mild symptoms are usually treated successfully with simple analgesics or antiinflammatory drugs. The severe pain and joint destruction of advanced Paget's disease, however, requires an effective interdisciplinary approach to care. Treatment does not cure the disease, but it can provide prolonged periods of remission. The primary provider monitors the patient's response to therapy and coordinates the activities of the health care team.

Drug Therapy

Aggressive treatment of Paget's disease typically involves the use of bisphosphonates. Alendronate (Fosamax) and pamidronate (Aredia) are the most frequently used medications. They cause a decrease of approximately 70% in levels of biochemical markers in one half of affected patients (Schneider and Hofmann, 2002). The recommended dosage of alendronate for treatment of Paget's disease is 40 mg daily for 6 months. If necessary, treatment may be reinstated after a break of 6 months. Pamidronate is given intravenously in a 60-mg dose over a 2- to 4-hour period for 2 or more days. Alternative dosing calls for 30 mg given over 4 hours on 3 consecutive days. Treatment may be reinstated at intervals as necessary. Disease activity remains low for months or years after cessation of these medications. Other bisphosphonates may also be prescribed for treatment of Paget's disease (see Table 26-2).

Secondary resistance to individual bisphosphonates can occur, so that the patient may have to be to switched from one medication to another during long-term treatment. Because bisphosphonates tend to be poorly absorbed, the patient must take them in the prescribed manner to avoid incomplete absorption. In addition, the patient must be carefully monitored, because prolonged use of any bisphosphonate can increase the risk of osteomalacia and pathologic fractures.

Calcitonin (Calcimar) also inhibits bone resorption, but it is not as powerful as bisphosphonates and does not suppress disease activity for as long after cessation of treatment. Calcitonin is available in both injectable and nasal spray forms, but only the injectable medication is approved for treatment of Paget's disease by the Food and Drug Administration.

Plicamycin (Mithracin), an antineoplastic antibiotic, has been shown to inhibit the effect of parathyroid hormone on osteoclasts. It has been used to treat symptoms of Paget's disease, but it has a high toxicity and is rarely used.

Pain directly related to Paget's disease is generally managed with one of the antiosteoclastic treatments described earlier. Some pain, however, may be due to muscle spasms associated with bone deformity, associated arthritis, or neurologic complications. Simple analgesics such as acetaminophen or NSAIDs may be prescribed for the management of nonskeletal pain.

Surgeon

Surgical procedures may occasionally be required to manage the symptoms and arthritic changes associated with the disease. Tibial osteotomy may be performed to realign the knee and relieve pain. Total joint arthroplasty and spinal decompression may be beneficial in alleviating the severe pain associated with Paget's disease. Surgery may also be indicated for delayed union of fractures.

Nurse

The main objectives for management of Paget's disease are to minimize the patient's symptoms, improve his or her physical function, slow the disease process, and prevent complications. The nurse plays an important role in helping the patient achieve each of these objectives by providing patient and family education and by encouraging the patient to adhere to the prescribed therapy.

According to the Paget Foundation (2002), the nurse should be aware that skeletal health, risk of complications, and safety of drug therapy are major sources of stress and anxiety for the individual who has been diagnosed with Paget's disease. Deformities are irreversible and can affect the patient's self-concept, but the patient is more likely to cope effectively with body image disturbances if the nurse is able to aid in the maintenance of independence and mobility. The nurse must help the patient address any self-care deficits and sexual dysfunction related to bone pain and deformity.

Effective health education promotes behaviors that increase the patient's ability to adhere to medical therapy, prevent injury, and participate in physical therapy. For example, the patient needs specific information regarding the risks and benefits of proposed medications, including side effects, cost, and duration of treatment. If subcutaneous calcitonin is prescribed, the patient also needs instruction in self-injection and site rotation. For the patient taking any of the oral bisphosphonates, the nurse must provide precise instructions in the method of administration to allow optimal absorption. To update the plan of care, the nurse also encourages the patient to provide feedback regarding the response to therapy. The nurse must emphasize the importance of the patient's long-term follow-up so that treatment can be reinstated if necessary.

Dietitian

Patients with Paget's disease should receive adequate amounts of calcium (1000 to 1500 mg daily) and vitamin D (400 IU daily). Patients should be encouraged to limit alcohol and caffeine intake because of their interference with calcium absorption. They should also be counseled to lose or maintain weight to decrease stress on affected joints and bones.

Physical Therapist

Exercise is recommended to maintain musculoskeletal health in patients with Paget's disease. Exercise programs must be carefully individualized, however, to prevent stress on affected bones. Simple strengthening and weight-bearing exercises may be initiated. The physical therapist can also offer advice on the use of walking aids, heel lifts, and other assistive devices to improve function and mobility. Strategies for fall and fracture prevention should also be discussed. An assessment of the home environment is especially helpful in decreasing the patient's risk for falls.

Medical Social Worker

If the patient lacks the financial resources for treatment of Paget's disease, the medical social worker may have to arrange assistance in the purchase of medication and possibly home care services. Progressive deformity and mobility impairment may affect the patient's ability to hold a job, and the medical social worker may have to assist the patient in accessing additional aid programs or obtaining alternate vocational training.

LOW BACK PAIN

Low back pain (LBP) has been documented as a human complaint since the times of the Egyptians 5000 years ago. After headache and fatigue, it is the third most common disorder discussed with health care providers. At any given time, 10% of adults have experienced activity restrictions over the previous 4 weeks due to LBP. Approximately 50% of all episodes of LBP resolve within a week, but recurrences after apparent resolution of symptoms are very common. Up to 20% of annual work loss among employed adults is related to LBP (Haigh and Clarke, 1999). A scientifically proven relationship exists between LBP and heavy physical work, lifting and forceful movements, bending and twisting, and whole-body vibrations.

Back injury and pain occur when the stress limits of the tissues are exceeded. Bone, cartilage, ligaments, and muscles may be injured by a direct trauma or a single strenuous event. They may also be affected over time by microtraumas or by repeated or sustained loading that lead to cumulative overloading. In most cases, LBP cannot be traced to a single specific incident of overexertion. In addition to being caused by strain or sprain, back pain can also occur as a result of degenerative disk disease, herniated disk, spinal stenosis,

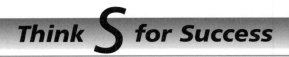

Think S for Success

Symptoms
■ Manage pain with medication.
■ Protect weakened bones from injury.
■ Minimize the impact of deformity on activities of daily living and role performance.

Sequelae
■ Maintain optimal function by instructing patient to follow exercise plan developed by physical therapist.

Safety
■ Teach patient and family the importance of the following:
　Adhering to administration requirements for prescribed medications
　Using mobility aids correctly
　Using assistive devices as needed for safe performance of activities of daily living

Support/Services
■ Assist with referrals for financial aid or community support.
■ Explore vocational alternatives for patient who is unable to continue in previous employment.

Satisfaction
■ Assess degree to which Paget's disease interferes with aspects of life patient considers important (e.g., role responsibilities, relationships, employment) and assist patient in developing a plan to reach or maintain optimal quality of life.

spondylolisthesis, or spondylolysis. Pain is characterized as chronic when symptoms last more than 3 months.

Pathophysiology

Low back strain is the most common cause of back pain (Rodts, 2002). It typically occurs following a change in activity but, as noted earlier, is not necessarily related to a significant traumatic event. Even a routine activity such as housecleaning can lead to strain and trigger an episode of LBP.

Other causes of LBP include several disorders that may be related both to overuse and to aging. Herniation can result when the outer fibrocartilaginous layer of the disk (annulus fibrosis) weakens, cracks, and loses its ability to contain the disk material (nucleus pulposus). The bulging disk puts pressure on neural structures, which often creates back and leg pain (Figure 26-4). Depending on the location of the defect and the relative amount of extruding nucleus pulposus, the patient may experience marked weakness and bowel or bladder difficulties. Surgical intervention may ultimately be needed. Men experience disk herniation more often than women, possibly due to occupational demands.

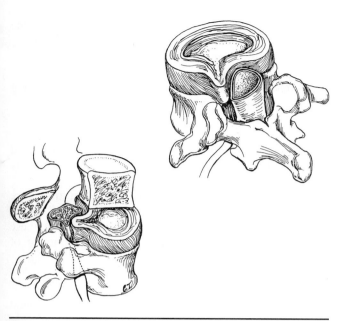

Figure 26-4 A herniated lumbar disc. (From Rodts MF: Disorders of the spine. In Maher AB, Salmond SW, Pellino TA, editors: *Orthopaedic nursing,* ed 3, Philadelphia, 2002, WB Saunders.)

Spondylolysis is a defect or break in the arch between the superior and inferior articulating processes of the vertebra. The point of union between these two areas is normally bone, but in spondylolysis it is composed instead of fibrocartilaginous tissue (Rodts, 2002). In many people the development of spondylolysis is due to a hereditary predisposition. However, the defect can be present without creating symptoms until participation in sports such as wrestling or gymnastics leads to repeated hyperextension stress.

Spondylolisthesis is a forward subluxation of one vertebra over another, most often in the lumbosacral region of the spine. This condition may actually develop at a fairly early age, but symptoms do not generally become apparent until later childhood or adolescence. Spondylolisthesis is typically described by using a classification system that grades the forward or downward slippage of the vertebrae.

Spinal stenosis is a narrowing of the spinal canal, nerve root canal, or intervertebral foramina. It can occur in any region of the spine. Congenital stenosis usually affects the entire spinal canal, whereas acquired stenosis is generally limited to one or several areas. The cervical and lumbar segments of the spine are the most commonly involved as a result of trauma, postoperative changes in the spinal canal, spondylolisthesis, or metabolic changes such as Paget's disease. A gradual shift in spinal alignment (kyphosis or lordosis) can also exacerbate stenosis.

Disk degeneration is generally considered a normal result of aging unless it is accompanied by back pain. A normal disk has enough viscoelasticity to allow optimal movement of the spine. A degenerated disk, however, can contribute to the development of pain, instability, or stenosis of the neural canal. It may be present and yet the patient may be asymptomatic until an unrelated traumatic event aggravates the condition.

Clinical Manifestations

With all spinal disorders, the patient's chief complaint is pain. Pain can occur acutely following a specific traumatic event, or the patient may reveal a long history of progressively worsening pain. Many patients try to treat the pain conservatively with heat and rest at home before seeking medical attention.

The type of pain resulting from disk herniation depends on the involved area of the spine. With lumbar herniation, LBP is often aggravated by standing, walking, bending, and coughing or sneezing—any activity that increases pressure in the affected area. Pain can also contribute to limitations in forward flexion of the spine, and the patient may list away from the affected side when standing or walking.

With spondylolysis and spondylolisthesis, LBP may be acute or may become a chronic condition that gradually worsens. LBP may or may not radiate into the legs. Lower extremity pain may contribute to a slow or waddling gait. The patient with spinal stenosis may describe a gradual onset of pain, usually over a period of years. Stenotic LBP and the frequent accompanying leg pain increase with standing or walking and decrease with sitting. Degenerative disk disease is also characterized by gradually increasing back pain and decreased, painful spinal movements.

In addition to pain, patients with lower back disorders may experience changes in a particular dermatome, which can cause diminished muscle strength, difficulty with heel or toe walking, and sensory deficits in the leg, foot, and toes. The Achilles and patellar reflexes may be diminished or absent. The patient with spinal stenosis will probably maintain a forward flexed posture to open the canal and alleviate pressure on the nerves. With more severe slips due to spondylolisthesis, the patient may show increased lumbar lordosis and a protruding abdomen. Changes in bowel and bladder function secondary to any low back disorder may require emergent evaluation and treatment.

Diagnosis

The majority of patients with LBP do not need radiographic evaluation, but spinal radiographs may be ordered to rule out any concomitant cause of LBP. They can also show the changes typical of each low back disorder.

MRI is the diagnostic tool of choice for demonstrating nerve root compromise due to disk herniation. Computed tomographic scanning with contrast dye can allow the visualization of the nerve roots and the subarachnoid space, but the invasive nature of the study has also made it less popular than MRI. Electromyography can be beneficial in demonstrating the specific nerve root level for a sensory deficit. Diskography, which can also be used to reproduce the patient's typical pain at the symptomatic disk level, is especially useful when the patient has multiple levels of involvement. All imaging results should be compared with the patient's signs and symptoms, because a large number of positive findings occur in asymptomatic individuals.

Interdisciplinary Care

Primary Provider (Physician/Nurse Practitioner)

The patient with mild symptoms can be treated conservatively, and full recovery is expected within a matter of weeks. Chronic LBP can be life altering, however, and requires an effective interdisciplinary approach to care. When conservative measures fail, the patient is referred to an orthopedist for evaluation and possible surgery.

Drug Therapy

Analgesia has been the mainstay of treatment for LBP. Simple analgesics such as acetaminophen have been as effective as all types of NSAIDs. NSAIDs are generally beneficial for uncomplicated short-term treatment but do not tend to work well for related sciatic nerve complaints. Muscle relaxants (e.g., cyclobenzaprine [Flexeril]), although effective in early stages of acute LBP, are impractical for use in chronic LBP because of their central nervous system side effects.

Although the use of epidural corticosteroids in the treatment of LBP is well established, it is still somewhat controversial because of contradictory evidence regarding efficacy. Corticosteroids are placed locally to reduce systemic side effects. They are often combined with a local anesthetic and injected into the epidural space. Complications are rare and relate largely to the technical aspects of needle placement (Box 26-9). Anticoagulation may be a contraindication to epidural injection because of the risk of hematoma formation. Facet joint and trigger point injections have also been advocated by some health care practitioners, but there is limited evidence to support their use.

Easily recognized side effects of corticosteroid injection include flushing, fever, fluid retention, and transient hyperglycemia.

Orthopedic Surgeon

When more conservative treatments have been unsuccessful in controlling symptoms of chronic back disorders, surgical intervention may be considered. See Box 26-10 for indications for back surgery. The type of surgery is based on the specific pathology, the presence or absence of spondylolisthesis, and the degree of spinal instability. Surgery is performed to relieve pain and neurologic symptoms and to allow the patient to regain independence in performing ADL.

Nurse

Patient education focuses initially on pain management and strategies to ensure that chronic pain interferes minimally with the patient's lifestyle (Box 26-11).

Illness behaviors and counterproductive attitudes are common in patients with chronic LBP. The nurse should help the family to avoid inadvertently reinforcing these behaviors because they may interfere with attainment of treatment goals.

Dietitian

Nutritional counseling may be beneficial for the overweight patient with LBP.

Physical Therapist

The physical therapist provides a program of stretching, flexibility, and strengthening exercises and offers instruction in proper body mechanics. In addition, aquatic therapy may be useful in decreasing the patient's pain. An aggressive exercise program improves physical function but also increases the patient's confidence in performing daily activities, which

---

Box 26-10   Indications for Back Surgery

- Decreased ability to perform activities of daily living
- Leg cramps that interfere with sleep
- Inability to walk more than 50 yd or sit longer than 30 minutes
- Motor weakness
- Bladder or bowel dysfunction

Box 26-11   Teaching Points Related to Pain Management Strategies

- Understand the purpose and proper administration of all medications being taken.
- Use analgesics and muscle relaxants safely.
- Modify activity to decrease pain.
- Perform self-care activities comfortably while wearing orthotics.
- Use orthotics only during periods of pain exacerbation.
- Perform prescribed exercises to decrease pain and improve function.
- Report any sensory and/or motor deficits or problems with bowel and bladder function.

Box 26-9   Complications of Epidural Corticosteroid Injection

- Dural puncture
- Headache
- Infection
- Hemorrhage
- Exacerbation of pain

ultimately decreases disability. Ultrasonographic and heat or cold therapies may be useful adjuncts to the prescribed exercise program.

The physical therapist may also be involved in the use of other modalities for symptom management in the patient with LBP. Transcutaneous electrical nerve stimulation is widely used for the treatment of LBP, but evidence regarding its effectiveness in chronic back disorders is contradictory.

Medical Social Worker

If the patient lacks the financial resources for prolonged treatment of lower back disorders, the medical social worker may have to arrange assistance in the purchase of medications and possibly home care services. Persistent pain and mobility impairment may affect the patient's ability to hold a job, and the medical social worker may have to assist the patient in accessing additional aid programs or obtaining alternate vocational training.

Complementary and Alternative Therapies

One of the most popular alternative treatment modalities for chronic LBP is chiropractic manipulation. Research has produced widely conflicting findings on the efficacy of chiropractic treatment. See Chapter 25 for additional discussion of chiropractic.

Behavioral therapies such as relaxation techniques and biofeedback may be particularly useful for the patient with chronic LBP. These interventions help the patient manage the mental fatigue associated with long-term illness and may also decrease symptom severity. Acupuncture and acupressure may have some benefit as well.

Ethical Considerations

The inadequate treatment of chronic LBP can be a health care concern. The patient with persistent symptoms and poor response to treatment may be labeled as a malingerer. If treatment includes long-term use of opioid analgesics, the patient is also often identified as a drug seeker. Later acute pain related to other conditions may be inadequately treated because of the health care provider's perception that the patient is "playing the system" to get medication. Health care providers need an increased understanding of the psychological impact of chronic pain and an open mind in accepting the patient's complaints at face value.

Family and Caregiver Issues

Box 26-12 lists family and caregiver issues that may arise in connection with musculoskeletal diseases.

Box 26-12 Family and Caregiver Issues for Musculoskeletal Diseases

- Difficulty in accepting changes in patient's role function due to disease
- Unwillingness to offer assistance with routine activities during periods of disease exacerbation, acute pain, or mobility impairment
- Encouragement of patient dependence by provision of too much assistance
- Loss of patience with long-term symptoms, limited response to treatment, and/or long-term rehabilitation
- Lack of understanding of the need to avoid the social isolation that may result from decreased self-esteem caused by the physical changes of the disease
- Lack of understanding of the impact of fatigue from coping with chronic disease on the patient's ability to participate in family activities, and of the need to modify activities

---

CASE STUDY
Patient Data
Mrs. G. is a 72-year-old widow who lives alone in a two-bedroom apartment in the suburbs of a large metropolitan area. Her 46-year-old daughter, an elementary school teacher, lives in the city about 5 miles from Mrs. G. Her three grandchildren, ages 14, 18, and 20, are frequent visitors to Mrs. G.'s home. Until recently, Mrs. G. has been able to attend many of their school and athletic activities. Mrs. G. has been an active member of her church for over 30 years but has not attended services in the last 3 months because of increasing disability from chronic back pain. She reports no other medical problems but notes that she did have a hysterectomy at age 32 for dysfunctional uterine bleeding. She takes a multivitamin with iron daily. Mrs. G.'s height and weight are recorded at the start of her clinic visit. Mrs. G. is 5 ft 3 inches tall and weighs 116 lb. She tells the nurse she was 5 ft 5 inches tall the last time she was measured a couple of years earlier. The nurse notes that Mrs. G. has hunched shoulders and marked kyphosis.

Diagnostic Findings
- Serum calcium level: 9 mg/dl
- Serum phosphorus level: 3.2 mg/dl
- Urinary calcium: 375 mg/day
- Spinal films, anteroposterior and oblique views: decreased intervertebral space with old fracture at T10, new fracture at T8

Thinking It Through
- What nursing diagnoses are appropriate for Mrs. G.?
- What complications are possible with osteoporosis?
- What are Mrs. G.'s concerns related to her persistent back pain? How would you as the nurse address them?
- What additional dietary supplements may be appropriate for Mrs. G. to take?
- What health care teaching should be extended to Mrs. G.'s daughter?

Case Conference
The interdisciplinary team that has gathered to discuss and plan Mrs. G.'s care includes her family practice physician, nurse, physical therapist, occupational therapist, Mrs. G., and her daughter.

Continued

CASE STUDY—cont'd

The physician has already reviewed the laboratory and radiologic findings with Mrs. G. and has explained that she has osteoporosis. The physician plans to order bone densitometry to determine her current bone mineral density. At this meeting, the physician provides prescriptions for alendronate (Fosamax) and ibuprofen (Motrin), and recommends calcium and vitamin D supplementation. The physician also plans to prescribe an exercise program based on recommendations from the physical therapist and to refer Mrs. G. to the occupational therapist for assistance in performing ADL.

The nurse has already spent some time talking with Mrs. G. and her daughter about the diagnosis of osteoporosis. The nurse will serve as case manager to coordinate the activities of the therapists. The nurse also teaches Mrs. G. the purpose of alendronate and the appropriate way to take the medication to achieve maximum benefit. The nurse ensures that Mrs. G. understands the possible side effects of ibuprofen use and the need to promptly report any signs of gastrointestinal bleeding. The nurse identifies an appropriate calcium and vitamin D supplement for her to take each day. The nurse also mentions the daughter's risk for osteoporosis and suggests early intervention to protect bone mineral density. The nurse provides some patient education brochures from the National Osteoporosis Foundation to help Mrs. G. and her daughter to understand the disease, its prevention, and its treatment. Mrs. G. says her grandchildren can help her find additional information on the Internet and at the public library. The nurse also suggests that, once Mrs. G. feels better, she consider involvement in an osteoporosis support group to learn how other patients live successfully with the disease.

Because Mrs. G. is interested in resuming her community activities, the physical therapist discusses safety strategies to avoid further bone injury. The therapist will meet with Mrs. G. twice a week for the next month to supervise her performance of exercises to help in muscle strengthening. In the meantime, the therapist suggests use of a quad cane to provide Mrs. G. greater stability as she ambulates. The therapist also discusses safe use of a heating pad at home to help with back pain.

The occupational therapist asks Mrs. G. about her ability to perform ADL. Mrs. G. describes some difficulty in activities that require reaching. The therapist will meet with Mrs. G. twice this week before her physical therapy visits to review the use of assistive devices for dressing and grooming.

The nurse asks Mrs. G. and her daughter if they have any questions. Mrs. G. mentions that she lives on a fixed income and is interested in cost-effective sources of dietary calcium. After receiving a food list from the nurse, Mrs. G. says she has no more questions at this time but would like to call the nurse if she finds something she does not readily understand in her reading. The nurse gives Mrs. G. her card and says she will follow up with Mrs. G. after her first week's therapy. The therapists confirm the schedule for this week's clinic visits.

Once the team meeting is over, the nurse develops a plan of care for Mrs. G.

■ What information from the team meeting should be included in the plan of care?

■ What short-term and long-term goals should be established with Mrs. G.?

■ What is the benefit of having both Mrs. G. and her daughter on the team?

Internet and Other Resources

American Fibromyalgia Syndrome Association: *http://www. afsafund.org*

Amputee Coalition of America: *http://www.amputee-coalition.org*

Amputee Resource Foundation of America, Inc.: *http://www. amputeeresource.org*

Amputees in Motion: local chapters

Arthritis Foundation: *http://www.arthritis.org*

International Osteoporosis Foundation: *http://www.osteofound. org*

International Rare Disease Support Network: *http://www. raredisorders.com*

Med Help International: *http://www.medhelp.org*

National Fibromyalgia Association: *http://www.fmaware.org*

National Fibromyalgia Partnership, Inc.: *http://www.fmpartner ship.org*

National Institute of Arthritis and Musculoskeletal and Skin Diseases: *http://www.niams.nih.gov*

National Institute of Neurological Disorders and Stroke: *http://www.ninds.nih.gov*

National Institutes of Health, Osteoporosis and Related Bone Diseases—National Resource Center: *http://www.osteo.org*

National Osteoporosis Foundation: *http://www.nof.org*

Orthotic and Prosthetic Assistance Fund: *http://www.opfund. org*

Paget Foundation: *http://www.paget.org*

REFERENCES

Agency for Healthcare Research and Quality: Osteoporosis in postmenopausal women: diagnosis and monitoring, Evidence Report/ Technology Assessment No. 28, AHRQ Pub No. 01-E031, 2001, Rockville, Md, The Agency, retrieved from *http://www.ahrq.gov/clinic/ epcsums/osteosum.htm* on April 26, 2003.

American College of Rheumatology: 1990 Criteria for the classification of fibromyalgia, *Arthritis Rheum* 33(2):160-72, 1990.

Burgess E, Nanes MS: Osteoporosis in men: pathophysiology, evaluation, and therapy, *Curr Opin Rheumatol* 14(4):421-8, 2002.

Carek PJ, Dickerson LM, Sack JL: Diagnosis and management of osteomyelitis, *Am Fam Physician* 63(12):2413-20, 2001.

Edwards AM, Blackburn L, David J: Food supplements in the treatment of primary fibromyalgia: a double-blind, crossover trial of anthocyanidins and placebo, *J Nutr Environ Med* 10:189-99, 2000.

Geier KA: Metabolic bone conditions. In Schoen DC, editor: *NAON core curriculum for orthopaedic nurses,* ed 4, Pitman, NJ, 2001, National Association of Orthopaedic Nurses, pp 341-59.

Haigh R, Clarke AK: Effectiveness of rehabilitation for spinal pain, *Clin Rehabil* 13(S1):63-81, 1999.

Kessenich CR: Alternative therapies in osteoporosis [Nursing Spectrum web site], 2002, retrieved from *http://nsweb.nursingspectrum.com/ce/ ce282.htm* on April 27, 2003.

Laeseke P: Treatment of osteomyelitis with hydroxyapatite, 2000, retrieved from *http://www.pharmacy.wisc.edu/courses/718-430/2000 presentation/ Laeseke.pdf* on April 27, 2003.

Lindberg L, Iwarsson S: Subjective quality of life, health, I-ADL ability and adaptation strategies in fibromyalgia, *Clin Rehabil* 16:675-83, 2002.

National Center for Complementary and Alternative Medicine: The efficacy of reiki in the treatment of fibromyalgia, 2003, retrieved from *http://www.clinicaltrials.gov/ct/gui/show/NCT00051428?order=1* on June 7, 2003.

National Institute of Arthritis and Musculoskeletal and Skin Disease: Questions and answers about fibromyalgia, 1999, retrieved from *http://www.niams.nih.gov/hi/topics/fibromyalgia/fibrofs.htm* on April 27, 2003.

National Osteoporosis Foundation: Osteoporosis and its most serious consequences, 2001, retrieved from *http://www.nof.org/news/press releases/background_hipfracture.htm* on April 26, 2003.

National Osteoporosis Foundation: America's bone health: the state of osteoporosis and low bone mass, 2002a, retrieved from *http://www.nof.org/advocacy/prevalence/index.htm* on April 26, 2003.

National Osteoporosis Foundation: Prevention: how can I prevent osteoporosis? 2002b, retrieved from *http://www.nof.org/prevention* on April 26, 2003.

National Osteoporosis Foundation: Prevention: who's at risk? 2002c, retrieved from *http://www.nof.org/prevention/risk.htm* on April 27, 2003.

Osteoporosis prevention, diagnosis, and therapy, *NIH Consens Statement Online* 17(1):1-36, March 27-29, 2000, retrieved from *http://consensus.nih.gov/cons/111/111_statement.htm* on April 26, 2003.

Ott S: Osteoporosis in males, University of Washington Online Continuing Medical Education, Osteoporosis and bone physiology, 1999, retrieved from *http://uwcme.org/site/courses/legacy/bonephys/opmale.html* on May 3, 2003.

Paget Foundation: A nurse's guide to Paget's disease of the bone, 2002, retrieved from *http://www.paget.org* on April 26, 2003.

Petras K: Boning up on calcium: what you need to know, 2002, retrieved from *http://www.earlymenopause.com/calcium* on June 8, 2003.

Roberto KA, Reynolds SG: The meaning of osteoporosis in the lives of rural older women, *Health Care Women Int* 22:599-611, 2001.

Roberts D: Arthritis and connective tissue disorders. In Schoen DC, editor: *NAON core curriculum for orthopaedic nursing,* ed 4, Pitman, NJ, 2001, National Association of Orthopaedic Nurses, pp 301-40.

Roberts D, Lappe J: Management of clients with musculoskeletal disorders. In Black JM, Hawks JH, Keene AM, editors: *Medical-surgical nursing: clinical management for positive outcomes,* ed 6, Philadelphia, 2001, WB Saunders, pp 551-85.

Rodts MF: Disorders of the spine. In Maher AB, Salmond JW, Pellino TA, editors: *Orthopaedic nursing,* ed 3, Philadelphia, 2002, WB Saunders, pp 515-50.

Salmond SW, Fine C: Infections of the musculoskeletal system. In Maher AB, Salmond SW, Pellino TA, editors: *Orthopaedic nursing,* ed 3, Philadelphia, 2002, WB Saunders, pp 734-78.

Schneider D, Hofmann MT: Diagnosis and treatment of Paget's disease of bone, *Am Fam Physician* 65(10):2069-72, 2002.

Sedlak CA, Doheny MO: Metabolic conditions. In Maher AB, Salmond SW, Pellino TA, editors: *Orthopaedic nursing,* ed 3, Philadelphia, 2002, WB Saunders, pp 423-67.

Undersea and Hyperbaric Medicine Society: Indications for hyperbaric oxygen therapy, 2003, retrieved from *http://www.uhms.org/Indications/indications.htm* on June 8, 2003.

Wirganowicz PZ: Aggressive surgical management of chronic osteomyelitis, *Univ Pa Orthop J* 12:7-12, 1999, retrieved from *http://www.uphs.upenn.edu/ortho/oj/1999/html/oj12sp99p7.html.*

World Health Organization: Osteoporosis: both health organizations and individuals must act now to avoid an impending epidemic, 1999, retrieved from *http://www.who.int/inf-pr-1999/en/pr99-58.html* on April 26, 2003.

CHAPTER 27

Living with Cancer

Sharron Guillett, PhD, RN

OBJECTIVES

After reading this chapter, you should be able to do the following:

- Define the term *cancer*
- Locate cancer in the experience of chronic illness and disability
- Cite the incidence and prevalence of cancer in the United States
- Describe the pathophysiology of cancer
- Describe the effects of cancer on the physiologic, psychosocial, emotional, and spiritual well-being of individuals and their family members
- Identify common treatment modalities for individuals with cancer
- Describe the effects of cancer treatment on the physiologic, psychosocial, emotional, and spiritual well-being of individuals and their family members
- Describe the role of each member of the interdisciplinary team in supporting individuals with cancer
- Describe the role of culture in the way that cancer is experienced
- Describe end-of-life care for patients with cancer

Cancer is a group of diseases that have been with us for centuries. In fact, the word *carcinoma* was first used by Hippocrates to describe a tumor that invaded surrounding tissues. Although the overall incidence of new cancers (with the exception of skin cancers) has been steadily declining since 1992, cancer continues to be the cause of significant morbidity and disability and is the second leading cause of death in the United States. According to the American Cancer Society (2003), one out of every two males and one out of every three females will have cancer at some time during their lives. The estimated number of new cases of cancer for 2003 is listed in Table 27-1.

Over 10 million Americans living in 2002 had a history of cancer, some of whom were considered to be "free of disease." The term *free of disease* or *no evidence of disease* is preferred to the term *cured*. The 5-year survival rate for cancer is about 62%; the figure could be as high as 95% for some cancers if early screening measures were taken.

As advances in detection and treatment improve survival rates, it becomes more important to view cancer as a chronic illness. Longer survival requires follow-up care that includes the recognition of chronic problems, the need for lifelong monitoring, and continued access to health care services (Leigh, 1998). Survivors and their families continue to deal with the aftermath of their cancer experience long after the individuals are considered free of disease. The disease process as well as the treatments used may interfere with normal physiologic functioning, alter physical appearance, impair mobility, and deplete resources. In addition, both living with and surviving cancer may have a profound impact on psychological, emotional, and spiritual well-being.

PATHOPHYSIOLOGY

Cancer is caused by inherited genetic mutations, external factors such as exposure to sunlight and the use of tobacco, and internal factors such as hormones and immune disorders. Most cancers are probably the result of a combination of these factors (Porth, 2002). Regardless of the cause, the pathologic process is one of inappropriate cellular growth and division.

Normally, the process of cellular growth and differentiation is well controlled. However, cancer cells are poorly controlled and continue to grow, sometimes at a very rapid rate. The mutation that is found in cancer cells probably occurs during the differentiation phase of cell development. Cancerous transformations that occur early in the growth cycle of the cell produce cancer cells that are less differentiated and more malignant than those that occur later in the process. Lack of differentiation interferes with the ability of the cell to carry out its normal functions. In addition, programmed cellular death (apoptosis) does not occur in cancer cells as it does in normal cells. Therefore, nonfunctional cancer cells proliferate and crowd out healthy cells until the latter are unable to carry out their intended functions. As the mass of cancer cells increases, it can obstruct other organs and/or apply pressure on vessels and nerves, which leads to erosion and necrosis. Cancer spreads by invading surrounding tissues, seeding cells into body cavities, and entering blood and lymphatic fluids, which carry cells to distant body sites. Some cancers release substances that produce conditions referred to as paraneoplastic syndromes (Box 27-1).

Table 27-1   Leading Sites of New Cancer and Cancer Deaths (2003 Estimates)

Estimated New Cases		Estimated Deaths	
Male	**Female**	**Male**	**Female**
Prostate 220,900 (33%)	Breast 211,300 (32%)	Lung and bronchus 88,400 (31%)	Lung and bronchus 68,800 (25%)
Lung and bronchus 91,800 (14%)	Lung and bronchus 80,100 (12%)	Prostate 28,900 (10%)	Breast 39,800 (15%)
Colon and rectum 72,800 (11%)	Colon and rectum 74,700 (11%)	Colon and rectum 28,300 (10%)	Colon and rectum 28,800 (11%)
Urinary bladder 42,200 (6%)	Uterine corpus 40,100 (6%)	Pancreas 14,700 (5%)	Pancreas 15,300 (6%)
Melanoma of the skin 29,900 (4%)	Ovary 25,400 (4%)	Non-Hodgkin's lymphoma 12,200 (4%)	Ovary 14,300 (5%)
Non-Hodgkin's lymphoma 28,300 (4%)	Non-Hodgkin's lymphoma 25,100 (4%)	Leukemia 12,100 (4%)	Non-Hodgkin's lymphoma 11,200 (4%)
Kidney 19,500 (3%)	Melanoma of the skin 24,300 (3%)	Esophagus 9900 (4%)	Leukemia 9800 (4%)
Oral cavity 18,200 (3%)	Thyroid 16,300 (3%)	Liver 9200 (3%)	Uterine corpus 6800 (3%)
Leukemia 17,900 (3%)	Pancreas 15,800 (2%)	Urinary bladder 8600 (3%)	Brain 5800 (2%)
Pancreas 14,900 (2%)	Urinary bladder 15,200 (2%)	Kidney 7400 (3%)	Multiple myeloma 5500 (2%)
All sites 675,300 (100%)	All sites 658,800 (100%)	All sites 285,900 (100%)	All sites 270,600 (100%)

Copyright 2003 American Cancer Society, Inc., Surveillance Research.
Excludes basal and squamous cell skin cancers and in situ carcinoma except of the urinary bladder.

The symptoms associated with each of these syndromes are related to the hormones, enzymes, or antigens secreted.

DIAGNOSIS

A variety of methods are used to diagnose cancer. The method selected depends on the type of cancer suspected as well as its location. Common diagnostic methods are listed in Box 27-2.

Once the presence of cancer is confirmed, the cancer is classified according to its histology and extent. Histology

---

Box 27-1   Paraneoplastic Syndromes

- Anemia
- Arthralgia
- Cushing's syndrome
- Gynecomastia
- Hypercalcemia
- Hyperglycemia
- Nephrotic syndrome
- Polycythemia
- Polymyositis
- Superior vena cava syndrome
- Syndrome of inappropriate secretion of antidiuretic hormone
- Tumor lysis syndrome

Box 27-2   Methods Commonly Used to Diagnose Cancer

- Biopsy
- Ultrasonography
- Radiologic studies
    Computed tomography
    Magnetic resonance imaging
    Angiography
    Intravenous pyelography
    Barium enema study
- Nuclear medicine scanning
    Positron emission tomography
    Bone scanning
    Thyroid scanning
- Laboratory studies
    Cytologic analysis
    Bence Jones protein test
    Cancer antigen 125 test
    Carcinoembryonic antigen test
    Papanicolaou test
    Prostatic specific antigen test
    Stool guaiac (test for occult blood)
    Liver enzyme levels
    Serum acid phosphatase level
    Complete blood count
    Urinalysis

is described in terms of a grade ranging from I to IV (Box 27-3) and extent is described in terms of a stage ranging from 0 to IV (Box 27-4). The International Union Against Cancer developed a standardized system for classifying cancer called the TNM classification system (Box 27-5). This system classifies tumors according to the size of the tumor (T), the degree of spread to regional lymph nodes (N), and absence or presence of distant metastases (M). A variety of classification systems exist that are specific to the type of cancer being categorized. For example, the Dukes classification system is used for colon cancer (see Chapter 32). These systems provide a standardized way to communicate the status of the cancer, facilitate research, develop a treatment plan, and evaluate its effectiveness.

Box 27-3   Tumor Grading System

- Grade I: Cells are slightly different from normal, well differentiated.
- Grade II: Cells are mildly abnormal, moderately differentiated.
- Grade III: Cells are very abnormal, poorly differentiated.
- Grade IV: Cells are immature and undifferentiated.

Box 27-4   Tumor Staging System

- Stage 0: Cancer in situ
- Stage I: Localized tumor growth in tissue of origin
- Stage II: Limited local spread
- Stage III: Extensive local and regional spread
- Stage IV: Metastases

Box 27-5   TNM Classification System

TUMOR (T)
- T_0: No evidence of tumor
- T_{is}: Tumor in situ
- T_{1-4}: Increasing degrees of tumor size

REGIONAL LYMPH NODES (N)
- N_0: No nodes involved
- N_{1-4}: Increasing numbers of nodes involved
- N_x: Unable to assess

METASTASES (M)
- M_0: No metastases
- M_1: Distant metastases
- M_x: Unable to determine

ASSESSMENT

Cancer affects functioning on many levels. On the micro level, it affects the functioning of virtually every body system, and on the macro level, it affects the functioning of individuals as people and therefore has an impact on the groups they belong to, their friends, and their families. Globally, cancer affects society as a whole in that enormous resources are expended on research and treatment annually. In the United States in 2002, overall costs of direct care for cancer and indirect costs related to morbidity were estimated at $171.6 billion (American Cancer Society, 2003).

Because the effects of cancer are multidimensional, assessments must also be multidimensional, as well as holistic and culturally relevant. Many scales have been devised to assess how well people with cancer are managing their illness and maintaining quality of life. The Karnofsky Performance Scale (Box 27-6) is widely used to assist in decision making regarding the advisability of available treatment options. Quality-of-life scales have also been developed to assess the impact of cancer using cancer-specific measures. When selecting a quality-of-life assessment tool, one must be sure that quality-of-life measures have been derived from patient-generated concepts, rather than being based on the developers' notions of what constitutes quality of life.

Additional assessment tools that may be used to evaluate health status and quality of life of individuals with cancer are listed in Box 27-7.

Functional health patterns (Box 27-8) provide a framework for assessing the effects of cancer from the individual's perspective. The data gathered from the health pattern

---

Box 27-6   Karnofsky Performance Scale

Normal, no complaints, no evidence of disease	100
Able to carry on normal activity, minor signs or symptoms of disease	90
Able to carry on normal activity with effort, some signs and symptoms of disease	80
Cares for self, unable to carry on normal activity or to do active work	70
Requires occasional assistance but is able to care for most needs	60
Requires considerable assistance and frequent medical care	50
Disabled, requires special care and assistance	40
Severely disabled, hospitalization is indicated although death is not imminent	30
Hospitalization is necessary, very sick, active supportive treatment necessary	20
Moribund fatal processes progressing rapidly	10
Dead	0

assessment contributes to problem identification and provides the basis for the plan of care.

CLINICAL MANIFESTATIONS

Cancer has both local and systemic effects. Clinical manifestations vary depending on the organs and systems affected by the cancer. For example, bowel cancer affects elimination patterns, whereas lung cancer affects respiratory function. However, most individuals find themselves in a state of physical, emotional, psychological, and perhaps spiritual upheaval (Wasteson et al, 2002).

People with cancer experience many of the same symptoms regardless of the tumor location or metastases. Fatigue, weakness, anxiety, depression, pain, and fear are examples of shared symptoms. Cachexia, a complex metabolic disturbance characterized by anorexia, weight loss, anemia, and asthenia, is also common among people with advanced cancer. The most common symptoms reported by patients with advanced cancer are listed in Box 27-9.

INTERDISCIPLINARY CARE

The treatments provided depend on the type, stage, and prognosis of the cancer as well as the individual's wishes regarding such treatment. Patients who are aggressively treating their cancer may be engaged in a variety of treatment modalities, including radiation, chemotherapy, and surgery. They may also be simultaneously exploring complementary and alternative therapies such as herbal remedies, acupuncture, and meditation. Other individuals may decide to stop treatment altogether or opt for palliative care. The health care team works closely with individuals and their families to explore what is possible and what is desired to develop a plan of care that supports individual and family goals and is culturally relevant, spiritually affirming, and consistent with best practices.

Primary Provider (Physician/Nurse Practitioner)

The primary provider is generally the professional who discovers the presence of the cancerous tissue. At the point at which the cancer diagnosis is confirmed, the primary provider shares the information with the patient and reviews treatment options with the patient and family. The management of the cancer is then transferred to an oncologist who specializes in the treatment of the specific cancer the patient has. The primary provider continues to follow the patient's progress and care and consults with the oncologist about the patient's overall health status and any comorbid conditions.

Specialists
Surgeon

The surgeon consults with the primary provider, oncologist, and radiation specialist to determine the goals of surgery and the procedure that will be of most value. Surgical interventions are the oldest and most commonly used treatment approaches to cancer. Surgical biopsies are used to assist in diagnosis and staging. Tumor excision and debulking are performed to bring about cure and provide palliation. Other surgical procedures may be undertaken to treat oncologic emergencies and provide pain relief.

In some instances, individuals who do not have cancer but have a strong genetic predisposition for cancer elect to have prophylactic surgery to reduce their risk. Examples of prophylactic surgery include mastectomy and oophorectomy to prevent breast and ovarian cancer, respectively.

Radiation Oncologist

Approximately 60% of cancer patients receive radiation therapy (RT) (Holland, 2002). RT is given for both curative and palliative purposes. The goal of curative RT is to eradicate the tumor or shrink it preoperatively, whereas the goal of palliative RT is to relieve obstructions and decrease pain. The radiation oncologist meets with the health care team and the patient to determine what the goals of therapy are and how they can best be met.

Ionizing radiation causes cellular death in all tissues exposed to the radiation. Some tissues are more susceptible to radiation than others. This susceptibility, termed *radiosensitivity,* is one of the factors considered in deciding whether radiation therapy is appropriate. Other factors that are taken into account include the patient's age and overall condition, the prognosis if radiation is used, the size and stage of the tumor, and the degree of metastases. Table 27-2 indicates the radiosensitivity of specific body organs.

Radiation is prescribed in units called rads or grays. A rad is the amount of radiation absorbed per dose and 1 gray (Gy) is equal to 100 rads. Radiation oncologists determine the most effective dose that can be safely given without damaging surrounding normal tissues. The radiation oncologist also determines the duration of a single exposure, the frequency of treatments, and length of therapy. Radiation can be delivered internally or externally using x-rays, artificially created radioactive isotopes, and naturally occurring radium.

Box 27-8   Functional Health Pattern Assessment for Cancer

HEALTH PERCEPTION/HEALTH MANAGEMENT
- Does the patient have a history of smoking or passive exposure to smoke?
- What screening studies have been done (e.g., stool guaiac)
- Has the patient been exposed to known carcinogens? Does the patient use sun screens?
- What is the patient's perception of his or her overall health?
- Is the patient aware of the diagnosis?
- What medications and therapies does the patient use, including over-the-counter drugs and alternative therapies?

NUTRITION/METABOLISM
- What is the patient's current weight? Has a recent unexplained weight loss or gain occurred?
- Is the patient on a special diet?
- What is the condition of the skin and mucous membranes?
- Is saliva production adequate? Does the patient have difficulty swallowing?
- What is the patient's typical dietary intake (daily)?
- Is nausea and/or vomiting present (if so, is it treatment related or anticipatory)?

ELIMINATION
- Have any changes occurred in bowel or bladder habits?
- Is the patient able to use toilet facilities?

ACTIVITY/EXERCISE
- Does the patient experience difficulty in walking, fatigue, or dyspnea on exertion? What are the patient's dyspnea management strategies?
- What are the patient's regular exercise activities and recreational activities?
- What mobility aids does the patient use?
- Is the patient able to perform regular and instrumental activities of daily living?
- Does the patient use supplemental oxygen?

SLEEP/REST
- How many hours of uninterrupted sleep does the patient get at night? Does the patient take naps or rest periods?
- Does the patient have orthopnea?
- What sleep aids are used?
- Is fatigue relieved by sleep?

COGNITION/PERCEPTION
- What are the nature, character, location, and duration of the pain? What factors aggravate and alleviate the pain?
- Is there bone involvement? Are paresthesias present?
- How effective are pain management strategies? What level of distress is associated with the symptoms?

- Are there any changes in mentation or level of consciousness; in taste or sense of smell, sight, or hearing; or in speech and communication patterns?

SELF-PERCEPTION/SELF-CONCEPT
- How does the patient describe himself or herself?
- How has the condition affected the patient's self-esteem?
- What changes have occurred in the patient's body image?
- How has the condition affected the patient's sense of self?

ROLES/RELATIONSHIPS
- What kind of work does the patient perform?
- What role does the patient play in the home and family?
- What changes have occurred in the patient's ability to carry out role functions?
- How satisfied is the patient with his or her current roles and relationships?
- How has the condition affected the patient's family and/or significant others? What changes have occurred in family organization and function?
- Who is the primary caregiver and how involved is this person in the patient's care?
- Who is the decision maker?

SEXUALITY/REPRODUCTION
- Is the patient sexually active?
- Have changes occurred in sexual performance?
- Is the patient satisfied with current sexual patterns?
- Has the patient experienced any changes in the menstrual cycle?

COPING/STRESS TOLERANCE
- What coping strategies does the patient use?
- What support systems are available to the patient?
- Can the patient manage the condition in the current setting?
- Is the patient aware of hospice and palliative care options? What level of hopefulness or despair is exhibited?
- What do the patient and family find comforting and meaningful?

VALUES/BELIEFS
- What constitutes good quality of life for the patient? What is important to the patient?
- What are the patient's spiritual beliefs; health beliefs, including beliefs about the use of medications for pain control; and cultural beliefs?
- To what degree does the individual participate in cultural traditions and the cultural community?
- What are the patient's views about locus of control?
- What are the patient's end-of-life concerns? Has the patient considered issues relating to advance directives and decisions? Does the patient want a spiritual leader, advisor, or counselor present?

External Radiation Therapy

External RT (teletherapy) may be used alone or with surgery for both cure and palliation. Before therapy is initiated, the patient goes through a simulation. During this time the patient lies on an x-ray table with an immobilization device in place while the treatment area is identified and isolated. Permanent markings are placed on the patient's skin to identify the area that is to receive the radiation. The patient must be

Box 27-9 Symptoms Most Frequently Experienced by Persons with Advanced Cancer

- Anorexia
- Constipation
- Dry mouth
- Dyspnea
- Early satiety
- Fatigue
- Weakness
- Weight loss

Box 27-10 Personal Care Related to Radiation Therapy

- Avoid using harsh soaps or perfumes because these irritate the skin. Cleanse the irradiated area with water or a mild soap and water, taking care not to remove the markings on the area (in most cases markings are tattooed, but some may be applied with inks or dyes that are not permanent). If soap is used, be sure to rinse thoroughly.
- Avoid rubbing the area with wash cloths or towels because the skin is fragile and may slough. Use gentle patting motions with soft cloths.
- Do not apply lubricants, emollients, talcs, or powders to the irradiated area while treatment is ongoing, because small particles of powder, oil, or lotion can disperse radiation and lessen treatment effectiveness.
- Be careful not to rub, bind, or irritate the irradiated area. Clothing should be soft and loose fitting.
- Avoid exposing the area to the sun. (This precaution should be followed for the remainder of the patient's life, because the adverse affects of irradiation may appear months to years after actual treatment.)
- Fatigue is a common side effect of radiation therapy. Take frequent naps or rest periods.
- Patients often report a decline in quality of life during treatment. This decline does not persist, and quality of life returns to normal within 4 to 6 weeks after treatment.
- Call the provider if any of the following occurs*:
  - Skin breakdown or drainage appears over radiation site. (Changes in skin color are normal.)
  - Radiation site becomes painful.

*Patients and their families should recognize that these symptoms can occur months after the treatment has concluded.

taught not to remove the markings and the proper care for the area being treated (Box 27-10). Simulations may take up to 2 hours, so a patient who has pain or finds it difficult to lie still for that long may require medication beforehand. Subsequent RT treatments generally last about 15 minutes. The treatments themselves do not produce any sensations; however, they do cause a number of side effects. The most common general side effects are skin irritation, changes in sense of taste, and fatigue.

Skin reactions vary depending on the area being treated, the dose of radiation, and the length of treatment. Initially, transient erythema develops, which over time becomes more noticeable and looks like sunburn. As radiation continues, cells begin to slough and the skin looks dry and flaky. This period of dry desquamation is followed by moist desquamation characterized by bright erythema and exudates. Today's linear accelerators are considered "skin sparing" and deliver the radiation primarily beneath the skin's surface (Holland, 2002). Skin reactions heal within 2 to 3 weeks, but complete return to normal may take months, and some skin reactions appear years after the original radiation. Hair loss occurs in the area irradiated and, although a local effect, may be permanent.

The fatigue associated with RT is unlike usual fatigue because it is not relieved by sleep. In fact, evidence is growing that exercise reduces cancer-related fatigue (Brown, 2002; Dimeo, 2002). Fatigue resolves within months following treatment, but it is one of the symptoms that patients report as most distressing (Holland, 2002). There are many nursing interventions that address fatigue, but it is essential to treat underlying causes such as anemia and poor nutrition as well as the fatigue itself.

External RT also produces site-specific side effects, some of which occur months to years after treatment. A list of these site-specific effects is found in Table 27-3. Secondary cancers such as lung cancer and breast cancer may occur as long as 5 years after treatment. Therefore, long-term follow-up of patients receiving external beam therapy is required.

Internal Radiation Therapy

In internal RT (brachytherapy), radioactive substances are placed directly into cancerous tissues. The radioactive

Table 27-2 Radiosensitivity of Specific Body Organs and Tissues

		Radiosensitivity		
High	Medium High	Medium	Medium Low	Low
Bone marrow	Skin	Growing bone and cartilage	Mature bone and cartilage	Muscle
Testes	Oral cavity	Vasculature	Kidney	Brain
Intestines	Esophagus		Liver	Spinal cord
	Vagina		Thyroid	
	Cervix			

Modified from Phipps WJ et al: *Medical-surgical nursing: health and illness perspectives,* ed 7, St Louis, 2003, Mosby.

Table 27-3 Site-Specific Side Effects of Radiation

Radiation Site	Side Effects	Nursing Considerations
Brain	Early: alopecia, earache, headache, dizziness Late: hearing loss, cataracts, brain necrosis	Explain potential side effects before treatment; hair loss is likely to be permanent. Provide pain management. Instruct patient in need for safety precautions Evaluate hearing and vision at follow-up visits.
Head and neck	Early: dysphagia, mucositis, loss of taste, weight loss Late: trismus, mandibular osteoradionecrosis, dental decay, hypothyroidism, xerostomia	Arrange nutrition consult, provide pain management with viscous lidocaine and narcotics. Prescribe stretching exercises for mouth and jaw; instruct patient to visit dentist prior to starting treatment and obtain frequent dental care. Encourage annual thyroid function studies. Advise patient to use sauces and gravies on foods, use artificial saliva or oral lubricants.
Lung, mediastinum, esophagus	Early: dysphagia, cough, esophagitis, carditis Late: pneumonitis, dyspnea, chronic cough	Give soft bland foods, provide pain management. Provide oxygen, treat with steroids.
Chest, breast	Early: dysphagia, cough, esophagitis, carditis Late: lymphedema, fibrosis of lung and esophagus	Give soft bland foods, provide pain management. Make early referral to physical therapy. Perform esophageal dilation for strictures.
Abdomen, pelvis	Early: anorexia, nausea, vomiting, diarrhea, dysuria, polyuria, nocturia Late: gastric atrophy and erosion, intestinal adhesions, perforations and obstructions, proctitis, impotency, sterility, vaginal stenosis, cystitis, incontinence	Provide antiemetics, nutrition consult. Provide low-residue diet, fluid replacement, antidiarrheals. Patient may be on H_2-blocking medications or metoclopramide (Reglan) to improve motility. Monitor bowel movements. Discuss procreation measures prior to treatment; sperm banking or egg harvesting may be desired. Perform vaginal dilation. Encourage fluids, incontinence management, skin care.
Extremities	Early: erythema, desquamation Late: ankylosis, necrosis, sarcomas	Provide good skin care. Sarcomas may occur as much as 5 yr after treatment; long-term follow-up required.

substances either can be sealed in molds, plaques, needles, wires, ribbons, or special applicators, or they can be unsealed and ingested or delivered in liquid form into a body cavity (Figure 27-1).

Patients who undergo brachytherapy with a substance that gives off gamma rays pose a radiation hazard to those around them. Therefore, precautions must be taken to limit exposure. Exposure can be controlled by using shielding, limiting the time spent with the patient, and increasing the distance from the radiation source. The intensity of the gamma rays given off follows the law of inverse squares. This means that the exposure of someone standing 3 ft away is one ninth the exposure of someone standing 1 ft away. Persons who care for individuals receiving brachytherapy must wear dosimeters so that the amount of exposure can be measured. Additional safety measures for the person caring for someone receiving brachytherapy are outlined in Box 27-11.

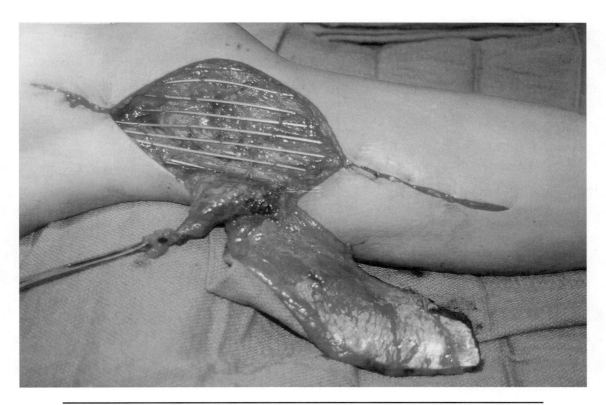

Figure 27-1 Brachytherapy radiation catheter implants with muscle flap. (Courtesy Kim Haynes, MS, RN, CS, ONC, ARNP, Mid-America Sarcoma Institute, Overland Park, Kan.)

Medical Oncologist

The medical oncologist is the patient's primary provider for cancer management. The oncologist assesses the status of the cancer and confers with the primary medical provider to discuss treatment options given the patient's overall health and wishes regarding such treatment. The oncologist also consults with the surgical and radiation team to develop a treatment plan.

Box 27-11 Safety Precautions When Caring for Patients Receiving Brachytherapy

- The patient should have private room and bath.
- Place a caution sign on the door of the patient's room.
- Pregnant women and children under the age of 16 should not be allowed to visit the patient.
- Visitors must remain 6 feet away from the radiation source.
- Limit visiting time to 30 minutes per visitor per day.
- Keep a lead container in the room in which to deposit radioactive source material should it become dislodged.
- Never touch a radioactive source with bare hands.
- Save all linens until the radioactive source has been removed to prevent accidental disposal of the source should it be unknowingly dislodged.

The plan may involve radiation, surgery, chemotherapy, biologic therapy, or some combination of these modalities. The oncologist follows the patient's response to treatment and recommends the next steps, which may include long-term follow-up, palliation, or hospice care.

Chemotherapy

Chemotherapy is given for cure, control, and palliation. The term *chemotherapy* is generally associated with cancer treatment, but chemotherapy is simply the treatment of disease through the use of chemical agents. The chemical agents used to treat cancer damage DNA, however, and therefore have toxic effects on healthy cells as well as cancerous cells. Individuals receiving chemotherapy experience severe side effects during treatment, some of which are life threatening. Some patients find the side effects intolerable and elect to discontinue treatment. Health care providers have the responsibility to ensure that the patient is well educated about the risks of stopping treatment versus the risks of continuing treatment so that an informed decision can be made. Once the decision has been reached, providers should support the patient and family in that decision. The most frequently experienced side effects of chemotherapy are bone marrow suppression, alopecia, nausea and vomiting, mucositis, and sterility. A list of chemotherapeutic agents frequently used to treat cancer and their common side effects appears in Table 27-4.

Table 27-4 Chemotherapeutic Agents and Their Side Effects

Chemotherapeutic Agent	Myelosuppression	Mucositis	Nausea and Vomiting	Alopecia	Vesication (V)/ Irritation (I)	Allergic Reaction	Other Specific Toxicities
Actinomycin D (Cosmegen)	+	+	+	+	+ (V)	0	Diarrhea
Aminoglutethimide (Cytadren)	±	−	+	−	−	−	Skin rash; sensory alterations, including lethargy, visual blurring, vertigo, ataxia, and nystagmus; hyponatremia, hyperkalemia, cortisol insufficiency
Amsacrine (m-AMSA)	+	0	+	0	+ (V)	0	Flulike syndrome, venoocclusive disease, hepatotoxicity
Bleomycin (Blenoxane)	±	+	±	+	0	+	Pulmonary toxicity, skin rash
Busulfan (Myleran)	+	0	±	0	0	0	Pulmonary fibrosis
Camptothecin-11 (CPT-11)	+	−	+	+	−	−	Diarrhea, pulmonary toxicity
Carboplatin (Paraplatin)	+	0	+	0	0	0	Pigmentation at injection site, hepatotoxicity, neurotoxicity, renal toxicity, pulmonary toxicity
Carmustine (BCNU)	+	+	+	0	+ (I)	0	Hepatotoxicity
Chlorambucil (Leukeran)	+	0	±	0	0	0	
Chlorodeoxyadenosine	+	0	0	0	0	0	Neurotoxicity, renal toxicity
Cisplatin (Platinol)	+	0	+	0	0	+	Nephrotoxicity, peripheral neuropathy, ototoxicity
Cladribine (Leustatin)	+	−	+	−	−	−	Fever, rash, diarrhea, constipation, cough, shortness of breath, tachycardia, edema
Cortisone	+	−	−	−	−	−	Gastric irritation, hyperglycemia, sodium and water retention, hypokalemia, hypocalcemia, behavioral changes
Cyclophosphamide (Cytoxan)	+	0	+	+	0	0	Sterile hemorrhagic cystitis, heart failure
Cytarabine (Cytosar, Ara-C)	+	+	+	+	0	0	Sterile hemorrhagic cystitis, heart failure
Dacarbazine (DTIC)	+	0	+	0	+ (I)	+	Hypotension
Diethylstilbestrol (DES)	0	0	+	0	0	0	Congestive heart failure
Doxorubicin (Adriamycin)	+	+	+	+	+ (V)	0	Cardiotoxicity, diarrhea
Estramustine (Emcyt)	+	−	+	−	+ (V)	0	Diarrhea, hepatotoxicity, hypocalcemia, hypophosphatemia, gynecomastia, congestive heart failure, thrombophlebitis, rash
Etoposide (VePesid)	+	0	+	+	+ (I)	±	Hepatotoxicity, neurotoxicity, hypotension
Floxuridine (FUDR)	+	+	+	+	0	0	Diarrhea, rash
Fludarabine (Fludara)	+	+	+	−	−	−	Pulmonary toxicity, pericardial effusion, neurotoxicity
5-Fluorouracil (5-FU)	+	+	±	±	0	0	Diarrhea, photosensitivity
Fluoxymesterone (Halotestin)	0	0	+	0	0	0	Masculinization
Gemcitabine (Gemzar)	+	−	+	−	−	−	Flulike symptoms
Hexamethylmelamine	+	0	+	±	0	0	Peripheral neuropathy
Hydroxyurea (Hydrea)	+	+	+	+	0	0	
Idarubicin (Idamycin)	+	+	+	+	+ (I)	0	Cardiomyopathy
Ifosfamide (Ifex)	±	0	±	+	0	0	Hematuria, neurotoxicity, hemorrhagic cystitis
L-Asparaginase (Elspar)	0	0	+	0	0	+	Major organ failure
Lomustine (CCNU)	+	+	+	±	0	0	Hepatotoxicity

Drug							Toxicity
Mechlorethamine (nitrogen mustard)	+	0	+	+	+(V)	0	Hemorrhagic cystitis
Megestrol (Megace)	0	0	0	+	0	0	Fluid retention
Melphalan (Alkeran)	+	±	±	+	0	0	Rarely pulmonary toxicity, secondary malignancy
6-Mercaptopurine (6-MP; Purinethol)	+	+	+	0	0	0	Hepatotoxicity
Methotrexate (MTX; Amethopterin)	+	+	±	±	0	0	Nephrotoxicity
Mithramycin (Mithracin)	+	+	+	0	+(V)	0	Hemorrhagic tendency
Mitomycin (Mutamycin)	+	+	+	+	+(V)	0	Nephrotoxicity, pulmonary toxicity
Mitotane (Lysodren)	−	−	+	−	−	−	Diarrhea, neurotoxicity, skin irritation or rash
Mitoxantrone (Novantrone)	+	+	+	+	0	0	Drug fever, diarrhea, increased liver enzymes
Oxaliplatin (Eloxatin)	+	−	+	−	−	−	Peripheral neuropathy
Oxymetholone (Anadrol-50)	0	0	0	0	0	0	Hepatotoxicity
Paclitaxel (Taxol)	+	0	+	±	0	±	Sensory neuropathy
Pentostatin (Nipent)	+	−	+	+	+(V)	−	Nephrotoxicity, hepatotoxicity, mental status changes, pulmonary toxicity, severe conjunctivitis
Prednisolone (Delta-Cortef)	0	0	0	0	0	0	Steroid side effects
Prednisone	0	0	0	0	0	0	Steroid side effects
Procarbazine (Matulane)	+	±	+	+	0	0	Monoamine oxidase inhibitor
Semustine (Methyl CCNU)	+	+	+	+	0	0	
Streptozocin (Zanosar)	+	0	+	±	+(I)	0	Nephrotoxicity
Tamoxifen (Nolvadex)	±	0	+	0	0	0	
Taxotere (Docetaxel)	+	−	−	+	−	+	Rash, fluid and electrolyte imbalance, peripheral edema, pleural effusion
Teniposide (Vumon)	+	−	+	+	+(I)	+	Hypotension, hepatotoxicity, cardiac arrhythmias, peripheral neuropathy
6-Thioguanine (6-TG)	+	+	+	0	0	0	Hepatotoxicity
Thiotepa	+	−	+	+	−	+	Sexual dysfunction, secondary malignancies, dizziness, headache, fever
Uracil mustard	+	0	+	±	0	0	
Vinblastine (Velban)	+	+	+	±	+(V)	0	Neurotoxicity
Vincristine (Oncovin)	0	0	0	+	+(V)	0	Neurotoxicity
Vindesine (Eldisine)	+	±	+	+	+(V)	−	Peripheral neuropathy, constipation, rash, diarrhea
Vinorelbine (Navelbine)	+	+	+	+	+(V)	−	Neurotoxicity, diarrhea, hepatotoxicity, injection site reaction, sexual/reproductive dysfunction

From Lewis SM, Heitkemper MM, Dirksen SR: *Medical-surgical nursing: assessment and management of clinical problems*, ed 5, St Louis, 2000, Mosby.

+, Common; ±, infrequent; 0, uncommon; −, no effect.

Most cancer chemotherapy is delivered intravenously, although it may be given via oral, intraarterial or intracavitary routes. Patients receiving chemotherapy over an extended period usually have venous access devices implanted to make drug administration easier and more comfortable. Regardless of the method of administration, providers must follow guidelines for safe handling of chemotherapeutic agents in institutional settings (Box 27-12) and in the home (Box 27-13).

Biotherapy

Biologic therapy or biotherapy is the use of agents that modify the body's response to cancer by interfering with tumor activities, modulating or restoring the individual's immune system functioning, or promoting stem cell differentiation. The indications for use of these agents are being investigated in clinical trials. The Food and Drug Administration has approved only a few of these agents, including interferon alpha, trastuzumab (Herceptin), granulocyte colony-stimulating factors, granulocyte macrophage-stimulating factors, erythropoietin (Epogen), and oprelvekin (Neumega) (Kee and Hayes, 2003).

The side effects produced by biologic response–modifying drugs are due to the body's inflammatory and immune response to the agents and therefore are somewhat different

---

Box 27-12 Safety Guidelines for Handling Chemotherapy Drugs

■ Prepare drugs in a restricted, preferably centralized, area within a biologic safety cabinet.

■ Post signs in this area restricting eating, grooming, and application of makeup.

■ Label prepared drugs in accordance with standard pharmacy labeling practices and use a distinctive warning label.

■ Make sure that spill kits, emergency skin and eye decontamination kits, and material safety data sheets for the drugs are kept in nursing stations where these drugs are administered.

■ Wear gowns, gloves, and goggles when preparing and administering drugs. (The Occupational Safety and Health Administration *recommends double gloving with latex gloves. The American Nurses Association recommends use of other synthetic gloves to decrease latex exposure.*) Pull gloves over the gown cuff and avoid contamination while removing them. Wash hands immediately afterward.

■ Do not completely fill prefilled syringes.

■ Prime intravenous tubing with non–drug-containing solution.

■ Use Luer-Lok fittings at connector sites to prevent leakage and place a plastic-backed absorbent pad under the tubing to catch any leakage.

■ Discard all unused drugs and contaminated waste in designated chemotherapy waste containers.

■ Place linens in labeled bags to alert laundry personnel.

Adapted from Worthington K: Chemotherapy on the unit. Protecting the provider as well as the patient, Am J Nurs 100(4):88, 2000.

Box 27-13 Management of Chemotherapy at Home

■ Have a spill kit available in the home.

■ Put all hazardous waste materials in leak-proof bags that can be sealed.

■ Use puncture-proof containers for needles and breakable items.

■ Place containers in an area away from the kitchen and where children and pets cannot get to them.

■ Make arrangements for proper disposal of waste.

■ Launder clothing or linen soiled with chemotherapy solutions or waste products immediately. Wear gloves to handle linens and do not launder with other clothes.

■ The person receiving chemotherapy should flush the toilet twice after use.

■ If urine or stool gets on the skin, the area should be cleansed immediately.

■ Wash hands after handling any chemotherapeutic product or waste.

Adapted from Brown K et al: Chemotherapy and biotherapy: guidelines and recommendations for practice, Pittsburgh, 2000, Oncology Nursing Society.

---

from those caused by traditional chemotherapeutic drugs. These side effects include flulike symptoms, central nervous system disturbances, orthostatic hypotension, and tachycardia. Patients are usually medicated with acetaminophen (Tylenol) before treatment and every 4 hours thereafter to prevent or reduce the severity of flulike symptoms. The four types of biologic response–modifying drugs approved by the Food and Drug Administration, along with their common side effects, are listed in Table 27-5.

Drug Therapy

Aside from the drugs used to treat the cancer itself, a number of other drugs are administered to manage symptoms resulting from both the disease process and the methods used to treat it. Table 27-6 lists classes of drugs employed to treat the most common symptoms encountered.

Nurses

Nurses assist the patient and family with all aspects of care coordination. A variety of care providers will enter and exit the patient's life as the cancer evolves and treatment modalities shift. Nursing presence is the constant in the experience of the patient and family. Nurses establish trusting relationships with the patient and family through open, honest communication. These relationships allow nurses to provide information and education as well as spiritual, physical, and emotional support and advocacy. Nurses conduct thorough assessments to make appropriate referrals and manage symptoms to the patient and family's satisfaction. Nurses help the family address end-of-life care issues such as the drafting of an advanced directive and are generally at the

Table 27-5 Biologic Response–Modifying Agents

Agent	Indication	Side Effect
Interferons		
Alpha and beta	Hairy cell leukemia Kaposi's sarcoma Chronic myelogenous leukemia	Fever, chills, malaise, fatigue Confusion, seizures, altered memory and concentration Proteinuria Nausea and vomiting, anorexia Leukopenia, anemia, thrombocytopenia Hypotension, tachycardia Alopecia, rash Photophobia, impotence
Interleukins		
Interleukin 2 (Proleukin)	Renal cell carcinoma	Fever, chills, malaise, fatigue, myalgia Confusion, seizures, altered memory and concentration, anxiety, agitation Oliguria, anuria, azotemia, hepatomegaly Lymphopenia, anemia, thrombocytopenia Hypotension, tachycardia, pulmonary edema, capillary leak syndrome Diffuse pruritic rash Decreased libido Arthralgia
Hematopoietic Growth Factors		
Sargramostim (Leukine)	Chemotherapy-induced leukopenia	Fever, chills, malaise, fatigue, headache, leukocytosis, dyspnea, rash, bone pain
Filgrastim (Neupogen)	Chemotherapy-induced neutropenia	Fever, chills, myalgia, headache, rash, bone pain
Epoetin alfa (Epogen)	Chemotherapy-induced anemia, fatigue, and renal failure	Hypertension (rare)
Oprelvekin (Neumega)	Chemotherapy-induced thrombocytopenia	Fluid retention, rash, blurred vision, exertional dyspnea, arrhythmias
Monoclonal Antibodies		
Trastuzumab (Herceptin)	Breast cancer	Fever, chills, malaise, fatigue, myalgia

bedside when death is imminent. This therapeutic presence is "an active intervention that can alleviate feelings of isolation and abandonment and sustain patients" at difficult moments (Scanlon, 2003, p. 50).

One aspect of cancer that is of particular concern to the individual and his or her family is pain management. Pain management at the end of life is considered later in this chapter. In all cases, the nurse must remember that pain is "whatever the patient says it is, experienced whenever the patient says he or she is experiencing it" (McCaffrey and Paseo, 1999). The patient who has physical reasons for discomfort but is unable to communicate the pain should be considered to have pain until proven otherwise. In this instance, it is also permissible to accept reports of friends or family members if they think the individual is experiencing pain.

Opioid therapy provides adequate pain relief for more than 75% of cancer patients and is therefore the first line of therapy (Lesage and Portenoy, 2002). Careful assessment of the patient's response to the drug and the amount of pain relief achieved is the hallmark of good pain management. The goal is to achieve a balance between analgesia and side effects, and therefore dosing is highly individualized. Medications for pain should be given on a fixed schedule around the clock, with "rescue" medications administered as needed. Other drugs may be given as adjuvant therapy depending on whether the pain is somatic, neuropathic, or psychogenic. Nonpharmacologic approaches such as positioning, diversion or distraction, comfort measures, therapeutic listening, spiritual support, relaxation techniques, music therapy, and therapeutic presencing may also be used. Alternative treatments such as meditation, therapeutic touch, and reiki may also be beneficial.

Table 27-6 Drugs Used to Manage Symptoms

Drug Classification	Hypersensitivity	Anxiety	Cough	Constipation	Depression	Diarrhea	Dyspnea	Fatigue	Nausea/Vomiting	Pain	Example
Antibiotics						X					Metronidazole (Flagyl)
											Penicillin
Anticholinergics			X				X				Atropine, hyoscine
Anticonvulsants		X									Clonazepam (Klonopin), midazolam (Versed)
										X	Carbamazepine (Tegretol)
										X	Gabapentin (Neurontin)
Antidepressants		X			X			X			Paroxetine (Paxil)
		X			X			X		X	Amitriptyline (Elavil)
Antihistamines	X	X							X		Diphenhydramine (Benadryl)
Anxiolytics		X			X		X				Buspirone (BuSpar)
Benzodiazepines		X					X		X		Lorazepam (Ativan)
Biologic response modifiers								X			Epoetin alfa (Epogen)
Bronchodilators							X				Albuterol (Proventil)
											Terbutaline (Brethine)
	X		X								Aminophylline (Theo-Dur)
Central nervous system depressants									X		Trimethobenzamide (Tigan)
Cough suppressants			X								Benzonatate (Tessalon Perles)
Diuretics							X				Furosemide (Lasix)
Expectorants			X								Guaifenesin (Robitussin)
Laxatives											
Bulk agents				X		X					Psyllium
Lubricants				X							Mineral oil
Softeners				X							Docusate (Colace), casanthranol with docusate (Peri-Colace)
Magnesium salts				X							Milk of Magnesia
Neuroleptics		X					X				Haloperidol (Haldol)
Opioids										X	Morphine
										X	Fentanyl (Duragesic)
										X	Codeine
										X	Methadone (Dolophine)
										X	Oxycodone (OxyContin)
										X	Hydromorphone (Dilaudid)

	Medications						
Osmotics	Sorbitol, lactulose					X	
Phenothiazines	Prochlorperazine (Compazine), chlorpromazine	X		X		X	
Serotonin antagonists	Ondansetron (Zofran), granisetron (Kytril)			X		X	
Somatostatins	Octreotide (Sandostatin)			X		X	
Steroids	Dexamethasone (Decadron)	X	X	X	X	X	X
	Methylprednisolone (Solu-Medrol), hydrocortisone (Solu-Cortef)			X			
Stimulants	Senna (Senokot)					X	
	Methylphenidate (Ritalin)	X			X		

In addition to dealing with the pain and fear caused by the disease process, nurses intervene to prevent and/or manage any complications associated with treatment. Studies have shown that effectively managing symptoms affects not only the individual's functional ability but also his or her will to live (Urie et al, 2000). Interventions related to treatment complications are described in Box 27-14.

One of the most serious complications that must be addressed is hypersensitivity. Hypersensitivity reactions vary from mild flare reactions at the site of drug administration

---

Box 27-14   Nursing Interventions for Treatment Complications

MUCOSITIS
- Encourage frequent oral hygiene.
- Have patient use toothpaste with sodium bicarbonate to reduce mouth acidity.
- Instruct patient to use soft-bristled narrow toothbrushes.
- Have patient rinse mouth with salt water, salt water and sodium bicarbonate combined, or half-strength hydrogen peroxide.
- Avoid commercial mouthwashes because they contain alcohol, which is drying.
- Provide room humidification.
- Advise patient to use topical anesthetics such as benzocaine or Orabase before eating to control pain.
- Instruct patient to avoid using alcohol and tobacco.
- Give analgesics 1.5 hours before eating.
- Instruct patient to increase oral fluid intake to 3000 ml/day if not contraindicated.
- Note that popsicles and cold fluids may be soothing.
- Assess for signs of infection and/or bleeding.

NAUSEA/VOMITING
- Treat anticipatory nausea and/or vomiting with distraction, relaxation techniques, and alternative therapies such as acupuncture.
- Serve meals at room temperature with clear fluids.
- Control unpleasant smells.
- Encourage patient to eat slowly and avoid large, high-bulk meals.
- Administer antiemetics as ordered.
- During chemotherapy give antiemetics before starting treatment.
- Assess effectiveness of antiemetic therapy.
- Encourage fluid intake.
- Monitor electrolyte levels.

BONE MARROW SUPPRESSION
Infection
- Monitor white cell counts.
- Maintain asepsis at all times.
- Teach patient to limit contact with individuals who have communicable illnesses.
- Encourage adequate fluid and nutritional intake.
- Keep fresh flowers and plants out of the patient's immediate environment if necessary.
- Inspect skin and mucous membranes frequently.
- Teach patient and family about signs of infection and actions to be taken.

Bleeding
- Monitor closely for hemorrhage.
- Monitor hemoglobin, hematocrit levels.

- Encourage consumption of foods high in vitamin K.
- Use protective measures to prevent trauma.
- Avoid intramuscular injections if possible.
- Monitor for occult as well as frank bleeding.
- Instruct patient and family about signs of bleeding and actions to take if it occurs.

XEROSTOMIA
- Encourage use of gravies and sauces on foods.
- Have patient use artificial saliva or oral lubricants.
- Consider the use of oral pilocarpine.
- Instruct patient to place oil or small pat of butter in mouth to provide comfort.
- Spray mouth with a fine mist of water.
- Keep patient's lips moist and lubricated.
- Note that sucking on sugarless candy or chewing sugarless gum sometimes stimulates saliva production.

ANOREXIA
- Offer small, frequent meals to increase oral intake.
- Give small portions on large plates so patient is not overwhelmed by portion sizes.
- Provide meals at times when symptoms are reduced.
- Maintain relaxed atmosphere.
- Encourage participation in family meals.
- Provide food with high nutritional value, particularly proteins.
- Consider administration of low-dose steroid medications to increase appetite (megestrol [Megace]) and prevent early satiety (metoclopramide [Reglan]).

FATIGUE
- Determine patient's and/or families' perceptions about causes of fatigue.
- Encourage verbalization of feelings about impact of fatigue on quality of life.
- Monitor nutritional intake.
- Monitor sleep-rest and activity pattern.
- Encourage exercise within patient tolerance.
- Monitor oxygen response to activity.
- Instruct patient and family to recognize signs of fatigue and adjust activity accordingly.
- Prepare patient and family for fatigue associated with radiation therapy and reassure that improvement generally occurs in the months following treatment.
- Provide or help patient plan for rest periods throughout day.
- Assist patient in identifying tasks that family and friends can perform in the home to prevent or relieve fatigue.

Modified from McCloskey JC, Bulechek GM, editors: *Nursing interventions classification (NIC),* ed 3, St Louis, 2000, Mosby.

to vascular collapse and death. Hypersensitivity reactions can be triggered by the medication, the diluent, or the base in which the medication is delivered. Reactions are more likely to occur with each subsequent treatment. Drugs associated with increased risk for hypersensitivity reactions are paclitaxel (Taxol), L-asparaginase (Elspar), and murine monoclonal antibodies (Brown et al, 2000). Other factors that place the patient at increased risk are a history of allergies and previous exposure to metals. Steps to take to prevent hypersensitivity reactions are listed in Box 27-15. If chemotherapy is given at home, the nurse should ensure that emergency medications are available. These include epinephrine, diphenhydramine (Benadryl), methylprednisolone (Solu-Medrol), aminophylline, dopamine, and dexamethasone (Decadron).

In addition to caring for the individual with cancer, the nurse must support the family. According to Yates (1999, p. 65), this support must be "based on processes that can assist families to find meaning in what will be extraordinarily devastating circumstances." Ways in which the nurse can be of benefit include communicating effectively by suggesting rather than telling so as to "co-create" solutions and enhance family self-esteem, mediating conflict, and assisting families to access support services to manage disruptions and sources of stress.

Dietitian

The dietitian assesses the nutritional needs of the patient and develops a diet prescription to meet those needs. Weight loss due to anorexia and cachexia is common among cancer patients. Continued weight loss contributes to fatigue and muscle wasting, which in turn interfere with mobility and recovery. The dietitian works with the patient and family to select foods that are nutritionally dense, palatable, and pleasing to the patient. The dietitian can also offer advice regarding supplements and foods that can help control side effects such as constipation or diarrhea. Although the use of enteral or parenteral nutrition has not been shown to reduce weight loss or increase survival rates (Urie et al, 2000),

---

Box 27-15   Prevention of Hypersensitivity Reactions

- Assess the patient for risk factors.
- Obtain vital signs.
- Give antihistamine or steroid medications as ordered.
- Make sure emergency equipment and medication are available.
- Perform a scratch test if this is the first dose or the patient is known to have adverse reactions.
- Infuse the drug slowly, observing for hives, itching, shortness of breath, and agitation.
- Stay with the patient for the first 15 minutes.
- If a localized reaction occurs, monitor vital signs every 15 minutes.
- If anaphylaxis occurs, stop infusion, maintain airway, and send for help.

---

these methods are appropriate for patients with dysphagia, and the dietitian discusses the feedings and fluids to be administered with other members of the health care team as well as with the patient and family.

Physical Therapist

The physical therapist works with the patient and family to help the patient improve, maintain, and recover functional mobility. The exact treatments and exercises prescribed vary with the part of the body affected. For example, the exercises prescribed after mastectomy are designed to reduce lymphedema and prevent contractures. These exercises include performing active range-of-motion movements with the arm on the affected side, slowly moving the hands up the wall until they are higher than the patient's head, and so on. When lower limbs are affected, the therapist may prescribe orthotics to reduce limb pain, work on gait or balance, teach ambulation with a prosthesis, and strengthen muscle groups for walking with assistive devices such as crutches and walkers.

Occupational Therapist

The occupational therapist works with the patient to reduce fatigue and manage the environment. Working with the patient and family, the occupational therapist assesses the living environment and suggests strategies for maximizing independence while minimizing exertion. When dyspnea is a major symptom, the therapist may make focused respiratory assessments, measuring oxygen saturation levels as the patient performs a number of basic activities. The occupational therapist may recommend ways to group activities to prevent exertional dyspnea as well as the use of supplemental oxygen. The occupational therapist can also assist the patient and family in obtaining adaptive equipment that allows the patient to be independent in feeding and dressing.

Medical Social Worker

The medical social worker informs the patient and family of federal, state, and community resources that can help them and very often serves as liaison between the family and the agencies supplying this assistance. Placement in a long-term or hospice care facility, in particular, is negotiated with the help of the medical social worker. The medical social worker also helps the family understand what insurance benefits are available and how to apply for government assistance programs. The social worker is very familiar with the type and quality of resources provided by the community, such as Meals on Wheels, respite care, and support groups, of which the patient and family may not be aware.

CULTURAL CONSIDERATIONS

The signs and symptoms described are experienced by individuals regardless of cultural or ethnic background, gender, or spiritual beliefs. However, each of these variables affects how those symptoms are interpreted and managed. Definitions of health and illness, attitudes toward cancer, adherence to treatment regimens, and coping strategies are all culturally bound (Navon, 1999).

It is essential for health care providers to be aware of other cultural beliefs. It is equally important for them to be aware of their own cultural biases to work effectively with people whose cultural perspectives are markedly different. A patient may be viewed as being nonadherent to the therapeutic regimen when in fact that person is being adherent to practices dictated by his or her cultural values. These values are neither right nor wrong. They are simply different. The issue of informed decision making provides an example of such difference. The values that underpin Western medicine and, consequently, beliefs about informed consent and decision making are the importance of autonomy, the sanctity of life, and the obligation to provide relief from suffering (Kagawa-Singer, 1998). Many non-Western cultures have opposing beliefs that value family decision making and view suffering as a valuable or even necessary experience (Mazanec and Tyler, 2003). In addition, many cultures believe that revealing a diagnosis of cancer or informing a person that he or she has a poor prognosis robs that person of hope and is at best tactless and possibly even cruel (Navon, 1999). Such a belief may be at odds with the provider's belief that the patient has a right to know his or her prognosis so that informed deci-

sions can be made. Decision making itself is culturally bound (Mazanec and Tyler, 2003), and providers are often uncomfortable to learn that the patient may not be the one who decides which treatment options are followed. Judgments must not be made about which perspective is right because such judgments interfere with therapeutic outcomes.

END-OF-LIFE CARE

The goal of end-of-life care is to facilitate a good death, which has been defined as a death "free of avoidable pain and suffering, in accord with the wishes of the patient and family and reasonably consistent with clinical, cultural and ethical standards" (Tolle et al, 2000, p. 310).

Interventions are aimed at managing symptoms, promoting meaningful interactions, maintaining quality of life, and ultimately facilitating a peaceful, dignified death. Providers' views about sustaining life may be different from those of the person being cared for. It is important to ascertain how the individual and family want to manage end-of-life care so that these desires can be honored and supported. The Patient Self-Determination Act, passed in 1990, requires all health care facilities that receive federal money to follow a patient's advance directive (Box 27-16). Yet research studies

---

Box 27-16   Concepts and Terminology Related to End-of-Life Decisions

LEGISLATION

Patient Self-Determination Act (1990)

■ This law requires health care facilities to inform patients in writing about their rights to either accept or refuse treatments before they become incapacitated.*

■ All 50 states and the District of Columbia have laws that comply with this act. Information about individual states can be obtained at the Partnership for Caring website *(http://www.partnership-forcaring.org).*

Uniform Health Decisions Act (1993)

■ This model was developed by uniform law commissioners to streamline state laws regarding advance directives. The model recognizes surrogates as valid decision makers and accepts both oral and written statements of patients as valid.

■ Not all states have adopted laws that support this act.

LEGAL DOCUMENTS

Living Will

■ The patient signs a written document describing the patient's wishes regarding treatment.

■ Usefulness may be limited by lack of specificity.

Durable Power of Attorney

■ The patient designates another individual to represent the patient in decision making.

■ The surrogate must base decisions on the patient's wishes.

ADVANCE DIRECTIVES

Death with Dignity

■ This is a term used in Oregon to describe physician-assisted suicide. Mentally competent residents of the state of Oregon with a terminal illness and less than 6 months to live may request a prescription for a life-ending medication from their physician. The medication must be self-administered. This is legal only in Oregon. Providers should use this term with care so as not to confuse the discussion of promoting a dignified death with this Oregon-specific practice.

Do Not Resuscitate Order

■ Documentation is placed in the medical record that no extraordinary measures are to be taken to sustain life.

■ Legal in all 50 states.

Double Effect

■ The physician orders pain medication in doses that may hasten death. Because the intention is comfort, this is not considered euthanasia.

■ Legal in all 50 states.

Euthanasia

■ Death is caused deliberately.

■ Often thought of as mercy killing.

■ Illegal in the United States.

Box 27-16 Concepts and Terminology Related to End-of-Life Decisions—cont'd

Refusal of Treatment
- Mentally competent adults may refuse life-sustaining treatments.
- Legal in all 50 states.

Terminal Sedation
- Mentally competent adults may consent to sedation to the point of unconsciousness.

- Death is usually the result of lack of hydration and nutrition.
- This is not considered euthanasia.

Withdrawal of Treatment
- Mentally competent adults may stop treatments if a physician agrees that the burdens are greater than the benefits.
- Legal in all 50 states.

---

*NOTE: Capacity and competence are not the same. Competence is decided by the courts. Capacity is a clinical judgment about the patient's ability to comprehend information and to make and communicate decisions. Capacity is assumed until there is evidence to the contrary (Scanlon, 2003).

continue to report that family wishes regarding withholding treatment are not honored and that pain management is inadequate (Tolle et al, 2000).

The Dying Person's Bill of Rights, (Box 27-17) was developed to address these concerns (Ferrell and Coyle, 2002). Providers must remember, however, that "rights" are culturally interpreted, and such documents may be best used

Box 27-17 The Dying Person's Bill of Rights

I have the right to be treated as a living human being until I die.

I have the right to maintain a sense of hopefulness; however, its focus may change.

I have the right to be cared for by those who can maintain a sense of hopefulness; however, its focus may change.

I have the right to express my feelings and emotions about my approaching death in my own way.

I have the right to participate in decisions concerning my care.

I have the right to expect continuing medical and nursing attention even if cure goals must be changed to comfort goals.

I have the right not to die alone.

I have the right to be free from pain.

I have the right to have my questions answered honestly.

I have the right not to be deceived.

I have the right to have help from and for my family in accepting my death.

I have the right to die with peace and dignity.

I have the right to retain my individuality and not to be judged for my decisions, which may be contrary to the beliefs of others.

I have the right to discuss and enlarge my religious and spiritual experiences, regardless of what they may mean to others.

I have the right to expect that the sanctity of the human body will be respected after death.

I have the right to be cared for by caring, sensitive, knowledgeable people who will try to understand my needs and will be able to gain some satisfaction from helping me face my death.

(Lansing, Mich, 1975)

Cited in Ferrell BR, Coyle N: An overview of palliative nursing care, *Am J Nurs* 102(5):26-32, 2002.

to guide discussions with patients and families about end-of-life care. Following the rites and traditions prescribed by an individual's culture or religion provides comfort for the family and facilitates a peaceful coming to terms with the end of life as it is understood and interpreted through those cultural values. Table 27-7 describes some generalized beliefs held by dominant cultural and religious groups in the United States. It is important to remember that individuals may or may not identify with their particular ethnic group or may follow some cultural practices and not others. The health care provider must assess the extent to which the individual identifies with and participates in cultural beliefs and practices.

Families need information about how they can provide support and comfort to their dying family member as well as information about what to expect in terms of the dying process and the decisions that must be made as that process unfolds (Jarr and Pierce, 2001) (Box 27-18). One of the first decisions that must be made and discussed is whether or not family members wish to be present at the time of death (Pitorak, 2003).

Palliative care can be continued or life-sustaining measures can be withdrawn. Some people want to die at home with hospice care; others would like hospice care but prefer that it occur in an institutional setting. Patients and families must understand the implications of these choices.

Individuals who eventually succumb to their cancer experience common end-of life symptoms (Box 27-19). The interdisciplinary care team addresses these symptoms specifically to alleviate patient suffering as understood in the broad sense, which extends beyond physical symptoms and includes the need to find meaning in life (Panke, 2002). Pain, in particular, is a complex phenomenon with physical, psychological, emotional, cultural, and spiritual components, and it both contributes to and is affected by suffering. Managing pain effectively at the end of life is one of the most important interventions that providers offer to patients and families (End-of-Life Nursing Education Consortium, 2002).

End-of-life pain is managed primarily through the use of opioids, although nonsteroidal antiinflammatory drugs may be used as adjuvant analgesics. Medication should be provided

Table 27-7 Cultural Beliefs Related to End-of-Life Care

Ethnic or Religious Group	Role of the Family	Traditions/Beliefs Related to End-of-Life Care
African American	Providers should talk with oldest family member. Strong sense of family loyalty is present. Families care for dying family members at home.	Some believe that dying at home brings bad luck. Distrust of medical system may exist. Hospice care is not used. Strong fears of addiction may interfere with management of end-of-life symptoms. Use of home remedies is common. Strong belief in spiritual life after death is present. Church and church leaders are an important source of support: primary religions are Protestant and Muslim. Organ donation is uncommon.
Chinese American	Family may not want patient to know diagnosis or prognosis. Affection between family members is not publicly displayed.	Saving face is important, so patient may not reveal information felt to be personal. Patient may not complain of pain because this shows disrespect for care provider. Some believe that dying at home brings bad luck, whereas others believe that the spirits of people who die in the hospital may get lost. Use of Chinese medicines and acupuncture is common. Religious practices vary widely. Autopsy and organ donation are uncommon.
Hispanic or Latino American	Family is of major importance and should always be inquired about. Family usually makes decisions. Family may not want patient to know diagnosis. Family members take turns staying around the clock with dying person.	Stoicism is valued. Pregnant women are not allowed to care for the dying. Some believe that dying at home brings bad luck, whereas others believe that spirits of people who die in the hospital may get lost. Folk remedies and the use of medallions are common. Predominant religion is Roman Catholic. Organ donation and autopsy are uncommon.
Native American	Families tend to avoid discussions of death. Families make care decisions. Some tribes believe contact with the dying should be avoided.	Use of traditional medicines is common. Many tribes with many different belief systems are found. Stoicism is common; patient may make vague references to not feeling "good" or "right."
Buddhism	Family may bring in food to support vegetarian diet. Shrine to Buddha may be placed in the room.	Awareness is valued, so pain medication may be refused. Patient may want to see a Buddhist monk. Death is accepted.
Christianity	Prayers are given privately and publicly at the dying person's bedside.	Subgroups and practices vary widely. Catholics anoint the sick and offer last rites that include Confession and Holy Communion. Protestants do not have last rites but some offer sacraments when requested. Jehovah's Witnesses do not accept blood transfusions. Christian Scientists and some charismatic groups believe in faith healing and reject medical care.

Table 27-7   Cultural Beliefs Related to End-of-Life Care—cont'd

Ethnic or Religious Group	Role of the Family	Traditions/Beliefs Related to End-of-Life Care
Hinduism	Priest or family may place sacred threads around the neck or wrist of the dying person, sprinkle the body with holy water, or place a basil leaf on the tongue. Family may bring in food to support vegetarian diet.	Death is accepted. Patient may want to see a Hindu priest. Providers should not remove any threads or wash the body.
Islam	Providers should talk to the second-degree male relatives (uncles or cousins). Families do not like to discuss death. Grief may be expressed by slapping or hitting the body.	Stopping treatment is seen as against Allah's will. Patient may wish to face Mecca (west or southwest in the United States). The head should always be higher than the body. After death, non-Muslims should wear gloves to avoid touching the body.
Judaism	Family may bring in food if patient follows a kosher diet. Family mourns the dead by "sitting Shiva" for 7 days. During this time mirrors are covered and men do not shave.	Everything must be done to prolong life, so terminating life support is not generally an option. The dying should not be left alone. Patient may want to have a rabbi present. After death, body is placed on floor and covered with a sheet. Sabbath is a day of rest and orthodox Jews are forbidden to do any work, including answering the telephone and turning lights and appliances on and off. If person dies at home on the Sabbath, he or she may not be moved until the following day.

Adapted from End-of-Life Nursing Education Consortium: *Continuing education for nurses: special end-of-life issue,* Sacramento, 2002, CME Resource; and Kirkwood NA: *A hospital handbook on multiculturalism and religion,* Australia, 1993, Millennium Books.

Box 27-18   Family Needs at the End of Life

- Open, honest information as early as possible
- Assistance in dealing with grief and regret
- Assistance in dealing with unfinished business such as forgiveness
- Instruction and support in how to talk with and care for their dying family member
- Understanding of the implications of decisions that must be made
- Understanding of the dying process
- Understanding of interventions designed to prolong life versus those that promote comfort
- Understanding of the family's role in providing comfort for the dying family member
- Personalized, rather than routine, care and conversations

Adapted from Jarr S, Pierce S: Nurses speak out to improve end-of-life care, *Adv Nurses,* April 23, 24, 2001.

Box 27-19   End-of-Life Symptoms

- Agitation
- Anorexia
- Anxiety
- Ascites
- Cachexia
- Confusion
- Cough
- Delirium
- Depression
- Dyspnea
- Fatigue
- Immobility
- Incontinence
- Mucositis
- Nausea and/or vomiting
- Weakness

Box 27-20   Barriers to Optimal End-of-Life Care

- Influence of managed care on end-of-life care
- Focus on acute care interventions
- Lack of continuity across settings
- Family members' avoidance of death
- Health care professionals' personal discomfort with death
- Lack of knowledge of health care providers
- Patients' and/or families' fears of addiction to pain-killing drugs
- Increased use of unlicensed assistive personnel in the care of the dying
- Legal restrictions placed on providers regarding prescription pain medication
- Cultural differences between provider and patient
- Avoidance of dying patients by health care providers
- Patients' avoidance or denial of death

---

around the clock via a sustained-release formulation. Immediate-release medication should also be available for any breakthrough pain that occurs. The amount of immediate-release medication administered is based on the amount of sustained-release medication given in 24 hours (usually 10% to 20% of the total dose). The breakthrough dose can be given every 1 to 2 hours as needed (End-of-Life Nursing Education Consortium, 2002). Pain levels may change as the individual moves through the dying process. Therefore, pain levels and the adequacy of pain relief measures must be continually reassessed. When medication begins to lose its effectiveness, dosages are increased or a different opioid drug is chosen. Medication is generally given orally but may be administered via other routes if necessary. Providers should check the equianalgesic dose for the particular medication being given to ensure that no decrease in effectiveness will occur with the switch to parenteral administration. As consciousness declines, nonverbal cues may indicate that pain is not being relieved. However, other sources of discomfort should be considered before medication dosages are increased. Even with aggressive pain management, end-of-life pain may not respond to opioid therapy. In these instances sedation should be considered (Wein, 2000).

Providers frequently report difficulty in rendering end-of-life care. Box 27-20 lists some barriers to end-of-life care that nurses encounter. Organizations established to improve provider care include the End-of-Life Nursing Education Consortium and the EPEC Project (Education on Palliative and End-of-Life Care).

Palliative Care

Palliative care is the active total care of patients whose disease is not responsive to curative therapy (World Health Organization, 1990). Unlike patients receiving hospice care, individuals receiving palliative care may not be facing imminent death. Thus, although the focus of palliative care is not on cure but on quality of life, palliation can occur concurrently with curative interventions (Farquhar et al, 2002) and should not be viewed as an isolated service offered only at life's end (Sheehan and Twaddle, 2002).

Hospice Care

Hospice care is a form of palliative care reserved for the last few months of life. The first hospice in America was established in Branford, Connecticut, in 1981 to provide home care for the terminally ill and their families. Over the past two decades, hospice care has grown to the extent that there are now over 2300 Medicare-certified hospices serving more than half a million people. In 2000, 60% of Medicare recipients who died of cancer received hospice care (Neigh, 2002).

Providers support both the individual who is dying and the family during the last days of illness. Families may ask questions about the physical and mental changes they are witnessing and may be concerned about pain or other discomfort. Providers should answer questions honestly while reassuring families that every effort is being made to keep their loved one comfortable.

Family members should be encouraged to speak with the dying person. Dying patients often communicate in ways that are symbolic and therefore seem confusing or nonsensical, and as a result are not attended to. It is important to respond to these statements and to help families understand that these communications are important, because they may be expressions of what the person is experiencing or needs (Pitorek, 2003). Families also should be aware that simply "being with" the dying person has as much significance as "doing for" the person.

When death occurs, providers should allow family members sufficient time to say goodbye to their loved one. Postmortem activities can wait until the family has gone. It is important that the providers present express sympathy or condolences to the family and respect their religious and cultural beliefs regarding handling the body. Families may ask the provider to join them in a moment of silence or prayer. Providers often feel awkward or uncomfortable at this time and are uncertain as to how to respond. Therapeutic presence and simple statements such as "I am sorry for your loss" convey compassion and caring (End-of-Life Nursing Education Consortium, 2002).

Ethical Concerns

A number of ethical issues have been discussed in this chapter (capacity, advance directives, respect for autonomy, disclosure of illness and prognosis information, etc.). Additional concerns include maintaining confidentiality and assisting patients and families to make decisions regarding resuscitation, use of life-sustaining treatments, and withdrawal of treatments (including intravenous lines and feeding tubes).

Internet and Other Resources

American Cancer Society: *http://www.cancer.org*

American Hospice Foundation: *http://www.americanhospice.org*

American Pain Foundation: *http://ampainsoc.org*

American Society of Pain Management Nurses: *http://www.aspmn.org*

City of Hope Pain/Palliative Care Resource Center: *http://www.cityofhope.org*

EPEC Project: Education on Palliative and End-of-Life Care: *http://www.epec.net*

GriefNet: *http://www.griefnet.org*

Last Acts: *http://lastacts.org*

National Cancer Institute: *http://www.nci.nih.gov*

Oncology Nursing Society: *http://www.ons.org*

Partnership for Caring: *http:/www.partnershipforcaring.org*

Robert Wood Johnson Foundation: *http://www.rwjf.org*

REFERENCES

American Cancer Society: Facts and figures 2003, retrieved from *http://www.cancer.org/docroot/STT/stt_0_2003.asp?sitearea=STT&level=1* on Feb 28, 2004

Brown JK: A systematic review of the evidence on symptom management of cancer-related anorexia and cachexia, *Oncol Nurs Forum* 29:517-30, 2002.

Brown K et al: *Chemotherapy and biotherapy: guidelines and recommendations for practice,* Pittsburgh, 2000, Oncology Nursing Society.

Dimeo F: Radiotherapy-related fatigue and exercise for cancer patients: a review of the literature and suggestions for further research. In Dörr W, Engenhart-Cabillic R, Zimmermann JS, editors: *Normal tissue reactions in radiotherapy and oncology,* New York, 2002, Karger, pp 49-56.

End-of-Life Nursing Education Consortium: Continuing education for nurses: special end-of-life issue, Sacramento, 2002, CME Resource.

Farquhar M et al: Defining patients as palliative: hospital doctors' versus general practitioners' perceptions, *Palliat Med* 16:247-50, 2002.

Ferrell BR, Coyle N: An overview of palliative nursing care, *Am J Nurs* 102(5):26-32, 2002.

Holland J: External beam radiation therapy, *Adv Nurses,* July 17-19, 2002.

Jarr S, Pierce S: Nurses speak out to improve end-of-life care, *Adv Nurses,* April 23-24, 2001.

Kagawa-Singer M: The cultural context of death rituals and mourning practices, *Oncol Nurs Forum* 55(10):1752-6, 1998.

Kee J, Hayes E: *Pharmacology: a nursing process approach,* ed 4, Philadelphia, 2003, WB Saunders.

Leigh SA: The long term cancer survivor: a challenge for nurse practitioners, *Nurse Pract Forum* 9(3):192-6, 1998.

Lesage P, Portenoy R: Trends in cancer pain management, *Cancer Control J* 6(2), 1999, retrieved from *http://www.moffitt.usf.edu/pubs/ccj/v6n2/article2.htm* on Dec 12, 2002.

Mazanec P, Tyler MK: Cultural considerations in end-of-life care, *Am J Nurs* 103(3):50-7, 2003.

McCaffrey M, Paseo S: Practical approaches to pain. In McCaffrey M, Paseo S, editors: *Pain: clinical manual,* ed 2, St Louis, 1999, Mosby, pp 399-427.

Navon L: Cultural views of cancer around the world, *Cancer Nurs* 22(1):39-45, 1999.

Neigh J: Hospices creatively expanding, *Caring* 21(10):5, 2002.

Panke J: Difficulties in managing pain at the end of life, *Am J Nurs* 10(7):26-35, 2002.

Pitorak E: Care at the time of death, *Am J Nurs* 10(7):42-52, 2003.

Porth C: *Pathophysiology: concepts of altered health states,* ed 6, Philadelphia, 2002, JB Lippincott.

Scanlon C: Ethical concerns in end-of life-care: when questions about advance directives and the withdrawal of life sustaining interventions arise, how should decisions be made? *Am J Nurs* 103(1):48-55, 2003.

Sheehan M, Twaddle M: Palliative care, *Caring* 2(10):10-11, 2002.

Tolle S et al: Family reports of barriers to optimal care of the dying, *Nurs Res* 49(6):310-7, 2000.

Urie J et al: Palliative care, *Pharm J* 265(7119):603-14, 2000.

Wasteson E et al: Daily assessment of coping in patients with gastrointestinal cancer, *Psychooncology* 11(1):1-11, 2002.

Wein S: Sedation in the imminently dying patient, *Oncology* 14(4):585-92, 2000.

World Health Organization: Cancer pain relief and palliative care, Technical Report Series 804, Geneva, 1990, The Organization.

Yates N: Family coping: issues and challenges, *Cancer Nurs* 22(1):63-71, 1999.

CHAPTER 28

Cancers of the Central Nervous System

Leslie Jean Neal, PhD, RN, FNP-C, and Julie Ries, MA, PT, GCS

OBJECTIVES

After reading this chapter, you should be able to do the following:

- Describe the pathophysiology of primary brain cancers and cancer of the spinal cord
- Describe the clinical manifestations of cancers of the brain and spinal cord
- Describe the functional health patterns affected by cancers of the brain and spinal cord
- Describe the role of each member of the interdisciplinary team involved in the care of persons with brain or spinal cord cancer
- Describe indications for use, side effects, and nursing considerations related to drugs used to treat brain or spinal cord cancer

Each year approximately 18,000 people in the United States are found to have primary malignant tumors of the central nervous system (CNS). Approximately 13,300 deaths, or 5 per 100,000 persons, occur annually. Tumors of glial cells (which provide protection, support, and nourishment to neurons [Ozuna, 2000]) comprise the majority of primary tumors of the CNS (50% to 60%), about 25% of primary tumors are meningiomas, and schwannomas account for 10%. Metastasis to the brain or spinal cord is more likely than development of a primary CNS malignancy (Sager and Israel, 2002).

In adults, spinal cord tumors comprise approximately 0.5% of all tumors and 10% to 15% of primary tumors of the CNS. Tumors of the thoracic spinal cord are most common, followed by cervical tumors and then lumbosacral tumors. Tumors of the spinal cord generally occur between the ages of 20 and 60 years, and males and females are affected equally (Shpritz, 2002).

ASSESSMENT

It is vital that the interdisciplinary team member conduct a thorough neurologic examination of all patients suspected of neurologic impairment. The literature is replete with descriptions of and tips for performing a neurologic assess-

ment. One example of a mnemonic that may be used to ensure that all of the elements required for a comprehensive assessment are evaluated is "Is Anybody Home?" (see Box 24-2).

Persons with cancer of the CNS are likely to be functionally impaired in almost every aspect of daily living depending on how advanced the cancer is and where it is located. Persons with brain cancer are likely to experience deficits that relate to the area of the brain affected by the malignancy. Persons with cancer of the spinal cord may be disabled by pain and limited range of motion or may be paralyzed. Box 28-1 lists the functional health patterns affected by CNS cancers and provides a framework for their assessment. The Karnofsky Performance Scale, which is often used to evaluate the functional ability of the patient with a CNS malignancy, is found in Box 27-6.

BRAIN TUMORS
Pathophysiology

Uncontrollable growth is one of the hallmarks that differentiate a benign brain tumor from a malignant tumor. Benign tumors may also become malignant as their cell composition changes. Some primary malignant brain tumors are called gliomas and originate in brain tissue. These tend to progress rapidly and generally lead to cerebral edema, increased intracranial pressure, obstruction of the flow of cerebrospinal fluid, deficits in neurologic function, and possibly pituitary dysfunction (Shpritz, 2002).

Primary tumors in adults are generally supratentorial, occurring in the dura within the area of the cerebral hemispheres that supports the occipital lobe. Tumors are typically named according to the cell type from which they originate and whether they originate in neurons or in neuroglial cells (Shpritz, 2002). Astrocytes, oligodendroglial cells, and ependymal cells are neuroglial cells (Shpritz, 2002).

Primary tumors of the brain can arise from any of three locations: the brain itself (astrocytoma [glioblastoma], oligodendroglioma, and ependymoma), the coverings of the brain (pineal or pituitary tumors or meningiomas), and the nerves (schwannomas and acoustic neuromas). Astrocytomas and glioblastomas are the most common primary malignancies of the brain (Turini and Redaelli, 2001) and occur most frequently in individuals in their forties to sixties (Shpritz,

---

Box 28-1   Functional Health Pattern Assessment for Central Nervous System Cancers

HEALTH PERCEPTION/HEALTH MANAGEMENT
- Is there a family history of central nervous system cancer?
- Has the patient been exposed to environmental chemical irritants?
- What is the patient's perception of his or her overall health?
- What medications, including over-the-counter drugs, does the patient take?
- What alternative therapies does the patient use?

NUTRITION/METABOLISM
- Has there been any unexplained recent weight gain or loss?
- Is the patient on any special diet?
- What is the condition of the skin and mucous membranes?
- Has the patient experienced nausea and/or vomiting related to treatment modalities?

ELIMINATION
- Have any changes occurred in bowel or bladder habits related to neurologic deficits?
- What medications or treatments does the patient use to manage these changes?

ACTIVITY/EXERCISE
- Does the patient have difficulty in moving, ambulating, or performing activities of daily living?
- Does the patient experience fatigue or malaise?
- Can the patient participate in instrumental and other activities of daily living?
- Is adaptive or assistive equipment needed?

SLEEP/REST
- How many hours of uninterrupted sleep does the patient get at night?
- Does the patient take naps or rest periods?
- What sleep aids are used?
- How effective are pain medications in allowing the patient to sleep?

COGNITION/PERCEPTION
- What are the nature, character, location, and duration of the pain? What factors alleviate and aggravate the pain?

- What alternative therapies does the patient use to manage the pain?
- Does the patient have paralysis, paresthesias, or depression?
- What changes have occurred that are related to focal neurologic deficits caused by the tumor or to the effects of treatment?

SELF-PERCEPTION/SELF-CONCEPT
- How does the patient describe himself or herself?
- How has the condition affected the patient's self-esteem?
- How has the condition changed the patient's body image?
- How has the condition affected the patient's sense of self?

ROLES/RELATIONSHIPS
- What kind of work does the patient perform?
- What role does the patient play in the home and family?
- What changes have occurred in the patient's ability to carry out role functions?
- How satisfied is the patient with his or her current roles and relationships?
- How has the condition affected the patient and others?

SEXUALITY/REPRODUCTION
- Is the patient sexually active?
- Have changes occurred in sexual activity?
- Is the patient satisfied with current sexual patterns?
- Have changes occurred in the menstrual cycle?

COPING/STRESS TOLERANCE
- What are the patient's coping strategies?
- What support systems are available to the patient?
- Can the patient manage the condition in the current setting?

VALUES/BELIEFS
- What constitutes quality of life for the patient?
- What is important to the patient?
- What are the patient's spiritual beliefs, health beliefs, and cultural beliefs?
- What is the patient's view regarding locus of control?

2002). Meningiomas, schwannomas, and acoustic neuromas tend to be benign. Ependymomas are discussed with spinal cord malignancies.

The cause of primary brain tumors remains uncertain. However, genetic, hereditary, and environmental factors are all strongly suspected to be possible contributors. Genetic abnormalities such as chromosomal aberrations have been linked to brain tumors. The genes that contribute to the development of primary brain malignancies can be categorized as tumor-suppressor genes or proto-oncogenes. DNA is lost on different chromosomes depending on the type of brain tumor involved. Rarely, amplification of specific genes occurs. Genetic aberrations differ for different types of glioma, and the abnormalities tend to accumulate over time.

Heredity may play a role through genetic predisposition or through the exposure of family members to similar causative environmental mechanisms. Certain syndromes characterized by genetic alterations result in the creation of gene products that have been associated with nervous system cancers (Sager and Israel, 2002).

Long-term exposure to several chemical agents is known to be highly correlated with the development of brain tumors. These agents include organic solvents, pesticides, lubricating oils, vinyl chloride, formaldehyde, N-nitroso compounds, polycyclic aromatic hydrocarbons, and phenols. The highest risk, however, appears to be associated with exposure to these agents in utero or in infancy. The mother's prenatal intake of adequate amounts of vitamins A,

C, E, and folic acid has been associated with a 50% reduction in the development of brain tumors in children under 5 years old (Turini and Redaelli, 2001). Exposure to ionizing radiation is the only risk factor for the development of primary malignancy of the brain whose effect has been thoroughly supported by research (Sager and Israel, 2002).

Astrocytomas are the most common primary brain malignancies and are derived from astrocytes located within the cerebral hemispheres. They are categorized by a grading system that was designed by the World Health Organization. Grade I tumors have an excellent prognosis, whereas grade IV tumors are aggressive. Astrocytomas may progress in grade over time. High-grade tumors are associated with a poor prognosis and a median survival time of 12 months among persons living in the United States. Prognosis is related to poor functional status and increased age as well as to less favorable pathology. Low-grade astrocytomas are more commonly seen in children and are not discussed here. In high-grade astrocytomas, neoplastic cells move from the tumor mass and infiltrate adjacent brain tissue. The cells frequently move along white matter pathways. The tumors have no distinct margins and are supratentorial (Sager and Israel, 2002).

Oligodendromas are associated with a longer survival time (10-year survival rate is 25% to 34%), are usually supratentorial (occurring particularly in the frontal lobe), and often contain a mixture of cells that appear astrocytic and oligodendroglial. If the tumor is mixed, it is called a mixed glioma. The more oligodendroglial the tumor appears, the more benign the course is likely to be, because such a tumor is less likely to infiltrate surrounding tissue than is an astrocytoma and is thus easier to resect surgically (Sager and Israel, 2002).

Germinomas are the most common type of germ cell tumor and tend to appear in the second decade of life within or around the third ventricle and the pineal region. They may be benign but are often invasive. Primary CNS cancers also include B-cell neoplasms that exist without evidence of systemic lymphoma. They are most often seen in immunocompromised patients and are associated with an Epstein-Barr virus infection of the neoplastic cells. B-cell neoplasms may arise in the meninges (Figure 28-1) or demonstrate ring enhancement on magnetic resonance imaging (MRI). The disease may extend into the eyes (Sager and Israel, 2002).

Gliomas are graded based on their differentiation from normal cells. Well-differentiated tumors are considered grade I tumors, tumors that are only moderately differentiated are grade II tumors, and poorly differentiated tumors are grades III and IV and carry a poor prognosis. Tumors initially classified as grade I or II may change to become grade III or IV (Shpritz, 2002). A grade III or IV astrocytoma is called glioblastoma multiforme, and life expectancy is less than 1 year even after surgery and radiotherapy (Cruickshank and Wilkinson, 1998; Wallace, 1999).

Clinical Manifestations

Primary malignant tumors of the brain are typically associated with one of three syndromes: "1) subacute progression of a focal neurologic deficit; 2) seizure; or 3) nonfocal neu-

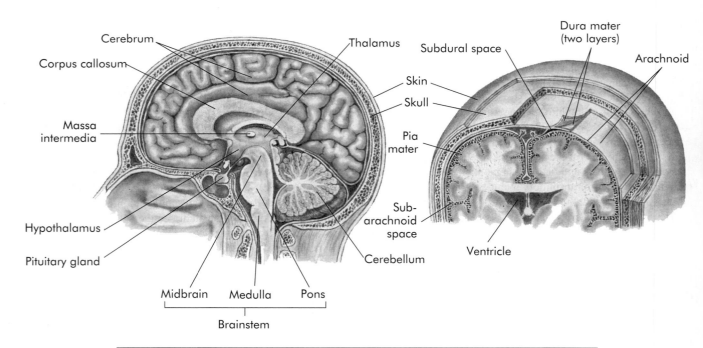

Figure 28-1   Meninges of the brain. (From Thompson JM: *Mosby's clinical nursing,* ed 5, St Louis, 2002, Mosby.)

rologic disorder such as headache, dementia, personality change, or gait disorder. The presence of systemic symptoms such as malaise, weight loss, anorexia, or fever, suggests a metastatic rather than primary brain tumor" (Sager and Israel, 2002, p. 2442).

Cerebral edema occurs with invasion of the tumor and leads to increased intracranial pressure, which ultimately causes compression of brain structures. Focal neurologic deficits occur depending on the area(s) of the brain involved. Compression of the pituitary gland can cause severe fluid and electrolyte imbalances, such as in diabetes insipidus or the syndrome of inappropriate secretion of antidiuretic hormone.

The presentation of a primary brain tumor might mimic the presentation of a cerebrovascular accident. When this occurs, the cause is likely to be hemorrhage and the tumor is probably a high-grade astrocytoma or metastatic melanoma. More commonly, however, the tumor produces a focal deficit as a result of compression of white matter tracts and neurons (Sager and Israel, 2002).

The individual with a primary brain tumor may develop seizure activity and more subtle symptoms such as dementia, depression, or a change in personality. The degree and severity of symptoms depend on the location of the tumor. Nonfocal deficits are typically manifested when there is hydrocephalus, increased intracranial pressure, or metastasis of the tumor into adjacent brain tissue (Sager and Israel, 2002).

Intracranial pressure or displacement or irritation of pain-sensitive brain tissue may cause headaches. A mass is typically manifested by a worsening headache, whereas a headache that results from intracranial pressure usually progresses from a few episodes a day to a continuous headache of varied intensity. The headaches develop rapidly, remain for approximately a half-hour, and then abate quickly. Valsalva's maneuvers such as sneezing may precipitate a headache, or the individual may be awakened from a sound sleep within 2 hours after going to bed. There may be associated vomiting or papilledema (Sager and Israel, 2002). Box 28-2 lists key features of common brain tumors.

Diagnosis

Unlike malignancies that metastasize from elsewhere in the body to the brain, primary brain tumors do not produce abnormalities detectable by serologic testing. Lumbar puncture and analysis of cerebrospinal fluid might indicate elevated protein levels, elevated opening pressure, or mild lymphocytic pleocytosis. Computed tomography and MRI may reveal neoplastic tissue and surrounding edema. Positron emission tomography and single-photon emission tomography can distinguish recurrence of the tumor from necrosis of tissue that can occur following radiation. Finally, electroencephalography can assist assessment of patients with seizures (Sager and Israel, 2002).

> ### Box 28-2   Key Manifestations of Common Brain Tumors
>
> **CEREBRAL TUMORS**
> - Headache (most common feature)
> - Vomiting
> - Changes in visual acuity and visual fields: diplopia (visual changes caused by papilledema)
> - Hemiparesis or hemiplegia
> - Hypokinesia
> - Hyperesthesia, paresthesia, decreased tactile discrimination
> - Seizures
> - Aphasia
> - Changes in personality and/or behavior
>
> **BRAINSTEM TUMORS**
> - Hearing loss (acoustic neuromas)
> - Facial pain and weakness
> - Dysphagia, decreased gag reflex
> - Nystagmus
> - Hoarseness
>
> **CEREBELLAR TUMORS**
> - Ataxia and dysarthria

From Shpritz DW: Interventions for critically ill clients with neurologic problems. In Ignatavicius D, Workman M, editors: *Medical-surgical nursing: critical thinking for collaborative care,* ed 4, Philadelphia, 2002, WB Saunders, p 1001.)

Interdisciplinary Care
Drug Therapy

Treatment of primary brain tumors includes the administration of glucocorticoids (dexamethasone 12 to 20 mg/day in divided doses, orally or intravenously) to reduce edema around the tumor and thereby improve neurologic function. Anticonvulsants are given to treat or to prevent seizures. Phenytoin, valproic acid, or carbamazepine is used. Anticoagulant prophylaxis may be initiated for persons with gliomas to prevent deep vein thrombosis and pulmonary embolism, because this therapy does not appear to increase the risk of intracranial hemorrhage (Sager and Israel, 2002). Table 28-1 lists drugs used for the symptomatic treatment of primary brain cancer along with their indications, side effects, and adverse reactions.

Surgery, Radiation, and Chemotherapy

If the tumor is localized, surgery is the treatment of choice for primary brain tumors. The purpose of surgery is to cure the cancer or, failing that, to remove as much of the tumor as possible. Surgery assists the physician in establishing a diagnosis based on biopsy and allows access for other therapies (Turini and Redaelli, 2001).

Radiotherapy may be given after surgery to kill any remaining cells or tumors, used as a substitute for surgery if

Table 28-1   Drugs Used to Treat Primary Brain Malignancy

Drug	Purpose	Side Effects	Adverse Reactions
Dexamethasone (Decadron)	Antiinflammatory	Insomnia Moon face Abdominal distention Increased sweating	Muscle wasting Osteoporosis Spontaneous fractures
Phenytoin (Dilantin)	Anticonvulsant	Drowsiness Lethargy Confusion	Status epilepticus if drug withdrawn abruptly Blood dyscrasias
Valproic acid (Depakene)	Anticonvulsant	Epilepsy Abdominal pain Irregular menses	Hepatotoxicity Blood dyscrasias
Carbamazepine (Tegretol)	Anticonvulsant	Drowsiness Dizziness Nausea and vomiting	Blood dyscrasias Cardiovascular disturbances Dermatologic effects

the tumor is inoperable or is more likely to respond to radiation than to surgery, or administered to alleviate symptoms and prevent metastasis (Turini and Redaelli, 2001). Studies have shown that a combination of therapies—radiotherapy and stereotactic radiosurgery (one-time high dose of radiation)—yields excellent results (Anonymous, 2001). Box 28-3 lists the various types of chemotherapy that may be used to treat brain tumors. See Chapter 27 for more detailed information on chemotherapy and radiation.

Nurse

The nurse provides pretreatment and preoperative teaching to prepare the patient and family. In addition, the nurse interprets the complex terminology used by other members of the health care team to the patient and family. While providing care, the nurse assesses and monitors the patient,

---

Box 28-3   Chemotherapeutic Methods for Treatment of Brain Tumors

■ Biological response modifiers
■ Blood-brain barrier disruption
■ Bone marrow or stem cell transplantation (after chemotherapy)
■ Combination chemotherapy
■ High-dose chemotherapy
■ Hormone therapies
■ Intracavitary and interstitial therapy
■ Lower-toxicity drugs
■ Drug-impregnated microspheres
■ Receptor-mediated permeabilizers
■ Drug delivery reservoirs

Adapted from Turini M, Redaelli A: Primary brain tumors: a review of research and management, *Int J Clin Pract* 55(7):471-5, 2001.

---

evaluates fluid and electrolyte balances, and uses strategies to detect treatment-related complications early.

The nurse cares for the patient postoperatively by positioning the patient according to orders, monitoring the dressing and laboratory test values, administering medications, and ventilating the patient as necessary. Analgesics may be ordered to prevent and reduce pain and antibiotics may be given prophylactically to prevent infection. The nurse plays a vital role in monitoring the patient to prevent postoperative complications such as increased intracranial pressure, fluid and electrolyte imbalance, wound infection, hematomas, meningitis, and respiratory problems (Shpritz, 2002).

The discharge planner is typically a nurse, who should have particular expertise in the unique requirements of the cancer patient. The discharge planner works to ensure that the home environment or the setting to which the patient will be discharged is appropriate and that there are sufficient resources to support the patient and family. Instruction to the patient and family regarding seizure precautions and treatment may be necessary. Reinforcement of the instructions given to the patient by the dietitian and therapist increases the likelihood that these recommendations will be followed.

The rehabilitation nurse may provide care both in inpatient and outpatient facilities as well as in the home setting. The rehabilitation nurse works with the patient and family to adapt the physical and emotional environment of the home to any lifestyle changes that will have to be made as a result of new disabilities. Also, the rehabilitation nurse works in conjunction with the therapists to prepare the patient to return to the work setting, if possible or to manage new strategies to enhance quality of life.

The oncology nurse will likely be involved in the patient's care and may provide chemotherapy treatments in the home setting. The nurse may recommend referral to hospice care and may provide that care within or outside the hospital setting. The hospice nurse coordinates a team that provides comfort and palliative measures to the patient and family and assists them in resolving end-of-life issues.

Primary Provider (Physician/Nurse Practitioner)

The primary care physician, nurse practitioner, or physician assistant may diagnose the primary brain tumor but will then work with a neurologist, surgeon, oncologist, and radiologist to design and carry out a plan of treatment. These physicians monitor the progression of the malignancy and manage drug and other therapies as needed.

Physical Therapist

The functional ability of the person with cancer may be limited by the effects of the tumor and of the treatment to eradicate or minimize the tumor. The person with a malignancy of the brain may have pain, nausea, fatigue and alterations in psychosocial function that contribute to disability.

The physical therapist (PT) works with the patient to assist the patient in navigating the environment safely and without undue pain. The PT may recommend a wheelchair, walker, or cane for ambulation and a hospital bed, tub seat, and possibly a Hoyer lift to make the patient more comfortable as mobility becomes more limited. Regardless of the patient's prognosis, the PT works with the patient and family to maximize the patient's involvement in his or her care and participation in activities of daily living (ADL).

Speech Pathologist

The speech pathologist may be called in to assess and treat the person with a brain tumor because the tumor and/or the treatment may alter speech and swallowing functions. A person with a brain tumor may experience speech difficulties similar to those experienced by persons with other types of neurologic deficits, such as stroke. Unlike the person with stroke, the person with a brain tumor is likely to be younger and to experience a gradual onset of speech difficulty. In addition, the deficit itself may change frequently with alterations in the size of the tumor, the treatment, and the side effects of medications (Cruickshank and Wilkinson, 1998). The speech pathologist works with the patient and family to improve the patient's communication skills and to provide adaptive equipment that can assist the patient should assistance with communication be needed. The speech pathologist also works with the patient if the patient experiences difficulty swallowing and may consult with the dietitian regarding foods that are most appropriate.

In addition, memory deficits may occur as a result of brain malignancies. The speech pathologist instructs the patient and family regarding adaptive devices and memory tools that may be of assistance.

Occupational Therapist

The occupational therapist (OT) works with the rest of the interdisciplinary team to assist the patient and family in learning adaptive ways of living to cope with any disability that may result from the tumor or its treatment. The OT specifically works with the patient's upper body to improve hand function and upper body mobility. The OT may recommend assistive devices for use when eating and performing ADL and may recommend computer programs to aid in functional substitution.

Dietitian

The dietitian may recommend particular vitamins and minerals to boost the immune system and to provide a foundation for healing. Calcium and magnesium, glutamine, vitamins E and C, beta-flavonoids, zinc, and beta-carotene might be among those recommended. In addition, sugar is thought by some to suppress the immune system and to feed cancer cells, so its avoidance might be recommended. The dietitian might recommend consumption of fish and flax for their omega-3 fatty acids, and melatonin, whey protein, and alkyl glycerols to maximize the effects of radiation and to protect healthy cells (Wallace, 1999). Vitamin supplements and herbal remedies should be prescribed and used in collaboration with the physician because of possible drug interactions that may adversely affect the patient's treatment.

Medical Social Worker

The medical social worker (MSW) assists the patient and family both within and outside of the inpatient facility. Frequently, the MSW is the discharge planner and works with the team to arrange for appropriate placement of the patient following hospital discharge. The MSW also assists the patient in obtaining necessary services and locating resources to pay for services, food, and medicine. In addition, the MSW may work with the nurse and psychologist or psychiatrist to help the patient and family accept the diagnosis and manage the emotions that may arise as the patient works to accept the prognosis for the disease.

Counselor and Psychotherapist

A person who is newly diagnosed with brain cancer and his or her family may experience fear and uncertainty as they move toward acceptance of the diagnosis and the need for palliative care. A counselor or psychotherapist may assist the other members of the interdisciplinary team in using a family-centered approach to move the patient and family through the stages in a supportive way (Leboeuf, 2000).

Complementary and Alternative Therapies

Some patients opt to try acupuncture and massage in conjunction with traditional medical therapy. A positive attitude and membership in a support group can offer comfort to the person with a brain tumor. Audiotapes for guided visualization or publications about people with cancer can motivate the patient to think of a positive outcome to the disease process. A natural substance called inositol hexaphosphate

Table 28-2   Alternative Therapies for Patients with Brain Cancer

Study	Therapy	Outcome
Sims (1986)	Back massage with rest	Improvement in symptoms or reduction of distress
Ferrell-Torry and Glick (1993)	Massage	Reduced pain perception and anxiety, increased feelings of relaxation
Meek (1993)	Back massage	Improvement in blood pressure and heart rate
Evans (1995)	Aromatherapy	Benefit derived for 80% of the subjects
Kite et al (1998)	Aromatherapy	Reported improvement in depression and anxiety in >50%
Hadfield (2001)	Aromatherapy	Reduction in respiratory rate, heart rate, and systolic and diastolic blood pressure suggesting relaxation

combined with inositol is thought by some people to inhibit tumor growth and stimulate the immune system.

A number of studies have been performed to determine whether alternative therapies help cancer patients. Table 28-2 lists some of these studies and their results.

SPINAL CORD CANCERS
Pathophysiology

Spinal cord cancers are typically extramedullary (intradural or epidural) or intramedullary (Figure 28-2). Extramedullary tumors, those that arise outside the cord but within the dura,

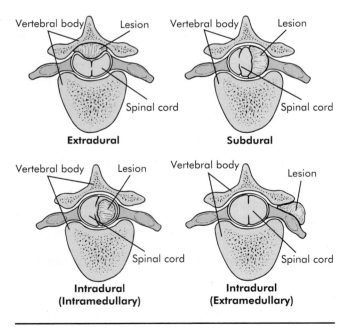

Figure 28-2 Types of spinal cord tumor. (From Lewis SM, Heitkemper MM, Dirksen SR: *Medical-surgical nursing: assessment and management of clinical problems,* ed 6, St Louis, 2004, Mosby.)

comprise the majority of spinal cord tumors. Intramedullary tumors begin in the gray matter of the spinal cord and are typically malignant. Tumors that are epidural or extradural develop between the spinal dura and the vertebrae and ultimately destroy the vertebral bodies. Intradural tumors arise from within the spinal dura (Shpritz, 2002).

Primary spinal tumors usually appear in the glial cells, epidural vessels, or spinal meninges and are of unknown etiology. Most frequently, spinal neoplasms in adults are epidural and are the result of metastasis. Metastases to the vertebrae involve the bone marrow. The likelihood of metastasis of a solid neoplasm to the vertebral column is higher than for some other locations because of the large amount of bone marrow located in the axial skeleton, especially in older persons. Cancers of the breast, prostate, lung, and kidney and lymphoma are the most likely cancers to metastasize to the vertebral column. However, almost any malignancy can spread to the spine. Except in the case of prostate or ovarian cancer, in which metastasis occurs in the lumbar and sacral vertebrae, the thoracic spinal column is most often affected (Hauser, 2002), followed by the lumbar and cervical areas (Shpritz, 2002).

Intradural tumors, the most common of which are meningiomas and neurofibromas, are usually benign and grow slowly. Meningiomas are tumors of the meninges and usually occur near the foramen magnum or behind the thoracic cord. Neurofibromas arise from the nerve sheath near the posterior root. Primary tumors that are intramedullary are unusual and are found in adults as low-grade astrocytomas, hemangioblastomas, or ependymomas. Metastatic intramedullary tumors are very uncommon. In general, the majority of spinal cord tumors are benign. However, the cord compression caused by the tumor contributes to symptoms and disability in patients with both benign and malignant spinal cord tumors.

Clinical Manifestations

Cord compression is responsible for most of the clinical manifestations of spinal cord tumors. Compression may disrupt nerve transmission, the vascular supply, or the flow of cerebrospinal fluid and may result in infarction of the spinal cord (Shpritz, 2002).

Malignancies that cause epidural compression typically produce sensory symptoms, neck or back pain, or alterations in bladder function, and can progress to paralysis. Aching, localized pain or pain that is sharp and radiates is typically the presenting symptom and results from the displacement of structures such as the meninges and periosteum. Movement and actions such as coughing or sneezing may precipitate the pain, which may become worse at night. In rare cases, no pain is present. However, when pain does occur, it usually begins before signs of spinal cord compression appear. Once cord compression develops, pain and the disease progress quickly (Hauser, 2002).

The rate of growth of the cancer determines the rate of cord compression and consequently the progression of neurologic symptoms. Box 28-4 lists common manifestations of spinal cord tumors.

Diagnosis

MRI is ideal for revealing the site and the extent of the malignancy and can often differentiate malignancy from nonmalignancy. It must be emphasized to the radiologist that the MRI is urgent, especially if the patient has signs of cord involvement. Persons with altered sensation or muscle weakness should be imaged on an emergency basis. The entire spine should be visualized because asymptomatic malignancy may be present elsewhere in the spinal cord in patients who have an epidural tumor. A biopsy is not usually performed if the individual has a known history of cancer because the previous cancer is likely to have metastasized to the spine (Hauser, 2002).

Interdisciplinary Care
Drug Therapy

In general, therapy must be initiated early before cord dysfunction is present if it is to be effective. Persons with paralysis must be treated within 48 hours if reversal of symptoms is to be likely. Dexamethasone 40 mg is given daily to reduce edema. Various pain management drugs and modalities are implemented in an effort to keep the patient as comfortable as possible (Hauser, 2002).

Chemotherapy is typically not used to treat primary spinal cord tumors. However, it may be used to control tumors that metastasize to the spinal cord from other areas of the body (Shpritz, 2002).

Anticoagulant therapy may be implemented to prevent deep vein thrombosis or pulmonary emboli, complications of immobility. In addition, stool softeners or antispasmodic medications may be prescribed to prevent constipation and urinary retention, which are associated with neurologic deficits in the bowel and bladder and with immobility.

Box 28-4   Key Manifestations of Spinal Cord Tumors

GENERAL
- Pain
- Sensory loss or impairment
- Motor loss or impairment
- Sphincter disturbance (bladder before bowel)

CERVICAL TUMORS
- High cervical
  Respiratory distress
  Diaphragm paralysis
  Occipital headache
  Quadriparesis
  Stiff neck
  Nystagmus
  Cranial nerve dysfunction
- Low cervical
  Pain in the arms and shoulders
  Weakness
  Paresthesia
  Motor loss
  Horner's syndrome
  Increased reflexes

THORACIC TUMORS
- Sensory loss
- Spastic paralysis
- Positive Babinski's sign
- Bowel and bladder dysfunction
- Pain in the chest and neck
- Muscle atrophy
- Muscle weakness in the legs
- Foot drop

LUMBOSACRAL TUMORS
- Low back pain
- Paresis
- Spastic paralysis
- Sensory loss
- Bladder and bowel dysfunction
- Sexual dysfunction
- Decreased to absent ankle and knee reflexes

From Shpritz DW: Interventions for critically ill clients with neurologic problems. In Ignatavicius D, Workman M, editors: *Medical-surgical nursing: critical thinking for collaborative care,* ed 4, Philadelphia, 2002, WB Saunders, p 943.

Primary Provider (Physician/Nurse Practitioner)

The physician, advanced practice nurse, or physician assistant orders the MRI scan to confirm the diagnosis and initiates a referral to an oncologist and/or neurologist for appropriate drug and radiation therapy. The physician or specialist may consider surgical options if radiation becomes less effective in controlling the signs of cord compression, if the maximum radiation dose has been delivered, or if a vertebral fracture worsens cord compression. Surgery may be aimed at decompression or resection of the vertebral body. Ambulatory patients have the best response to radiotherapy and may recover some motor function. However, persons who have become paraplegic or tetraplegic do not respond to surgery or radiation therapy (Hauser, 2002).

Nurse

The nurse may be the first health care provider to detect that the patient has pain or sensory changes that should be investigated. The nurse may then refer the patient to a neurologist via the primary care practitioner. Nurses provide preoperative, perioperative, and postoperative care to the patient with spinal cord cancer. Monitoring for drainage of cerebrospinal fluid, signs of respiratory compromise, and signs of infection is particularly important postoperatively (Shpritz, 2002).

In addition, the nurse assists the patient and family to manage the effects of radiation, brachytherapy, and drug therapy. (See Chapter 27 for detailed discussions of radiation therapy, brachytherapy, and drug therapy.) Within the inpatient facility, the nurse positions the patient frequently and observes the skin for signs of pressure ulcers. Persons who are immobilized either postoperatively or because of the tumor compression of the spinal cord are at increased risk for pressure ulcers and deep vein thrombosis and, consequently, for pulmonary emboli. The nurse implements preventive measures including good skin care, a turning and positioning schedule, and the placement of sequential compression devices or administration of anticoagulant medication.

The nurse addresses bowel, bladder, and sexuality issues with the patient and may refer the patient to a gastroenterologist, urologist, or sex therapist. The nurse working with the patient in the community setting, either in an extended nursing care facility or at home, teaches the patient to use medications effectively and to try other strategies to increase bowel, bladder, and sexual effectiveness. Box 28-5 lists some of these strategies. Chapter 23 provides a detailed explanation of the teaching provided by the nurse and the rest of the interdisciplinary team to patients with spinal cord damage.

Therapists

The PT and OT work with the individual with a spinal cord tumor using strategies similar to those used with a patient following spinal cord injury. See Chapter 23 for a detailed discussion of the care provided by therapists to the person with injury to the spinal cord.

Box 28-5 Basic Strategies for Management of Bowel, Bladder, and Sexual Dysfunction

BOWEL DYSFUNCTION
- Bowel cleansing before initiation of bowel program
  Manual disimpaction
  Laxatives
  Cleansing enemas (will not work in persons with loss of sphincter function)
- Regulation of timing
  Scheduled time of day for bowel program (usually time of bowel movement before morbidity)
  Consistent time for elimination
- Management of diet and fluid intake
  High-fiber diet
  Increased fluid intake (2-3 qt/day)
- Encouragement of exercise
  Assistance to allow patient to participate in activities of daily living as much as possible
- Provision of privacy
- Proper positioning
  Maintain patient in upright position whenever possible.
  Avoid use of bedpans unless absolutely necessary.
  Use incontinence pad in bed if patient is unable to sit on toilet.

Position the patient on his or her right side if inserting suppository or performing manual disimpaction. This will aid elimination.
Perform abdominal massage from right groin up and across to left groin.
Have patient take slow, deep breaths and contract the abdomen (Valsalva's maneuver)
- Suppositories and medications
- Digital stimulation

BLADDER DYSFUNCTION
- Increase in fluid intake
- Toileting assistance
- Reduction of functional deficits (ability to reach toilet)
- Timed or prompted voiding (voiding at specific intervals)
- Positive reinforcement
- Pelvic muscle rehabilitation
- Vaginal weight training
- Biofeedback
- Electrical stimulation
- Intermittent catheterization
- Indwelling catheter

Box 28-5   Basic Strategies for Management of Bowel, Bladder, and Sexual Dysfunction—cont'd

BLADDER DYSFUNCTION—cont'd
- Medications
  Anticholinergics
  Estrogen replacement
  Antispasmodic agents
  α-Adrenergic agents

SEXUAL DYSFUNCTION
- Education of patient and partner
- Alternative techniques
- Pharmacologic agents

- Penile implants
- Compensation for motor dysfunction
- Compensation for sensory dysfunction
- Pain control
- Continence management
- Medication management
- Consideration of reproductive issues
- Interventions for activity intolerance
- Interventions for body image disturbance and low self-esteem

Adapted from Gender AR: Bowel elimination and regulation. In Hoeman SP, editor: *Rehabilitation nursing,* ed 3, St Louis, 2002, Mosby, pp 422-44; Pires M: Bladder elimination and continence. In Hoeman SP, editor: *Rehabilitation nursing,* ed 3, St Louis, 2002, Mosby, pp 383-421; and Greco SB: Sexuality education and counseling. In Hoeman SP, editor: *Rehabilitation nursing,* ed 3, St Louis, 2002, Mosby, pp 507-41.

Medical Social Worker

The MSW works with the patient and family in much the same way as for the person with brain cancer. The MSW may participate in planning for discharge from the acute care facility and assist in finding an appropriate placement for the patient following discharge. The MSW works with other team members to help the patient and family accept the diagnosis and work through the stages of grief to acceptance. In addition, the MSW garners resources and instructs the patient and family regarding financial and vocational issues that may result from the changes in lifestyle associated with reduced mobility and pain.

Complementary and Alternative Therapies

Persons faced with spinal cord cancer may consider using alternative therapies in conjunction with conventional medicine. Types of therapy from which to choose include the following (Eliopoulos, 1999):
- Mind-body interventions (such as biofeedback, hypnosis, meditation, progressive relaxation, yoga, and guided imagery)
- Nonbiomedical systems of healing (such as acupuncture, homeopathy, and ayurvedic medicine)
- Manual healing methods (such as chiropractic, massage, and therapeutic touch)
- Herbal medicine (internal or external)
- Diet and nutritional therapies

END-OF-LIFE ISSUES

For the person with CNS cancer, acceptance that the condition is likely to be terminal is important for both the patient and family. See Chapter 27 for a detailed discussion of end-of-life issues for persons with cancer.

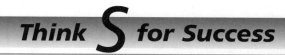
Think S for Success

Symptoms
- Manage pain and changes in neurologic function with symptom-specific strategies.

Sequelae
- Prevent or minimize disability by reinforcing plan designed by rehabilitation nurse, physical and occupational therapists, and speech pathologist.
- Provide palliative care as needed.
- Provide psychosocial support to patient and family and prepare them for hospice care.

Safety
- Teach patient and family about correct use of medications, new ways to design the environment so that patient can navigate it safely, and correct use of adaptive and assistive equipment.

Support/Services
- In conjunction with the medical social worker, assist patient in obtaining needed resources, managing finances and reintegrating into the community.

Satisfaction
- Determine degree to which the condition is interfering with important aspects of patient's life and develop a plan to help patient reach desired quality of life.

FAMILY AND CAREGIVER ISSUES

The person diagnosed with brain or spinal cord cancer is the recipient of devastating news. Although the prognosis may be good depending on the location and extent of the tumor, it is most likely that the patient will face a terminal disease. The family members and caregivers are a vital support system for the patient and for each other. The implementation of treatment may be swift once the diagnosis is made, and events may occur before the patient or those who care for the patient have had a chance to emotionally absorb the news. The family and caregivers will be relied on heavily to assist the patient in dealing with and accepting the diagnosis and in providing emotional support while the patient undergoes treatment for the condition. At the same time, those close to the patient also need assistance in accepting the diagnosis. Changes in neurologic function have a profound effect on the patient as the ability to participate in instrumental and other ADL decreases or otherwise changes. Cognitive deficits such as memory loss may occur. Bowel, bladder, and sexual dysfunction precipitate changes in the lifestyle of the spouse or significant other as well as that of the patient. Caring for the patient at home may be difficult without outside assistance or changes to the home environment.

ETHICAL CONSIDERATIONS

Ethical considerations for persons with CNS cancer are likely to be the same as those for all persons with a life-threatening illness. It is important that the patient have a living will and medical power of attorney specifying his or her wishes regarding end-of-life care and following death. The decision as to whether to accept treatment with its often limited ability to prolong life and the possibility of associated pain and disfigurement or to decline treatment is perhaps the most significant and difficult ethical dilemma in medicine. Frequently, treatment is palliative and may relieve pain and other symptoms to allow the patient better quality of life for a time. The decision to pursue palliative treatment and to forego attempts at cure is a difficult one. Often, patients do not enter hospice care until very limited time is left to provide patients and families with the specialized care and comfort hospice can offer. See Chapter 27 for further discussion of this topic.

CASE STUDY

Patient Data
Ms. B. is a 45-year-old single woman who entered the health care system through the intensive care unit after losing consciousness while out grocery shopping. She fell hard on the floor of the store and hit her head. She was taken by ambulance to the hospital emergency department and then to the intensive care unit. A tumor was discovered during testing. Two days after the admission, Ms. B. underwent brain surgery and most of the tumor was removed.

Ms. B. has no children and no relatives who live in the area. She is involved in her local synagogue and helps out at community charitable events. Most of her friends are from work because she has no time to cultivate friendships outside of work. She works at a women's shelter in the city and lives in an apartment in the same building as the shelter. The rent for the apartment is paid partially by the organization that sponsors the shelter.

Diagnostic Findings
In the emergency department, the computed tomographic scan revealed a hemorrhaging brain tumor the size of a lemon. After surgery, the pathology report revealed that the tumor was a glioblastoma multiforme grade IV.

Thinking It Through
■ What symptoms is Ms. B. likely to have as the remaining tumor continues to grow?
■ What methods will probably be used to treat the tumor?
■ What nursing diagnoses are likely to pertain to Ms. B.?
■ How can the health care team contribute to Ms. B.'s quality of life?
■ What are Ms. B.'s concerns likely to be? How would you address them?

Case Conference
Ms. B. is discharged to her home following recovery from brain surgery. She has experienced speech deficits and right-sided hemiparesis as a result of the surgery. The interdisciplinary team gathers to discuss a plan of care. The team includes the home health registered nurse, the primary care physician (PCP), the oncologist, the dietitian, the MSW, the PT, the OT, and the speech pathologist. Ms. B. and her mother are also in attendance.

The surgeon has reported via telephone that she provided a prescription for narcotic pain medication to Ms. B. and plans to see Ms. B. for follow-up in 2 weeks. The PCP and the oncologist have reviewed Ms. B.'s medical history and data relevant to this recent hospitalization. The oncologist has prescribed chemotherapy, which will begin shortly. Ms. B. has declined radiation treatment because the oncologist has informed her that the rate of success of radiation treatment with this type of tumor is low.

The home health registered nurse will act as case manager while Ms. B. receives home care services. He will coordinate the services of the therapists, the dietitian, and the MSW and will report to the primary care physician, the oncologist, and the surgeon as needed. He has already discussed with Ms. B. the impact of the diagnosis on Ms. B.'s lifestyle and has worked with the MSW to recruit members of Ms. B.'s synagogue to help her at home.

The MSW spoke with Ms. B.'s family in another state and explained the diagnosis at Ms. B.'s request. Ms. B.'s mother has arrived from out of state and is present at the case conference, and she and Ms. B.'s sister plan to stay with Ms. B. alternately to help care for her. The MSW has already visited the patient and her mother in Ms. B.'s home to begin to provide counseling to reduce Ms. B.'s fear of the diagnosis and prognosis. The MSW has previously reported that, as yet, she detects no symptoms of depression in either Ms. B. or her mother or any need for medication to reduce depression or anxiety at this time. Ms. B.'s mother speaks up and states that Ms. B. has had trouble sleeping the last few nights since she has been home from the hospital. The PCP explains that he can give her a prescription for a sleeping pill to aid her sleep, and Ms. B. nods her head to show her agreement.

The dietitian explains to Ms. B. and her mother that she will meet with them to outline a nutritional plan to help maximize Ms. B.'s energy and to facilitate brain tissue healing. The PT explains that Ms. B.'s hemiparesis has made ambulation slow and awkward, and she has suggested the use of a quad cane to Ms. B. and has prescribed some strengthening exercises. The OT is working with Ms. B. to strengthen her upper body and explains that she

CASE STUDY—cont'd

plans to bring some adaptive devices to the home to assist with feeding. The OT and the MSW are working with Ms. B. and her employer to enable Ms. B. to work at home part time using her computer.

The speech pathologist is concerned about Ms. B.'s expressive aphasia and is working with Ms. B. to develop and implement a plan to improve Ms. B.'s speech. The speech pathologist will also help Ms. B. obtain an adaptive device for her telephone to facilitate oral communication.

Individually, the team members express their concern for Ms. B. and her family and explain that they are available to her by telephone at any time to address any questions or concerns she or her family might have. The oncologist reiterates that he wants Ms. B. to be comfortable and to participate in her daily activities as much as she is able and that he will prescribe medication as needed to reduce any side effects from the chemotherapy or pain that she might experience. The PCP explains that he will

remain involved, although the oncologist will manage Ms. B.'s care, and that he will be happy to prescribe antianxiety or antidepressant medications as required or to refer Ms. B. to a psychologist or psychiatrist if the need arises.

After Ms. B. and her mother leave, the team remains briefly to discuss future plans for conferencing, which will take place via telephone calls. Each agrees to reinforce the teaching that will be provided by other team members in their specialty areas.

- What new information was provided that would assist the nurse in developing and revising the plan of care?
- What strengths do the individual team members bring to the team?
- What strengths and/or weaknesses does Ms. B. bring to her plan of care?
- What team members might be added or dropped from the team as time goes on?
- Identify two collaborative problems that the plan of care should address.

Internet and Other Resources

American Spinal Cord Injury Association: telephone 312-908-3425; 250 East Superior Street, Suite 619, Chicago, IL 60611

Brain Research Foundation: telephone 312-782-4311; 208 LaSalle Street, Chicago, IL 60604

Brain Tumor Information Line, National Brain Tumor Foundation: *http://www.braintumor.org;* telephone 510-839-9777 or 800-934-2873; 414 Thirteenth Street, Suite 700, Oakland, CA 94612-2603

Brain Tumor Research Center: telephone 415-476-2805; University of California, San Francisco, San Francisco, CA 94143

Brain Tumor Society: *http://www.tbts.org;* telephone 800-770-8287; 124 Watertown Street, Suite 3-H, Watertown, MA 02472

National Family Brain Tumor Registry, The Johns Hopkins Oncology Center: telephone 301-955-3071; 600 North Wolfe Street, Room 132, Baltimore, MD 21287

Spinal Cord Society: *http://members.aol.com/scsweb/private/scshome.htm;* telephone 218-739-5252; 19051 County Highway 1, Fergus Falls, MN 56537

REFERENCES

Anonymous: Combined modalities aid brain cancer survival, *QI/TQM* 11(12):140-1, 2001.

Cruickshank GS, Wilkinson SC: Speech and language services for patients with malignant brain tumours: a regional survey of providers, *Health Bull* 56(3):659-66, 1998.

Eliopoulos C: *Integrating complementary and alternative therapies,* St Louis, 1999, Mosby.

Evans B: An audit into the effects of AM and the cancer patient in palliative and terminal care, *Complement Ther Med* 3:239-41, 1995.

Ferrell-Torry AT, Glick OJ: The use of therapeutic massage as a nursing intervention to modify anxiety and the perception of cancer pain, *Cancer Nurs* 16(2):93-101, 1993.

Hadfield N: The role of aromatherapy massage in reducing anxiety in patients with malignant brain tumours, *Int J Palliat Nurs* 7(6):279-85, 2001.

Hauser SL: Diseases of the spinal cord. In Braunwald E et al, editors: *Harrison's principles of internal medicine,* ed 15, New York, 2002, McGraw-Hill, pp 2425-34.

Kite M et al: Development of an aromatherapy service at a cancer centre, *Palliat Med* 12:171-80, 1998.

Leboeuf I: Impact of a family-centred approach on a couple living with a brain tumour: a case study, *Axone* 22(1):24-31, 2000 (Tumour Foundation award paper).

Meek SS: Effects of slow back massage on relaxation in hospice clients, *Image J Nurs Sch* 25:17-21, 1993.

Ozuna JM: Neurologic system. In Lewis SM, Heitkemper MM, Dirksen SR, editors: *Medical-surgical nursing,* ed 5, St Louis, 2000, Mosby, pp 1581-607.

Sager SM, Israel MA: Primary and metastatic tumors of the nervous system. In Braunwald E et al, editors: *Harrison's principles of internal medicine,* ed 15, New York, 2002, McGraw-Hill, pp 2442-52.

Shpritz DW: Interventions for critically ill clients with neurologic problems. In Ignatavicius D, Workman M, editors: *Medical-surgical nursing: critical thinking for collaborative care,* ed 4, Philadelphia, 2002, WB Saunders, pp 973-1008.

Turini M, Redaelli A: Primary brain tumours: a review of research and management, *Int J Clin Pract* 55(7):471-5, 2001.

Wallace JM: Battling a brain tumor, *Total Health* 21(3):22-3, 1999.

CHAPTER 29

Cancers of the Head and Neck

Marcia H. Krugler, MSN, APRN, BC, and Deyann D. Davis, MSN, RN

OBJECTIVES

After reading this chapter, you should be able to do the following:

- List the risk factors for head and neck cancer
- Identify the six types of head and neck cancer by anatomic classification
- Describe the clinical manifestation of chronic conditions associated with head and neck malignancies
- Describe nursing interventions for the chronic complications of cancer of the head and neck
- Discuss nursing interventions specific to caring for patients with a laryngectomy
- Describe the role of each member of the interdisciplinary team involved in the care of patients with head and neck cancer
- Discuss the role of the nurse in the interdisciplinary team
- Discuss the use of opioids in the treatment of patients with head and neck cancer

Cancers of the head and neck are a diverse class of debilitating and disfiguring malignancies involving different structures of the head and neck. The high incidence of cancer recurrence and the multiple chronic problems associated with head and neck cancers mandate careful and long-term monitoring for quality health care. These complications and the chronic side effects of treatment require diligent follow-up by an interdisciplinary health care team. This team may include the surgeon, radiation oncologist, medical oncologist, pathologist, prosthodontist, dentist, nurse, registered dietitian, speech therapist, physical therapist, and social worker to achieve optimal management of the disease (National Cancer Institute, 2002).

Head and neck cancers account for 3% of all cancers in the United States and up to 2% of all cancer deaths (Taneja et al, 2002). Approximately 38,000 men and women were projected to develop head and neck cancers in 2002 (National Cancer Institute, 2002). Low-income groups and African Americans have the highest incidence of advanced-stage cancer at the time of diagnosis. For oral and pharyn-geal cancers, incidence is greater and mortality is higher for African Americans than for any other racial group (Hoffman et al, 1998).

The highest incidence of head and neck cancers occurs among those between the ages of 60 and 69 years. Affected males outnumber affected females 1.5:1 (Hoffman et al, 1998). An exception is oral cancer, for which the incidence in men is two to four times higher than in women. More frequent presence of risk factors for oral cancer is considered to be largely responsible for the higher incidence in men. The risk is higher for males than for females across all ethnic groups; therefore, Table 29-1 provides a comparison by race for men only.

The overall 5-year survival rate is 64% for head and neck cancers (Hoffman et al, 1998). Lip cancer has the best survival rate (91.1%), and hypopharyngeal cancer has the worst survival rate (31.4%) (Hoffman et al, 1998). Patients with laryngeal and hypopharyngeal malignancies are more likely to have advanced disease at the time of diagnosis (Carvalho et al, 2002). In general, the more posterior and inferior the tumor site, the worse the outcome for squamous cell carcinoma of the head and neck (Hoffman et al, 1998).

The primary risk factors for head and neck cancers are smoking, chewing smokeless tobacco, and using alcohol. This is particularly true for cancers of the oral cavity, oropharynx, hypopharynx, and larynx. The combination of alcohol consumption and cigarette smoking is an established risk factor. These lifestyle activities interact synergistically to increase risk (National Cancer Institute, 2002; Miller et al, 1996). Approximately 30% of head and neck cancer patients who are unwilling to change smoking behaviors will have recurrent cancer (Otto, 2001).

Tobacco use and/or use of alcohol accounts for over 95% of head and neck cancers (Mood, 1997). The tumor site is related to the placement of tobacco. Cigarette smoking increases the risk of lung and laryngeal cancer, pipe smoking increases the risk of lip and oral cancer, and smokeless tobacco use increases the risk of tumors of the cheek and gums (Feber, 2000). Radiation exposure, exposure to industrial toxins, and viral infections are also implicated in the development of head and neck cancer. The causes of head and neck cancer are outlined in Table 29-2.

Table 29-1 Ethnic Differences in the Incidence of Head and Neck Cancers

Type	Groups with Highest Incidence (Males)
Oral cavity cancer	African Americans
	Whites
	Vietnamese
	Hawaiians
Nasopharynx	Chinese
	Filipinos
	Vietnamese
	African Americans
	Hispanics
	Whites
Laryngeal	African Americans
	Whites
	Hispanics
	Chinese
	Japanese
	Filipino

Adapted from Miller BA et al, editors: Racial/ethnic patterns of cancer in the United States 1988-1992, National Cancer Institute, NIH Pub No. 96-4014, Bethesda, Md, 1996; and National Cancer Institute: Seer program: larynx, 2002, retrieved from *http://www.seer.cancer.gov/publications/ethnicity/larynx.pdf* on Nov 27, 2002.

PATHOPHYSIOLOGY

Cancerous tumors are caused by the unregulated growth of cells that form into a mass of tissue. Masses of cancerous tissue are considered to be malignancies. The majority of head and neck cancers (55.8%) are squamous cell carcinomas (epithelial tumors) that begin in the squamous epithelial cells of the head and neck. Tumors that arise in glandular cells are adenocarcinomas and comprise 19.4% of all tumors. Malignancies of the lymph nodes account for 15.1% of head and neck cancers (Hoffman et al, 1998).

Cancers of the head and neck can spread (metastasize) either from the primary site to adjacent sites via lymphatic drainage to lymph nodes, or to other locations in the body by blood circulation. As a result, malignant lymph nodes are a common occurrence in head and neck cancers.

The presence of distant metastases to other organs in the body is related to the location and number of cancerous nodes involved. The risk of distant metastases is higher for cancerous lymph nodes located in the lower neck (Radiological Society of North America, 2004). Taneja et al (2002) note that although progress has been made in the control of local oropharyngeal tumors, the incidence of distant metastases has unfortunately doubled for this type of cancer.

Cancers of the head and neck are categorized according to the region in which they originate (Figure 29-1) and do not include tumors of the brain, eye, thyroid, scalp, skin, muscle, and bones of the head and neck (National Cancer Institute, 2002). Table 29-3 shows the classification of head and neck malignancies by anatomic location and clinical features.

At the time of diagnosis, most patients have symptoms such as a lump, a change or hoarseness in the voice, or a sore throat that does not resolve. In general, head and neck cancer symptoms differ depending on the location of the cancer. Although these symptoms may arise from other noncancerous conditions, patients should be carefully screened for the presence of malignancies of the head and neck (National Cancer Institute, 2002). It is of vital importance that patients receive health education reinforcing the need to seek medical attention if they are experiencing such symptoms.

ASSESSMENT

Assessment for chronic complications of head and neck cancer involves the frequent monitoring of symptoms, development of a plan of care, and continuous reevaluation of the plan to improve the patient's comfort and well-being. Because complications or recurrence of the cancer can appear months or years after treatment, this population must be followed up on a regular basis.

There are several areas of functional assessment that should be monitored to identify chronic problems and determine overall quality of life. Areas of interest include pain, eating, nutrition, sensory deprivation, self-image, skin integrity, and sleep patterns. Box 29-1 provides assessment guidelines to assist nurses in the identification of these problematic areas.

DIAGNOSIS

Diagnosis depends on medical history, physical examination, and diagnostic tests. Physical examination may include visual inspection of the oral and nasal cavities, throat, and tongue, and palpation for lumps in the neck, lips, gums, and cheeks. Diagnostic tests may include endoscopy, blood and urine analysis, radiography, computed tomography (CT), and magnetic resonance imaging (MRI). Analysis of a biopsy specimen of the tumor tissue is the definitive test to determine malignancy and type of cancer. This may be done either by incisional biopsy, by endoscopy with biopsy, or by fine needle aspiration (National Cancer Institute, 2002a).

Laryngeal and hypopharyngeal cancers are diagnosed using fiberoptic scopes put through the nose and mouth because the larynx and hypopharynx are deep within the neck and not easily seen. In addition, a barium swallow test may be indicated to evaluate the esophagus and view the hypopharynx. A chest radiograph is also routinely taken to check for lung cancer and emphysema (American Cancer Society, 2004).

Diagnosis of chronic conditions consists of assessment of persistent or recurrent symptoms of head and neck cancer months after the completion of surgical, chemotherapy, or

Table 29-2   Causes of Head and Neck Cancers by Site

Site	Carcinogens/Hazardous Occupations	Other Factors
Skin	Inorganic arsenics in drugs, water, or occupational environment Ultraviolet rays of sun, ionizing radiation Polycyclic aromatic hydrocarbons (coke ovens) Gas industry work	Burns Riboflavin deficiency Syphilis (lip cancer)
Nose and sinuses	Radiochemicals (Thorotrast) Mustard gas Isopropyl oil BCME (bis[chloromethyl]ether), alkylating agent (produces esthesioneuroepithelioma in animals) Wood dust (furniture industry) Shoe industry work (leather manufacturing) Textile industry work Nickel refining work Radium dial painting and chemical industry work (osteogenic sarcomas) Cigarette smoke	Chronic sinusitis
Nasopharynx	Nitrosamines (N-nitrosodimethylamine)	Epstein-Barr virus infection Genetics: Chinese from Kwantung province 25 times more susceptible Vitamin C deficiency Salted fish consumption
Oral cavity	Cigarette smoke, reverse smoking Snuff, chewing tobacco, betel nut Ethyl alcohol Polycyclic aromatic hydrocarbons (coke ovens) Textile industry work Leather manufacturing work	Syphilis (tongue cancer) Vitamin B (riboflavin) deficiencies
Hypopharynx, larynx	Cigarette smoke Asbestos (ship building) Mustard gas Polycyclic aromatic hydrocarbons (coke ovens) Ethyl alcohol Wood exposure	Riboflavin deficiency
Esophagus	Ethyl alcohol Cigarette smoke Nitrosamine	Riboflavin deficiency Race and nationality: higher rates in Eskimos, Iranians, blacks
Thyroid	Radiation	Iodine deficiencies Genetics
Salivary glands	Radiation	Genetics: higher rates in Eskimos

Adapted from Jesse TC: Etiology of head and neck cancer. In Suen JW, Myers EN, editors: *Cancer of the head and neck,* New York, 1981, Churchill Livingstone.

radiation treatment. Education of patients and families about chronic complications helps to ensure that symptoms are reported to the health care professional in a prompt manner. In the event that cancer recurs after prior successful treatment, a CT scan or MRI scan and biopsy may be performed to evaluate the type and stage of cancer. A new plan of care is then developed and implemented in consultation with the patient and health care team.

CLINICAL MANIFESTATIONS

Head and neck cancers and the methods used to treat them cause many symptoms that can become chronic (Table 29-4). These problems may be the result of surgery, chemotherapy, or radiation treatment, or they may be related to tumor recurrence and/or metastases requiring additional treatment. With radiation therapy, for instance, side effects of treatment typically occur within the first 3 years after the beginning of

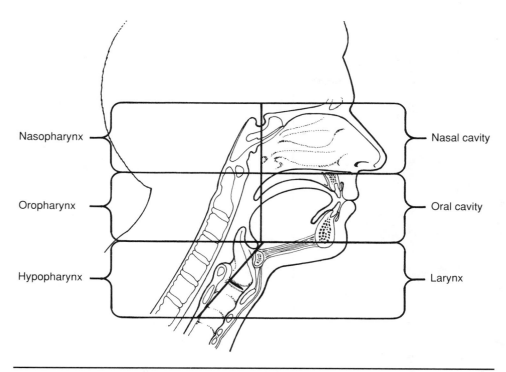

Figure 29-1   Regions of the head and neck. (From Otto SE, editor: *Oncology nursing,* ed 4, St Louis, 2001, Mosby.)

radiation therapy, although some effects may appear at a much later time (Trotti and Mocharnuk, 2001). Patients must be advised at the beginning of treatment of the potential long-term complications and the appropriate management of such complications.

CHRONIC COMPLICATIONS OF HEAD AND NECK CANCERS

Lymphedema

Surgical lymph node dissection can impair lymph drainage and cause lymphedema. Lymphedema is a condition in which interstitial fluid accumulates in the tissues as a result of obstruction of lymph vessels. Chronic lymphedema is caused by scarring and fibrosis in the lymphatic channels. Acute lymphedema can develop quickly after surgery, but chronic lymphedema can appear months to years after cancer treatment has ended. Lymphedema may even develop as long as 5 to 10 years after surgery (Yarbro, Frogge, and Goodman, 1999).

Chronic lymphedema can be caused by surgery and/or radiation therapy for orofacial tumors. Older adults (over 60 years of age) are at increased risk for lymphedema, possibly because of the aging of lymphatic processes (Yarbro, Frogge, and Goodman, 1999). In particular, bilateral surgical removal of cervical lymph nodes or bilateral radiation of cervical lymph nodes can cause severe lymphedema that is difficult to manage (Feber, 2000).

Facial lymphedema can be extremely deforming, can have distressing psychosocial consequences, and can cause functional problems (Feber, 2000). Box 29-2 lists some of the problems associated with lymphedema. The nurse must assist the patient with the management of lymphedema. Teaching the patient to perform light massage of the skin surface (manual lymphatic drainage) to promote fluid movement is very important (Piso et al, 2001). The goal of manual lymphatic drainage therapy is to increase lymphatic transport capacity and to remove excess protein from the tissue (Williams and Venables, 1996). Gentle exercise and range-of-motion movements of the affected parts can be also beneficial (Yarbro, Frogge, and Goodman, 1999). In addition, use of customized compression garments (as used by burn patients) assists in reducing lymphedema. The compression garments cannot be worn by patients with edematous eyelids, however. In these cases, more intensive manual lymphatic drainage is recommended (Piso et al, 2001).

Good skin care is also crucial in the management of lymphedema (Box 29-3). Dry skin, contact dermatitis, fungal infections, cellulitis (acute inflammation of the skin), and hyperkeratosis can occur with lymphedema (Williams and Venables, 1996). The goals of good skin care are to keep the skin supple, moisturized, and free of infection (Feber, 2000).

Table 29-3 Major Subdivisions of the Aerodigestive Tract and Clinical Features of Related Cancers

Site	Function	Anatomic Relationships	Clinical Features of Cancer
Oral cavity	Maintains oral competency for swallowing, articulation	Sensory and motor innervation of tongue is bilateral; comprises central chamber of salivary system; sensory innervation is mediated by lingual nerve (V); motor innervation to muscles is mediated by hypoglossal nerve (XII).	Early symptoms: painless "white spot," persistent ulcerations, difficulty with denture fit, difficulty swallowing, blood-tinged sputum
Oropharynx	Mouth and pharynx perform together in alimentary functions of swallowing and emesis, and respiratory functions of crying, speaking, coughing, and yawning	Boundaries include soft palate, tonsils, tonsillar fossa, and base of tongue; glossopharyngeal nerve (IX) mediates motor and sensory innervation to pharynx and posterior one third of tongue; soft palate and pharynx are innervated by vagus nerve (X).	Irregular ulcerations of mucosal surfaces, painless growth, dysphagia, pain on swallowing, otalgia, persistent sore throat Late symptoms: speech difficulties, resultant palatal incompetence with nasal regurgitation, dysphagia with or without aspiration, trismus
Nasal cavity	Conditions affecting inspired air before entrance: olfaction, humidification, temperature control, cleansing, antibacterial and antiviral protection	First cranial nerve (olfactory) innervates mucous membranes to mediate sense of smell. Drains into submandibular nodes.	Similar to those of chronic sinusitis
Nasopharynx	Serves as anatomic boundary that lies behind nasal cavities and above soft palate	Open space situated just below base of skull behind nasal cavity; inferior wall bordered by soft palate, pharyngeal orifice of eustachian tube, abducens nerve (VI), oculomotor nerve (III), trochlear nerve (IV), and optic nerve (II). Behind eustachian tube lies internal carotid artery, internal jugular vein, and glossopharyngeal (IX), vagus (X), spinal accessory (X), and hypoglossal (XII) nerves. Lymph node chain that drains these areas is posterior cervical triangles, supraclavicular nodes, and jugular chain.	Persistent poorly localized frontal headaches; temporal, parietal, and orificial pain; decreased hearing, tinnitus; multiple nerve palsies, sensory losses Blood in postnasal drip Profuse epistaxis an infrequent presenting symptom
Paranasal sinuses	Consists of air-filled cavities within bones of skull lined by mucous membranes that drain into nasal cavities	Four pairs of maxillary, ethmoid, and frontal sphenoid sinuses drain into submaxillary, retropharyngeal, and jugular lymph nodes.	Chronic sinusitis, bump on hard palate, swelling, numbness and/or pain of cheek, swollen gums, toothache, increased lacrimation, visual changes (diplopia, exophthalmos), persistent unilateral rhinorrhea (epistaxis)
Hypopharynx	Serves as anatomic boundary extending from tip of epiglottis to lower border of cricoid cartilage Structures important for swallowing and airway protection	Lower subdivision of oropharynx, also called laryngopharynx, divided into pyriform sinuses and posterior cricoid area; posterior and lateral pharyngeal walls. Pharyngeal constrictions are innervated by glossopharyngeal (IX) and vagus (X) nerves. Lymphatic drainage is primarily along internal jugular vein and retropharyngeal and paratracheal nodes.	Painless enlarged cervical lymph nodes, odynophagia accompanied by progressive dysphagia and rapid weight loss, otalgia on same side as tumor, hoarseness, dysphagia

Structure	Function	Anatomic characteristics	Signs and symptoms
Larynx	Serves for speech production, maintenance of airway, and airway protection	Located directly below hypopharynx; sensory innervation is supplied from internal laryngeal branch of superior laryngeal nerve of vagus and recurrent laryngeal nerve. Divided into three anatomic sites: (1) supraglottic, (2) glottic, and (3) subglottic. Lymph drainage is to anterior jugular nodes.	Persistent hoarseness; change in quality, pitch of voice; pain; hemoptysis; dysphagia; cough; aspiration
Salivary glands	Produce saliva	Divided into major glands: paired parotid, submandibular, sublingual, and minor salivary glands. Lymphatic drainage is usually to deep jugular or intraglandular or paraglandular lymph nodes. Innervation of this area includes mandibular branch of seventh cranial, lingual, and hypoglossal (XII) nerves.	Painless, rapidly growing mass with or without associated nerve paralysis
Thyroid gland	Serves an endocrine function	Highly vascular gland located in anterior and lower part of neck; composed of small central part, isthmus, and two lobes; isthmus covers second, third, and fourth tracheal rings; thyroid is related medially to esophagus and recurrent laryngeal nerve and laterally to carotid sheath, containing carotid artery; internal jugular vein, and vagus nerve. Lymphatic drainage of thyroid gland is mainly through lymphatic vessels that accompany arterial blood supply.	Neck pain, tightness or fullness in neck, hoarseness, dysphagia, dyspnea

Modified from Otto SE, editor: *Oncology nursing,* ed 4, St Louis, 2001, Mosby.

Box 29-1 Functional Health Pattern Assessment for Head and Neck Cancers

HEALTH PERCEPTION/HEALTH MANAGEMENT
- Is there a family history of head and neck cancer?
- Has the patient been exposed to risk factors such as alcohol use and smoking?
- What medications, including over-the-counter drugs, does the patient take?
- What alternative therapies does the patient use?
- What is the patient's perception of his or her overall health?

NUTRITION/METABOLISM
- Does the patient have dysphagia?
- What is the patient's current weight? Has there been any recent weight loss?
- Does the patient follow a modified diet? What eating methods are used?
- Has the patient experienced any loss of smell and/or taste?
- Does the patient have mouth ulcers?

ELIMINATION
- Have any changes occurred in bowel or bladder habits?
- Does the patient experience any pain or difficulty in urinating?

ACTIVITY/EXERCISE
- Does the patient experience fatigue or malaise?
- What are the patient's regular exercise activities?
- Is the patient able to perform regular and instrumental activities of daily living?

SLEEP/REST
- How much uninterrupted sleep does the patient get at night?
- Does the patient take naps or rest periods?
- What sleep aids are used?
- Is rest interrupted by pain?

COGNITION/PERCEPTION
- What are the nature, character, location, and duration of the pain? What factors aggravate and alleviate the pain?
- Is sensation impaired?
- Have there been mental status changes?
- Are speech patterns impaired?

SELF-PERCEPTION/SELF-CONCEPT
- How does the patient describe himself or herself?
- How has the condition affected the patient's self-esteem?
- Have there been changes in body image related to disfigurement and disability?
- How is the person coping with being a cancer patient?

ROLES/RELATIONSHIPS
- Is the patient employed?
- What role does the patient play in the home and family?
- What changes have occurred in the patient's ability to carry out role functions?
- How satisfied is the patient with his or her current roles and relationships?
- How has the condition affected the patient's family and/or significant others?
- Have changes in social interactions or isolation been noted?

SEXUALITY/REPRODUCTION
- Is the patient sexually active?
- Have changes occurred in sexual performance because of disfigurement and disability?
- Is the patient satisfied with current sexual patterns?

COPING/STRESS TOLERANCE
- What coping strategies does the patient use?
- What support systems are available to the patient?
- Can the patient manage the condition in the current setting?

VALUES/BELIEFS
- What constitutes quality of life for the patient? What is important to the patient?
- What are the patient's spiritual beliefs, health beliefs, and cultural beliefs?
- What are the patient's views regarding locus of control?
- What are the patient's goals for life with disease?

Nurses should educate patients in the careful monitoring and care of the skin to prevent complications.

Alterations in Skin

Radiation therapy can cause alterations in skin that may appear months to years after treatment. Skin atrophy, glossy appearance, and dryness due to lack of oil from dysfunctional sebaceous glands may occur. A late effect of radiation is the development of tiny varicose veins (telangiectasia). This condition is caused by capillary dilation in the skin and is characterized by small reddish or purplish focal lesions with a spidery appearance. The incidence and severity of telangiectasia are related to the radiation technique and the total radiation dose (Feber, 2000).

The oral mucosa is particularly at risk for erosion and trauma to the epithelium (mucositis) 2 weeks after the initiation of radiation treatment (Feber, 2000). During the cellular repair process following mucosal ulceration, however, oral tissues that have been subjected to scarring and vascular compromise become very susceptible to damage from even minor trauma. Serious chronic mucositis can continue from months to even a year after treatment (Yarbro, Frogge, and Goodman, 1999). The nurse may use the interventions listed in Chapter 27 to assist the patient in coping with this difficult problem.

Table 29-4   Chronic Complications of Head and Neck Cancers

Cancer Type	Complications
Sinus (paranasal, nasal cavity)	Trismus
	Vision deficits
	Olfactory impairment
	Pituitary and hypothalamus dysfunction
Oral	Dental caries
	Chronic mucositis
	Osteoradionecrosis
	Alterations in taste
	Disfigurement
Salivary glands	Xerostomia
	Alterations in taste
	Dental caries
	Eye and facial problems
Nasopharynx	Trismus
	Olfactory impairment
	Vision deficits
	Hearing loss
	Pituitary and hypothalamic dysfunction
	Temporal lobe necrosis
Oropharynx	Trismus
Hypopharynx	Hypothyroidism
Larynx	Hypothyroidism
	Olfactory impairment
	Alterations in taste
	Aspiration risk
	Disfigurement
	Loss of speech
	Compromised airway
Lymph nodes	Lymphedema
	Disfigurement

Adapted from Feber T: *Head and neck oncology nursing,* Philadelphia, 2000, Whurr.

Box 29-2   Problems Associated with Lymphedema

- Difficulty with the use of artificial voice devices if the neck is swollen
- Patient fear of tumor recurrence if there is firm, submental lymphedema after laryngeal irradiation
- Impaired airway if edema occludes the tracheostomy
- Facial disfigurement
- Speech and swallowing problems
- Feeling of dull tension in the skin
- Impaired vision if the eyelids are swollen

Adapted from Feber T: *Head and neck oncology nursing,* Philadelphia, 2000, Whurr, p 256; and Piso DU et al: Early rehabilitation of head-neck edema after curative surgery for orofacial tumors, *Am J Phys Med Rehabil* 80:261-9, 2001.

Box 29-3   Basic Skin Care for Lymphedema

- Clean the skin daily with soap substitutes or bath oils and water, pat dry, and then apply moisturizer.
- Assess the condition of the skin frequently.
- Decrease the risk of skin damage from shaving, sunburn exposure, and insect bites.
- Immediately treat skin injury with antiseptics.
- Wear clothing that fits loosely.
- If skin problems are present, use dermatologic medications as required.

Adapted from Williams A, Venables J: Skin care in patients with uncomplicated lymphedema, *J Wound Care* 5:223-6, 1996.

Fungating Tumors

Fungating tumors are wounds caused by cancerous cells that infiltrate the epidermis of the skin, mucosa, or lymph and blood vessels. They may arise from either local tumors or from metastases from a primary tumor. These tumors are visible, grow rapidly, and have a funguslike form. They frequently progress to necrotic, infected, purulent, fragile, and foul-smelling lesions (Yarbro, Frogge, and Goodman, 1999).

Fungating tumors also cause complications by forming fistulas (abnormal passages or openings between organs or between organs and the surface of the body). For instance, fistulas from the interior of the oral cavity to the exterior of the cheek can be very distressing because it becomes almost impossible to eat, drink, and speak. Another distressing consequence of orocutaneous fistulas is the continuous leakage of saliva. In tracheostomy, tumor recurrence around the stoma can impair the airway, cause tracheoesophageal fistula, and invade major blood vessels. Carotid hemorrhage caused by tumor erosion is the one traumatic event in head and neck cancer that is viewed with great trepidation. The extraordinary and dramatic blood loss is very distressing for patients, families, and health care personnel (Feber, 2000).

These chronic lesions require nursing interventions that include complex skin care and psychological and emotional support (Feber, 2000). Care is centered on provision of comfort and minimization of symptoms rather than on wound healing. Management of odor, pain, and exudate (wound discharge of fluids and cellular materials due to inflammation) are primary concerns in dealing with fungating tumors (Bryant, 2000). Table 29-5 outlines the assessment of fungating wounds.

As Feber (2000) notes, "A fungating lesion severely affects the quality of life, often alienating and isolating an individual from normal life. It is a constant visible reminder of cancer. It often gives a sense of lingering death, 'rotting away'" (p. 307). Management of these tumors may require palliative radiation and chemotherapy to reduce the size of the lesions and surgical excision of lymph nodes to decrease

Table 29-5   Assessment of Fungating Wounds

Assessment Parameter	Description
Appearance	Necrosis, slough, bleeding ulceration
Odor	Sweet, foul (offensive)
Drainage or exudates	Clear, thick, thin; low, moderate, copious amount
Presence of infection	Increased drainage; fever, leukocytosis
Periwound skin	Erythema, maceration, edema, tenderness, maculopapular rash
Size and shape of site	Interference with dressing application

Adapted from British Columbia Cancer Agency: Guidelines for the care of chronic ulcerating malignant skin lesions, Cancer management manual, 1997, retrieved from *http://www.bccancer.bc.ca/cmm/ulcerating-lesions?01.shtml* on Feb 3, 2004; and Moody M, Grocott P: Let us extend our knowledge base: assessment and management of fungating malignant wounds, *Prof Nurse* 8(9):586, 1993.

the risk of additional fungating tumors. In end-stage cancer, however, good wound care may be the only treatment available (Feber, 2000).

Malodorous tumors are the result of tissue hypoxia (lack of oxygen) and the presence of anaerobic bacteria that thrive in necrotic tissue. This problem is typical of fungating tumors (Collier, 1997) and can be extremely difficult to bear, even stimulating nausea and loss of appetite in patients. The unpleasant smell of end-stage disease can cause self-consciousness, emotional distress, embarrassment, and social isolation at a time when the patient most needs the support of family and friends. Malodor can also have a negative impact on intimacy and sexual function (Price, 1996). Management of odor includes wound cleansing, control of exudate, maintenance of clean dressings, use of wound deodorizers, débridement (removal of necrotic tissue), and topical application of antimicrobials to treat infection (Bryant, 2000). Table 29-6 lists nursing interventions for fungating wounds.

Xerostomia

Xerostomia (dry mouth) is a common side effect of radiation treatment in head and neck cancer patients. This condition can become permanent due to salivary gland fibrosis (Robbins and Gosselin, 2002). The predictor of xerostomia is the daily dose of radiation administered (Otto, 2001). Other causes of xerostomia include oxygen use, dehydration, mouth breathing, and drugs (Feber, 2000). Examples of drugs that can cause xerostomia are anticonvulsants, antidepressants, antihistamines, antipsychotics, diuretics, hypotensives, opioids, and tranquilizers, including benzodiazepines.

Xerostomia is a problem because the patient's saliva may become thick and sticky, which impairs swallowing and speaking. Food may adhere to the teeth or throat, or the patient may have a burning sensation when eating spicy foods (Robbins and Gosselin, 2002). An excessively dry mouth can lead to oral fungal infections, mouth ulcers, dental caries (cavities) caused by aerobic organisms, and salivary gland

Table 29-6   Interventions for Fungating Wounds

Pain Management	Odor Management	Exudate Control
Nontraumatic Dressing Changes ■ Contact layer ■ Gauzes, nonadherent or coated ■ Foam ■ Protective barrier films ■ Nontraumatic tapes **Control of Bleeding** ■ Hemostatic dressings ■ Nonadherent gauze ■ Alginates ■ Silver nitrate sticks **Periwound Skin Management** ■ Nontraumatic tapes ■ Skin sealants (alcohol free) ■ Barrier ointment or cream ■ Hydrocolloid wafer	**Wound Cleansing** ■ Ionic cleansers ■ Sodium-impregnated gauze ■ Antimicrobials ■ Polysaccharide beads **Deodorizers** ■ Charcoal dressings ■ Chloromycetin solution **Débridement** ■ Dry, hard, necrotic tissue: hydrogel, enzymatic débriders ■ Wet, sloughy tissue: polysaccharide beads, starch, copolymer dressing **Reduction of Bacterial Burden** ■ Irrigation with ionic cleansers ■ Antimicrobial dressings and creams ■ Absorptive dressings ■ Sodium-impregnated gauze ■ Oral antimicrobials	**Exudate Collection and Containment** ■ Foam, alginates, hydrofiber dressings, hydrofibers, absorptive powders ■ Wound drainage pouch **Dressing Changes at Appropriate Time Interval** ■ When pooling on intact skin occurs ■ When strikethrough occurs

From Bryant RA: *Acute and chronic wounds: nursing management,* ed 2, St Louis, 2000, Mosby.

enlargement (Stack and Papas, 2001). A decrease in saliva promotes rapid tooth decay, so frequent monitoring by a dentist and good dental care are extremely important (Robbins and Gosselin, 2002). An interdisciplinary approach that includes patient education and interventions to correct problems in oral care and nutrition is required for proper dental management (Stack and Papas, 2001).

Quality of life may be greatly affected by xerostomia. The patient may need to take frequent sips of fluids while eating and may avoid eating with others because of embarrassment. Wearing dentures can be uncomfortable because saliva is necessary for their retention in the mouth, and the resulting poor fit may cause difficulty in chewing. Xerostomia can also cause alterations in the taste of food. Both of these problems contribute to nutritional deficiencies.

Sleep may be impaired because the patient must drink water frequently during the night to avoid waking with his or her tongue adhered to the roof of the mouth. Public speaking, airplane travel, or talking for long periods on the telephone may be difficult as a result of the abnormally dry mouth and lack of moisture. The curtailing of normal social and daily activities due to difficulty speaking or swallowing can have a detrimental affect on the patient's quality of life (Yarbro, Frogge, and Goodman, 1999). The nurse should encourage the patient to verbalize his or her emotions concerning this serious and life-altering problem. Box 29-4 lists nursing interventions to help the patient cope with xerostomia.

Loss of Smell

The sense of smell (olfaction) is important for safety in the environment (to smell fires and gas leaks) and for the enjoyment of food flavor. Impairment of olfaction decreases the enjoyment of taste and eating, which may have negative consequences on dietary habits (van Dam et al, 1999) and can increase the risk of malnutrition, especially in the elderly (Murphy et al, 2002).

Absence of smell (anosmia) and distortion of smell (dysosmia) can be caused by age, smoking, malnutrition, vitamin deficiency, medications, radiation of the head and neck, chemotherapy, and olfactory nerve dysfunction secondary to craniofacial surgery (Bromley, 2000; Feber, 2000; Murphy et al, 2002; Schiffman, 1983; Weinstein et al, 2001). Ho et al (2002) noted a significant decrease in olfactory function 1 year after radiation therapy for nasopharyngeal cancer. In addition, anosmia can occur after laryngectomy because breathing is accomplished through the tracheostomy and not through the nose (Feber, 2000). Box 29-5 lists various nursing interventions that assist the patient in coping with loss of smell.

Alterations in Taste

Cancer patients frequently experience taste alterations, which can cause food aversions and impaired nutritional status (Sherry, 2002). Radiation therapy may cause taste alterations that can continue for up to 6 months after treatment is concluded (Robbins and Gosselin, 2002).

Box 29-4   Nursing Interventions for Xerostomia

- Use artificial saliva or other oral lubricants.
- Oral pilocarpine may help patients with residual salivary function.
- Encourage use of gravies and sauces on soft foods and frequent drinking of fluids.
- Use oil or a small pat of butter in the mouth to provide comfort, especially during sleep to avoid frequent awakening with a dry mouth.
- Spray the mouth with a fine mist of water from a bottle.
- Sucking on sugarless candies or chewing sugarless gum can stimulate saliva production. Keep lips moist with lip balm.
- Avoid lemon glycerin products, which can cause further drying and irritation.
- Advise the patient to avoid alcohol and tobacco use because they contribute to dryness and irritation of the oral mucosa.
- A solution of meat tenderizer or crushed papain tablets in water, rinsed in the mouth and expectorated before meals, can help to liquefy thick saliva.
- Use a room humidifier.
- Ensure that the patient has a dental evaluation for proper denture fit.

Adapted from Otto SE, editor: *Oncology nursing,* ed 4, St Louis, 2001, Mosby; Robbins M, Gosselin TK: Symptom management in radiation oncology, *Am J Nurs* 102(suppl 4):32-6, 2002; and Yarbro CY, Frogge MH, Goodman M: *Cancer symptom management,* ed 2, Sudbury, Mass, 1999, Jones and Bartlett.

Taste dysfunction includes absence of taste (ageusia), decreased taste acuity (hypoageusia), and abnormal taste sensation (dysgeusia). Alteration in taste can be caused by many factors, including older age (Bromley, 2000), use of certain drugs, chemotherapy, oral fungal infections, laryngectomy (van Dam et al, 1999), and radiation damage to the taste buds (Ahne et al, 2000; Gaziano, 2002). To compensate, patients may increase consumption of sugar and salt in an effort to improve the taste of food (Feber, 2000).

Box 29-5   Nursing Interventions for Loss of Smell

- Teach safety precautions such as checking for gas leaks, installing smoke alarms.
- Instruct the patient to clearly label all prepared foods with the date and to discard expired foods.
- Instruct the patient to clearly label toxic substances such as cleaning products, insecticides, and gas in containers.
- Make the patient aware that loss of smell can greatly impair taste sensation.

Adapted from Feber T: *Head and neck oncology nursing,* Philadelphia, 2000, Whurr, pp 265-6.

Taste dysfunction may result in poor appetite and malnutrition (Ahne et al, 2000). To address this nutritional problem, the nurse should encourage the patient to experiment with different foods, to monitor nutritional intake, and to obtain a nutritional consult (Robbins and Gosselin, 2002). Patients can also be advised to try different food textures and to pay attention to food temperature, aroma, and color. The nurse may also suggest options such as liquefying or pureeing foods, adding spices for improved taste, thickening liquids with commercial thickeners, or using creative cooking methods to increase taste or change food consistency.

Caregivers should be advised that cooking for patients with taste alterations can be problematic and that there are complex psychosocial issues associated with eating. Eating is a pleasurable experience. It is not just a nutritional requirement for health; rather, it is an emotional, social, and sensory event (Feber, 2000).

Alterations in Nutrition

Nutrition plays a critical role in the care of head and neck cancer patients. Cancer patients have the highest incidence of malnutrition of any hospitalized patients. Otto (2001) notes that 60% of head and neck cancer patients have malnutrition. Gaziano (2002) found that the severity of malnutrition is often related to the patient's precancer nutritional state, the type of tumor, and the treatments given for the cancer. Therefore, it is critical that patients at risk for nutritional deficits be carefully monitored.

Patients with head and neck cancers may experience significant and chronic dysphagia (difficulty swallowing). Estimates are that 37% to 46% are unable to eat a solid diet, and 79% have significant eating problems that interfere with their quality of life (Yarbro, Frogge, and Goodman, 1999). Surgical interventions for oral and oropharyngeal cancer can create multiple nutritional problems. Surgical removal of parts of the tongue result in swallowing problems. Likewise, mandibular resection and maxillary surgery can cause severe functional deficits in chewing and swallowing (Rogers, 2001). In addition, if a patient is unable to resume oral feedings, lifelong tube feedings may be necessary (Gaziano, 2002). Box 29-6 lists the various psychosocial difficulties experienced by patients coping with dysphagia.

Dysphagia can contribute to malnutrition, dehydration, aspiration pneumonia, impaired wound healing, and a decreased response to medical treatments. The size and location of the tumor, the amount and location of surgical dissection and reconstruction, the presence of cranial nerve damage, and the side effects of treatment all affect the level of dysphagia experienced. Surgery to the base of the tongue and soft palate usually causes more severe dysphagia because the tongue plays a critical role in the process of swallowing. Surgical resections of the pharynx and larynx can also cause significant dysphagia. The goals of swallowing rehabilitation are to prevent aspiration, malnutrition, and dehydration (Gaziano, 2002). A speech therapist should be

---

Box 29-6 Psychosocial Issues Related to Dysphagia

■ Changes in dining-out habits and inability to participate in mealtimes as before, which leads to social isolation
■ Avoidance of social meal consumption related to increased amount of time required to ingest a meal, decreased availability of food choices, and need for special food preparation
■ Concerns related to ingestion of food in a socially acceptable manner
■ Anxiety related to having to use adaptive equipment, special foods, or feeding tubes
■ Altered family relationships because of significant lifestyle changes
■ Concern over the financial burden of special meal preparation and cost of tube feedings, equipment, and food supplements

Adapted from Gaziano JE: Evaluation and management of oropharyngeal dysphagia in head and neck cancer, *Cancer Control* 9(5):23-9, 2002.

---

consulted to determine what the patient can safely swallow (Feber, 2000).

In patients receiving radiation therapy, nutritional deficits may arise prior to, during, or up to 6 months after completion of treatment. This may result in anorexia (loss of appetite) and cachexia (the inability to absorb the nutritional value of the food eaten) (Robbins and Gosselin, 2002). Reirradiation of head and neck cancer patients, especially the elderly, can cause late complications such as esophageal stricture and ulcers that necessitate the permanent use of a liquid diet (Ohizumi et al, 2002). In addition, tumors of the head and neck can cause pain on eating, produce dysphagia, and result in poorly fitting dentures that compromise chewing and swallowing (Feber, 2000).

Patients who undergo partial laryngectomy (removal of half of the larynx, one true and one false vocal cord, and half of the thyroid cartilage) usually do not have swallowing problems. However, aspiration can become a problem in patients who undergo a horizontal laryngectomy (removal of the false vocal cords, epiglottis, and hyoid bone) (McGuire, 1999). Advanced laryngeal cancers are treated with a total laryngectomy (removal of entire larynx, hyoid bone, true and false vocal cords, and two or three tracheal rings), which does not result in aspiration problems because the digestive tract and upper airway are then completely separate (Cyr, Higgins, and McGuire, 1998).

Treatment of cancers of the oropharynx and nasopharynx can result in swallowing and aspiration problems. Patients undergoing pharyngolaryngoesophagectomy for advanced hypopharyngeal cancers do not have swallowing problems but are at risk for postprandial dumping syndrome. These patients must be taught to eat small, frequent meals and to sit upright for 1 hour after eating to prevent regurgitation, because the esophageal sphincter has been removed (McGuire, 2000). It is important for nurses to help patients and families find practical strategies for coping with nutritional problems.

Alteration in Dental Status

Poor oral health has multiple negative consequences. It can decrease quality of life, compromise nutritional intake, cause chronic pain and discomfort, hinder personal relationships, and negatively affect self-image (Ritchie, 2002). All problems related to poor oral health and alterations in smell and taste must be rigorously addressed by the health care team to maximize the patient's quality of life.

Head and neck cancer patients have a high risk of dental caries associated with radiation therapy and xerostomia. A dentist should evaluate patients regularly before and after radiation treatment. Careful attention should be paid to dental hygiene, and patients should be instructed to decrease sugar intake and to use sugarless gum (Otto, 2001).

Radiation-induced caries can be caused by xerostomia, excessive sugar consumption, and poor oral hygiene. Irradiated teeth are susceptible to fracture, so postradiation extraction of carious teeth is not recommended. Good oral care of the head and neck cancer patient includes assessment prior to cancer treatments, provision of periodontal care, education in good oral hygiene and the need to decrease sugar intake, and daily fluoride application (Otto, 2001). The dentist should fit the patient with a customized appliance that holds fluoride gel. The patient bites down into the tray and holds it in place for up to 15 minutes a day (Robbins and Gosselin, 2002).

Poorly fitting dentures can cause tissue breakdown, so the use of denture liners may be necessary to cushion the dentures against the gums. A dentist must evaluate the stability of the dentures and assist with the installation of a liner to improve denture fit (Yarbro, Frogge, and Goodman, 1999). Properly fitting dentures are necessary to decrease the risk of trauma and irritation, which may cause osteoradionecrosis (Jansma et al, 1992). The nurse should instruct the patient to soak dentures daily in a chlorhexidine gluconate solution to decrease the risk of microbial growth and infection in the mouth (Otto, 2001).

Osteoradionecrosis

Osteoradionecrosis (bone death) may occur at any time after radiation therapy, even years later. Osteoradionecrosis is a condition in which bony structures become necrotic because of lack of blood flow to the area (Robbins and Gosselin, 2002). Radiation and trauma to blood vessels and bone cause vascular insufficiency (Otto, 2001). Osteoradionecrosis is considered one of the most devastating complications of radiation treatment. It most frequently affects the mandible (jawbone) and is often accompanied by soft tissue necrosis, infection, pathologic fractures, pain, and formation of oral-cutaneous (mouth to cheek) fistulas (Otto, 2001). Osteoradionecrosis of the mandible is diagnosed when exposed bone (in the absence

of tumor) does not heal over an extended period of time despite treatment (Hunter and Scher, 2003). Dental demineralization is also a late effect of radiation and results in bone fracture and impaired bone healing (Dunne-Daly, 1995).

Management of osteoradionecrosis relies on high doses of antibiotics, local irrigation, surgical removal of the necrotic bone tissue (Otto, 2001), and dental management prior to radiation. Necrotic bone is surgically replaced by vascularized bone transfers (Celik et al, 2002). Hunter and Scher (2003) note that more than half of patients with mandibular osteoradionecrosis will require surgical treatment for this problem. Hyperbaric oxygen therapy to increase tissue oxygenation in ischemic wounds has demonstrated some success in treating osteoradionecrosis.

High radiation dose, anatomic location of tumor near bone, and poor dental status predispose the patient to osteoradionecrosis (Celik et al, 2002). Other predisposing factors include brachytherapy (the insertion of radioactive sources into tumor sites), irradiation of a large amount of mandibular bone, biopsy, postradiation dental extractions, trauma to the bone, impaired wound healing that results in infection, and alcohol and tobacco use. Because tooth removal after radiation therapy increases the risk of osteoradionecrosis, it is advised that tooth extractions for dental cavities be performed prior to therapy (Hunter and Scher, 2003). A minimum of 10 days between extraction and therapy is required to prevent complications in healing (Feber, 2000). Prompt identification of dental problems reduces the need for the difficult treatments required for osteoradionecrosis. Therefore, early detection improves the quality of life for the irradiated patient (Celik et al, 2002).

Muscle Trismus

Trismus is due to the scarring and fibrosis of the masticatory (chewing) muscles caused by tumor obstruction, radiation, or surgery. This problem results in restriction of the movement of the temporomandibular joint and difficulty opening the mouth. Box 29-7 lists complications related to muscle trismus.

Box 29-7 Complications of Muscle Trismus

- Eating difficulties
- Speech difficulties
- Inadequate oral care
- Instability of dentures
- Impaired body image
- Impaired ability to socialize
- Weight loss
- Pain
- Dental problems

Adapted from Feber T: *Head and neck oncology nursing*, Philadelphia, 2000, Whurr, p 138; and Giuliano J, Rudy S: Nursing care of the patient with trismus, *ORL Head Neck Nurs* 13(1):23-30, 1995.

Assessment is accomplished easily by asking the patient to perform the "three finger test." This is done by inserting three fingers vertically into the mouth between the central incisors. If the patient has dentures that are not in place, four fingers can be inserted into the mouth. If fewer than three or four fingers can be inserted, then trismus is present (Giuliano and Rudy, 1995).

The best treatment for this disorder is prevention. If trismus is not prevented, surgery may be required (Feber, 2000). Surgery is the treatment of last resort because irradiated bone and tissue are at risk for poor healing and infection (Otto, 2001). Prevention is accomplished through exercises that are designed to stretch the jaw using a stack of wooden tongue depressors placed in the mouth three to four times a day for 15 minutes per session. Use of nonsteroidal antiinflammatory drugs, warm moist heat over the temporomandibular joints, massage, and ultrasound treatment prior to exercises can be helpful. A physical therapist may be required to assist with treatments (Feber, 2000). In addition, opening the mouth wide and closing it 20 times in a row, 3 times a day is recommended to decrease muscle fibrosis and stricture (Otto, 2001).

The patient with trismus must adopt coping mechanisms to deal with significant oral problems. If chewing is impaired, then nutritional status must also be assessed. Liquefied food can be given through large straws or syringes with tubing attached. Using a small toothbrush, irrigating the mouth with a syringe, and performing oral care immediately after stretching exercises can facilitate oral hygiene. The nursing care plan should also include assessment for pain, altered body image, impaired speech patterns, and ineffective airway clearance related to restricted mouth opening (Giuliano and Rudy, 1995). A dentist and speech therapist should be consulted for jaw and mouth problems and difficulty with speech (Feber, 2000).

Hearing Loss

Patients who undergo surgery or radiation therapy for tumors of the ear are at risk for hearing loss, tinnitus, and equilibrium problems. Chapter 5 describes assessment methods used to determine hearing loss. The chemotherapy drug cisplatin can also cause hearing deficits (Yarbro, Frogge, and Goodman, 1999).

Irradiation of nasopharyngeal cancers can cause chronic bilateral hearing loss because the ears are in the radiation field (Low and Fong, 1998). Postradiation symptoms may include hearing deficits, ear soreness, crusting of the ear canal, and infection (serous otitis media). The incidence of hearing loss in nasopharyngeal cancer appears to be age related, with patients over 50 years of age having the highest risk for this problem (Kwong et al, 1996).

Hearing loss and impaired communication are stressful for the patient and family and can cause social isolation. Hearing loss may elicit emotions such as grief, anger, frustration, sadness, and depression. The nurse should explore these feelings with the patient and assist in the development of new coping methods. All patients with hearing loss should be referred to an audiologist for assessment and fitting of hearing aids, if possible (Feber, 2000). Refer to Chapter 5 for nursing interventions that may assist the patient with persistent hearing loss.

Impaired Vision

Impaired vision can be caused by many factors related to head and neck cancer. Tumors of the paranasal sinuses can cause edema that interferes with the opening of the eye or can directly invade the orbit. Tumors, surgery, or radiation therapy may cause damage to the optic nerve. Nasopharyngeal tumors can affect motor and sensory nerves, which can result in decreased eye movement and vision impairment (Feber, 2000).

Surgery for cancer of the nose and sinuses can cause monocular vision, misalignment of the eyes (dystopia), double vision (diplopia), excessive tearing of the eye (epiphora), and depression of the eye into the socket (enophthalmos) (Mathong et al, 1997). Surgery of the parotid gland can cause trauma to the facial nerve that leads to unilateral facial droop, inability to close the eye, and impaired tear production. Inflammation of the eye (exposure keratitis) may result from these problems (Anderson et al, 1996). Radiation can impair lacrimal gland function, leading to "dry eye" (Feber, 2000), and can increase the risk of cataracts (Brady and Davis, 1988). Refer to Chapter 4 for nursing interventions to assist the patient who is coping with vision deficits.

Hypothyroidism

Hypothyroidism can be a long-term complication of treatment of head and neck cancers. The average time for hypothyroidism to appear is approximately 8 months after treatment. Among patients undergoing advanced head and neck surgery who are treated with surgery and radiation, approximately 15% will develop hypothyroidism. Patients treated with laryngectomy, thyroid lobectomy, and radiation have a 61% risk of hypothyroidism (Sinard et al, 2000).

Abnormal thyroid function typically develops within the first year after treatment. It is advisable to test thyroid function levels in patients prior to cancer treatment to determine baseline levels and to continue testing for up to 2 years after treatment. Management consists of thyroid supplementation with drugs such as levothyroxine (Sinard et al, 2000).

Disfigurement

Head and neck cancer and its corresponding treatments can cause permanent alterations in appearance and function. The emotional consequences of a highly visible deformity and the interference in normal, basic functions such as eating and breathing can threaten personal identity (Albino, 2002). Therefore, head and neck cancer affects self-image and self-esteem, and has a profound impact on psychosocial well-being. These patients may feel stigmatized by their altered appearance. Because a pleasing physical appearance is socially important, being different from the perceived norm is difficult at best (Feber, 2000).

In addition to coping with demanding cancer treatments and the possibility of suffering and death, these patients must also face the prospects of disfigurement and loss of identity. This increases the risk of psychological problems and social isolation from friends and family (Albino, 2002). Newell and Marks (2000) note that facially disfigured patients can be vulnerable to the development of social phobic avoidance behaviors, which can include anxiety, depression, and agoraphobia (intense, irrational fear of being in open spaces or public places).

Head and neck cancer patients often experience grief and loss related to functional deficits. Some of these devastating effects include the loss of speech, inability to eat properly, loss of an appealing facial appearance, loss of normal vision and hearing, loss of previous social roles, and loss of future expectations (Feber, 2000).

Laryngectomy also results in a conspicuous abnormality because the patient has a stoma and possibly a tracheotomy appliance. The person with a laryngectomy must learn to cope with many major psychological and social challenges. The individual must cope not only with the consequences of having cancer but also with the need to breathe through a hole (stoma) in the neck (Stam, Koopmans, and Mathieson, 1991).

Nurses can assist the patient by supporting the patient through the painful process of adjusting to disfigurement and loss. They can assist the patient by referring the person to good role models and by supporting the patient's expectations of a better future. Nurses must be aware that some patients' coping abilities may not be adequate for the adjustment process and these individuals may require psychological counseling (Feber, 2000).

Sleep Disorders

Obstructive sleep apnea (OSA), which is caused by a partially obstructed upper airway that collapses during sleep, is a common chronic problem in head and neck cancer patients. The detection of this problem is important for improving the quality of life of these patients. Box 29-8 lists symptoms of OSA and impaired sleep patterns.

Head and neck cancer patients already have numerous reasons for fatigue and sleep disorders; cancer treatments, poor dietary habits, anxiety, depression, and pain can lead to sleep disturbances and fatigue. Therefore, OSA should not be considered a normal consequence of cancer and its treatments.

The incidence of OSA in this population is 91%, compared with only 9% in the general population. A paralyzed vocal cord or narrowed larynx, hypopharynx, or pharynx may cause OSA. Anatomic changes from cancer treatments, impaired healing from radiation, overall debility, and fear of a recurrence of cancer preclude the use of surgical interventions to clear the obstructed upper airway. Treatment options

are limited. Continuous positive airway pressure and tracheostomy are considered the best alternatives for these patients (Friedman et al, 2001).

Problems Associated with Laryngectomy

Problems can occur in patients who have undergone laryngectomy, and patients should be advised at the time of surgery of potential chronic complications (Figure 29-2). They should be apprised of the physical adjustment required to breathe through a stoma in the neck and the psychosocial impact of a radically altered appearance (Feber, 2000).

> **Box 29-8   Symptoms of Obstructive Sleep Apnea and Impaired Sleep Patterns**
>
> - Restless sleep
> - Fatigue
> - Snoring
> - Sleepiness
> - Impaired alertness during the day
> - Irritability
> - Forgetfulness
> - Alterations in mood or behavior
> - Anxiety or depression
> - Morning headaches
> - Loss of libido
>
> Adapted from Friedman M et al: The occurrence of sleep-disordered breathing among patients with head and neck cancer, *Laryngoscope* 111:1917-9, 2001.

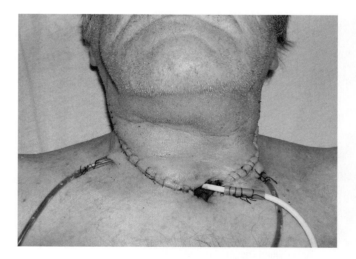

Figure 29-2   Patient after total laryngectomy. No tracheotomy appliance was used and a transesophageal feeding tube was placed during surgery. (Photograph courtesy of W. Brundage, MD, M. Zavod, MD, and E.R. Anderson, MD, University of Vermont College of Medicine, Burlington, Vermont.)

Laryngectomy can also impair basic human functions such as smell, speech, taste, swallowing, coughing, and kissing (Papadas et al, 2002). In addition, Ackerstaff et al (1994) found that laryngectomy can cause respiratory complaints such as coughing, problems with sputum and expectoration, dyspnea, and nasal discharge. Rehabilitation of laryngectomy patients using an interdisciplinary team approach is extremely important to maximize the quality of life in the face of such extreme disability (Papadas et al, 2002). Box 29-9 lists the various problems associated with laryngectomy.

Patients should be taught as early as possible about self-care of their tracheostomy. Care of the stoma, cleaning of the tracheotomy tube, and expectoration of mucus to avoid suctioning should be encouraged. Box 29-10 shows interventions the nurse can implement to assist laryngectomy patients in managing self-care.

The disfiguring appearance of a stoma can have a significantly negative effect on a patient's willingness to socialize and is considered to have the greatest impact on the patient's quality of life compared with other sequelae of laryngectomy (Weinstein et al, 2001). The ability to speak also greatly influences the patient's view of his or her social acceptability. If the patient has acquired satisfactory esophageal speech, then the patient is more likely to feel positive about social acceptance. Although the majority of patients find that their social and outdoor activities may be compromised, most say they remain independent despite their physical challenges (Jay, Ruddy, and Cullen, 1991).

INTERDISCIPLINARY CARE

Quality of life is greatly affected by the diagnosis and treatment of head and neck cancers and by rehabilitation after

treatment. Long-term problems with chewing, eating in public, and disfigurement lower patients' views of the quality of their lives. The definition of quality of life used in this text comes from the Canadian Health Promotion Model, which states that quality of life is the extent to which a person can enjoy the important possibilities of his or her life (Centre for Health Promotion, 2003). Many scales or instruments are available that are specifically designed to measure quality of life over time for head and neck cancer patients (Box 29-11). Considering the patient's perspective is crucial when using any quality-of-life scale. The following sections discuss the roles of the interdisciplinary care team members, with a focus on quality of life in the various domains represented by the team.

Primary Provider (Physician/Nurse Practitioner)

Primary care providers can include physicians, advanced practice nurses, and physician assistants. The initial diagnosis is made by the primary care provider, who is very involved at the outset in the patient's care and then becomes involved again as needed if there is a recurrence of the disease. Specialists include the medical oncologist, otolaryngologic surgeon, radiation oncologist, and pathologist. Because the current trend in treatment is organ preservation, most patients undergo radiation therapy first and then have surgery after radiation therapy. This means that for most patients both the otolaryngologic surgeon and the radiation oncologist are involved in their care from the beginning of treatment.

Dentist

Most chronic head and neck cancer patients have undergone radiation therapy and thus require regular dental care. The

---

Box 29-9 Complications of Laryngectomy

- Impaired lung function and oxygen saturation caused by loss of airflow resistance from the nares to the upper trachea, which ordinarily prevents alveolar collapse and maintains proper lung ventilation
- Difficulty in using bronchodilator and corticosteroid inhalers due to the lack of airtight seal
- Hypoxia (oxygen deprivation) due to suctioning
- Lung collapse (atelectasis) caused by negative pressure during suctioning
- Bradycardia (slow heart rate) and hypotension (low blood pressure) caused by cardiac hypoxia and stimulation of the vagus nerve when suctioning
- Inability to shower, bathe, or swim without use of appliances to protect the airway

- Dysphagia
- Formation of scar tissue at the base of the tongue, which results in swallowing problems and need for a liquid diet
- If a tracheotomy appliance is present, interference with laryngeal function, which causes difficulty swallowing
- Loss of nasal function (anosmia)
- Difficulty sniffing and blowing the nose, and on occasion chronic running of the nose
- Increased frequency of chest infection
- Alterations in intraabdominal pressure caused by loss of laryngeal function, which can lead to difficulty with urination, defecation, and weight lifting
- Stoma degradation
- Pharyngocutaneous fistula

Adapted from Feber T: *Head and neck oncology nursing,* Philadelphia, 2000, Whurr, pp 113-4, 118, 159; Jay S, Ruddy J, Cullen RJ: Laryngectomy: the patient's view, *J Laryngol Otolaryngol* 105:934-8, 1991; and Yarbro CY, Frogge MH, Goodman M: *Cancer symptom management,* ed 2, Sudbury, Mass, 1999, Jones and Bartlett, p 213.

Box 29-10   Nursing Interventions for Laryngectomy and Tracheotomy

- Teach the patient to wash hands well before and after all tracheotomy care.
- Provide extra moisture through a nebulizer or humidifier because the nose and mouth, which filter warm and moistened air, are bypassed. Clean the humidifier regularly to avoid bacterial growth.
- Encourage the frequent drinking of fluids to keep the airway moist.
- Instruct the patient to avoid over-the-counter antihistamines (cold medications) because they may dry the airway and secretions.
- Advise the patient that pink or blood-tinged sputum may indicate excessive dryness of the airway.
- Teach the patient proper suctioning technique: Take four or five deep breaths before gently inserting the suction catheter into the stoma. Do not suction for more than 10 seconds, rotating the catheter as it is withdrawn. Do not suction for more than three times in a session. Take 5- to 10-minute rest periods between suctioning sessions and breathe deeply after each suctioning attempt.
- Teach the patient proper catheter care: Clean catheters in hot, soapy water and rinse with tap water. Soak catheters in equal parts of white vinegar and tap water for 1 hour and rinse with saline solution. Allow to dry on a clean towel and store in a clean, covered container. Wash suction bottle and tubing daily with hot, soapy water.
- Instruct the patient to keep the stoma clean and dry. Cotton-tipped swabs or a damp wash cloth may be used to remove dried secretions around the stoma. Application of a thin film of petrolatum ointment to the outside of the stoma may be helpful in preventing crusting.

- Instruct the patient to cover the stoma with a stoma shield or gauze squares to prevent inhalation of dust, insects, or foreign matter. A high-necked sweater or shirt, or a scarf may also be worn as a stoma cover.
- Teach the patient to cover the stoma when bathing or showering and not to swim. Powders and aerosol sprays should not be used, and dust, smoke, and lint from facial tissues should be avoided. The patient should not smoke.
- Instruct the patient to make plans to obtain assistance in case of an emergency, especially if talking is difficult. The patient should wear a Medic Alert bracelet or necklace.
- Because of the loss of taste and smell, the patient will not be as aware of mouth odor. Encourage daily mouth care.
- Instruct the patient to increase fiber in the diet and/or use laxatives to help with constipation, which may result because of the inability to hold the breath and bear down during defecation.
- Instruct the patient to advise the nurse and physician of problems such as difficulty breathing or noisy breath sounds, mucous plugs or bloody secretions, chest discomfort, increased sputum, thick malodorous secretions, fever, decreased stoma size, redness or skin breakdown around the stoma, and dysphagia.
- If a tracheotomy appliance is used, instruct the patient to change the twill tape tie when wet, dirty, or frayed. Someone should assist if the appliance is dislodged. The tube should be changed once a week. The tube should be cleaned with mild soap and water or equal parts of hydrogen peroxide and water. It should be rinsed well, air dried, and stored in a clean, covered container.

Adapted from Dawson C, Fitzpatrick K: Part V, nursing protocols. In Hoffman HT et al, editors: *Iowa head and neck protocols: surgery, nursing and speech pathology,* San Diego, Calif, 2000, Singular, pp 629-41.

dentist and dental hygienist can provide important teaching regarding oral care to prevent or lessen the side effects of radiation therapy as well as to catch problems early. It is ideal for the patient to visit the dentist before beginning

Box 29-11   Quality-of-Life Scales for Use with Patients with Head and Neck Cancers

- The M.D. Anderson Dysphagia Inventory (Chen et al, 2001)
- The Performance Status Scale for Head and Neck Cancer Patients (List et al, 1996)
- The Functional Assessment of Cancer Therapy-Head and Neck Scale (List et al, 1996)
- The Head and Neck Radiotherapy Questionnaire (Browman et al, 1993)
- The University of Michigan Head and Neck Quality of Life Questionnaire (Terrell, Fisher, and Wolf, 1998)
- The European Organisation for Research and Treatment of Cancer Core Quality of Life Questionnaire (Hammerlid et al, 1997)

radiation therapy. If this is not possible or has not occurred in the chronic head and neck cancer patient, then a visit to the dentist as soon as possible is critical (National Oral Health Information Clearing House, 2002).

Drug Therapy

One of the major problems faced by the patient with head or neck cancer is pain. Pain can be an issue at the time of initial diagnosis, throughout treatment, and sometimes for the rest of the patient's life (Thompson, 2000). Pain is a subjective experience, and its treatment must be individualized as well. The nurse must be armed with the facts based on scientific evidence, rather than fear or misinformation, to adequately treat the patient experiencing pain. Many different classes of drug are used to treat patients with head and neck cancer, including tricyclic antidepressants, antiseizure drugs, and drugs that treat pain.

Opioids have been and remain the drug class of choice for the treatment of moderate to severe head and neck cancer pain. This class of drug includes a variety of agents that can be given by various routes, do not have a maximum dose (a ceiling effect), have predictable and manageable side effects, and, except for meperidine, lack dangerous toxicities. Morphine is the prototype of the opioids. Unfortunately, pain in head and neck cancer patients is sometimes undertreated. In addition, because many patients who develop head and neck cancers have a history of alcohol and nicotine abuse, these patients may also be substance abusers. Therefore, the nurse must understand the appropriate use of opioids for the aggressive management of pain and the need for diligent monitoring in these patients, in the hopes of improving their quality of life (Thompson, 2000).

Opioids have unique pharmacologic properties: they do not damage organs, they do not have a ceiling effect, they rarely cause respiratory depression in opioid-tolerant patients, and, although they do cause physical dependence, they do not cause addiction. It bears repeating that although tolerance and physical dependence are to be expected in long-term opioid use, this does not mean the patient is addicted to the drug (Thompson, 2000). Tolerance means that higher doses of the opioid are required over time to maintain pain relief. Physical dependence means that if the patient were to stop taking the opioid suddenly, he or she would experience withdrawal symptoms. Thus, if an opioid is to be discontinued, the dosage is tapered to avoid putting the patient into a withdrawal state.

For the head and neck cancer patient who is also a substance abuser, treatment of chronic pain can present challenges. Initially, such a patient is to be treated as is any non–substance abusing patient. The patient's complaint of pain is to be believed. The use of a behavioral contract regarding the appropriate use of opioids can be useful in this population (Thompson, 2000). If over time, however, the nurse and other members of the interdisciplinary team note drug-seeking behaviors, a referral to a drug treatment program may be in order.

Dietitian

For head and neck cancer patients, a proactive stance regarding nutritional status is taken prior to initial treatment because it is known that difficulties with swallowing and chewing will most likely appear after treatment. In the chronic stages of the illness, the patient with an advanced tumor and oral defects or swallowing problems caused by treatments and surgeries may have continuing problems maintaining an adequate nutritional status (Mood, 1997). "Nutritional failure is a significant morbidity factor in head and neck cancer patients, stemming from both poor eating habits that are common among heavy drinkers and a high incidence of cachexia" (Mood, 1997, p. 279). Therefore, the patient's nutritional status must continue to be evaluated at regular intervals long after treatment.

Assessment should address weight changes, dietary intake, functional status, symptoms affecting nutrition, physical examination findings, and nutritional problems that might be projected to occur with continued treatment and/or disease progression (Brown, 2002). Biochemical indicators (laboratory tests) of nutritional status include levels of albumin, prealbumin, transferrin, and retinol-binding protein (Brown, 2002). The consistency of food may have to be changed. Liquids can be thickened with commercial thickeners if necessary. Food preparation may have to be altered with a focus on how the food tastes (Feber, 2000). When patients are identified as malnourished or at risk for malnourishment, a dietary consult is in order. Not only does malnutrition have physical consequences in this population, but the ability to eat normally and with family and friends affects the patient's experience of quality of life (Cremonese, Bryden, and Bottcher, 2000).

Nurse

In addition to performing the specific nursing interventions already mentioned in previous sections of this chapter, the nurse has a crucial role to play in the ongoing care of the patient with chronic head and neck cancer. Because so many different health care professionals are required for the care of this population, it is the nurse's responsibility to coordinate and evaluate the patient's complex treatment plan. It is also the nurse's responsibility to help the patient understand what roles the other members of the interdisciplinary team play and why each member of the team is critical to the plan of care for that specific patient. As a patient educator, the nurse helps the patient prepare for and manage the side effects of treatments. The nurse assists the patient in managing pain, caring for wounds if present, following eating regimens, and dealing with emotional issues (Mood, 1997) and makes referrals to other members of the team as necessary. The nurse reinforces what other members of the team have already taught the patient. Regardless of the setting, the nurse is also responsible for coordinating the teaching done in multiple settings (Padberg and Padberg, 2000). For instance, the home care nurse must know what teaching has already occurred in the inpatient setting so that the appropriate continuity and reinforcement can occur.

The goal of patient education is to effect some change in the learner (Padberg and Padberg, 2000). Because many head and neck cancer patients use alcohol and nicotine, patient education and referral to substance abuse programs to help patients quit the use of these substances is a priority. Another area of education in which the nurse can be instrumental is that of exercise. Exercise has also been shown to increase quality of life; improve functional capacity, muscle strength, body composition, and hematologic indicators; and reduce nausea, fatigue, diarrhea, anxiety, and depression in cancer patients (Brown, 2002).

Speech Therapist

One of the primary rehabilitation goals for the head and neck cancer patient is the restoration and/or preservation of swallowing. The speech therapist, radiation oncologist, and advanced practice nurse conduct a swallowing evaluation collaboratively. Swallowing function is evaluated with video-fluoroscopy and a modified cookie barium swallow test using both pastes and liquids. The presence or absence of aspiration is noted. The amount of pharyngeal residue after swallowing and the transit time are measured. Acceptable swallowing function must be present for the patient to resume normal feedings. Alternative methods of using the tongue must be taught to the patient if tongue function in propelling the bolus of food to the back of the mouth is in any way impaired. Patients with impaired pharyngeal reflexes or impaired inferior laryngeal sphincter function do not adapt as well to alternative methods of transporting food in the mouth (Harris, 2000). These patients may need prolonged use of alternative methods of receiving nutrition, such as enteral delivery of nutrition through a gastrostomy tube.

Patients who have undergone partial laryngectomies require speech therapy to strengthen the remaining portions of the voice box to improve voice quality and strength. In addition, these patients must learn to compensate for reduced laryngeal closure in an effort to avoid aspiration (Harris, 2000).

Patients who have undergone total laryngectomy are unable to speak. However, restorative speech methods are available that will compensate for this loss. An artificial larynx is an electronic vibrating device that resonates sound into the oral cavity and generates mechanical, robotlike speech. This method is easy to learn. Production of esophageal speech requires that the patient learn to swallow air into the esophagus and burp up this air at the moment of articulation. This method requires no equipment but can take up to 6 months to learn. Finally, in tracheoesophageal puncture, a one-way plastic valve prosthesis is placed surgically that provides airflow from the lung to the esophagus to the mouth when the stoma is occluded. This method of speech restoration allows fluent, easy-to-learn speech and prevents aspiration. It requires that the patient have an adequate stoma size, an intact cricopharyngeal muscle, and good hand-eye coordination and bimanual dexterity. The patient must learn to clean, maintain, and insert the prosthesis (Harris, 2000).

Medical Social Worker

Typically, the functional variables of breathing, speaking, and eating are taken into account in planning the treatment of the head and neck cancer patient. However, because the treatments for these diagnoses can involve significant disfigurement, distortion of features, and functional impairments, psychosocial variables also influence overall quality of life and outcomes (D'Antonio et al, 1998; Harris, 2000; Mood, 1997). In patients with long histories of smoking and drinking, the sense of having caused their malignancy adds to their stress and anxiety, which can hinder their recovery (Harris, 2000).

Depression, which is associated with anger and anxiety, can be a factor in treatment nonadherence (Harris, 2000). Malnutrition and poor self-care may also be symptoms of depression (Mood, 1997). The social worker can refer such a patient for counseling and put the patient in touch with other patients who have undergone the same treatments. These have been found to be effective rehabilitative strategies (Mood, 1997).

Although sadness is an expected response to a cancer diagnosis, if that sadness lasts for 2 weeks or longer, depression must be considered (Lovejoy et al, 2000). In the depressed patient with chronic head and neck cancer, ongoing psychotherapy and antidepressant treatment may be called for to enhance nutritional status and self-care ability, as well as to improve overall quality of life. If the social worker suspects depression in a patient, a referral to a psychiatrist is in order. Lovejoy et al (2000) suggest cognitive behavioral therapy as a viable means of promoting recovery from cancer-related depression. The social worker is also instrumental in connecting both the patient and family with community resources.

COMPLEMENTARY AND ALTERNATIVE THERAPIES

Complementary and alternative medicine (CAM) is highly sought after in the general cancer population (National Cancer Institute, 1999). Of 26 National Cancer Institute–designated centers in the United States, 88% have CAM staff members at the institution and 54% offer CAM programs for patients. Currently, a variety of CAM modalities are popular with patients with cancer. These include dietary protocols (macrobiotics, the Gerson method) (Cunningham and Herbert, 2000), guided imagery, meditation and relaxation, art therapy, biofeedback, music therapy, acupuncture, and yoga, among others. CAM therapies used by the general population in the United States also include herbal medicine, folk medicine, energy healing, and homeopathy (Eisenberg et al, 1998).

According to the Oncology Nursing Society (2000), the most important aspect of CAM use is that the patient be comfortable disclosing the use of CAM modalities to the health care providers and that health care providers seek to establish evidence for CAM use. This means that the patient's choices must be accepted while, at the same time, evidence-based information is provided so that the patient can make an educated and intelligent choice regarding care. In the head and neck cancer population, patients who sought out CAM modalities were found to be younger, more affluent, and better educated than those who did not (Warrick et al, 1999).

PALLIATIVE CARE

Palliative care may be required for patients with advanced head and neck cancer that is resistant to treatment. Cancer that continues to spread (locally and/or to distant sites) despite treatment may require a shift from curative care to palliative care. Symptoms related to incurable head and neck cancers, such as increasing dysphagia, weight loss, chronic pain, fistulas, and fungating tumors, require palliative interventions to promote comfort.

Radiation may be given palliatively to reduce pain and other symptoms in incurable cancer. This treatment usually entails giving a moderate dose of radiation over a short time to shrink the tumor while reducing the side effects of the radiation (Radiological Society of North America, 2002). Another radiation therapy approach may be necessary to treat a patient who has a recurrence of a tumor in a previously irradiated area, which limits the possibility for another full-course treatment (Schleicher, Andreopoulos, and Ammon, 2001).

Multimodal therapy for locally advanced squamous cell carcinoma of the head and neck may also be used for organ preservation and palliation. This therapy, however, may result in undesirable side effects such as severe mucositis, neutropenia, and renal toxicity (Poole et al, 2001). The benefits of palliative treatments versus the burdens of treatments in a terminally ill patient must be given careful consideration. The overriding question must be whether the treatments will contribute to the patient's quality of life.

END-OF-LIFE CARE

Referral of the patient with end-stage head and neck cancer to hospice care should be considered. If curative measures are no longer effective, death appears inevitable, and the patient and family wish that comfort measures only be provided, then a referral to hospice care is appropriate. The hospice interdisciplinary team consists of a physician, nurse, social worker, chaplain, and volunteers who provide specialized palliative measures to ensure the best quality of life for the patient until death. Excellent pain and symptom management and emotional and spiritual supports are hallmarks of good end-of-life care.

In hospice care, the patient and family are considered to be one integral unit, because the impending death greatly affects not only the patient but all family members as well. Because most end-stage cancer patients are cared for in the home by the family, it is critical that the hospice team instruct the patient and family in how to provide comfort measures and support in the face of the multitude of challenges presented by disease progression and the dying process. See Box 29-12 for issues facing the family as caregiver. Continual assessment, development of a plan of care, and its implementation and evaluation by the hospice team are needed to provide the best physical, emotional, and spiritual care possible during this end-of-life stage.

ETHICAL CONSIDERATIONS

Decisions to treat head and neck cancer often involve a threat to a person's sense of intactness because of the resulting disfigurement and dysfunction. Can the patient tolerate such a fundamental change in personal identity? "Patients with head and neck cancers may be more vulnerable with their values

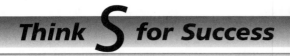

Think S for Success

Symptoms
- Treat symptoms with a focus on increased function and quality of life.
- Symptoms include trismus, vision deficits, dental caries, chronic mucositis, alterations in taste, xerostomia, olfactory impairment, hypothyroidism, risk of aspiration, lymphedema, disfigurement, osteoradionecrosis, alterations in skin, obstructive sleep apnea.

Sequelae
- Encourage adherence to the treatment regimen, which includes ongoing evaluations by members of interdisciplinary health care team.

Safety
- Teach patient and family the importance of proper nutrition and wound care.
- Assess for depression.
- Prevent aspiration, ensure proper mouth care.

Support/Services
- Assist patient in obtaining counseling and peer support, locating cancer survivor groups, and reintegrating into the community.
- Help patient with health insurance as needed.
- Refer to substance abuse groups if needed.

Satisfaction
- Determine degree to which patient's functional status and/or disfigurement is interfering with quality of life and take measures to help patient reach desired quality of life.

far more at stake than patients with other serious diseases" (Schenck, 2002, p. 1). Ethical considerations involve quality-of-life issues such as "self-image, coping abilities, social relationships, performance and functional abilities ..." (Schenck, 2002, p. 2). Other patient issues include autonomy, the meaning of life-threatening disease, the question of informed consent in highly vulnerable patients, and the line between physician persuasion and coercion (Schenck, 2002).

Box 29-12   Family and Caregiver Issues

- Difficulty adjusting to family member's disfigurement and lifestyle changes
- Fear of cancer recurrence and death
- Financial strain
- Changes in role expectations
- Physical and emotional exhaustion
- Challenges related to food preparation and eating
- Potential alcohol and tobacco withdrawal

CASE STUDY
Patient Data
Mr. K. is a 62-year-old retired factory worker. He lives with his wife, age 58, and one unmarried adult daughter in a small two-bedroom house in an urban area. They have another married daughter who lives out of the state. Mr. K.'s wife works at a local grocery store, and his daughter is living with them because of a recent divorce and the resulting financial difficulties.

Mr. K. is currently experiencing many problems related to the total laryngectomy he underwent 6 months earlier, which was preceded by a full course of radiation therapy. He is having difficulties coping with his altered body image and the need to breathe through a hole in his neck. Managing the care of the stoma is difficult for him, and he is having problems with excessive secretions. In addition, he is experiencing some weight loss secondary to a decreased sense of smell that impairs his enjoyment of food and some difficulty swallowing because of a "feeling of tightness in his throat." He struggles with not being able to smoke and he is no longer drinking alcohol.

His greatest frustration, however, is with his loss of speech. Mr. K. is unhappy with the electrolarynx appliance and speech clarity. He feels that the speech produced with the device is "robotic" and that he cannot make himself understood by others. He writes on a tablet, "My life is so miserable now, I have nothing left that I can enjoy. It is so depressing." He indicates that he has stopped socializing with others outside of his family because of these embarrassing and stressful problems. His wife and daughter are at a loss to help him. His daughter, in particular, finds the stoma and excessive secretions repulsive.

Mr. K. has a history of smoking two packs of cigarettes per day for the past 40 years. He typically had three to four beers each night after he returned from his factory job. Once he retired, he changed his drinking habits to two drinks of hard liquor each evening before dinner. At times he would have another drink before bedtime because it "helped me to sleep." At retirement, Mr. K. was of normal weight for his size and had no previous history of pathology.

Nine months earlier Mr. K. began to experience difficulty swallowing and had a persistent sore throat and hoarseness. He lost 15 lb over 2 months. His wife insisted that he seek medical attention. Initially he was resistant, saying, "If something is wrong, I don't want to know about it." He finally agreed when his difficulty swallowing became more severe.

Diagnostic Findings
■ A palpable mass was found in the lower neck.
■ Radiography and laryngoscopy revealed a tumor in the larynx.
■ Incisional biopsy of the tumor indicated a malignant, poorly differentiated, high-grade tumor.

■ MRI revealed regional lymph node involvement.
■ No distant metastasis was noted.

After consultation with the radiation oncologist and otolaryngologic surgeon, Mr. K. received a full series of radiation therapy and then underwent a total laryngectomy and removal of metastatic regional lymph nodes. Treatment was concluded 6 months ago, and there has been no tumor recurrence at this time.

Thinking It Through
■ What nursing diagnoses pertain to Mr. K.?
■ What is the psychosocial impact of being a cancer patient and having a tracheotomy?
■ What are the physical challenges of laryngectomy?
■ How can the interdisciplinary health care team improve Mr. K.'s quality of life?
■ What physical and emotional challenges must Mr. K. overcome? How would you as the nurse assist Mr. K. in coping with these problems?

Case Conference
Attending the team conference are Mr. and Mrs. K., the physician, nurse, social worker, speech therapist, and dietitian. Mrs. K. shares with the team the problems Mr. K. is exhibiting at home. She expresses her concerns regarding his episodes of difficulty breathing, periodic choking, isolation of himself, and refusal to participate in any family activities or even leave the house.

The physician refers Mr. K. to a psychiatrist for assessment and pharmacologic management of his depression. The social worker makes an appointment to meet with Mr. K. to begin a course of cognitive-behavioral therapy. The social worker also refers Mr. K. to a peer support group of other laryngectomy patients and provides Mrs. K. with a videotape that was made especially to help families learn to adjust and cope with a family member who has undergone a laryngectomy.

Arrangements are made for a number of home nursing visits so the nurse can assess Mr. K.'s ability to care for his stoma. Reteaching can occur as needed in the home with the materials Mr. K. usually uses. The speech therapist also plans a home visit with Mr. K. to review his electrolarynx speech and help him learn to use this equipment better to make himself more easily understood. Because Mr. K.'s weight has dropped since surgery, the dietitian makes suggestions to Mrs. K. about enhancing the flavor of cooked foods with stronger spices and the use of nutritional supplements. Although Mr. K. does not seem very enthusiastic at the end of the team conference, he agrees to keep these appointments. Mrs. K. seems relieved that help and support are available.

Internet and Other Resources

American Cancer Society: *http://www.cancer.org*
Cancer Information Services: 800-4-Cancer
Cancerfax: fax-on-demand service, 800-624-2511
CancerMail Service: E-mail *cancermail@cips.nci.nih.gov*
HNCancer.com: *http://www.hncancer.com*
Let's Face It USA: *http://www.faceit.org*
Memorial Sloan-Kettering Cancer Center: *http://www.mskcc.org*
National Cancer Institute: *http://www.cancer.gov*
National Coalition for Cancer Survivorship: *http://www.cancer advocacy.org*
Oncology Channel, Head and Neck Cancer: *http://www.oncology channel.com/headneck/*

People Living with Cancer: *http://www.peoplelivingwithcancer.org*
Support for People with Oral and Head and Neck Cancer (SPOHNC): *http://www.spohnc.org*

REFERENCES

Ackerstaff AH et al: Complications, functional disorders and lifestyle changes after total laryngectomy, *Clin Otolaryngol* 19:295-300, 1994.

Ahne et al: Assessment of gustatory function by means of tasting tablets, *Laryngoscope* 110(8):1396-401, 2000.

American Cancer Society: How are laryngeal and hypopharyngeal cancer diagnosed? 2004, retrieved from *http://www.cancer.org/docroot/CRI/CRI_2_1X.asp?dt=23* on Aug 12, 2002.

Albino JE: A psychologist's guide to oral diseases and disorders and their treatment, *Prof Psychol Res Pr* 33(2):176-82, 2002.

Andersen PE et al: Management of the orbit during anterior fossa craniofacial resection, *Arch Otolaryngol Head Neck Surg* 122:1305-7, 1996.

Brady L, Davis L: Treatment of head and neck cancer by radiation therapy, *Semin Oncol* 15(1):29-38, 1988.

Bromley SM: Smell and taste disorders: a primary care approach, *Am Fam Physician* 61:427-36, 2000.

Browman GP et al: The Head and Neck Radiotherapy Questionnaire: a morbidity/quality of life instrument for clinical trials of radiation therapy in locally advanced head and neck cancer, *J Clin Oncol* 11:863-72, 1993.

Brown JK: A systematic review of the evidence on symptom management of cancer-related anorexia and cachexia, *Oncol Nurs Forum* 29:517-30, 2002.

Bryant RA: *Acute and chronic wounds: nursing management,* ed 2, St Louis, 2000, Mosby.

Carvalho AL et al: Predictive factors for diagnosis of advanced-stage squamous cell carcinoma of the head and neck, *Arch Otolaryngol Head Neck Surg* 128:313-8, 2002.

Celik N et al: Osteoradionecrosis of the mandible after oromandibular cancer surgery, *Plast Reconstr Surg* 109:1875-81, 2002.

Centre for Health Promotion, University of Toronto: The quality of life model, 2003, retrieved from *http://www.utoronto.ca/qol/concepts.htm* on May 25, 2003.

Chen AY et al: The development and validation of a dysphagia-specific quality-of-life questionnaire for patients with head and neck cancer. The M. D. Anderson dysphagia inventory, *Arch Otolaryngol Head Neck Surg* 127:870-6, 2001.

Collier M: The assessment of patients with malignant fungating wounds: a holistic approach, *Nurs Times* 93(44)A, 93(45)B, 1997 (Professional Update insert).

Cremonese G, Bryden G, Bottcher C: An interdisciplinary team approach to preservation of quality of life for patients following oral cancer surgery, *ORL Head Neck Nurs* 18(2):7-11, 2000.

Cunningham RS, Herbert V: Nutrition as a component of alternative therapy, *Semin Oncol Nurs* 16(2):163-9, 2000.

Cyr M, Higgins T, McGuire M: Laryngeal, hypopharyngeal conditions and care. In Harris L, Huntoon M, editors: *Core curriculum for otorhinolaryngology and head and neck nursing,* New Smyrna Beach, Fla, 1998, Society of Otorhinolaryngology and Head-Neck Nurses, pp 275-90.

D'Antonio LL et al: Quality of life and functional status measures with head and neck cancer, *Arch Otolaryngol Head Neck Surg* 122:482-7, 1996.

D'Antonio LL et al: Relationship between quality of life and depression in patients with head and neck cancer, *Laryngoscope* 108:806-11, 1998.

Dunne-Daly CF: Potential long-term and late effects from radiation therapy, *Cancer Nurs* 18:(1):67-79, 1995.

Eisenberg DM et al: Trends in alternative medicine use in the United States 1990-1997: results of a follow-up national survey, *JAMA* 280:1569-75, 1998.

Feber T: *Head and neck oncology nursing,* Philadelphia, 2000, Whurr.

Friedman M et al: The occurrence of sleep-disordered breathing among patients with head and neck cancer, *Laryngoscope* 111:1917-9, 2001.

Gaziano JE: Evaluation and management of oropharyngeal dysphagia in head and neck cancer, *Cancer Control* 9(5):23-9, 2002.

Giuliano J, Rudy S: Nursing care of the patient with trismus, *ORL Head Neck Nurs* 13(1):23-30, 1995.

Hammerlid E et al: Prospective, longitudinal quality-of-life study of patients with head and neck cancer: a feasibility study including the EORTC QLQ-C30, *Otolaryngol Head Neck Surg* 116:666-73, 1997.

Harris L: Head and neck malignancies. In Yarbro CH et al, editors: *Cancer nursing: principles and practice,* ed 5, Sudbury, Mass, 2000, Jones and Bartlett, pp 1210-43.

Ho W et al: Change in olfaction after radiotherapy for nasopharyngeal cancer: a prospective study, *Am J Otolaryngol* 23(4):209-14, 2002.

Hoffman HT et al: The national cancer data base report on cancer of the head and neck, *Arch Otolaryngol Head Neck Surg* 124:951-62, 1998.

Hunter SE, Scher RL: Clinical implications of radionecrosis to the head and neck surgeon, *Otolaryngol Head Neck Surg* 11(2):103-6, 2003.

Jansma J et al: Protocol for the prevention of treatment of oral sequelae resulting from radiation therapy, *Cancer* 70:2171-3, 1992.

Jay S, Ruddy J, Cullen RJ: Laryngectomy: the patient's view, *J Laryngol Otolaryngol* 105:934-8, 1991.

Kwong DL et al: Sensorineural hearing loss in patients treated for nasopharyngeal cancer: a prospective study of the effect of radiation and cisplatin treatment, *Int J Radiat Oncol Biol Phys* 36(2):281-9, 1996.

List MA et al: The performance status scale for head and neck cancer patients and the functional assessment of cancer therapy-head and neck scale, *Cancer* 77:2294-301, 1996.

Lovejoy NC et al: Cancer-related depression: part I—neurologic alterations and cognitive-behavioral therapy, *Oncol Nurs Forum* 27:667-78, 2000.

Low WK, Fong WK: Long term hearing status after radiotherapy for nasopharyngeal carcinoma, *Auris Nasus Larynx* 25(1):21-4, 1998.

Mathong RH et al: Rehabilitation of patients with extended facial and craniofacial resection, *Laryngoscope* 107(1):30-9, 1997.

McGuire M: Current trends in management of head and neck cancer, *Dev Support Cancer Care* 3:30-9, 1999.

McGuire M: Nutritional care of surgical oncology patients, *Semin Oncol Nurs* 16(2):128-34, 2000.

Miller BA et al, editors: Racial/ethnic patterns of cancer in the United States 1988-1992, National Cancer Institute, NIH Pub No. 96-4014, Bethesda, Md, 1996.

Mood DW: Cancers of the head and neck. In Varricchio C, editor: *A cancer source book for nurses,* ed 7, Atlanta, Ga, 1997, American Cancer Society, pp 271-83.

Murphy C et al: Prevalence of olfactory impairment in older adults, *JAMA* 228:2307-12, 2002.

National Cancer Institute: Complementary and alternative medicine resources at NCI–designated cancer centers, Survey results, 1999, retrieved from *http://cpen.nci.nih.gov/planning_resources/cam_survey_results.* on Feb 23, 2004.

National Cancer Institute: Head and neck cancer: questions and answers, 2002, retrieved from *http://www.cancer.gov/cancer_information/cancer_type/head_and_* on Feb 23, 2004.

National Oral Health Information Clearing House: Radiation treatment and your mouth, 2002, from *http://www.nohic.nidcr.nih.gov/campaign/rad_bro.htm* retrieved on Aug 12, 2002.

Newell R, Marks I: Phobic nature of social difficulty in facially disfigured people, *Br J Psychiatry* 176:177-81, 2000.

Ohizumi Y et al: Complications following re-irradiation for head and neck cancer, *Am J Otolaryngol* 23(4):215-21, 2002.

Oncology Nursing Society: Oncology Nursing Society position on the use of complementary and alternative therapies in cancer care, *Oncol Nurs Forum* 27:749, 2000.

Otto SE, editor: *Oncology nursing,* ed 4, St Louis, 2001, Mosby.

Padberg LF, Padberg RM: Patient education and support. In Yarbro CH et al, editors: *Cancer nursing: principles and practice,* ed 5, Sudbury, Mass, 2000, Jones and Bartlett, pp 1609-31.

Papadas T et al: Rehabilitation after laryngectomy: a practical approach and guidelines for patients, *J Cancer Educ* 17(1):37-9, 2002.

Piso DU et al: Early rehabilitation of head-neck edema after curative surgery for orofacial tumors, *Am J Phys Med Rehabil* 80:261-9, 2001.

Poole MD et al: Chemoradiation for locally advanced squamous cell carcinoma of the head and neck for organ preservation and palliation, *Arch Otolaryngol Head Neck Surg* 127:1446-50, 2001.

Price E: The stigma of smell, *Nurs Times* 92(20):70-1, 1996.

Radiological Society of North America: Head and neck cancer, 2004, retrieved from *http://www.radiologyinfo.org/content/therapy/thera%2Dhd%5Fneck* on Feb 23, 2002.

Ritchie CS: Oral health, taste and olfaction, *Clin Geriatr Med* 18:709-17, 2002.

Robbins M, Gosselin TK: Symptom management in radiation oncology, *Am J Nurs* 102(suppl 4):32-6, 2002.

Rogers SN: Surgical principles and techniques for functional rehabilitation after oral cavity and oropharyngeal oncologic surgery, *Otolaryngol Head Neck Surg* 9(2):114-9, 2001.

Schenck DP: Ethical considerations in the treatment of head and neck cancer, *Cancer Control* 9:410-9, 2002, retrieved from *http://www.medscape.com/viewarticle/442599_print*.

Schiffman S: Taste and smell in disease, *N Engl J Med* 308:1275-9, 1983.

Schleicher UM, Andreopoulos D, Ammon J: Palliative radiotherapy in recurrent head and neck tumors by a percutaneous superfractionated treatment schedule, *Int J Radiat Oncol Biol Phys* 50(1):65-8, 2001.

Sherry VW: Taste alterations among patients with cancer, *Clin J Oncol Nurs* 6(2):73-7, 2002.

Sinard RJ et al: Hypothyroidism after treatment for nonthyroid head and neck cancer, *Arch Otolaryngol Head Neck Surg* 126:652-7, 2000.

Stack KM, Papas AS: Xerostomia: etiology and clinical management, *Nutr Clin Care* 4(1):15-21, 2001.

Stam HT, Koopmans JP, Mathieson CM: The psychosocial impact of laryngectomy: a comprehensive assessment, *J Psychosoc Oncol* 9(3):37-58, 1991.

Taneja C et al: Changing patterns of failure of head and neck cancer, *Arch Otolaryngol Head Neck Surg* 128:324-7, 2002.

Terrell JE, Fisher SG, Wolf GT: Long-term quality of life after treatment of laryngeal cancer, *Arch Otolaryngol Head Neck Surg* 124:964-71, 1998.

Thompson AR: Opioids and their proper use as analgesics in the management of head and neck cancer patients, *Am J Otolaryngol* 21:244-54, 2000.

Trotti A, Mocharnuk RS: Management of radiation-induced toxicity in patients with head and neck cancer, 2001, *Medscape Hematology-Oncology eJournal* 4(2), retrieved from *http://www.medscape.com*.

van Dam FS et al: Deterioration of olfaction and gustation as a consequence of total laryngectomy, *Laryngoscope* 109(7, pt 1):1150-5, 1999.

Warrick PD et al: Use of alternative medicine among patients with head and neck cancer, *Arch Otolaryngol Head Neck Surg* 125:573-9, 1999.

Weinstein GS et al:. Laryngeal preservation with supracricoid partial laryngectomy results in improved quality of life when compared with total laryngectomy, *Laryngoscope* 111(2):191-9, 2001.

Williams A, Venables J: Skin care in patients with uncomplicated lymphedema, *J Wound Care* 5:223-6, 1996.

Yarbro CY, Frogge MH, Goodman M: *Cancer symptom management,* ed 2, Sudbury, Mass, 1999, Jones and Bartlett.

CHAPTER 30

Cancer of the Breast

Fatma Youssef, DNSc, RN

OBJECTIVES

After reading this chapter, you should be able to do the following:

- Describe the epidemiology and etiology of breast cancer
- Describe the pathophysiology of breast cancer
- Describe the clinical manifestations of breast cancer
- Compare and contrast chronic implications of breast cancer treatment modalities
- Describe the functional health patterns affected by breast cancer
- Describe the therapeutic approaches and nursing management in the care of patients with breast cancer
- Describe the role of each member of the interdisciplinary team involved in the care and follow-up of breast cancer survivors
- Describe the indications for use, side effects, and nursing considerations related to drugs recently used to treat and support breast cancer survivors
- Compare issues of survivorship in the three seasons of survival

Breast cancer accounts for one out of every three cancer diagnoses in the United States and is the leading cause of death for women between the ages of 45 and 50 years. It is second in frequency only to skin cancer among American women. The lifetime risk for breast cancer is 12%, which means that one in eight women will be affected. In 2002, approximately 203,500 women were diagnosed with invasive breast cancer nationally; about 77% of these were older than age 50 years. An estimated 40,000 died from the disease in 2002 (American Cancer Society, 2003).

Despite advances in detection and treatment, breast cancer statistics remain daunting because breast cancer affects women of all ages, races, ethnicity, socioeconomic strata, and geographic areas. Breast cancer is expected to continue to be the most common cancer diagnosed in women. It is the most frequently diagnosed cancer among women in nearly every social and ethnic group, including African Americans, Alaskan Natives, Native Americans, Chinese, Filipinos, Hawaiians and Pacific Islanders, Hispanics, Japanese, and Koreans (Brinker and Winston, 2001).

Breast cancer among men accounts for about 1% of all breast cancer cases. Approximately 1500 cases of breast cancer and 400 deaths from the disease occurred in men in 2002 (Vogel, 2003). Although men are at low risk of developing breast cancer, they should be aware of risk factors, especially family history, and report any changes in their breasts to a health care provider.

According to Jackson (2002), more than 2 million breast cancer survivors are living in the United States today. Recently, there has been an apparent increase in the incidence of breast cancer due to the adoption of early detection measures. More than 90% of those with breast cancer survive for 5 years after diagnosis. For all cancer survivors, what begins as a crisis involving diagnosis and treatment gradually becomes a chronic illness characterized by lifelong follow-up medical care, permanent psychological effects, and changes in social and employment relationships (Hoskins, Harber, and Budin, 2001; Susan G. Komen Breast Cancer Foundation, 2001).

Based on recent data (Ries et al, 2001), survival rates for women diagnosed with breast cancer are as follows:

- 86% at 5 years after diagnosis
- 76% after 10 years
- 58% after 15 years
- 53% after 20 years

The 5-year survival rates for breast cancer increase with age at diagnosis until age 75 (Box 30-1). Researchers speculate that younger women have lower survival rates because their tumors may be more aggressive and less responsive to hormonal therapies (American Cancer Society, 2002). In addition, the 5-year relative survival rate is lower for women with a more advanced stage of disease at diagnosis (Ries et al, 2001).

African American women with breast cancer are less likely than white women to survive for 5 years (72% versus 87%). This difference can be attributed to the fact that the disease is at a later stage at detection and that tumors are more aggressive and less responsive to treatment in African American women (Greenlee et al, 2001). A lack of health insurance is associated with lower survival rates among breast cancer patients. Moreover, patients with a low income have lower 5-year survival rates than higher-income patients. Low-income African American women are three times more likely than

Box 30-1   Factors That Influence Survival after Breast Cancer

- Time since diagnosis
- Age at diagnosis
- Stage at diagnosis
- Race/ethnicity
- Socioeconomic status

Box 30-3   Stages of Breast Cancer

- Stage 0: Cancer is confined
- Stage I: Cancer is localized
- Stage II: Limited spread has occurred
- Stage III: Tumor is larger and has spread to lymph nodes
- Stage IV: Cancer has spread to other parts of the body

higher-income African American women to be diagnosed with advanced disease (American Cancer Society, 2002).

PATHOPHYSIOLOGY

Breast cancer, an outgrowth of neoplastic cells of the breast, is life threatening and, when diagnosed, a life-altering disease. Now that women are living longer, the threat of breast cancer is increasing. When cells grow abnormally, these cells divide more than they should and form lumps known as tumors. Cancerous tumors can interfere with the function of normal tissues. Cells may break away from the original tumors and travel to other parts of the body by way of the bloodstream or the lymph system. Lymph nodes located in the armpit help to block the spread of cells to other parts of the body. There are several different types of breast cancer. The most common kinds are ductal carcinoma and lobular carcinoma (Box 30-2). Ductal carcinoma, which accounts for about 80% of all breast cancers, occurs in the lining of the breast ducts. Stages of breast cancer are defined in Box 30-3.

The precise cause of breast cancer is unknown. However, the etiology of the disease appears to be multifactorial, related to genetics, environmental factors, and the use of hormones. Researchers are investigating the possibility that some breast cancers are caused by inherited genetic mutations. It is believed that some breast tumors can be linked to changes in breast cancer 1 (BRCA1) and breast cancer 2 (BRCA2) genes. Mutations in these genes may interfere with the body's ability to suppress tumors. BRCA-related cancers tend to occur at a younger age (i.e., younger than age 50), and carriers tend to have tumors that are estrogen receptor negative. BRCA1 or BRCA2 mutation can impart a 60% to 85% lifetime risk for breast cancer (King et al, 2001).

Some proven risk factors for breast cancer as well as others that are suspected risk factors have now been identified (Box 30-4).

CLINICAL MANIFESTATIONS

The female breast is closely linked with womanhood, not only in the American culture but also in most other cultures.

Box 30-2   Types of Breast Cancer

NONINVASIVE BREAST CANCERS
- Ductal carcinoma in situ
  Most common type of noninvasive breast cancer
  Confined to ducts
  Does not spread through walls of the ducts
- Lobular carcinoma in situ
  Begins in lobules but does not penetrate lobule walls
  Marker of increased risk of invasive cancer in either breast

INVASIVE BREAST CANCERS
- Infiltrating ductal carcinoma
  Accounts for 80% of all breast cancers
  Starts in duct
  Invades the breast's fatty tissues
- Infiltrating lobular carcinoma
  Accounts for 10% to 15% of invasive breast cancers
  Starts at glands
  Can spread

Box 30-4   Risk Factors for Breast Cancer

PROVEN RISK FACTORS
- Female gender: more than 99% of breast cancers occur in women
- Older age: risk increases as age increases
- Early menstruation (before age 12 years)
- Late menopause (after age 55 years)
- Family history: close relative with breast cancer
- Carrier of BRCA1 or BRCA2 mutation
- Physical inactivity
- Overweight/obesity
- Use of hormone replacement therapy

POSSIBLE RISK FACTORS
- Consumption of too much alcohol
- Consumption of high-fat diet
- Never breast feeding
- Use of birth control pills

Therefore, the loss or injury of the breast is potentially psychologically devastating to a woman. The initial signs and symptoms of breast cancer are sometimes ignored (Box 30-5).

Women who discover that they have breast cancer often feel extremely uncertain about the future, which affects how well they and their families adjust to the disease both physically and emotionally. Invasive or infiltrating cancer moves beyond the original site and invades other parts of the breast. Infiltrating ductal carcinomas account for about 80% of invasive breast cancers. Infiltrating lobular cancers account for only 10% to 15% of invasive cancers (see Box 30-2).

According to Ferrell et al (1997), long-term survivors of breast cancer are challenged to direct their energy from issues of cancer treatment and early side effects toward issues of long-term survivorship, such as premature menopause, infertility, fear of recurrence, family distress, and uncertainty.

DIAGNOSIS

Screening tests for breast cancer are performed regularly when no unusual symptoms have occurred. These include mammography, clinical breast examination, and breast self-examination (Figure 30-1). Diagnostic tests are performed after a suspicious condition has been found. Such testing may include a diagnostic mammogram, ultrasonography, and/or biopsy (Figure 30-2).

If a lump is detected through mammography, its size and the nature of its growth must be assessed. Ultrasonography or biopsy may be recommended for further testing. Ultrasonographic examination generally can distinguish between a liquid-filled cyst and a solid lump in the breast. If the lump is solid, biopsy options are discussed with the patient (Box 30-6).

Newer imaging techniques may be used to obtain information about a tumor detected by another method. These techniques generate a computerized image that the physician then analyzes for the presence of an abnormal breast lump. These methods include digital mammography and positron emission tomography (PET).

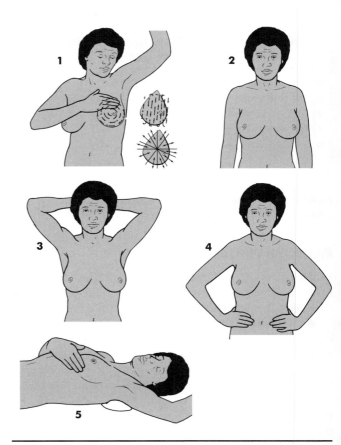

Figure 30-1 Breast self-examination and patient instructions. *1,* While in the shower or bath, when the skin is slippery with soap and water, examine your breasts. Use the pads of your second, third, and fourth fingers to firmly press every part of the breast. Use your right hand to examine your left breast, and use your left hand to examine your right breast. Using the pads of the fingers on your left hand, examine the entire breast by making small circular motions in a spiral or in an up-and-down motion so that the entire breast is examined. Repeat the procedure using your right hand to examine your left breast. Repeat pattern of palpation under the arm. Check for any lump, hard knot, or thickening of the tissue. *2,* Look at your breasts in a mirror. Stand with your arms at your sides. *3,* Raise your arms overhead and check for any changes in the shape of your breasts, dimpling of the skin, or changes in the nipple. *4,* Place your hands on your hips and press down firmly, tightening the pectoral muscles. Observe for asymmetry or changes, keeping in mind that your breasts probably do not exactly match. *5,* While lying down, feel your breasts as described in step 1. When examining your right breast, place a folded towel under your right shoulder and put your right hand behind your head. Repeat the procedure while examining your left breast. Mark your calendar that you have completed your breast self-examination; note any changes or unique characteristics you want to check with your health care provider. (From Lewis SM, Heitkemper MM, Dirksen SR: *Medical-surgical nursing: assessment and management of clinical problems,* ed 6, St Louis, 2004, Mosby.)

Box 30-5 Signs and Symptoms of Breast Cancer

- A breast lump that may or may not be painful
- An unusual increase in the size or shape of one breast
- A change in the texture of the skin of the breast (scaliness, pitting, etc.)
- An unusual swelling of the upper arm or enlargement of the lymph nodes
- A change in the appearance of the nipple (scaling, inversion, etc.)
- An unusual discharge from the nipple

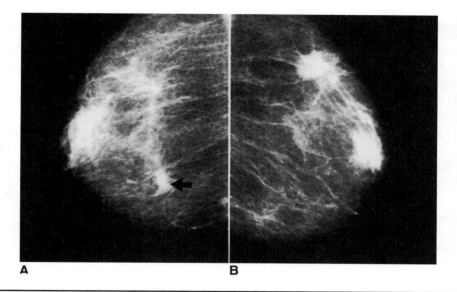

Figure 30-2 Mammogram showing bilateral invasive ductal carcinoma. **A,** Left breast. The larger left mass was palpable. The smaller right mass *(arrow)* was not palpable. **B,** Right breast. Multiple masses are seen. (From Powell DE, Stelling CB: *The diagnosis and detection of breast disease,* St Louis, 1993, Mosby.)

Digital Mammography

Digital mammography is magnetic resonance imaging that generates a precise image of the inside of the body, including tissues and fluids. Magnetic resonance imaging can also be used to determine if a silicone breast implant has leaked or ruptured.

Positron Emission Tomography

The use of PET imaging is growing, and reimbursement coverage for the technique is expanding as more and more oncology groups across the country order PET scanners. PET can be used to discriminate between benign and malignant tumors in women for whom mammography is not effective, to stage newly discovered breast cancer, to detect distant metastases, and to evaluate tumor response to therapy.

Box 30-6   Types of Biopsy

■ Needle biopsy: The surgeon may use fine needle or core needle (stereotactic) breast biopsy. The procedure is done to detect whether the lesion is benign or malignant.
■ Open biopsy
  Excisional (lumpectomy): This is the most common type of open biopsy and the most accurate way to diagnose breast cancer.
  Incisional: In this procedure, only a portion of the lump is removed. This method is most often used when the tumor is too large to be removed through excisional biopsy.

Whereas mammography can only detect suspicious masses, PET, as noted, can also help in staging the tumor—determining if the cancer is early or advanced—and identifying spread and recurrences. Mammography is less effective for women with dense or fibrous breasts and for women with breast implants.

When a breast biopsy is performed, the cells are examined by a pathologist to make a diagnosis and to provide information on the stage of breast cancer.

ASSESSMENT

Critical components of assessment include a thorough patient and family history, physical examination, and diagnostic tests. Family history encompasses both a shared genetic component and a shared environmental component. The history may include, but is not limited to, occupational and chemical exposures, region of residence, and lifestyle factors. Assessment of chronic complications of breast cancer requires the frequent monitoring of symptoms, development of a plan of care, and continuous evaluation of the plan to improve the patient's comfort and well-being. Because complications or recurrence of the cancer can appear months or years after treatment, it is essential that these individuals be followed on a regular basis.

Several areas of functional health patterns should be monitored. Areas of interest include health perception and health management, ongoing recovery, eating, nutrition, self-image, and quality of life (Box 30-7).

Box 30-7   Functional Health Pattern Assessment for Breast Cancer

HEALTH PERCEPTION/HEALTH MANAGEMENT
- Is there a family history of breast cancer?
- Does the patient have risk factors?
- What is the patient's perception of his or her overall health?

NUTRITION/METABOLISM
- What is the patient's current weight? Has there been any recent weight loss?
- Is the patient on a modified diet?
- What are the patient's eating patterns?

ELIMINATION
- Has the patient experienced any changes in bowel or bladder habits?
- Does the patient experience any pain or difficulty urinating or defecating?
- Does the patient have any unusual bleeding or discharge?

ACTIVITY/EXERCISE
- Does the patient experience fatigue or malaise?
- What are the patient's regular exercise activities?
- Is the patient able to perform the activities of daily living?

SLEEP/REST
- How many hours of uninterrupted sleep does the patient get at night?
- Does the patient take naps or rest periods?
- What sleep aids are used?
- Is rest interrupted by pain?

COGNITION/PERCEPTION
- What are the nature, character, location, and duration of the pain? What factors aggravate and alleviate the pain?
- Is sensory perception impaired?
- Have changes in mental status occurred?

SELF-PERCEPTION/SELF-CONCEPT
- How does the patient describe himself or herself?

- How has the condition affected the patient's self-esteem?
- Has the patient experienced changes in body image related to disfigurement and disability?
- What is the patient's perception of her or his current quality of life?

ROLES/RELATIONSHIPS
- What kind of work does the patient perform?
- What role does the patient play in the home and family?
- What changes have occurred in the patient's ability to carry out role functions?
- How satisfied is the patient with his or her current roles and relationships?
- How has the condition affected the patient's family and/or significant others?
- Have changes in social interactions or isolation been noted?

SEXUALITY/REPRODUCTION
- Is the patient sexually active?
- Have changes occurred in sexual performance because of disfigurement and disability?
- Is the patient satisfied with current sexual patterns?

COPING/STRESS TOLERANCE
- What coping strategies does the patient use?
- What support systems are available to the patient?
- Can the patient manage the condition in the current setting?
- How is the individual coping with being a breast cancer patient?

VALUES/BELIEFS
- What constitutes good quality of life for the patient?
- What is important to the patient with regard to spirituality, health beliefs, and cultural and religious beliefs?
- What are the patient's beliefs related to this condition?
- To what extent do the patient's cultural/spiritual beliefs influence decision making related to this condition?

Assessment of Functional Limitations

Although the incidence of severe arm and shoulder disorder after mastectomy has declined sharply because radical procedures are now seldom performed, minor nerve damage may still occur. This may affect arm and shoulder mobility. Moreover, lymphedema (swelling of the arm) may occur after surgery or radiotherapy. The loss of function can affect an individual's ability to perform. This can be especially true with respect to sexual functioning, because body image problems can interfere with any phase of the sexual response cycle. During the diagnosis and treatment of breast cancer, women often experience actual or potential loss of independence, social mobility, and capacity to work, and may experience pain and disfigurement (Ebright and Lyon, 2002).

Assessment of physical changes and alterations in body image is essential. Many patients tend to become depressed when tired or in pain. One third experience a desire to die when their condition is poor. Another third experience occasional irritability, loneliness, and aversion toward the disease. Eleven percent of patients report feelings of anger, mostly toward themselves and their helplessness (Henry, 2002).

Assessment of Body Image Problems

Many problems or conflicts arise when an individual's body image is threatened as a result of a chronic illness such as breast cancer. Although it is not unusual for disturbances to develop, a conflict is more likely to occur when the individual has difficulty accepting and adapting to the changes. Physical disfigurement is one of the problems that may be caused by this chronic illness. The patient must cope not only with personal feelings about the disfigurement but also with the responses of others, especially the patient's partner. The inability to adjust to a changed body image may be manifested by a variety of physical and/or psychological symptoms. Physical symptoms can include pain and chronic fatigue. Psychological problems may be as varied and as frequent as physical complaints and may include anger, frustration, or resentment focused on the partner, family, or health care provider. Finally, an individual with poor adjustment to body image changes may withdraw from previously enjoyed social interactions and experience depression.

Assessment of Recurrence of Breast Cancer and Quality-of-Life Issues

You may have to fight a battle more than once to win it.—*Margaret Thatcher*

After bravely enduring one or more types of treatment, even the most noble of fighters may be faced with the devastating news that the cancer has recurred. Breast cancer may recur as a tumor growth at the site of the original cancer, in either the remaining breast tissues, the skin, the chest wall, or nearby lymph nodes. It may also be a metastasis, a cancer that has spread through the blood and/or lymph system to other parts of the body such as the bones, liver, lungs, or brain. Some of the original cancer cells may not have been destroyed by the first round of treatment but may have lain dormant for several months or even years before beginning regrowth (Brinker and Winston, 2001).

The lasting repercussions of cancer can take their toll on quality of life and health for survivors of breast cancer. Mullen (1985) conceptualized the cancer experience for the individual as "seasons of survival." These seasons include acute survival, extended survival, and permanent survival (Figure 30-3).

In extended survival, the survivor of cancer is dealing with the uncertainty of treatment and possible recurrence. During the phase of permanent survival, a number of variables including self-esteem, social support, and sociodemographic

status affect breast cancer survivors. Also, these variables continue to affect the health-related quality of life (HRQL) of long-term survivors (Padilla, Grant, and Ferrell, 1992).

The concept of HRQL is multidimensional and subjective and includes social well-being, not merely the absence of disease (Pedro, 2001). HRQL for the survivor of breast cancer has been broadened to include not only the extension of life but also the patient's perceived quality of survival at each stage of the experience. More recently, the spiritual domain has been included in the framework of HRQL studies.

Zuckerman (2002) concluded that breast cancer patients who are considering reconstructive surgery following a mastectomy may not always receive the information regarding safety and quality of life that they need to make a truly informed decision about breast implants. Two recent studies by the National Cancer Institute found that women with silicone or saline breast implants were more likely to develop cancer than other women their age and were more likely to die from brain cancer, lung cancer, or suicide than were other plastic surgery patients (Brinton et al, 2001).

REHABILITATION ISSUES

Ferrell et al (1997) analyzed women's scores on the Cancer Rehabilitation Evaluation System and found that global quality of life, sexual functioning, and marital functioning declined significantly between the 1-year and 3-year evaluations. Breast cancer survivors reported a number of important and severe rehabilitation problems that persisted beyond 1 year after primary treatment. Especially frequent were problems associated with physical and recreational activities, body image, and sexual function. A number of aspects of quality of life as well as rehabilitation problems were reported to be worse after that time.

Measurement of quality of life in persons with breast cancer is essential. The central focus of nursing in empowering chronically ill persons with breast cancer is to maintain and enhance the quality of life. Studies have shown that a perception of lack of control over aspects of one's life interferes with achieving good quality of life (Nissen, Swenson, and Kind, 2002).

Maximizing the patient's power resources has been found to improve the patient's ability to cope with breast cancer. An individual's power resources include physical strength, psychological stamina, social support, positive self-concept, energy, knowledge, motivation, and belief system and hope. Persons living with breast cancer may have deficits in some of these power resources (Wyatt and Friedman, 1996).

Physical strength and energy affect the patient's power and ability to cope with demands. For example, individuals who are undergoing long-term therapy with immunosuppressive drugs have less energy reserve to fight infection than do others.

Social support and its effect on cancer patients' adjustment to diagnosis, treatment, and long-term survival have been

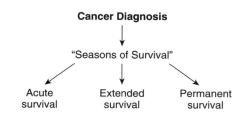

Figure 30-3 Conceptual framework of cancer survival. Modified from Mullan F: Seasons of survival: reflections of a physician with cancer, *N Engl J Med* 313[4]:270-3, 1985.)

studied extensively. Nissen, Swenson, and Kind (2002) pointed out that the perception of support is associated with positive outcomes, such as improved emotional adjustment and better coping. Social support has been found to be related to coping effectiveness, quality of life, and adaptation. Maintaining intact social support systems and supporting the family in coping with the burden of caring for and worrying about their family member is a challenge for nursing.

Self-concept is the individual's total thoughts and feelings about herself or himself (Rosenberg, 1979). It includes the physical self (body image), functional self (role performance), and personal self (moral self, self-ideal, and self-expectations).

Being diagnosed with and living with breast cancer affect the individual's self-concept. Having the illness may promote a feeling of being permanently different or of having less worth as an individual (Miller, 2000).

TREATMENT AND INTERDISCIPLINARY CARE

The treatment of breast cancer depends on a number of factors, including the type and stage of cancer. Treatment options for breast cancer are (1) surgery, (2) removal of lymph nodes, (3) chemotherapy, (4) radiation therapy, (5) hormonal therapy, (6) biologic therapy (immunotherapy), (7) breast reconstruction, and (8) complementary therapies.

An interdisciplinary team approach is the hallmark of the modern management of breast cancer. The participation of many different health care professionals is required for the ongoing care of the breast cancer patient. Team members include the primary care provider, oncologist, surgeon, nurse, radiologist, physical therapist, occupational therapist, dietitian, psychologist, and social worker. One of the nurse's responsibilities is to coordinate the patient's complex treatment plan. It is also the nurse's responsibility to help the patient understand what the roles of the other members of the interdisciplinary team are and why each member of the team is important to the plan of care. The plan must provide for the comprehensive care of the patient to meet the patient's physical, social, emotional, economic, and vocational needs.

Primary Provider (Physician/Nurse Practitioner)

The primary provider is generally the first practitioner to suspect or discover the lump. A thorough assessment, including clinical breast examinations, alerts the provider to the possibility of a pathologic process. Diagnostic testing is ordered. If the lesion is cancerous, the individual is referred to specialists for further interventions and treatment.

Surgeon

Today the breast cancer patient may be given a choice of either surgery that preserves the breast (lumpectomy with radiation therapy) or surgery that removes the whole breast (mastectomy). The choice of surgery and follow-up treatments depends on the type and stage of the breast cancer. Other considerations are the patient's age, overall health, and willingness to accept certain side effects.

Important factors to know about breast cancer are the following: (1) the size and extent of the primary tumor, (2) whether cancer cells have spread to the lymph nodes, and (3) the characteristics of the cancer cells as determined by microscopic or histologic examination.

Some breast cancers may require a mastectomy. A mastectomy is a non–breast conserving approach in which the breast is removed to effectively eliminate the cancer (Box 30-8).

Types of Surgery

- **Lumpectomy:** The surgeon removes the breast cancer and some normal tissue around it (to obtain clear margins). This procedure usually results in removal of all the cancer while leaving the breast looking much the same as it did before surgery.
- **Partial or segmental mastectomy:** The surgeon removes the cancer, some of the breast tissue, the lining over the chest muscles below the tumor, and usually some of the lymph nodes under the arm. In most cases, radiation therapy follows.
- **Total or simple mastectomy:** The surgeon removes the entire breast. Some lymph nodes under the arm may also be removed.
- **Modified radical mastectomy:** The surgeon removes the breast, some of the lymph nodes under the arm, the lining over the chest muscles, and sometimes part of the chest wall muscles.
- **Radical mastectomy:** The surgeon removes the breast, chest muscles, and all the lymph nodes under the arm. This procedure was the standard operation for many years, but it is now used only when the tumor has spread to the chest muscles. Fisher et al (2002) released an update on a trial of radical mastectomy versus less extensive surgery that showed no difference in survival or breast cancer recurrence after 25 years of follow-up (Health Canada, 2003).

Box 30-8 Indications for Mastectomy

- Tumor is larger than 4 cm.
- Breast is small or shaped in such a way that a lumpectomy would leave little tissue or a very deformed breast.
- Cancer is found in more than one part of the breast.
- The woman chooses not to have radiation therapy.
- The woman prefers a mastectomy.
- There has been prior radiation to the breast.

Reconstruction

Two types of breast reconstruction are used (Box 30-9). Reconstruction can be performed at the same time as the mastectomy or delayed until after mastectomy (National Comprehensive Cancer Network and American Cancer Society, 1999). If reconstruction—for example, placement of an implant—is done and then chemotherapy is given afterward, complications such as infection sometimes arise. The suggestion has been made that the reconstruction be delayed until the patient finishes chemotherapy and sometimes until radiation therapy is completed. Then the reconstruction can be undertaken. The decision to have breast reconstruction depends on the woman's preferences.

Twenty-nine women were interviewed to explore the psychosocial consequences of breast cancer on their health and lives. This study demonstrated that breast reconstruction failed to meet the expectations of women with breast cancer, because the women identified disjunctures between social expectations and their own interests in health and well-being (Kasper, 1995).

Side Effects of Surgical Treatment

As is true after any kind of surgery, there is a risk of infection, poor wound healing, or bleeding following surgery for breast cancer. Fluid may collect under the skin, or tingling, numbness, stiffness, weakness, or swelling of the arm (lymphedema) may occur.

Lymphedema

Recently, despite the less extreme nature of current surgical techniques for breast cancer, greater numbers of patients are getting lymphedema, usually manifested as the swelling of the arm, that is caused by the buildup of lymph. The type of lymphedema that occurs months or years after cancer treatment can be quite painful (Burt and White, 1999). The lymphatic system can be impaired in a variety of ways: by surgery, radiotherapy, injury, infection, or simply as a result of genetic tendencies.

Box 30-9   Breast Reconstruction Methods

SALINE IMPLANT

At the time of mastectomy, an expander is inserted that slowly enlarges the implant area to create enough space for the prosthetic implant. Later, the expander is removed and the saline implant is inserted.

TRAM FLAP

In a TRAM flap (transverse rectus abdominis myocutaneous flap) procedure, some of the woman's own muscle tissue is taken from the lower abdomen or upper buttock and is used to reconstruct the breast (Rowland et al, 2000).

The patients who are at risk for lymphedema are those who have undergone radiation therapy or who have had underarm lymph nodes removed after mastectomy. Lymphedema can have distressing psychological consequences and can cause functional problems. According to Swirsky and Nannery (1998), there is no cure for lymphedema at this time. Because it is a lifelong condition, management, not cure, is the ultimate goal.

How lymphedema is treated depends on how serious the problem becomes. Options include wearing an elastic sleeve, using an arm pump, massaging the arm, and bandaging the arm. Exercise and diet are also important. The nurse should assist in the management of lymphedema. Teaching the patient massage of the skin surface to promote fluid movement to bypass the lymph obstruction is important for good care of this difficult problem (Williams, 1997). The patient should also be taught how to exercise the affected area to stimulate muscle contraction. Good skin care is highly recommended for management of lymphedema. The patient should be taught to perform skin care and monitoring to prevent further complications.

Oncologist

The oncologist manages the therapeutic regimen by consulting with the surgical team and a radiation oncologist. Which drugs the patient takes depends on the type and stage of cancer, where it is located in the breast, how much or how fast it has grown, and how it is affecting the patient. The use of adjuvant therapy is common in the treatment of breast cancer. Adjuvant therapy is a treatment given in addition to surgery for breast cancer. Chemotherapy, radiation therapy, and hormone therapy are all types of adjuvant therapy. This therapy is administered to minimize the risk of cancer reoccurrence.

Localized adjuvant therapy is the recommended treatment following breast-conserving surgery such as lumpectomy. It is administered directly to the breast to destroy any cancer cells that may remain. It is also administered to the lymph nodes under the axilla.

Chemotherapy

Chemotherapy uses anticancer drugs that travel throughout the body to slow the growth of cancer cells or kill them. Often, the drugs are injected into the bloodstream through the intravenous route. Some drugs are given orally. Treatment can last as little as a few months or as long as 2 years.

Throughout chemotherapy, the oncologist and the nurse monitor the patient and the patient's response to therapy. Physical examinations and blood tests are performed frequently. The current practice in adjuvant therapy is based on the results of about 400 clinical trials encompassing more than 22,000 women (Hortobagyi, 1998). The addition of chemotherapy and hormonal therapy to local surgical treatment or radiation appears to reduce the incidence of cancer recurrence. Combination chemotherapy is more effective than single-drug therapy in decreasing the annual risk of death (Box 30-10). Although the benefits of combination chemotherapy are more marked in women younger than 60 years, especially those who are premenopausal when the therapy is begun, its effectiveness has been clearly demonstrated up to the age of 69 years (National Comprehensive Cancer Network, 1999).

A discussion of chemotherapeutic drugs is found in Chapter 27.

Side Effects of Chemotherapy

Chemotherapy can cause short-term and long-term side effects that are different for each patient, depending on the drugs used. The most common short-term side effects that appear during chemotherapy include loss of appetite, nausea, vomiting, diarrhea, constipation, fatigue, infections, bleeding, weight change, mouth sores, and throat soreness. Some of these problems may continue for some time after chemotherapy ends.

Serious long-term side effects may include weakening of the heart, damage to the ovaries, infertility, early menopause, and development of secondary cancers such as leukemia (cancer of the blood). These side effects may not appear until later, some time after chemotherapy is completed. Chemotherapy treatments affect the stomach and intestines. Nausea may occur in the first days following the treatment. New antinausea medications can help control this uncomfortable side effect. Hair loss is another side effect of chemotherapy. This hair loss may include not only scalp hair but also eyebrows, lashes, and other body hair. The patient may want to wear a wig. The hair loss is a temporary phenomenon. The Look Good, Feel Better Program, with affiliates located throughout the country, helps patients enhance their self-image during adjuvant therapy.

Hormone Therapy

Hormone therapy is used to prevent the growth, spread, or recurrence of breast cancer. One of the most common drugs used for hormone therapy for breast cancer is tamoxifen. Tamoxifen treatment is often recommended as another type of adjuvant therapy and has been shown to be an effective treatment for both early and advanced stages of breast cancer. It is widely used in patients who have had breast cancer in one breast to reduce the chances of developing cancer in the opposite breast and as a preventive therapy for individuals who are at high risk for breast cancer.

Tamoxifen is taken daily in pill form and works by preventing estrogen from binding to estrogen receptors in estrogen receptor–positive breast cancers. The oncologist determines the dosage and length of treatment in keeping with current research findings. Studies have shown that, for patients with estrogen receptor–positive breast cancer, taking tamoxifen for 5 years significantly reduces the risk of recurrence of breast cancer and the risk of dying from breast cancer.

Side Effects of Hormone Therapy

Common side effects of hormone therapy include hot flashes, vaginal dryness, and vaginal discharge. A few women may experience mild nausea, weight gain, fatigue, or depression. Because tamoxifen is an antiestrogen drug, its side effects may be similar to the symptoms of menopause. In addition to the side effects that have already been listed, mood swings and a decrease in white blood cells and platelets can occur. Tamoxifen may also increase the risk for uterine cancer. Therefore, women taking tamoxifen should be monitored by a gynecologist and should undergo ultrasonographic testing once or twice a year for 5 years. Frequent blood tests and physical examinations are necessary while a woman is taking hormonal therapy.

Radiation Oncologist

In radiation therapy after a lumpectomy, radiation is delivered to the affected breast and, in some cases, to the lymph nodes under the arm or at the clavicle. Radiation is given because breast cancer can occur in the breast in different places at the same time. Radiation therapy may be necessary to treat patients who have a recurrence of tumors in areas that were previously irradiated, so that the possibility for a full-course treatment is limited. Radiation therapy may also be given palliatively to reduce pain and other symptoms in incurable breast cancer. The actual treatment, which is given by a radiation therapist, takes only a few minutes each day. The usual schedule for radiation therapy is 5 days a week for 5 to 6 weeks. Sometimes an additional "boost" or higher dose of radiation is given to the area where the cancer was found. The radiation oncologist plans the specific treatment based on a physical examination, mammogram results, pathology and laboratory reports, and the patient's medical history (Radiological Society of North America, 2002).

Side Effects of Radiation Therapy

The side effects of radiation therapy are generally less intense than those of chemotherapy and are related to the radiation technique, the individual dose levels, and the total radiation dose given. Side effects include skin problems such as itchiness, redness, soreness, peeling, darkening, or shininess of the skin; greater fatigue than usual; and decreased sensation in the breast.

Box 30-10   Most Common Drug Combinations for Treatment of Breast Cancer

- Cyclophosphamide, methotrexate, and fluorouracil (CMF)
- Cyclophosphamide, doxorubicin (Adriamycin), and fluorouracil (CAF)
- Doxorubicin (Adriamycin) and cyclophosphamide (AC), with or without paclitaxel (Taxol)
- Doxorubicin (Adriamycin) followed by CMF

Possible long-term changes include changes in the shape and color of the treated breast and a feeling of heaviness in the breast.

Occasionally the patient may develop some radiation-related effects in the lungs because they are right behind the breast. Changes in the breast tissue and skin usually disappear in 6 to 12 months. Radiation of axillary lymph nodes can also cause lymphedema.

New Treatment Approaches

New approaches to the treatment of breast cancer include biologic therapy (immunotherapy), peripheral blood cell transplantation (PBCT), bone marrow transplantation (BMT) or bone marrow stem cell transplantation, and alternative and complementary therapies

Biologic Therapy (Immunotherapy)

Biologic treatments are designed to repair, stimulate, or increase the body's natural ability to fight infections and cancer. Researchers are investigating many types of biologic therapy that use and boost the substances produced naturally by the body's own cells. They are also creating new substances that can imitate or assist the body's natural immune system in working against infection and disease. These treatments are being used in clinical trials as adjuncts to chemotherapy and radiation therapy.

Peripheral Blood Cell Transplantation

In PBCT, a certain type of stem cell is removed from the patient's blood. The removed stem cells are frozen and stored while the patient is treated with high-dose chemotherapy. After chemotherapy ends and the drugs are gone from the body, the stem cells are returned to the patient through a vein. The healthy stem cells can begin to grow and produce all types of blood cells that the patient needs to survive. PBCT has fewer side effects, shorter hospitalization, and lower cost than BMT.

Bone Marrow Transplantation

BMT is an accepted breast cancer treatment to stimulate a more functioning marrow or to replace marrow. BMT is given as an intravenous infusion of bone marrow cells from donor to patient.

Complementary and Alternative Therapies

The use of alternative therapies is becoming more common in the treatment of a wide range of diseases, including breast cancer. In addition to medical treatment, some breast cancer patients want to try complementary therapies. There is evidence that one in three patients in the United States routinely uses alternative therapies and that 60% of these users do not discuss these practices with their primary physicians (Carlson, 2003). The National Institutes of Health now has an office dedicated to the study of complementary and alternative medicine. These modalities include guided imagery, meditation and relaxation, art and music therapy, biofeedback, acupuncture, yoga, herbal medicine, energy healing, and use of nutritional supplements and vitamins. Some breast cancer patients feel that they benefit from some of these therapies.

Many people are using therapies such as guided imagery (imagining the patient's body fighting the cancer and healing itself), aromatherapy (using fragrances to help the patient feel calm, relaxed, or energized), and art therapy (having patients express their feelings through art). Healing touch methods use human touch to promote healing. These include massage and chiropractic, acupressure (using touch to stimulate certain points on the patient's body), and therapeutic touch (rebalancing the body's energy fields through touch). Refer to Chapter 3 for in-depth discussion of complementary and alternative therapies.

Nurse

The nurse has a crucial role to play in the ongoing care of the breast cancer patient. Nursing care of the patient with breast cancer includes patient education regarding the disease process, treatment and possible complications, possibility of treatment failure, self-care after treatment, and importance of follow-up care. As a patient educator, the nurse helps the patient prepare for potential problems and manage current side effects of treatments. The nurse assists the patient in managing pain and dealing with emotional issues and makes referrals to the rest of the team as needed. The nurse also reinforces what other members of the team have taught (Padberg and Padberg, 2000).

Because good skin care is highly recommended for lymphedema, the nurse should teach the patient how to perform skin care and how to exercise the affected area to stimulate muscle contraction.

Breast implant patients should be encouraged to report any pain, lumps, loss of size or shape, or other symptoms of a problem. Because the implant can interfere with the detection of a tumor during mammography, the patient should insist on having a specially trained technician conduct the test.

Each patient is culturally and psychosocially unique. Cultural traditions affect how patients and families relate physically and emotionally to the nurse. Familiarity with the characteristics of a patient's cultural group as well as the patient's preferences can help the nurse to provide truly individualized care. The nurse should provide culturally sensitive counseling (the patient's family usually needs support as well, and an appropriate referral should be made). The patient should be assured that past misdeeds, family sins, or improper health does not cause individuals to develop breast cancer; however, the nurse should be mindful that individuals of some cultures may continue to hold this belief. The nurse should help the patient look for inner resources of strength. This will help the patient to cope with fear, anxiety, and impaired self-image.

The home care nurse should keep in mind that using a cooperative and interactive team approach in caring for the patient is vital. The nurse should encourage family support and make a referral to a support group such as Reach to Recovery or to a counselor, or talk with the patient about how difficult it has been for the person so far. Also, the home care nurse should provide the patient with continuity of care and should reinforce the teaching that occurred in the hospital setting.

Role of the Nurse in Follow-up Care

The follow-up regimen for survivors who have had chemotherapy varies and depends on the response to the drugs received. Survivors may be given tamoxifen for 2 to 5 years with follow-up every 6 months. The nurse teaches the survivors the following:

- Those who receive tamoxifen should have a physical examination every 3 to 4 months for the first 5 years, with a complete blood count twice yearly and a chest radiograph and mammogram annually. Endometrial evaluation should be performed routinely.
- Survivors of breast-conservation procedures who are symptomatic are often requested to have mammography every 6 months for the first 2 to 3 years after radiation therapy.
- Patients who decide to undergo breast reconstruction with implants may ask the provider's advice about when the surgery should be performed. It can take place at the time of tumor removal or months or years afterward.

Dietitian

The dietitian teaches breast cancer survivors to eat a variety of healthful foods, with an emphasis on foods from plant sources.

- Eat five or more servings of vegetables and fruits each day.
- Choose whole grains rather than processed (refined) grains and sugars.
- Limit consumption of red meats, especially high-fat or processed meats.

Survivors should maintain a healthy weight throughout the rest of their lives. In addition, they should limit alcohol consumption (American Cancer Society, 2002).

Physical Therapist

The use of an appropriate prosthesis is an important aspect of physical rehabilitation after mastectomy and can also strongly influence psychological rehabilitation. A light temporary prosthesis can be used for the first 2 weeks until the wound has healed. A suitable permanent prosthesis can be selected from the wide range available, according to the required size, shape, and degree of adherence to the chest wall. Many hospitals have a nurse or physical therapist trained in the use of breast prostheses.

Few studies have been done to find out whether physical activity affects survival after cancer treatment. Studies have shown that moderate exercise (walking, biking, and swimming) for about 30 minutes every day can have the following benefits:

- Reduces anxiety and depression
- Improves mood
- Boosts self-esteem
- Reduces symptoms of fatigue, nausea, pain, and diarrhea

During recovery, it is important that the patient start an exercise program slowly and increase activity over time, working with a specialist (such as a physical therapist) if needed.

The effect of a comprehensive lymphedema management program was assessed in 25 patients in whom moderate to severe lymphedema had developed after surgery and/or radiotherapy for carcinoma of the breast. Intensive treatment (4 weeks) involved massage and compression bandaging with an adjunct program of education to provide skills in exercise, massage, bandaging, and containment garment use. A significant reduction in limb circumference and volume was observed, and improvement continued over 12 months of self-management. Quality of life generally remained high and stable throughout the 12 months. Perceived comfort and strength of the lymphedematous limb improved, and perceived size decreased. The study confirmed that the combination of multimodal physical therapy and education for self-management reduces lymphedema and its adverse subjective consequences and maintains the improvement thus achieved (Mirolo et al, 1995).

Occupational Therapist

Occupational therapists contribute to the well-being of the patient because they offer ways that promote independence. They provide education and skills training. They help in obtaining assistive technology, tools, and devices. These strategies allow patients to continue their self-care activities and have a sense of control.

Medical Social Worker

Being a breast cancer survivor can affect the patient's job, health insurance, finances, and other practical matters. Often, the social worker can be a good source for answers to the survivor's questions. Resources may be available in the community that can help the survivor get the services needed. Research shows that breast cancer survivors who continue to work are as productive on the job as other workers. Returning to work can help cancer survivors feel that they are getting back to the life they had before being diagnosed with breast cancer.

Some survivors may find themselves changing jobs after cancer treatment. If survivors decide to look for new employment after treatment, they should not try to do more—or settle for less—than they are able to handle. Whether survivors go back to their old jobs or begin new ones, some are treated unfairly when they return to the workplace. Employers and employees may have doubts about breast cancer survivors' ability to work. Information on the legal rights of survivors should be provided.

The medical social worker should discuss with the patient ways of handling problems that may be encountered at work. The patient should be provided with the following information:

- If necessary, ask the employer to adjust to your needs. For example:
  - Start by talking informally with the supervisor, personnel office, employee assistance counselor, shop steward, or union representative.
  - Ask for a change that will make it easier for you to keep your job (e.g., flexible hours, working at home).
- Get your doctor to write a letter to your employer or personnel office explaining how, if at all, the cancer may affect your work or work schedule.
- If necessary, contact your local breast cancer support organization or local bar association for the names of qualified lawyers who specialize in antidiscrimination law.

Clergy

Members of the clergy are trained to counsel patients on issues of concern that relate to feeling alone, searching for meaning, doubts about faith, and fear of death.

PALLIATIVE CARE

End-of-life care is changing because people are living longer. Only 10% of the population will die from acute illness; the other 90% will face a steady decline with a long period of fragility at the end of life (Jossi, 2003). Butler and Ferris (2003) describe palliative care as helping to smooth out the peaks and valleys that occur with chronic illness. Palliative care for patients with breast cancer requires a multidisciplinary team to address the patient's needs, which may include pain management, nutritional assessment, and spiritual support. Multicultural aspects of care must also be taken into consideration. Although palliative care evolved from hospice care, there are some distinctions. Whereas hospice patients are not expected to survive beyond 6 months, patients may receive palliative care for many years and may receive aggressive treatment at the same time (Jossi, 2003). Although palliative care encompasses end-of-life care, it is not necessary to wait until death is imminent to begin palliative care. The importance of providing palliative care as early as possible should be emphasized.

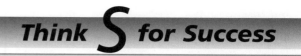
Think S for Success

Symptoms
- Treat symptoms, with a focus on increased function and quality of life.
- Provide management and follow-up for lymphedema, cancer recurrence, anxiety, depression, and low self-concept (self-esteem and body image).

Sequelae
- Promote early detection of recurrence.
- Manage symptoms using medications.
- Address feelings of inability to cope.

Safety
- Teach patient and family and/or significant others the importance of the following:
  Maintenance and promotion of self-esteem to increase quality of life
  Compliance with schedule for follow-up visits
  Adherence to therapeutic regimens
  Reporting of any side effects related to drug therapy; identification and reporting of symptoms of depression

Support/Services
- Provide assistance with finances and help in locating free or discounted referral services if necessary. Help patient secure health insurance coverage, obtain counseling, and locate support groups. These are all crucial elements in rehabilitation.

Satisfaction
- Determine degree to which living with breast cancer interferes with daily activities, roles, and relationships, all of which are important aspects of patient's quality of life.
- Develop a plan to help patient reach or maintain desired quality of life.

FAMILY AND CAREGIVER ISSUES

Family and caregiver issues include difficulty adjusting to the patient's disfigurement; changes in lifestyle and role expectation, fear of cancer recurrence, physical and emotional strains, and financial strains.

During treatment, breast cancer patients focus on getting their health insurance plan to approve the treatment and pay for their care. After treatment is over, many survivors have questions about how their cancer will affect their insurance coverage. Resources for finding out more or getting help are listed at the end of this chapter.

CASE STUDY

Patient Data

Mrs. R. is a 56-year-old cancer survivor. After discovering a large tumor in her left breast that turned out to be cancer, she had a mastectomy. Her lymph nodes tested negative for breast cancer, and the tumor itself was determined to be estrogen receptor positive. She has been a survivor for 8 years. After her surgery, her husband worked a lot of hours and was not able to help out with the household chores. She did not call on him during that time and resented it in some ways. A few months after the surgery, her husband left her. She states, "He would not even touch me, and never wanted to talk about my cancer. I wonder if I can ever trust again. A woman wants to feel like a woman and wants to be feminine. I felt like I am less than a woman."

At times Mrs. R. feels angry, tense, sad, or blue. When she goes for her checkups, she feels very nervous and scared. Two years after the surgical removal of her left breast, a lump was found in the right breast. She states, "I still have that fear every time I go for checkup. I am so scared the cancer is going to come back. It is all I think about every day, the possibility of recurrence."

She has thought about joining a support group but says she is not really a group person.

She is seeing her primary provider today because she found a lump in her right breast.

Diagnostic Findings

■ Physical examination reveals a large lump in the right breast.
■ A mammogram shows a tumor of 2.8 cm.
■ Results of incisional biopsy of the tumor indicate a malignant tumor of stage II.
■ Lymph nodes test negative for breast cancer.
■ No distant metastases are noted.

After consultation with the oncologist and surgeon, Mrs. R. is scheduled for a mastectomy of the right breast. The plan of care calls for several months of multimodal therapy. Currently, she is taking tamoxifen.

Thinking It Through

■ What are Mrs. R.'s concerns likely to be? How would you as the nurse address them?
■ What is the psychosocial impact of being a breast cancer patient and having a mastectomy?
■ How can the health care team improve Mrs. R.'s quality of life?
■ What physical and emotional challenges must Mrs. R. overcome?
■ What strengths does Mrs. R. bring to the team?
■ What barriers to therapy must be overcome?
■ How would you as the nurse assist Mrs. R. in coping with these problems?

Case Conference

The nurses and the other members of the team who are involved in breast cancer care must utilize expert communication skills. This will help the patient and her family to attain an optimal quality of life and achieve the psychological adjustment they need to cope with the experience.

The team meets for a case conference. The team members include the nurse, oncologist, primary care provider, dietitian, physical therapist, medical social worker, counselor, occupational therapist, and clergy member.

The oncologist explains that Mrs. R. will have frequent follow-up and that the team members will work together to help her to manage her pain and other symptoms.

The nurse tells Mrs. R. that lifestyle is not a written prescription that never changes; it is a dynamic process. The first and biggest step for Mrs. R. is to care enough for herself, and that means self-care. There are organizations that provide toll-fee telephone numbers and 24-hour help lines. These lines are staffed by either breast cancer survivors or health care professionals, who should be able to answer many of Mrs. R.'s questions and respond to her concerns.

The physical therapist and occupational therapist recommend an exercise program for Mrs. R. It is an aerobic exercise program consisting of continuous movement using her legs and arms at a moderate to high level of intensity for at least 20 minutes. The therapists explain that the benefits of aerobic exercise include the following:

■ Increased energy
■ Reduced risk of lymphedema
■ Sleep promotion
■ Improved cardiovascular fitness
■ Improved mood
■ Strengthened bones
■ Reduction in hot flashes
■ Weight maintenance
■ Regularity of the gastrointestinal tract

The dietitian explains that a nutritious, well-balanced diet will help Mrs. R. to feel more energetic and will improve her overall sense of well-being.

The nurse and the medical social worker tell Mrs. R. the following:

■ People have found that when they express strong feelings like anger or sadness, they are more able to let go of these feelings. Some people sort out their feelings by talking to friends or family, to other cancer survivors, or to a counselor.
■ Being involved in her health care, keeping her appointments, and making changes in her lifestyle are among the things Mrs. R. can control.

Mrs. R. may find that the following activities are useful to reduce stress:

■ Exercise
■ Dance or movement
■ Sharing of personal stories: Telling and hearing stories about living with breast cancer can help people learn, solve problems, feel more hopeful, air their concerns, and find meaning in what they have been through
■ Music and art

The clergy member tells Mrs. R. that it is normal to feel somewhat cut off from other people—even family and friends—after breast cancer. Often friends and family want to help, but they don't know how. To assist Mrs. R. in dealing with depression and its symptoms, the medical social worker encourages her to be alert for signs of depression (i.e., emotional signs and body changes) and instruct her to contact her health care provider if she experiences these signs for more than 2 weeks.

Emotional signs of depression are the following:

■ A sense of being worried, anxious, blue, or depressed that does not go away
■ A sense of guilt or worthlessness
■ Helplessness or hopelessness
■ Difficulties in concentrating, or frequent crying
■ Inability to enjoy things that were once pleasurable, such as food, sex, or socializing
■ Suicidal thoughts or a feeling that one is "losing it"

CASE STUDY—cont'd
The primary care provider describes the body changes that may signal depression:
- Poor sleeping patterns
- Racing heart, dry mouth, increased perspiration, upset stomach, and diarrhea
- Physically slowing down
- Fatigue that does not go away
- Headaches or other aches and pains

The nurse and social worker encourage Mrs. R. to join support groups and tell her where to find them. Support services offered over the telephone or Internet can help her feel better during the lonely times.

Internet and Other Resources

American Cancer Society: *http://www.cancer.org;* telephone 800-ACS-2345; National Office, 1599 Clifton Road NE, Atlanta, GA 30329

American Institute for Cancer Research: *http://www.aicr.org;* telephone 800-843-8114; 1759 R Street NW, Washington, DC 20009

American Medical Women's Association: *http://www.amwa-doc.org;* telephone 703-838-0500; 801 North Fairfax Street, Suite 400, Alexandria, VA 22314

Cancer Care, Inc.: *http://www.cancercare.org;* telephone 800-813-4673

Cancer Information Service: *http://cancernet.nci.nih.gov;* telephone 800-4-CANCER (800-422-6237); NCI Public Inquiries Office, Building 31, Room 10A03, 31 Center Drive, MSC 2580, Bethesda, MD 20892-2580

Living Beyond Breast Cancer: *http://www.lbbc.org;* telephone 888-753-LBBC or 610-645-4567, 10 East Athens Avenue, Suite 204, Ardmore, PA 19003

National Coalition for Cancer Survivorship: *http://www.canceradvocacy.org/;* telephone 877-NCCS-YES (877-622-7937); 1010 Wayne Avenue, Suite 770, Silver Spring, MD 20910-5600

Rise Sister Rise: telephone 202-463-8040

Sisters Network National Headquarters: telephone 713-781-0255

Susan G. Komen Breast Cancer Foundation: *http://www.komen.org;* telephone 800-IM-AWARE, 972-855-1600; 5005 LBJ Freeway, Suite 250, Dallas, TX 75244

Y-ME National Organization for Breast Cancer: *http://www.y-me.org;* telephone 800-221-2141; 212 West Van Buren, 5th Floor, Chicago, IL 60607-3908

Health Insurance and Legal Rights

Centers for Medicare and Medicaid Services (CMS): *http://cms.hhs.gov/* (click on HIPAA); telephone 877-267-2323

National Cancer Institute: *http://www.cancer.gov* (click on clinical trials area); telephone 800-4-CANCER (1-800-422-6237)

U.S. Department of Labor, Employee Benefits Security Administration: *http://www.dol.gov/ebsa* (COBRA and ERISA); telephone 866.444.3272; rights under COBRA and ERISA (federal laws about pensions and keeping of insurance when you change jobs)

REFERENCES

American Cancer Society: Cancer statistics 2000, *CA Cancer J Clin* 50(1):7-33, 2002.

American Cancer Society: *Breast cancer facts and figures,* Atlanta, 2003, ACS Publications.

Brinker N, Winston C: *Winning the race: taking charge of breast cancer,* Irving, Tex, 2001, Tapestry.

Brinton L et al: Cancer risk at sites other than the breast following augmentation mammoplasty, *Epidemiology* 11(4):248, 2001.

Burt J, White G: *Lymphedema: a breast cancer patient's guide to prevention and healing,* Alameda, Calif, 1999, Hunter House.

Butler A, Ferris A: Palliative care—peaks and valleys, *Nurs Spectrum* 13(3):12, 2003.

Carlson J: *Complementary therapies and wellness: practice essentials for holistic care,* Englewood Cliffs, NJ, 2003, Prentice Hall.

Ebright R, Lyon B: Understanding hope and factors that enhance hope in women with breast cancer, *Oncol Nurs Forum* 29(3):561-7, 2002.

Ferrell B et al: Quality of life in breast cancer survivors as identified by focus groups, *Psychooncology* 6(1):13-23, 1997.

Fisher B et al: Twenty-year follow-up of randomized trial comparing total mastectomy, lumpectomy, and lumpectomy plus radiation for the treatment of invasive breast cancer, *N Engl J Med* 347:233-41, 2002.

Greenlee RT et al: Cancer statistics, *CA Cancer J Clin* 51:15-36, 2001.

Health Canada: It's your health: reducing the risk of breast cancer, retrieved from *http://www.hc-sc.gc.ca/english/iyh/diseases/breast_cancer.html* on April 2, 2003.

Henry B: How to give psychological support to patients with cancer, *Nurs Spectrum* 12(20):16-8, 2002.

Hortobagyi GN: Treatment of breast cancer. Review of drug therapy, *N Engl J Med* 339:974-84, 1998.

Hoskins C, Harber J, Budin W: *Breast cancer: journey to recovery,* New York, NY, 2001, Springer.

Jackson L: After breast cancer, *Adv Nurses* 14:27-8, 2002.

Jossi K: Palliative care, *Nurs Spectrum* 13(3):13, 2003.

Kasper A: The social construction of breast loss and reconstruction, *Womens Health* 1(3):197-219, 1995.

King M et al: Tamoxifen and breast cancer incidence among inherited mutations in BRCA1 and BRCA2: breast cancer prevention trial, *JAMA* 286:2251-6, 2001.

Miller J: *Coping with chronic illness: overcoming powerlessness,* ed 3, Philadelphia, 2000, FA Davis.

Mirolo B et al: Psychological benefits of post mastectomy lymphedema therapy, *Cancer Nurs* 18(3):197-205, 1995.

Mullan F: Seasons of survival: reflections of a physician with cancer, *N Engl J Med* 313(4):270-3, 1985.

National Comprehensive Cancer Network and American Cancer Society: *Breast cancer treatment guidelines for patients,* 1999.

Nissen M, Swenson K, Kind E: Quality of life after postmastectomy breast construction, *Oncol Nurs Forum* 29(3):547-53, 2002.

Padberg L, Padberg R: Patient education and support. In Yarbo CH et al, editors: *Cancer nursing: principles and practice,* ed 5, Sudbury, Mass, 2000, Jones and Bartlett.

Padilla G, Grant M, Ferrell B: Nursing research and quality of life, *Life Res* 1:341-8, 1992.

Pedro LW: Quality of life for long term survivors of cancer, *Cancer Nurs* 24(1):1-11, 2001.

Radiological Society of North America: RadiologyInfo: breast cancer, retrieved from *http://www.radiologyinfo.org/content/therapy/therabreast.htm* on Dec 15, 2002.

Ries L et al, editors: SEER cancer statistics review 1973-1998, Bethesda, Md, 2001, National Cancer Institute.

Rosenberg M: *Conceiving the self,* New York, NY, 1979, Barie Books.

Rowland J et al: Role of breast reconstructive surgery in physical and emotional outcomes among breast cancer survivors, *J Natl Cancer Inst* 92(17):1422-9, 2000.

The Susan G. Komen Breast Cancer Foundation: Mission news from the front, *Mission Newsletter* Summer:3, 2001.

Swirsky J, Nannery S: *Coping with lymphedema,* Garden City Park, NY, 1998, Avery.

Vogel W: The advanced practice role in a high risk breast cancer clinic, *Oncol Nurs Forum* 30(1):115-21, 2003.

Williams A: Lymphedema, *Prof Nurse* 12(9):645-8, 1997.

Wyatt G, Friedman L: Long term female cancer survivors: quality of life issues and clinical implications, *Cancer Nurs* 19(1):1-7, 1996.

Zuckerman D: The breast cancer information gap, *RN* 66(2):39-42, 2002.

CHAPTER 31

Cancer of the Lung

Sharron Guillett, PhD, RN

Lung cancer is the leading cause of cancer-related death not only in the United States but across the world. With a 5-year survival rate of only 14%, lung cancer accounts for more deaths than all other cancers combined (Chandy, Lesser, and Rashid, 2001). This is due in part to the fact that most cancers of the lung are not detected until they are at an advanced stage when metastasis is present (only 15% are localized at diagnosis) and treatment options are limited. The incidence of cancer is slightly higher in men: approximately 91,000 cases occurred in men in 2001 compared with 79,000 cases in women.

Because of the poor prognosis associated with lung cancer, the treatment focus is on prevention. Estimates are that 85% of lung cancers could be prevented by eliminating smoking. Smoking cessation strategies should be discussed with all patients (Box 31-1).

ETHNIC VARIATIONS

Lung cancer is more common among African Americans than among whites (American Cancer Society, 2001). African Americans also have lower survival rates. There is considerable evidence that the differences in survival rate are linked to socioeconomic factors and not to biologic factors (Greenwald et al, 1998). Socially and economically disadvantaged groups tend to have poorer health in general, engage in unhealthy behaviors such as smoking, and have less access to health care services, which may account for differences in both incidence and survival rates.

ASSESSMENT

Because cancer deaths are related to delayed diagnosis, all patients should be assessed for risk factors and warning signs associated with lung cancer during routine physical evaluation regardless of the reason for the patient's visit. In particular, patients should be asked about occupational hazards such as exposure to asbestos, radiation, or coal dust, and about smoking history. The number of packs of cigarettes smoked per day and the number of years of smoking are used to compute the pack-year history. There is a direct dose-response relationship between smoking and the risk of developing lung cancer, and the risk decreases when smoking stops. Patients should be asked about exposure to sidestream smoke, because passive exposure to smoking also increases the risk of developing lung cancer.

Many of the symptoms associated with lung cancer are common to other respiratory disorders or other diseases. For example, shortness of breath occurs with chronic bronchitis, emphysema, and some cardiac conditions as well. The patient with such a chronic disorder may have experienced these symptoms for some time, so it is important to evaluate when symptoms began and whether any change has occurred in the way the symptoms are experienced. Other warning signs of lung cancer include hoarseness, persistent cough, hemoptysis, and weight loss. The provider should ask specifically about chest pain or tightness, chest pressure, or subscapular pain. Box 31-2 lists the warning signs of lung cancer.

Once the diagnosis of lung cancer has been made, a careful assessment of the individual's response to both the diagnosis and the illness is very important because it forms the basis for the plan of care. The symptoms manifested and the extent to which they interfere with functional health patterns depend on the size and location of the tumor and the extent of metastasis. Box 31-3 identifies areas that should be

---

Box 31-1   Smoking Cessation Strategies

■ Set goals.
■ Set a quit date and stick to it.
■ Find out what help is available in your community.
■ Get rid of all ashtrays and lighters after you smoke your last cigarette.
■ Keep healthy snacks, gum, or mints on hand to substitute for tobacco.
■ Get support from your health care provider, friends, and family.
■ Join a support group for people quitting smoking.
■ Get counseling (individual, group, or telephone) or attend a class to help you quit smoking.
■ Decide what you are going to do instead of smoking.
■ Avoid situations and places where you are tempted to smoke.
■ Start an exercise program, begin a hobby, or find other ways to stay busy.
■ Get and use medication.
■ Be prepared for relapse.
■ Reward yourself for meeting goals.
■ Remind yourself that every smoking-free day makes you healthier.
■ Plan to try again.

---

included in the assessment of these health patterns. In addition, the provider must evaluate not only the presence of symptoms but the level of distress caused by these symptoms for the individual and family. Several studies have shown that very intense symptoms, for example, fatigue, are often not the symptoms that are most distressing (Tishelman, Degner, and Mueller, 2000). Therefore, when a symptom is found to be present, the provider should explore the meaning of that symptom. Questions such as "What is that like for you?" or "How distressing is this?" help the provider understand the patient's distress, coping strategies, and priorities. Involving the family in discussions of distress level is beneficial in determining the type of services that will be needed in the home.

Box 31-2   Warning Signs of Lung Cancer

■ Bloody sputum
■ Change in cough
■ Chest pain
■ Dyspnea
■ Hoarseness
■ Persistent cough
■ Recurrent bronchitis or pneumonia
■ Rust-colored sputum
■ Shoulder pain
■ Weight loss
■ Wheezing

PATHOPHYSIOLOGY

Chronic irritation and inflammation of lung tissues, primarily as a result of inhaled carcinogens, causes lung cells to mutate and lose their ability to function normally. These cells divide and grow rapidly, producing neoplasms that are classified according to their cell type. The two main categories of lung cancer are small cell lung cancer (SCLC) and non–small cell lung cancer (NSCLC). NSCLC both occurs and recurs more frequently. These cancers include squamous cell carcinomas, large cell carcinomas, and adenocarcinomas (Figure 31-1). Of these, adenocarcinomas are the most common and the most likely to metastasize. The majority of lung cancers originate in the bronchial epithelium. Tumors that occur in the bronchial tubes can partially or completely obstruct them. Tumors in other areas of the lung can compress airways, nerves, blood vessels, and the heart.

Metastasis occurs by direct tumor extension and by invasion of pulmonary lymph nodes and blood vessels. Lung cancer is known to spread to the bones, liver, brain, adrenal glands, and abdomen.

Small cell tumors produce conditions referred to as paraneoplastic syndromes. The symptoms associated with each of these syndromes are related to the hormones, enzymes, or antigens secreted (see Box 27-1).

Some studies have suggested a hereditary link for cancer susceptibility unrelated to smoking. Other studies have shown a genetic predisposition to lung cancer in some women smokers. Women who smoked who were missing a specific gene were more likely to develop lung cancer than were men who did not have the gene (Tang et al, 1998).

CLINICAL MANIFESTATIONS

The clinical signs and symptoms of lung cancer are nonspecific and are often attributed to other conditions such as bronchitis. The particular symptoms experienced depend on the type and location of the tumor. Airway obstruction causes shortness of breath, altered respiratory patterns, use of accessory muscles, sternal retraction, chest pain, and chest tenderness. Cough, fever, and chills may be present if there is an infection. Sputum may be purulent and plentiful or blood tinged, although hemoptysis occurs late in the disease process.

Breath sounds change according to the tumor location. Decreased or absent breath sounds indicate airway obstruction, whereas wheezes indicate only partial obstruction. A change in the timbre of the voice indicates that lung tissues are either compressed or consolidated. On palpation, fremitus is absent if the bronchus is obstructed and present when air spaces are obstructed. Due to the proximity of the heart and lungs, many patients have cardiac manifestations as well, such as dysrhythmias, digital clubbing, and circumoral cyanosis.

As with all cancers, patients develop generalized symptoms such as fatigue, anorexia, and weight loss. With metastasis, patients will manifest symptoms related to the systems

Box 31-3 Functional Health Pattern Assessment for Lung Cancer

HEALTH PERCEPTION/HEALTH MANAGEMENT

■ Does the patient have a history of smoking or exposure to passive smoke?

■ What is the patient's perception of his or her overall health?

■ What medications, including over-the-counter drugs, does the patient take?

■ What alternative therapies does the patient use?

NUTRITION/METABOLISM

■ What is the patient's current weight? Has there been any recent unexplained loss or gain of weight?

■ Is the patient on any special diet?

■ What is the condition of the skin and mucous membranes?

■ Is saliva production adequate?

■ Does the patient have difficulty swallowing?

■ What is the patient's typical dietary intake (daily)?

ELIMINATION

■ Have any changes occurred in bowel or bladder habits?

■ Is the patient able to use toilet facilities?

ACTIVITY/EXERCISE

■ Does the patient experience difficulty in walking, fatigue, or dyspnea on exertion? What strategies does the patient use to manage dyspnea?

■ What are the patient's regular exercise activities and recreational activities?

■ What mobility aids does the patient use?

■ Is the patient able to perform regular and instrumental activities of daily living?

■ Does the patient use supplemental oxygen?

SLEEP/REST

■ How many hours of uninterrupted sleep does the patient get at night?

■ Does the patient take naps or rest periods?

■ What sleep aids are used?

■ Does the patient experience orthopnea?

COGNITION/PERCEPTION

■ What are the nature, character, location, and duration of the pain? What factors aggravate and alleviate the pain?

■ Is there bone involvement? Does the patient have paresthesias?

■ How effective are current pain management strategies?

■ What level of distress is associated with the patient's symptoms?

SELF-PERCEPTION/SELF-CONCEPT

■ How does the patient describe himself or herself?

■ How has the condition affected the patient's self-esteem?

■ How has the condition changed the patient's body image?

■ How has the condition affected the patient's sense of self?

ROLES/RELATIONSHIPS

■ What kind of work does the patient perform?

■ What role does the patient play in the home and family?

■ What changes have occurred in the patient's ability to carry out role functions?

■ How satisfied is the patient with his or her current roles and relationships?

■ How has the condition affected the patient's family and/or significant others?

■ Who is the primary caregiver? How involved is this person in the patient's care?

SEXUALITY/REPRODUCTION

■ Is the patient sexually active?

■ Have changes occurred in sexual performance?

■ Is the patient satisfied with current sexual patterns?

■ Has the patient experienced any changes in the menstrual cycle?

COPING/STRESS TOLERANCE

■ What coping strategies does the patient use?

■ What support systems are available to the patient?

■ Can the patient manage the condition in the current setting?

■ Are the patient and family aware of hospice care and palliative care options?

VALUES/BELIEFS

■ What constitutes good quality of life for the patient? What is important to the patient?

■ What are the patient's spiritual beliefs? What are the patient's health beliefs, including beliefs about the use of medications for pain control? What are the patient's cultural beliefs?

■ What are the patient's views regarding locus of control?

■ What are the patient's views on end-of-life concerns, including the question of do-not-resuscitate orders?

■ To what extent do the patient's cultural/spiritual beliefs influence decision making related to this condition?

---

in which the metastasis occurs, such as fractures, confusion, and nausea.

DIAGNOSIS

Radiologic examinations identify the presence of tumors in the lung, but the diagnosis of cancer is made by directly examining cancer cells. Cells are retrieved via sputum collection, thoracentesis, bronchoscopy, thoracoscopy, needle aspiration, or surgical biopsy. Once the diagnosis of cancer is confirmed, nuclear medicine scans are performed to determine if metastasis has occurred. Based on the findings of these diagnostic studies, the cancer is staged using the TNM classification described in Chapter 27.

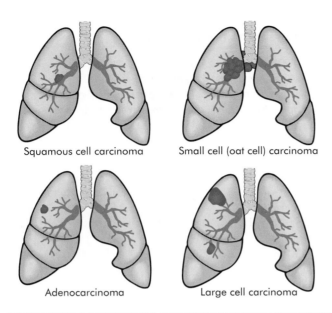

Squamous cell carcinoma

Small cell (oat cell) carcinoma

Adenocarcinoma

Large cell carcinoma

Figure 31-1 Predominant sites of various types of lung cancer. (From Lewis SM, Heitkemper MM, Dirksen SR: *Medical-surgical nursing: assessment and management of clinical problems,* ed 6, St Louis, 2004, Mosby.)

INTERDISCIPLINARY CARE

The goals of care for patients with lung cancer are directed at curing the cancer if possible, increasing survival time if cure is not possible, and maintaining or improving quality of life in either case.

Surgery

Surgery is the preferred treatment for NSCLC in early stages. If possible, the entire tumor is resected. This may involve removal of a lung or a portion of lung. If the tumor cannot be resected, it is debulked. The type of surgery chosen depends on the cell type and stage of the tumor. Among people with NSCLC, the 5-year survival rate is 75% for those with stage I tumors and 45% for those with stage II tumors with surgery alone. The poor 5-year survival rate overall (14%) is due to the fact that patients come for treatment when the cancer is too advanced for surgery to be effective (Knippel, 2001). The average age at diagnosis is 70 years for whites and 65 years for African Americans, ages at which the presence of comorbidities is likely. Therefore, the overall health of the individual is an important consideration when surgical options are weighed (Smith and Glynn, 2000).

Radiation Therapy

Radiation therapy is used for both curative and palliative treatment of lung cancers. For intrathoracic tumors radiation can be an effective primary treatment. However, it is most effective

when used as an adjuvant treatment to chemotherapy and/or surgery. When used as a curative measure, radiation treatments are given daily for approximately 6 weeks. Palliative radiation therapy is given for shorter periods (depending on the symptoms being treated) at higher dose levels. Teaching for the patient undergoing radiation therapy is outlined in Box 27-10.

Drug Therapy
Chemotherapeutic Agents

Drug therapy for lung cancer includes chemotherapeutic agents to treat the cancer as well as pharmacologic agents to treat the symptoms caused by both the disease and the chemotherapy. Radiation and surgical interventions are not recommended for SCLC because of its aggressive nature and poor prognosis. Therefore, chemotherapy is the mainstay of treatment for SCLC. Among NSCLC tumors, adenocarcinomas respond fairly well to chemotherapy, and chemotherapeutic agents may be used palliatively for squamous cell carcinomas. Chemotherapeutic agents are toxic to normal cells, however, and produce a variety of side effects. To minimize these untoward effects, a combination of agents is used. Combination therapy provides a broader range of action at lower dosages. The chemotherapy protocol selected depends on the nature of the tumor and the overall health of the patient. Some commonly used chemotherapeutic agents and their side affects are listed in Table 31-1. Research on the use of combination chemotherapy to treat lung cancer is ongoing. Recent discoveries in genetics suggest that anticancer gene therapy may produce improved cure rates with lower toxicity for individuals with NSCLC (Tong et al, 2001). For a more complete discussion of chemotherapeutic agents, refer to Chapter 27.

Antiemetics

Two of the most common side effects of chemotherapy are nausea and vomiting. Antiemetics are usually administered before and after the chemotherapy is given and should be available as needed as well, because the nausea and vomiting continue for 1 to 2 days after treatment and in some cases may persist for up to a week. In addition to the commonly prescribed phenothiazines such as prochlorperazine (Compazine) and central nervous system depressants such as trimethobenzamide (Tigan), serotonin antagonists are very effective in managing nausea and vomiting related to chemotherapy. However, serotonin antagonists can cost over $100 per dose, whereas the older drugs cost less than $1. The health care team must work with patients and families to develop treatment regimens that are effective and use resources wisely. For example, combining antiemetics or using alternative therapies in conjunction with antiemetics may be a cost-effective way to achieve the desired outcome.

Colony-Stimulating Factors

Chemotherapeutic agents are cytotoxic and therefore kill healthy cells as well as malignant ones. One of the most

Table 31-1 Chemotherapy Drugs Commonly Used to Treat Lung Cancer

Drug Classification	Drug	Side Effects
Alkylating agents	Cyclophosphamide (Cytoxan)	Hemorrhagic cystitis, renal failure, alopecia, nausea, vomiting, stomatitis, impotence, cardiotoxicity, hepatotoxicity, bone marrow suppression
	Ifosfamide (Ifex)	Hemorrhagic cystitis, cardiotoxicity, nausea, vomiting, bone marrow suppression
	Mechlorethamine (Mustargen)	Nausea, vomiting, anorexia, diarrhea, gastrointestinal upset, leukopenia, hemorrhagic cystitis
Antimetabolites	Methotrexate (MTX; Amethopterin)	Rash, bone marrow suppression, nausea, vomiting, alopecia, diarrhea
	Procarbazine (Matulane)	Same as above
Antitumor antibiotics	Bleomycin (Blenoxane)	
	Doxorubicin (Adriamycin)	Vesication, nausea, vomiting, anemia, esophagitis, alopecia, hyperpigmentation of nails and oral mucosa, stomatitis, bone marrow suppression
	Mitomycin-C (Mutamycin)	Vesication, pneumonitis, pulmonary fibrosis
Plant alkaloids (mitotic inhibitors)	Etoposide (VePesid)*	Alopecia, nausea, vomiting, bone marrow suppression
	Vinblastine (Navelbine)	Vesication, alopecia, nausea, vomiting, bone marrow suppression, jaw pain, neuropathies
	Vinorelbine (Velban)	Same as above
Miscellaneous	Cisplatin* (Platinol)	Nausea, vomiting, stomatitis, tinnitus, bone marrow suppression, renal tubular damage, peripheral neuropathies

*Commonly used in combination for treatment of lung cancer.

serious side effects of chemotherapy is immunosuppression, which places the patient at risk for infections that may overwhelm the patient and ultimately prove fatal. Severe immunosuppression results in interruption of treatment. Colony-stimulating factors are given to stimulate bone marrow to produce white cells, red cells, and platelets (Table 31-2). By strengthening the immune system, these agents enable the patient to continue treatment and lower the risk of infection, and the patient often experiences increased energy and functionality.

Narcotics

Individuals with lung cancer may experience chest pain that radiates to the arm and shoulder and bone pain as a result of metastasis. Opioid analgesics are given around the clock to manage the pain associated with both the primary cancer and metastasis. Opioids are also used to manage dyspnea, which may become extreme in the advanced stages of the disease. Narcotics can be delivered transdermally or by aerosol when swallowing becomes difficult and noninvasive methods are preferred.

Table 31-2 Colony-Stimulating Factors

Factor	Cells Stimulated	Dosage
Sargramostim (Leukine, Prokine)	Granulocytes, macrocytes, macrophages	IV 250 µg/m^2/day as a 2-hour infusion for 21 days
Filgrastim (Neupogen)	Neutrophils	IV/SC 5 µg/kg/day
Epoetin alfa (Epogen, Procrit)	Erythrocytes	IV/SC 50-100 U/kg 3 times/week
Oprelvekin (Neumega)	Thrombocytes	50 µg/kg daily up to 21 days based on platelet counts

IV, Intravenously; *SC,* subcutaneously.

Other Drugs

Other drugs that may be given to manage symptoms include bronchodilators, mucolytics, and steroids.

Nurse

The primary role of the nurse in any terminal illness is that of maintaining an optimal quality of life for the patient. Quality of life among patients with NSCLC was shown to be positively correlated with survival rate (Cooley, 1998). Helping the individual maintain an acceptable quality of life is accomplished in part by providing physiologic and psychologic comfort to both patient and family.

Pain Management

Although reports of pain intensity vary among lung cancer patients, older individuals, males, persons with three or more comorbidities, and those who underwent treatments within the previous month most frequently reported pain (Given et al, 2001). This may indicate that women or younger patients underreport pain, experience pain differently, or attach a different level of significance to the pain experienced. Pain assessment is essential for all patients with cancer, and effective pain management is critical, especially in the later stages of the disease. As stated previously, opioids are generally given around the clock orally, intravenously, or transdermally. Assessing and evaluating the effectiveness of the pain management regimen is the nurse's responsibility. It is also helpful to offer alternative comfort measures and to teach these measures to others. Teaching others involved in the patient's care to provide nonpharmacologic comfort measures is valuable for a number of reasons. Aside from easing the patient's pain, use of such measures increases intimacy and gives significant others an opportunity to contribute to the comfort of their loved one. Comfort care is satisfying for all parties involved.

Dyspnea Management

Individuals with lung cancer experience a great deal of fear related to the poor prognosis as well as the fear and anxiety that normally accompany illnesses that produce profound dyspnea. Dyspnea is reported to have a negative effect on quality of life (Smith et al, 2001), and therefore dyspnea management is a key focus area for the chronic care nurse. However, dyspnea is a very complex problem that requires complex, individualized management strategies (Connolly and O'Neill, 1999). The nurse should encourage and support activities that help clear airways and reduce energy demands. Increased fluid intake, frequent rest periods, and supplemental oxygen make the work of breathing easier. Many patients experience panic when they become breathless, which increases their dyspnea. Panic management and breathing retraining can help these individuals deal with episodes of breathlessness more successfully. Patients usually find it easier to sleep and rest in semi-Fowler's position. Hospital beds can be rented from medical equipment suppliers, but many patients find sleeping in a recliner preferable to sleeping in a bed. Most patients with end-stage disease use supplemental oxygen. Chemotherapy, radiation, pleurodesis, and the use of aerosol morphine are effective palliative care modalities that should be considered (Focus on Oncology Nursing, 2001).

Weight Loss

Weight loss and fatigue are also important areas for nursing interventions. It is important to monitor nutritional intake and note changes in the ability to tolerate meals and fluids. Changes in weight should be noted and documented. The nurse and the dietitian collaborate to develop interventions to keep weight as stable as possible.

Fatigue

Fatigue, often related to weight loss and the loss of protein stores, is one of the symptoms most frequently reported by individuals with lung cancer. Although fatigue is rated high in terms of intensity, it may or may not produce significant distress for either the patient or the family. Fatigue must be assessed for both its intensity and its importance to the patient. Likely causes must be identified and addressed. For example, fatigue may be related to anemia secondary to bone marrow suppression, to decreased pulmonary function, or to malnutrition. Measures are taken to correct the fatigue based on the suspected cause. The fatigue itself is managed using the Nursing Interventions Classification strategies identified in Box 31-4.

Box 31-4   Nursing Interventions for Energy Management

- Determine the causes of fatigue.
- Determine the patient's and family's and/or significant others' perception of the causes of fatigue.
- Encourage verbalization of feelings about limitations.
- Monitor nutritional intake to ensure adequate energy resources.
- Consult with the dietitian about ways to increase the intake of high-energy foods.
- Monitor and record the patient's sleep pattern and number of hours of sleep.
- Assist the patient in scheduling rest periods.
- Avoid performing care activities during scheduled rest periods.
- Plan activities for periods when the patient has the most energy.
- Monitor the patient's oxygen response (e.g., pulse rate, cardiac rhythm, and respiratory rate) to self-care or nursing activities.
- Instruct the patient and family and/or significant others to recognize signs and symptoms of fatigue that require reduction in activity.
- Assist the patient to identify tasks that family and friends can perform in the home to prevent or relieve fatigue.

From McCloskey JC, Bulechek GM, editors: *Nursing interventions classification (NIC),* ed 3, St Louis, 2000, Mosby.

Medical Social Worker

The social worker works with the patient and family to decide what care setting is most beneficial and to arrange for needed services and equipment. The social worker can make arrangements for hospice care and make referrals for home care and respite services.

The social worker helps the family understand what services the patient and family are eligible for and who pays for these services. In addition, the social worker is familiar with the volunteer agencies in the surrounding communities and can link the family with resources of which they may not be aware. For example, the local affiliates of the American Lung Association or American Cancer Society may have information, support groups, or equipment loan programs.

Dietitian

The dietitian works with families to prevent malnutrition and correct weight loss. Although weight loss may not be preventable, it can be minimized. Controlling weight loss in cancer patients is important because weight loss is thought to be associated with increased morbidity, decreased quality of life, and decreased survival time (Brown and Radke, 1998). A thorough assessment, which includes a nutritional history as well as a physical examination (with measurement of anthropometric dimensions), is conducted to identify the most appropriate strategies for each individual. For example, interventions for patients with anorexia differ from those for patients who have difficulty swallowing or are depressed.

In addition to providing supplements and encouraging intake, the care provider may find it desirable to give the patient an appetite stimulant or artificial saliva product.

Physical Therapist

The physical therapist is most likely to be involved in the care of the patient postoperatively to prevent frozen shoulder syndrome. A patient who has undergone a thoracotomy must be encouraged to maintain normal functioning of the arm and shoulder on the affected side. Range-of-motion and gentle stretching exercises are generally taught to the family or significant others so that the exercises can be continued at home. The patient should not lift heavy objects for up to 6 months after surgery, and the therapist teaches the patient proper body mechanics and ways to use the affected limbs safely while carrying out daily activities.

END-OF-LIFE CARE

Individuals with terminal illnesses should be made aware of the options available to them for end-of-life care. Open discussions of the patient's concerns, fears, and wishes related to death and dying should be encouraged. The individual may not want to voice his or her feelings in front of family members initially. Similarly, family members may find it too painful to talk about their loved one's death. However, care providers must gently encourage such discussions so that

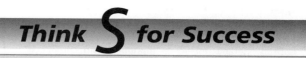

Think S for Success

Symptoms
- Assess level of symptom distress associated with symptom and develop a plan with patient that prioritizes care on that basis.
- Manage dyspnea with supplemental oxygen, positioning, and energy conservation strategies.
- Manage pain with opioids given around the clock.

Sequelae
- Prevent malnutrition and control weight loss.
- Use range-of-motion exercises for arm and shoulder if surgery was performed.
- Remind patient to undergo follow up screening every 4 to 6 months during the first 2 years after treatment.

Safety
- Assess for suppression of respiration related to medications.

Support/Services
- Refer patient and family to community organizations, support groups, respite care, hospice care.
- Assess family coping skills and degree family wishes to be involved in providing physical care and emotional support.
- Teach strategies for meeting needs of both patient and caregivers.

Satisfaction
- Determine how illness has interfered with ability of patient and family to enjoy the important aspects of their lives. Encourage patient to continue to engage in those activities that are meaningful and to avoid social isolation.

the best care possible can be given during the time the patient has left to live. The health care team must have a clear understanding of how the patient and family members feel about resuscitative efforts and whether the patient and family agree on that issue. The family must understand the options and the difference between hospice care and palliative care. Very often the individual wants to live long enough to achieve some personal goal or participate in some important life event, such as the birth of a grandchild or a wedding. Palliative care is designed to keep the patient alive as long as possible and as comfortable as possible. Therefore, palliative care includes the provision of treatments that may be invasive to manage symptoms that interfere with comfort and longevity. For example, thoracentesis may be performed repeatedly to remove fluid and improve breathing. Box 31-5 lists procedures that may be undertaken for palliation.

Hospice care, on the other hand, is provided when the patient's focus shifts from prolonging life at any cost to living as comfortably as possible and dying with dignity under circumstances over which the patient still has control. In addition, fostering discussions about end of life very often opens the

---

Box 31-5   Palliative Care Treatments

- Drug therapy, including treatment with bronchodilators, mucolytics, steroids, and analgesics
- Laser therapy to treat obstruction
- Oxygen therapy
- Pleurodesis
- Radiation therapy to treat hemoptysis, dysphagia, obstruction, and bone pain
- Thoracentesis

---

door for family members to resolve old hurts and disappointments, express feelings of love, and share joys and memories of the life that has been lived. Family members often find great solace in knowing that there was no "unfinished business" or things left unsaid. Such conversations are difficult but are made less so by the presence of a sincerely concerned professional.

FAMILY AND CAREGIVER ISSUES

Family members may be angry with the patient, especially if smoking caused the cancer. By the same token, there may be feelings of guilt if the family members are also smokers or felt that they did not provide encouragement or support for smoking cessation efforts. Individuals who have extreme dyspnea may be afraid to be left alone or in the care of a stranger and thus may attempt to keep their family members near or make them feel guilty for going out. This behavior, even if understood by family members on an intellectual level, can create resentment. Families must normalize activities as much as possible. Providers should assess family dynamics, distribution of caregiving tasks, and coping mechanisms, and offer support and anticipatory guidance.

ETHICAL CONSIDERATIONS

The ethical considerations related to the treatment of lung cancer are the same as those for all cancers and include decisions about withdrawal of treatment and resuscitation efforts, and the high cost of end-of-life care. Unlike for other cancers, prevention of lung cancer raises ethical questions about the production and sale of tobacco, a carcinogen known to cause lung cancer; advertising campaigns aimed at inducing people to smoke; and the rights of smokers versus nonsmokers.

CASE STUDY

Patient Data

Mr. S., a 73-year-old retired toolmaker, sees his physician for his annual physical. He reports increasing hoarseness and shortness of breath over the previous few months. He has had a cough in the morning for several years but didn't think too much about it because he has been a cigarette smoker since the age of 12 and thought it was just "smoker's cough." Mr. S. is married to a woman 20 years younger than himself who is also a smoker. He has two grown children from a previous marriage and five grandchildren. His wife has one adult child from a previous marriage. Mr. S. reports drinking alcoholic beverages weekly and smoking one to two packs of cigarettes a day for 60 years.

On examination Mr. S. appears thin, with good skin color. Vital signs are blood pressure 146/82 mm Hg, heart rate 82 beats per minute, respiration rate 22 breaths per minute, and temperature 98.8° F. He is alert and oriented and in no acute distress. A chest radiograph shows evidence of a mass and a computed tomographic scan is ordered. The computed tomographic scan shows a large pulmonary mass with subclavicular nodes. Cytologic analysis of sputum shows bronchogenic oat cell carcinoma.

Thinking It Through

- What is the prognosis for Mr. S.?
- What treatment options are available to him?
- What nursing diagnoses pertain to Mr. S. and his family?
- How can the health care team contribute to Mr. S.'s quality of life?
- What are Mrs. S.'s concerns likely to be? How would you as the nurse address them?
- What are Mr. S.'s concerns likely to be? How would you as the nurse address them?

Case Conference

Mr. S. has been made aware of his diagnosis. Due to the size, cell type, and location of the tumor, surgery is not considered an option for Mr. S. The health care team is meeting to discuss options with Mr. and Mrs. S. and to develop a plan of care based on their decision.

The physician explains that Mr. S. is not a good candidate for surgery and introduces him to the oncologist who will oversee his care should Mr. S. opt for chemotherapy. The oncologist outlines the course of chemotherapy that would be most beneficial for Mr. S. and explains what the side effects of the chemotherapy are likely to be. He also explains what Mr. S. can expect in terms of disease progression with and without treatment.

Mr. and Mrs. S. have anticipated that chemotherapy would be recommended. They are not, however, prepared for the news that the outlook is so bleak. They had decided initially that Mr. S. should have the chemotherapy and, in light of the prognosis, feel it is their only hope.

The nurse explains what Mr. S. can expect while receiving treatments and outlines some measures that Mr. and Mrs. S. can take to reduce the unpleasant side effects associated with therapy. He explains that he will be coordinating the care and plans to visit them in their home to assess their needs for home care services. He also introduces the topic of advance directives and gives Mr. and Mrs. S. printed information to look over and discuss when they are home. The nurse senses that too much information is being delivered at this time for Mr. and Mrs. S. to process it and make informed decisions, but he wants them to be thinking about the future. He gives them his card and encourages them to call if they have questions or concerns about treatment issues.

CASE STUDY—cont'd

The social worker explains that there are agencies that provide financial and emotional support for patients with cancer and gives Mr. and Mrs. S. a list of resources that they might find helpful. She indicates that, although her services may not be needed immediately, she is available should they need help navigating the health care system in the future.

The dietitian expresses concern regarding Mr. S.'s weight loss and discusses the importance of maintaining adequate nutrition to minimize fatigue and increase resilience during the prescribed treatment regimen. She asks Mr. S. to keep a diet diary for 3 days and indicates that she will make an appointment to review his diet and offer some suggestions for maintaining nutrition and minimizing weight loss. She plans to visit him during the course of his treatment and will be available for consultation should the need arise.

Mr. S. has remained calm and matter of fact throughout the discussion, but Mrs. S. has been tearful and distressed. When they are asked if they have questions about the plan of care, she asks, "Is he going to die?" After a brief moment of uncomfortable silence, the physician says that she is hopeful that the treatment prescribed will prolong Mr. S.'s life for a number of years but that, as in any illness situation, there are no guarantees. The nurse offers to stay after the team meeting to discuss Mr. and Mrs. S.'s concerns about the future. Mr. S. states that this won't be necessary, that he can handle whatever comes along. He laughs and says, "She's just worried that I won't leave her anything in my will." The nurse encourages Mr. and Mrs. S. to discuss their concerns with each other and with their children.

Mrs. S. looks angry but says nothing. Mr. S. says that his only question is how soon he can start treatment. Mrs. S. asks if she will have to quit smoking now. The nurse explains that quitting smoking is always a good idea and that it would certainly be helpful to Mr. S. if the environment were smoke free. He gives her some information about smoking cessation programs.

Arrangements are made for Mr. S. to begin his chemotherapy the following week and the team conference is concluded. The nurse prepares to visit Mr. and Mrs. S. in their home.

- What are the care priorities for Mr. S.?
- What role is Mrs. S. likely to play in Mr. S.'s care?
- Was the nurse right in his decision to delay the discussion of advance directives?
- What resources should the team begin to assemble in anticipation of Mr. S.'s disease course?

Internet and Other Resources

Alliance for Lung Cancer Advocacy, Support, Education: *http://www.alcase.org*

American Cancer Society: *http://www.cancer.org*

American Hospice Foundation: *http://www.americanhospice.org*

American Lung Association: *http://lungusa.org*

American Pain Foundation: *http://www.painfoundation.org*

City of Hope, Pain/Palliative Care Resource Center: *http://www.cityofhope.org/prc*

Last Acts: *http://www.lastacts.org*

Lungcancer.org: *http://www.lungcancer.org*

REFERENCES

American Cancer Society: Cancer facts and figures—2001, Atlanta, 2001, The Society.

Brown JK, Radke KJ: Nutritional assessment, intervention, and evaluation of weight loss in patients with non-small cell lung cancer, *Oncol Nurs Forum* 25(3):547-53, 1998.

Chandy D, Lesser M, Rashid A: Lung cancer: early intervention is the key, *Patient Care* 35(20):12-4, 17-8, 21-2, 2001.

Connelly M, O'Neill J: Teaching a research based approach to the management of breathlessness in patients with lung cancer, *Eur J Cancer Care* 8(1):30-6, 1999.

Cooley ME: Quality of life in persons with non-small cell lung cancer: a concept analysis, *Cancer Nurs* 21(3):151-61, 1998.

Focus on oncology nursing, *Oncol News Int* 10(3):21-2, 2001.

Given CW et al: Predictors of pain and fatigue in the year following diagnosis among elderly cancer patients, *J Pain Symptom Manage* 21(6):456-66, 2001.

Greenwald HP et al: Social factors, treatment, and survival in early stage non-small cell lung cancer, *Am J Public Health* 88(11):1681-4, 1998.

Knippel S: Surgical therapies for lung carcinomas, *Nurs Clin North Am* 36(3):517-25, 2001.

Smith EL et al: Dyspnea, anxiety, body consciousness and quality of life in patients with lung cancer, *J Pain Symptom Manage* 21(4):323-9, 2001.

Smith R, Glynn T: Epidemiology of lung cancer, *Radiol Clin North Am* 38:458-70, 2000.

Tang D: Association between both genetic and environmental biomarkers and lung cancer: evidence of greater risk of lung cancer in women smokers, *Carcinogenesis* 19(11):1949-53, 1998.

Tishelman C, Degner LF, Mueller B: Measuring symptom distress in patients with lung cancer, *Cancer Nurs* 23(2):82-90, 2000.

Tong AW et al: Potential clinical application of antioncogene ribozymes for human lung cancer, *Clin Lung Cancer* 2(3):220-6, 2001.

CHAPTER 32

Cancers of the Abdomen

Sharron Guillett, PhD, RN

Cancers of the abdomen include colorectal, gastric, pancreatic, and hepatobiliary cancers as well as cancers of the urinary bladder, kidney, and reproductive organs. Cancers of the reproductive system are covered in Chapter 33. Table 32-1 lists the cancers of the abdomen discussed in this chapter, along with their incidence and etiologic factors. Combined, these cancers accounted for over 125,000 deaths in 2000 (Dienstag and Isselbacher, 2001; Jensen, 2001; Mayer, 2001a; Scher and Motzer, 2001).

ASSESSMENT

Cancer has both local and systemic effects. The health care team must thoroughly assess the physiologic effects of the cancer on the organ(s) involved as well as the impact on the patient's and family's functional status and ability to cope. Box 32-1 provides a functional health pattern assessment guide for cancers of the abdomen. Other assessment instruments are listed in Chapter 27.

GASTRIC CANCER

The incidence and mortality rates for gastric cancer have declined markedly over the past 50 years. However, among the common causes of cancer-related deaths, gastric carci-

noma still ranks fourteenth overall and fifth among minority populations. This may be due to the fact that the risk of gastric cancer is increased among persons with low socioeconomic status. Native Americans and African Americans are twice as likely as whites to develop the disease.

Mortality rates have been reduced from 28 to 5 per 100,00 in men and from 27 to 2.3 per 100,000 in women (Mayer, 2001a). However, 21,000 new cases were diagnosed in 2000.

Assessment

In addition to assessing functional health patterns and conducting a physical examination, the provider performs a focused evaluation to determine the presence of known risk factors, use of tobacco and alcohol, and family history of the disorder, although familial occurrence is rare. The patient is also queried regarding any history of gastric surgery, atrophic gastritis, pernicious anemia, or infection with *Helicobacter pylori*.

Diagnosis

An upper gastrointestinal radiographic series with contrast is generally ordered to detect ulcers and masses. Computed tomographic (CT) scans are then used to further evaluate any lesions found on radiographs and to determine the extent of any metastasis. The definitive diagnosis is made by direct visualization and biopsy via endoscopy.

Pathophysiology

The majority of gastric lesions are adenocarcinomas that arise in either the distal or proximal third of the stomach. Only 20% of gastric cancers arise in the midsection of the stomach. Adenocarcinomas of the stomach can be either diffuse or intestinal as a result of intestinal metaplasia or atrophic gastritis.

Gastric cancers spread by direct extension through the gastric wall into the lymphatic system and adjacent organs. Hematogenous spread via systemic circulation results in metastasis to lungs and bones. Seeding into the peritoneum and omentum can also occur.

Clinical Manifestations

Early symptoms such as indigestion, abdominal discomfort, and epigastric pain often go unrecognized because they are

Table 32-1 Abdominal Cancers

Organ Affected	Incidence (per year)	Risk Factors
Stomach	Men: 13,400 Women: 8300	Atrophic gastritis Intestinal metaplasia Chronic infection with *Helicobacter pylori* bacteria Long-term ingestion of nitrates Consumption of partially decayed foods Blood type A (incidence is higher for persons with type A than for those with type O)
Bowel	Men: 50,000 Women: 57,300	Diets high in calories and animal fat Hereditary syndromes Inflammatory bowel disease Tobacco use
Liver	Men: 10,700 Women: 5500	Chronic liver disease Long-term administration of androgenic steroids
Pancreas	Men: 14,200 Women: 15,000	Cigarette smoking Obesity Diabetes mellitus Chronic pancreatitis Genetic mutations
Urinary bladder	Men: 42,200 Women: 15,200	Cigarette smoking Diet rich in meat and fat Certain drugs (phenacetin) Exposure to external beam radiation and cyclophosphamide
Kidney	Men: 18,700 Women: 12,100	Cigarette smoking Obesity Acquired cystic disease of the kidney

commonplace. As the cancer progresses, the symptoms become more intense and more difficult to manage, and the individual may experience nausea, vomiting, pronounced weight loss, and fatigue. Palpable masses may be found in the epigastric region and are suggestive of liver involvement. Hard, enlarged nodes in other locales may indicate metastasis (Box 32-2).

Interdisciplinary Care
Primary Provider (Physician/Nurse Practitioner)

As is the case in the majority of cancers, the person who first suspects that the patient's symptoms are indicative of cancer and warrant referral to a surgeon or oncologist is the primary provider. If this suspicion is proven correct, the role of the primary provider then becomes one of consultation in the management of comorbidities. Many times the primary provider has been caring for the patient for a considerable length of time and has established a relationship with the patient and family that can support them through the challenges of the newly diagnosed life-threatening illness.

Specialists

The type of treatment selected depends on the stage of the cancer when it is diagnosed. Surgery is the preferred treatment and the only hope for cure. When there is evidence of distant metastasis, however, the opportunity for cure has passed. Most individuals in the United States are diagnosed at the point of advanced disease when options are limited and the prognosis is poor. In these cases surgery is used for palliation. There is no evidence that chemotherapy affects survival rate, although single-drug and combination therapies are being used. Radiation is effective, but its use is limited when metastasis has occurred.

Surgeon

The surgeon performs either a total or subtotal gastrectomy depending on the location of the tumor. If the proximal third of the stomach is involved, the entire stomach is removed and the esophagus is anastomosed to the jejunum in a procedure called the Roux-en-Y esophagojejunostomy. If a partial gastrectomy is performed, either a Billroth I or Billroth II procedure is done (Figure 32-1). In the Billroth I procedure, the distal part of the stomach is removed and the remainder is anastomosed to the duodenum. In the Billroth II procedure, the lower stomach is removed and the body of the stomach is anastomosed to the jejunum.

Box 32-1 Functional Health Pattern Assessment for Cancers of the Abdomen

HEALTH PERCEPTION/HEALTH MANAGEMENT
- Does the patient have a history of smoking? Does the patient use alcohol? Has the patient been exposed to known carcinogens? Does the patient use drugs containing phenacetin?
- What screening studies (e.g., stool guaiac) have been done?
- Is there a family history of cancer or predisposing genetic conditions?
- What medications and therapies does the patient use, including over-the-counter drugs and alternative therapies?
- What is the patient's perception of his or her overall health?
- Is the patient aware of the diagnosis?

NUTRITION/METABOLISM
- What is the patient's current weight? Has there been any recent loss or gain of weight?
- Is the patient on a special diet?
- What is the condition of the skin and mucous membranes?
- Is saliva production adequate? Does the patient experience difficulty swallowing?
- What is the patient's typical dietary intake (daily)?
- Does the patient experience nausea and/or vomiting? If present, is it treatment related or anticipatory?

ELIMINATION
- Have any changes occurred in bowel or bladder habits?
- What are the color, frequency, and caliber of stools? Is tenesmus present?
- Is there a history of irritable bowel disease?
- What are the color and character of the urine? Is dysuria or hematuria present?

ACTIVITY/EXERCISE
- Does the patient experience difficulty in walking, fatigue, or dyspnea on exertion? What strategies are used to manage dyspnea?
- What are the patient's regular exercise activities and recreational activities?
- What mobility aids does the patient use?
- Can the patient perform instrumental and other activities of daily living?
- Does the patient use supplemental oxygen?

SLEEP/REST
- How many hours of uninterrupted sleep does the patient get at night?
- Does the patient take naps or rest periods?
- What sleep aids are used?
- Does the patient have orthopnea?
- Is fatigue relieved by sleep?

COGNITION/PERCEPTION
- What are the nature, character, location, and duration of the pain? What factors aggravate and alleviate the pain?
- Is there bone involvement? Does the patient experience paresthesias?
- How effective are pain management strategies? What level of distress is associated with the symptoms?
- Have changes occurred in mentation or level of consciousness, in the sense of taste or smell, sight, or hearing, or in speech and communication patterns?

SELF-PERCEPTION/SELF-CONCEPT
- How does the patient describe himself or herself?
- How has the condition affected the patient's self-esteem?
- What changes have occurred in the patient's body image?
- How has the condition affected the patient's sense of self?

ROLES/RELATIONSHIPS
- What kind of work does the patient perform?
- What role does the patient play in the home and family?
- What changes have occurred in the patient's ability to carry out role functions?
- How satisfied is the patient with his or her current roles and relationships?
- How has the condition affected the patient's family and/or significant others?
- Have changes occurred in family organization and function?
- Who is the primary caregiver and how involved is this person in the patient's care?
- Who is the decision maker?

SEXUALITY/REPRODUCTION
- Is the patient sexually active?
- Have changes occurred in sexual performance?
- Is the patient satisfied with current sexual patterns?
- Does the patient have concerns about potential changes in sexual performance or sexuality
- Has the patient experienced any changes in the menstrual cycle?

COPING/STRESS TOLERANCE
- What coping strategies does the patient use?
- What support systems are available to the patient?
- Can the patient manage the condition in the current setting?
- Is the patient with a terminal condition aware of hospice and palliative care options?
- What is the patient's level of hopefulness or despair?
- What do the patient and family find comforting and meaningful?

VALUES/BELIEFS
- What constitutes good quality of life for the patient? What is important to the patient?
- What are the patient's spiritual beliefs? What are the patient's health beliefs, including beliefs about the use of medications for pain control?
- What are the patient's cultural beliefs? To what degree does the individual participate in cultural traditions and the cultural community?
- What are the patient's views regarding locus of control?
- What are the patient's views on end-of-life concerns, including issues and decisions regarding advance directives? Does the patient want a spiritual leader, advisor, or counselor present?

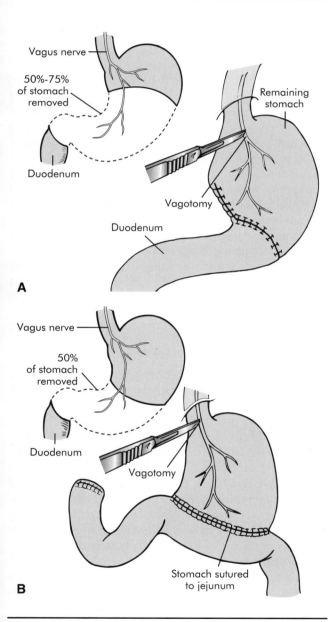

Figure 32-1 A, Billroth I procedure (subtotal gastric resection with gastroduodenostomy anastomosis). **B,** Billroth II procedure (subtotal gastric resection with gastrojejunostomy anastomosis). (From Lewis SM, Heitkemper MM, Dirksen SR: *Medical-surgical nursing: assessment and management of clinical problems,* ed 6, St Louis, 2004, Mosby.)

Nurse

Nursing care of patients with gastric carcinoma includes all of the care commonly given to patients with cancer (see Chapter 27). In addition, a major focus of nursing care is on overcoming debilitation and restoring nutritional balance. The nurse and dietitian work closely together to teach the individual and family about methods for improving nutritional status. Box 32-3 lists measures to prevent and manage postprandial distention (dumping syndrome) caused by decreased gastric capacity.

The nurse also evaluates nutritional status by monitoring weight and energy levels. Patients may become anemic and require vitamin B_{12} injections. Laboratory values for complete blood counts and levels of iron, folate, and serum proteins should be closely monitored.

Recurrence of gastric cancer is common. Therefore, nurses often become case managers, making sure that community resources are provided as needed to help with activities of daily living (ADL), home care, emotional support, and hospice if needed. End-of-life care is discussed in Chapter 27.

Dietitian

The dietitian works closely with the individual and the family to develop a diet plan that will support healing, restore nutritional balance, and avoid complications such as regurgitation or postprandial distention. Vitamins and minerals as well as protein supplements must be added to the diet to promote healing and correct the deficits present at the time of surgery.

Although the dietitian attempts to include foods that the patient enjoys, certain foods should be used with caution and some should be avoided altogether (Box 32-4). In general, foods that are high in animal proteins and fats and low in carbohydrates are encouraged. The dietitian reviews the diet plan carefully with the individual and family, explaining the rationale for limiting or excluding certain foods. Recording calorie counts and measuring intake and output might also be requested to confirm adherence to the plan and determine the plan's effectiveness.

Physical Therapist

For the patient who is severely debilitated, the physical therapist provides an exercise program aimed at restoring the

---

Box 32-4   Dietary Restrictions after Gastric Resection

LIMITED FOODS
- Foods made with milk
- Whole-grain breads
- Gas-producing vegetable
- Unsweetened fruit, fruit juice
- Beverages containing caffeine
- Diet carbonated beverages (if tolerated)
- Salted, smoked, or pickled foods

EXCLUDED FOODS
- Sweetened beverages, including juices, malts, shakes, carbonated beverages
- Alcohol
- Spicy foods, including spicy soups, potatoes, meats, or meat substitutes
- Breads with frosting or jelly
- Sweet rolls, coffee cake, doughnuts
- Cakes, pies, cookies, candy, ice cream, sherbet
- Honey, syrup, molasses

---

patient's strength and energy to overcome any deconditioning that has occurred as a result of the disease process.

Occupational Therapist

The occupational therapist assesses the patient's ability to manage ADL and remain productive. Large tasks are broken down into simpler ones that are more manageable to conserve energy. The occupational therapist also attempts to find means to keep the individual active and productive by exploring ways that professional or leisure interests can still be pursued.

COLORECTAL CANCER

Colorectal cancer ranks third as a cause of both cancer and cancer-related deaths in the United States. It occurs equally often in men and in women, most commonly after the age of 50 years. Cancer deaths related to this disease are on the decline because of increased rates of early detection; however, a significant number of deaths occur annually.

Assessment

In addition to assessing functional health patterns, the nurse reviews the health history for the presence of specific risk factors and any changes in bowel patterns.

The physical assessment focuses on auscultation and palpation of the abdomen, digital rectal examination, and procurement of a small amount of stool for occult blood analysis.

Diagnosis

The definitive method for diagnosis of colorectal cancer is a colonoscopy. This procedure allows direct visualization of the entire colon and permits the removal of polyps and tissue samples for analysis. Colonoscopy is recommended as a screening examination for all individuals older than age 50 years (Table 32-2). Individuals with a positive genetic history of the disease may be asked to undergo a colonoscopy at a much younger age.

Pathophysiology

Ninety-five percent of colon cancers are adenocarcinomas arising from the glandular epithelium of the bowel.

Clinical Manifestations

Colorectal cancer is usually asymptomatic. The signs and symptoms that do occur vary with the location of the tumor. As stool passes through the intestine, it becomes more solid and therefore more difficult to move past a space-occupying lesion. The most common symptoms are abdominal cramping and a change in either the frequency or character of bowel movements. Cancers of the left side of the bowel are easier to detect because stool becomes either difficult to pass or thin and pencil shaped. Right-sided cancers generally produce vague symptoms such as pain or discomfort in the lower right quadrant or umbilical region. Whereas rectal cancers are more likely to produce frank blood in the stool, right-sided cancers can ulcerate the bowel, which causes dark or mahogany-colored blood to appear in the stool.

Interdisciplinary Care
Primary Provider (Physician/Nurse Practitioner)

As with other cancers, the primary provider is generally the first to suspect the presence of the cancer. In the case of colorectal cancer, however, the primary provider plays a major role in early detection and screening.

All individuals should have annual rectal examinations and testing for fecal occult blood (FOBT). Because conditions other than cancer and some medications can produce false-positive results, the provider questions the individual regarding the presence of hemorrhoids and the use of salicylates, steroids, and nonsteroidal antiinflammatory drugs. Positive FOBT findings warrant follow-up assessment. The patient is instructed to avoid meats, horseradish, and beets and to stop taking antiinflammatory medications for 48 hours, and then the test is repeated. If the FOBT results remain positive, further studies such as sigmoidoscopy, barium enema testing, and/or colonoscopy may be ordered.

The primary provider has the responsibility of teaching and counseling the patient about the necessity of follow-up and the importance of long-term screening. Many patients who have no family history of colorectal cancer are reluctant to schedule the screening examinations, especially those requiring the use of enemas and cathartics for preparation.

Table 32-2 American Cancer Society Screening Recommendations for Colorectal Cancer

Degree of Risk	Age to Begin Screening	Examination	Frequency
Average	50 yr	Fecal occult blood test	Annually
		Flexible sigmoidoscopy	Every 5 yr
		Colonoscopy	Every 10 yr
Increased			
Single adenoma <1 cm	3-6 yr after polypectomy	Colonoscopy	If normal, every 10 yr
Polyp >1 cm, multiple polyps, or high-grade dysplasia	Within 3 yr after polypectomy	Colonoscopy	If normal, in 3 yr; if again normal, every 10 yr
Personal history of resection for colon cancer	1 yr after resection	Colonoscopy	If normal, in 3 yr; if again normal, every 5 yr
History of colorectal cancer or adenomas in any first-degree relative before age 60 or in two or more first-degree relatives of any age	Age 40 or 10 yr before age of earliest case in first-degree relative	Colonoscopy	Every 5-10 yr
High			
Family history of familial adenomatous polyposis	Puberty	Endoscopy and genetic counseling	If test result is positive, colectomy is indicated
Family history of hereditary nonpolyposis colon cancer	Age 21	Colonoscopy and genetic counseling	Every 1-2 yr until age 40, then annually
Inflammatory bowel disease	8 yr after pancolitis or 12-15 yr after left-sided colitis	Colonoscopy	Every 1-2 yr

Adapted from American Cancer Society: ACS cancer detection guidelines, 2004, retrieved from *http://www.cancer.org/docroot/PED/content/PED_2_3y_ACS_ Cancer_Detection_Guidelines_36.asp?sitearea=PED* on Mar 8, 2004.

The primary provider stresses the value of early detection and carefully explains the procedures and the measures taken to ensure safety and comfort. Suggested screening schedules are listed in Table 32-2.

Specialists

Surgeon

The type of surgery performed depends on the location and the stage of the cancer. Small cancers that have not penetrated the bowel wall may be locally excised. Others require either a hemicolectomy with reanastomosis, a colon resection with a colostomy (which may be temporary), or an abdominoperineal resection in which the sigmoid colon, rectosigmoid colon, rectum, and anus are removed. The latter procedure generally requires the creation of a colostomy unless the rectal sphincter is spared.

Oncologist

The oncologist prescribes chemotherapy for the patient with advanced cancer (stage IV) and as an adjuvant to surgery for individuals with stages II or III carcinoma. The preferred treatment is combination therapy using 5-fluorouracil (5-FU) with either leucovorin or irinotecan (Camptosar). This combination of drugs has been shown to improve response rates and increase survival time.

Oxaliplatin, an analog of platinum, has shown promise in Europe and is in clinical trials in the United States. Oxaliplatin is given either every 2 weeks or every 3 weeks depending on the dose prescribed and is infused intravenously over 1 hour. It is incompatible with sodium chloride and alkaline solutions. Therefore, if it is given with 5-FU, an alkaline solution, the oxaliplatin must be given first and the line flushed thoroughly before the 5-FU is administered. In addition, aluminum degrades oxaliplatin, so care must be taken to prevent contact with aluminum needles and equipment (Wilkes, 2002).

Oxaliplatin acts as an alkylating agent, and its side effects are similar to those of other drugs in this category, especially cisplatin. The dose-limiting side effects are neurologic, and acute neurotoxicity is common, occurring in up to 90% of individuals (Wilkes, 2002). Symptoms of neurotoxicity occur within 1 to 5 days after infusion and are usually precipitated by exposure to cold. The symptoms are mild, involve paresthesias of the mouth, throat, and distal extremities, and usually resolve spontaneously in a matter of minutes. It is important to inform the patient that these side effects may occur and that they usually resolve quickly. The patient should report the symptoms to his or her provider. Symptoms produced by exposure to cold can be avoided by teaching the patient the self-care strategies listed in Box 32-5.

Box 32-5   Self-Care Strategies to Prevent Cold-Induced Paresthesias

■ Avoid going out in cold weather.
■ Wear gloves when reaching into the freezer.
■ Avoid cold foods and fluids.
■ Use a drinking straw with all fluids.
■ Do not use the air conditioner in the home or car.

Modified from Wilkes G: New therapeutic options in colon cancer: focus on oxaliplatin, *Clin J Oncol Nurs* 6(3):131-51, 2002.

Box 32-6   Nursing Interventions Involving Grief Work Activities

■ Identify the loss.
■ Encourage expression of feelings about the loss.
■ Encourage identification of fears related to the loss.
■ Assist in identifying personal strengths and coping strategies.
■ Involve family members in discussion as appropriate.
■ Identify sources of community support.

Modified from McCloskey JC, Bulechek GM: *Nursing interventions classification (NIC),* ed 3, St Louis, 2000, Mosby.

Radiation Oncologist

No evidence exists that radiation therapy can successfully treat colorectal cancer or improve survival. It may be used for palliation to manage pain, hemorrhage, or obstruction. For cancers confined to the rectum, however, radiation is routinely used as adjuvant therapy.

Nurse

In addition to management of symptoms associated with cancer treatment (nausea, vomiting, pain, anxiety, etc.), nursing care of the patient with colorectal cancer focuses on maintenance of bowel function, stoma care, perineal wound care, and self-image issues. Stoma care is discussed in detail in Chapter 16.

The perineal wound may continue to drain serosanguineous fluid for up to 2 months after abdominoperineal resection, and complete healing may take as long as 9 months. The wound is a potential source of infection and abscess and must be closely monitored. In addition, it causes great discomfort for the patient. Comfort measures include the use of sitz baths, pain medications, side-lying positions while in bed, and soft pillows while seated (Knowles, 2002).

The nurse encourages the individual to look at the stoma if present and to learn to manage the care of the stoma independently. The nurse should help the patient explore feelings about the change in appearance and its impact on roles and self-image. The individual with a stoma or perineal wound will have concerns about sexuality and the resumption of sexual activity. The nurse must address these in an open, factual manner. If the patient does not pose any questions related to sexual activity, the nurse should open a discussion on the topic. If the patient is unable or unwilling to have such discussions with the nurse, a referral should be made to a counselor or psychologist. Grief reactions are common among individuals undergoing body-altering surgery, and these may have to be addressed before the individual can consider resuming prior role functions. Nursing Interventions Classification (NIC) grief work activities are listed in Box 32-6.

Enterostomal Therapist

The enterostomal therapist (ET) specializes in the management of stomas, including care of the stoma, the surround-

ing skin, ostomy pouch systems, and bowel elimination. The ET generally sees the patient in the hospital and teaches the patient and family how to care for the stoma, apply drainage devices, care for the underlying skin, control odor, avoid problem foods, and detect complications.

The ET continues to follow the patient's progress during office or clinic visits, but home management of the stoma is reinforced and evaluated by the nurse (Box 32-7). If complications arise or care of the stoma requires specialized problem solving, the ET can also visit the patient at home.

Medical Social Worker

The medical social worker (MSW) works with the individual to obtain the necessary equipment and supplies to maintain the stoma and manage drainage and elimination needs once the patient resumes work or other public activities. The MSW also makes sure that the patient and family are aware of the multitude of resources available nationally and in the local community. The United Ostomy Association and Ostomates are two self-help organizations for people with ostomies. Both organizations have publications to which one can subscribe and offer information via the Internet.

CANCER OF THE LIVER

Most often, when cancer is found in the liver, it is the result of metastasis from some other organ. Such cancer is named for

---

Box 32-7   Home Care of the Patient with a Colostomy

■ Assess bowel functioning.
■ Assess nutritional status.
■ Assess the stoma.
■ Assess the skin surrounding the stoma.
■ Assess the ability of the individual and/or family to care for the stoma.
■ Assess for changes in self-esteem.
■ Assess for signs of social isolation.

the primary site and is referred to as metastatic. For example, lung cancer that has metastasized to the liver is still called metastatic lung cancer even though it is found in the liver.

Primary liver cancer affects about 16,000 people annually in the United States. The majority of individuals have an advanced stage of cancer at the time of diagnosis. Therefore, the 5-year survival rate is about 10%. Close to 14,000 people die from liver cancer annually.

Hepatocellular cancer has a strong association with hepatitis and cirrhosis. Consequently, it is one of the most common cancers in the world, with the highest rates occurring in regions with a high incidence of hepatitis B and hepatitis C (primarily Asia and sub-Saharan Africa). In the United States peak incidence is in the sixth and seventh decades.

Diagnosis

Diagnosis of liver cancer is made using imaging studies such as ultrasonography, CT, and magnetic resonance imaging (MRI). Laboratory tests commonly demonstrate an increase in levels of alkaline phosphatase and α-fetoprotein. Levels of α-fetoprotein higher than 500μg/L are strongly suggestive of liver cancer.

Staging

Liver cancer can be staged using the TNM classification system, the Okuda system, or the Cancer of the Liver Italian Program (CLIP) system (Ueno, 2001). The widely used Okuda system predicts clinical course based on four criteria: tumor size greater than 50% of the liver, presence of ascites, bilirubin level higher than 3 mg/dl, and albumin level higher than 3 g/dl. A score of 1 point is assigned for each of these factors that is present. Points are then totaled to determine stage and prognosis (Table 32-3).

Clinical Manifestations

The primary presenting symptom of cancer of the liver is right upper quadrant abdominal pain. Because most patients who develop liver cancer already have underlying liver disease, the cancer generally goes undetected until a mass is palpated. Jaundice is uncommon unless the mass obstructs the bile ducts.

Treatment

If untreated, individuals with liver cancer will die of the disease within 6 months. Most tumors are not resectable at the time of diagnosis; however, if the tumor is discovered early enough for resection to be possible, survival can be extended to up to 2 years after resection. Some countries in which there are high incidences of hepatitis B or hepatitis C have begun serial screening in an effort to detect the cancer early enough to improve survival rates. However, to date, no studies with a randomized design have demonstrated a survival benefit with early screening (Dienstag and Isselbacher, 2001).

Treatment options for unresectable cancer of the liver are limited because the cancer is not responsive to chemotherapy and the liver cannot tolerate high doses of radiation. The focus of the interdisciplinary team, then, is on managing symptoms, assisting individuals and families to maintain good quality of life, and helping the patient ultimately to experience a peaceful, dignified death.

Interdisciplinary Care
Primary Provider (Physician/Nurse Practitioner)

The primary provider may have been treating the individual for nonmalignant liver disorders for some time. In these instances the primary provider continues to manage any related disorders such as hypertension, fluid imbalance, and nutritional deficits. Once liver functioning is impaired, drug regimens must be carefully assessed and adjusted to maintain therapeutic doses of medications and avoid overtaxing the organ.

Specialists

Surgeon

Surgical resection is the only treatment that offers any hope of long-term survival (Chan et al, 2002). Most patients are not candidates for surgery, however, because their cancer is advanced. Cryosurgery in which select tumors are ablated with liquid nitrogen has yielded some improvement in long-term survival rates. A new approach called radiofrequency ablation uses radio waves to destroy the tumors. Ligating or tying off the hepatic artery is another surgical treatment that may be performed but is dangerous in patients who have underlying liver disease such as cirrhosis.

Oncologist

Liver cancer is resistant to most chemotherapy regimens. Doxorubicin (Adriamycin) and cisplatin (Platinol) have been successful in shrinking tumors but have not been able to prolong life.

Many patients receive chemotherapy via hepatic arterial catheters that may be connected to a port or implanted pump.

Drug Therapy

The use of medication by the patient with liver cancer is complex because the liver detoxifies drugs. Therefore, all medications should be evaluated carefully and dosages and routes altered as appropriate.

Table 32-3 Okuda Staging System for Liver Cancer

	Stage I	Stage II	Stage III
Score*	0	1 or 2	3 or 4
Life expectancy without treatment	8 months	2 months	<1 month

*See text for method of determining score.

Medications used in the treatment of liver cancer are directed at managing symptoms. (See Chapter 27.)

Nurse

Nursing care of the patient with liver cancer is primarily supportive. The individual and family need assistance in coping with the terminal nature of the disease. Referral to hospice care may be warranted. Advance directives should be addressed. See Chapter 27 for a more thorough discussion of end-of-life issues.

Care of patients with hepatic ports or implanted pumps includes maintaining the pump and assessing for infection or erosion around the pump site (Martin, 2002) (Figure 32-2 and Box 32-8).

Dietitian

A special diet is not required. However, maintaining adequate nutrition is important, and strategies such as giving small frequent feedings may improve nutrient intake.

CANCER OF THE PANCREAS

Approximately 28,000 people are diagnosed with pancreatic cancer annually, more than 98% of whom do not survive. Pancreatic cancer ranks eleventh in cancer incidence and fifth as a cause of cancer-related mortality (Mayer, 2001b).

The two biggest risk factors for the development of pancreatic cancer are smoking and advanced age (Magee et al, 2002). The highest incidence rates are in the seventh decade of life. Alcohol and coffee consumption, once thought to be risk factors, are not related to the development of pancreatic cancer, although persons with chronic pancreatitis are at increased risk. Obesity and diabetes mellitus are being considered as possible risk factors.

Assessment

In addition to performing a functional health pattern assessment, the provider should carefully inspect the skin and mucous membranes and conduct a thorough abdominal evaluation, palpating for organomegaly and percussing for dullness that indicates the presence of ascites.

Diagnostic studies include CT, endoscopic retrograde cholangiopancreatography, and needle aspiration biopsy. There are no laboratory tests specific for pancreatic cancer, although carcinoembryonic antigen levels are elevated in 80% to 90% of cases and the tumor marker CA19-9 (carbohydrate antigen 19-9) is present. The vagueness of symptoms and poor sensitivity of blood assays combine to make early diagnosis difficult. By the time jaundice appears, the cancer is usually well advanced.

Clinical Manifestations

The symptoms of pancreatic cancer are related, in part, to the area of the pancreas involved. Jaundice is associated with cancer of the head of the pancreas, whereas pain more

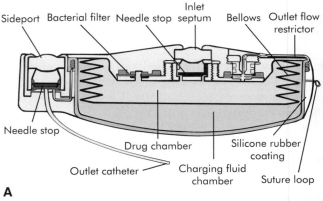

A

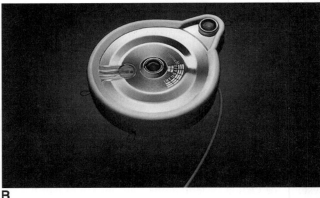

B

Figure 32-2 A, Cross section of implantable pump for drug delivery displaying its two chambers: the drug chamber (inner) and the charging fluid chamber (outer). As the drug chamber is filled, the bellows expand, compressing the charging fluid in the outer chamber. The resulting increased pressure in the outer chamber forces the drug through a membrane filter and preset flow restrictor and thus ensures a nearly constant flow. **B,** Infusaid pump. (**A** from Lewis SM, Heitkemper MM, Dirksen SR: *Medical-surgical nursing: assessment and management of clinical problems,* ed 6, St Louis, 2004, Mosby; **B** courtesy Strato/Infusaid, Inc., Norwood, Mass.)

often occurs when the body and tail of the pancreas are involved. Other symptoms of pancreatic cancer are listed in Box 32-9.

Interdisciplinary Care
Primary Provider (Physician/Nurse Practitioner)

The primary provider is the first to suspect pancreatic involvement and orders the initial diagnostic studies. A referral to a gastroenterologist may be made at the time diagnostic studies are ordered to expedite treatment. Unfortunately, the median survival time for the 80% of individuals whose cancer is nonresectable is 6 months. Therefore, it is unlikely that the primary provider will have contact with the patient once the referral to a specialist is made.

Box 32-8   Care of the Patient with an Implanted Hepatic Arterial Infusion Device

- Never leave the system open to air.
- Always use aseptic technique.
- Assess for excessive movement of the pump under the skin.
- Assess for local (pouch or skin pocket) and systemic infection.
- Assess for hematoma at the site.
- Assess for signs of extravasation (pain, burning, swelling, leakage).
- Assess for ease of entry into the port.
- Do not allow the pump to become empty.
- When accessing the pump, do the following:
  Insert the needle at a 90-degree angle.
  Do not rock the needle back and forth during insertion.
  Flush with 10 ml of saline before instilling medications.
  Use the secondary port for bolus medications.
  Always use syringes of at least 10 ml to avoid applying excessive pressure.

Specialists

Surgeon

Complete resection of the pancreatic tumor(s) is the only cure. However, fewer than 15% of cases of pancreatic cancer are diagnosed early enough for cure to be possible. In addition, even among individuals who have a complete resection, the 5-year survival rate is about 10% (Mayer, 2001b). The procedure of choice is a pancreaticoduodenectomy, because this preserves exocrine function and prevents the development of brittle diabetes.

Tumors are also resected for palliation. The choice of a surgeon is critical: the experience of the surgeon is the most important variable determining mortality rate, which can be

Box 32-9   Clinical Manifestations of Pancreatic Cancer

- Jaundice
- Gnawing epigastric pain
  May radiate to back
  Improves on leaning forward
- Fatigue
- Nausea and vomiting
- Anorexia
- Weight loss
- Dark urine
- Clay-colored stools
- Palpable liver, gallbladder
- Ascites
- Thrombophlebitis
- Glucose intolerance

as high as 15% because of the complex vascular anatomy and the numerous anastomoses required (Magee et al, 2002).

Other palliative surgical procedures that may be performed include placement of stents to relieve obstructive jaundice and obstructions of the duodenum.

Oncologist

External beam radiation may be considered for palliative treatment. Radiation does shrink the tumor, which may lessen pain, but it does not increase survival time.

Although chemotherapy has not been shown to be effective in the treatment of pancreatic cancer, combining external beam radiation therapy with chemotherapy using 5-FU has prolonged survival in some individuals.

Drug Therapy

The focus of pharmacologic intervention is pain management. High doses of opioid analgesics are generally given on a fixed schedule around the clock. The cytotoxic agent gemcitabine (Gemzar) is routinely given to reduce the size of the tumor, which aids in pain management.

Nurse

The nurse works with the patient and family to plan and coordinate the care required. The goals of care for the patient with resectable disease include improving nutritional status and preventing skin breakdown. Diarrhea and frequent defecation are common symptoms related to impaired digestion and absorption of fats. The nature and frequency of stool make skin care an important consideration. The anal region should be cleansed after each stool and an emollient or skin barrier should be applied to protect the skin. In addition, individuals with jaundice may have pruritus that causes them to scratch and abrade the skin. Box 32-10 lists interventions to manage pruritus. Most individuals need assistance with ADL until they have gained sufficient strength to manage independently. Consideration must be given to toileting, and bedside commodes should be ordered if necessary.

The focus areas for the patient with nonresectable disease are maintaining quality of life for the time that remains and ensuring a peaceful, dignified death (see Chapter 27 for a

Box 32-10   Strategies to Manage Pruritus

- Avoid hot baths or showers.
- Pat, rather than rub, skin dry.
- Humidify room.
- Apply emollients.
- Stay well hydrated.
- Take antihistamines.
- Use alternatives to scratching, such as rubbing with knuckles, pinching the skin.
- Keep fingernails short and clean.

discussion of end-of-life care). In addition to meeting the physical and emotional needs of the patient, the nurse must support family members and caregivers to ensure that they remain physically and emotionally healthy throughout the difficult period after the diagnosis is made. This is a particularly stressful time because the prognosis is generally poor and the time within which to address that fact is relatively short. An advance directive must be discussed and the appropriate legal documents prepared. Depending on the overall health of the patient, the nurse may suggest hospice care.

Dietitian

Diet teaching focuses on restriction of rich, fatty foods and consumption of small, frequent meals. Individuals with pancreatic cancer typically experience anorexia and significant weight loss. The weight loss is due in part to the disruption in the exocrine function of the pancreas. Therefore, pancreatic supplements must be given with meals to enhance digestion and absorption. Individuals and family members are instructed to report signs of abdominal distention, cramping, or frothy, fatty stools, because these indicate the need for an increase in the amount of replacement enzymes. Teaching regarding the proper way to take pancreatic enzymes is outlined in Box 32-11.

COMPLEMENTARY AND ALTERNATIVE THERAPIES

Individuals with cancer often look to other treatment modalities when traditional care fails to offer a hope for cure. Providers must ask about the use of herbal, homeopathic, and other therapies because they might interfere with the treatment plan. Some complementary strategies that can be suggested are balanced nutrition, relaxation techniques, and exercise.

FAMILY AND CAREGIVER ISSUES

The diagnosis of abdominal cancer related to the bowel or digestive organs creates a major upheaval in family functioning. Because of the poor prognosis and limited time for adjustment, families often do not know what to do first. They are grieving for their own potential losses and require

---

Box 32-11 Teaching Points Related to the Use of Pancreatic Enzymes

- Take with meals and/or snacks.
- Do not take with antacids or H_2 receptor blockers.
- Do not crush enteric-coated preparations.
- Prevent irritation to the mouth and lips by swallowing tablets whole and wiping lips after taking.
- Mix powdered forms with juice; do not mix with milk or other protein-containing foods.

---

emotional support at the same time that they are needed to support the affected family member. Many families are in a state of shock and denial and need help mobilizing resources to manage the illness and its treatment. There may be a sense of hopelessness and panic as things move swiftly out of control. Families also need support and assistance in obtaining resources for an unwanted future. Discussions about advance directives and financial preparation are essential. Relationships between family members may be strained as each attempts to deal with grief and continue with "life as usual." Complementary therapies that enhance relaxation can help reduce anxiety. Participation in support groups can improve quality of life and in some instances has been shown to prolong life (Dest, 2000).

Think S for Success

Symptoms
- Assess level of distress associated with symptoms and develop a plan with patient that prioritizes care on that basis.
- Prevent dumping syndrome by offering frequent small meals and avoiding dairy products, gas-producing foods, and liquids with meals.

Sequelae
- Prevent malnutrition and monitor weight loss. Manage nutritional deficits by controlling nausea, ascertaining food preferences, offering small, frequent meals, and providing supplements as needed (e.g., pancreatic enzymes).
- Maintain normal bowel pattern, manage intestinal diversions to prevent constipation, provide meticulous skin care to stoma sites.
- Assess stoma frequently for signs of complications.

Safety
- Assess for life-threatening side effects while patients are receiving chemotherapy, especially cytokines.

Support/Services
- Refer patient and family to community organizations, support groups, respite care, hospice care, sex therapists, counselors.
- Assess family's coping skills and degree to which family wishes to be involved in providing physical care and emotional support.
- Teach strategies for meeting the needs of both patient and caregiver.

Satisfaction
- Determine how illness has interfered with the ability of patient and family to maintain roles and enjoy the important aspects of their lives.
- Develop a plan to maintain quality of life.

RENAL CELL CARCINOMA

A number of tumors can develop in the kidney, including renal sarcoma, angiomyolipoma, Wilms' tumor, and renal cell adenoma. The most common type of kidney cancer is renal cell carcinoma. Approximately 30,000 cases of renal cell cancer are diagnosed each year, the majority of which occur in men between the ages of 40 and 70 years.

Smoking is the most significant risk factor for renal cell cancer. Obesity and exposure to cancer-producing chemicals such as asbestos are also risk factors. There is some evidence that people who eat well-cooked meat are more likely to develop renal cancer, whereas people who eat the recommended amounts of fruits and vegetables have lower risk (American Cancer Society, 2003).

Assessment

The early signs and symptoms of renal cancer are nonspecific and include complaints of generalized weakness and fatigue. The provider uses the functional health pattern assessment to uncover any changes in elimination patterns. Patients may complain of back or flank pain. Although frank hematuria is a late sign of kidney cancer, urinalysis should be ordered for all persons who come for treatment with difficulties in urinary elimination. Physical assessment may reveal a palpable mass in the area of the kidney.

Diagnosis

Several imaging techniques are used to detect the presence of renal tumors, including ultrasonography, CT, and MRI. The study that is most useful for detecting and evaluating renal cancer is the intravenous pyelogram with nephrotomography.

Pathophysiology

Renal cell cancer originates in the renal cortex for reasons that remain unclear. Current research is focusing on DNA mutations and their causes to understand how renal cancer develops. The hypothesis is that, because the kidney filters blood, toxic substances found in the blood reach concentrations in the kidney high enough to damage cellular DNA.

Renal carcinoma spreads by direct extension. Several staging systems are used to aid in diagnosis and treatment of the disease. The oldest is Robson's staging system. Robson's system relies solely on the extent of metastasis, whereas the TNM system considers tumor size, lymph node involvement, and the presence of metastasis to stage the disease (Box 32-12). In either case, higher stages indicate more advanced cancer and more limited treatment options.

Clinical Manifestations

Kidney cancer is usually diagnosed late in the course of the disease because there are no initial signs or symptoms. Individuals who are diagnosed incidentally while some other ailment is being investigated generally have no pain, discomfort, or difficulty with elimination.

The classic manifestations of renal cancer are hematuria and flank pain, although these signs and symptoms are present in other conditions as well. Signs and symptoms that should prompt further testing are listed in Box 32-13.

Box 32-12   Staging Systems for Renal Cell Carcinoma

TNM STAGES

I   Tumor is about 7 cm or less and limited to the kidney.

II   Tumor is larger than 7 cm but still limited to the kidney.

III   Tumor has spread to a nearby lymph node but not to distant nodes or organs.
or
Tumor has spread to fatty tissue or large veins but not to any lymph nodes.

IV   Tumor has spread through fatty tissue and fascia or there is distant metastasis.

ROBSON'S STAGES

I   Tumor is confined to the kidney.

II   Cancer has spread to fatty tissue or adrenal gland.

III   Cancer has spread to nearby nodes and/or blood vessels.

IV   Cancer has spread to a nearby organ or there is distant metastasis.

Interdisciplinary Care
Primary Provider (Physician/Nurse Practitioner)

The primary provider assesses overall health status, collects routine urine samples, and is alert to complaints that, in light of the patient's history, indicate the need for follow-up. People who have hereditary conditions such as von Hippel-Lindau disease or who require dialysis to treat other conditions should have frequent screening examinations to detect for renal masses. The latter will probably have a nephrologist as their primary provider.

Once cancer is detected, the individual is referred to a surgeon for staging of the disease and removal of either the tumor or the kidney.

Specialists

Surgeon
Surgical resection is the treatment of choice and the only curative measure available. The type of surgery performed is

---

Box 32-13   Clinical Manifestations of Renal Cancer

- Hematuria
- Flank pain
- Unilateral low back pain not associated with injury
- Weight loss
- Fatigue
- Anemia
- Persistent fever
- Abdominal mass
- Pedal edema

based on the stage of the cancer. Individuals with stage I or II cancer will undergo partial or radical nephrectomy. The survival rate is better than 90% for those with stage I cancers and between 65% and 75% for those with stage II cancers. Adjuvant therapy is not recommended for these individuals.

The most common treatment for patients with stage III cancer is radical nephrectomy along with regional lymphadenectomy. Many variations in the size and spread of cancer are seen at this stage, so the 5-year survival rate varies greatly, ranging from 40% to 70%. Patients with stage IV cancers are generally not candidates for surgery because of the presence of distant metastases. In some cases, however, if the metastatic tumors are few and resectable, surgery may be attempted. Nevertheless, the 5-year survival rate is less than 10%.

Oncologist

Neither radiation nor chemotherapy has been shown to be successful in treating renal cell cancer. The oncologist today is more likely to use immunotherapy or a combination of immunotherapy and chemotherapy with 5-FU. In immunotherapy, cytokines such as interleukin 2 (Proleukin) and interferon alpha (Roferon-A) are given to activate the immune system.

These substances have significant side effects that include heart attack, pleural effusion, and intestinal bleeding. Therefore, the American Cancer Society (2003) recommends that patients seek out providers who have expertise in the administration of these drugs. Cytokines are also injected into cells that have been removed from the patient's bloodstream. The immune-activated cells are then returned to the patient's bloodstream to seek out and kill cancer cells.

Nurse

Renal cell cancer is usually unilateral, and the individual who has undergone nephrectomy generally returns to previous roles and activities. The nurse encourages the patient to adopt healthy behaviors such as managing the weight, decreasing the amount of red meat in the diet, and stopping smoking to reduce the risk for developing cancer in the remaining kidney. In addition, the individual and family members are informed about the importance of follow-up and are provided with a list of community resources to help them deal with residual fear and anxiety related to the diagnosis of cancer. For the individual with advanced disease, the role of the nurse is primarily one of supporting end-of-life care (see Chapter 27).

CANCER OF THE URINARY BLADDER

Bladder cancer accounts for 1 out of every 20 cancers diagnosed in the United States. It is three times more common in men and most often occurs in the sixth to seventh decade.

The three main types of cancer that affect the bladder are urothelial carcinoma (also known as transitional cell carcinoma), squamous cell carcinoma, and adenocarcinoma. Urothelial carcinoma is the most common form of bladder cancer and accounts for more than 90% of cases.

Assessment

A complete physical examination, health history, and functional health assessment are performed. In addition, urine is examined for the presence of neoplastic cells sloughed off from the bladder surface and/or bladder cancer antigens.

Diagnosis

Imaging techniques such as CT, MRI, intravenous pyelography, and ultrasonography are used to determine if masses are present in the bladder. The diagnosis of cancer is confirmed by direct visualization via cystoscopy and biopsy. Cancer stage is determined by evaluating the depth of the invasion (Box 32-14).

Cancer in situ and cancers at stages O and A are considered superficial cancers. Cancers at stages B and C are considered invasive, and cancers at stage D are metastatic. Bladder cancer is also graded according to the amount of cell differentiation present. Cancers with well-differentiated cells are classified as grade I. The lower the grade and stage, the better the prognosis.

Pathophysiology

Urothelial tumors are categorized into several subtypes depending on whether they are noninvasive or invasive and whether their shape is papillary or flat. Noninvasive cancers involve only the innermost layer of the bladder, the urothelium, whereas invasive cancers have spread from the urothelium to the deeper layers of the bladder wall. It is very important to determine exactly how far into the bladder wall the cancer has invaded. Invasion of the thick muscle layer of the bladder is much more serious than invasion that is limited to the superficial connective tissue or thin muscle layers.

Papillary tumors have slender, fingerlike projections that grow into the hollow center of the bladder. Papillary urothelial tumors that grow only toward the center of the bladder are called *noninvasive papillary urothelial tumors*. Papillary carcinomas that grow both inward toward the center and

Box 32-14	Staging System for Bladder Cancer
STAGE	**TISSUE INVOLVED**
O	Mucosa
A	Submucosa
B	Muscle
C	Perivesical fat
D	Lymph nodes

outward into the bladder wall are called *invasive papillary urothelial carcinomas.* Papillary urothelial carcinomas are papillary tumors showing variable degrees of abnormality in the shape, size, and arrangement of cells. Those with relatively slight abnormality are termed *low grade.* Although they rarely invade the bladder wall, they often return after surgery. Carcinomas with greater abnormalities, called *high-grade carcinomas,* are more likely to invade the bladder wall or spread to other parts of the body.

Flat urothelial carcinomas do not grow toward the hollow part of the bladder at all. Some of these involve only the layer of cells closest to the inside or hollow part of the bladder. These are called *noninvasive flat urothelial carcinomas.* Another name for noninvasive flat urothelial carcinomas is *flat carcinoma in situ.*

Clinical Manifestations

Gross hematuria is the presenting symptom in over 80% of individuals. Other symptoms include frequency, urgency, and dysuria.

Interdisciplinary Care

Urothelial carcinomas, squamous cell carcinomas, and adenocarcinomas respond differently to radiation and chemotherapy. Treatment recommendations are influenced by the type of carcinoma, but the goal of treatment is to preserve the bladder if possible.

Primary Provider (Physician/Nurse Practitioner)

The primary provider thoroughly interviews and examines the patient to determine the potential cause of the patient's symptoms. Once cancer is diagnosed, the individual is referred to a surgeon for staging and treatment.

Specialists

Surgeon
Surgical resection is curative if the cancer is detected early. A variety of procedures are performed based on the location and invasiveness of the disease. The tumor can be resected transurethrally through a cystoscope or photocoagulated with laser beams. In come cases segments of the bladder may be resected or a radical cystectomy with urinary diversion may be performed.

Oncologist
Chemotherapy and radiation are primarily palliative. External beam radiation may be ordered to shrink tumors preoperatively or given as an adjunct to cystectomy.

If chemotherapy is used in combination with radiation, the drugs commonly given are cisplatin (Platinol), vinblastine (Velban), and doxorubicin (Adriamycin).

Some oncologists may suggest intravesical instillation of chemotherapy drugs if the cancer is noninvasive. In these cases, the drug is instilled into the patient's bladder weekly for 6 to 12 weeks. The most commonly used agents are bacille

Calmette-Guérin, a strain of mycobacterium used to stimulate the immune system, and thiotepa, an alkylating agent. Although patients who receive these drugs intravesically do not experience the common side affects associated with chemotherapy, they may have dysuria, hemorrhagic cystitis, and flulike symptoms.

Nurse

Unless the patient has undergone urinary diversion, the nursing care of the patient with bladder cancer focuses on education and support. The individual should be encouraged to quit smoking and should be reminded to increase fluid intake and keep follow-up appointments.

A patient who has undergone a urinary diversion needs support to accept the changes in the way the body functions and appears. The patient and his or her family require reassurance that, once the individual has recovered, he or she can resume most normal work and leisure activities. They also must be given specific instruction about the care of the stoma, surrounding skin, and appliances, and about self-catheterization. Urinary diversions may be continent or incontinent, depending on the type of procedure performed. A stoma is created in both types, but the continent diversion allows urine to be collected in an internal reservoir. Intermittent catheterization is required with a continent diversion. An incontinent diversion drips urine constantly and requires the use of an appliance and meticulous skin care. In addition, the appliance or reservoir must be emptied every 2 or 3 hours to prevent backflow and subsequent infection. Monitoring of output is an important aspect of care, because a decrease in output can be a sign of obstruction or internal leakage. Box 32-15 lists nursing interventions related to care of a patient with a urinary stoma.

Box 32-15   Nursing Interventions for the Patient with a Urinary Stoma

- Encourage high oral intake of fluids.
- Assess for changes in self-esteem and coping.
- Assess the concerns of the individual and his or her partner regarding sexual patterns.
- Discourage the wearing of tight-fitting clothing or binders over the stoma.
- Teach the patient and family the following:
  Need to monitor output as appropriate
  Signs of infection
  Stoma care
  Method of assessing stoma for complications
  Correct method for applying pouches and drainage devices
  Correct method for self-catheterization

Enterostomal Therapist

The ET generally meets with the individual prior to surgery and then again postoperatively in the hospital, clinic, and at home if home visits are warranted. The ET works with the patient and family to determine the best appliance system and to fit the appliance to the stoma. Because the stoma shrinks over time, the individual may have to be refitted. The opening of the appliance should be more than 2 to 3 mm larger than the stoma. The ET also teaches self-care techniques and prevention and management of skin problems. Table 32-4 lists skin problems commonly encountered and interventions to address them.

Medical Social Worker

The MSW works with the individual to obtain the necessary supplies and equipment and seeks financial aid for the purchase of such items if the individual is eligible. If the person is unable to manage the care of the stoma independently, the MSW may be called on to find an extended care facility or long-term care placement for that person.

Family and Caregiver Issues

Individuals with urinary diversions must attend to elimination and skin care needs several times a day. This may interfere with the ability to maintain employment and perform functional roles within the family. The individual may become absorbed with self-care and withdraw from social situations. Changes in roles and usual activities can alter family dynamics and strain family relationships. Individuals and families should be encouraged to discuss their concerns openly. These discussions can be facilitated by providers, who can help families express their feelings and identify both positive and negative coping behaviors.

Think **S** for Success

Symptoms
- Assess level of distress associated with symptoms and develop a plan with patient that prioritizes care on that basis. Manage stoma complications with good skin care and appropriate fitting of appliance.

Sequelae
- Prevent urinary tract infection by encouraging consumption of up to 2 L of fluid daily, ensuring that appliance or reservoir is emptied every 2 to 3 hours during the day and that the drainage bag is in dependent position during sleep.
- Reinforce need to use sterile or clean technique with self-catheterization.
- Stress importance of follow-up to screen for recurrence.

Safety
- Instruct patient with nephrectomy to inform all providers of that fact. Use care with nephrotoxic drugs, etc.
- Arrange for renal laboratory tests to be done annually to monitor function of remaining kidney.

Support/Services
- Refer patient and family to community organizations, support groups, respite care, hospice care, counselors.
- Assess family's coping skills and degree to which family wishes to be involved in providing physical care and emotional support.
- Teach strategies for meeting needs of both patient and caregiver.

Satisfaction
- Determine how illness has interfered with the ability of patient and family to maintain roles and enjoy important aspects of their lives.
- Develop a plan to maintain quality of life.

Table 32-4 Stoma-Related Skin Problems and Treatments

Problem	Treatment
Erythema	Check pouch for leakage. May have to refit opening or change appliance for better seal.
Allergic reaction	Change pouch systems or products. See dermatologist if reaction persists.
Candidal infection	Apply antifungal powders.
Excoriations	Make sure appliance is fitted properly and positioned so as to lessen drag on skin. Replace only as necessary. Loosen adhesive using solvent when replacing permanent appliances.
Encrustation	Keep skin around stoma clean and dry. Keep urine acidic.

CASE STUDY
Patient Data

Mr. C. is a 57-year-old man who comes to see his primary provider because he has been experiencing rectal bleeding for about 1 month. Mr. C. did not want to come to the doctor because he thinks this bleeding is due to his hemorrhoids, but his wife insisted that he see a doctor or nurse practitioner. He states that he feels fine except for being tired. He reports no nausea, vomiting, bloating, rectal or abdominal pain, weight loss, or anorexia. His physical examination is unremarkable with the exception of a positive result on the FOBT.

Mr. C. has no history of diverticulosis, irritable bowel disease, or diagnosed hemorrhoids. He also reports no family history of colorectal cancer or polyps. He is an ex-smoker with a 20 pack-year history. He has not had any screening tests for colorectal cancer, and his last visit to the doctor was 3 years earlier.

CASE STUDY—cont'd

The provider discusses the positive FOBT result with Mr. and Mrs. C. and explains the need for a colonoscopy, which is subsequently scheduled and reveals an ulcerated lesion in the sigmoid colon. The biopsy results indicate that the lesion is a poorly differentiated invasive carcinoma.

Thinking It Through

■ What additional tests or studies should be ordered for Mr. C.?

■ What type of procedure will most likely be performed? Will he have a colostomy?

■ What are the nursing priorities at this time?

■ What disciplines should be brought together to provide Mr. and Mrs. C. with comprehensive health care. What will each team member contribute?

Case Conference

Mr. C. has undergone surgical removal of his sigmoid colon with anastomosis. The resected margins are free of cancer, but several local nodes were found to be positive. Mr. C.'s cancer is determined to be stage III. Therefore, adjuvant treatment with a combination of 5-FU and leucovorin is recommended. The treatment is scheduled to begin in 3 weeks and will continue on a weekly basis for 6 months.

Mrs. C. asks about the side effects of the chemotherapy medication because she has heard "horror stories about how sick it makes you." The nurse tells Mrs. C. that there are typical side effects that they can expect. Most often patients receiving 5-FU experience nausea and vomiting, but they may also have diarrhea, mild hair loss, hyperpigmentation, and photosensitivity. Mr. C. looks a little worried by this, but he is quickly reassured that excellent drugs are available now to manage these symptoms and that he will be given medication to manage the nausea before the treatment even begins.

The MSW asks about the type of insurance they have, because some of the newer medications are quite expensive. Working with the insurance case manager up front may make financing the health care easier. He also inquires about the status of Mr. C.'s employment and the arrangements being made for them to continue receiving an income. The MSW also asks Mrs. C. whether she plans to accompany her husband to treatments and what impact this illness is having on her role and responsibilities. Transportation can be arranged to and from treatment sessions if necessary. Mrs. C. says that they have two children in the area who have offered to help.

The nurse notices that Mr. C. did not have advance directives in place until the time of the surgery. She encourages Mr. and Mrs. C. to discuss their feelings about these directives with their children and make sure their wishes are understood and documented in legal fashion. Mrs. C. looks alarmed and says, "I thought he was going to be okay!" The nurse reassures her that all patients are encouraged to have advance directives and that Mrs. C. herself should think about her own advance directives now, while she is relatively young and healthy.

The registered dietitian wants to know if Mr. C. is able to tolerate a regular diet and determines his food preferences. She sets up a time to visit him at home once chemotherapy has started to evaluate his nutritional status and needs. She provides him with a list of foods that are helpful in controlling diarrhea should that occur.

The nurse recognizes that the C.'s are probably overwhelmed at this point, and the case conference is ended. Mr. and Mrs. C. are asked if they have questions. They are instructed to call the outpatient clinic to set up the first treatment, and a series of home visits by the nurse, social worker, and dietitian is arranged. Mr. and Mrs. C. are encouraged to call the nurse, who will be the case manager, if they have additional questions or concerns.

■ What are the nursing diagnoses related to this case?

■ To what resources might the C.'s be referred?

■ What is the 5-year survival rate for this type of cancer?

■ Do you think the nurse should have brought up the subject of advance directives at this meeting?

■ Is there a role here for an occupational or physical therapist?

Internet and Other Resources

American Cancer Society: *http://www.cancer.org*
American Liver Foundation: *http://www.liverfoundation.org*
Colon Cancer Alliance: *http://www.ccalliance.org*
National Cancer Institute: *http://www.nci.nih.gov*
Pancreas.org: *http://www.pancreas.org*
Society of Urologic Nurse and Associates: *http://www.Suna.org*
United Ostomy Association: *http://www.uoa.org*

REFERENCES

American Cancer Society: Cancer reference information, 2003, retrieved from *http://www.cancer.org* on May 2, 2003.

Chan ES-Y et al: Neoadjuvant and adjuvant therapy for operable hepatocellular carcinoma, *Cochrane Library* 1, 2002, retrieved from *http://www.cochrane.de/cochrane/revabstr/ab001199.htm* on Feb 22, 2004

Dest V: Colorectal cancer, *RN* 6(7):53-60, 2000.

Dienstag J, Isselbacher K: Tumors of the liver and biliary tract. In Braunwald E et al, editors: *Harrison's principles of internal medicine,* New York, 2001, McGraw-Hill, pp 588-90.

Jensen RT: Endocrine tumors of the GI tract and pancreas. In Braunwald E et al, editors: *Harrison's principles of internal medicine,* New York, 2001, McGraw-Hill, pp 593-8

Knowles G: The management of colorectal cancer, *Nurs Standard* 16(17):47-59, 2002.

Magee C et al: Update on pancreatic cancer, *Hosp Med* 63(4):100-6, 2002.

Martin R: Use of hepatic lines, *J Infus Nurs* 25(2):127-33, 2002.

Mayer RJ: GI tract cancer. In Braunwald E et al, editors: *Harrison's principles of internal medicine,* New York, 2001a, McGraw-Hill, pp 578-88.

Mayer RJ: Pancreatic cancer. In Braunwald E et al, editors: *Harrison's principles of internal medicine,* New York, 2001b, McGraw-Hill, pp 591-3.

Scher H, Motzer R: Bladder and renal cell carcinomas. In Braunwald E et al, editors: *Harrison's principles of internal medicine,* New York, 2001, McGraw-Hill, pp 604-8.

Ueno S et al: Discrimination value of the western prognostic system (CLIP score) for hepatocellular carcinoma in 662 Japanese patents, *Hepatology* 34(3):529-34, 2001.

Wilkes G: New therapeutic options in colon cancer: focus on oxaliplatin, *Clin J Oncol Nurs* 6(3):131-51, 2002.

CHAPTER 33

Cancers of the Reproductive System

Judith Rogers, RNC, MSN, PhD(c)

The cancers of the reproductive system discussed in this chapter include cancers of the uterus, vagina, cervix, vulva, and testes, and prostate. (Cancer of the breast is discussed separately in Chapter 30.) Combined, these cancers accounted for over 100,000 deaths in 2002.

Sexuality and reproductive ability, critical components of the experience of being human, may be affected negatively by the biologic processes of cancer and cancer treatment. Therefore, the sense of sexuality and body image as well as the ability to be sexually intimate and to bear children are major concerns of patients with cancers of the reproductive organs.

Psychological and psychosexual issues may exacerbate infertility and sterility and the inability to have intercourse. These issues include alteration in body image, fear of abandonment, diminishing self-esteem, changes in sexual identity, and concerns about self (Yarbo et al, 2000) (Box 33-1).

Patients coping with reproductive organ cancer often have concerns about sexual functioning and responsiveness and may experience varying degrees of alteration in sexual functioning depending on the type of cancer, the stage of the disease, and the type of intervention. Patients at risk for difficulty in adjustment may benefit from early assessment and referral to professionals.

Surgical procedures may cause dysfunction through removal or alteration of reproductive organs or through damage to nerves that enervate sexual organs. Invasive and disfiguring surgery may also contribute to sexual dysfunction by causing individuals to be self-conscious or to feel less desirable. Removal of the ovaries may cause vaginal dryness, inelasticity of the vagina, and dyspareunia due to the loss of estrogen. Men may experience absence of erection, absence of ejaculation, or inability to penetrate. Decreased libido due to loss of testosterone may also occur.

Chemotherapy may create partial or total impotence and ejaculatory difficulties as well as a decrease in desire, arousal, and orgasmic ability. In women, chemotherapy contributes to menopausal symptoms and increased risk of urinary tract infection, vaginal irritation, and exacerbation of genital herpes and human papillomavirus infection. Patient and family education and provision of information regarding the drug regimen used is critical for patients receiving chemotherapy (see Chapter 27).

Similarly, radiation therapy contributes to sterility or transient infertility and may cause a decrease in sexual enjoyment, ability to attain orgasm, libido, frequency of intercourse, and sexual dreams. Women may experience vaginal stenosis or shortening as well as vaginal dryness and irritation and are at increased risk of infection.

Nausea, vomiting, and diarrhea can decrease energy, sexual desire, and feelings of desirability. Inflammation, pain, and limited range of motion may make sexual activity uncomfortable or impossible, and treatment-related fatigue can limit all activity. The use of energy conservation strategies, medication, lubricants, dilators, and sexual devices may prove helpful.

Extensive disease, mutilating treatments, and unavailability of reconstructive surgery increase the likelihood of sexual morbidity. Other factors such as depression, anxiety about cancer diagnosis, and relationship difficulties may also influence sexual functioning.

Box 33-1   Stress Related to Cancer of the Reproductive System

- Feelings of helplessness and uncertainty
- Requirement to redefine goals and expectations
- Need for family support to maintain good quality of life
- Negative impact on work, relationships, and ability to enjoy life
- Perceived loss of gender role functioning, such as loss of femininity or virility
- Concerns regarding sexual functioning and responsivity
- Anxiety related to loss of fertility

ASSESSMENT

In addition to assessing the physiologic effects of the cancer on the organ(s) involved and the impact on the patient's and family's functional status, the health care team must thoroughly assess sexual functioning and the patient's ability to cope with alterations in sexual functioning or body image.

Assessment of sexual functioning requires sensitive interviews by health care providers to gather information about sexual health history. The PLISSIT model (Box 33-2) of sexual counseling identifies different levels of discussion at which providers and patients can explore important sexual and body image concerns. The provider can be most effective by communicating permission to express these critical concerns. Patients may benefit from receiving limited information about sexual anatomy, response cycle, or changes to be expected. Specific suggestions such as use of alternative positioning and techniques, use of devices, and medical interventions to restore function may also be helpful. Patients who require intensive therapy should be referred to a trained professional. Box 33-3 provides a framework for functional health pattern assessment for reproductive cancers.

CANCER OF THE OVARIES

Cancer of the ovaries is called the "silent killer." It is often asymptomatic and has a poor prognosis. According to the National Ovarian Cancer Coalition (2002), almost 70% of women with common epithelial ovarian cancer are not diagnosed until the disease is in its advanced stage. Recent

---

Box 33-2   PLISSIT Model for Sexual Counseling

P	Permission giving
LI	Limited information
SS	Specific suggestions
IT	Intensive therapy

---

progress in treatment includes advanced cytoreductive surgery and more accurate staging of the disease. Specific and sensitive tests to detect the disease must be developed and become widely available to provide effective population-wide, screening programs. Currently no diagnostic tests are available to help detect the disease in the early stages.

Most ovarian cancers are sporadic and are not influenced by heredity. However, 5% to 10% of women who develop ovarian cancer have an inherited genetic susceptibility to the disease. The risk of developing ovarian cancer increases as the number of family members affected by ovarian cancer increases. Having a first-degree relative affected by ovarian cancer increases a woman's lifetime risk from 1.4% to 3.1%.

In comparison with other female reproductive organ cancers, ovarian cancer is by far the most lethal. Ovarian cancer accounts for 4% of cancers among women and ranks fifth as a cause of cancer-related death. The 5-year survival rate is 15% to 20% for advanced-stage cancer compared with 90% for stage I disease.

Pathophysiology

The most common type of ovarian cancer develops predominantly from the malignant transformation of a single cell type, surface epithelial cells. There are five types of epithelial ovarian cancers: serous, mucinous, endometrioid, clear cell, and Brenner tumors (Ausperg et al, 1998). Serous and mucinous tumors account for the vast majority of all ovarian tumors and may be benign, especially in women under the age of 40 years. Malignant tumors are usually found in women over 40 years of age. They are generally found as solid masses with areas of necrosis and hemorrhage.

The disease spreads by direct extension after penetrating the capsule of the ovary and invading nearby structures. Ovarian cancer metastasis can affect any organ and shows two patterns: lymphatic and direct. Most frequently, metastasis occurs to the intestines and bladder. In addition, cancer cells in peritoneal fluid can cause spread to the intestines, bladder, and mesentery. This is termed peritoneal seeding. Cells can also spread systematically through the lymphatic system and the blood to organs such as the liver, the diaphragm, and the lungs. Many risk factors for ovarian and other reproductive organ cancers have been identified (Table 33-1).

The monthly ovulatory cycle affects the ovarian epithelium. Because of this, the number of ovulatory cycles in a woman's life span has a significant influence on the likelihood of developing ovarian cancer. Nulliparous women have uninterrupted cell division with regeneration of ovarian epithelium. This provides an opportunity for mutation. Pregnancy, parity, and lactation have a protective effect.

Taking combined oral contraceptives also decreases the risk of ovarian cancer. The progestin in oral contraceptives induces damaged ovarian cells to die before malignancy can occur. Women who have low levels of follicle-stimulating hormone and luteinizing hormone, who have a history of

---

Box 33-3   Functional Health Pattern Assessment for Cancers of the Reproductive System

HEALTH PERCEPTION/HEALTH MANAGEMENT
- Is there a family history of cancer of the reproductive organs?
- Does the patient participate in screening programs such as regular Pap smear testing, breast self-examination, or testicular self-examination?
- What risk factors are present?

NUTRITION/METABOLISM
- What is the patient's current weight? Has there been any unexplained recent weight loss?
- How is the patient's appetite?
- Does the patient experience nausea and vomiting or a sensation of bloating?

ELIMINATION
- Have any changes occurred in bowel or bladder habits?
- Does the patient experience pain or difficulty in urination?
- Does the patient have a stoma or urinary diversion device?

ACTIVITY/EXERCISE
- Does the patient experience fatigue or malaise?
- What are the patient's regular exercise activities and activity habits?
- Can the patient perform the activities of daily living?

SLEEP/REST
- Is there any disruption of sleep patterns?

COGNITION/PERCEPTION
- What are the nature, character, location, and duration of the pain? What factors alleviate and aggravate the pain?
- Is there pain with sexual intercourse?

SELF-PERCEPTION/SELF-CONCEPT
- How has the condition affected the patient's personal identity?
- How has the condition affected the patient's self-esteem?
- What alterations have occurred in body image related to disfigurement and/or sexual dysfunction?
- What is the patient's perception of his or her sexual attractiveness?
- What are the patient's feelings about fertility?

ROLES/RELATIONSHIPS
- What kind of work does the patient perform?
- What role does the patient play in the home and family?
- What changes have occurred in sexual patterns?
- What changes have occurred in the patient's ability to carry out role functions (especially sexual role functions)?

- Has the opportunity for a future parenting role in the relationship been lost?
- How satisfied is the patient with his or her current roles and relationships, including sexual role?
- How has the condition affected the patient's family and/or significant others?
- How has the condition affected the sexual relationship of the patient and his or her partner?
- Have there been changes in the patient's social interaction or isolation?

SEXUALITY/REPRODUCTION
- At what age was the onset of menses? Is the menstrual cycle normal? Have changes occurred in the menstrual cycle or menstrual flow? Is discharge present?
- Is the patient sexually active? What is the frequency of intercourse? How many sexual partners has the patient had?
- What is the nature of the patient's sexual activity? Have there been any changes in this activity?
- Is the patient satisfied with current sexual patterns?
- Have there been any changes in sexual performance related to disfigurement, dysfunction, or disability?
- Has the patient experienced any changes in libido, erectile or orgasmic dysfunction, or alterations of sexual enjoyment?
- What are the patient's concerns regarding fertility?

COPING/STRESS TOLERANCE
- What coping strategies does the patient use?
- What support systems are available to the patient?
- Does the patient participate or wish to participate in a counseling program or receive sexual advice or therapy?
- Does the patient engage in any self-help efforts toward body-image enhancement?
- Does the patient want sexual device instruction?

VALUES/BELIEFS
- What constitutes good quality of life for the patient?
- What is important to the patient?
- What are the patient's beliefs about sexual norms?
- What are the patient's spiritual beliefs, health beliefs, and cultural beliefs?
- What are the patient's beliefs about the value of sexual performance, sexual enjoyment, and sexual fulfillment to an individual's life experience?

---

polycystic ovary syndrome with elevated androstenedione levels, and who experience endometriosis and associated hormone and immunologic abnormalities are at increased risk for ovarian cancer.

Tubal ligation or hysterectomy physically interrupts the utero-ovarian circulation and decreases the risk of ovarian cancer. These surgical procedures diminish exposure to exogenous toxins, which results in decreased risk for ovarian cancer.

A family history of ovarian cancer dramatically influences an individual's risk of developing ovarian cancer. The closer the relative and the younger the age at diagnosis, the higher the risk is. Women who have mutations of the BRCA1 tumor suppressor gene have increased susceptibility to

Table 33-1 Risk Factors Associated with Cancer of the Reproductive Organs in Women

Risk Factor	Type of Cancer				
	Ovarian	Cervical	Endometrial	Vulvar	Vaginal
Nulliparity	X		X		
Use of infertility drugs	X				
History of pelvic inflammatory disease	X				
Low serum gonadotropin levels	X				
Use of talc	X				
Family history of breast or ovarian cancer	X		X	X	
Residence in an industrialized Western country	X				
Jewish heritage	X				
Lower socioeconomic status		X			X
Exposure to occupational carcinogenics		X			
Sexual activity before age 17 years		X			
Sexual relations with a large number of partners		X		X	
Maternal use of diethylstilbestrol during pregnancy		X			X
Multiparity		X			
Smoking		X		X	
Immunosuppressed status		X		X	
Older age			X	X	X
Obesity			X		
Estrogen overproduction or estrogen replacement therapy			X		
Human papillomavirus infection		X		X	X
Herpes simplex virus type 2 infection		X		X	X
Genital warts		X		X	X
Chronic vulvar disease				X	
Previous radiation therapy					X

ovarian cancer. Several ethnic differences are seen in the incidence of ovarian cancer (Friedlander, 1998) (Box 33-4).

None of the currently available screening strategies alone or in combination is sufficiently sensitive or specific to screen the whole population. Although the CA-125 (cancer antigen 125) serum marker is highly specific to epithelial ovarian cancer, CA-125 is present in only about 50% of primary ovarian carcinomas confined to the ovary. Thus early studies, although encouraging, suggest that levels of this marker are not sufficiently sensitive or specific to merit recommending CA-125 determination as a single test for pop-ulation screening, particularly among premenopausal women (Bast, Xu, and Yu, 1998).

Clinical Manifestations

The initial signs and symptoms of ovarian cancer, although subtle and often ignored, are persistent and usually increase over time (Box 33-5).

Assessment

Critical components of assessment include a thorough patient and family history, physical examination, and diagnostic tests. Patient history must include both menstrual and reproductive history. An assessment of functional health patterns allows the provider to collect data about how the cancer is affecting the individual as a whole as well as what coping strategies are being employed (see Box 33-3). The physical examination reveals an enlarged, boggy uterus or the presence of a defined mass.

Diagnosis

A variety of diagnostic studies are used to detect ovarian cancer. These include computed tomography, colonoscopy, measurement of serum CA-125 levels, Doppler flow studies, and ultrasonography. Transvaginal ultrasonography provides superior visualization of the ovaries. The procedure

---

Box 33-4 Ethnic Differences in the Incidence of Ovarian Cancer

- The highest rates of ovarian cancer are found in North America, Scandinavian countries, and Israel.
- The lowest incidence is in Japan and in developing countries.
- In the United States, the incidence is slightly higher among the whites and native Hawaiians.
- Intermediate incidence is found among African Americans, Hispanics, and Asian Americans.
- Native Americans have the lowest incidence.

Box 33-5   Signs and Symptoms of Ovarian Cancer

EARLY
- Abdominal bloating, a feeling of fullness, gas, distention
- Frequent or urgent urination
- Nausea, indigestion, constipation, diarrhea
- Menstrual disorders, pain during intercourse
- Fatigue
- Lower abdominal pressure
- Back pain
- Increasing waist circumference

LATE
- Ascites
- Pleural effusion
- Anorexia
- Nausea and vomiting
- Abdominal, pelvic, ovarian, omental mass

---

allows measurement of ovarian size, can detect small masses, and is efficient and comfortable. However, ultrasonography cannot distinguish between benign and malignant ovarian masses (Ozols, 1997).

Over 30 types of ovarian cancer exist, classified by cell of origin. Staging of the disease is based on both surgical and histologic evaluation.

Interdisciplinary Care

The patient with reproductive organ cancer requires care by members of several different medical disciplines. The interdisciplinary team may include the primary care provider, surgeon, infertility specialist, radiation and medical oncologists, pathologist, nurse, dietitian, physical and occupational therapists, social worker, and counselor who specialize in relationships and sexual counseling.

Primary Provider (Physician/Nurse Practitioner)

The primary provider is generally the first practitioner to suspect the presence of ovarian cancer. Although early signs and symptoms may be dismissed by the individual, careful listening and thorough assessment (including pelvic examination) alert the provider to the possibility of a pathologic process. Diagnostic studies are ordered, and if results are positive for ovarian cancer, the individual is referred to specialists for treatment (Young and Pecorelli, 1998).

Surgeon

Surgery is considered the critical, core treatment. Referral to a gynecologic surgical oncologist is recommended. The aim of surgery is to provide a definitive diagnosis, stage the cancer, remove as much tumor as possible, improve survival prognosis, and relieve symptoms (Boente, Chi, and Hoskins,

1998). Common surgical procedures for early and advanced ovarian cancer are listed in Box 33-6.

Oncologist

Chemotherapy

The oncologist manages the therapeutic regimen by consulting with the surgical team and the radiation oncologist. Chemotherapy is aimed at remission rather than cure. Combination regimens including cyclophosphamide and cisplatin may be used. Altretamine (Hexalen) is used for palliative treatment of persistent, recurrent ovarian cancer. Paclitaxel (Taxol) and topotecan (Hycamtin) are used to treat metastatic ovarian cancer. The most significant toxic effects of these drugs include bone marrow destruction and renal damage. Patients undergoing maintenance therapy may develop drug-resistant tumors or recurrent disease, both of which indicate poor prognosis.

Radiation Therapy

Radiotherapy is often effective in shrinking tumors and may be used alone or in conjunction with surgery. Radiation may be delivered intraperitoneally or by external beam (Lanciano et al, 1998).

After the initial treatments, patients are followed closely for evidence of recurrence. Although elevated levels of CA-125 serum tumor marker are predictive of recurrence, there is no evidence that immediate chemotherapy is beneficial as long as the patient is asymptomatic and the pelvic examination is normal and without evidence of definitive disease. Therapeutic measures for recurrent disease often produce only a brief response. Salvage therapy includes repeating the original treatments or trying new chemotherapeutic agents. Use of investigational drugs and clinical trial

---

Box 33-6   Surgical Procedures for Early and Advanced Ovarian Cancer

EARLY
- Total abdominal hysterectomy
- Bilateral salpingo-oophorectomy
- Peritoneal cytologic analysis
- Omentectomy
- Scraping of the undersurface of the right diaphragm
- Multiple peritoneal biopsies
- Pelvic and paraaortic lymph node sampling

ADVANCED
- Interval debulking
- Cytoreductive surgery
- Second-look surgery
- Laparoscopic surgery
- Palliative surgery

participation is recommended (Roland et al, 1998). Those most likely to benefit from salvage therapy include patients with small-volume disease, good performance status, long disease-free period, favorable serous histologic analysis, and a low number of disease sites. When determining whether or not an individual should receive additional treatment, the provider considers the patient's age, prior response to treatment, quality of life, comorbidities, and toxicity profile as well as the patient's preference.

Nurse

Depending on the type of cancer, stage of the disease, type of surgical intervention, and chemotherapeutic and radiation regimen, patients may experience varying degrees of alteration in sexual functioning. Key nursing interventions include patient education regarding what to expect and strategies for response. Patients at risk for difficulty in adjustment benefit from early assessment and referral to trained professionals.

Advanced ovarian cancer can cause dysfunction in many different systems. Women may experience a multitude of gastrointestinal problems, including ascites, intestinal obstruction, malnutrition, pleural effusion, and lymphedema. Nursing management of patients with advanced disease focuses on the management of these problems (Box 33-7).

CANCER OF THE CERVIX

Cervical cancer is a significant cause of morbidity and mortality for women worldwide. In the United States, 13,000 women developed cervical cancer in 2002, and 4100 women died from the disease. Cervical cancer is the twelfth most common cancer in women and the fourteenth most common cause of cancer death. Cure rates are greatly improved by early detection.

Cervical cancer often occurs during the reproductive years. The majority of women are diagnosed in the preinvasive stages of the disease (National Cervical Cancer Coalition, 2002). The cause of cervical cancer has not been determined, but several risk factors (see Table 33-1) and ethnic factors (Box 33-8) increase the likelihood of the disease (Cadman, 1998). The presence of viral infections such as infection with human immunodeficiency virus, human papillomaviruses, and herpes simplex virus 2 is significantly correlated with the occurrence of cervical cancer. Smoking has also been linked to the likelihood of contracting cervical cancer, as has experiencing early first coitus and having a large number of sexual partners (Ross, 1998).

Pathophysiology

About 80% to 90% of cervical cancers are squamous cell tumors. The remaining 10% to 20% are adenocarcinomas. Prognosis is related to tumor size and metastasis to the lymph nodes.

Cancer of the cervix is the culmination of a progressive disease than begins as a neoplastic alteration of the squamocolumnar junction (junction of the endocervix and the exocervix at the cervical os, also called the transformation zone). Over time these abnormal cells progress to involve the full thickness of the epithelium and invade the stromal tissue of the cervix.

Squamous cell cancers spread by direct extension to adjacent structures such as the vagina, pelvic wall, bladder, and rectum. Metastasis is most often confined to the pelvis, but distant metastasis occurs through the lymphatic system. The most common sites are the lungs, mediastinal and supraclavicular nodes, liver, and bone. Metastasis may also occur through hematogenous spread and intraperitoneal implantation.

The initial preinvasive or premalignant changes are called *cervical intraepithelial neoplasia*. Each step in the cervical disease process merges imperceptibly into the next.

Clinical Manifestations

Preinvasive and early-stage cancer is usually asymptomatic. Symptoms are often subtle, persistent, and usually increase over time (Box 33-9).

Assessment

Critical components of assessment include a thorough patient and family history including both menstrual and reproductive history, physical examination, and diagnostic studies. The most effective screening mechanism for detection of cervical cancer is an annual pelvic examination with Papanicolaou (Pap) smear testing. The Pap smear analysis screens for cervical intraepithelial neoplasia as well as cervical cancer. In addition, the test can assess the patient's hormonal status and screen for the presence of sexually transmitted diseases. Current research also suggests that screening for the presence of human papillomavirus may facilitate early detection of cervical cancer.

Cancer of the cervix is categorized either as a squamous intraepithelial lesion or as invasive disease. The assessment, therapeutic approach, and nursing responsibilities differ depending on the diagnosis.

Diagnosis

If the results of the screening Pap test show atypical cells, the test should be repeated. Various classification systems are used to report Pap test results. If results of the repeat Pap test show abnormal cells, the patient is referred for biopsy, colposcopy, and/or treatment. In advanced disease, clinical examination under anesthesia is recommended, as are cervical biopsies, endocervical curettage, cystoscopy, and proctosigmoidoscopy.

Diagnostic tests to detect tumor spread include chest radiography, skeletal radiography, intravenous pyelography, barium enema study, complete blood count and blood chemistry tests, liver scan, lymphangiography, computed tomography, magnetic resonance imaging, and node biopsy.

Box 33-7   Nursing Interventions for Advanced Cancer of the Ovaries, Cervix, and Endometrium

ASCITES
- Instruct the patient and/or family to measure weight or abdominal girth daily.
- Caution the patient to notify the provider if fluid starts to reaccumulate.
- Advise the patient to alternate activity with rest periods to conserve energy.
- Encourage the patient to lie on the left side with the feet elevated to alleviate pressure on internal organs, improve vascular return from the lower extremities, facilitate lymphatic flow, and improve diuresis.
- Instruct the patient to eat small, frequent meals to avoid discomfort.
- Ensure that the patient maintains fluid restrictions if imposed to minimize recurrence of ascites.
- Assist the patient in taking an active part in the management of ascites to lessen anxiety, help restore a sense of control, promote self-esteem, improve body image, and increase the ability to function.

INTESTINAL OBSTRUCTION
- Manage the gastrostomy tube.
- Facilitate adequate hydration by giving small, low-residue meals.
- Manage total parental nutrition.
- Restrict oral intake if bowel obstruction is not surgically managed.
- Give small amounts of clear liquids after several hours of bowel rest and slowly advance diet.
- Encourage consumption of a low-fiber diet because of profound narrowing of the small or large intestine.

MALNUTRITION
- Instruct patient to keep a food diary.
- Instruct patient to weigh daily.
- Provide information on how to maintain a well-balanced, high-calorie diet.
- Enlist the support of a dietitian.
- Consider the use of nutritional supplements.
- Design menus incorporating the patient's favorite foods.
- Avoid foods with disturbing odors or tastes.
- Manage symptoms that are interfering with appetite.
- Assess food intake every 4 weeks, allowing 8 to 12 weeks for weight gain.
- Manage total parental nutrition.
- Use pharmacologic management, including the following medications:
  Corticosteroids to produce short-term improvement in appetite
  Megestrol (Megace)
  Dronabinol (Marinol)

LYMPHEDEMA
- Instruct the patient and caregiver to report early swelling or problems with edema.

- Provide the patient with strategies to manage the discomfort of edema.
- Support the patient in coping with limitation of mobility.
- Teach the patient meticulous skin care of affected edematous limbs.
- Use pharmacologic management, including the following medications:
  Antibiotics for concurrent infections
  Diuretics (may provide limited benefit)
- Enlist the support of a physical therapist for manual lymphatic drainage, bandaging, exercise, and use of a compression garment on the affected extremity.

PLEURAL EFFUSION
- Observe for pain, increased respiration rate, dyspnea, increased pulse rate, vertigo, and uncontrollable cough.
- Provide the patient with palliative measures for severe dyspnea, including instructions to sit upright and lean forward over a table or rest the elbows on the knees.
- Instruct the patient in relaxation techniques, including controlled breathing, listening to relaxing music, massage, and range-of-motion exercises.

NAUSEA AND VOMITING
- Assess duration and frequency of vomiting and nature of vomitus, and identify aggravating and alleviating factors.
- Assess for dehydration and administer intravenous fluids if ordered.
- Maintain an accurate record of intake and output.
- Encourage the patient to take small sips of fluid as tolerated.
- Monitor laboratory results indicating electrolyte balance.
- Remove visual stimuli and sources of odors.
- Provide mouth care.
- Use diversional activities.
- Maintain a quiet environment.
- Encourage the patient to limit visitors when fatigued.
- Avoid unnecessary procedures or activities.
- Assess the patient's interest in food.
- Encourage resumption of eating by providing bland, nonirritating foods and proceed cautiously.
- Use pharmacologic management (antiemetics).
- Instruct the patient in deep breathing.
- Prevent sudden changes in position.
- Keep the head of the bed elevated.

PAIN
- Instruct the patient to evaluate pain frequently using a quantitative pain scale.
- Provide comfort measures such as touch.
- Encourage the support of family members.
- Use pharmacologic management (analgesics with evaluation of their efficacy).

Interdisciplinary Care
Primary Provider (Physician/Nurse Practitioner)

As with ovarian cancer, the primary provider generally detects cervical cancer. Unlike ovarian cancer, however, cervical cancer is likely to be detected early because of the widespread practice of performing annual Pap smear testing. If the primary provider is a gynecologist, treatment may be provided by that physician. If the primary provider is an internal medicine or family practice provider, the patient is referred for treatment.

The choice of therapy is based on the extent of the disease, the patient's age and general medical condition, the patient's preference with regard to preservation of ovarian and reproductive function, the presence of any complicating abnormalities, and the physician's recommendation (Yarbo et al, 2000) (Box 33-10).

Surgeon

Gynecologists specialize in medical and surgical treatment of gynecologic conditions. Surgery, including direct cervical biopsy, is the critical first intervention to determine the extent of the cervical cancer. Together with colposcopy, laser surgery may prove effective when the cancer is limited to the cervical epithelium. Electrocautery and cryosurgery cause necrosis and sloughing of endometrial tissue and can be effective treatments for noninvasive lesions. Conization, the surgical removal of a cone-shaped portion of the cervix, is used to treat microinvasive carcinoma of the cervix when colposcopy cannot define the limits of the invasion.

Hysterectomy or radical hysterectomy is performed for invasive lesions. A pelvic exenteration (removal of all pelvic contents, including the bowel, vagina, and bladder) is undertaken in cases of disease recurrence without involvement of the lymphatic system.

Oncologist
Chemotherapy

Individuals who have recurrent disease or metastasis are referred to an oncologist for chemotherapy. Chemotherapy has not proven useful as initial therapy for women who are at high risk for recurrence. However, the use of neoadjuvant therapy to shrink tumors before surgery or radiotherapy can be an effective strategy, especially in the management of advanced cervical cancer.

Many different chemotherapeutic drugs are used and are often given in combination for several months. The most common drug regimens include cisplatin, but other drugs such as 5-fluorouracil (5-FU), hydroxyurea (Hydrea), ifosfamide (Ifex), and paclitaxel (Taxol) may also be used. The selection of a drug regimen is based on the current overall health status, personal values and goals of therapy, and tolerance.

Radiation Therapy

Radiation therapy is used to treat invasive cervical cancer. External beam radiation is used to decrease tumor size, whereas radioactive implants are used to treat tumors that have metastasized beyond the pelvic wall. Radiation is also used for palliation in patients who have very advanced cancer to ease symptoms.

Nurse

Nursing care of the patient undergoing a local therapy such as laser surgery, cryosurgery, and electrocautery includes patient education regarding the disease process, treatments and possible complications, possibility of treatment failure, self-care after treatment, and importance of follow-up care.

Nursing care of the patient receiving radiation therapy focuses on education regarding treatment procedure, side effects of therapy, and mobility restrictions with intracavity and interstitial radiotherapy (see Chapter 27).

Education for the patient receiving chemotherapy should include the rationale for the therapy, an explanation of side effects and signs of toxicities, and information about clinical trials.

The patient who has undergone radical surgery needs assistance with changes in elimination and instruction in stoma care (Box 33-11 and Figure 33-1). The nurse must also address concerns related to sexual function, changes in body image or self-image, anxiety, and depression, and psychological issues associated with sexually transmitted diseases such as guilt, blame, and mistrust (Box 33-12). Nursing care for recurrent or persistent disease involves assisting the patient in dealing with the physical and psychological effects of a life-threatening illness and entails regular follow-up. The patient must be instructed that long-term follow-up with health care specialists will be required. Grief counseling may prove helpful. The patient should be encouraged to participate in self-care activities, including everyday activities and sexual functioning to the extent possible and practical.

CANCER OF THE ENDOMETRIUM

Endometrial cancer is the most common gynecologic cancer in the United States and the fourth leading cause of cancer in women. Estimates are that about 35,000 new cases of endometrial cancer occur every year in the United States, resulting in 4000 to 5000 deaths per year (Oncology Channel, 2002). Endometrial cancer may be the most curable cancer when diagnosed early. The majority of women with

---

Box 33-11 Nursing Interventions for Altered Elimination

URINARY INCONTINENCE
- Assess for bladder distension by palpation.
- Encourage the use of the toilet every 2 hours while awake and every 3 to 4 hours at night.
- Focus the patient on the need to urinate with direct command.
- Assist the patient with mobility and clothing removal.
- Schedule the majority of fluid intake during daytime hours.
- Encourage the patient to use the customary positioning for urinating.

FECAL INCONTINENCE
- Establish a regular time to defecate.
- Do not delay defecation.
- Use suppositories or "mini-enemas" to help reestablish a regular elimination pattern.
- Maintain skin integrity by washing, rinsing, and drying the skin and using protective barriers.
- Help the patient use devices such as drainage tubes or catheters, continence briefs, or perianal pouching.

STOMA CARE
- Prevent injury to the stoma.
- Encourage fluid intake to promote adequate output and to flush ileal conduit or continent diversion.
- Facilitate meticulous skin care around stoma site.
- Assess for peristomal skin problems, including the following:
  Yeast infection
  Product allergies
  Excoriations caused by a shearing effect
  Poorly fitting appliances
- Encourage acceptance of the surgery and of alterations in body image.
- Address patient concerns, including the following:
  Fear of offending others with the stoma
  Fear of alterations in sexual, personal, professional, and recreational activities

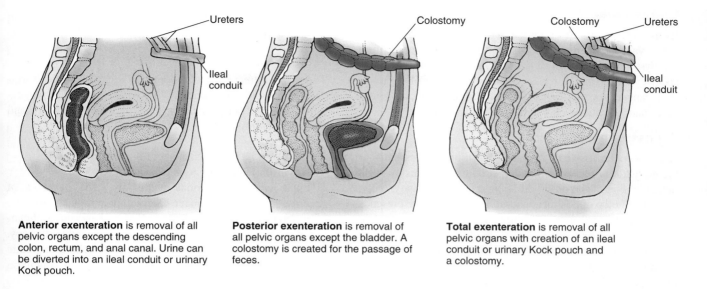

Anterior exenteration is removal of all pelvic organs except the descending colon, rectum, and anal canal. Urine can be diverted into an ileal conduit or urinary Kock pouch.

Posterior exenteration is removal of all pelvic organs except the bladder. A colostomy is created for the passage of feces.

Total exenteration is removal of all pelvic organs with creation of an ileal conduit or urinary Kock pouch and a colostomy.

Figure 33-1   Pelvic exenteration. (Ignatavicius DD, Workman ML, editors: *Medical-surgical nursing: critical thinking for collaborative care,* ed 4, Philadelphia, 2002, WB Saunders.)

endometrial cancer have already gone through menopause, although the disease can occur in younger women as well (Yamada and McGonigle, 1998).

The use of unopposed estrogen therapy has been linked to an increased incidence of endometrial cancer. This problem can be virtually eliminated through the use of combined or cyclic estrogen and progesterone. Either exogenous or endogenous estrogen may lead to endometrial hyperplasia.

Tamoxifen, which functions as an antiestrogen in breast tissue, has been associated with thickening of the endometrium and changes from polyps to hyperplasia and cancer. Data regarding the relationship of tamoxifen treatment to endometrial cancer are conflicting, however.

Although smoking has been associated with risk reduction, the risk of developing lung cancer and other health problems from smoking negates any potential benefit. A healthy lifestyle of a low-fat diet, regular physical activity, and main-

tenance of normal weight may contribute to risk reduction and health promotion.

Use of oral contraceptives containing mostly progesterone provides significant protection against endometrial cancer. Early treatment of endometrial hyperplasia, particularly the atypical type, can prevent progression to cancer. Multiple risk factors for endometrial cancer have been identified (see Table 33-1). Ethnicity plays little role (Box 33-13).

Pathophysiology

Endometrial hyperplasia, primarily the atypical type, is a premalignant cytologic change that can progress to malignancy. The majority of endometrial cancers are adenocarcinomas (Yarbo et al, 2000).

Cancer generally starts in the fundus and may spread to involve the entire endometrium. The cancer spreads to the myometrium, endocervix, cervix, fallopian tubes, and ovaries.

Metastasis usually occurs to pelvic and paraaortic lymph nodes. Less common sites of metastasis include the vagina, peritoneal cavity, omentum, and inguinal lymph nodes. Hematogenous spread often involves lung, liver, bone, and brain (Boente, Chi, and Hoskins, 1998).

Box 33-12   Nursing Interventions Related to Sexual Function, Body Image, and Psychological Function

■ Discuss the effect of the illness on sexuality and sexual function.
■ Discuss necessary modifications in sexual activity, if any.
■ Encourage the patient to ask questions and verbalize concerns.
■ Discuss alternative forms of sexual activity, as appropriate.
■ Include the spouse or significant other in counseling if possible.
■ Determine the amount of sexual guilt and the factors that cause it.
■ Avoid prematurely terminating the discussion of guilt, even if the guilt seems unreasonable.

Box 33-13   Ethnic Features in the Incidence of Endometrial Cancer

■ Endometrial cancer is one of the five most frequent cancers in women regardless of race or ethnicity (except in Korean, Vietnamese, and Native Alaskan women).

Clinical Manifestations

Even early stages of endometrial cancer can cause symptoms. Vaginal bleeding in a postmenopausal woman is often the first symptom of the disease. Other symptoms are less specific and do not always suggest a diagnosis of endometrial cancer. As the size of the tumor increases, different signs and symptoms may appear (Box 33-14).

Assessment

A thorough discussion of the patient's symptoms is essential to the evaluation of suspected endometrial cancer. This includes determination of the onset, duration, amount, intensity, color, and consistency of postmenopausal bleeding and the presence of concurrent cramping. Identification of risk factors (see Table 33-1) and a review of systems to identify advanced-stage symptoms such as abdominal pain, changes in bowel or bladder function, and weight loss is critical. Investigation of family or personal history of cancer—especially breast, ovarian, endometrial, and colorectal cancer—is necessary.

Physical examination of the lymph nodes with particular attention to the supraclavicular and inguinal nodes is important. In addition, the lungs and abdomen should be assessed for organomegaly. A complete pelvic examination is required to evaluate the external genitalia, vagina, cervix, uterus, and adnexa. A bimanual examination should be conducted to examine the rectovaginal space.

Diagnosis

Pap smear analysis alone does not always detect endometrial cancer. A more reliable test is endometrial biopsy, which permits histologic evaluation. Endometrial cancer is staged surgically when the patient's medical condition and intraabdominal location of the disease make surgical treatment an option.

Interdisciplinary Care

The goal of treatment for stage I and II endometrial cancer is cure. Surgery is the most common therapy choice. Treatment for stage III and IV cancer and for recurrent disease focuses on control of the disease and palliative care. The type of therapy given depends on the specific site of recurrence. Although surgery or radiation may be used in certain cases, chemotherapy is the primary treatment for advanced disease.

Surgeon

The surgical treatment of endometrial cancer includes surgical staging, total abdominal hysterectomy, bilateral salpingectomy, selective pelvic and paraaortic lymphadenectomy, and omentumectomy.

Oncologist

Hormonal Therapy and Chemotherapy

Synthetic progestational agents are used in cases of recurrent endometrial cancer. Chemotherapeutic agents have a limited role in the treatment of advanced endometrial cancer in women who have not responded to hormonal therapy. Drugs that have been effective in primary chemotherapeutic treatments include doxorubicin (Adriamycin), cisplatin (Platinol), ifosfamide (Ifex), and paclitaxel (Taxol).

Radiation Therapy

Use of radiation therapy for early endometrial cancer is determined by stage, histologic findings, and cytologic findings. Candidates for pelvic external beam radiation therapy include patients with localized pelvic disease, a high-grade tumor, or greater than 50% myometrial invasion. Intracavity radiation therapy or whole-pelvis, paraaortic, or possibly whole-abdominal radiation may be selected as the cancer advances.

Nurse

The majority of women with early endometrial cancer are cured with primary surgery. The patient must be encouraged to adhere to the treatment plan and schedule regular follow-up visits. For the patient with advanced disease, the focus of care varies depending on the extent of disease and associated symptoms. Nursing care of the patient with advanced disease focuses on resource mobilization, case management, ambulatory care access, home care support, social work, and participation in support groups, and spiritual counseling.

CANCER OF THE VULVA

Cancer of the vulva is uncommon. Approximately 4000 new cases occur each year in the United States. Vulvar and vaginal cancers usually occur in older, postmenopausal women. Both types of cancer are often preceded by a preinvasive intraepithelial neoplasia and both are curable when diagnosed early.

The etiology of vulvar intraepithelial neoplasia and invasive vulvar cancer is not known. There is significant evidence to suggest a relationship between sexually transmitted diseases, particularly human papillomavirus infection, and vulvar cancer.

Annual examination with Pap smear testing, including examination of the vulva and the biopsy of any existing lesion, is critical to early detection of vulvar and vaginal cancer.

Box 33-14   Signs and Symptoms of Endometrial Cancer

- Vaginal bleeding in a postmenopausal woman
- Abnormal vaginal bleeding (bleeding in between periods or heavier or longer-lasting menstrual bleeding)
- Vaginal discharge
- Pelvic or back pain
- Pain on urination
- Pain with sexual intercourse
- Blood in the stool or urine

Pathophysiology

The premalignant phase of vulvar squamous cell cancer has several different names: carcinoma in situ, vulvar intraepithelial neoplasia grade III (VIN III), severe dysplasia, and Bowen's disease. This condition is diagnosed by analysis of a tissue biopsy specimen and is characterized by a full-thickness disorder of maturation of the squamous epithelium. It is usually symptomatic, with itching and burning, and can be present for years (Nash and Curry, 1998).

Squamous cell cancer of the vulva usually causes pain, soreness, and itching. An obvious growth on the skin or an ulcerated area is usually present. Diagnosis is by simple biopsy. Vulvar cancer often appears as discoloration of the vulva with white, gray, red, or brown lesions. Lesions may be exophytic (proliferating outwardly), endophytic (proliferating inwardly), ulcerative, or verrucous (resembling a wart). Most vulvar tumors are squamous cell carcinomas; few are other types of neoplasm.

The primary site of vulvar cancer is usually the labia majora, but the cancer may be found on the labia minora, clitoris, or perineum. VIN is divided into three categories: VIN I (mild), VIN II (moderate), and VIN III (carcinoma in situ).

The most common route of metastatic spread is through direct extension or dissemination to regional lymph nodes. The pattern of lymphatic spread is from superficial inguinal lymph nodes to deep inguinal and femoral nodes and then to pelvic lymph nodes.

Clinical Manifestations

Many women with VIN are asymptomatic. The signs and symptoms of cancer of the vulva may be subtle (Box 33-15).

Assessment

Taking a thorough patient history is critical, and information should be obtained on the duration and severity of signs and symptoms, previous malignancies, cigarette smoking, number of sexual partners, and family history of cancer. Additional components of the assessment include a physical examination, biopsy, and diagnostic tests. The patient's report of any itching, burning, sore, or lesion on the vulva warrants careful inspection and biopsy of any lesion found.

Box 33-15   Signs and Symptoms of Cancer of the Vulva

- Vulvar pruritus
- Vulvar burning
- Presence of a vulvar lesion
- Vulvar bleeding
- Discharge
- Dysuria

Diagnosis

An excisional biopsy specimen is analyzed to establish the diagnosis. The staging of vulvar cancer is based on surgical and histologic examination of the primary tumor and the presence of metastases to adjacent organs and inguinal lymph nodes.

Interdisciplinary Care
Primary Provider (Physician/Nurse Practitioner)

The goal of care is to eradicate the lesion and reduce the risk of recurrence. The provider develops a treatment plan based on the stage of the cancer, the patient's age, the location and extent of disease, and the psychosocial consequences of treatment procedures.

Surgeon

Surgery is by far the most common treatment for vulvar cancer. Local treatment with cautery, laser surgery, or cryosurgery is the treatment of choice for noninvasive lesions. The advantages of this type of treatment are the sparing of surrounding tissue, minimal scarring, and the opportunity to manage the patient on an outpatient basis. Wide local excision of the lesion(s) helps maintain sexual and reproductive function.

Simple or radical vulvectomy has historically been reserved for patients with advanced disease (Table 33-2). Major complications after radical surgery include groin wound infection and skin breakdown. Late-onset complications of radical surgery include chronic leg edema, cellulitis, urinary stress incontinence, genital prolapse, and numbness and paresthesia over the anterior thigh caused by nerve damage.

Oncologist
Chemotherapy

The chemotherapeutic regimen may include 5-FU for noninvasive lesions. For invasive tumors, a combination of

---

Table 33-2   Surgical Treatment for Invasive Cancer of the Vulva According to Stage

Stage	Treatment
I	Wide local excision with ipsilateral inguinofemoral lymphadenectomy
II	Radical vulvectomy with removal of the labia minora, labia majora, and clitoris and bilateral node dissection
III	Radical vulvectomy with removal of a portion of the distal urethra or vagina and possibly excision of a portion of the anus
	Radiation therapy with chemotherapy
IV	Pelvic exenteration (removal of the vagina, uterus, ovaries, fallopian tubes, bladder, and rectum) with radical vulvectomy if the bladder or rectum is involved
	Possible creation of a urinary conduit and colostomy

5-FU, cisplatin (Platinol), and mitomycin C (Mutamycin) may be helpful.

Radiation Therapy

Radiation therapy is reserved for invasive cancer and is used in combination with surgery to reduce the need for extensive radical surgery. The use of radiation may decrease the recurrence rate of the cancer. Postoperatively, radiation treatment may be combined with chemotherapy for locally advanced cancer. Complications include severe erythema and swelling, radiation cystitis, and vulvar fibrosis, atrophy, or necrosis.

Nurse

Nursing care of the patient with vulvar cancer focuses on the patient's concerns regarding pain and suffering related to surgery and treatments. Loss of sexual function is also a critical patient concern. Care includes patient education, including explanation of the type of treatment recommended, self-care and home care instructions, and discussion regarding sexual satisfaction and approaches to maintaining sexual activity. Close and long-term follow-up care is critical.

Advanced or recurrent disease often appears within the first 2 years after initial treatment. Physical symptoms can be distressing. Tumors may be large and painful. Nursing care focuses on symptom management (Box 33-16).

CANCER OF THE VAGINA

Cancer is classified as vaginal only when the primary site of tumor growth is in the vagina. Carcinomas of the vagina are uncommon tumors that account for only 1% to 2% of gynecologic malignancies and are rare in women under 40 years of age. Secondary spread from sites such as the cervix, vulva, endometrium, ovary, and rectum occurs more frequently than primary carcinoma.

Incidence of squamous cell cancer of the vagina increases with age and is significantly linked to existing or previous viral infection. Prevention measures focus on protection against sexually transmitted disease and exposure to vaginal infection.

Pathophysiology

The histologic distinction between squamous cell carcinoma and adenocarcinoma of the vagina is important because the two types represent distinct diseases, each with a different pathogenesis and natural history. Squamous cell vaginal cancers account for about 85% of tumors. This type of tumor initially spreads superficially within the vaginal wall and later extends into paravaginal tissues. Lesions may appear red, white, or gray and have an ulcerated appearance.

Adenocarcinoma is present in about 15% of cases of vaginal cancer and differs from squamous cell carcinoma in that it is associated with a higher incidence of pulmonary metastases and supraclavicular and pelvic node involvement. Rarely, a primary vaginal cancer is a melanoma or sarcoma.

Lymphatic drainage is the primary mechanism of disease spread. The lymphatics drain to the inguinal and femoral nodes. All the lymph nodes of the pelvis may at one time or another serve as sites of drainage from the vagina.

Vaginal cancers occur most commonly in the upper third of the vagina. The tumor may spread along the vaginal wall to involve the cervix or vulva. Anterior vaginal lesions can penetrate into the vesicovaginal septum during the early stages of the disease. Posterior lesions can invade the rectum. The incidence of lymph node metastasis is proportional to the stage of the vaginal cancer. In squamous cell carcinoma, metastasis to the lungs or supraclavicular nodes tends to occur in the more advanced stages. In clear cell carcinoma, metastasis to the lungs and supraclavicular nodes occurs frequently.

Clinical Manifestations

The most common initial symptom of invasive vaginal cancer is abnormal bleeding after sexual intercourse (Box 33-17).

Assessment

Taking an extensive patient and family history is the necessary first step in assessing a patient with vaginal cancer. Important considerations include in utero exposure to diethylstilbestrol, history of previous cancer, history of exposure to human papillomavirus or herpes simplex type 2, and any genetic predisposition. Physical examination and diagnostic tests help to determine the type of vaginal cancer and influence decisions about the treatment plan.

Box 33-16   Nursing Care in Advanced or Recurrent Vulvar Cancer

PATIENT AND FAMILY EDUCATION ABOUT SURGERY
- Extent of surgery
- Changes to expect
- Patient participation in postoperative care

SYMPTOM MANAGEMENT
- Pain management regimen
- Infection prevention
- Meticulous skin care
- Management of leg edema with elastic stockings if necessary
- Massage and exercise to help relieve leg discomfort
- Skin moisturization
- Identification of patients at risk for ineffective coping

EXTENDED CARE
- Referrals as needed using a multidisciplinary approach
- Continued education and reassurance to facilitate effective coping
- Sexual and reproductive counseling
- Coordination of care between home and hospital

Diagnosis

Physical examination should include careful visual inspection and palpation of the vagina. Pap smear analysis may be helpful for evaluation of squamous cell carcinoma. Colposcopy may be indicated for directed biopsy.

Interdisciplinary Care

Primary Provider (Physician/Nurse Practitioner)

Although routine population-wide screening is not warranted given the low incidence of vaginal cancer, inspection of the vagina should be part of a routine health examination. There are no molecular markers for vaginal cancer. For women who have a history of vaginal intraepithelial neoplasia (VAIN) follow-up examination and colposcopy by a gynecologist (if the primary provider is not a gynecologist) is recommended.

Therapeutic alternatives depend on the stage of the disease. Surgery or radiation therapy is highly effective in early stages, whereas radiation therapy is the primary treatment in more advanced stages. Chemotherapy has not been shown to be curative for advanced vaginal cancer, and there are no standard drug regimens.

Women with VAIN I (Box 33-18) do not usually need treatment, whereas women with VAIN II may respond to laser ablative treatment or application of 5-FU cream. Complications of laser therapy include watery discharge for 2 to 3 weeks after the procedure.

VAIN III is considered premalignant. A local excision is appropriate for one or several lesions in cluster. For multifocal lesions or recurrent disease, or in poor surgical candidates, the treatment of choice is brachytherapy.

Women with stage III and IV disease have a high recurrence rate. In advanced disease, therapeutic interventions are directed at symptom management. Symptoms depend on the location of the tumor. Anterior tumors often cause urinary problems such as hematuria and urinary tract infections. Palliative radiotherapy can reduce hematuria caused by an ulcerating lesion. The patient may need continuous bladder irrigation. Repeated urinary tract infections may be indicative of fistula formation. Urinary incontinence, dysuria, and painful bladder spasms are common. Surgery may be indicated to close fistulas. Symptomatic treatment with appropriate antibiotics and antispasmodics is common. For large fistulas, a urinary-vaginal prosthesis can be used to divert drainage and maintain skin integrity.

Posterior tumors are often associated with constipation and blood in the stool. Stool softeners and laxatives may be helpful for mild constipation. Rectovaginal fistulas may cause fecal incontinence. Vaginal tampons can help to control fistula discharge. For large fistulas, a loop colostomy may be considered.

Surgeon

The patient undergoing surgery for vaginal cancer requires extensive preoperative and postoperative education, preoperative counseling, and postoperative care and rehabilitation. Depending on the stage of the disease, radical vaginectomy, radical hysterectomy, or pelvic exenteration may be indicated. Vaginal reconstructive surgery may be possible after therapeutic surgical management.

Oncologist

Chemotherapy

Chemotherapy may provide an option when vaginal cancer is metastatic or recurrent or when surgery or radiation therapy cannot be used. Cisplatin (Platinol) and 5-FU are the chemotherapeutic agents most commonly used in combination with radiation therapy. Mitomycin C (Mutamycin) has also proven helpful.

Radiation Therapy

Radiation therapy is the most widely used treatment modality for all stages of vaginal cancer. Complications include desquamation of the skin, which requires patient education about the need for meticulous skin care. Corticosteroids and antibiotic creams may prove helpful in managing inflammation and infection. Vaginal fibrosis and scarring with loss of blood supply and elasticity may also occur. Frequent intercourse and use of vaginal dilators with lubricants may be helpful in addressing this problem.

Nurse

Nursing care of the woman diagnosed with VAIN focuses on emphasizing the importance of regular follow-up visits. During radiation therapy, education that addresses changes in body image, alterations in sexuality, and specific coping mechanisms can be helpful. A critical nursing function is the facilitation of communication between in-patient facilities and home care agencies. After extensive surgical therapy, the development with the patient and family of a specific plan to address the implications of the surgery is critical to postoperative recovery.

Major problems associated with advanced disease include hematuria, urinary tract infections, urinary and fecal incontinence, loss of skin integrity, constipation, and fistula formation. Nursing care focuses on the management of these symptoms (Box 33-19).

CANCER OF THE TESTES

Germ cell tumors are the most common solid malignancy in men aged 15 to 35 years, and testicular cancer is the most common of these malignancies. Germ cell tumors are composed of seminomatous and nonseminomatous cell types. Seminoma is the most singular cell type. Testicular cancer is rare. The incidence of testicular cancer has increased slowly. However, deaths due to this type of cancer have decreased significantly since the 1960s as a result of early diagnosis and intervention, which are directly correlated with lower cancer stage at the time of detection.

The etiology of germ cell tumors is unknown, but several risk factors have been identified. These risk factors include prior history of testicular cancer, cryptorchidism, genetic predisposition, familial environmental factors, and increased hormone levels (Box 33-20). Young men have a significantly higher likelihood of acquiring the disease than older men. Several ethnic patterns are seen in the incidence of testicular cancer (Box 33-21).

Testicular self-examination should be performed routinely. Any man who experiences infertility problems should be evaluated for testicular cancer. Cure rates are highest with early-stage disease management. Educational programs beginning during adolescence should provide specific instruction on how to perform testicular self-examination.

Pathophysiology

As noted earlier, germ cell tumors are divided into two main histologic categories: seminomas and nonseminomas. Seminomas include classic and spermatocytic tumors, whereas nonseminomas include embryonal tumors, yolk sac tumors, choriocarcinomas, and teratomas. Germ cell tumors begin with the transformation of a single cell and develop as the abnormal growth pattern continues.

Box 33-19 Nursing Interventions in Advanced Vaginal Cancer

HEMATURIA
- Irrigate bladder to decrease bleeding.

CONSTIPATION
- Increase dietary fiber intake to 20 to 30 g daily.
- Have the patient drink 3 qt of fluids per day.
- Ensure that the patient gets regular exercise.
- Establish a regular time to defecate.
- Do not delay defecation.
- Ask the patient to keep a bowel elimination diary.
- Avoid the use of laxatives and enemas unless absolutely necessary.

URINARY TRACT INFECTIONS
- Monitor vital signs.
- Administer antipyretics and antibiotics as ordered.
- Ensure adequate hydration.
- Monitor input and output.
- Assess pain at regular intervals and administer medications as ordered.
- Use nonpharmacologic comfort measures such as appropriate positioning and heating pads.
- Observe urine for color, odor, amount, and frequency to evaluate effectiveness of treatment.

FISTULA
- Assist the patient with perineal hygiene.
- Give warm sitz baths.
- Change perineal pads frequently.
- Encourage consumption of fluids to promote urinary output.

Box 33-20 Risk Factors for Testicular Cancer

- History of testicular cancer
- Undescended testes (cryptorchidism)
- Familial tendency for the development of testicular cancer
- Use of diethylstilbestrol by mother during pregnancy
- Increased levels of gonadotropins
- Klinefelter's syndrome
- Down syndrome
- Testicular feminization syndrome
- Hermaphroditism

Box 33-21 Ethnic Differences in the Incidence of Testicular Cancer

- Testicular cancer is rare in African Americans and Asians.
- Incidence is rapidly rising among men in Scandinavia, Germany, and New Zealand.

The spread of germ cell tumors is generally predictable. Initially, the disease spreads to the retroperitoneal lymph nodes. Once the cancer cells have entered the lymphatic system, vascular dissemination routinely follows. The lungs are the most common distant organ affected by metastasis. Additional sites include the central nervous system and the contralateral testicle.

Clinical Manifestations

The most common presenting clinical manifestation of testicular cancer is a painless swelling or enlargement of the testis (Box 33-22). This is often ignored or attributed to recent trauma. Painful scrotal enlargement initially may be treated as epididymitis or testicular torsion. This misdiagnosis may result in delayed diagnosis of testicular cancer. As the disease progresses, individuals often develop cough, dyspnea, chest pain, and shortness of breath.

Assessment

Taking a complete patient and family history is critical for determining the plan of care. Prior history of testicular cancer, history of trauma, cryptorchidism, epididymitis, gynecomastia, back pain, and infertility require evaluation. There is a significant familial risk for the development of cancer of the testes.

Diagnosis

Thorough inspection of the scrotum is crucial to detect the presence of a mass. Transillumination is indicated to diagnose a hydrocele. Examination of the lymph nodes and examination of the breasts for gynecomastia should also be performed.

Levels of serum markers such as β-human chorionic gonadotropin and α-fetoprotein are elevated in 85% of individuals with disseminated nonseminomatous germ cell tumors. Several systems have been devised for the classification and staging of testicular cancer, and different classification systems are used in Europe and in the United States.

Interdisciplinary Care
Primary Provider (Physician/Nurse Practitioner)

The primary provider is likely to be either the person who discovers the testicular mass or the person to whom the patient takes his complaint of discomfort or swelling. It is important to explore the possibility of testicular cancer so that misdiagnosis and treatment delay are avoided.

Box 33-22   Signs and Symptoms of Testicular Cancer

- Painless testicular swelling
- Enlargement of the testis
- Back pain
- Gynecomastia
- Elevated levels of β-human chorionic gonadotropin

Surgeon

Early disease is managed primarily with surgical intervention (Gospodarowicz, Sturgeon, and Jewett, 1998). Advanced stages of disease are managed with a cisplatin (Platinol)-based chemotherapy regimen and postsurgical resection of remaining tumor. Surgical treatment includes retroperitoneal lymph node dissection following orchiectomy. Men who undergo full bilateral lymphadenectomy universally lose emission and the ability to ejaculate and therefore lose fertility. Modified retroperitoneal lymph node dissection preserves the nerves necessary for ejaculation and may be substituted for the radical procedure in certain cases. An alternative treatment approach includes active surveillance after orchiectomy and chemotherapeutic intervention only in cases of reoccurrence. Complications of surgery include postoperative paralytic ileus. Men who have received bleomycin (Blenoxane) are also at risk for pulmonary fibrosis with subsequent respiratory failure.

Oncologist
Chemotherapy

Advances in chemotherapeutic approaches are one of the primary reasons for increased cure and survival rates. After orchiectomy, cisplatin-based chemotherapy is recommended for cytoreduction. The most widely used combination is BEP (bleomycin [Blenoxane], etoposide [VePesid], and cisplatin [Platinol]). In men with advanced or bulky disease, chemotherapy is the treatment modality of choice.

Radiation Therapy

Seminomas are extremely sensitive to radiation therapy. Side effects of radiation include gastrointestinal complications such as diarrhea, nausea and vomiting, and peptic ulcers as well as fatigue, impaired fertility, myelosuppression, and bladder irritation. Advanced and recurrent disease is treated with a combination of radiation therapy and chemotherapy.

Nurse

Nursing care of the patient with testicular cancer includes psychosexual assessment and counseling. Recent changes in the health care delivery system have influenced approaches to the care of the patient with testicular cancer. Hospitalizations have been shortened and chemotherapy management has shifted from an inpatient to an outpatient setting. The role of home care has become increasingly important. Home care focuses on hydration management, phlebotomy, management of nausea, and wound care. Nursing care and the educational needs of the patient receiving chemotherapy for testicular cancer are specific to the type of chemotherapeutic agent used (Box 33-23).

CANCER OF THE PROSTATE

Prostate cancer is the sixth most common cancer in the world and the most common type of cancer found in American men,

---

Box 33-23   Nursing Interventions for Patients Receiving Chemotherapy for Testicular Cancer

NAUSEA AND VOMITING
- Administer prophylactic antiemetics.
- Record schedule of antiemetic regimen.
- Encourage and maintain adequate fluid intake.
- Consider supplemental intravenous hydration.
- Consider use of music and relaxation therapy.

CONSTIPATION
- Assess bowel function prior to drug administration.
- Encourage intake of fluids and consumption of a high-fiber diet.
- Monitor bowel sounds.
- Instruct the patient to report significant bowel changes.
- Administer stool softeners and laxatives.

MYELOSUPPRESSION
- Monitor results of complete blood count.
- Instruct the patient to report signs of infection, fever, bleeding, shortness of breath, severe weakness, or tachycardia.
- Instruct the patient to avoid crowds and individuals with active infection, take bleeding precautions, and use good hand-washing technique.
- Inform the patient with advanced disease that blood or platelet transfusion may be necessary.
- Monitor incisions, wounds, catheters, and sites of infection.
- Obtain blood and urine culture specimens and chest radiograph prior to administering antibiotics.
- Administer antibiotics as prescribed or instruct the patient to take the full course of antibiotics.

NEPHROTOXICITY
- Monitor levels of serum electrolytes, creatinine, and blood urea nitrogen as well as daily intake and output.
- Provide aggressive hydration before and after treatments and have the patient increase oral intake of fluids.
- Avoid using aminoglycosides for the treatment of granulocytopenic fever when the patient is receiving cisplatin (Platinol).

HEMORRHAGIC CYSTITIS
- Order urinalysis daily; if results show more than 10 red blood cells per high-power field, alert the physician.

- Provide aggressive hydration before and after treatments and have the patient increase oral intake of fluids.

INTEGUMENTARY CHANGES
- Prepare the patient for hair loss and reinforce that it is temporary.
- Alert the patient to the possibility of skin hyperpigmentation and nail changes.

REPRODUCTION
- Arrange for sperm banking if possible prior to chemotherapy.
- Reinforce that ejaculation and erectile function will not change.
- Inform the patient that reduced zoospermia will occur for at least 12 months, with normal spermatogenesis returning in 50% of men within 2 years.

NEUROLOGIC CHANGES
- Instruct the patient to report any numbness or tingling of the hands and feet (Raynaud's phenomenon).
- Advise the patient to wear gloves and dress warmly in cold weather.
- Instruct the patient to report hearing changes.
- Obtain baseline and serial audiometric measurements in patients at high risk.

PULMONARY CHANGES
- Assess for bibasilar rales, inspirational lag, and cough.
- Evaluate patients at high risk for fibrosis (i.e., men who smoke, have decreased renal function, or previously underwent chest irradiation).

BODY IMAGE CHANGES
- Encourage the patient to verbalize feeling about hair loss and changes in appearance.
- Teach the patient self-care activities related to body image disturbance.
- Reinforce any verbalization of feeling about actual or perceived loss.
- Provide consultation with a hair stylist or barber.

---

other than skin cancer (Klingman, 2002; American Cancer Society, 2004). Prostate cancer is the second leading cause of cancer death in men, exceeded only by lung cancer.

Because prostate cancer is more prevalent in certain ethnic backgrounds, genetic and hormonal variances have been suggested as causes of the disease. About 5% to 10% of prostate cancers are linked to changes in the structure of DNA. High levels of androgens may play a part in prostate cancer risk in some men. Also, some researchers have noted that men with high levels of the hormone IGF-1 are more likely to get prostate cancer. Although the exact cause of

prostate cancer is unknown, certain risk factors are linked to the disease. Box 33-24 lists the factors that place men at increased risk

Ethnic Variations

Prostate cancer is most common in North America and in Scandinavian countries. It is less common in Asia, Africa, Central America, and South America. African American men are more likely to have prostate cancer and to die of it than are white or Asian men. The reasons for this are unknown.

Pathophysiology

The prostate is divided into peripheral, central, and transitional zones. Most cancers develop in the peripheral zone. Both stromal and epithelial tissues depend on androgens for growth, and both are involved in the development of primary and metastatic cancer sites (Scher, 2001). Most cancers (>95%) are adenocarcinomas.

Clinical Manifestations

Prostate cancer is one of the slowest growing cancers, and many men with prostate cancer never develop symptoms. According to Scher (2001) more than 70% of men who died in their seventh decade of life for reasons other than prostate cancer were found on autopsy to have prostate cancer.

Difficulty urinating could be a sign of prostate cancer. Symptoms of advanced prostate cancer include trouble having or maintaining an erection, blood in the urine, and pain in the pelvis, spine, hips, or ribs.

Diagnosis

According to the American Cancer Society (2004), the most effective screening measures for prostate cancer are the digital rectal exam (DRE) and the prostate-specific antigen (PSA) test. Screening remains controversial, however, because it has not been proven effective in clinical trials (Scher, 2001).

PSA is a protein made by prostate cells. Although PSA levels are elevated in prostate cancer, they are also elevated in other conditions such as benign prostatic hypertrophy and prostatitis. Additionally, a significant percentage of men who have cancer of the prostate do not have elevated PSA levels. Therefore, PSA is not diagnostic and should be used only in addition to the DRE. PSA levels under 4 ng/ml are usually considered normal, whereas results between 4 and 10 ng/ml indicate a 25% chance of prostate cancer. PSA levels aid in treatment decisions and are also used to detect recurrence. Serum acid phosphatase levels are elevated in clients with advanced disease, and elevated levels of alkaline phosphatase signal possible metastasis to bone.

If cancer is present, the DRE will reveal a gland that is hard, nodular, and irregular. These findings warrant histologic examination of the gland.

A core needle biopsy is performed to analyze several tissue specimens taken from the prostate. These samples are analyzed for cancer cells and graded according to the Gleason system. In the Gleason system samples from two areas of the prostate are graded from 1 to 5, and the numbers are added to give a Gleason score. A lower number indicates a slower growing cancer and a better prognosis. Scores of 2 through 4 are considered low, and scores of 7 to 10 are considered high. The tumor is also staged using a modification of the TNM classifications system (see Chapter 27). Computed tomography, magnetic resonance imaging, and bone scans are used to assist in staging the tumor.

Interdisciplinary Care
Primary Provider (Physician/Nurse Practitioner)

The primary provider plays an important role in early screening and detection. Although screening is controversial, providers should talk to men about the benefits and risks of testing. Men who do not have any serious medical problems should have the PSA blood test and DRE offered to them annually beginning at age 50. Men at high risk should begin testing at age 45. If cancer is suspected, the client will be counseled about his options. If he chooses "expectant therapy," also called "watchful waiting," he will in all likelihood continue to be followed up by the primary provider. Otherwise he will be referred for surgery or radiation. Cytotoxic chemotherapy has not been shown to be effective (Scher, 2001).

Surgeon

Surgery is the standard treatment for prostatic cancer. The two most common operations are radical prostatectomy and transurethral resection of the prostate (TURP). Radical prostatectomy is done when there is no evidence of metastasis. The risk of impotence and incontinence after surgery depends on whether the surgeon was able to spare the nerves controlling these functions. Bilateral orchiectomy may be performed to interrupt the influence of testosterone.

Radiation Therapy

External beam radiation therapy is used curatively when the cancer is locally contained. It is also used as adjuvant and palliative therapy. Side effects can include diarrhea with or without blood in the stool. Between 30% and 60% of men become impotent within 2 years of having external beam radiation therapy.

Brachytherapy is a cost-effective method of treating prostate cancer in the early stages. Radioactive pellets are implanted in the prostate and remain in place until the radiation is dissipated Although this treatment is well tolerated, the client may experience localized pain and may have red-brown urine. Brachytherapy can also cause impotence, urinary incontinence, and bowel problems.

Nurse

Nursing care focuses on working with the client and his partner to adjust to the changes created by the cancer and/or its treatment. Men who elect "watchful waiting" often experience high levels of anxiety (Wallace, 2003); men who undergo treatment must deal with incontinence and changes in sexual experience and perhaps sexual identity. As with other cancers of the reproductive system, the nurse must do a careful psychosexual assessment and offer information and support as appropriate. Nurses can facilitate return of urinary control by teaching perineal exercises. If incontinence continues, the nurse should offer support and encourage the patient to discuss his concerns. Rondorf-Klym and Colling (2003) found that quality of life after prostate surgery was related to social support and self-esteem and only indirectly influenced by issues related to urinary function.

Drug Therapy

The drugs used to treat cancer of the prostate are primarily estrogens and gonadotropin-releasing hormone agonist analogs such as leuprolide acetate (Lupron) and flutamide (Eulexin). Hormonal treatment produces many unpleasant side effects, including hot flashes, breast tenderness, gynecomastia, osteoporosis, anemia, loss of muscle mass, and weight gain. Cancer that is no longer responding to hormone therapy may respond to ketoconazole (Nizoral), megestrol (Megace), or diethylstilbestrol (DES).

Alternative Therapy

Alternative therapies should be used with caution. Even the use of vitamins can be contraindicated. Vitamin E appears to have a protective effect, but excessive amounts of vitamin A may actually increase cancer risk. PC-SPES, a mixture of saw palmetto and Chinese herbs widely used by men with advanced prostate cancer, was taken off the market in 2002 because capsules were found to contain other drugs that could cause serious health problems.

Foods that have been suggested as protective include those high in lycopene, such as tomatoes, grapefruits, and watermelons.

CASE STUDY

Patient Data

Mrs. M. is a 35-year-old married woman who has arrived for her annual visit to her gynecologist. Mrs. M. lives with her husband, has never been pregnant, and has been taking infertility drugs to conceive for the last year. She is not employed outside the home but earns extra income by baby-sitting for two neighborhood children. This income is critical to the family's ability to meet their monthly expenses. She is also active in her local synagogue and volunteers at the Jewish Community Center's elder care program.

While the nurse is taking Mrs. M.'s vital signs, Mrs. M. shares that she has recently begun to experience nausea, indigestion, constipation, and abdominal distention. She has no history of medical problems. She had pelvic inflammatory disease when she was a teenager. She has attempted to treat her symptoms with over the counter medications but they have not helped.

During the pelvic examination, the physician palpates a mass on the right ovary. She orders a transvaginal Doppler ultrasonographic study and measurement of baseline CA-125 level along with a complete blood count and abdominal ultrasonography. She also refers Mrs. M. to a gynecologic oncologist.

Diagnostic Findings

Hemoglobin level: 9 g/dl
Hematocrit: 28%
White blood count: 10.2/mm^3
CA-125 (cancer antigen 125) level: 75 U/ml
Vaginal Doppler ultrasonography: High flow rate
Abdominal ultrasonography: 12-cm mass on right ovary

Thinking It Through

■ What nursing diagnoses pertain to Mrs. M.?
■ What type of surgical, radiation, and chemotherapeutic treatment will most likely be recommended for Mrs. M. and what will be the primary aim of this treatment?
■ What role will the gynecologic oncologist play in Mrs. M.'s care?
■ What comfort measures can the nurse recommend to assist Mrs. M. with the management of her symptoms?

■ What are Mrs. M.'s support needs likely to be? How would you as the nurse address them?

Ethical Considerations

Mrs. M. is informed of her diagnosis of advanced ovarian cancer by the gynecologic oncologist. She insists that she will not let this stop her from continuing to take her fertility drugs. She believes that she will "beat this cancer" and that she cannot afford to delay having a baby while she waits for a regimen of chemotherapy. She will not accept her physician's advice to have surgery and she refuses drug or radiation therapy. She has read about "safe" herbal therapies for certain cancers and she plans to explore this strategy.

■ What are the responsibilities and ethical obligations of the nurse and/or physician regarding Mrs. M.'s statements? Is there an ethical conflict inherent in Mrs. M.'s decisions?
■ If there is an ethical or moral dilemma here, what are the facts of the dilemma and who are the stakeholders in the outcome?
■ What are the ethical principles involved when Mrs. M. suggests that she will refuse treatment? What ethical and moral viewpoint theories could be used to evaluate and interpret her refusal?
■ What are the issues related to medical and scientific futilities in this situation based on the evidence in the literature?

Case Conference

The nurse in whom Mrs. M. confided suggests that Mrs. M. discuss her plans with the people who can best advise her about the important issues relevant to her decision. Mrs. M. agrees, and an interdisciplinary team assembles to address Mrs. M.'s decision to decline surgical, chemotherapeutic, and radiation therapy. The members of the team include the gynecologic oncologist, the nurse, the dietitian, the social worker, and the respiratory therapist. Mr. M. is also in attendance.

The gynecologic oncologist has already communicated the diagnosis of advanced ovarian cancer to Mrs. M. based on the findings of the diagnostic testing and physical examination. The purpose of this meeting is to discuss what the implications of Mrs. M.'s decision are and how to best manage the symptoms

CASE STUDY—cont'd

associated with ovarian cancer, which have begun to cause significant discomfort for Mrs. M. The nurse will serve as the person responsible for the continuity of Mrs. M.'s care, including coordination of services, provision of referrals, and patient education.

Mrs. M. communicates that the most disturbing symptom is her loss of appetite caused by feelings of abdominal bloating. The dietitian responds by asking Mrs. M. to review her favorite foods so that a meal plan including these foods can be developed. She encourages Mrs. M. to eat frequent, small meals to avoid discomfort and to choose caloric beverages to supplement food selections in order to provide sufficient calories and avoid weight loss. She reminds Mrs. M. to drink adequate fluids but suggests that fluids may have to be restricted if abdominal ascites becomes a problem. Mrs. M. agrees to review her diet with the dietitian and to keep a food journal for a week to see how best to adapt her diet. She will participate in telephone consultations with the dietitian weekly and will E-mail her dietary preferences and food journal when complete.

Mrs. M. inquires about food supplements she has heard about that are suggested to "cure" cancer. The dietitian tells Mrs. M. that none of the suggested "cure" diets has ever been found effective in treating cancer. She explains that nutritional alteration can have a significant effect on patients with cancer and emphasizes that it is vital that Mrs. M. commit to a sound nutritional plan. Mrs. M. responds by saying that she just does not believe that food supplements or herbs will not be able to correct this problem. She starts to cry, raises her voice, and tells the members of the team that they are lying to her.

Mr. M. becomes clearly disturbed by this interaction and asks his wife please to reconsider her decision. She refuses to look at him and suggests that he is not supportive of her decision. After watching this exchange, the social worker comments that it is common for communication problems to arise when family processes are disrupted by a diagnosis of cancer. She suggests that Mrs. and Mr. M. will need time and an opportunity to discuss caregiving issues and the emotional implications of the diagnosis. Facilitated communication can help to foster mutual support in the couple. Mr. and Mrs. M. agree to set up a weekly appointment with a counselor to discuss the changes in their lives and the implications of Mrs. M.'s illness. The social worker also notes that many support groups exist whose members have

shared experiences similar to those of the M.'s and she recommends exploring participation.

Throughout the discussion, the nurse observes that Mrs. M. seems to be having difficulty breathing. She appears short of breath. The nurse inquires if this is a recent problem for Mrs. M. and Mrs. M. confirms that it is. The respiratory therapist offers suggestions for managing this dyspnea. He instructs Mrs. M. to sit upright, lean over a table, or rest her elbows on her knees whenever symptoms are present. He recommends instruction on relaxation exercises and controlled breathing to foster relaxation. He also recommends massage therapy. Mrs. M. agrees that this will help "her nerves," and the nurse suggests that she and Mrs. M. select among several providers who offer these services.

The nurse asks if Mr. and Mrs. M. have any questions. Mrs. M. has one. She wonders if she will have any pain. The gynecologic oncologist responds by saying that there are "pain experts," doctors and nurses who are specialists in managing people's pain. He tells Mrs. M. that any and all pain will be aggressively managed and that reducing and eliminating her pain will be the focus of the pain management team who works with her. He gives the nurse a consultation form to forward to the hospital pain management team so that Mrs. M. can meet with them to discuss pain management strategies immediately. The nurse agrees to contact the pain management team at once and to coordinate an appointment for Mrs. M.

Mr. and Mrs. M. rise to leave. They thank everyone for their time and support. The nurse makes certain that Mr. and Mrs. M. know how to contact the other members of the team and gives them her card with instructions to call her in the morning so that the process of coordinating appointments and scheduling can begin.

Once the team meeting is over, the nurse reviews the process and considers the experience as she continues to develop her plan of care for Mrs. M.

■ What are the most significant barriers to therapy demonstrated during the conference?

■ What issues regarding Mrs. M.'s body image disturbance and coping difficulties became evident during the conference?

■ What are the responsibilities of the nurse and other interdisciplinary team members in responding to Mrs. M.'s interest in trying unproven methods of cancer treatment?

Internet and Other Resources

General

Cancer Link: *http://www.cancerlink.org*
MEDLINEplus: *http://www.nlm.nih.gov/medlineplus/*
National Cancer Institute: *http://www.cancer.gov*
OncoLink: *http://www.oncolink.com*
Women's Cancer Network: *http://www.wcn.org*
Ovarian Cancer
Gilda's Club: *http://www.gildasclub.org*
National Ovarian Cancer Coalition: *http://www.ovarian.org*
Ovarian Cancer National Alliance: *http://www.ovariancancer.org*
Cervical Cancer
Center for Disease Control and Prevention, National Breast and Cervical Cancer Early Detection Program: *http://www.cdc.gov/cancer/nbccedp*
National Cervical Cancer Coalition: *http://www.nccc-online.org*

Vulvar Cancer
Cancer Information and Support International: *http://www.cancer-info.com/vulvarcancer*
Vaginal and Endometrial Cancer
National Cancer Institute: *http://www.cancer.gov/cancerinfo/pdq/treatment/endometrial/patient*
Testicular Cancer
Testicular Cancer Resource Center: *http://tcrc.acor.org/*
Urology Channel: *http://www.urologychannel.com/testicularcancer*

REFERENCES

American Cancer Society: Can prostate cancer be found early?, 2004, retrieved from *http://www.cancer.org/docroot/CRI/content/CRI_2_4_3x_Can_prostate_cancer_be_found_early_36.asp?sitearea=* on Mar 8, 2004.

Ausperg N et al: The biology of ovarian cancer, *Semin Oncol* 25:281-304, 1998.

Bast R, Xu F, Yu Y: CA 125: the past and the future, *Int J Biol Markers* 13:179-87, 1998.

Boente M, Chi D, Hoskins W: The role of surgery in the management of ovarian cancer in the United States, *J Clin Oncol* 15:3408-15, 1998.

Cadman L: Lifelong protection from cervical cancer, *Community Nurse* 3:12-3, 1998.

Friedlander M: Prognostic factors in ovarian cancer, *Semin Oncol* 25:305-14, 1998.

Gospodarowicz M, Sturgeon F, Jewett M: Early stage and advanced seminoma: role of radiation, therapy, surgery, and chemotherapy, *Semin Oncol* 25:160-73, 1998.

Klingman L: Interventions for male clients with reproductive problems. In Ignatavicius DD, Workman ML, editors: *Medical-surgical nursing: critical thinking for collaborative care,* ed 4, Philadelphia, 2002, WB Saunders.

Lanciano R et al: Update on the role of radiotherapy in ovarian cancer, *Semin Oncol* 25:361-71, 1998.

Nash J, Curry S: Vulvar cancer, *Surg Oncol Clin North Am* 7:335-46, 1998.

National Cervical Cancer Coalition: Worldwide cervical cancer issues, retrieved from *http://nccc-online.org/worldcancer.htm* on Sep 20, 2002.

National Ovarian Cancer Coalition: What is ovarian cancer?, 2002, retrieved from *http://www.ovarian.org/pages.asp?page=what%20is%20it* on April 10, 2004.

Oncology Channel: Endometrial cancer, retrieved from *http://www. oncologychannel.com/endometrialcancer/* on Nov 21, 2002.

Ozols RF: Ovarian cancer practice guidelines, *Oncology* 11:95-105, 1997.

Roland P et al: Response to salvage treatments in recurrent ovarian cancer treated initially with paclitaxel and platinum based combination regimens, *Gynecol Oncol* 68:178-82, 1998.

Rondorf-Klym LM, Colling J: Quality of life after radical prostatectomy, *Oncol Nurs Forum* 30(2):E24-E32, 2003.

Ross S: Cervical cancer prevention, *Nurs Spectrum* 7:12-14, 1998.

Scher H: Hyperplastic and malignant diseases of the prostate. In Braunwald E et al, editors: *Harrison's principles of internal medicine,* ed 15, New York, 2001, McGraw-Hill, pp 608-16.

Wallace M: Uncertainty and quality of life of older men who undergo watchful waiting for prostate cancer, *Oncol Nurs Forum* 30(2):303-9, 2003.

Yamada S, McGonigle K: Cancer of the endometrium and corpus uteri, *Curr Opin Obstet Gynecol* 10:57-60, 1998.

Yarbo C et al: *Cancer nursing: principles and practice,* ed 5, Sudbury, Mass, 2000, Jones and Bartlett.

Young R, Pecorelli S: Management of early ovarian cancer, *Semin Oncol* 25:335-9, 1998.

CHAPTER 34

Cancers of the Musculoskeletal System

Kimberly Haynes, MS, RN, CS, ONC, ARNP

OBJECTIVES

After reading this chapter, you should be able to do the following:

- Describe the pathophysiology of tumors of the musculoskeletal system, which include primary bone and soft tissue sarcomas
- Describe the clinical manifestations and typical presentation of sarcomas
- Describe the role of each member of the interdisciplinary team involved in the care of patients with tumors of the musculoskeletal system
- Describe the treatment regimen for patients with sarcomas
- Describe the nursing considerations involved in the treatment of cancers of the musculoskeletal system
- Discuss rehabilitation issues for patients with tumors of the musculoskeletal system as well as family and/or caregiver issues
- Describe end-of-life issues and ethical considerations for terminally ill patients and their family members

Malignant tumors of the musculoskeletal system include sarcomas, metastatic carcinomas, and multiple myeloma. The distinguishing factor in these cancers is the cell of origin.

Sarcomas are rare, malignant tumors that originate in the connective tissue of the body. Approximately 10,700 new sarcomas were diagnosed in 2002 (Jemal et al, 2002). Of those, 2400 were primary bone tumors and 8300 were primary soft tissue tumors.

Primary bone tumors enlarge, cause pain, and weaken the bone. In contrast, soft tissue sarcomas are usually painless. They can cause local destruction of the adjacent bone or invade nearby soft tissue structures, such as muscles, nerves, and blood vessels. Sarcomas can be very debilitating functionally, physiologically, and psychologically.

The etiology of bone and soft tissue sarcomas is unknown, but several factors are associated with their development, including trauma or past injury, oncogenic viruses, immunologic factors, and genetic factors.

This chapter discusses the diagnosis and treatment of bone and soft tissue sarcomas.

ASSESSMENT

Sarcomas are usually discovered when an individual seeks treatment related to an injury. Assessment includes taking a medical history, determining the onset of symptoms, and evaluating changes in functionality. The functional health pattern assessment (Box 34-1) should include questions related to the presence of hereditary musculoskeletal conditions, because these inherited bone and soft tissue tumor conditions can predispose the person to sarcomas (Box 34-2).

DIAGNOSIS

Diagnostic testing is needed when a soft tissue tumor or bone tumor is suspected. Diagnostic studies may include imaging examinations such as magnetic resonance imaging (MRI), computerized axial tomography or computed tomography (CT), nuclear medicine bone scanning, angiography, and plain radiography (Table 34-1). Imaging is done before biopsy to provide the surgeon with the information needed to perform the biopsy correctly. Because placement and orientation of the biopsy site can be the deciding factor in whether limb salvage surgery or amputation is performed, proper selection of the biopsy site is crucial.

There are no laboratory tests to detect sarcomas. Diagnosis of a malignant soft tissue tumor or bone tumor is ultimately confirmed by the results of a tissue biopsy, which should be performed by an orthopedic oncologist. The pathology report indicates the grade of the tumor, which describes the aggressiveness of the tumor. A low-grade tumor has a lower propensity to spread to the lungs but may be locally aggressive. A high-grade tumor has a greater chance of recurring locally and metastasizing to the lungs. The pathology report may also state whether the tumor is well differentiated or poorly differentiated. When a sarcoma is classified as well differentiated, it is usually a low-grade tumor, whereas a poorly differentiated sarcoma is more likely to be a high-grade tumor (Enzinger and Weiss, 1995).

The surgical margin is the tissue surrounding the tumor when it is removed. Surgical margins are described as *clear* (free of tumor cells), *close* (abnormal tumor cells are seen microscopically within 1 to 2 mm of the edge of the tumor specimen), or *positive* (the tumor is found at the edge of the surgical resection and tumor cells may still be left in the

---

Box 34-1 Functional Health Pattern Assessment for Musculoskeletal Tumors

HEALTH PERCEPTION/HEALTH MANAGEMENT
- Is there a family history of cancer?
- What is the patient's perception of his or her overall health?
- What medications and therapies does the patient use, including over-the-counter drugs, herbal treatments, and other alternative therapies?
- Does the patient have any allergies?

NUTRITION/METABOLISM
- What is the patient's current weight? Has a recent unexplained weight loss or gain occurred?
- What is the condition of the skin and mucous membranes?
- Does the patient have any metabolic or endocrine disorders?

ELIMINATION
- Does the patient experience difficulty with urination or urinary frequency?
- Does the patient have hematuria, kidney stones, bladder infections, constipation, or diarrhea?

ACTIVITY/EXERCISE
- Does the patient participate in a regular exercise program?
- Does the patient experience shortness of breath with exertion or pain with ambulation or movement?
- Does the patient require assistive devices for ambulation or activities of daily living?
- Does the patient have degenerative joint disease? Is there a fracture or impending fracture? Has there been a recent injury?

SLEEP/REST
- How many hours of uninterrupted sleep does the patient get at night?
- Does the patient take naps or rest periods?
- Does the patient take medications to induce sleep or use relaxation techniques?

COGNITION/PERCEPTION
- Are there any sensory deficits?
- What is the patient's educational level?
- Can the patient express himself or herself clearly and logically?
- Does the patient have any diseases that affect cognitive functioning or metastatic disease to the brain?
- What are the nature, character, location, and duration of the pain? What factors aggravate and alleviate the pain? What pain medication is used?

SELF-PERCEPTION/SELF-CONCEPT
- How does the patient perceive himself or herself?
- How has the condition affected the patient's self-esteem?
- How has the condition changed the patient's body image?
- Is the patient comfortable with his or her appearance?
- What is the patient's affect?

ROLES/RELATIONSHIPS
- Is the patient married?
- What kind of work does the patient perform?
- What role does the patient play in the home and family?
- What changes have occurred in the patient's ability to carry out role functions?
- How has the condition affected the patient's family and/or significant others?
- What is the patient's financial situation?
- Does the patient have a good family support system? Does the patient have supportive friendships and work relationships?

SEXUALITY/REPRODUCTION
- Is the patient sexually active?
- Have changes occurred in sexual performance? Does the patient have concerns about the ability to perform sexually?
- Is the patient satisfied with current sexual patterns?
- How many children does the patient have? Is the patient or the patient's partner trying to conceive?
- Has the patient experienced any changes in the menstrual cycle?

COPING/STRESS TOLERANCE
- What coping strategies does the patient use?
- What family and friend support systems are available to the patient?
- Can the patient manage the condition in the current setting?
- Is the patient currently seeking mental health treatment through counseling or medication?

VALUES/BELIEFS
- What constitutes good quality of life for the patient?
- What are the patient's spiritual beliefs? What are the patient's health beliefs? What are the patient's cultural beliefs?
- To what ethnic group does the patient belong? Are there support systems in the community?

---

wound bed, although they may be microscopic). If the resection margins are close or positive, then radiation treatment is considered.

SARCOMAS
Pathophysiology

A malignant neoplasm of the musculoskeletal system is called a sarcoma. As noted earlier, sarcomas are further subdivided into primary soft tissue sarcomas and primary bone sarcomas. A sarcoma is differentiated from a carcinoma by the cell of origin. Sarcomas arise from the mesoderm that forms the connective tissue of the body, such as muscle, fat, cartilage, bone, and fascia. Carcinomas arise from endodermal and ectodermal tissues; common carcinomas are lung, breast, prostate, kidney, and thyroid carcinomas. The cells that form the nervous system also arise from the ectoderm, but malignant nerve tumors, because of their aggressive behavior, are categorized as sarcomas, not as carcinomas.

There are approximately 40 different types of soft tissue sarcoma. Soft tissue sarcomas may develop from fat, striated and smooth muscle, nerves, and fibrous tissue.

Primary bone sarcomas include osteosarcoma, chondrosarcoma, and Ewing's sarcoma. The most common of these is osteosarcoma.

Clinical Manifestations
Primary Soft Tissue Sarcomas

The patient may come to the primary care physician complaining of an enlarging painless mass or the patient may have suffered an injury to the area and noticed a lump. Soft tissue tumors, whether malignant or benign, rarely cause pain; therefore, patients frequently delay seeking treatment. Soft tissue masses can occur throughout the body. According to Enzinger and Weiss (1995), the primary locations for soft tissue sarcomas are the extremities. Soft tissue sarcomas can also occur in the retroperitoneum and are associated with a less favorable outcome when in this location. High-grade soft tissue sarcomas will metastasize to the lungs if not treated.

Soft tissue tumors that are deep to the underlying fascia and larger than 5 cm raise concern that the mass may be a malignancy. The most common soft tissue tumor is a malignant fibrous histiocytoma.

Table 34-1   Radiologic Examinations for Diagnostic Tumor Workup

Tumor Type	Plain Radiograph	MRI Scan	CT Scan	Full-Body Bone Scan	Arteriogram
Bone	X	X	X	X	
Soft tissue		X			X

CT, Computed tomographic; *MRI,* magnetic resonance imaging.

Primary Bone Sarcomas

Approximately 2400 primary bone sarcomas are diagnosed each year. Bone tumors, like soft tissue tumors, are most often detected after trauma or injury. Occasionally a primary bone tumor is found incidentally. Symptoms such as generalized weakness and malaise, significant weight loss, fever, or fracture may also prompt the patient to seek treatment.

The most common age range for diagnosis of an osteosarcoma is between 10 and 25 years. Osteosarcoma is slightly more prevalent in males. Adult patients seek treatment from their primary care physician because of a slow onset of pain or pain precipitated by an injury.

Interdisciplinary Care

Treatment for sarcomas consists of surgery, chemotherapy, and radiation therapy and usually follows a national protocol. The combination of treatments used depends on many factors, including the age and general health of the patient, the size and location of the tumor, and the presence of metastatic disease to the lungs. Another important factor is whether the tumor is responsive to chemotherapy and radiation. The order of treatments can vary. Surgery is considered the primary treatment for sarcomas. A general guide for treatment of sarcomas is presented in Table 34-2.

All malignant bone tumors must be treated aggressively with surgery. Bone tumors will metastasize to the lungs and will cause local destruction of the bone and joint if not treated. The surgery involves removal of all neoplastic tissue, including bone and soft tissue involved with the tumor. Reconstruction with a custom metal prosthesis is one method used when the tumor is near the joint. Chemotherapy and radiation may be used as adjuvant therapy (see Table 34-2). Long-term follow-up and monitoring of the patient with a sarcoma is imperative. Sarcomas can recur locally or metastasize to the lungs. Early diagnosis of a recurrence or metastatic disease improves the chances for regaining control of the disease. A local recurrence of the tumor will be surgically excised if possible. Metastatic disease to the lungs is what ultimately causes death. Removal of lung nodules (metastasectomy) may be possible depending on the number and location of the nodules. The use of chemotherapy and radiation for a local recurrence or metastatic disease is considered even if these treatments were used when the tumor was originally diagnosed. However, the total amount of chemotherapy and radiation a person can receive during his or her lifetime is limited. Therefore, early diagnosis of local recurrence or distant metastases is desired.

Radiologic monitoring for local recurrence and metastatic disease to the lungs is performed at regular intervals for several years. For high-grade sarcomas, the interval may be every 2 months for the first year, then every 3 months for the second year. Monitoring during years 3 to 5 may require imaging every 4 to 6 months. MRI scans are used to monitor for local recurrence of the tumor in both bone and soft tissue. CT scans of the lungs are used to monitor for pulmonary

Table 34-2   General Treatments for Sarcomas

Tumor (Bone)	Neoadjuvant Chemotherapy	Surgery	Adjuvant Chemotherapy	Radiation Therapy
Bone Tumors				
Osteosarcoma	Yes	Yes	Yes	No
Ewing's sarcoma	Yes	Yes	Yes	Yes
Extremity tumor	Yes			
Pelvic tumor	No			
Chondrosarcoma	No	Yes	No	No
Soft Tissue Tumors				
Malignant fibrous histiocytoma	Yes	Yes	Yes	Depends on grade of tumor and surgical margins (clear, close, or positive)
Liposarcoma (low grade)	No	Yes	No	No
Liposarcoma (high grade)	Yes	Yes	Yes	Yes
Liposarcoma (myxoid) (depends on grade)	No	Yes	No	Yes
Fibrosarcoma (depends on grade)	Yes	Yes	Yes	Depends on grade of tumor and surgical margins (clear, close, or positive)
Neurofibrosarcoma	Yes	Yes	Yes	Depends on grade of tumor and surgical margins (clear, close, or positive)
Leiomyosarcoma (depends on grade)	Yes	Yes	Yes	No
Synovial sarcoma	Yes	Yes	Yes	Yes
Rhabdomyosarcoma	Yes	Yes	Yes	Yes
Angiosarcoma	Yes	Yes	Yes	No

nodules. CT scanning of the abdomen and pelvis may also be performed to monitor for the spread of the tumor to the retroperitoneum. The interval between examinations increases as the years progress without a local recurrence or metastatic disease. Monitoring practices vary by institution and by physician. Usually after 5 years the patient is monitored once a year.

Primary Provider (Physician/Nurse Practitioner)

An orthopedic oncologist is the primary physician in charge of the treatment plan for patients with sarcomas; however, many health care professionals are involved throughout the treatment process. The team includes surgical, medical, and radiation oncologists, nurses, social workers, and physical and occupational therapists.

The decision as to whether to offer neoadjuvant chemotherapy or radiation first or to perform the definitive surgical procedure first is usually made at a multidisciplinary tumor conference or by the team of physicians caring for the patient. The options are discussed with the patient and the final treatment plan is agreed upon.

Surgical Oncologist

The orthopedic oncologist performs the biopsy and definitive surgical procedure for sarcomas. As previously mentioned, proper biopsy incision placement is crucial in determining whether limb salvage surgery can be performed. Therefore the orthopedic oncologist or the treating physician should per-

form the initial biopsy and definitive surgery. The surgeon may choose to use one of the following techniques: fine needle aspiration, core needle biopsy, open or incisional biopsy, or excisional biopsy. Many factors must be considered in deciding on the appropriate biopsy technique, such as what the location, size, and depth of the mass are and whether the mass is a bone tumor or soft tissue tumor.

The ability to treat these tumors adequately and appropriately has been revolutionized by technologic advances as well as by advances in chemotherapy, radiation, and surgical techniques. Mapping out the surgical procedure with MRI scans and three-dimensional CT scans and searching for metastases with CT scans of the chest, abdomen, and pelvis are the current standard of care.

Prior to the late 1970s amputation was the standard treatment for sarcomas of the extremities. Currently limb salvage surgery is the treatment of choice. The surgical goal is complete eradication of the tumor while maintaining function in the limb. If the tumor cannot be completely excised (i.e., excised with clear surgical margins) with preservation of limb function, then amputation may be necessary. Customized megaprostheses or alloprostheses (Figure 34-1) are used in adults with bone tumors or destructive soft tissue tumors around or within a joint.

Surgical treatment for a soft tissue sarcoma is radical resection. Radical resection includes removal of the tumor with a cuff of normal tissue surrounding it, usually muscle, fascia, and subcutaneous fat. For a primary bone sarcoma of

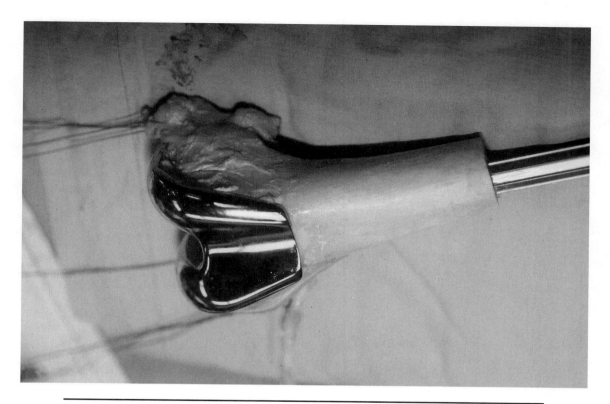

Figure 34-1 Alloprosthesis. Allograft and prosthesis composite. (Courtesy Kim Haynes, MS, RN, CS, ONC, ARNP, Mid-America Sarcoma Institute, Overland Park, Kan.)

an extremity such as osteosarcoma or Ewing's sarcoma, the surgical procedure performed is radical resection of the portion of the bone affected by the tumor. This generally involves resection of the distal, proximal, or mid-shaft portion of the bone. The defect left in the bone is replaced. When the defect is near a joint, the joint is replaced with a large metal prosthesis (Figure 34-2). After removal of a tumor of the diaphysis of the bone, a cadaver allograft and/or metal rod may be used for the reconstruction.

If the tumor is a chondrosarcoma and is confined to the intramedullary canal of the bone, then curettage, or scraping of the tumor out of the inside of the bone (Figure 34-3), followed by cryosurgery and bone grafting is one method of treatment. Cryosurgery is the use of liquid nitrogen as an adjuvant therapy. The liquid nitrogen is poured into the cavity formed by curetting or scraping the inside of the bone. The liquid nitrogen freezes the cavity, killing any remaining microscopic tumor cells. Bone graft is used to fill the cavity. The use of the cryosurgical technique increases the risk of fracture to the bone; therefore, prophylactic internal fixation with a metal plate and screws or an intramedullary rod may be used to help support the bone until the bone graft has matured and the defect has filled in with good bone.

Treatment of an impending fracture or pathologic fracture due to a sarcoma of bone is surgical and emergent.

Surgery is performed for stabilization and pain management as well as for resection of the tumor. Surgical treatment varies depending on where the impending fracture is located. Surgical procedures may include a partial or total hip replacement, hip pinning, curettage, bone grafting, and internal fixation with plates and screws or an intramedullary rod.

Medical Oncologist

Clinical trials and protocols for chemotherapy have been established nationally, and treatment is implemented before surgical resection (neoadjuvant therapy) or postoperatively (adjuvant therapy). Once the diagnosis of a sarcoma is confirmed, a medical oncologist discusses the use and administration of chemotherapy.

The use of chemotherapy for the treatment of soft tissue sarcomas is controversial. It has not been shown to provide significant benefit in controlling the disease either locally or systemically (Brennan, Alektiar, and Maki, 2001). However, clinical trials testing different chemotherapy drugs and dosages are being performed continuously with the goal of finding the right combination of drugs to aid in controlling metastatic disease.

Chemotherapy for bone sarcomas such as osteosarcoma and Ewing's sarcoma has been shown to help cure or at least

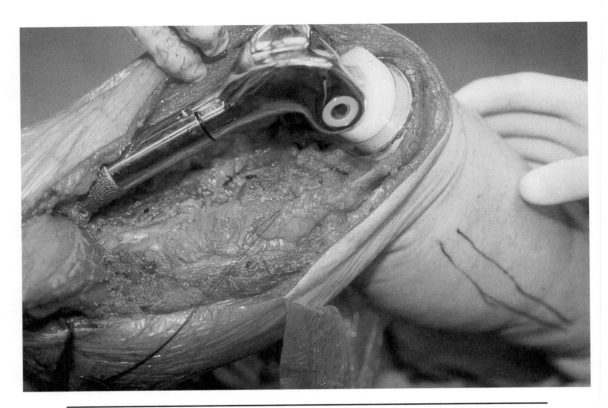

Figure 34-2 Distal femoral replacement prosthesis. (Courtesy Kim Haynes, MS, RN, CS, ONC, ARNP, Mid-America Sarcoma Institute, Overland Park, Kan.)

control local recurrence and metastatic disease. The success of chemotherapy is evaluated by examining the specimen after surgery to determine the amount of tumor necrosis. Generally, if tumor necrosis is more than 95%, the response is considered good and the chemotherapy regimen remains the same. If the necrosis is less than 95%, then the drugs and dosages used may be adjusted. Table 34-3 lists the chemotherapy drugs most commonly used in the treatment of sarcomas.

Radiation Oncologist

Radiation therapy is used in conjunction with surgery and chemotherapy to treat sarcomas and to assist in cure, palliation, and pain control. The side effects of radiation are caused by damage to normal cells in the area to which the radiation was delivered. Side effects of radiation include skin damage and blistering and soft tissue damage such as fibrosis and scarring. Another side effect is an increased risk for developing a cancer in the area of the radiation.

Radiation therapy used as an adjuvant treatment for sarcomas can be administered in several ways. The radiation oncologist discusses the principles and administration techniques available. The most commonly used method is external beam radiation therapy. It can be delivered before the surgical removal of the tumor (neoadjuvantly) to help shrink the tumor and make surgical resection easier or it can be given postoperatively to help prevent local recurrence. External beam radiation therapy is delivered every day, and treatments may last up to 6 weeks. A break in the treatment schedule may be required if skin problems occur.

The second method for radiation delivery is brachytherapy. In this technique, plastic catheters are implanted in the surgical wound bed immediately after the tumor has been removed. Three to 5 days postoperatively, the catheters are loaded with radioactive isotopes, which allows a high dose of radiation to be delivered directly to the surgical wound bed. During the interim between surgery and the loading of the catheters, the patient may be discharged home. However, the patient must be hospitalized while the radiation seeds are inside the catheters, and strict radiation precautions must be followed (see Chapter 27). During this time the patient is in isolation and in a lead-lined room or in a room at the end of the hall, depending on hospital policy and procedure. Visitors are not allowed because of the risk of radiation exposure. Nurses and other health care professionals are allowed in the room for only a limited amount of time each shift and wear dosimeter badges to monitor the amount of radiation exposure. The period over which the patient receives the specified dose of radiation is 3 to 5 days.

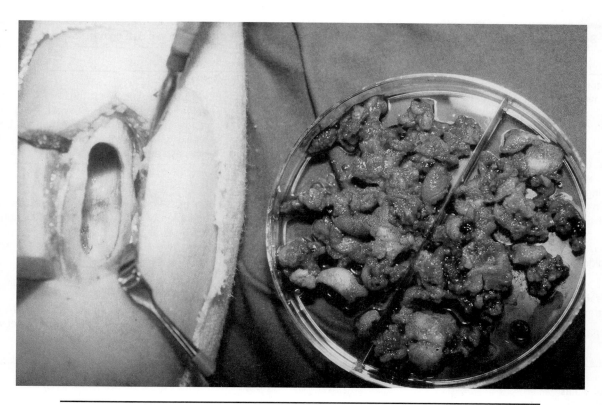

Figure 34-3   Curettage of bone tumor. (Courtesy Kim Haynes, MS, RN, CS, ONC, ARNP, Mid-America Sarcoma Institute, Overland Park, Kan.)

The third method of delivering radiation is known as intraoperative radiation therapy. Use of this technique requires a special operating room equipped with a linear accelerator, and this is usually found in large radiation or cancer centers. In this method the dose of radiation is delivered directly to the wound bed after removal of the tumor. The benefit of this method is the ability to direct the radiation to specific areas of concern.

Nurse

Nursing care for cancer patients is multifaceted and can be divided into two stages: acute phase and treatment phase. During the acute phase, initial diagnosis by surgical biopsy and treatment planning take place.

The second stage is the treatment phase. During this phase neoadjuvant chemotherapy and radiation are given. This phase may start as soon as 2 weeks after the biopsy is performed. Neoadjuvant chemotherapy lasts for approximately 3 months and includes three courses or rounds of chemotherapy depending on the protocol being followed. External beam radiation therapy may last up to 6 weeks depending on the total amount of radiation being delivered prior to surgery. If brachytherapy is being used, then the length of hospitalization required is approximately 3 to 5 days. Patient care issues critical during this time include

knowledge deficit related to chemotherapy and radiation side effects, and fear and anxiety related to a cancer diagnosis and having a potentially fatal illness.

During chemotherapy the patient and family need constant education and reinforcement regarding the side effects of the drugs used. The main side effects of chemotherapy in general include myelosuppression, nausea and vomiting, mucositis, diarrhea, cardiotoxicity, alopecia, and infection. The side effects can be very debilitating and are generally dose dependent. Table 34-4 lists the most common side effects of chemotherapy, surgery, and radiation therapy.

When the patient is hospitalized to receive chemotherapy or admitted for a side effect such as neutropenia (low white blood cell count) or intractable nausea and vomiting, supportive measures for infection control are in order. See Chapter 27 for detailed discussion of the care of the patient with cancer.

Nursing care of the patient receiving radiation therapy includes careful monitoring of the skin at the radiation site as well as education regarding the expected outcomes and side effects. When the patient is hospitalized for brachytherapy, all nursing and hospital staff, as well as visitors, follow radiation precautions. As noted earlier, the patient is placed in a special lead-lined private room or a room at the end of the hall to decrease radiation exposure of others. Radiation precautions may vary among institutions. Nursing interventions

Table 34-3   Chemotherapy Drugs Commonly Used in the Treatment of Sarcoma

Agent	Route	Action
Antitumor Antibiotics Actinomycin d (Dactinomycin) Bleomycin (Blenoxane) Doxorubicin (Adriamycin)	IV SC, IM, IV IV	Bind to DNA to inhibit synthesis of RNA and DNA. Formation of toxic oxygen-free radicals results in single- and double-stranded DNA breaks with subsequent inhibition of DNA synthesis and function.
Alkylating Agents Cisplatin (Platinol) Cyclophosphamide (Cytoxan) Dacarbazine (DTIC) Ifosfamide (Ifex)	IV PO, IV IV IV	Form cross-links with DNA, which results in inhibition of DNA synthesis and function. Act in all phases of the cell cycle. Ifosfamide is activated by the liver cytochrome P-450 system.
Antimetabolites Methotrexate (MTX)	PO, IM, IV, IT	Folic acid analog that interferes with DNA and RNA synthesis by inhibiting enzyme activity; acts on rapidly dividing cells that are synthesizing DNA.
Plant Alkaloids Vincristine (Oncovin) VP-16	IV IV	Bind to substance necessary for formation of mitotic spindles, preventing cell division. They work on cells in the mitosis phase, during which the parent cell divides into two new daughter cells.

Adapted from Chu E, DeVita VT: *Physician's cancer chemotherapy drug manual 2003*, Sudbury, Mass, 2003, Jones and Bartlett.
IM, Intramuscularly; *IV*, intravenously; *IT*, intrathecally; *PO*, orally; *SC*, subcutaneously.

for knowledge deficit and fear or anxiety are listed in Boxes 34-3 and 34-4, respectively.

After neoadjuvant chemotherapy and radiation is completed, surgical resection of the tumor takes place. Surgical resection of the tumor occurs approximately 2 to 3 weeks after completion of the neoadjuvant chemotherapy to allow the patient's immune system to recover. Surgery also occurs 3 weeks after radiation therapy to allow healing of the

Table 34-4   General Side Effects of Surgery, Chemotherapy, and Radiation Therapy

	Surgery	Chemotherapy	Radiation Therapy
Side effects	Pain, immobility, nausea, vomiting, constipation, wound complications (infection or dehiscence)	Nausea, vomiting, diarrhea, neutropenia, stomatitis, fatigue, hair loss, infection	Burning and blistering of skin Muscle fibrosis Radiation exposure to entire body
Duration of treatment or of side effects	Severe pain: 3-5 days; mild to moderate pain: 2-3 wk Immobility: up to 3 mo or more on crutches or walker Nausea, vomiting, diarrhea: up to 1 wk or longer depending on narcotic use. Infection: 1-2 wk Wound dehiscence: could last several weeks if left to close by secondary method	3-12 mo or longer depending on treatment protocol	Length of treatment: varies with mode of delivery External beam—up to 6 wk Intraoperative radiation therapy—one-time dose during surgery Brachytherapy—3-5 days Skin reaction: can last several days; treatment stops to allow skin to heal Muscle fibrosis: can be permanent

patient's skin. During the postoperative hospitalization, the nursing interventions should cover pain management and prevention of wound complications. Wound complications may include blistering, superficial or deep wound infection, or wound dehiscence because of the patient's compromised skin integrity and immune system. Proper nutrition must be encouraged to help the patient regain strength and to promote wound healing. Early mobilization is necessary to prevent blood clots and promote bowel function. The patient should be assisted with ambulation and range-of-motion exercises according to the physical therapy care plan formulated under the physician's orders during each shift. Common nursing interventions for wound care are listed in Box 34-5.

Once the patient's wound is healed, further chemotherapy may be necessary depending on treatment protocol. Adjuvant (postoperative) chemotherapy begins approximately 2 to 3 weeks after surgery to allow maximum time for complete healing of the surgical wound. The entire course of chemotherapy may last for up to 1 year. Nursing care during this time again addresses knowledge deficit, fear, and anxiety on the part of the patient as well as pain management, and infection prevention.

Box 34-3   Nursing Interventions for Knowledge Deficit

- Assess the level of understanding of the disease and treatment process by asking the patient to verbalize the current situation and treatment.
- Assess the views and beliefs of the patient and family members about cancer.
- Explain the common or standard anticancer therapies.
- Educate the patient about the specific type of cancer, the prognosis, and the treatment plan.
- Instruct the patient regarding the desired outcome of the treatment plan.
- Provide the patient with written information regarding treatment.
- Initiate referrals to other health team members as needed.
- Advise the patient and family of the side effects of each chemotherapy drug to be given.
- Advise the patient and family of the potential side effects of radiation treatment, such as blistering of the skin and muscle fibrosis.

Box 34-4   Nursing Interventions for Fear and Anxiety Related to Having a Potentially Fatal Illness

- Evaluate for the presence of anxiety, depression, fear, and anger.
- Answer questions calmly and allow sufficient time for the patient to verbalize feelings and queries.
- Provide reassurance regarding the patient's behavior.
- Initiate referral to a psychiatric advanced practice nurse.

Box 34-5   Nursing Interventions for Prevention of Wound Complications

- Follow proper hand-washing protocol and teach the patient and family members the importance of hand washing.
- Monitor the wound each shift for signs of infection, including redness and drainage.
- Teach the patient and family members how to change the dressing and what signs and symptoms to report to the physician.
- Change the dressing only as needed to prevent further skin irritation from tape.
- Administer antibiotics per the physician's order.

Physical and Occupational Therapists

The physical therapist and occupational therapist assist the patient in maintaining the ability to perform the activities of daily living during hospitalization and at home. These two specialists are used on a regular basis to restore the patient to the presurgery level of functioning. Therapy is initiated in the hospital and then continued on an outpatient basis after the patient is discharged. Using practitioners knowledgeable about sarcomas and the therapy and modalities needed postoperatively helps provide continuity of care for these cancer patients.

Depending on the type of surgery performed, a return to full function may not be possible or desirable. If a metal prosthesis is used for a tumor of the distal femur or proximal tibia, touchdown weight bearing is initiated after surgery and continued for approximately 6 weeks. Theoretically the metal prosthesis is as strong as it will ever be immediately after surgery, but the restricted weight bearing allows the soft tissues to heal. During this time physical therapy consists of gait training and occupational therapy focuses on practicing activities of daily living. After 6 weeks, if the radiograph reveals evidence of callus formation at the interface between the host bone and the prosthesis, and if soft tissue swelling has resolved, then range-of-motion and strengthening exercises begin. The goal is to achieve at least a 90-degree flexion at the knee. Further flexion may be achieved but is not necessary for daily functioning such as sitting in a chair or riding in cars or airplanes. Return to full flexion at the knee joint is not desired, because flexion of greater than 90 degrees can put extra stress on the prosthesis, which may cause early loosening of the metal implant.

As weight bearing and strength increase, the patient progresses from a walker or crutches to a cane. In general, a patient with a prosthesis is allowed to bear partial weight on the extremity for the first 6 weeks and then to progress to full weight bearing during the next 6 weeks. When the patient is able to bear full weight and safely ambulate, the patient may walk without assistive devices. This usually occurs by 3 months. Activities that put strain and stress on the prosthesis, such as hard running and jumping and activities that require planting and twisting of the knee, are restricted. Therefore, sports activities such as basketball, running, football, and tennis are not allowed. Cycling and swimming are encouraged for aerobic exercise and enjoyment. Prosthesis failure may occur due to metal fatigue and loosening. The prosthesis may last 12 to 15 years or longer before loosening occurs. The key is to allow the patient a full life but to restrict some activities so that the prosthesis does not wear out too soon. A prosthesis revision is inevitable in a young person if the individual survives the cancer.

When tumors involve the upper extremities, range of motion and lifting are restricted. An occupational therapist is consulted to develop an upper extremity program. If a proximal shoulder replacement or total shoulder replacement has been performed, then gentle range-of-motion exercises may begin in 2 weeks and strengthening exercises may begin in 6 weeks depending on the treating physician's protocol. If a curettage and bone graft with or without internal fixation has been performed on the humerus, then strengthening will not begin for at least 6 to 8 weeks or until the radiographs show evidence of healing and good consolidation of the bone graft.

If an amputation is performed, gait training and exercises related to the activities of daily living will be used to meet the needs of the patient. Factors affecting the exercise program include level of amputation, general health of the patient, site of the amputation (upper or lower extremity), and age of the patient. A physiatrist (a physician specializing in rehabilitation) takes over monitoring of the patient's progress and the ordering and maintenance of the prosthesis if applicable.

Medical Social Worker

The social worker is consulted for assistance with home health and long-term care planning. The social worker plays an integral role in the care of the sarcoma patient. Such a patient requires extensive treatment involving chemotherapy, home care, special equipment, and possibly placement in a skilled nursing or long-term care facility. Working with the patient's insurance company and acquiring authorization for certain treatments takes time, planning, and the negotiating skills that the social workers possesses.

Complementary and Alternative Therapies

Alternative and complementary therapies may play an important role in the treatment of cancer patients. Complementary treatments such as massage, biofeedback, reflexology, meditation, yoga, and guided imagery can benefit the patient. Other forms of complementary treatment used by patients include music, art, play therapy, laughter, and prayer.

Concern arises when a patient wants to bypass conventional treatment (surgery, chemotherapy, or radiation) and try to treat or cure cancer through unproven methods such as use of shark cartilage, consumption of megadoses of vita-

mins or herbal formulations, or use of cleansing enemas. This occasionally happens at the time of diagnosis but occurs more frequently when the patient is informed that the disease is terminal. At this point some patients and their families want to try any possible treatment in an attempt to cure the disease. It is important for health care professionals

---

Think S for Success

Symptoms
- Manage postoperative pain and side effects of chemotherapy with medication.
- Treat side effects of radiation with extremity mobility and massage.

Sequelae
- Prevent disability by administering pain medication appropriately and encouraging and assisting with physical therapy and mobility.
- Prevent nausea and vomiting by administering antiemetics appropriately.
- Prevent infection by using clean and sterile technique and good hand washing when giving care to the patient; encourage family and friends to follow same procedures.
- Encourage extremity mobility and use massage to decrease muscle stiffness and fibrosis caused by radiation.

Safety
- Teach patient and family the importance of the following:
  Using pain medication appropriately and properly
  Monitoring for side effects such as constipation and oversedation
  Avoiding use of other pain medications in conjunction with a narcotic unless instructed to do so by the physician
  Avoiding use of alcohol during narcotic use
  Requesting antiemetics as needed during chemotherapy
  Eating frequent small meals or foods that are high in protein to promote wound healing
  Following infection control practices at all times
  Following radiation safety protocols while radiation is being administered
  Monitoring the wound

Support/Services
- Arrange for assistance at home for patient and/or family by home health and/or hospice care as needed.
- Arrange for emotional support for patient and/or family through counselors or cancer support groups as needed.

Satisfaction
- Determine degree to which cancer is interfering with patient's quality of life and develop a plan to help patient and family achieve desired quality of life; refer patient and family to hospice care if desired.

to openly discuss these treatments with their patients and to encourage their patients to report any treatments they may be using at home. Providers must educate patients and family members about the side effects and potentially lethal effects that may occur if these treatments are used alone or in combination with prescription medications. This may be the time to discuss participation in experimental clinical trials and to provide patients and families with information regarding these studies.

FAMILY AND CAREGIVER ISSUES

The patient with terminal cancer and his or her family and caregivers need support and guidance throughout the end stage of the disease process. Management of the patient's pain is crucial. The initial goal is to keep the patient comfortable enough to tolerate diagnostic and therapeutic procedures during active treatment. When the disease has advanced, the pain management goals shift to those of controlling the pain enough to allow the patient to function at the level the individual has chosen and making death as pain free as possible (Foley, 2001).

Other issues that must be addressed during end-stage cancer include those involving physical, psychological, social, and spiritual care (Ferrell, Virani, and Grant, 1998). Financial concerns such as estate planning and funeral planning must be discussed. The patient, family members, and caregivers can also benefit from education regarding the death event and what to expect or anticipate. Hospice care programs offer excellent services but remain underused.

ETHICAL CONSIDERATIONS

Ethical issues are inherent in the care of the terminally ill patient. Issues that may have to be dealt with include do-not-resuscitate status, a decision to forgo feeding and hydration, assisted suicide, conflicts among medical colleagues, and pain control. The most important consideration for nurses in these situations is to be knowledgeable and informed. (See Chapter 27.)

CASE STUDY

Patient Data

Mrs. K. is a 30-year-old nursing student. She lives with her husband. She has one little girl who is 3 years old and attends preschool 2 days a week. She lives in a two-story home with a large yard. She does not work outside the home and attends school full time. She is in her final semester of nursing school. Her husband is an attorney. Her parents are still alive and live 2 hours away. She has two sisters and one brother who live in the area. She is active in her church and participates in a weekly Bible study group. She teaches Sunday school and participates in couples Sunday school with her husband. She is a runner and currently runs at least four times a week. Approximately 8 weeks ago she noticed a small lump on her left anterior thigh. This was not precipitated by any antecedent trauma or change in activity. She noticed the lump while stretching after running. She attributed the mass to a pulled muscle even though it was not painful. Over the next 2 months the mass doubled in size and started to cause pain. She sought treatment through her primary care physician, who ordered an MRI scan. The scan revealed a $10 \times 5 \times 5.5$ cm mass with a differential diagnosis of soft tissue sarcoma. An open biopsy was scheduled, and the pathologic analysis revealed a high-grade myxoid malignant fibrous histiocytoma. Further diagnostic workup included a CT scan of her chest, abdomen, and pelvis and laboratory work. All results were negative.

At her initial postoperative office visit, the disease process and treatment plan are discussed thoroughly. Mrs. K. is notably anxious and upset and tearful at times. Her husband is very supportive. Mrs. K. voices numerous concerns about the long-term prognosis and if and how she is going to be able to finish school and care for her daughter. It is suggested that neoadjuvant chemotherapy and radiation be given, followed by the definitive surgical removal of the tumor. The patient's case is to be presented at the musculoskeletal tumor conference for discussion. Arrangements are made for the patient to see a medical oncologist for chemotherapy and a radiation oncologist for radiation therapy in anticipation of beginning the treatment plan that will be formulated at the tumor conference.

Diagnostic Findings

MRI scan: $10 \times 5 \times 5.5$ cm soft tissue mass
CT scans of chest, abdomen, and pelvis with contrast: negative for metastatic disease
Chest radiograph: normal
Complete blood count with differential, chemistry profile, prothrombin time, partial thromboplastin time, culture results: within normal limits

Thinking It Through

- What nursing diagnoses pertain to Mrs. K.?
- What can you do as a nurse to address her fears about her prognosis?
- What can you do as a nurse to address her concerns regarding care of her daughter?
- What assistive services can be offered Mrs. K. during her treatment that will help her manage her home situation?
- What concerns will Mr. K. have regarding his wife's treatment and prognosis?
- How can the health care team assist Mrs. K. during her treatment?

Case Conference

The musculoskeletal tumor conference meets and discusses Mrs. K.'s case. The multidisciplinary team present at the conference includes the orthopedic surgical oncologist, medical oncologist, radiation oncologist, pathologist, radiologist, advanced practice nurse for the surgeon, and medical oncologist. A social worker who specializes in hospice care, a physical therapist, and an occupational therapist are also present. This conference is a teaching conference in which the health care team shares data and statistics and a plan of treatment is formulated. Therefore, the patient and her husband are not present.

The surgeon describes the nature and natural history of this type of tumor and discusses the patient's history. The radiologist shows the MRI scan of the thigh and describes the size of the tumor and its imaging characteristics. The pathologist gives a Power Point computer presentation showing actual histologic slides of the tumor cells and discusses the implications of the cell

Continued

CASE STUDY—cont'd

pattern and the number of mitoses present per high-power field. The pathologist then gives the diagnosis and the grade of the tumor.

The team agrees on a treatment plan. Three rounds of chemotherapy and 6 weeks of radiation therapy will be given first. The goal of the chemotherapy is to kill the tumor in the thigh as well as any tumor cells that may be circulating in the bloodstream. The goal of radiation is to shrink the tumor. The mass will then be surgically resected, and the pathologist will check the entire specimen for viable tumor. Further chemotherapy or other treatment may be ordered depending on the final pathologic findings regarding the amount of viable tumor present in the resected specimen.

The medical oncologist states that the main side effects from the chemotherapy will be neutropenia, nausea and vomiting, and hair loss. The side effects from radiation will be restricted to the demarcated area on the left thigh and will include possible skin burning and blistering. The physical therapist states that an exercise program that includes range-of-motion and strengthening exercises will be useful after the definitive surgical resection takes place. The services of an occupational therapist will be used if needed. The social worker states that she will be involved in planning for any necessary home services such as home nursing care, nutritional counseling, and physical therapy if needed. Hospice care is not needed at this time.

The surgeon calls Mrs. K. after the conference and confirms the treatment plan with her. The advanced practice nurse overhears the conversation. It is obvious that Mrs. K. is very anxious but is willing to get started with the treatment. The advanced practice nurse answers Mrs. K.'s questions and encourages her to call the office at any time if she has questions. The nurse proceeds to her office and formulates a plan of care for Mrs. K., keeping in mind the following concerns.

■ How will the patient's education level affect her ability to cope with her cancer?
■ How important does Mrs. K.'s running appear to be and what kind of exercise program will she be able to continue?
■ Will psychological support through counseling or drug therapy likely be needed to control Mrs. K.'s anxiety?
■ List two problems that the plan of care should address.

Internet and Other Resources

American Cancer Society: *http://www.cancer.org*
CancerGuide: *http://cancerguide.org*
Look Good...Feel Better: *http://www.lookgoodfeelbetter.org/*
National Cancer Institute: *http://www.nci.nih.gov*
OncoLink: *http://www.oncolink.upenn.edu/*
Washington Musculoskeletal Tumor Center (Sarcoma.org): *http://www.sarcoma.org*

REFERENCES

Brennan M, Alektiar K, Maki R: Sarcomas of the soft tissue and bone. In DeVita V, Hellman S, Rosenberg S, editors: *Cancer: principles and practice of oncology,* ed 6, Philadelphia, 2001, Lippincott Williams & Wilkins, pp 1841-91.

Enzinger F, Weiss S: *Soft tissue tumors,* ed 3, St Louis, 1995, Mosby.

Ferrell B, Virani R, Grant M: HOPE: home care outreach for palliative care education, *Cancer Pract* 6(2):79-85, 1998.

Foley KM: Supportive care and quality of life. In DeVita V, Hellman S, Rosenberg S, editors: *Cancer: principles and practice of oncology,* ed 6, Philadelphia, 2001, Lippincott Williams & Wilkins, pp 2977-3011.

Jemal A et al: Cancer statistics, 2002, *CA Cancer J Clin* 52:23-47, 2002.

CHAPTER 35

Living with HIV and AIDS

Diana Jordan, MS, RN, ACRN, Rosalyn Cousar, MSN, RN, AACRN, and Juna Mackey-Padilla, PhD, MSN, RN

OBJECTIVES

After reading this chapter, you should be able to do the following:

- Describe the pathophysiology and epidemiology of human immunodeficiency virus (HIV) infection and identify special populations affected by this disease
- Describe the clinical manifestations of HIV disease, including opportunistic infections, coinfections, and other complications
- Describe the indications for use, side effects, and nursing considerations related to antiretroviral medications
- Describe the functional health patterns affected by HIV disease
- Describe the role of each member of the interdisciplinary team involved in the care of patients with HIV infection

The spread of human immunodeficiency virus (HIV) infection and acquired immunodeficiency syndrome (AIDS) has reached pandemic proportions, devastating multitudes of individuals, families, and communities. According to the Joint United Nations Programme on HIV/AIDS and the World Health Organization (WHO) (Joint United Nations Programme, 2003), an estimated 40 million people worldwide were living with HIV/AIDS at the end of 2003, and an estimated 14,000 people become infected every day. Globally 95% of people with HIV infection live in low- and middle-income countries. In the United States, approximately 900,000 people are estimated to be living with HIV/AIDS, and 40,000 individuals were newly infected with HIV in 2003. Worldwide in 2003, about 3.1 million people died as a result of AIDS. According to WHO and UNAIDS (Joint United Nations Programme, 2003) statistics, between 12,000 and 15,000 of those deaths occurred in the United States.

Women, adolescents, and people of color, especially African Americans and Latinos, are disproportionately affected by HIV/AIDS. The poor, the undereducated, and those without regular access to health services are overrepresented among those with the disease and are increasingly at risk for acquiring HIV/AIDS.

Factors that perpetuate the spread of HIV/AIDS include migration, economic instability, social and environmental determinants, drug use, mental illness, increased rates of sexually transmitted diseases, and poverty. Social stigma and discrimination continue to cause some of the most painful consequences of HIV/AIDS, which lead to feelings of rejection and isolation and thus create barriers to the effective prevention and treatment of HIV/AIDS. A plan of care developed for the treatment of individuals living with HIV/AIDS must include an assessment of these factors in addition to a comprehensive review of the physical symptoms of the disease.

Drug therapy has brought about a significant decrease in the AIDS death rate and has made it possible for the potentially fatal consequences of HIV/AIDS to be managed as a chronic condition. How well the individual can live his or her life while also living with HIV/AIDS is an important focus as individuals living with the disease make choices to manage their illness with drug therapy, in spite of all of the adverse effects of the medications, and/or other complementary and alternative treatment methods.

ETHNIC VARIATIONS

AIDS was first discovered as an illness among gay white men. In the United States, people who identify themselves as men who have sex with men, lesbians, bisexuals, and transgendered individuals have represented the largest subgroup affected by HIV disease since its existence. However, the HIV infection rate among minorities has risen rapidly and disproportionately. African Americans and Hispanics represent 24.8% of the United States population but make up 51% of the cases of AIDS (Centers for Disease Control and Prevention [CDC], 2002). Infection rates are also increasing among injection drug users, women, adolescents, young men who have sex with men, and the elderly.

Another consideration is the individual's travel history. The complexity of this disease, in combination with migration patterns, ethnic and cultural values and beliefs, and physiologic and behavioral norms, has led to the development of diverse strains of HIV throughout the world. Complementary and alternative therapies and folk medicine are part of ethnic cultures and should be considered when developing a plan of care.

ASSESSMENT

HIV disease affects physical, mental, and emotional well-being. Periodic assessment of functional health patterns (Box 35-1) helps providers to develop and adjust the plan of care.

PATHOPHYSIOLOGY

Two types of HIV have been isolated. HIV-1 is the type identified in the majority of cases in the United States. HIV-2 has been isolated predominantly from individuals in West Africa. HIV-1 has several different subtypes. Ninety-eight percent of HIV-1 infections in the United States are caused by class B. Most infections with non-B subtypes and with HIV-2 are acquired in other countries.

Box 35-1   Functional Health Pattern Assessment for HIV/AIDS

HEALTH PERCEPTION/HEALTH MANAGEMENT
- What is the patient's perception of his or her overall health?
- What is the patient's perception and use of medication? Has the patient received all necessary immunizations?
- What alternative therapies does the patient use?
- Is the patient able to adhere to the treatment regimen and keep medical appointments?

NUTRITION/METABOLISM
- What is the patient's current weight? Has there been any unexplained recent weight gain or loss?
- Is the patient on any special diet?
- What are the patient's dietary needs?
- What is the condition of the skin and mucous membranes?
- Does the patient experience nausea and vomiting? Have there been any oral, gastrointestinal, and/or esophageal changes?
- What are cultural and traditional foods for the patient?

ELIMINATION
- Have any changes occurred in bowel or bladder habits?
- Does the patient experience any pain or difficulty in urinating?
- Have any rectal changes occurred?
- Does the patient have diarrhea? What is the number of stools daily?

ACTIVITY/EXERCISE
- Does the patient experience difficulty in walking, fatigue, malaise, or joint stiffness?
- What are the patient's regular exercise activities?
- What mobility aids does the patient use?
- Is the patient able to perform the activities of daily living?
- Does the patient have neuropathy, edema, shortness of breath, or muscle wasting?

SLEEP/REST
- How much uninterrupted sleep does the patient get at night?
- Does the patient take naps or rest periods?
- Does the patient have insomnia or nightmares? What sleep aids are used?

COGNITION/PERCEPTION
- Does the patient have pain or paresthesias?
- How does patient describe character, location, duration, and exacerbating and remitting aspects of pain?
- Have there been any changes in mental status?

SELF-PERCEPTION/SELF-CONCEPT
- How does the patient describe himself or herself?
- How has the condition affected the patient's self-esteem?
- What changes have occurred in the patient's body image?
- How has the condition affected the patient's sense of self?
- Does the patient have any dermatologic manifestations of the disease?

ROLES/RELATIONSHIPS
- What kind of work does the patient perform?
- What role does the patient play in the home and family?
- What changes have occurred in the patient's ability to carry out role functions?
- How satisfied is the patient with his or her current roles and relationships?
- How has the condition affected the patient's family and/or significant others?
- What is the patient's disability status?

SEXUALITY/REPRODUCTION
- Is the patient sexually active?
- Have changes occurred in sexual performance?
- Does the patient have a history of sexually transmitted disease (other than HIV infection) or currently have such a disease?
- What are the patient's sexual practices? Does the patient use safer sex strategies?
- Have changes occurred in the menstrual cycle?
- Is the patient pregnant?

COPING/STRESS TOLERANCE
- What coping strategies does the patient use?
- What support systems are available to the patient?
- Can the patient manage the condition in the current setting?

VALUES/BELIEFS
- What constitutes good quality of life for the patient? What is important to the patient?
- What are the patient's spiritual beliefs, health beliefs, and cultural beliefs?
- What are the patient's views regarding locus of control?
- To what extent do patient's cultural and spiritual beliefs influence decision making?

HIV infects and induces cell death in T helper lymphocytes that express the cell marker CD4, also known as CD4 cells. CD4 cells become steadily depleted from peripheral blood in most untreated persons with HIV infection. AIDS is an end point of HIV infection resulting from severe immunologic damage and loss of an effective immune response to specific opportunistic pathogens and tumors. HIV infection causes a wide range of symptoms and clinical conditions that indicate differing levels of immune dysfunction. The most widely used HIV/AIDS classification system in the United States was pub-lished by the CDC in 1992 (Table 35-1). In the CDC classification system, HIV infection and AIDS are divided into categories based on two types of information: peripheral blood CD4 cell counts and clinical manifestations. CD4 cell counts are grouped into three levels, ranging from relatively normal counts (more than 500 cells/mm^3) to severe CD4 cell depletion (fewer than 200 cells/mm^3). The clinical manifestations of HIV infection and AIDS are also placed into three categories, generally in accordance with the level of immunologic dysfunction associated with the various symptoms.

Table 35-1   1993 Revised Classification System for HIV Infection and Expanded Surveillance Case Definition for AIDS Among Adults and Adolescents

CD4 Cell Category	Clinical Category A	Clinical Category B	Clinical Category C
(1) ≥500 cells/mm^3 (≥29%)	A1	B1	C1
(2) 200-499 cells/mm^3 (14% to 28%)	A2	B2	C2
(3) <200 cells/mm^3 (<14%)	A3	B3	C3

Category A Conditions	Category B Conditions	Category C Conditions
■ No symptoms ■ Acute HIV infection (resolves) ■ Generalized lymphadenopathy	■ Bacillary angiomatosis ■ Oropharyngeal candidiasis ■ Vulvovaginal candidiasis: persistent, frequent or poorly responsive to therapy ■ Cervical intraepithelial neoplasia II or III ■ Constitutional symptoms: fever, diarrhea >1 mo ■ Oral hairy leukoplakia ■ Herpes zoster: multiple episodes or involving >1 dermatome ■ Idiopathic thrombocytopenic purpura ■ Listeriosis ■ Pelvic inflammatory disease, particularly if complicated by tubo-ovarian abscess ■ Peripheral neuropathy	■ Candidiasis of bronchi, trachea, lungs, or esophagus ■ Invasive cervical cancer ■ Coccidioidomycosis, disseminated or extrapulmonary ■ Cryptococcosis, extrapulmonary ■ Cryptosporidiosis (intestinal infection >1 mo duration) ■ Cytomegalovirus disease (excluding liver, spleen, or lymph nodes) ■ HIV-related encephalopathy ■ Herpes simplex: chronic ulcer >1 mo duration, or bronchitis, pneumonitis, or esophagitis ■ Histoplasmosis: disseminated or extrapulmonary ■ Isosporiasis: >1 mo duration ■ Kaposi's sarcoma ■ Burkitt's lymphoma ■ Immunoblastic lymphoma ■ Primary lymphoma of the brain ■ *Mycobacterium avium-intracellulare complex* or *Mycobacterium kansasii* infection: disseminated or extrapulmonary ■ *Mycobacterium. tuberculosis* infection: any site ■ *Mycobacterium* infection with other species or unknown species, disseminated or extrapulmonary ■ *Pneumocystis carinii* pneumonia ■ Recurrent pneumonia: >2 episodes in 12 mo ■ Progressive multifocal leukoencephalopathy ■ *Salmonella* septicemia, recurrent ■ Toxoplasmosis of an internal organ ■ Wasting syndrome due to HIV

From Centers for Disease Control: 1993 Revised classification system for HIV infection and expanded surveillance case definition for AIDS among adolescents and adults, *MMWR Recomm Rep* 41(RR-17):1-19, 1992.
All patients with diseases categorized as A3, B3, and C1 through C3 are defined as having AIDS based on the presence of an AIDS-defining condition and/or a CD4 cell count below 200 cells/mm^3.

Category A disease is characterized by normal clinical findings, clinical findings that do not indicate immune injury (including absence of symptoms), generalized lymphadenopathy, or resolved acute HIV infection. Category B includes conditions that indicate the presence of a defect in cell-mediated immunity or conditions that appear to be worsened by HIV infection. Category C includes conditions that are considered AIDS defining even in the absence of a CD4 cell count of fewer than 200 cells/mm³. All patients with disease categorized as A3, B3, and C1 through C3 are defined as having AIDS based on the presence of an AIDS-defining condition and/or a CD4 cell count below 200 cells/mm³.

CLINICAL MANIFESTATIONS

Signs of immune system compromise in HIV/AIDS include low white cell counts, lymphadenopathy, and fatigue. As the immune system fails, opportunistic infections develop, giving rise to a host of symptoms that depend on the specific invading organism. In addition, individuals with HIV/AIDS are prone to develop malignancies, dementia, and wasting. General manifestations of HIV/AIDS are listed in Box 35-2. A more detailed discussion of opportunistic infections, malignancies, and complications follows (Table 35-2).

Opportunistic Infections
Mycobacterium Avium-Intracellulare Complex Infection

Mycobacterium avium-intracellulare complex (MAI or MAC) is an infectious agent that can cause serious disease in immunocompromised individuals. The organisms are commonly found in food, water, animals, birds, and soil. Infection is acquired by ingesting or inhaling the bacteria. *M. avium-intracellulare complex* can cause infection in the liver, spleen, lymph nodes, bone marrow, and gastrointestinal tract (DeLorenzo and Ingram, 2001). Diagnosis is made by culturing sputum, bronchial wash, or stool; acid-fast bacillus blood culture; bone marrow aspiration; or tissue biopsy.

Optimal treatment is a combination of two or three drugs. The most effective therapy is clarithromycin (Biaxin) or azithromycin (Zithromax) with ethambutol (Myambutol) with or without rifabutin (Mycobutin) (Kirton, 2003; Murphy and Flaherty, 2003).

Tuberculosis

Tuberculosis (TB) is caused by *Mycobacterium tuberculosis* (MTB), an acid-fast bacillus transmitted through droplet nuclei that become aerosolized via talking, laughing, coughing, or singing. Droplets can remain airborne for 48 hours (Kirton, 2003). (See Chapter 9 for a comprehensive discussion of TB.)

There is a bidirectional interaction between MTB infection and HIV infection, so it is critical to assess all HIV-infected patients for TB and all TB patients for HIV disease. MTB is inhaled and the organisms penetrate the lung parenchyma. The infection can be detected in 2 to 10 weeks with a tuberculin skin test (Kirton, 2003).

TB can be diagnosed through purified protein derivative (tuberculin) testing, chest radiograph, sputum smear analysis, and sputum culture.

Drug treatment of active cases of TB varies based on current use of antiretroviral therapy. If the patient is not taking a protease inhibitor or nonnucleoside reverse transcriptase inhibitor (NNRTI), the first-choice regimen consists of combinations of drugs such as isoniazid (INH), rifampin (Rifadin), pyrazinamide (Tebrazid), and ethambutol (Myambutol). If the patient is taking protease inhibitors or NNRTIs, rifabutin (Mycobutin) or streptomycin is used in place of rifampin. Treatment for persons exposed to isoniazid- and/or rifampin- or rifabutin-resistant TB should be based on relative risk for exposure to resistant organisms. These regimens can induce multiple drug interactions with antiretroviral drugs (Murphy and Flaherty, 2003).

Candidiasis

Candida albicans is the causative agent of candidiasis (thrush, yeast infection). The organism is found in soil and food, on inanimate objects, and in hospital environments. *Candida* organisms are fungi (yeasts). *Candida* species cause the most frequently reported fungal infections in patients with HIV disease. *C. albicans* is part of the normal flora of the teeth, gingiva, skin, vagina, oropharynx, and large intestines. The level of immunosuppression is inversely related to the development of candidiasis in HIV disease. Dehydration, poor nutrition, or altered skin integrity can also contribute to the development of candidiasis.

Box 35-2   General Clinical Manifestations Associated with HIV/AIDS

- Dry skin
- Poor wound healing
- Skin lesions
- Mucositis
- Fever
- Night sweats
- Dry cough
- Shortness of breath
- Fatigue
- Diarrhea
- Weight loss
- Nightmares
- Confusion
- Memory loss
- Personality changes
- Seizures
- Headache
- Visual changes

Table 35-2 Clinical Manifestations Associated with Opportunistic Infections and Other HIV-Related Conditions

Infection/Condition	Manifestations
Mycobacterium avium-intracellulare complex infection	Persistent fever, weight loss, night sweats, chronic diarrhea, weakness, fatigue, anemia, neutropenia, abdominal discomfort
Tuberculosis	Fever, cough, night sweats, hemoptysis, shortness of breath, fatigue, headache, chills, mental status changes, lymphadenopathy, nausea and vomiting, weight loss
Candidiasis	Oropharyngeal 　White plaques; smooth red patches on the palate, buccal mucosa, or tongue; erythema, cracks and fissure at the corners of the mouth Esophageal 　Dysphagia, odynophagia, substernal chest pain, feelings of obstruction or heartburn Vulvovaginal 　Marked itching, watery to cottage cheese–like discharge, vaginal erythema with adherent white discharge, swelling of the labia and vulva
Cryptococcosis	Headache, fever, malaise, cough, dyspnea, pleuritic-type chest pain, stiff neck, focal deficits, seizures, nausea, dizziness, confusion, irritability, low-grade fever, nonproductive cough, dyspnea, weight loss, fatigue
Cryptosporidiosis	Frequent stools (6-26 bowel movements daily), fever, watery diarrhea, right upper quadrant abdominal pain and cramping, flatulence, nausea and vomiting, anorexia, weight loss, malaise
Cytomegalovirus infection	Floaters, scotomata (blind spots), loss of peripheral vision, chorioretinitis, headaches, difficulty concentrating, sleepiness, encephalitis, mouth ulcerations, dysphagia or odynophagia, abdominal pain or bloody diarrhea, weight loss, rectal ulcers, persistent fever, fatigue, weight loss, adrenalitis, shortness of breath, dyspnea on exertion, dry cough, pneumonia (rare in AIDS patients), bilateral lower extremity weakness, urinary retention, incontinence or spasticity, low back pain, especially back pain radiating to perianal area, polyradiculopathy, confusion, apathy, lethargy, withdrawal, personality changes, encephalitis
Toxoplasmosis	Dull constant headache, visual changes, altered mental status, disorientation, seizures, changes in gait, aphasia, hemiparesis, cranial nerve palsies
Herpes simplex (genital herpes)	Fever, malaise, adenopathy, painful ulcerative lesions, prodromal symptoms of paresthesias, itching or tingling at the site of impending eruption, possible presence of papules that rapidly evolve into fluid-filled vesicles
Herpes zoster (shingles)	Unilateral vesicular eruption with dermatomal distribution, anorexia, fever, cough, burning or stabbing pain, postherpetic neuralgia
Kaposi's sarcoma	Multicentric skin lesions varying from brown to red to purple; asymptomatic visceral involvement, especially in the oral cavity and gastrointestinal tract; swelling and pain in lower extremities, penis, scrotum, or face
Non-Hodgkin's lymphoma	Nodal swelling, night sweats, weight loss, persistent fevers, gastrointestinal bleeding, persistent perirectal pain, jaundice or light-colored stools Confusion, lethargy, memory loss, hemiparesis, aphasia, seizures, headaches, cranial nerve palsies
Progressive multifocal leukoencephalopathy	Changes in speech and/or gait, limb weakness, altered mental status, hemiparesis, personality changes, seizures, visual changes, cranial nerve palsies, dysphagia
HIV-associated dementia	Impaired concentration, depressed mood, paranoia, other psychotic features, spasticity, motor weakness, memory loss, global cognitive dysfunction, agitation, ataxia, parkinsonism
Wasting syndrome	Fatigue, fever, nausea and vomiting, abdominal pain, pain or discomfort while eating, diarrhea

Candidiasis of the bronchi, trachea, lungs, or esophagus is an AIDS-defining criterion (see Table 35-1).

Mucosal candidiasis is often the first clinical sign of CD4 T lymphocyte impairment. Vaginal candidiasis is the most common initial clinical manifestation of HIV infection in women. Diagnosis is made by inspection, culture, and endoscopy if appropriate. The diagnosis is confirmed by positive results in cultures of the lesions.

Candidiasis may be treated with antifungals, including clotrimazole (Femcare) or nystatin (Mycostatin) and ketoconazole (Nizoral). Fluconazole (Diflucan) and amphotericin B (Fungizone) are used for recurrences of candidiasis or severe cases (Kirton, 2003; Murphy and Flaherty, 2003).

Cryptococcosis

Infection with *Cryptococcus neoformans* occurs when the organism is inhaled. This fungus is present in soil, fruit, fruit juices, and pigeon droppings. The primary site of infection is the central nervous system, but spores enter through the pulmonary system. Cryptococcosis is the most prevalent life-threatening fungal infection seen in people with HIV infection.

The diagnosis is made by detection of cryptococcal capsular antigens in the cerebrospinal fluid or positive findings on India ink stain or blood culture, computed tomography (CT), or magnetic resonance imaging (MRI) (DeLorenzo and Ingram, 2001; Kirton, 2003).

Treatment is with fluconazole (Diflucan) or intravenous amphotericin B (Fungizone). Lifelong suppressive treatment is also necessary unless immune reconstitution occurs when the patient receives highly active antiretroviral therapy (HAART).

Pneumocystis Carinii Pneumonia

Pneumocystis carinii is a fungus that invades the epithelium of the lung. *P. carinii* pneumonia has been the most frequent AIDS-defining diagnosis in the United States (DeLorenzo and Ingram, 2001). A disease with airborne transmission, it is usually confined to the pulmonary system but can involve the skin, meninges, eye, lymph nodes, heart, spleen, and liver.

Diagnosis is based on chest radiograph, analysis of specimens obtained through sputum induction or bronchoscopy, gallium scan, measurement of lactate dehydrogenase levels and arterial blood gas concentrations, and/or pulmonary function tests (Kirton, 2003).

Trimethoprim-sulfamethoxazole (TMP-SMZ or Bactrim) is the recommended treatment and prophylactic agent. Adverse reactions to medication can occur, and there are guidelines to indicate when to lower the dosage, discontinue therapy, or use alternative medications such as Dapsone, pyrimethamine (Daraprim), leucovorin (Wellcovorin), aerosolized pentamidine (Nebupent), or atovaquone (Mepron) (CDC, 2002).

Cryptosporidiosis

Cryptosporidium, an enteric protozoon, can cause debilitating diarrhea and weight loss in patients with advanced HIV disease. Cryptosporidia have been found in the small intestines, stomach, esophagus, rectum, appendix, bladder, pancreas, and lungs (DeLorenzo and Ingram, 2001). The modes of transmission of cryptosporidiosis include direct contact with infected adults, diaper-aged children, and infected animals; drinking of or contact with contaminated water; and consumption of contaminated foods (CDC, 2002). Diagnosis is by stool testing for ova and parasites (Kirton, 2003).

Most patients experience symptom improvement or remission with HAART. Rifabutin (Mycobutin) or clarithromycin (Biaxin), when taken for *M. avium-intracellulare complex* prophylaxis, can protect against cryptosporidiosis. Spiramycin and paromomycin (Humatin) have been used against this parasite to decrease diarrhea (Kirton, 2003).

Cytomegalovirus Infection

Cytomegalovirus (CMV) is a double-stranded DNA herpesvirus that is found in semen, cervical secretions, saliva, urine, blood, and organs (Kirton, 2003). Modes of transmission include perinatal transmission, sexual contact, blood exchange, and transplantation of infected organs or tissues. The prevalence of CMV is higher among homosexual men with HIV infection than among any other HIV patients (DeLorenzo and Ingram, 2001). CMV infection can result in several clinical illnesses in patients with HIV infection, including pneumonia, esophagitis, colitis, encephalitis, chorioretinitis, polyradiculopathy, adrenalitis, and hepatitis (Health Resources Service Administration [HRSA], 2003). CMV infection causes retinitis in 80% to 85% of AIDS patients and gastrointestinal disease in 12% of 15% of AIDS patients (Anderson, 2001).

Ganciclovir (Cytovene), foscarnet (Foscavir), or cidofovir (Vistide) can be used for treatment or long-term suppression. For retinitis, intraocular devices can be inserted surgically to slowly release small amounts of ganciclovir directly into the vitreous (Murphy and Flaherty, 2003). Lifelong suppressive therapy may be warranted.

Toxoplasmosis

Toxoplasma gondii is a protozoon that infects the central nervous system of immunodeficient patients. It is carried by mammals as oocysts, tachyzoites, or bradyzoites in the gastrointestinal system and eliminated in fecal matter (HRSA, 2003). Contact with cat feces, in particular, can result in infection. The organism can also be transmitted by ingestion of undercooked or raw meat. The most common sites for the organisms to be found in meat are the brain, heart, and striated muscle (Kirton, 2003). Toxoplasmosis usually develops when patients have a CD4 cell count of fewer than 100 cells/mm^3. Perinatal transmission of toxoplasmosis has been reported (DeLorenzo and Ingram, 2001).

Toxoplasmosis is definitively diagnosed by examination of a brain biopsy specimen. More commonly, however, a *Toxoplasma* serum antibody test, MRI scan, or CT scan is used to guide treatment. The therapy of choice is some combination of clindamycin (Cleocin), Dapsone, azithromycin (Zithromax), atovaquone (Mepron), clarithromycin (Biaxin), and folic acid for treatment and prophylaxis. *Toxoplasma*-seropositive patients with a CD4 cell count of fewer than 100 cells/mm^3 should receive prophylaxis using the preventive regimen for *P. carinii* pneumonia. Seronegative individuals should be monitored for antibodies to *Toxoplasma*. Prophylaxis can be discontinued if the patient has responded to

HAART and the CD4 count has been above 200 cells/mm^3 for at least 3 months. It should be reintroduced if the CD4 count drops below 200 cells/mm^3 (CDC, 2002).

Herpes Simplex (Genital Herpes)

Herpes simplex virus (HSV) is a member of the herpesvirus group. There are two types of HSV: HSV-1, which is acquired via infected droplets in childhood, and HSV-2, which can be acquired by sexual activity. Transmission is from person to person when lesions that are shedding contact mucosal surfaces or breaks in the skin (Kirton, 2003). Virions then travel from the site of inoculation to corresponding nerve root ganglia where the infection is permanently established (Kirton, 2003). Most often, infection is accompanied by a vesicular eruption of the oral or perioral area, vulva, mucous membranes, perianal skin, and occasionally inguinal or buttock areas (HRSA, 2003). Blisters rupture, ulcerate, and generally crust over and heal in 7 to 14 days. They may be pruritic and painful. Reaction or recurrence may be triggered by a variety of stimuli (e.g., stress, trauma, ultraviolet light) (Kirton, 2003). As immunosuppression progresses in patients with HIV infection, the lesions may recur more often and take longer to heal (HRSA, 2003). Definitive diagnosis is obtained by culturing HSV from the base of lesions. The presence of severe lesions or ulcers for longer than 4 weeks is an AIDS-defining illness.

Recurrent genital herpes can be suppressed by therapy with oral antiviral agents such as acyclovir (Zovirax), valacyclovir (Valtrex), and famciclovir (Famvir). If the use of antiherpes drugs results in the development of drug-resistant HSV strains, intravenous foscarnet (Foscavir) can be given.

Herpes Zoster (Shingles)

Human herpesvirus 3, or varicella-zoster virus (VZV), causes shingles. Shingles is a skin or mucosal infection that occurs along a dermatome. VZV infection results in two clinically distinct entities: primary infection or chickenpox and reactivation of latent infection or herpes zoster (shingles) (Kirton, 2003). The infection may be particularly painful, necrotic, and hemorrhagic in patients with HIV disease (HRSA, 2003). Disseminated infection usually involves the skin and the visceral organs. Outbreaks involving more than two dermatomes are considered disseminated. Diagnosis is by culture of samples from freshly opened vesicles or examination of biopsy specimens from the border of a lesion. Acyclovir (Zovirax), foscarnet (Foscavir), varicella-zoster immune globulin (VZIG), or ganciclovir (Cytovene) is used to treat VZV infection (Kirton, 2003; Bartlett and Gallant, 2001).

AIDS-Related Malignancies and Conditions

Other conditions may occur in HIV disease that produce a variety of symptoms, including dermatologic, neurologic, gastrointestinal, oral, psychiatric, and sleep-related symptoms, and that may or may not be associated with an opportunistic infection. These conditions add to the complexity of the clinical manifestations and treatment for HIV infection.

HIV-Associated Dementia

HIV-associated dementia (HAD) or AIDS dementia complex is the most frequent single neurologic complication of AIDS, affecting 40% to 60% of all AIDS patients. Most patients with AIDS experience some degree of HAD. HAD often occurs in patients who have had an opportunistic infection or malignant tumor. HAD primarily involves damage to the white matter of the brain, spinal cord, and/or subcortical gray matter. It is characterized by cognitive, motor, and behavioral disturbances (DeLorenzo and Ingram, 2001).

Diagnosis is based on a thorough history taking; CT and MRI scans, which show cerebral atrophy; or analysis of spinal fluid.

If a patient is on a HAART regimen, improvements in cognitive and motor functions should be noted. There is no other identified treatment for these neurologic complications.

Kaposi's Sarcoma

Kaposi's sarcoma (KS) is an endothelial neoplasm of the skin, mucosal surfaces, and/or internal organs. It is the most common tumor seen in HIV infection (HRSA, 2003). It primarily affects gay and bisexual men and is fairly uncommon in women and injection drug users. Researchers believe it is caused by human herpesvirus 8 (HRSA, 2003; Kirton, 2003).

Mucocutaneous KS can usually be diagnosed by inspection, but a biopsy specimen showing typical spindle-shaped cells provides the definitive diagnosis of KS. Mucocutaneous KS may be treated using several modalities, including intralesional administration of vincristine (Oncovin) or vinblastine (Velban), radiation therapy, and topical application of retinoids. Gastrointestinal lesions can be cauterized endoscopically. Visceral disease requires systemic chemotherapy (Kirton, 2003).

Non-Hodgkin's Lymphoma

Non-Hodgkin's lymphomas (NHLs) are a heterogeneous group of malignant neoplasms (HRSA, 2003). (See Chapter 11 for a detailed discussion of lymphomas.) If a person is diagnosed with primary lymphoma of the brain, it is an AIDS indicator. NHL is more likely to occur in persons with immunosuppression (CD4 count of fewer than 200 cells/mm^3) and a history of an AIDS-defining illness. Epstein-Barr virus infection has been implicated in the pathogenesis (Kirton, 2003). HAART has helped produce a decline in the incidence of lymphoma but not as significant as that seen for opportunistic infections in general. The incidence of bone marrow, gastrointestinal, and liver involvement is high. NHL is diagnosed by analysis of biopsy specimens, bone marrow, and aspirates obtained by lumbar puncture, which look for disseminated disease. Diagnosis of central nervous system (CNS) lymphoma is by examination of brain biopsy specimens, CT, or MRI. For CNS lymphoma, it is important to rule out toxoplasmosis, cryptococcosis, and mycobacterial, other bacterial, or fungal disease. No standard effective cytotoxic chemotherapy exists for this disease, and radiation therapy is considered palliative. The signs and symptoms will depend on the location of the disease. Survival after diagnosis of CNS lymphoma is usually limited. Treatment options for other NHLs include chemotherapy, radiation therapy, and immunotherapy (interferon) (Kirton, 2003).

Progressive Multifocal Leukoencephalopathy

Progressive multifocal leukoencephalopathy (PML) is an end-stage complication of HIV disease. It usually manifests as a focal neurologic deficit. PML is caused by JC virus, a human papillomavirus, which can be detected by polymerase chain reaction testing of cerebrospinal fluid. PML is rare and occurs most frequently in people whose immunity is compromised by HIV infection and whose CD4 cell count is below 100/mm^3. It is rapidly progressive. Definitive diagnosis can be made by examination of a brain biopsy specimen or positive results on polymerase chain reaction testing (Anderson, 2001). There is no specific proven therapy for this condition (Anderson, 2001; HRSA, 2003). However, clinical remission has occurred for patients started on potent combination antiretroviral therapy. Prognosis was very poor before the availability of antiretroviral therapy, but now some patients have lived more than a year after diagnosis (Anderson, 2001).

Wasting Syndrome

HIV wasting syndrome is defined as a weight loss of more than 10% of the baseline body weight (Figure 35-1) accompanied by low-grade fever (maximum of 100.6° F) on most days

for 1 month or longer and/or diarrhea with two or more loose stools per day in the absence of concurrent illness (HRSA, 2003). Medications should be administered to treat nausea, vomiting, and diarrhea. Anorexia may be managed with the use of appetite stimulants such as megestrol (Megace) and dronabinol (Marinol). Anabolic agents such as nandrolone (Androlone-D), oxandrolone, and oxymetholone (Anadrol) as well as growth hormone and testosterone have the potential to improve muscle mass and strength (DeLorenzo and Ingram, 2001). Supplements such as Sustacal, Boost, or milkshakes are also used. Total parental nutrition is a last choice.

DIAGNOSIS

In many chronic diseases, diagnosis is prompted by the patient's symptoms. With HIV infection, this is not always the case. Ideally, individuals will become aware of their HIV infection before symptoms develop. To accomplish this goal, health care providers must assess their patients for risk behaviors that can result in HIV infection. Taking a thorough history that includes specific yet nonjudgmental questions about sexual behaviors and drug use is vital to identify individuals who could benefit from HIV testing. In addition, testing should be encouraged for individuals who are pregnant or have been diagnosed with sexually transmitted diseases or TB.

In many individuals, the initial clinical manifestations of HIV disease serve as the impetus for testing. HIV infection should be considered in the differential diagnosis of young adults with shingles, women with refractory or recurrent vaginal candidiasis, and individuals with opportunistic conditions suggestive of defective cell-mediated immunity.

HIV antibody testing is the primary means of diagnosing HIV infection and can be performed on blood, oral mucosal transudate, or urine. A positive or reactive test result consists of a repeatedly reactive finding on enzyme immunoassay (EIA) confirmed by a Western blot (WB) test result showing the presence of antibodies to gp120/160 and either gp41 or p24, or a reactive result on immunofluorescent assay. Used in combination, these standard serologic tests are highly accurate.

Tests giving rapid results such as the Single Use Diagnostic System for HIV-1 manufactured by Abbott-Murex Diagnostics and the OraQuick Rapid HIV-1 Antibody Test manufactured by OraSure Technologies provide preliminary results in 20 to 107 minutes. These tests are based on EIA methodology. Because of the high sensitivity of these tests, negative results may be reported as definitive; however positive results must be confirmed with standard serologic testing.

Most individuals develop antibodies to HIV within 3 to 4 weeks after infection; the range is 2 weeks to 6 months. The time lag between HIV infection and the development of detectable levels of antibodies (known as "seroconversion") is commonly called the "window period." Thus, to rule out

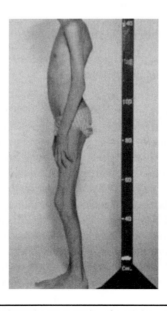

Figure 35-1 Clinical appearance of patient with wasting syndrome. (From Taylor PK: *Diagnostic picture tests in sexually transmitted disease,* London, 1994, Mosby-Wolfe.)

HIV infection, a test result must be negative 6 months after the individual's last possible exposure to the virus.

Indeterminate test findings consisting of a reactive EIA result and an indeterminate WB result (showing any band pattern other than gp120/160 and either gp41 or p24) occur infrequently. Common causes of indeterminate results include recent HIV infection with seroconversion in progress; the presence of cross-reacting nonspecific antibodies, such as are seen in collagen vascular or autoimmune diseases; and technical or clerical error. If the indeterminate test result is due to incomplete seroconversion, the WB test result will usually become reactive within 1 month. A variety of antigen-based tests directly detect HIV or components of the virus. These methods include polymerase chain reaction and branched DNA tests, p24 antigen assays, and viral culture. These testing methods may be used to clarify an indeterminate antibody test result or to detect HIV infection before antibodies have developed, such as when primary infection is suspected.

HIV testing has many implications for the person at risk for infection. HIV prevention counseling is a critical element in helping the individual to take the next step to address risk and obtain needed services. Although this type of counseling may include information about HIV transmission and testing, its focus is on risk reduction. A patient-centered counseling approach is useful for improving the individual's self-perception of risk and identifying realistic incremental behavioral changes to reduce that risk. This approach is appropriate whether or not an individual decides to take an HIV test and applies regardless of HIV status. Key elements of patient-centered HIV infection prevention counseling are listed in Box 35-3.

When an individual tests positive for HIV infection, counseling and support are crucial to ensure integration of the information and movement toward addressing health needs. Clear, simple language is most useful in helping the individual to understand the test results. The individual's emotional response must be attended to before other issues are considered. Assessing the individual's coping strategies enhances safety and provides a springboard for making referrals that can support coping. The psychosocial needs of the newly diagnosed individual vary greatly from person to person and may include mental health counseling, crisis intervention, substance abuse treatment, pastoral counseling, and participation in support groups. In addition, the individual needs referrals for medical evaluation and may require assistance in talking to sexual and/or needle-sharing partners about the diagnosis. Local health departments can provide partner counseling and referral services that maintain confidentiality while ensuring access to HIV testing and counseling for exposed partners.

Reporting of HIV infection is required in 46 states, the District of Columbia, and the territories of Puerto Rico, Guam, and the U.S. Virgin Islands. Although the majority of states and territories use a traditional name-based reporting

---

> ### Box 35-3 Elements of HIV Prevention Counseling
>
> ■ Keep the session focused on HIV risk reduction. Each counseling session should be tailored to address the personal HIV risk of the patient rather than provide a predetermined body of information.
>
> ■ Include an in-depth, personalized risk assessment.
>
> ■ Acknowledge and support positive steps already made. This approach increases the patient's belief that he or she can successfully take further HIV risk reduction steps. For some patients, simply agreeing to take an HIV test is an important step in reducing risk.
>
> ■ Clarify critical rather than general misconceptions. Tailor the information provided to the individual's risk reduction needs.
>
> ■ Negotiate a concrete, achievable behavior change that will reduce HIV risk.
>
> ■ Seek flexibility in the prevention approach and counseling process. Avoid a one-size-fits-all prevention message (e.g., "Always use condoms").
>
> ■ Provide skill-building opportunities. Depending on patient needs, the counselor can demonstrate or ask the patient to demonstrate problem-solving strategies such as the following:
>
>   Communicating safer sex commitments to new or continuing sex partners
>
>   Using male latex condoms properly
>
>   Trying alternative preventive methods (e.g., female condoms)
>
>   Cleaning drug-injection equipment if clean syringes are unavailable
>
>   Communicating safer drug-injection commitments to persons with whom the patient shares drug paraphernalia

Adapted from Centers for Disease Control and Prevention, Revised guidelines for HIV counseling, testing, and referral and revised recommendations for HIV screening of pregnant women, *MMWR Morb Mortal Wkly Rep* 50(RR-19), 2001, retrieved from *http://www.cdc.gov/mmwr/preview/mmwrhtml/rr5019al.htm* on Feb 29, 2004.

---

system, some have opted for code-based or name-to-code–based systems in which coded identifiers are substituted for names at some point in the process. California, Georgia, New Hampshire, and Pennsylvania do not have HIV reporting requirements. State and local health departments can provide specific reporting requirements for their areas.

INTERDISCIPLINARY CARE
Primary Provider (Physician/Nurse Practitioner)

The primary care provider plays a key role in optimizing the health of the HIV-infected person. In many care settings, nurse practitioners and physician assistants as well as physicians fill this role. As the medical management of HIV disease has become increasingly complex, the primary care provider has been required to master a broader range of knowledge. Studies have shown that patients cared for by providers who are experienced in the treatment of HIV infection (those who see more than 50 HIV-infected patients per year) have better clinical outcomes.

The HIV-infected person whose primary care provider treats a lower number of HIV-infected patients can benefit from consultation with a more experienced provider, usually an infectious disease specialist. An infectious disease physician often guides the strategic use of combination antiretroviral therapy to optimize viral suppression and minimize resistance.

Specialists

Other specialty care may be needed depending on the different clinical manifestations present. Treatment of most opportunistic infections and some coinfections requires the expertise of an infectious disease physician. Treatment of malignancies such as lymphoma or Kaposi's sarcoma requires an oncologist's care. As people live longer with HIV infection because of the effectiveness of combination antiretroviral therapy, other health problems may become more pressing. Hyperglycemia and dyslipidemia, which can be caused by protease inhibitors, may require consultation with an endocrinologist or cardiologist, respectively. Maintaining optimal viral suppression while minimizing adverse effects of treatment requires close collaboration between the primary care provider and all specialty providers.

Nursing

Nursing care has a major impact on the quality of life of the person living with HIV infection. In many care settings, the nurse serves as the case manager ensuring continuity of care. This has become increasingly important because HIV-infected individuals are living longer and must learn to cope with HIV as a chronic illness. Patient teaching is a critical nursing responsibility that helps the individual and family understand the disease and implement wellness strategies, which may include consumption of a healthy diet, exercise, sexual risk reduction, harm reduction for addiction, stress management, and steps to safeguard the immune system (Box 35-4).

Educating the patient about medications, adverse reactions, and management of potential side effects is an essential part of nursing management for all individuals and is especially important for the individual with HIV/AIDS. Maximizing adherence to the treatment regimen is critical to achieving viral suppression through antiretroviral therapy. Although supporting adherence is the responsibility of the entire multidisciplinary team, the nurse plays a central role in helping the individual develop strategies to ensure that antiretroviral medications are taken consistently and correctly. The nurse's role in the adherence support process can be described by the acronym ADHERE (Jordan and Mealy, 2000):

Box 35-4 Patient Strategies for Preventing Infection

- Avoid crowds.
- Do not share personal grooming articles.
- Bathe or shower daily with an antibacterial soap.
- Clean toothbrush daily by rinsing it in laundry bleach.
- Avoid raw fruits and vegetables and undercooked meat.
- Wash hands before and after eating.
- Do not drink water that has been standing longer than 15 minutes.
- Do not share drinking or eating utensils.
- Wash dishes and glasses in hot soapy water.
- Do not change pet litter boxes or scoop pet waste material.
- Do not care for indoor or garden plants.
- Take all medications.
- Get all recommended immunizations.

- **A**ssess the individual's readiness for HAART.
- **D**etermine the individual's health priorities and goals.
- **H**elp the individual to implement strategies to enhance adherence.
- **E**licit feedback from the individual and the multidisciplinary team.
- **R**eview adherence measures.
- **E**valuate the adherence plan and adjust strategies as needed.

For the individual receiving HAART, supporting adherence to treatment becomes central to the plan of care and therefore should be included at each visit.

The nurse also works with the individual and family to promote comfort and adequate rest and nutrition. Most people with HIV infection experience some level of fatigue. The nurse helps the individual group activities and conserve energy. Periods of activity should be alternated with rest periods and scheduled to avoid fatigue at mealtime. Every effort should be made to maintain adequate nutrition because this will help to improve immune system function.

Should the patient develop an opportunistic infection, the nurse assists the individual and family in managing the associated symptoms (Table 35-3). The nurse also helps the individual and family to manage the symptoms related to malignancies and other conditions the individual is likely to experience (Table 35-4).

The individual with HIV/AIDS and his or her family also experience a variety of emotions, including fear, loneliness, anxiety, and guilt. The nurse works with family members as they explore and express these feelings. Referral to a psychologist or counselor may be warranted. Strategies to help families cope include empowering the patient and family to make decisions and participate in care; incorporating spirituality and cultural values, beliefs, and norms into care; providing individual and/or family counseling and education; and referring the patient and family to support groups.

Table 35-3 **Nursing Interventions for Opportunistic Infections**

Opportunistic Infection	Intervention
Mycobacterium avium-intracellulare complex infection	Observe skin carefully to detect any changes. Monitor laboratory results for anorexia, neutropenia. Monitor nutrition and hydration.
Tuberculosis	Instruct patient to contact provider if a rash or itching occurs. Teach patient to avoid alcohol while taking medications. Ensure that all patients have an annual tuberculin skin test. Teach patient that topical creams help to control pruritus and pain and analgesics. Implement directly observed therapy if possible.
Candidiasis	Educate patient to maintain good oral hygiene. Instruct patient to rinse mouth of all food before using lozenges or suspensions. Teach women with vaginal candidiasis to avoid tight-fitting underwear and pantyhose, douching, and consumption of high-sugar foods. Encourage patient to eat yogurt to adjust intestinal flora. Provide nutritional assessment and intervention if needed.
Cryptococcosis	Provide hydration. Monitor blood urea nitrogen level, creatinine level, platelet count, liver function test results.
Pneumocystis carinii pneumonia	Monitor for side effects or adverse effects of medicines, such as rash or photosensitivity, peripheral neuropathy, liver function abnormalities, hepatotoxicity, nephrotoxicity. Evaluate all rashes. Advise patient not to consume dairy products for 2 hr before or 1 hr after taking a sulfa drug.
Cryptosporidiosis	Monitor for side effects or adverse effects of medicines, such as rash or photosensitivity, peripheral neuropathy, and liver function abnormalities. Monitor fluid and electrolyte levels and replace as needed. Medicate with antidiarrheals: diphenoxylate with atropine (Lomotil), loperamide (Imodium), antiemetics. Provide skin care, especially in perianal region. Provide nutritional support.
Cytomegalovirus infection	Routinely monitor for visual changes. Ensure that patient undergoes an ophthalmologic examination every 6 mo. Monitor for side effects or adverse effects of medicines. Educate patient about the need for suppressive therapy for life to prevent blindness. Address safety concerns related to possible limited vision. Monitor laboratory test results Teach intravenous line care if patient has an indwelling venous access line.
Toxoplasmosis	Teach memory reminder strategies. Instruct patient to eat only completely cooked or cured meats and to wash fruits and vegetables before eating. Advise patient to wash hands and kitchen surfaces thoroughly after handling raw meat. Teach patient pet safety and maintenance strategies (patient should not handle litter boxes, etc.).
Herpes simplex	Instruct patient to avoid sexual contact when genital lesions are visible. Teach patient that herpes simplex virus can be transmitted when no lesions are present. Teach patient that there is no cure; outbreaks may occur for the rest of patient's life. Teach patient the importance of stress management and adequate rest to decrease the possibility of recurrence due to low immunity.
Herpes zoster	Teach patient to use a separate cloth to clean affected areas to prevent autoinoculation and dissemination. Teach patient that topical creams and analgesics help to control pruritus and pain.

Table 35-4   Nursing Interventions for AIDS-Related Conditions

Condition/Syndrome	Intervention
HIV-associated dementia	Check gait by asking patient to walk rapidly. Complete dementia screening. Educate patient with gait changes or ataxia regarding safety. Enlist support of family and/or significant others.
Kaposi's sarcoma	Provide education about signs and symptoms of pulmonary or gastrointestinal involvement and treatment options. Educate patient regarding the importance of nutrition and rest when undergoing treatments. Discuss skin integrity and lesion care. Discuss social supports and impact on body image.
Non-Hodgkin's lymphoma	Identify support system or caregiver because prognosis for HIV-related non-Hodgkin's lymphoma is usually poor. Discuss terminal care with patient and/or caregiver. Provide safety. Discuss potential for cognitive deficits and lack of motor coordination. Manage pain. Provide and teach comfort measures.
Progressive multifocal leukoencephalopathy	Provide supportive care because prognosis is poor. Emphasize safety measures.
Wasting syndrome	Do a stool workup. Ensure adequate hydration. Educate patient regarding nutrition, exercise, and strength building. Instruct patient to report fever, chills, night sweats, cough, diarrhea, and other symptoms of infection.

Drug Therapy

Zidovudine (AZT), the first medication used to treat HIV infection, was approved in 1987. Since then, HIV treatment has evolved dramatically. With the advent of protease inhibitors in 1995, combination therapy became a successful treatment strategy that has resulted in decreased AIDS-related morbidity and mortality. Combinations of three or more antiretroviral medications (commonly called HAART for highly active antiretroviral therapy) have been shown to be effective in suppressing viral replication and thereby facilitating immune reconstitution.

Table 35-5 lists Food and Drug Administration–approved antiretroviral medications and gives the drug names (generic, trade, and abbreviation), drug classes, usual dosages, food restrictions, side effects, and other special considerations. Other medications used for the treatment of opportunistic infections and malignancies were discussed previously (see the section on clinical manifestations).

New medications to treat HIV infection are continually being developed. One aim of drug research has been to find new medications or new formulations of existing medications that can be administered once a day. The advantages of once-a-day dosing in terms of adherence to the drug regimen make this an attractive alternative for patients and providers. Development of new drugs or new formulations of existing medications to reduce pill burden, enhance bioavailability, and improve tolerance has been another goal of researchers.

Antiretroviral therapy is indicated for the treatment of chronic HIV infection in specific clinical circumstances. Because the optimal time to initiate therapy is not known, multiple factors including CD4 cell count, viral load (plasma HIV RNA level), and clinical presentation are assessed to determine whether treatment is indicated. Each factor, along with the individual's readiness to start and adhere to the treatment regimen, is considered in the decision. Table 35-6 summarizes the clinical features used to make treatment decisions.

Just as debate exists over the ideal time to start therapy, opinions vary as to the best initial regimen. Generally an initial HAART regimen includes a protease inhibitor or an NNRTI or abacavir, a nucleoside reverse transcriptase inhibitor (NRTI), plus two compatible NRTIs. Table 35-7 categorizes treatment regimen choices based on currently available data from clinical trials, expert opinion, information on toxicity, and other factors. In addition, the choice of specific agents must take into account the regimen's pill burden, dosing frequency, food requirements, convenience, toxicity, and drug interaction profile to ensure that the regimen is compatible with the individual's needs and preferences.

Because of its high rate of replication and propensity for mutations, HIV is able rapidly to develop resistance to antiretroviral medications. When a HAART regimen effectively reduces viral load below the level of detection, chances of the development of resistance are minimized. If little or no

Table 35-5 Antiretroviral Medication Chart

Drug Name	Usual Dose and Frequency*	No. Pills/Day	Special Considerations/Side Effects
Nucleoside Reverse Transcriptase Inhibitors Side effects of this class may include mitochondrial toxicity, lactic acidosis. Fat redistribution (lipodystrophy) may be associated with this class of medications.			
Abacavir (ABC; Ziagen)	1 × 300-mg tablet BID	2	Watch for hypersensitivity reaction. *Do not rechallenge.*
Didanosine (DDI; Videx)	2 × 100-mg tablets BID (preferred); or 2 × 200-mg tablets QD	2-4	Should be taken on empty stomach; delavirdine or indinavir should be taken at least 1 hr before; nelfinavir should be taken 1 hr after; tenofovir should be taken 2 hr before or 1 hr after. Side effects include peripheral neuropathy and pancreatitis.
Videx EC (unbuffered) formulation	1 × 400-mg capsule QD if body weight ≥60 kg 1 × 250-mg capsule QD if body weight <60 kg	1	Same as above. (Preferred dosing schedule is twice daily with Videx in liquid or tablet form.)
Lamivudine (3TC; Epivir)	1 × 150-mg tablet BID	2	Active against hepatitis B.
Stavudine (D4T; Zerit)	1 × 40-mg capsule BID	2	Should not be taken with zidovudine. Side effects include peripheral neuropathy.
Zalcitabine (DDC; Hivid)	1 × 0.375-0.75-mg tablet TID	3	Should not be taken with antacids.
Zidovudine (AZT; Retrovir)	1 × 300-mg tablet BID	2	Should not be taken with stavudine. Taking with food may minimize stomach discomfort. Side effects include nausea, headache, and rarely anemia.
Combination Nucleoside Reverse Transcriptase Inhibitors			
Lamivudine + zidovudine (Combivir)	1 co-formulated tablet BID	2	See information for individual drugs.
Lamivudine + zidovudine abacavir (Trizivir)	1 co-formulated tablet BID	2	Should not be taken if weight is <90 lb. See information for individual drugs.
Nucleotide Reverse Transcriptase Inhibitor			
Tenofovir (Viread)	1 × 300 mg tablet QD	1	Should be taken with a meal. Should be taken 2 hr before or 1 hr after didanosine. Shows in vitro activity against hepatitis B. Side effects include GI discomfort and flatulence.
Nonnucleoside Reverse Transcriptase Inhibitors			
Nevirapine (Viramune)	1 × 200-mg tablet BID	4	Lead-in dose 1 × 200 mg QD for 14 days. Side effects include rash, GI discomfort, increased LFT, and rarely hepatotoxicity.
Efavirenz (Sustiva)	1 × 600-mg capsule QD (at bedtime)	3	Should be taken on an empty stomach. Side effects include rash, increased LFT values, central nervous system effects including vivid dreams.
Delavirdine (Rescriptor)	2 × 200-mg tablets TID	6	Should be taken 1 hr before or after antacids or didanosine. Side effects include rash, increased LFT values.

Continued

Table 35-5 Antiretroviral Medication Chart—cont'd

Drug Name	Usual Dose and Frequency*	No. Pills/Day	Special Considerations/Side Effects
Protease Inhibitors			
Side effects of this class may include elevated blood glucose and fat levels, and fat redistribution (lipodystrophy).			
Amprenavir (Agenerase)	8 × 150-mg capsules BID	16	Should be taken 1 hr before or after antacids or didanosine. High-fat meal should be avoided with dose. Vitamin E supplements should be avoided. Side effects include rash, diarrhea, nausea, vomiting, and oral tingling or numbness.
Indinavir (Crixivan)	2 × 400-mg capsules every 8 hr	6	Should be taken on empty stomach or with low-fat snack. Patient should drink at least 1.5 L of fluid/day. Store in original container. Side effects include rash, diarrhea, nausea, vomiting, kidney stones.
Lopinavir + ritonavir (ABT-378r; Kaletra)	3 × co-formulated capsules BID	6	Should be taken with food. Refrigeration preferred; if not, keep at <77° F and use within 2 mo. Side effects include diarrhea, nausea, vomiting.
Nelfinavir (Viracept)	5 × 250-mg capsules BID	10	Should be taken with food. Side effects include diarrhea, nausea, increased LFT values.
Ritonavir (Norvir)	6 × 100-mg capsules BID	12	Used at lower doses as pharmacokinetic enhancer of other protease inhibitors. Refrigeration of capsules recommended. Side effects include increased LFTs, diarrhea, nausea, vomiting and oral tingling or numbness.
Entry Inhibitors			
Main identified side effect of this class is injection site reactions.			
Enfuvirtide (T-20; Fuzeon)	90 mg (1 ml) by SQ injection BID	SQ injection	Extensive patient education is needed to teach proper drug reconstitution and injection technique. Store at controlled room temperature (77° F); excursions permitted to 59-86° F. Reconstituted solution must be refrigerated and used within 24 hr.

NOTE: Indications, safety, and efficacy may vary.
BID, Twice a day; *GI,* gastrointestinal; *LFTs,* liver function tests; *QD,* once a day; *SQ,* subcutaneously; *TID,* 3 times a day.
*Alternative dose and frequency schedules are available for many of these medications. Please refer to the complete prescribing information for each medication for details.

viral suppression is achieved, the presence of the partially effective medication exerts selective pressure for the development of resistant strains of virus. Factors that contribute to the development of resistance include reduced potency of a regimen, reduced drug delivery due to poor absorption or drug interactions, and decreased adherence with the treatment regimen. A very high level of adherence (around 95%) is necessary to provide the best opportunity for a regimen to fully suppress HIV replication and achieve an undetectable viral load. For the typical regimen, this means missing less than one dose per week. In the treatment of chronic HIV infection, antiretroviral therapy is considered lifelong.

Clearly a strong commitment is necessary for an individual to receive maximal benefit from HAART.

Response to antiretroviral therapy is monitored by assessing viral load, CD4 cell count, and clinical response. Viral load testing provides the quickest feedback on response to HAART. A rapid and significant decline in viral load (of 50% or 0.3 log unit or more) is expected after the initiation of an effective regimen. After a new regimen is begun, viral load should be checked at 2 to 4 weeks, 12 to 16 weeks, and again at 16 to 24 weeks, at which time maximum antiviral effect is expected. CD4 cell count is generally monitored every 3 to 6 months. If viral suppression is

Table 35-6   Indications for the Initiation of Antiretroviral Therapy in the Patient with Chronic HIV-1 Infection

Clinical Category	CD4 Cell Count	Plasma HIV RNA	Recommendation
Symptomatic (AIDS, severe symptoms)	Any value	Any value	Treat
Asymptomatic, AIDS	CD4 cell count <200/mm³	Any value	Treat
Asymptomatic	CD4 cell count >200/mm³ but <350/mm³	Any value	Treatment should generally be offered, although controversy exists.
Asymptomatic	CD4 cell count >350/mm³	>55,000 (by bDNA or RT-PCR testing)	Some experts would recommend initiating therapy because the 3-yr risk of developing AIDS among untreated patients is >30%; some would defer therapy and monitor the CD4 cell count and level of plasma HIV RNA more frequently.
Asymptomatic	CD4 cell count >350/mm³	<55,000 (by bDNA or RT-PCR testing)	Many experts would defer therapy and observe because the 3-yr risk of developing AIDS among untreated patients is <15%.

Adapted from the Panel on Clinical Practices for Treatment of HIV Infection, Department of Health and Human Services: Guidelines for the use of anti-retroviral agents in HIV-1–infected adults and adolescents, Nov 10, 2003, retrieved from *http://www.aidsinfo.nih.gov/guidelines/adult/AA_111003.html* on Feb 23, 2004
bDNA, Branched DNA, *RT-PCR,* reverse transcriptase polymerase chain reaction.

achieved, CD4 count can increase significantly. In addition to viral load and CD4 cell count, complete blood counts and chemistry panels are routinely ordered to assist in detection of medication toxicities.

Antiretroviral therapy may have to be changed if medication toxicities occur or if a therapeutic effect is lacking, which is most often evidenced by suboptimal viral suppression. In cases in which viral suppression is suboptimal, resistance testing is a powerful tool that can guide the choice of medications to use in the next regimen.

Two forms of resistance testing are available: genotypic testing and phenotypic testing. Genotypic testing reports specific viral mutations that may correlate with resistance. Its advantages are that it is simpler to perform, less expensive, and quicker than phenotypic testing. Its disadvantages are the degree of expertise needed to interpret the results correctly and the indirect nature of this measure of susceptibility. Phenotypic testing measures susceptibility directly in a method analogous to that used in traditional antimicrobial sensitivity tests. Unfortunately, phenotypic testing is more expensive and results take longer to obtain. Both types of test should be performed in the presence of the antiretroviral agents in question before therapy is changed or discontinued. A viral load of at least 500 to 1000 copies/ml is required to perform the tests.

For individuals with extensive HIV treatment histories, multidrug resistance becomes a serious problem. One approach to this problem is called multidrug rescue or salvage therapy (also known as mega-HAART). In this approach, the patient is usually treated with six or more antiretroviral medications, some of which the individual may have been given before. Because an individual is unlikely to be infected with a virus strain resistant to all drugs, and because resistant virus tends to replicate less efficiently than wild-type virus, some success has been reported with this therapy. Unfortunately the cost, toxicity, side effects, and drug interactions make this type of therapy difficult for individuals to tolerate. Preventing drug resistance through strategic treatment planning and provision of support in adherence to the treatment regimen is preferred to the rigors of salvage therapy.

Chemoprophylaxis, the administration of medications in advance to prevent opportunistic infections, has become an effective tool against these infections. In the second decade of the HIV/AIDS epidemic, it has become evident that antiretroviral therapy is also a useful treatment to decrease the replication of the virus and restore immune function. Since the development of HAART, chemoprophylaxis for opportunistic infections no longer need be lifelong because, as the immune system is restored, opportunistic infections become less prevalent and remain so until the function of the immune system begins to decrease once more.

In 1999, many experts suggested that it may be safe to stop primary or secondary prophylaxis for some opportunistic infections if HAART has led to an increase in CD4 T-lymphocyte counts above specified threshold levels. However, no data are available to indicate when to restart prophylaxis for opportunistic infections when the CD4 cell

Table 35-7 Antiretroviral Regimens Recommended for Treatment of HIV-1 Infection in Antiretroviral Naïve Patients

Regimens	No. of Pills Per Day
NNRTI-Based Regimens	
Preferred	
Efavirenz + lamivudine + (zidovudine or tenofovir DF or stavudine*)—except for pregnant women or women with pregnancy potential†	**3-5**
Efavirenz + emtricitabine + (zidovudine or tenofovir DF or stavudine*)—except for pregnant women or women with pregnancy potential†	3-4
Alternative	
Efavirenz + (lamivudine or emtricitabine) + didanosine—except for pregnant women or women with pregnancy potential†	3
Nevirapine + (lamivudine or emtricitabine) + (zidovudine or stavudine* or didanosine)	4-5
PI-Based Regimens	
Preferred	
Lopinavir/ritonavir (coformulated as Kaletra) + lamivudine + (zidovudine or stavudine*)	**8-10**
Alternative	
Amprenavir + ritonavir‡ + (lamivudine or **emtricitabine**) + (zidovudine or stavudine*)	12-14
Atazanavir + (lamivudine or emtricitabine) + (zidovudine or stavudine*)	4-5
Indinavir + (lamivudine or emtricitabine) + (zidovudine or stavudine*)	8-10
Indinavir + ritonavir‡ + (lamivudine or **emtricitabine**) + (zidovudine or stavudine*)	8-11
Lopinavir/ritonavir (coformulated as Kaletra) + emitricitabine + (zidovudine or stavudine*)	8-9
Nelfinavir§ + (lamivudine or **emtricitabine**) + (zidovudine or stavudine*)	6-14
Saquinavir (soft or hard gel capsule)/ritonavir‡ + (lamivudine or **emtricitabine**) + (zidovudine or stavudine*)	14-16
Triple NRTI Regimen (only when an NNRTI- or a PI-based regimen cannot or should not be used as first-line therapy)	
Only as Alternative to NNRTI- or PI-Based Regimen	
Abacavir + lamivudine + zidovudine (or stavudine*)	2-6

From the Panel on Clinical Practices for Treatment of HIV Infection, Department of Health and Human Services: Guidelines for the use of antiretroviral agents in HIV-1–infected adults and adolescents, Nov 10, 2003, retrieved from *http://www.aidsinfo.nih.gov/guidelines/adult/AA_111003.html* on Feb 23, 2004.

This table is a guide to treatment regimens for patients who have no previous experience with HIV therapy. Regimens should be individualized based on the advantages and disadvantages of each combination, such as pill burden, dosing frequency, toxicities, and drug-drug interactions, and patient variables, such as pregnancy, comorbid conditions, and level of plasma HIV RNA. Preferred regimens are in bold type; regimens are designated as preferred for use in treatment of naïve patients when clinical trial data suggest optimal and durable efficacy with acceptable tolerability and ease of use. Alternative regimens are those for which clinical trial data show efficacy but that are considered alternative due to disadvantages compared with the preferred agent in terms of antiviral activity, demonstrated durable effect, tolerability, or ease of use. In some cases, based on individual patient characteristics, a regimen listed as alternative in the table may actually be the preferred regimen for a selected patient. Clinicians initiating antiretroviral regimens in the HIV-1–infected pregnant patient should refer to *Recommendations for Use of Antiretroviral Drugs in Pregnant HIV-1–Infected Women for Maternal Health and Interventions to Reduce Perinatal HIV-1 Transmission in the United States* at *http://aidsinfo.nih.gov/guidelines.*

NRTI, Nucleoside reverse transcriptase inhibitor; *NNRTI,* nonnucleoside reverse transcriptase inhibitor; *PI,* protease inhibitor.

*Higher incidence of lipoatrophy, hyperlipidemia, and mitochondrial toxicities reported with stavudine than with other NRTIs.

†"Women with pregnancy potential" implies women who want to conceive or those who are not using effective contraception.

‡Low-dose (100 to 400 mg) ritonavir.

§Nelfinavir available in 250 mg or 625 mg tablets.

count again decreases to levels at which the patient is likely to be at risk for such infections. Nevertheless, it is clear that HAART has slowed the number of deaths associated with AIDS-defined illnesses and opportunistic infections, and it has greatly affected the management of HIV infection.

Nutritional Therapy

HIV infection presents many nutritional challenges. Nutrition therapy in HIV disease includes early assessment and treatment of nutrient deficiencies, maintenance and restoration of lean body mass, and support for activities of daily living and quality of life. Thorough and ongoing nutritional assessment is key to timely intervention. Factors to be considered in a nutritional evaluation are included in Box 35-5.

Consistent evaluation of anthropometric measures such as height, weight, and waist circumference as well as body composition measures such as bioelectrical impedance values is useful in detecting early changes associated with wasting and lipodystrophy. As noted earlier, wasting is the loss of lean body mass resulting in an involuntary decrease

Box 35-5   Elements of Nutritional Evaluation

- Diet history: includes 24-hour recall of intake, eating frequency, food diaries, enteral or parenteral intake, supplement intake, food behaviors
- Physical examination: includes anthropometric measurements, other body composition measures, fat deposition patterns, and clinical signs of nutrient deficiency or toxicity
- Laboratory tests: include albumin, prealbumin, triglycerides, cholesterol, high-density lipoprotein, low-density lipoprotein, and glucose levels; transferrin level and total iron-binding capacity; measurement of hydration indicators; liver function tests; pancreatic function tests; measurement of anemia indicators; HIV viral load; CD4 cell count; nutrient levels
- Medical profile: includes history and current presence of infection, neoplasm, or wasting; additional disease diagnoses; medications or other therapies used; and substance abuse
- Assessment of psychosocial and economic factors: includes cultural background, language and literacy levels, caregiver support, family and friend dynamics that support or interfere with maintenance of nutritional status, and access to medical care, food, and other resources

Adapted from American Dietetic Association and Dieticians of Canada: Nutrition intervention needed in care of persons with HIV infection—position of the American Dietetic Association and Dieticians of Canada, *J Am Diet Assoc* 100:78, 708-17, 2000.

in weight of more than 10% of the baseline value. This problem becomes increasingly common in advanced HIV disease and is associated with decreased survival. Current treatment strategies include enteral feedings; administration of appetite stimulants, anabolic steroids, or testosterone; resistance exercise; cytokine suppression; and growth hormone therapy.

Lipodystrophy is characterized by changes in the distribution of body fat, which generally include central obesity and peripheral fat wasting. The incidence of this problem has increased since the advent of protease inhibitor therapy. Some experts believe that mitochondrial toxicity associated with the use of NRTIs may contribute to the problem. Optimum management of lipodystrophy is unclear. Therapy change to an NNRTI-based regimen has been tried with mixed results.

Many treatment modalities have been used to treat wasting with varying levels of success. Cosmetic surgery has been performed to replace buccal fat pads and mitigate the very apparent symptom of facial wasting.

Several other side effects of antiretroviral treatment require nutritional intervention. Elevated blood lipid levels may occur with lipodystrophy or independently of it in association with protease inhibitor therapy. Fasting serum triglyceride levels and cholesterol levels should be monitored regularly when the

individual is receiving protease inhibitor therapy, especially when other cardiovascular risk factors are present. Although a low-fat diet and lipid-lowering drugs may be used, response to these interventions varies. Care must be exercised in the selection of lipid-lowering medications to avoid interactions with some antiretrovirals, because statins share the cytochrome P-450 metabolic pathway with many protease inhibitors and NNRTIs. Some individuals respond to discontinuation of protease inhibitor therapy, but this decision requires a careful risk-benefit analysis. Hyperglycemia, including new-onset diabetes mellitus or exacerbation of existing diabetes, has been associated with protease inhibitor therapy. Treatment of this condition includes use of a diabetic diet and medical management. Some individuals experience a normalization of glucose level when protease inhibitors are discontinued; however, data on reversibility are limited. For both hyperglycemia and hyperlipidemia, switching to a HAART regimen without protease inhibitors, when feasible, is an option to consider. Diarrhea is a common side effect of many antiretroviral medications, especially protease inhibitors. Dietary management includes changing to a bland, low-residue diet and consuming small, frequent meals. Soluble-fiber supplements and the amino acid glutamine have shown some effectiveness in the treatment of protease inhibitor–related diarrhea. Glutamine is available as a food supplement at many health food retailers. If dietary intervention alone is unable to control protease inhibitor–related diarrhea, antidiarrheal agents can be quite effective. Dose titration is key so that the minimum amount of medication is used to control the symptom. Infectious causes of diarrhea must be ruled out before antidiarrheal medications are administered.

Patient education and counseling is a vital component of the nutritional management of HIV infection. Box 35-6 specifies key areas that should be addressed.

Physical Therapy

The physical rehabilitation needs of people with HIV disease vary greatly and depend largely on the clinical manifestations experienced. Opportunistic infections such as toxoplasmosis-related encephalitis can result in neuromuscular impairment. Wasting and progression of HIV disease can cause general debilitation and loss of strength. Physical therapy is beneficial in rebuilding gross motor skills and overall strength during the recuperative phase of these kinds of manifestations.

Occupational Therapy

Occupational therapy needs also vary depending on the HIV-related complications present. Peripheral neuropathy is a common side effect of some antiretroviral medications and in some instances is a direct consequence of HIV infection. Its impact on fine motor control and activities of daily living can be minimized through occupational therapy. CMV retinitis can result in substantial loss of vision, which may require extensive rehabilitation and retraining.

Box 35-6   Nutritional Education and Counseling in HIV Disease

Specific counseling guidelines and recommendations should address the following areas as appropriate for the individual patient:

- Healthful eating principles to ensure adequate nutrient intake
- Food and water safety issues related to food shopping, storage, preparation, and dining away from home
- Nutritional strategies for management of symptoms such as anorexia, early satiety, dysphagia, thrush, nausea and vomiting, diarrhea, food intolerances, and other barriers to food intake
- Food-medication interactions, including meal timing for optimal medication efficacy, supplementation, and foods to emphasize or avoid to reduce unwanted interactions (such as reduced medication absorption, nutrient depletion, or altered laboratory test values)
- Psychosocial and economic issues that may prevent appropriate nutrient intake; referral and access to community resources that help to support nutrition and health, such as parenting classes or other support groups, may be appropriate
- Alternative feeding methods (supplementation, tube feeding, or parenteral nutrition)
- Additional therapies that support nutrition, including physical activity and exercise, and medications for symptom management, inflammation reduction, hormonal modulation, and disease treatment
- Guidelines for the evaluation of nutrition information and claims for special diets, individual vitamin and mineral supplementation, and other complementary nutritional practices
- Strategies for treatment of altered fat metabolism and deposition, including diet and exercise, lipid-lowering medications, glycemic control, hormonal normalization, and anabolic medications

---

Medical Social Work

HIV infection challenges people in many different ways. Virtually every aspect of life is affected, including physical functioning, social acceptance, financial stability, and sexual relationships. Mental health challenges are prevalent, and more than 50% of HIV-infected patients demonstrate primary psychiatric disorders other than substance use and personality disorder. Addiction is prevalent and is associated with transmission of HIV and other infections. Depression is common and has been shown to adversely affect adherence to the treatment regimen and other aspects of disease management. The medical social worker is instrumental in assessing and enhancing coping strategies and implementing a variety of interventions for psychosocial support, which can range from arranging individual mental health therapy to organizing peer support opportunities. HIV infection disproportionately affects those of lower economic status. The life challenges faced by indigent populations are magnified by the demands of HIV disease. It is difficult for an individual to address HIV-related needs if basic human needs such as food, shelter, or clothing are going unmet. When working with patients from lower income and disenfranchised populations, the medical social worker must be prepared to deal with practical support issues. Financial assistance, housing, and transportation must be addressed to help individuals meet the health challenges of HIV. The costs of HIV-related medical care and treatment are astronomical. Access to government-supported HIV care and medications is available in many localities. The social worker must learn about these local resources so that appropriate referrals can be made.

COMPLEMENTARY AND ALTERNATIVE THERAPIES

A wide variety of alternative or complementary health practices are used by people with HIV infection. Modalities such as acupuncture and massage can enhance quality of life, especially when combined with allopathic approaches (Mealy and Jordan, 2000). Other strategies such as the use of certain herbal therapies require caution. Studies show that garlic and St. John's wort (also known as *Hypericum*) can interact with some protease inhibitors and may decrease their effectiveness, which increases the risk for resistance. Individuals with HIV must be educated about both the risks and benefits of any complementary therapy they may choose and about the need to inform their health care provider regarding their use of such therapies.

REHABILITATION

The availability of HAART changed HIV infection from an unremitting terminal illness into a chronic disease. With currently available antiretroviral therapies, many individuals will live out their normal life spans. For individuals diagnosed in the pre-HAART era (before 1995), this represents a drastic change. Individuals who had come to grips with the reality of premature disability and death have now experienced significant improvement and a return to preillness levels of functioning. This transition has been dubbed the "Lazarus syndrome." Successful immune reconstitution has allowed some people to move from receiving permanent disability benefits to working full time. Although these changes are exceedingly positive, they require significant adjustment for the individual experiencing them. Counseling, support, and vocational rehabilitation are very useful in facilitating adaptation.

As people with HIV infection have begun to live longer, healthier lives, the need for targeted prevention strategies that address their specific needs and circumstances has increased. Although early prevention efforts focused on keeping uninfected people from acquiring HIV, the focus has broadened to include interventions that keep infected people from transmitting HIV or acquiring additional strains of the virus and other coinfections. These include individual and group-level interventions that reinforce sexual risk reduction and other harm-reduction measures such as safer injection practices and substance use reduction through education, counseling, and behavioral support.

Although many people have benefited from HAART, for others the burdens of treatment outweigh the benefits. Side effects and toxicities can be difficult to tolerate and even unbearable. The burden of daily pill taking is unmanageable for some. Some individuals have chosen to forgo antiretroviral therapy. For some, this becomes a delicate weighing of quantity versus quality of life.

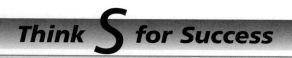

Think S for Success

Symptoms
- Manage symptoms with rest, fluids, nutrition, and comfort measures.

Sequelae
- Prevent transmission of HIV, acquisition of additional strains of HIV, and other sexually transmitted diseases through sexual education.
- Prevent unplanned pregnancy.
- Teach strategies to prevent infection.

Safety
- Teach individual importance of safer sex practices, which include the following:
  Use of latex condoms consistently and correctly
  Negotiation of risk reduction with partners
  Choice of a family planning method to prevent unplanned pregnancy
- Institute safety precautions for individuals with neurologic changes.

Support/Services
- Offer ongoing prevention counseling.
- Reinforce all risk reduction measures attempted.
- Teach importance of adherence to treatment regimen.
- Support family caregivers.

Satisfaction
- Reassess individual's sexual behavior patterns at each visit.
- Determine impact of risk reduction practices on individual's sexual relationships. Assess impact of sexual relationships on quality of life.

END-OF-LIFE AND PALLIATIVE CARE CONSIDERATIONS

With improved antiretroviral therapy, the use of prophylaxis for opportunistic infections, and treatment by providers who are knowledgeable about HIV/AIDS, some patients can look forward to living longer and healthier lives. This is not the case for other patients with HIV/AIDS who suffer from a more episodic course of illness with end points that are very difficult to predict. Generally speaking, it is best to weave palliative care into the overall HIV/AIDS treatment plan from the time of diagnosis.

HIV/AIDS is an incurable disease, and eventually many patients will die of complications of the illness. It is important for health care providers to make patients and their families and loved ones aware of the prognosis and assist them in addressing issues such as the drafting of an advance directive and durable power of attorney.

The level of medical intervention, extraordinary measures, and comfort measures desired should be discussed with the patient. The patient can also identify someone to be his or her durable power of attorney to make decisions when the patient can no longer do so. All decisions should be outlined and written in a legal document such as a living will or advance directive. For the patient with children, it is very important to address custody issues, discuss who will raise the children, and consider the legal implications of these decisions sooner rather than later in the disease course. Dealing with these issues early in the disease helps the patient to remain in control and make his or her own choices.

Symptom management is an important element of palliative care. Fatigue, pain, and insomnia are several of the more common symptoms experienced by patients with HIV/AIDS over the course of the disease and occur with greater intensity as the disease progresses toward death. Management of individual symptoms is based on a thorough understanding of the symptom and education of the patient and family to allow for appropriate planning in anticipation of crisis episodes. A multidisciplinary perspective is required. The ultimate goal is to help the patient feel as much as possible in control of the symptoms and consequently of the illness, so that the patient and the family do not feel abandoned but feel supported and can experience closure at the end of life.

Although overall prognosis may be difficult to determine, certain signs indicate advanced disease or failure of the immune system. Situations such as repeated episodes of opportunistic infection, repeated hospitalizations, and uncontrollable weight loss signify that the patient is not doing well. Once this decline begins and drug therapy is no longer effective or the patient does not wish any further treatment, it is best to focus on psychosocial and spiritual issues related to life closure.

FAMILY AND CAREGIVER ISSUES

A major concern for many families is how to safely care for the HIV-infected person at home. Providers must teach standard precautions for the handling of sharps, body waste, and body fluids (as well as anything soiled with body waste and fluids) and reassure family members that if these precautions are followed they should not become infected. Box 35-7 lists infection control measures that should be followed in the home.

Box 35-7 Infection Control Measures in the Home for Caregivers

- Wash hands thoroughly and frequently.
- Wear gloves when handling body fluids, body wastes, and linens or garments that have been soiled with body fluids or wastes.
- When cleaning up body fluids (blood, vomitus, stool, etc.), wash the area with soap and water and dispose of the fluids or excreta, as well as the cleaning solution, by flushing them down the toilet.
- After cleaning up the body fluids, disinfect the area with a solution of 1 part household bleach and 10 parts water. Soak rags, mops, sponges, etc., in a similar solution.
- Clean bathrooms with regular cleansing agents and then disinfect with the bleach solution.
- Wash dishes in hot soapy water.
- Launder soiled linens in hot water and bleach.
- Store soiled clothes in a plastic bag until they are laundered.
- If using needles or other sharps at home, store them in a sturdy container that is puncture proof and has a lid. When the container is full, disinfect sharps with bleach solution and then seal and tape the container. Place it in a paper bag and dispose of it with regular trash.
- Contaminated paper products, dressings, disposable equipment, and gloves should be placed in tied plastic bags and disposed of with regular trash.

From Ignatavicius DD, Workman ML, editors: *Medical-surgical nursing: critical thinking for collaborative care,* ed 4, Philadelphia, 2002, WB Saunders.

Family members should also be reminded that displays of affection such as embracing, touching, and even kissing (if saliva is not exchanged) are permissible and desirable. Other concerns that family members may have are identified in Box 35-8.

Box 35-8 Family Issues and Concerns

- Adherence to medication regimen and appointment schedule
- Acceptance or isolation because of stigma associated with HIV disease
- Confidentiality
- Costs associated with disease management
- Grief and loss
- Lack of education about disease, prevention, management, and treatment
- Lack of support systems
- Safety and exposure precautions related to needle sticks, prevention of sexual transmission
- Quality of life (i.e., patient's ability to maintain duties and responsibilities in the family)

ETHICAL CONSIDERATIONS

Because of the sensitive nature of HIV infection and AIDS, health care workers will likely confront ethical dilemmas and problems in the care and treatment of persons living with the disease (Fry and Veatch, 2000).

Three main principles in bioethics apply to the clinical management and treatment of individuals living with HIV/AIDS. These principles include respect for the person, beneficence, and justice. Respect for the individual entails accepting the choices and decisions of an autonomous person regarding treatment or nontreatment. Beneficence requires that the health care provider do good and act in the best interests of the patient at all times. Justice requires that all individuals be treated equitably so that benefits and burdens are distributed equally and fairly within society.

In clinical situations, specific ethical issues also arise that are related to the confidentiality of HIV-related medical information and informed consent (for HIV testing) and that may present unique challenges in the management and treatment of individuals living with HIV/AIDS.

In the United States, all medical information is generally considered confidential and is protected under law. Recently implemented federal legislation, the Health Insurance Portability and Accountability Act, provides for increased protection of patient medical information. Because of the sensitive nature of HIV-related information, many states already have laws that provide additional protection for HIV-related medical records. Exempted from the confidentiality requirements for HIV medical records are health care providers in the United States who have a duty to report HIV infections and AIDS cases to public health authorities. In most states health care providers may, without legal consequences, disclose a patient's HIV status to persons at risk of infection (e.g., spouses, sexual partners) but are not required to do so. There is much debate about whether providers should disclose such information and whose rights the provider must protect and is ethically bound to support.

HIV-infected health care workers are another exception to the general rule of confidentiality for HIV-related information. U.S. government policy recommends that the case of an HIV-infected health care worker who performs exposure-prone invasive procedures be reviewed by a panel of experts, who will decide whether the worker can continue to practice the procedures and whether patients must be informed of the worker's HIV infection. States are required to adopt this policy or its "equivalent." Because states are not compelled to adopt the actual policy, state laws vary widely with regard to HIV-infected health care workers, and some states do not require disclosure of HIV status by such workers.

HIV testing is different from other blood tests because of the psychosocial risks associated with positive test results (e.g., rejection by family members, discrimination in access to health care, housing, employment, and in other areas).

To help safeguard against these risks, special procedures such as pretest counseling and specific informed consent related to HIV testing are required as part of HIV testing. Some states allow HIV testing without informed consent under certain circumstances, such as in the event of an occupational exposure to HIV by health care workers.

Mother-to-child transmission of HIV can be significantly reduced if antiretroviral therapy is implemented as soon as possible during the pregnancy. The Institute of Medicine has recommended that all pregnant women be tested for HIV as a part of routine prenatal care. Women would be informed that an HIV test is to be performed with other prenatal blood tests, but specific consent for the HIV test would not be required. The American College of Obstetrics and Gynecology and the American Academy of Pediatrics also support routine universal prenatal HIV testing.

Ethical concerns related to these recommendations include the woman's ability and right to make autonomous choices related to HIV testing, the substantial psychosocial impact of a positive HIV test result without adequate pretest counseling, the rights of the unborn child, and other difficult questions.

CASE STUDY

Patient Data

Ms. S. is a 29-year-old mother of two boys, aged 5 years and 18 months. Ms. S. was diagnosed with HIV infection during her second pregnancy. Both children are uninfected. Ms. S. took antiretroviral therapy during her second pregnancy to prevent perinatal transmission. She had a difficult time tolerating the medication because of nausea and vomiting. At her last checkup, Ms. S.'s CD4 cell count was 310/mm^3 and her viral load was 48,000 copies/ml. She has had some recurrent vaginal candidiasis but no other HIV-related symptoms. Ms. S. is ambivalent about starting medication at this time. She demonstrates a high degree of understanding about HIV infection and the benefits of treatment. At the same time, she is concerned that the side effects of treatment will interfere with her ability to care for her two young, active children. Ms. S. has recently started a new job and does not have any sick leave. She is a single parent and is the sole support for her children. Ms. S. identifies her ability to care and provide for her children as her highest priority.

Ms. S.'s strengths include her knowledge of HIV disease and its treatment and her strong motivation to care for her children. She receives emotional support from her mother, who is aware of Ms. S.'s HIV status. Ms. S. is engaged in her health care and views her health care team as a resource on which she can call to meet her physical, emotional, and practical needs. She has a particularly close bond with her social worker, with whom she has been working since her diagnosis. Ms. S.'s current health needs include slowing HIV disease progression while maintaining her ability to work and parent. Although she perceives some conflict between these goals, after discussion with her physician, she realizes they are not mutually exclusive. She is willing to consider starting HAART.

Diagnostic Findings

CD4 cell count: 310/mm^3
Viral load: 48,000 copies/ml
History of recurrent vaginal candidiasis

Thinking It Through

■ What barriers to treatment adherence does Ms. S. face?

■ Is Ms. S. ready to start HAART?
■ What strengths does Ms. S. demonstrate that may enhance her ability to adhere to treatment?
■ How can the health care team support Ms. S.'s treatment decision making? her ability to adhere to the therapy regimen?

Case Conference

A case conference is set up to determine whether Ms. S. is ready to begin HAART. Ms. S.'s social worker, physician, and nurse are in attendance. Ms. S. is encouraged to bring her mother with her, but unfortunately her mother has to work and is unable to attend. Ms. S.'s physician sets the stage by reviewing her recommendation that Ms. S. start HAART based on her CD4 cell count, viral load, and recurrent vaginal candidiasis. She discusses treatment options less likely to cause nausea and vomiting. Ms. S. likes the idea of choosing medications without those side effects but is concerned that any medication can cause some discomfort. Ms. S.'s nurse points out that, once a regimen is selected, probable side effects can be anticipated and managed proactively. Again Ms. S. is receptive but is concerned about the impact the medications will have on her daily routine. She expresses concern about all the challenges she is currently facing. Her oldest boy has just started kindergarten. Her new job schedule conflicts with that of her day care provider, so she must find a new placement for her younger child. The baby's father has not paid any child support for 8 months and finances are tight. Ms. S.'s social worker commits to helping her explore subsidized day care options and food stamps, and can provide a referral for assistance in getting the child support to which Ms. S. is entitled. The social worker asks Ms. S. what she most needs to feel ready to start treatment. Ms. S. answers that all the support offered sounds good but that she is just feeling overwhelmed. She asks if it would be possible to wait on treatment for now. Her physician responds that, with ongoing monitoring of CD4 cell count and viral load, there is little risk of a serious disease complication in the next few months. Agreement is reached on a plan to recheck laboratory results in 3 months and reevaluate initiating HAART at that time.

Internet and Other Resources

AIDSinfo (sponsored by the U.S. Department of Health and Human Services): *http://www.aidsinfo.nih.gov/*

HIV InSite (sponsored by the University of California San Francisco School of Medicine): *http://hivinsite.ucsf.edu/*

Joint United Nations Programme on HIV/AIDS (UNAIDS) and World Health Organization (WHO): *http://www.unaids.org/*

New Mexico AIDS InfoNet: *http://www.aidsinfonet.org/*; patient education materials in Spanish and English

REFERENCES

Anderson JR, editor: A guide to the clinical care of women with HIV, Rockville, Md, 2001, HIV/AIDS Bureau, Health Resources and Services Administration.

Bartlett JG, Gallant JE: 2001-2002 Medical management of HIV infection, Baltimore, Md, 2001, Johns Hopkins University, Division of Infectious Diseases.

Centers for Disease Control and Prevention: 1993 Revised classification system for HIV infection and expanded surveillance case definition for AIDS among adolescents and adults, *MMWR Recomm Rep* 41(RR-17):1-19, 1992.

Centers for Disease Control and Prevention: Sexually transmitted diseases treatment guidelines, *MMWR Morb Mortal Wkly Rep* 51(RR-6), 2002.

DeLorenzo L, Ingram C: *Nursing care of the HIV-infected patient,* Brockton, Mass, 2001, Western Schools.

Fry ST, Veatch RM: HIV/AIDS care. In *Case studies in nursing ethics,* ed 2, Boston, 2000, Jones and Bartlett, pp 274-300.

Health Resources Services Administration: Clinical management of the HIV-infected adult: a manual for midlevel clinicians, Chicago, 2003, The Administration.

Joint United Nations Programme on HIV/AIDS and World Health Organization, AIDS epidemic update, December 2003, retrieved from *http://www.unaids.org/epidemicupdate/reportdec03/* on Feb 29, 2004.

Jordan D, Mealy R: Demonstrating the effectiveness of community based adherence support, XIII International AIDS Conference abstracts, abstract ThPpD1511, 2000, retrieved from *http://www.iac2000.org/abdetail.asp?ID=ThPpD1511* on Dec 11, 2002.

Kirton C: *ANAC's core curriculum for HIV/AIDS nursing,* ed 2, New York, 2003, Sage Publications.

Mealy R, Jordan D: The impact of complementary therapy on quality of life for people living with HIV and AIDS, XIII International AIDS Conference abstracts, abstract ThPeB5049, 2000, retrieved from *http://www.iac2000.org/abdetail.asp?ID=ThPeB5049* on Dec 11, 2002.

Murphy RL, Flaherty JD: *Contemporary diagnosis and management of HIV/AIDS infections,* ed 2, Newtown, Penn, 2003, Handbooks in Health Care.

Index

A

Abacavir (ABC, Ziagen), for HIV/AIDS, 577t
ABC (abacavir), for HIV/AIDS, 577t
ABCDE assessment format, for skin cancer, 63, 69f
Abdomen
    cancers of, 516-531
        assessment of, 516, 518b
        colorectal cancer as, 520-522
        complementary and alternative therapies for, 526
        family and caregiver issues on, 526
        gastric cancer as, 517-518, 520
        incidence of, 517t
        liver cancer as, 522-524
        pancreatic cancer as, 524-526
        renal cell carcinoma as, 526-528
        risk factors for, 517t
        urinary bladder cancer as, 528-530
    radiation side effects on, 442t
ABI. *See* Ankle-brachial index (ABI).
Absorbent dressings, in wound care, 92
ABT-378r (lopinavir + ritonavir), for HIV/AIDS, 578t
Acarbose (Precose), for diabetes mellitus, 291t
Accolate (zafirlukast), for chronic obstructive pulmonary disease, 115t
Accupril (quinapril), for hypertension, 188t
Accutane (isotretinoin), side effects and nursing considerations for, 73t
Acebutolol (Sectral), for hypertension, 186t
Aceon (perindopril), for hypertension, 188t
Acetaminophen (Tylenol), for joint and connective tissue disorders, 398t
Acetazolamide (Diamox), side effects and nursing considerations for, 45t
Acetylcholine (Miochol), side effects and nursing considerations for, 46t
Aciphex (rabeprazole), for gastroesophageal reflux disease and peptic ulcer, 217t
Achromycin (tetracycline), side effects and nursing considerations for, 72t
Aciphex (rabeprazole), for *Helicobacter pylori* infection, 223t
Acne, 76
Acoustic neuroma, 53
Acquired immunodeficiency syndrome (AIDS), 565-586. *See also* HIV/AIDS.
Acromegaly, 307-311
    clinical manifestations of, 309, 309t
    diagnosis of, 309-310
    drug treatment for, 310, 310t
    interdisciplinary care for, 310-311
    pathophysiology of, 307-309
    progression of, 308f
    skin signs associated with, 64t
Actinic keratoses, 79
Actinomycin D (Cosmegen, Dactinomycin)
    for sarcomas, 560t
    side effects of, 444t

Actonel (risedronate), for osteoporosis, 415, 416t, 417
Actos (pioglitazone), for diabetes mellitus, 292t
Acyclovir (Zovirax), side effects and nursing considerations for, 73t
Adapalene (Differin), side effects and nursing considerations for, 72t
Addison's disease, 305-307
    clinical manifestations of, 302t
    skin signs associated with, 64t
Adipex-P (phentermine), for weight loss, 210t
Adrenal cortex, hormones of, effects of, 285t
Adrenal cytotoxic drugs, for cortisol excess/deficiency, 304t
Adrenal gland dysfunction, 300-307
    Addison's disease as, 305-307
    Cushing's syndrome as, 301-305. *See also* Cushing's syndrome.
    pathophysiology of, 301
Adrenergic inhibitors, for hypertension, 185-186t
Adriamycin (doxorubicin)
    for lung cancer, 511t
    for sarcomas, 560t
    side effects of, 444t
Advance directives, on end-of-life care, 452b
Advil (ibuprofen)
    for headaches, 319t
    for joint and connective tissue disorders, 397t
AeroBid (flunisolide), for chronic obstructive pulmonary disease, 114t
Aerolate, (theophylline), for chronic obstructive pulmonary disease, 114t
AF. *See* Atrial fibrillation (AF).
African Americans, end-of-life care and, 454t
Agenerase (amprenavir), for HIV/AIDS, 578t
Ageusia, complicating head and neck cancers, 479
Aging
    hearing loss associated with, 54
    macular degeneration related to, 40
    ocular changes associated with, 37b
    skin changes related to, 65b
Agnosia, Alzheimer's disease and, by stage, 352t
Aides
    in interdisciplinary team, 18
    in liver disease care, 252
    in neuromuscular disorder care, 382
AIDS (acquired immunodeficiency syndrome), 565-586. *See also* HIV/AIDS.
Airways, obstructive disease of, 107-125. *See also* Obstructive airway disease.
AK-Dex (dexamethasone), side effects and nursing considerations for, 45t
AK-Dilate (phenylephrine), side effects and nursing considerations for, 46t
Albuterol (Proventil, Ventolin), for chronic obstructive pulmonary disease, 114t
Alcohol use, assessment tools for, 242t
Aldactone (spironolactone), for hypertension, 185t
Aldomet (methyldopa), for hypertension, 186t
Alendronate (Fosamax), for osteoporosis, 415, 416t, 417

Page numbers followed by *f* indicate figures; *t*, tables; *b*, boxes.

Aleve (naproxen)
for headaches, 319t
for joint and connective tissue disorders, 397t
Alexander technique, 31
Alkaloids, plant
for lung cancer, 511t
for sarcomas, 560t
Alkeran (melphalan), side effects of, 445t
Alkylating agents
for lung cancer, 511t
for sarcomas, 560t
Allopurinol (Zyloprim), for joint and connective tissue disorders, 398t
Alpha hydroxyl acids 15-80%, 72t
α-adrenergic agonists, for urinary incontinence, 278t
α-adrenergic antagonists, for urinary incontinence, 278-279t
α-adrenergic blockers, for migraines, 320t
$α_1$-adrenergic blockers, for hypertension, 186t
$α_2$-agonists, for brain disorders, 321t
$α_1$-antitrypsin, for chronic obstructive pulmonary disease, 115t
α-glucosidase inhibitors, for diabetes mellitus, 291t
ALS (amyotrophic lateral sclerosis), 390
Altace (ramipril), for hypertension, 188t
AlternaGEL (aluminum hydroxide), for gastroesophageal reflux disease and peptic ulcer, 216t
Aluminum hydroxide (AlternaGEL, Amphojel)
for gastroesophageal reflux disease and peptic ulcer, 216t
with magnesium hydroxide (Maalox, Mylanta), for gastroesophageal reflux disease and peptic ulcer, 216t
Alupent (metaproterenol), for chronic obstructive pulmonary disease, 114t
Alzheimer's disease. *See also* Dementias.
case study on, 361
clinical manifestations of, 351, 351f, 352-353t
pathophysiology of, 348, 349f
Amaryl (glimepiride), for diabetes mellitus, 292t
Amerge (naratriptan), for migraines, 320t
Amethopterin (methotrexate)
for lung cancer, 511t
side effects of, 445t
Amicar (aminocaproic acid), for hemophilia, 145t
Amikacin (Amikin), for tuberculosis, 131t
Amikin (amikacin), for tuberculosis, 131t
Amiloride (Midamor), for hypertension, 185t
Aminocaproic acid (Amicar), for hemophilia, 145t
Aminoglutethimide (Cytadren), side effects of, 444t
Aminoglycosides, for tuberculosis, 131t
Aminosalicylates, for Crohn's disease, 231
Amitriptyline (Elavil)
for brain disorders, 321t
for musculoskeletal disorders, 417t
Amlodipine (Norvasc), for hypertension, 188t
Amnesia, Alzheimer's disease and, by stage, 352t
Amoxicillin, for *Helicobacter pylori* infection, 223t
Amphojel (aluminum hydroxide), for gastroesophageal reflux disease and peptic ulcer, 216t
Amprenavir (Agenerase), for HIV/AIDS, 578t
Amsacrine (m-AMSA), side effects of, 444t
Amyotrophic lateral sclerosis (ALS), 390
AN. *See* Anorexia nervosa (AN).
Anadrol-50 (oxymetholone), side effects of, 445t
Analgesics
for joint and connective tissue disorders, 398t
opiate, for migraine rescue, 322t
Androgens
deficiency of, skin signs associated with, 64t
excess of, skin signs associated with, 64t
in osteoporosis care, 415, 416t
Anemia, 135, 136-141
care of, 139-141
clinical manifestations of, 138-139
complementary and alternative therapies for, 141
diagnosis of, 139

Anemia *(Continued)*
laboratory tests for, 140t
iron deficiency, 136
macrocytic, 137-138
microcytic, 136-137
nutritional, 204-205
pathophysiology of, 136-138
sickle cell, 142-143
signs and symptoms of, 139b
skin signs associated with, 65t
treatment of, 139-141
Anesthetics, topical, nursing considerations for, 45t
Aneurysm, types of, 330f
Angina, in coronary artery disease, 162-163
Angiosarcoma, general treatments for, 556t
Angiotensin-converting enzyme (ACE) inhibitors
for brain disorders, 321t
for congestive heart failure, 170
for coronary artery disease, 166
for hypertension, 188t
Angiotensin II receptor blockers, for hypertension, 188t
Angiotensin inhibitors, for hypertension, 188t
Ankle-brachial index (ABI), in venous stasis disease diagnosis, 97, 97t
Anorexia, complicating cancer treatment, nursing interventions for, 450b
Anorexia nervosa (AN), 198, 200-202
demographic characteristics of, 198b
educational topics for, 201b
Anosmia, complicating head and neck cancers, 479
Antacids
for cirrhosis, 248b
for gastroesophageal reflux disease and peptic ulcer, 216t
Anthra-Derm (anthralin), side effects and nursing considerations for, 73t
Anthralin (Anthra-Derm), side effects and nursing considerations for, 73t
Anti-Parkinson agents, for traumatic brain injury, 340t
Antiandrogens, for urinary incontinence, 279t
Antianxiety agents, for traumatic brain injury, 340t
Antibacterials, 72t
nursing considerations for, 45t
Antibiotics
antitumor
for lung cancer, 511t
for sarcomas, 560t
for cancer symptom management, 448t
for chronic obstructive pulmonary disease, 115t
for cirrhosis, 248b
for *Helicobacter pylori* infection, 223t
side effects and nursing considerations for, 72t
Antibody(ies), monoclonal
for cancer, indications and side effects of, 447t
for neuromuscular disorders, 383t, 384t
Anticholinergics
for cancer symptom management, 448t
for chronic obstructive pulmonary disease, 114t
for Crohn's disease, 231
for neuromuscular disorders, 383t
for traumatic brain injury, 340t
for urinary incontinence, 277t
Anticholinesterase agents, for neuromuscular disorders, 383t
Antichorea agents, for neuromuscular disorders, 383t
Anticoagulants, for brain disorders, 321t
Anticonvulsants
for cancer symptom management, 448t
for traumatic brain injury, 340t
Antidepressants
for brain disorders, 321t
for cancer symptom management, 448t
for chronic obstructive pulmonary disease, 115t
for neuromuscular disorders, 383t, 384t
for traumatic brain injury, 340t
tricyclic. *See* Tricyclic antidepressants (TCAs).

Antieczematous agents, side effects and nursing considerations for, 72t
Antiemetics
for brain disorders, 322t
in lung cancer care, 510
side effects and nursing considerations for, 57t
Antiepileptic drugs, 319t, 327b
Antifungals, side effects of, 45t
Antihistamines
for cancer symptom management, 448t
for neuromuscular disorders, 383t
side effects and nursing considerations for, 57t, 72t
Antihyperlipidemic agents, for coronary artery disease, 166
Antihypertensives
for brain disorders, 320t
for traumatic brain injury, 340t
Antiinfectives, nursing considerations for, 45t
Antiinflammatories, side effects and nursing considerations for, 45t
Antilipidemics, for brain disorders, 321t
Antimalarials, for joint and connective tissue disorders, 397t
Antimetabolites
for lung cancer, 511t
for sarcomas, 560t
Antineoplastic agents, for musculoskeletal disorders, 417t
Antioxidants
foods rich in, 257t
for neuromuscular disorders, 383t
Antiplatelet medications, for coronary artery disease, 166
Antipruritics, side effects and nursing considerations for, 72t
Antipsoriatic agents, side effects and nursing considerations for, 73t
Antipsychotics, for neuromuscular disorders, 383t
Antiretroviral therapy
highly active, for HIV/AIDS, 570, 571, 574, 576, 578, 579-580
for HIV/AIDS, 576, 577-578t
regimens for, 580t
Antismoking medications, for chronic obstructive pulmonary disease, 115t
Antispasmodics, for neuromuscular disorders, 383t
Antitumor antibiotics
for lung cancer, 511t
for sarcomas, 560t
Antivert (meclizine)
side effects and nursing considerations for, 57t
for traumatic brain injury, 340t
Antivirals
nursing considerations for, 45t
side effects and nursing considerations for, 73t
Antrizine (meclizine), side effects and nursing considerations for, 57t
Anturane (sulfinpyrazone), for joint and connective tissue disorders, 398t
Anxiolytics
for brain disorders, 322t
for cancer symptom management, 448t
Aortic valve disorders, 175f, 176
Aphasia, Alzheimer's disease and, by stage, 352t
Apnea, sleep, obstructive, complicating head and neck cancers, 483, 483b
Apraxia, Alzheimer's disease and, by stage, 352t
Apresoline (hydralazine), for hypertension, 187t
Aquatab (benzthiazide), for hypertension, 185t
Ara-C (cytarabine), side effects of, 444t
Aralen (chloroquine), for joint and connective tissue disorders, 397t
Arava (leflunomide), for joint and connective tissue disorders, 397t
Aredia (pamidronate), for musculoskeletal disorders, 416t
Arfonad (trimethaphan), for hypertension, 188t
Aricept (donepezil), for Alzheimer's disease, 351
Aristocort (triamcinolone)
for chronic obstructive pulmonary disease, 114t
for joint and connective tissue disorders, 398t
Aromatherapy, 29-30, 30t
Arterial occlusive disease, chronic, 189-190
Arterial ulcers, 101-103, 102f, 189-190

Arteriosclerosis, skin signs associated with, 65t
Arthritis
metabolic disease associated with, 408-409
rheumatoid, 401-404. *See also* Rheumatoid arthritis (RA).
Arthropan (choline salicylate), for joint and connective tissue disorders, 397t
Aspiration, after stroke, interventions to prevent, 335b
Aspirin
for brain disorders, 321t
for coronary artery disease, 166
for headaches, 319t
for joint and connective tissue disorders, 397t
Astemizole (Hismanal), side effects and nursing considerations for, 72t
Asthma, chronic, 118-124
clinical manifestations of, 118-119
diagnosis of, 119
interdisciplinary care of, 119-121
management plan for, 122f
pathophysiology of, 118
severity of, classification of, 121t
symptoms suggestive of, 118b
triggers of, interventions for, 119t
Astrocytomas, 460
Atacand (candesartan), for hypertension, 188t
Atarax (hydroxyzine), 72t
Atelectasis, secondary to spinal cord injury, 370
Atenolol (Tenormin), for hypertension, 186t
Atherosclerosis, 189-190
Ativan (lorazepam)
for brain disorders, 322t
side effects and nursing considerations for, 57t
Atopic dermatitis, 75-76
Atrial fibrillation (AF), 171, 173-175
Atro-Pen (atropine), for chronic obstructive pulmonary disease, 114t
Atropine (Atro-Pen)
for chronic obstructive pulmonary disease, 114t
for neuromuscular disorders, 383t
Atrovent (ipratropium), for chronic obstructive pulmonary disease, 114t
Attorneys, elder law, in dementia care, 359-360
Audiologist, in hearing loss care, 55-56
Auranofin (Ridaura), for joint and connective tissue disorders, 397t
Aurothioglucose (Solganal), for joint and connective tissue disorders, 397t
Autonomic dysreflexia, secondary to spinal cord injury, 371, 371f
Autonomic neurogenic bladder, 273
Avandia (rosiglitazone), for diabetes mellitus, 292t
Avapro (irbesartan), for hypertension, 188t
Axid (nizatidine), for gastroesophageal reflux disease and peptic ulcer, 217t
Ayurveda, 26-27
Azathioprine (Imuran)
for Crohn's disease, 231
for joint and connective tissue disorders, 397t
for ulcerative colitis, 232
Azelaic acid (Azelex), 72t
Azelex (azelaic acid), 72t
Azopt (brinzolamide ophthalmic solution 1%), side effects and nursing considerations for, 45t
AZT (zidovudine), for HIV/AIDS, 576, 577t
Azulfidine (sulfasalazine)
for Crohn's disease, 231
for joint and connective tissue disorders, 397t

B

Bacitracin (Neosporin), 72t
Back, low, pain in, 430-433. *See also* Low back pain (LBP).
Bactroban (mupirocin), 72t
Barbiturates, for brain disorders, 319t
Bard EndoCinch System, for gastroesophageal reflux disease, 219

Barrett's esophagus
  characteristics of, 215b
  complicating gastroesophageal reflux disease, 214
Basal cell carcinoma, 79
Bathing, Alzheimer's disease and, by stage, 352t
BCNU (carmustine), side effects of, 444t
Beclomethasone (Beclovent), for chronic obstructive pulmonary
    disease, 114t
Beclovent (beclomethasone), for chronic obstructive pulmonary
    disease, 114t
Bedsores, 84-95. *See also* Pressure ulcers.
Behavioral functions, Alzheimer's disease and, by stage, 353t
Behavioral interventions, for cardiac rehabilitation, 178
Behavioral therapist, in bladder disorder care, 276-277
Behaviorist, in traumatic brain injury care, 339
Behaviors, difficult, managing, guidelines for, 359b
Benadryl (diphenhydramine), 72t
Benazepril (Lotensin), for hypertension, 188t
Bendroflumethiazide (Naturetin), for hypertension, 185t
Benemid (probenecid), for joint and connective tissue disorders,
    398t
Benicar (olmesartan), for hypertension, 188t
Benign paroxysmal positional vertigo, 56-57
  Dix-Hallpike test for, 58, 58b
Benzac (benzoyl peroxide), 72t
Benzodiazepines
  for cancer symptom management, 448t
  for seizure disorders, 319-320t
  side effects and nursing considerations for, 57t
Benzoyl peroxide (Benzac), 72t
Benzthiazide (Aquatab, Exna), for hypertension, 185t
β-agonists, for neuromuscular disorders, 383t, 384t
β-blockers
  for brain disorders, 320t
  for chronic obstructive pulmonary disease, 114t
  for coronary artery disease, 166
  for hypertension, 186-187t
  for hyperthyroidism, 298, 299t
  side effects and nursing considerations for, 46t
β-hydroxy-β-methylglutaryl-coenzyme A reductase inhibitors, for
    coronary artery disease, 166
Betagan Liquifilm (levobunolol), side effects and nursing considerations
    for, 46f
Betaxolol (Betoptic, Kerlone)
  for hypertension, 186t
  side effects and nursing considerations for, 46t
Bethanechol (Urecholine)
  for neuromuscular disorders, 383t
  for urinary incontinence, 279t
Betoptic (betaxolol), side effects and nursing considerations
    for, 46t
Biaxin (clarithromycin), for *Helicobacter pylori* infection, 223t
Bicozene (resorcinol), 72t
Biguanides, for diabetes mellitus, 291t
Biliary tract obstruction, skin signs associated with, 64t
Bill of Rights, Dying Person's, 453b
Billroth I procedure, 517, 519f
Billroth II procedure, 517, 519f
Binge eating disorder, 203-204
  case study on, 211
  demographic characteristics of, 198b
Biologic response modifiers
  for cancer symptom management, 448t
  for joint and connective tissue disorders, 398t
Biologic therapy, for breast cancer, 501
Biological-based therapy, 29-30
Biopsy, in breast cancer diagnosis, 494, 495b
Biotherapy, for cancer, 446, 447t
Bismuth subsalicylate (Pepto-Bismol)
  for gastroesophageal reflux disease and peptic ulcer, 216t
  for *Helicobacter pylori* infection, 224t
Bisoprolol (Zebeta), for hypertension, 186t
Bisphosphonates, in osteoporosis care, 415, 416t, 417

Bladder, urinary
  cancer of, 528-530
    skin signs associated with, 64t
  disorders of, 271-283
    assessment of, 271, 272b
    case study on, 282-283
    clinical manifestations of, 272-274
    complementary and alternative therapies for, 282
    diagnosis of, 274
    ethnic variations in, 271
    interdisciplinary care for, 276-282
    pathophysiology of, 271-272
  dysfunction of, in spinal cord tumor, management strategies
      for, 466b
  incidence of, 517t
  neurogenic, 273
  paralytic, 273-274
  retention in, 274
    differential diagnosis of, 276t
    medications contributing to, 281b
  risk factors for, 517t
Blenoxane (bleomycin)
  for lung cancer, 511t
  for sarcomas, 560t
  side effects of, 444t
Bleomycin (Blenoxane)
  for lung cancer, 511t
  for sarcomas, 560t
  side effects of, 444t
Blepharitis, nursing considerations for, 47t
Blindness
  definition of, 35
  legal, definition of, 35
Blocadren (timolol)
  for brain disorders, 320t
  for hypertension, 187t
Blood cells, development of, 150f
Blood disorders, 135-160
  anemia as, 136-141. *See also* Anemia.
  assessment of, 135, 137b
  case study on, 147-148
  end-of-life issues on, 147
  ethical considerations on, 136b, 147
  family and caregiver issues on, 147
  hemochromatosis as, 143-146
  hemophilia as, 143, 144t
  interdisciplinary care for, 146-147
  long-term care for, 147
  malignant, 149-160. *See also* Malignancy(ies), of blood.
  overview of, 135
  polycythemia as, 141-142
Blood pressure
  classification of, for adults, 183t
  elevated, 181-189. *See also* Hypertension (HTN).
Blood vessel disorders, 181-196. *See also* Vascular disorders.
BN. *See* Bulimia nervosa (BN).
Body-based therapies, 30-33
Bone(s)
  affected by Paget's disease, 427t
  infection of, 423-427. *See also* Osteomyelitis.
  sarcomas of, primary, 555
  tumors of, general treatments for, 556t
Bone marrow suppression, complicating cancer treatment, nursing
      interventions for, 450b
Bone marrow transplantation
  allogenic, for chronic myelogenous leukemia, 152
  for breast cancer, 501
Bonine (meclizine), side effects and nursing considerations for, 57t
Bontril (phendimetrazine), for weight loss, 210t
Boric acid (Ear-Dry), nursing considerations for, 57t
Bouchard's nodes, in osteoarthritis, 395
Bowel
  cancer of

Bowel *(Continued)*
    incidence of, 517t
    risk factors for, 517t
  dysfunction of, in spinal cord tumor, management strategies
    for, 466b
Bowel elimination, altered, secondary to spinal cord injury, 370
Brachytherapy, 441-442
  safety precautions for, 443b
Braden scale risk assessment tool, for pressure ulcers, 86, 88-89t
Brain
  disorders of, 314-347
    assessment of, 314, 315b, 316b
    epilepsy as, 323-328. *See also* Epilepsy.
    headache as, 314-323. *See also* Headache.
    medications for, 319-322t
    persistent vegetative state as, 341-343
    stroke as, 328-336
    traumatic brain injury as, 336-341. *See also* Traumatic brain
      injury (TBI).
  healthy, nutrients for, 359b
  meninges of, 460f
  radiation side effects on, 442t
  tumors of, 458-464
    case study on, 468-469
    clinical manifestations of, 460-461, 461b
    complementary and alternative therapies for, 463-464, 464t
    diagnosis of, 461
    interdisciplinary care for, 461-463
    pathophysiology of, 458-460
Brainstem tumors, key manifestations of, 461b
Breast(s)
  cancer of, 492-506
    assessment of, 495-497, 496b
      for body image problems, 496-497
      for functional limitations, 496
      for recurrence and quality-of-life issues, 497
    case study on, 504-505
    clinical manifestations of, 493-494
    complementary and alternative therapies for, 501
    diagnosis of, 494-495, 495f
    family and caregiver issues in, 504
    interdisciplinary care for, 498-503
    palliative care for, 503
    pathophysiology of, 493
    rehabilitation issues for, 497-498, 503
    risk factors for, 493b
    signs and symptoms of, 494b
    skin signs associated with, 64t
    stages of, 493b
    survival after, factors influencing, 493b
    survival rates for, 492
    treatment of, 498-503
    types of, 493b
  radiation side effects on, 442t
  reconstruction of, 499
  self-examination of, 494f
Brethine (terbutaline), for chronic obstructive pulmonary disease,
  114t
Brevibloc (esmolol), for hypertension, 187t
Brinzolamide ophthalmic solution 1% (Azopt), side effects and nursing
  considerations for, 45t
Bromocriptine (Parlodel), for acromegaly, 310, 310t
Bronchitis, chronic, 109-111
Bronchodilators
  for cancer symptom management, 448t
  for chronic obstructive pulmonary disease, 114t
Brown-Séquard syndrome, 363f, 365
Buddhism, end-of-life care and, 454t
Budesonide (Rhinocort), for chronic obstructive pulmonary disease, 114t
Buerger's disease, 191-192
  skin signs associated with, 65t
Bulimia nervosa (BN), 202-203
  demographic characteristics of, 198b

Bulla, 68t
Bumetanide (Bumex), for hypertension, 185t
Bumex (bumetanide), for hypertension, 185t
Bupropion (Wellbutrin), for chronic obstructive pulmonary
  disease, 115t
Burow's solution, 72t
Busulfan (Myleran), side effects of, 444t

C

C-reactive protein level, high-sensitivity, in coronary artery disease
  diagnosis, 165t
CAD. *See* Coronary artery disease (CAD).
Calan (verapamil), for brain disorders, 321t
Calcimar (calcitonin), for musculoskeletal disorders, 416t
Calcipotriene (Dovonex), side effects and nursing considerations
  for, 73t
Calcitonin, for musculoskeletal disorders, 416t, 417
Calcium, recommended daily allowance for, 419t
Calcium alginate, in wound care, 91t
Calcium carbonate (Rolaids, Titralac, Tums)
  for gastroesophageal reflux disease and peptic ulcer, 216t
  for osteoporosis, 417-418
Calcium channel blockers
  for brain disorders, 321t
  for hypertension, 188t
Calm-X (dimenhydrinate), side effects and nursing considerations
  for, 57t
Caloric testing, for vertigo, 58-59
Camphor, side effects and nursing considerations for, 72t
Camptothecin-11 (CPT-11), side effects of, 444t
Canadian Centre for Health Promotion (CHP) model, 3, 3f
Cancer(s), 436-564
  of abdomen, 516-531. *See also* Abdomen, cancers of.
  assessment of, 438-439, 440b
  of breast, 492-506. *See also* Breast(s), cancer of.
  of central nervous system, 458-469
    assessment of, 458, 459b
    brain tumors as, 458-464. *See also* Brain, tumors of.
    case study on, 468-469
    end-of-life issues in, 467
    ethical considerations on, 468
    family and caregiver issues in, 467-468
    spinal cord cancers as, 464-467. *See also* Spinal cord, cancers of.
  of cervix, 537-540. *See also* Cervix, cancer of.
  clinical manifestations of, 439
  colorectal, 520-522
    case study on, 530-531
  diagnosis of, 437-438, 437b
  of endometrium, 540-542
  grading systems for, 438b
  of head and neck, 470-491. *See also* Head and neck, cancers of.
  interdisciplinary care for, 439-451
  leading sites of, 437t
  of liver, 522-524
  living with, 436-457
    cultural considerations on, 451-452
  of lung, 507-515. *See also* Lung(s), cancer of.
  of musculoskeletal system, 553-564. *See also* Musculoskeletal system,
    cancers of.
  of ovaries, 533-537. *See also* Ovary(ies), cancer of.
  of pancreas, 524-526
  pathophysiology of, 436-437
  of prostate, 547-550. *See also* Prostate, cancer of.
  of reproductive system, 532-552. *See also* Reproductive system,
    cancers of.
  skin signs associated with, 64t
  of stomach, 517-518, 520
  of testes, 546-547, 548b
  of vagina, 544-546
  of vulva, 542-544
Candesartan (Atacand), for hypertension, 188t
Candidiasis, in HIV/AIDS, 568-570, 569t
  nursing interventions for, 575t

Cannulas, for oxygen administration, 116t
Capastat Sulfate (capreomycin), for tuberculosis, 131t
Capoten (captopril)
    for brain disorders, 321t
    for hypertension, 188t
Capreomycin (Capastat Sulfate), for tuberculosis, 131t
Capsaicin cream, for joint and connective tissue disorders, 398t
Captopril (Capoten)
    for brain disorders, 321t
    for hypertension, 188t
Carbachol (Miostat), side effects and nursing considerations
        for, 46t
Carbamazepine (Tegretol)
    for brain disorders, 320t
    for brain tumors, 462t
Carbamide peroxide (Debrox), nursing considerations for, 57t
Carbidopa, for neuromuscular disorders, 384t
Carbohydrates, foods containing 15 grams of, 292b
Carbonic anhydrase inhibitors, side effects and nursing considerations
        for, 45t
Carboplatin (Paraplatin), side effects of, 444t
Carcinoma
    basal cell, 79
    renal cell, 526-528
    squamous cell, 79-80
Cardene (nicardipine), for hypertension, 188t
Cardiac catheterization, in coronary artery disease diagnosis, 164t
Cardiologist, in coronary artery disease care, 165-166
Cardiology, nuclear, in coronary artery disease diagnosis, 164t
Cardiopulmonary disorders, secondary to spinal cord injury,
        368-370
Cardiovascular disorders
    secondary to spinal cord injury, 368
    skin signs associated with, 65t
Cardizem (diltiazem)
    for hypertension, 188t
    for thyroid disorders, 299t
Cardura (doxazosin)
    for hypertension, 186t
    for urinary incontinence, 279t
Care settings, 11-20
    case management and, 19
    community-based, 13-14
    home care in, 12t, 14-15
    hospice care in, 14
    interdisciplinary team in, 15-19
    long-term, 11-12, 12t
    public health care in, 14
    rehabilitation facility as, 12-13, 12t
    skilled nursing, 13
    subacute, 11, 12t
Caregiver(s)
    for abdominal cancer patients, issues of, 526
    for blood disorder patients, issues on, 147
    for blood malignancy patients, issues for, 158b
    for breast cancer patients, issues of, 504
    for Buerger's disease patients, issues of, 192
    for central nervous system cancer patients, issues of, 467-468
    in chronic illness and disability, caring for, 9b, 10
    for chronic kidney disease patients, issues for, 269
    for chronic liver disease patients, issues of, 258
    for dementia patients, 354
    for diverticular disease patients, issues of, 236
    for eating disorder patients, issues of, 204
    for head and neck cancer patients, issues for, 488b
    for HIV/AIDS patients, issues on, 583-584, 584b
    for inflammatory bowel disease patients, issues of, 234
    for irritable bowel syndrome patients, issues of, 238
    for joint and connective tissue disorder patients, issues of, 409
    for lung cancer patients, issues of, 514
    for malabsorption syndrome patients, issues of, 239
    for malnourished patients, issues of, 208
    for neuromuscular disorder patients, issues of, 391

Caregiver(s) (*Continued*)
    for obstructive airway disease patients, issues of, 123
    for pancreatic disease patients, issues for, 258
    for persistent vegetative state patients, issues of, 341-342
    for sarcoma patients, issues of, 563
    for skin disorder patients, issues of, 81
    for spinal cord injury patients, issues of, 374-375
    for stroke patients, issues on, 336
    for traumatic brain injury patients, issues of, 341
    for tuberculosis patients, issues of, 133
Carmustine (BCNU), side effects of, 444t
Carteolol (Cartol), for hypertension, 186t
Cartol (carteolol), for hypertension, 186t
Carvedilol (Coreg), for hypertension, 186t
Case management, 19
CAT. *See* Complementary and alternative therapy (CAT).
Catapres (clonidine)
    for brain disorders, 321t
    for hypertension, 185t
Cataracts, 40-41
    case study on, 48
    removal of, postoperative instructions for, 42b
Catheterization
    for bladder emptying, 280
    cardiac, in coronary artery disease diagnosis, 164t
Cauda equina syndrome, 363f, 365
CCNU (lomustine), side effects of, 444t
Celebrex (celecoxib)
    for headaches, 319t
    for joint and connective tissue disorders, 397t
Celecoxib (Celebrex)
    for headaches, 319t
    for joint and connective tissue disorders, 397t
Central cord syndrome, 363f, 365
Central nervous system (CNS)
    cancers of, 458-469
        assessment of, 458, 459b
        brain tumors as, 458-464. *See also* Brain, tumors of.
        case study on, 468-469
        end-of-life issues in, 467
        ethical considerations on, 468
        family and caregiver issues in, 467-468
        spinal cord cancers as, 464-467. *See also* Spinal cord,
                cancers of.
    depressants of, for cancer symptom management, 448t
    disorders of, vertigo in, 56
Central poststroke pain, 331
Centrilobar emphysema, 111
Cerebellar tumors, key manifestations of, 461b
Cerebral edema, in stroke, 330-331
Cerebral tumors, key manifestations of, 461b
Cerebrovascular accident (CVA), 328-336. *See also* Stroke.
Cerebyx (fosphenytoin), for seizure disorders, 319t
Certified nurse's aide, in neuromuscular disorder care, 382
Ceruminolytics, nursing considerations for, 57t
Cervical tumors, manifestations of, 465t
Cervix, cancer of, 537-540
    advanced, nursing interventions for, 538b
    assessment of, 537
    clinical manifestations of, 537, 539b
    diagnosis of, 537
    incidence of, ethnic differences in, 539b
    interdisciplinary care for, 539-540
    pathophysiology of, 537
    signs and symptoms of, 539b
    treatment for, 539b
Cetirizine (Zyrtec), nursing considerations for, 72t
Chelation therapy, 29
Chemical-based therapy, 29-30
Chemoprophylaxis, in HIV/AIDS, 579
Chemotherapy, 443, 446
    agents and side effects of, 444-445t
    for brain tumors, 462, 462b

Chemotherapy (Continued)
for breast cancer, 499-500
for cervical cancer, 539-540
drugs for, handling safety guidelines for, 446b
for endometrial cancer, 542
home management of, 446b
for lung cancer, 510, 511t
for multiple myeloma, 157
for ovarian cancer, 536
for sarcomas, 557-558, 560t
side effects of, 560t
for testicular cancer, 547
nursing interventions for, 548b
for vaginal cancer, 545
for vulvar cancer, 543-544
Chest
radiation side effects on, 442t
radiograph of, in coronary artery disease diagnosis, 163t
Chinese Americans, end-of-life care and, 454t
Chinese medicine, traditional, 27-28
Chiropractor
in osteoarthritis care, 399
in vestibular disorder care, 60
Chloasma, 78
Chlorambucil (Leukeran)
for chronic lymphocytic leukemia, 153
side effects of, 444t
Chloramphenicol (Chloromycetin), nursing considerations for, 45t
Chlorodeoxyadenosine, side effects of, 444t
Chloromycetin (chloramphenicol), nursing considerations for, 45t
Chloroquine (Aralen), for joint and connective tissue disorders, 397t
Chlorothiazide (Diuril), for hypertension, 185t
Chlorpropamide (Diabinese), for diabetes mellitus, 292t
Chlorthalidone (Hygroton), for hypertension, 185t
Cholelithiasis, 252-254
demographic differences in, 244t
Cholesterol profile, in coronary artery disease diagnosis, 164-165t
Choline salicylate (Arthropan), for joint and connective tissue disorders, 397t
Cholinergic urticaria, clinical features of, 75t
Cholinergics
for neuromuscular disorders, 383t
side effects and nursing considerations for, 46t
for urinary incontinence, 279t
Cholinesterase inhibitors
for neuromuscular disorders, 384t
side effects and nursing considerations for, 46t
Chondrosarcoma, general treatments for, 556t
CHP model. See Canadian Centre for Health Promotion (CHP) model.
Christianity, end-of-life care and, 454t
Chronic arterial occlusive disease, 189-190
case study on, 195-196
Chronic illness and disability
alternative approaches and therapies for, 21-34. See also Complementary and alternative therapy (CAT).
care settings for, 11-20. See also Care settings.
caring for caregiver in, 9b, 10
Healthy People 2010 focus areas on, 1b
impact of, 5-10
on families, 8
on person, 6-7
on society, 8-9
nature of, impact on person and, 6-7
practice models on, 2-5
role of health care provider in, 9
understanding, 1-10
Chronic obstructive pulmonary disease (COPD), 109-117
assessment of, instruments for, 109b
case study on, 124
chronic bronchitis as, 109-111
classification of severity of, 107t
complementary and alternative therapies for, 117

Chronic obstructive pulmonary disease (Continued)
diagnosis of, 111-112
emphysema as, 111
ethnic variations in, 108-109
interdisciplinary care of, 112-117
Chronicity, 2
Cierny-Mader staging system, for osteomyelitis, 423b
Ciloxan (ciprofloxacin), nursing considerations for, 45t
Cimetidine (Tagamet), for gastroesophageal reflux disease and peptic ulcer, 217t
Cipro (ciprofloxacin), for tuberculosis, 131t
Ciprofloxacin (Ciloxan, Cipro)
nursing considerations for, 45t
for tuberculosis, 131t
Cirrhosis, 245-252
causes of, 246t
clinical manifestations of, 247f
demographic differences in, 244t
diagnosis of, 247, 248b
interdisciplinary care for, 247-252
medications for, 248b
pathophysiology of, 245-246
treatment focus for, 248t
Cisplatin (Platinol)
for lung cancer, 511t
for sarcomas, 560t
side effects of, 444t
Cladribine (Leustatin), side effects of, 444t
Clarithromycin (Biaxin), for Helicobacter pylori infection, 232t
Claritin (loratadine), nursing considerations for, 72t
Claudication
in arterial ulcers, 101
intermittent, in chronic arterial occlusive disease, 189
Clemastine (Tavist), nursing considerations for, 72t
Cleocin (clindamycin), side effects and nursing considerations for, 72t
Clergy
in breast cancer care, 503
in interdisciplinary team, 18-19
Clindamycin (Cleocin), side effects and nursing considerations for, 72t
Clinoril (sulindac)
for headaches, 319t
for joint and connective tissue disorders, 397t
Clonazepam (Klonopin), for seizure disorders, 319t
Clonidine (Catapres)
for brain disorders, 321t
for hypertension, 185t
Clopidogrel (Plavix), for brain disorders, 321t
Clorazepate (Tranxene), for seizure disorders, 320t
Clotting disorders, skin signs associated with, 65t
Cluster headache, 315
clinical manifestations of, 317
Coal tar (Estar, psoriGel), side effects and nursing considerations for, 73t
Coal tar solution, side effects and nursing considerations for, 72t
Cobalamin deficiency, anemia in, 137-138
clinical manifestations of, 139
Codeine
with acetaminophen or aspirin (Tylenol No. 3, No. 4, Empirin No. 3, No. 4), for joint and connective tissue disorders, 398t
for Crohn's disease, 231
Cognitive functions, Alzheimer's disease and, by stage, 352-353t
Colace, for neuromuscular disorders, 384t
Colchicine (Novocolchine), for joint and connective tissue disorders, 398t
Cold urticaria, clinical features of, 75t
Colitis
granulomatous, 228, 230-231
spastic, 236-238
ulcerative, 231-234. See also Ulcerative colitis.
Collagens, in wound care, 91t

Colon
  cancer of, skin signs associated with, 64t
  spastic, 236-238
Colony-stimulating factors, for lung cancer, 510-511, 511t
Colorectal cancer, 520-522
  case study on, 530-531
Colostomy, home care for, 522b
Communication
  after stroke, strategies to enhance, 334b
  in dementia, guidelines for, 359b
Community-based care, 13-14
Complementary and alternative therapy (CAT), 21-34
  for abdominal cancers, 526
  for anemia, 141
  for asthma, 121
  biological- and chemical-based, 29-30
  for bladder disorders, 282
  body-based, 30-33
  for brain tumors, 463-464, 464t
  for breast cancer, 501
  for chronic liver disease, 252
  for chronic obstructive pulmonary disease, 117
  for chronic pancreatitis, 257-258
  for diabetes mellitus, 295
  ethical considerations on, 33
  for fibromyalgia, 422
  for gastroesophageal reflux disease, 225
  for head and neck cancers, 487
  for headache, 323
  for hearing loss, 56
  for heart disorders, 178-179
  for HIV/AIDS, 582
  for low back pain, 433
  manipulative, 30-33
  mind-body, 28-29
  for neuromuscular disorders, 384
  for obesity, 210
  for osteoarthritis, 301b, 399-400
  for osteomyelitis, 426
  for osteoporosis, 419
  for peptic ulcer disease, 225
  practitioners of
    assessment criteria or, 22b
    licensing of, 22
  for prostate cancer, 550
  reasons for using, 26b
  resources on, 33
  for sarcomas, 562-563
  for skin disorders, 71b, 74b
  for spinal cord cancers, 467
  for spinal cord injury, 374
  systems for, 23, 26-28
  for vascular disorders, 194-195
  for vestibular disorders, 60-61
Complete blood count, in coronary artery disease diagnosis, 164t
Compression therapy, types of, comparison of, 98-99t
COMT inhibitors, for neuromuscular disorders, 383t
Congestive heart failure (CHF), 169-171, 172-173b
  case study on, 179-180
Conjugated estrogen (Premarin), for urinary incontinence, 278t
Connective tissue diseases, diffuse, 401-408
  assessment of, 393, 394b
  drugs for, 397-398t
  ethnic variations in, 395b
  rheumatoid arthritis as, 401-404. *See also* Rheumatoid arthritis (RA).
  systemic lupus erythematosus as, 404-406, 405f
  systemic sclerosis as, 406-408
Connective tissue disorders, skin signs associated with, 64t
Contact dermatitis, 75, 76b
Contact layer, in wound care, 91t
Contracture, secondary to spinal cord injury, 372
Conus medullaris syndrome, 363f, 365
Copaxone, for neuromuscular disorders, 383t

Coping, impaired, secondary to spinal cord injury, 370
Coreg (carvedilol), for hypertension, 186t
Corgard (nadolol)
  for hypertension, 186t
  for thyroid disorders, 299t
Coronary artery disease (CAD), 161-169
  clinical manifestations of, 162-163
  diagnosis of, 163-165t
  dietary recommendations for, 167-168t
  drug therapy for, 166
  ethnic differences in, 162b
  interdisciplinary care for, 165-166
  nursing considerations on, 166, 169
  pathophysiology of, 161
  risk factor modification in, 166
Cortaid (hydrocortisone), for chronic obstructive pulmonary disease, 114t
Cortef (hydrocortisone), for cortisol excess/deficiency, 304t
Corticosteroids
  for chronic obstructive pulmonary disease, 114t
  commonly used, 74b
  for cortisol excess/deficiency, 304t
  epidural injection of, complications of, 432b
  for joint and connective tissue disorders, 398t
  for migraines, 322t
  for neuromuscular disorders, 383t
  for rheumatoid arthritis, 403
  side effects and nursing considerations for, 73t
  for ulcerative colitis, 232
Cortisol, excess/deficiency of, drug treatment for, 304t
Cortisone (Cortone)
  for chronic obstructive pulmonary disease, 114t
  for cortisol excess/deficiency, 304t
  side effects of, 444t
Cortone (cortisone)
  for chronic obstructive pulmonary disease, 114t
  for cortisol excess/deficiency, 304t
  side effects of, 444t
Cosmegen (actinomycin D), side effects of, 444t
Cough suppressants, for cancer symptom management, 448t
Coumadin (warfarin)
  for atrial fibrillation, 174
  for brain disorders, 321t
Counseling
  HIV prevention, elements of, 573b
  sexual, PLISSIT model for, 533b
Counselor
  in anorexia nervosa care, 201-202
  in binge eating disorder care, 204
  in brain tumor care, 463
  in irritable bowel syndrome care, 237
  in malnutrition care, 206
Coup and contrecoup brain injury, 336, 337f
Cozaar (iosartan), for hypertension, 188t
CPT-11 (camptothecin-11), side effects of, 444t
Credé's method, of bladder emptying, 280
Creutzfeldt-Jakob disease, pathophysiology of, 349
Crixivan (indinavir), for HIV/AIDS, 578t
Crohn's disease, 228, 230-231
  demographic differences in, 229t
  skin signs associated with, 64t
Crolom (cromolyn), for chronic obstructive pulmonary disease, 114t
Cromolyn (Crolom), for chronic obstructive pulmonary disease, 114t
Crust, 68t
Cryoglobulinemia, manifestations of, in hepatitis C, 245b
Cryoprecipitate, for hemophilia, 145t
Cryptococcosis, in HIV/AIDS, 569t, 570
  nursing interventions for, 575t
Cryptosporidiosis, in HIV/AIDS, 569t, 570
  nursing interventions for, 575t

Cultural considerations
  on end-of-life care, 454-455t
  on living with cancer, 451-452
Cuprimine (penicillamine), for joint and connective tissue disorders, 397t
Cushing's syndrome, 301-305
  clinical manifestations of, 301-302, 301f, 302t
  diagnosis of, 302-303
  interdisciplinary care for, 303-305
  skin signs associated with, 64t
CVA (cerebrovascular accident), 328-336. *See also* Stroke.
Cyclobenzaprine (Flexeril), for musculoskeletal disorders, 417t
Cyclophosphamide (Cytoxan)
  for joint and connective tissue disorders, 397t
  for lung cancer, 511t
  for sarcomas, 560t
  side effects of, 444t
Cyclosporine A, for ulcerative colitis, 232
Cyclosporine (Sandimmune), for joint and connective tissue disorders, 397t
Cystic fibrosis, skin signs associated with, 64t
Cystourethroscopy, 274
Cytadren (aminoglutethimide), side effects of, 444t
Cytarabine (Cytosar, Ara-C), side effects of, 444t
Cytomegalovirus infection, in HIV/AIDS, 569t, 570
  nursing interventions for, 575t
Cytomel (liothyronine), for hypothyroidism, 298-299
Cytosar (cytarabine), side effects of, 444t
Cytoxan (cyclophosphamide)
  for joint and connective tissue disorders, 397t
  for lung cancer, 511t
  for sarcomas, 560t
  side effects of, 444t

D

Dacarbazine (DTIC)
  for sarcomas, 560t
  side effects of, 444t
Dactinomycin (actinomycin D), for sarcomas, 560t
Daranide (dichlorphenamide), side effects and nursing considerations for, 45t
Darvocet (propoxyphene with acetaminophen), for joint and connective tissue disorders, 398t
Darvon (propoxyphene with aspirin), for joint and connective tissue disorders, 398t
DDAVP (desmopressin), for hemophilia, 145t
DDC (zalcitabine), for HIV/AIDS, 577t
DDI (didanosine), for HIV/AIDS, 577t
Death, with dignity, 452b
Débriding agents, in wound care, 92t
Debrox (carbamide peroxide), nursing considerations for, 57t
Decadron (dexamethasone)
  for brain tumors, 462t
  for cortisol excess/deficiency, 304t
  for joint and connective tissue disorders, 398t
  for migraines, 322t
Decerebrate posturing, from traumatic brain injury, 337, 337f
Decibel scale, 54t
Decision making
  Alzheimer's disease and, by stage, 353t
  in dementia, issues in, 359b
Decongestants, side effects and nursing considerations for, 57t
Decorticate posturing, from traumatic brain injury, 337, 337f
Decubiti, 84-95. *See also* Pressure ulcers.
Deep vein thrombosis, secondary to spinal cord injury, 368
Delavirdine (Rescriptor), for HIV/AIDS, 577t
Delta-Cortef (prednisolone), side effects of, 445t
Deltasone (prednisone)
  for chronic obstructive pulmonary disease, 114t
  for joint and connective tissue disorders, 398t
Demadex (torsemide), for hypertension, 185t
Demecarium (Humorsol), side effects and nursing considerations for, 46t

Dementias, 348-361
  alternative therapies for, 360
  assessment of, 349, 350b, 351b
  case study on, 361
  clinical manifestations of, 351, 351f, 352-353t
  decision making in, issues in, 359b
  diagnosis of, 349, 351
  eating strategies in, by stage, 35-358t
  HIV-associated, 569t, 571
    nursing interventions for, 576t
  interdisciplinary care for, 351, 354-360
  pathophysiology of, 348-349
  task organization aids for, 360b
  types of, descriptive terms for, 349b
Demerol (meperidine), for migraine rescue, 322t
Demographic differences
  in liver, gallbladder, and pancreatic disorders, 244t
  in lower gastrointestinal tract disorders, 229t
  in nutritional and eating disorders, 198b
  in upper gastrointestinal tract disorders, 214t
Denavir (penciclovir), side effects and nursing considerations for, 73t
Dental status, alterations in, complicating head and neck cancers, 481
Dentist, in head and neck cancer care, 484-485
Depakene (valproate, valproic acid)
  for brain disorders, 320t
  for brain tumors, 462t
Depakote (valproate), for brain disorders, 320t
Depen (penicillamine), for joint and connective tissue disorders, 397t
Depression, secondary to spinal cord injury, 370
Dermatitis, 75-76, 76b
  perioral, 76-77
Dermatographic urticaria, symptomatic, clinical features of, 75t
Dermatologist, 69
  in skin disorder care, 69
Dermatomyositis, skin signs associated with, 64t
DES (diethylstilbestrol), side effects of, 444t
Desmodium, for hepatitis C, 253t
Desmopressin (DDAVP), for hemophilia, 145t
Detrol (tolterodine), for urinary incontinence, 277t
Detrusor hyperreflexia, 272
Dexamethasone (AK-Dex, Decadron)
  for brain tumors, 462t
  for cortisol excess/deficiency, 304t
  for joint and connective tissue disorders, 398t
  for migraines, 322t
  side effects and nursing considerations for, 45t
DHE (dihydroergotamine), for migraines, 320t
DiaBeta (glyburide), for diabetes mellitus, 292t
Diabetes mellitus, 286-295
  case study on, 311-312
  clinical manifestations of, 288
  complementary and alternative therapies for, 295
  diagnosis of, 288, 288b
  drug therapy for, 290, 291-292t, 292
  education curriculum for, 288b
  ethnic variations in, 286
  health promotion measures for, 290b
  interdisciplinary care for, 289-294
  monitoring in, 289
  pathophysiology of, 286-288
  skin signs associated with, 64t
  treatment of, 288-289
Diabetic foot ulcer, 102f, 103-105
Diabetic retinopathy, 41-43, 43f
Diabinese (chlorpropamide), for diabetes mellitus, 292t
Dialysis
  daily short, 268
  nocturnal, 267-268
  trends in, 266-268

Diamox (acetazolamide), side effects and nursing considerations for, 45t
Diazepam (Valium)
  for brain disorders, 322t
  for seizure disorders, 320t
  side effects and nursing considerations for, 57t
Diazoxide (Hyperstat), for hypertension, 187t
Dichlorphenamide (Daranide), side effects and nursing considerations for, 45t
Diclofenac (Voltaren)
  for headaches, 319t
  for joint and connective tissue disorders, 397t
  side effects and nursing considerations for, 45t
Didanosine (DDI, Videx), for HIV/AIDS, 577t
Didronel (etidronate), for musculoskeletal disorders, 416t
Diet
  in atrial fibrillation management, 174, 174t
  in congestive heart failure management, 170
  in coronary artery disease management, 167-168t
  in hypertension management, 184
  in valvular heart disease management, 176
Diethylpropion (Tenuate, Tenuate Dospan), for weight loss, 210t
Diethylstilbestrol (DES), side effects of, 444t
Dietitian
  in Addison's disease care, 306
  in anorexia nervosa care, 201
  in asthma care, 121
  in blood disorder care, 146
  in blood malignancy care, 158
  in brain tumor care, 463
  in breast cancer care, 502
  in cancer care, 451
  in cardiac rehabilitation, 178
  in cholelithiasis care, 254
  in chronic obstructive pulmonary disease care, 116-117, 117b
  in chronic pancreatitis care, 257
  in Crohn's disease care, 231
  in Cushing's syndrome care, 303
  in dementia care, 354
  in diabetes mellitus care, 292-293
  in diabetic foot ulcer care, 105
  in diverticular disease care, 235
  in fibromyalgia care, 422
  in gastroesophageal reflux disease care, 220
  in gout care, 409
  in head and neck cancer care, 486
  in interdisciplinary team, 18
  in irritable bowel syndrome care, 237
  in liver cancer care, 524
  in liver disease care, 252
  in low back pain care, 432
  in lung cancer care, 513
  in malabsorption syndrome care, 239
  in malnutrition care, 206
  in neuromuscular disorder care, 382
  in obesity care, 210
  in osteoporosis care, 418
  in Paget's disease care, 430
  in pancreatic cancer care, 526
  in peptic ulcer disease care, 224-225
  in pressure ulcer care, 95
  in spinal cord injury care, 373
  in stroke care, 333
  in systemic sclerosis care, 407
  in thyroid disorder care, 300
  in traumatic brain injury care, 340
  in tuberculosis care, 132
  in wound care, 95
Differin (adapalene), side effects and nursing considerations for, 72t
Diffuse axonal injury (DAI), 336, 337

Diflunisal (Dolobid)
  for headaches, 319t
  for joint and connective tissue disorders, 397t
Digital mammography, in breast cancer diagnosis, 495
Digoxin, for congestive heart failure, 170
Dihydroergotamine (DHE, Migranal), for migraines, 320t
Dilantin (phenytoin)
  for brain tumors, 462t
  for seizure disorders, 319t
Diltiazem (Cardizem)
  for hypertension, 188t
  for thyroid disorders, 299t
Dimenhydrinate (Calm-X, Dimetabs, Dramamine), side effects and nursing considerations for, 57t
Dimetabs (dimenhydrinate), side effects and nursing considerations for, 57t
Diovan (valsartan), for hypertension, 188t
Diphenhydramine (Benadryl), 72t
Dipivefrin (Propine), side effects and nursing considerations for, 46t
Dipyridamole (Persantine), for brain disorders, 321t
Disability, 2
  chronic illness and. See Chronic illness and disability.
Disease-modifying antirheumatic drugs (DMARDs), for rheumatoid arthritis, 403
Disfigurement, complicating head and neck cancers, 482-483
Disk
  degeneration of, low back pain from, 431
  herniation of, low back pain from, 430, 431f
Ditropan, for neuromuscular disorders, 383t
Ditropan (oxybutynin), for urinary incontinence, 277t
Diuretics
  for cancer symptom management, 448t
  for cirrhosis, 248b
  for congestive heart failure, 170
  for hypertension, 185t
Diuril (chlorothiazide), for hypertension, 185t
Diverticular diseases, 234-236
Diverticulitis, signs and symptoms of, 230t
Diverticulitis/diverticulosis, demographic differences in, 229t
Diverticulosis, 234-236
Dix-Hallpike test, for benign paroxysmal positional vertigo, 58, 58b
Dizziness, 54
  vertigo differentiated from, 56
DMARDs (disease-modifying antirheumatic drugs), for rheumatoid arthritis, 403
Do Not Resuscitate Order, 452b
Docetaxel (taxotere), side effects of, 445t
Dolobid (diflunisal)
  for headaches, 319t
  for joint and connective tissue disorders, 397t
Donepezil (Aricept), for Alzheimer's disease, 351
Dopamine agonists, for acromegaly, 310, 310t
Dopaminergic agents, for neuromuscular disorders, 383t
Dorzolamide (Trusopt), side effects and nursing considerations for, 45t
Double effect, 452b
Dovonex (calcipotriene), side effects and nursing considerations for, 73t
Doxazosin (Cardura)
  for hypertension, 186t
  for urinary incontinence, 279t
Doxepin (Sinequan)
  for musculoskeletal disorders, 417t
  for urinary incontinence, 277t
Doxorubicin (Adriamycin)
  for lung cancer, 511t
  for sarcomas, 560t
  side effects of, 444t
Dramamine (dimenhydrinate), 57t
Dressing, Alzheimer's disease and, by stage, 352t
Dressings, in wound care, 92t

Dronabinol (Marinol), for malnutrition, 206
Drug(s)
　for acromegaly, 310, 310t
　for Addison's disease, 304t, 306
　in anorexia nervosa management, 201
　for asthma, 120-121
　for atrial fibrillation, 173-174
　in binge eating disorder management, 204
　for brain tumors, 461, 462t
　for cancer, 443, 444-445t, 446
　　in symptom management, 448-449t
　causing photosensitivity, 71t
　for chronic ear disorders, 57t
　for chronic kidney disease, 266
　in chronic obstructive pulmonary disease management, 113,
　　114-115t
　for chronic pancreatitis, 255-256
　for congestive heart failure, 170
　contributing to urinary retention, 281b
　for Crohn's disease, 231
　for Cushing's syndrome, 303, 304t
　for dementia, 351, 354
　for diabetes mellitus, 290, 291-292t, 292
　for diverticular disease, 235
　for epilepsy, 326-327, 327b
　for fibromyalgia, 421
　for gastroesophageal reflux disease and peptic ulcer,
　　216-217t
　for gout, 409
　for head and neck cancers, 485-486
　for headache, 318, 319-322t
　for hemophilia, 145t
　in HIV/AIDS management, 576-580, 577-578t, 579t
　for hypertension, 184, 185-188t
　for irritable bowel syndrome, 237
　for liver cancer, 523-524
　　implantable pump for, 524f, 525b
　for low back pain, 432
　for lung cancer, 510-512, 511t
　for malabsorption syndrome, 239
　for malnutrition, 206
　for neuromuscular disorders, 382, 383-384t
　for obesity, 210, 210t
　for osteoarthritis, 396, 397-398t
　for osteomyelitis, 425
　for osteoporosis, 415, 416-417t, 417-418
　ototoxic, 53
　for Paget's disease, 429
　for pancreatic cancer, 525
　for peptic ulcer disease, 222, 223-224t, 224
　for prostate cancer, 550
　for rheumatoid arthritis, 403
　sensitivity to, skin signs associated with, 64t
　for skin disorders, 70-71, 72-73t
　for spinal cord cancers, 465
　for spinal cord injury, 373
　for stroke, 332
　for systemic lupus erythematosus, 405-406
　for systemic sclerosis, 407
　for thyroid disorders, 298-300, 299t
　for traumatic brain injury, 339-340, 340t
　for tuberculosis, 130-131, 130t, 131t
　for ulcerative colitis, 232
　for urinary incontinence, 277t
　for valvular heart disease, 176
Dry eye syndromes, nursing considerations for, 47t
D4T (stavudine), for HIV/AIDS, 577t
DTIC (dacarbazine)
　for sarcomas, 560t
　side effects of, 444t
Dumping syndrome, management strategies for, 519b
Durable Power of Attorney, 452b
Dying Person's Bill of Rights, 453b

DynaCirc (isradipine), for hypertension, 188t
Dyrenium (triamterene), for hypertension, 185t
Dysgeusia, complicating head and neck cancers, 479
Dysosmia, complicating head and neck cancers, 479
Dysphagia, complicating head and neck cancers, 480, 480b
Dysplastic nevi syndrome, 79
Dyspnea, in lung cancer, management of, 512

E

E-Mycin (erythromycin), side effects and nursing considerations
　　for, 72t
Ear(s)
　disorders of, 50-62
　　chronic, drugs for, 57t
　　functional health pattern assessment for, 52b
　　hearing loss in, 50-56. *See also* Hearing loss.
　　vestibular disorders as, 56-61. *See also* Vestibular disorders.
　irrigation of, 51b
Ear-Dry (boric acid), nursing considerations for, 57t
Eating, Alzheimer's disease and, by stage, 352t
Eating disorders, 197-205. *See also* Nutritional disorders.
　anorexia nervosa as, 198, 200-202
　binge eating disorder as, 203-204
　bulimia nervosa and purging as, 202-203
　caregiver issues associated with, 204
　demographic differences in, 198b
　diagnosis of, 198
　diagnostic criteria for, 200b
　family issues associated with, 204
　nursing interventions for, 201b
ECG. *See* Electrocardiogram (ECG).
Echocardiogram, two-dimensional, in coronary artery disease
　　diagnosis, 164t
Echothiophate (Phospholine Iodide), side effects and nursing
　　considerations for, 46t
Econopred (prednisolone acetate), side effects and nursing
　　considerations for, 45t
Edecrin (ethacrynic acid), for hypertension, 185t
Education
　on chronic liver disease, 250t
　on diabetes mellitus, curriculum for, 288b
　on lifestyle modifications for gastroesophageal reflux disease,
　　218-219, 219t
　on pancreatitis, 256t
　on upper gastrointestinal tract disorders, 218t
Efavirenz (Sustiva), for HIV/AIDS, 577t
Elavil (amitriptyline)
　for brain disorders, 321t
　for musculoskeletal disorders, 417t
Eldisine (vindesine), side effects of, 445t
Electrocardiogram (ECG), in coronary artery disease diagnosis,
　　163t
Electronystagmography, for vertigo, 59
Elimination, altered, nursing interventions for, 540b
Eloxatin (oxaliplatin), side effects of, 445t
Elspar (L-asperginase), side effects of, 444t
Embolus, pulmonary, secondary to spinal cord injury, 368
Emcyt (estramustine), side effects of, 444t
Emgel (erythromycin), side effects and nursing considerations
　　for, 72t
Emollients, side effects and nursing considerations for, 73t
Emphysema, 111
　pathophysiology of, 109f
Empirin No. 3, No. 4 (codeine with aspirin), for joint and connective
　　tissue disorders, 398t
Enalapril (Vasotec)
　for brain disorders, 321t
　for hypertension, 188t
Enalaprilat (Vasotec Injection), for hypertension, 188t
Enbrel (etanercept), for joint and connective tissue disorders, 398t
End-of-life care, 452-456
　in HIV/AIDS, 583
　hospice, 456

End-of-life care *(Continued)*
  in lung cancer, 513-514
  optimal, barriers to, 456b
  palliative, 456
End-of-life issues
  on blood disorders, 147
  on blood malignancies, 159b
  on Buerger's disease, 191-192
  on cancer, 452-456
    of central nervous system, 467
  on chronic kidney disease, 269
  on chronic liver disease, 251b
  concepts and terminology related to, 452-453b
  cultural beliefs related to, 454-455t
  on head and neck cancers, 488
  on neuromuscular disorders, 391
  on obstructive airway disease, 123
  on stroke, 336
End-of-life symptoms, 455b
Endocrine disorders, 284-313
  acromegaly as, 307-311. *See also* Acromegaly.
  adrenal gland dysfunction as, 300-307. *See also* Adrenal
    gland dysfunction.
  altered thyroid function as, 295-300. *See also* Thyroid
    disorders.
  assessment of, 284-285, 287b
  case study on, 311-312
  diabetes mellitus as, 286-295. *See also* Diabetes mellitus.
  major, 286t
  pathophysiology of, 284
  skin signs associated with, 64t
  treatment of, 285
Endometrium, cancer of, 540-542
  advanced, nursing interventions for, 538b
Enduron (methyclothiazide), for hypertension, 185t
Energy conservation tips, 252b
Energy management, in lung cancer, nursing interventions for,
  512b
Enteritis, regional, 228, 230-231
Enterostomal therapist
  in colorectal cancer care, 522
  in urinary bladder cancer care, 530
Enzymes, pancreatic
  for cirrhosis, 248b
  teaching points related to, 526b
Epidural injection, of corticosteroids, complications of,
  432b
Epifrin (epinephrine), side effects and nursing considerations
  for, 46t
Epilepsy, 323-328
  assessment of, 324
  clinical manifestations of, 324-326
  diagnosis of, 324
  ethical considerations on, 328
  interdisciplinary care for, 326-328
  interviewing person with, guide for, 327b
  pathophysiology of, 324
  seizures in
    classification of, 325t
    triggers for, 324b
  sudden unexpected death in, 325
Epinephrine (Epifrin, Glaucon), side effects and nursing
  considerations for, 46t
Epivir (lamivudine), for HIV/AIDS, 577t
Eplerenone (Inspra), for hypertension, 185t
Epoetin alfa (Epogen, Procrit)
  for cancer, indications and side effects of, 447t
  for lung cancer, 511t
Epogen (epoetin alfa)
  for cancer, indications and side effects of, 447t
  for lung cancer, 511t
Eprosartan (Teveten), for hypertension, 188t
Ergot alkaloids, for brain disorders, 320t

Erythromycin (E-Mycin, Emgel, Romycin)
  nursing considerations for, 45t
  side effects and nursing considerations for, 72t
Esidrix (hydrochlorothiazide), for hypertension, 185t
Esmolol (Brevibloc), for hypertension, 187t
Esomeprazole (Nexium)
  for gastroesophageal reflux disease and peptic ulcer,
    217t
  for *Helicobacter pylori* infection, 223t
Esophagus
  Barrett's
    characteristics of, 215b
    complicating gastroesophageal reflux disease, 214
  disorders of, 213-220
    gastroesophageal reflux disease as, 213-220. *See also*
      Gastroesophageal reflux disease (GERD).
    hiatal hernia as, 220, 221f
  dysfunction of, secondary to spinal cord injury, 370
  radiation side effects on, 442t
Estar (coal tar), side effects and nursing considerations for,
  73t
Estramustine (Emcyt), side effects of, 444t
Estrogen (Vivelle, Premarin, Prempro, Premphase)
  in osteoporosis care, 415, 416t
  for urinary incontinence, 278t
Etanercept (Enbrel), for joint and connective tissue disorders,
  398t
Ethacrynic acid (Edecrin), for hypertension, 185t
Ethambutol (Myambutol), for tuberculosis, 130t
Ethical considerations
  on blood disorders, 147
  on blood malignancies, 158b
  on Buerger's disease, 192
  on central nervous system cancer, 468
  on chronic kidney disease, 269
  on chronic liver disease, 248b
  on complementary and alternative therapy, 33
  on end-of-life care, 456
  on epilepsy, 328
  on head and neck cancers, 488
  on hearing impairment, 61
  on heart disorders, 179-180
  on HIV/AIDS, 584-585
  on joint and connective tissue disorders, 410
  on low back pain, 433
  on lung cancer care, 514
  on neuromuscular disorders, 391, 391b
  on osteomyelitis, 427
  on sarcomas, 563
  on spinal cord injury, 375
  on tuberculosis, 122
Ethnicity
  bladder disorders and, 271
  blood disorders and, 136b
  blood malignancies and, 149
  cervical cancer incidence and, 539b
  chronic kidney disease and, 262
  chronic obstructive pulmonary disease and, 108-109
  coronary artery disease and, 162b
  endometrial cancer incidence and, 541b
  head and neck cancers and, 471t
  HIV/AIDS and, 565-566
  joint and connective tissue diseases and, 395b
  lung cancer and, 507
  ovarian cancer and, 535b
  prostate cancer incidence and, 548
  stroke and, 328-329
  testicular cancer incidence and, 546b
  tuberculosis and, 126
Ethosuximide (Zarontin), for seizure disorders, 319t
Ethotoin (Peganone), for seizure disorders, 319t
Etidronate (Didronel), for musculoskeletal disorders,
  416t

Etoposide (VePesid)
    for lung cancer, 511t
    side effects of, 444t
Etretinate (Tegison), side effects and nursing considerations
      for, 73t
Euthanasia, 452b
Euthyroid sick syndrome, 296
Evista (relosifene), for musculoskeletal disorders, 416t
Ewing's sarcoma, general treatments for, 556t
Executive function, Alzheimer's disease and, by stage,
      352t
Exelon (rivastigmine), for Alzheimer's disease, 351
Exenteration, pelvic, for cervical cancer, 539, 541f
Exercise(s)
    in dementia, 360
    pelvic muscle, for urinary incontinence, 276-277
    in skin disorder management, 66
    for weight loss, 210
Exercise treadmill test, in coronary artery disease diagnosis,
      163t
Exna (benzthiazide), for hypertension, 185t
Exophthalmos, in hyperthyroidism, 300f
Expectorants, for cancer symptom management, 448t
Extremity(ies)
    lower, ulcers of, 95-105
    radiation side effects on, 442t
    tumors of, general treatments for, 556t
    ulcers of. *See also* Ulcer(s), lower extremity.
Eye drops, instillation of, 47b
Eyes
    changes in, with aging, 37b
    disorders of, 35-49
      age-related macular degeneration as, 40
      assessment of, 35-36, 36f, 37b, 39b
      cataracts as, 40-41
      chronic, 47t
      clinical manifestations of, 36, 39b
      diabetic retinopathy as, 41-43, 43f
      diagnosis of, 36
      family issues and concerns for, 39-40
      glaucoma as, 43-44
      interdisciplinary care for, 36-39
      medications for, 45-46t
      systemic diseases/syndromes associated with, 37b

F

Family
    of abdominal cancer patient, issues of, 526
    of blood disorder patient, issues on, 147
    of blood malignancy patient, issues for, 158b
    of breast cancer patient, issues of, 504
    of Buerger's disease patient, issues of, 192
    of central nervous system cancer patient, issues of,
      467-468
    of chronic kidney disease patient, issues for, 269
    of chronic liver disease patient, issues of, 258
    of chronic pancreatitis patient, education for, 256t
    of diverticular disease patient, issues of, 236
    of eating disorder patient, issues of, 204
    education for, on peginterferon and ribavirin therapy,
      251t
    end-of-life needs of, 455b
    of gastroesophageal reflux disease patient, education of,
      218t
    of head and neck cancer patient, issues for, 488b
    of hearing impaired patient, issues and concerns of, 61
    of HIV/AIDS patient, issues on, 583-584, 584b
    impact of chronic illness and disability on, 8
    of inflammatory bowel disease patient, issues of, 234
    of irritable bowel syndrome patient, issues of, 238
    of joint and connective tissue disorder patient, issues of,
      409
    of liver disease patient, education for, 250t

Family *(Continued)*
    of low vision patient, issues and concerns for, 39-40
    of lung cancer patient, issues of, 514
    of malabsorption syndrome patient, issues of, 239
    of malnourished patient, issues of, 208
    of neuromuscular disorder patient, issues of, 391
    of pancreatic disease patient, issues for, 258
    of patient with obstructive airway disease, issues of, 123
    of persistent vegetative state patient, issues of, 341-342
    of sarcoma patient, issues of, 563
    of skin disorder patient, issues of, 81
    of spinal cord injury patient, issues of, 374-375
    of stroke patient, issues on, 336
    of traumatic brain injury patient, issues of, 341
    of tuberculosis patient, issues of, 133
Famotidine (Pepcid), for gastroesophageal reflux disease and
      peptic ulcer, 217t
Fastin (phentermine), for weight loss, 210t
Fatigue
    complicating cancer treatment, nursing interventions for,
      450b
    in lung cancer, 512
Fatty acids, essential, deficiency of, skin signs associated with,
      64t
Feldene (piroxicam)
    for headaches, 319t
    for joint and connective tissue disorders, 397t
Felodipine (Plendil), for hypertension, 188t
Fenoprofen (Nalfon)
    for headaches, 319t
    for joint and connective tissue disorders, 397t
Fiber
    in diverticular disease care, 235-236
    in selected foods, 236t
Fibrillation, atrial, 171, 173-175
Fibromyalgia syndrome (FS), 420-422
Fibrosarcoma, general treatments for, 556t
Filgrastim (Neupogen)
    for cancer, indications and side effects of, 447t
    for lung cancer, 511t
Finasteride (Proscar), for urinary incontinence, 279t
Flagyl (metronidazole), for *Helicobacter pylori* infection,
      223t
Flexeril (cyclobenzaprine)
    for musculoskeletal disorders, 417t
    for neuromuscular disorders, 383t
Flomax (tamsulosin), for urinary incontinence, 279t
Flonase (fluticasone), for chronic obstructive pulmonary disease,
      114t
Florinef (fludrocortisone), for cortisol excess/deficiency,
      304t
Floxin (ofloxacin), for tuberculosis, 131t
Floxuridine (FUDR), side effects of, 444t
Fludara (fludarabine), side effects of, 444t
Fludarabine (Fludara), side effects of, 444t
Fludrocortisone (Florinef), for cortisol excess/deficiency,
      304t
Flunisolide (AeroBid), for chronic obstructive pulmonary disease,
      114t
Fluoroquinolones, for tuberculosis, 131t
5-Fluorouracil (5-FU), side effects of, 444t
Fluoxetine (Prozac)
    for brain disorders, 322t
    for musculoskeletal disorders, 417t
Fluoxymesterone (Halotestin), side effects of, 444t
Flurbiprofen (Ocufen), side effects and nursing considerations
      for, 45t
Fluticasone (Flonase), for chronic obstructive pulmonary disease,
      114t
Foams, in wound care, 91t
Folic acid
    for cirrhosis, 248b
    deficiency of, anemia in, 137

Folic acid *(Continued)*
    clinical manifestations of, 139
      treatment of, 139-140
Food(s)
    antioxidant-rich, 257t
    with carbohydrates (15 grams), 292b
    fiber content of, 236t
    high in vitamin K, 174t
    high-sodium, 172t
Food Guide Pyramid, 207f
    for vegetarian diet, 207f
Food security, 205
Foradil (formoterol), for chronic obstructive pulmonary
      disease, 114t
Formoterol (Foradil), for chronic obstructive pulmonary
      disease, 114t
Fosamax (alendronate), for osteoporosis, 415, 416t, 417
Fosinopril (Monopril), for hypertension, 188t
Fosphenytoin (Cerebyx), for seizure disorders, 319t
Fractures, secondary to spinal cord injury, 372
Friction, pressure ulcers and, 85
Fröhlich's syndrome, skin signs associated with, 64t
FS (fibromyalgia syndrome), 420-422
5-FU (5-fluorouracil), side effects of, 444t
FUDR (floxuridine), side effects of, 444t
Fungating tumors, complicating head and neck cancers,
      477-478, 478t
Furosemide (Lasix), for hypertension, 185t

G

GABA antagonists, for neuromuscular disorders, 383t,
      384t
Gabapentin (Neurontin), for brain disorders, 320t
Galantamine (Reminyl), for Alzheimer's disease, 351
Gallbladder, disorders of, cholelithiasis as, 252-254
Gallstones, 252-254
    secondary to spinal cord injury, 370
Ganglionic blockers, for hypertension, 188t
Garamycin (gentamicin), nursing considerations for, 45t
Gastric cancer, 517-518, 520
Gastroesophageal reflux disease (GERD), 213-220
    assessment of, 213
    case study on, 225-226
    clinical manifestations of, 214-215
    complementary and alternative therapies for, 225
    demographic differences in, 214t
    diagnosis of, 215-216
    interdisciplinary care of, 216-220
    pathophysiology of, 213-214
    surgical intervention for, preparation for, 219-220
Gastrointestinal tract
    disorders of
      secondary to spinal cord injury, 370
      skin signs associated with, 64t
    lower, disorders of, 228-240
      assessment of, 228, 229-230b
      demographic differences in, 229t
      diagnosis of, 228, 230b
      diverticular diseases as, 234-236
      inflammatory bowel disease as, 228, 230-234. *See also*
        Inflammatory bowel disease (IBD).
      irritable bowel syndrome as, 236-238
      malabsorption syndromes as, 238-239
      signs and symptoms of, 230t
      ulcerative colitis as, 231-234. *See also* Ulcerative colitis.
    upper, disorders of, 213-227
      complementary and alternative therapies for, 225
      gastroesophageal reflux disease as, 213-220. *See also*
        Gastroesophageal reflux disease (GERD).
      hiatal hernia as, 220
      peptic ulcer disease as, 220-225. *See also* Peptic ulcer
        disease.
GBS (Guillain-Barré syndrome), 386

Gemcitabine (Gemzar), side effects of, 444t
Gemzar (gemcitabine), side effects of, 444t
Genital herpes, in HIV/AIDS, 569t, 571
Genitourinary disorders, secondary to spinal cord injury, 370
Genotypic testing, in HIV/AIDS, 579
Gentamicin (Garamycin), nursing considerations for, 45t
Germinomas, 460
Ginger, for hepatitis C, 253t
Ginkgo biloba, for dementia, 360
Gland(s)
    salivary, function, anatomic relationships, and cancer features
      of, 475t
    thyroid, function, anatomic relationships, and cancer features
      of, 475t
Glasgow Coma Scale, 337, 338t
Glaucoma, 43-44
    case study on, 48
Glaucon (epinephrine), side effects and nursing considerations
      for, 46t
Gleevec (imatinib), for chronic myelogenous leukemia,
      152-153
Glimepiride (Amaryl), for diabetes mellitus, 292t
Gliomas, 460
Glipizide (Glucotrol), for diabetes mellitus, 292t
Glucocorticoids
    for cortisol excess/deficiency, 304t
    excess of, skin signs associated with, 64t
Glucophage (metformin), for diabetes mellitus, 291t
Glucose, blood level of, hemoglobin A_{1C} and, relation between,
      289t
Glucotrol (glipizide), for diabetes mellitus, 292t
Glyburide (DiaBeta, Micronase), for diabetes mellitus, 292t
Glycerin, side effects and nursing considerations for, 46t
Glyset (miglitol), for diabetes mellitus, 291t
G_{M1} ganglioside, for neuromuscular disorders, 383t
Gold salts, for joint and connective tissue disorders, 397t
Gold sodium thiomalate (Myochrysine), for joint and connective
      tissue disorders, 397t
Gout, 408-409
    drugs for, 398t
Granisetron (Kytril), for brain disorders, 322t
Granulomatous colitis, 228, 230-231
Grief work, nursing interventions involving, 522b
Guanabenz (Wytensin), for hypertension, 186t
Guanadrel sulfate (Hylorel), for hypertension, 186t
Guanethidine (Ismelin), for hypertension, 186t
Guanfacine (Tenex), for hypertension, 186t
Guillain-Barré syndrome (GBS), 386

H

H2 receptor blockers, for gastroesophageal reflux disease and
      peptic ulcer, 27t
HAART (highly active antiretroviral therapy), for HIV/AIDS,
      570, 571, 574, 576, 578, 579-580
Halotestin (fluoxymesterone), side effects of, 444t
Hashimoto's thyroiditis, 296
HD (Huntington's disease), 388-389
Head and neck
    cancers of, 470-491
      assessment of, 471, 476b
      case study on, 489
      causes of, by site, 472t
      clinical manifestations of, 472-473
      complementary and alternative therapies for, 487
      complications of, 473-484, 477t
        dental status alterations as, 481
        disfigurement as, 482-483
        fungating tumors as, 477-478, 478t
        hearing loss as, 482
        hypothyroidism as, 482
        loss of smell as, 479, 479b
        lymphedema as, 473, 476
        muscle trismus as, 481-482

Head and neck *(Continued)*
    nutrition alterations as, 480-481, 480b
    osteoradionecrosis as, 481
    skin alterations as, 476
    sleep disorders as, 483
    taste alterations as, 479-480
    vision impairment as, 482
    xerostomia as, 478-479, 479b
  diagnosis of, 471-473
  drug therapy for, 485-486
  end-of-life care for, 488
  ethical considerations on, 488
  ethnic differences in, 471t
  family and caregiver issues on, 488b
  interdisciplinary care for, 484-487
  laryngectomy in, problems associated with, 483-484, 484b
  palliative care for, 487-488
  pathophysiology of, 471
  quality-of-life scales for patients with, 485b
  radiation side effects on, 442t
  regions of, 473f
Headache, 314-323
  assessment of, 314, 316b, 317b
  causes of, 317b
  clinical manifestations of, 315, 317
  cluster, 315
  complementary and alternative therapies for, 323
  interdisciplinary care for, 318-323
  migraine, 315
  pathophysiology of, 314, 315
  symptom profile for, 317b
  tension-type, 314-315
Healing, wound, nutrients and, 86t
Health care providers
  implications of complementary and alternative therapy for, 33
  regulation of, 24-25t
  role of, in chronic illness and disability, 9
Healthy People 2010, on chronic illness and disability, 1b
Hearing aid, care of, 56b
Hearing loss, 50-56
  assessment of, 50-52
  clinical manifestations of, 54
  communication with, strategies to improve, 55b
  complementary and alternative therapy for, 56
  complicating head and neck cancers, 482
  conductive, 53
  drug therapy for, 56
  ethical concerns for, 61
  family concerns and considerations on, 61
  interdisciplinary care of, 54-56
  noise-induced, 54
  pathophysiology of, 53-54
  sensorineural, 53
Heart
  disease of
    ischemic, 161-169. *See also* Coronary artery disease (CAD).
    rheumatic, skin signs associated with, 65t
    valvular, 175-176
  disorders of, 161-180
    assessment of, 161, 162b
    case study on, 179-180
    complementary and alternative therapies for, 178-179
    ethical considerations on, 179
    rehabilitation for, 177-178
  failure of, congestive, 169-171, 172-173b
Heberden's nodes, in osteoarthritis, 395, 396f
Helicobacter pylori infection, peptic ulcer disease and, 220, 221b
Hematologic disorders, skin signs associated with, 65t
Hematopoiesis, 135

Hematopoietic growth factors, for cancer, indications and side effects of, 447t
Hemochromatosis, 135, 143-146
  case study on, 147-148
  clinical manifestations of, 144-145
  diagnosis of, 145-146, 145t
  pathophysiology of, 143-144
  treatment and care of, 146
Hemodialysis, 268f
Hemoglobin A_{1C}, average blood glucose level and, relation between, 289t
Hemophilia, 135, 143, 144t
  drugs for, 145t
Hemorrhagic strokes, 329-330
Hepatitis, viral, 242-245
  case study on, 258-259
  cirrhosis from, 245
  clinical manifestations of, 244-245
  cryoglobulinemia manifestations in, 245b
  demographic differences in, 244t
  diagnosis of, 245, 246t
  epidemiology of, 244b
  herbal therapies for, 253t
  interdisciplinary care for, 247-252
  medications for, adverse reactions to, 249b
  pathophysiology of, 242-244
  risk factors for, 244b
  treatment for, responses to, 248b
Herbal therapies, for hepatitis C, 253t
Herceptin (trastuzumab), for cancer, indications and side effects of, 447t
Hernia, hiatal, 220, 221f
Herniation, disk, low back pain from, 430, 431f
Herpes simplex, in HIV/AIDS, 569t, 571
  nursing interventions for, 575t
Herpes zoster, in HIV/AIDS, 569t, 571
  nursing interventions for, 575t
Herplex Liquifilm (idoxuridine), nursing considerations for, 45t
Heterotopic ossification, secondary to spinal cord injury, 372
Hexamethylmelamine, side effects of, 444t
Hiatal hernia, 220, 221f
High-technology private duty care, 15
Highly active antiretroviral therapy (HAART), for HIV/AIDS, 570, 571, 574, 576, 578, 579-580
Hinduism, end-of-life care and, 455t
Hismanal (astemizole), side effects and nursing considerations for, 72t
Hispanic Americans, end-of-life care and, 454t
Histiocytoma, fibrous, malignant, general treatments for, 556t
HIV. *See* Human immunodeficiency virus (HIV).
HIV/AIDS, 565-586
  assessment of, 566, 566b
  case study on, 585
  classification system for, 567t
  clinical manifestations of, 568-572, 568b, 569t
  complementary and alternative therapies for, 582
  diagnosis of, 572-573
  end-of-life care in, 583
  ethical considerations on, 584-585
  ethnic variations in, 565-566
  family and caregiver issues on, 583-584, 584b
  interdisciplinary care for, 573-582
  opportunistic infections in, 568-571, 569t
  palliative care for, 583
  pathophysiology of, 566-568
  prevention counseling for, elements of, 573b
  rehabilitation for, 582-583
Hives, 74-75
Hivid (zalcitabine), for HIV/AIDS, 577t
HMS Liquifilm (medrysone), side effects and nursing considerations for, 45t

Hodgkin's disease, 154, 155t
skin signs associated with, 64t
treatment of, 154-155
Holter monitoring, in coronary artery disease diagnosis, 163t
Home care, 12t, 14
Homemaker, in liver disease care, 252
Homeopathy, 23
Homocysteine level, in coronary artery disease diagnosis, 165t
Hormonal therapy
for breast cancer, 500
in endometrial cancer care, 542
Hormones
disorders of, 284-313. *See also* Endocrine disorders.
major, effects of, 285t
for musculoskeletal disorders, 415, 416t
thyroid, 295. *See also* Thyroid disorders.
Hospice care, 14
end-of-life, 456
Huang qi, for hepatitis C, 253t
Human immunodeficiency virus (HIV)
infection with, 565-586. *See also* HIV/AIDS.
tuberculosis coinfection with, 129
drug therapy for, 131
Humorsol (demecarium), side effects and nursing considerations for, 46t
Huntington's disease (HD), 388-389
Hydralazine (Apresoline), for hypertension, 187t
Hydrea (hydroxyurea), side effects of, 444t
Hydrochlorothiazide (Esidrix, HydroDIURIL, Oretic), for hypertension, 185t
Hydrocodone, with acetaminophen or aspirin (Lorcet, Vicodin), for joint and connective tissue disorders, 398t
Hydrocolloids, in wound care, 91t
Hydrocortisone (Cortaid, Cortef, Solu-Cortef)
for chronic obstructive pulmonary disease, 114t
for cortisol excess/deficiency, 304t
for joint and connective tissue disorders, 398t
HydroDIURIL (hydrochlorothiazide), for hypertension, 185t
Hydrogels, in wound care, 92t
Hydroxychloroquine (Plaquenil), for joint and connective tissue disorders, 397t
Hydroxyurea (Hydrea)
for chronic myelogenous leukemia, 152
for polycythemia, 142
side effects of, 444t
Hydroxyzine (Vistaril, Atarax), 72t
Hygroton (chlorthalidone), for hypertension, 185t
Hylorel (guanadrel sulfate), for hypertension, 186t
Hypercalcemia, immobilization, secondary to spinal cord injury, 372
Hyperpigmentation, 78
Hyperpituitarism, skin signs associated with, 64t
Hypersensitivity reactions, prevention of, 451b
Hyperstat (diazoxide), for hypertension, 187t
Hypertension (HTN), 181-189
chronic kidney disease and, 263
clinical manifestations of, 183-184
diagnosis of, 184, 184t
diet for, 184
drug therapy for, 184, 185-188t
interdisciplinary care for, 184
nursing considerations on, 184, 189
pathophysiology of, 181-183, 183f
Hyperthyroidism
clinical manifestations of, 296, 296f
diagnosis of, 298t
drug therapy for, 298, 299t
hypothyroidism compared with, 297t
pathophysiology of, 295-296
skin signs associated with, 64t
Hypervitaminosis A, skin signs associated with, 64t
Hypnotherapy, 28-29
Hypnotism, for weight loss, 210

Hypoageusia, complicating head and neck cancers, 479
Hypoglycemia, signs and symptoms of, 293b
Hypoparathyroidism, skin signs associated with, 64t
Hypopharynx, 473f
function, anatomic relationships, and cancer features of, 474t
Hypopigmentation, 78
Hypopituitarism, skin signs associated with, 64t
Hypothalamus, hormones of, effects of, 285t
Hypothyroidism
clinical manifestations of, 296, 296f
complicating head and neck cancers, 482
diagnosis of, 298t
drug therapy for, 298-300, 299t
hyperthyroidism compared with, 297t
pathophysiology of, 296
skin signs associated with, 64t
Hytrin (terazosin)
for hypertension, 186t
for urinary incontinence, 278t

I

IBD. *See* Inflammatory bowel disease (IBD).
IBS. *See* Irritable bowel syndrome (IBS).
Ibuprofen (Advil, Motrin)
for headaches, 319t
for joint and connective tissue disorders, 397t
Idamycin (idarubicin), side effects of, 444t
Idarubicin (Idamycin), side effects of, 444t
Idoxuridine (Herplex Liquifilm), nursing considerations for, 45t
Ifex (ifosfamide)
for lung cancer, 511t
for sarcomas, 560t
side effects of, 444t
Ifosfamide (Ifex)
for lung cancer, 511t
for sarcomas, 560t
side effects of, 444t
Illness, in foreground of shifting perspectives model, 5
Imatinib (Gleevec), for chronic myelogenous leukemia, 152-153
Imipramine (Tofranil), for urinary incontinence, 277t
Imitrex (sumatriptan), for migraines, 320t
Immobility, pressure ulcers and, 85
Immobilization hypercalcemia, secondary to spinal cord injury, 372
Immune disorders, skin signs associated with, 64t
Immunomodulators
for neuromuscular disorders, 383t
for ulcerative colitis, 232
Immunosuppressants, for joint and connective tissue disorders, 397t
Immunotherapy, for breast cancer, 501
Imuran (azathioprine)
for Crohn's disease, 231
for joint and connective tissue disorders, 397t
for ulcerative colitis, 232
Incontinence, urinary
functional, 273
medications associated with, 276b
medications for, 277-279t, 277-280
overflow, 273
stress, 272-273
case study on, 282-283
urge, 272
Inderal (propranolol)
for brain disorders, 320t
for hypertension, 187t
for thyroid disorders, 299t
Indinavir (Crixivan), for HIV/AIDS, 578t
Indocin (indomethacin)
for headaches, 319t
for joint and connective tissue disorders, 397t

Indomethacin (Indocin)
    for headaches, 319t
    for joint and connective tissue disorders, 397t
Infection(s)
    of bone, 423-427. *See also* Osteomyelitis.
    cytomegalovirus, in HIV/AIDS, 569t, 570
        nursing interventions for, 575t
    HIV, 565-586. *See also* HIV/AIDS.
    Mycobacterium avium-intracellulare complex, in HIV/AIDS,
        568, 569t
        nursing interventions for, 575t
    opportunistic, in HIV/AIDS, 568-571, 569t
    of urinary tract, secondary to spinal cord injury, 370
Inflamase (prednisolone NA phosphate), side effects and nursing
        considerations for, 45t
Inflammatory bowel disease (IBD), 228, 230-234
    Crohn's disease as, 228, 230-231
    demographic differences in, 229t
    signs and symptoms of, 230t
Infliximab (Remicade), for Crohn's disease, 231
INH (isoniazid), for tuberculosis, 130t
Inhalers
    effective use of, procedure for, 123b
    estimating fullness of, 123f
Inspra (eplerenone), for hypertension, 185t
Insulin, for diabetes mellitus, 290, 291t, 292
Interdisciplinary team (IDT), 15-19
    aides in, 18
    dietitian in, 18
    for eye disorders, 36-39
    function of, 19
    medical social worker in, 18
    nurse practitioner in, 16
    occupational therapist in, 17-18
    pastor/clergy in, 18-19
    patient in, 15-16
    physical therapist in, 16-17
    physicians in, 16
    significant others in, 15-16
Interferon(s)
    for cancer, indications and side effects of, 447t
    for polycythemia, 142
Interleukins, for cancer, indications and side effects of,
        447t
131Iodine therapy, for hyperthyroidism, 298, 299t
Ionamin (phentermine), for weight loss, 210t
Iosartan (Cozaar), for hypertension, 188t
Ipratropium (Atrovent), for chronic obstructive pulmonary
        disease, 114t
Irbesartan (Avapro), for hypertension, 188t
Iron, for cirrhosis, 248b
Iron deficiency anemia, 136
    treatment of, 139
Irritable bowel syndrome (IBS), 236-238
    demographic differences in, 229t
Ischemic heart disease, 161-169. *See also* Coronary artery
        disease (CAD).
Ischemic strokes, 329
Islam, end-of-life care and, 455t
Ismelin (guanethidine), for hypertension, 186t
Ismotic (isosorbide ophthalmic), side effects and nursing
        considerations for, 46t
Isolation, social, 7
Isoniazid (INH, Lanizid, Nydrazid), for tuberculosis,
        130t
Isoptin (verapamil), for hypertension, 188t
Isopto Carpine (pilocarpine), side effects and nursing
        considerations for, 46t
Isopto Eserine (physostigmine), side effects and nursing
        considerations for, 46t
Isopto Tears, side effects and nursing considerations for, 46t
Isosorbide ophthalmic (Ismotic), side effects and nursing
        considerations for, 46t

Isotretinoin (Accutane), side effects and nursing considerations
        for, 73t
Isradipine (DynaCirc), for hypertension, 188t

J

Joint(s)
    degenerative diseases of, 393-400
        assessment of, 393, 394b
        drugs for, 397-398t
        ethnic variations in, 395b
        osteoarthritis as, 393-400. *See also* Osteoarthritis (OA).
    protecting, tips for, 399b
Judaism, end-of-life care and, 455t

K

Kaletra (lopinavir + nitonavir), for HIV/AIDS, 578t
Kanamycin (Kantrex), for tuberculosis, 131t
Kantrex (kanamycin), for tuberculosis, 131t
Kaposi's sarcoma, AIDS-related, 569t, 571
    nursing interventions for, 576t
Karnofsky Performance Scale, 438b
Kegel exercises, for urinary incontinence, 276-277
Keratoconus, nursing considerations for, 47t
Keratolytics, side effects and nursing considerations for, 72t
Keratoplastics, side effects and nursing considerations for, 72t
Keratoses, actinic, 79
Kerlone (betaxolol), for hypertension, 186t
Kidney(s)
    cancer of, 526-528
        skin signs associated with, 64t
    disease of, chronic, 261-270
        assessment of, 261-262, 262b
        case study on, 270
        classification of, 264t
        clinical action plans for, 267t
        clinical manifestations of, 263, 265
        complications of, 265-266
        definition of, 263b
        diagnosis of, 265
        dialysis for, trends in, 266-268
        end-of-life issues in, 269
        ethical issues in, 269
        ethnic variations in, 262
        family and caregiver issues in, 269
        interdisciplinary care for, 266
        management goals for, 267t
        pathophysiology of, 262-263
        prevalence of individuals at risk for, 263t
        risk factors for, kidney disease type and, 264t
        transplantation for, 268-269
    disorders of, skin signs associated with, 65t
    failure of, chronic, skin signs associated with, 65t
    incidence of, 517t
    risk factors for, 517t
    transplantation of, 268-269
Klonopin (clonazepam), for seizure disorders, 319t
Kytril (granisetron), for brain disorders, 322t

L

L-Asperginase (Elspar), side effects of, 444t
Labetalol (Normodyne, Trandate), for hypertension, 187t
Laboratory studies, in coronary artery disease diagnosis,
        164-165t
Labyrinthitis, pathophysiology of, 57
Lacri-Lube, side effects and nursing considerations for, 46t
Lactulose, for cirrhosis, 248b
Lamictal (lamotrigine), for seizure disorders, 320t
Lamivudine (3TC, Epivir), for HIV/AIDS, 577t
Lamotrigine (Lamictal), for seizure disorders, 320t
Lanizid (isoniazid), for tuberculosis, 130t
Lansoprazole (Prevacid)
    for gastroesophageal reflux disease and peptic ulcer, 217t
    for *Helicobacter pylori* infection, 223t

Laryngectomy
    complications of, 484b
    nursing interventions for, 485b
    problems associated with, 483-484, 484b
Larynx, 473f
    function, anatomic relationships, and cancer features
        of, 475t
Lasix (furosemide), for hypertension, 185t
Latino Americans, end-of-life care and, 454t
Laxatives, for cancer symptom management, 448t
LBP. *See* Low back pain (LBP).
Leflunomide (Arava), for joint and connective tissue
        disorders, 397t
Legal documents, related to end-of-life decisions, 452b
Legislation, on end-of-life decisions, 452b
Leiomyosarcoma, general treatments for, 556t
Leukemia, 150-153
    chronic lymphocytic, 153
    chronic myelogenous, 150-153
        case study on, 159-160
        clinical manifestations of, 151-152
        diagnosis of, 152b
        pathophysiology of, 150
        treatment of, 152-253
    overview of, 149
Leukeran (chlorambucil), side effects of, 444t
Leukine (sargramostim)
    for cancer, indications and side effects of, 447t
    for lung cancer, 511t
Leukoencephalopathy, progressive multifocal, AIDS-related,
        569t, 572
Leukotriene modifiers, for chronic obstructive pulmonary
        disease, 115t
Leustatin (cladribine), side effects of, 444t
Levaquin (levofloxacin), for tuberculosis, 131t
Levatol (penbutolol), for hypertension, 186t
Levobunolol (Betagan Liquifilm), side effects and nursing
        considerations for, 46t
Levodopa, for neuromuscular disorders, 384t
Levofloxacin (Levaquin), for tuberculosis, 131t
Levothyroxine (Synthroid), for hypothyroidism, 298-300, 299t
Lewy body disease, pathophysiology of, 349
Licorice root, for hepatitis C, 253t
Lifestyle modifications, for gastroesophageal reflux disease,
        education on, 218-219, 219t
Liothyronine (Cytomel), for hypothyroidism, 298-299
Lipidoses, skin signs associated with, 64t
Lipitor (torvastatin), for brain disorders, 321t
Lipodystrophy, in HIV/AIDS, 581
Lipoprotein, low-density, recommended levels of, based on risk,
        333t
Liposarcomas, general treatments for, 556t
Lisinopril (Prinivil, Zestril)
    for brain disorders, 321t
    for hypertension, 188t
Liver
    cancer of, 522-524
        incidence of, 517t
        risk factors for, 517t
    disease of, skin signs associated with, 64t
    disorders of, 241-252
        assessment of, 241, 242t, 243t
        cirrhosis as, 245-252
        end-stage, 245-252
            causes of, 246t
        energy conservation tips for, 252b
        ethical considerations in, 248b
        patient and family education on, 250t
        viral hepatitis as, 242-245. *See also* Hepatitis, viral.
Living Will, 452b
Lomustine (CCNU), side effects of, 444t
Long-term care, for blood disorder patients, 147
Long-term care settings, 11-12, 12t

Loniten (minoxidil), for hypertension, 187t
Loop diuretics, for hypertension, 185t
Loperamide, for Crohn's disease, 231
Lopinavir + ritonavir (ABT-378r, Kaletra), for HIV/AIDS, 578t
Lopressor (metoprolol), for hypertension, 186t
Loratadine (Claritin), nursing considerations for, 72t
Lorazepam (Ativan)
    for brain disorders, 322t
    side effects and nursing considerations for, 57t
Lorcet (hydrocodone with acetaminophen), for joint and connective
        tissue disorders, 398t
Lotensin (benazepril), for hypertension, 188t
Low back pain (LBP), 430-433
    clinical manifestations of, 431
    complementary and alternative therapies or, 433
    diagnosis of, 431-432
    ethical considerations on, 433
    interdisciplinary care for, 432-433
    pathophysiology of, 430-431
Low vision specialist
    in age-related macular degeneration care, 40
    in diabetic retinopathy care, 43
    in eye disorder care, 38
Lower extremity ulcers, 95-105. *See also* Ulcer(s), lower extremity.
Lubricants, ophthalmic, side effects and nursing considerations
        for, 46t
Lumbosacral tumors, manifestations of, 465t
Luminal (phenobarbital), for brain disorders, 319t
Lumpectomy, 498
Lung(s)
    cancer of, 507-515
        assessment of, 507-508, 509b
        case study on, 514-515
        clinical manifestations of, 508-509
        diagnosis of, 509
        end-of-life care in, 513-514
        ethical considerations on, 514
        ethnic variations in, 507
        family and caregiver issues on, 514
        interdisciplinary care for, 510-513
        pathophysiology of, 508
        skin signs associated with, 64t
        warning signs of, 508
    obstructive disease of, chronic, 109-117. *See also* Chronic
        obstructive pulmonary disease (COPD).
    radiation side effects on, 442t
Lupus erythematosus, systemic, 404-406, 405f
    skin signs associated with, 64t
Lymphedema
    after breast cancer treatment, 499
    complicating head and neck cancers, 473, 476
    problems associated with, 477b
    skin care for, 477b
Lymphocytic leukemia, chronic, 153
Lymphoma(s), 153-156
    Ann Arbor staging system for, 155b
    clinical manifestations of, 154
    diagnosis of, 154
    non-Hodgkin's, AIDS-related, 569t, 571-572
        nursing interventions for, 576t
    overview of, 149
    pathophysiology of, 153-154
    skin signs associated with, 64t
    T-cell, 80-81
    treatment of, 154-156
Lysodren (mitotane)
    for cortisol excess/deficiency, 304t
    side effects of, 445t

M

M-AMSA (amsacrine), side effects of, 444t
Maalox (aluminum hydroxide with magnesium hydroxide), for
        gastroesophageal reflux disease and peptic ulcer, 216t

Macrocytic anemia, 137-138
Macular degeneration, age-related, 40
Macule, 67t
Magnesium hydroxide, with aluminum hydroxide (Maalox, Mylanta),
  for gastroesophageal reflux disease and peptic ulcer, 216t
Magnesium salts, for cancer symptom management, 448t
Malabsorption syndromes, 238-239
  demographic differences in, 229t
  skin signs associated with, 64t
Malignancy(ies)
  AIDS-related, 569t, 571-572
  of blood, 149-160
    assessment of, 149-150
      functional health pattern, 151b
    case study on, 159-160
    end-of-life issues on, 159b
    ethical issues on, 158b
    ethnic variations in, 149
    family and caregiver issues on, 158b
    interdisciplinary care for, 158-159
    leukemia as, 150-153. *See also* Leukemia.
    lymphomas as, 153-156. *See also* Lymphoma(s).
    multiple myeloma as, 156-157, 157b
    overview of, 149
Malignant fibrous histiocytoma, general treatments for, 556t
Malignant melanoma, 80, 80b
Malnutrition, 205-208
  assessment of, 206
  clinical manifestations of, 205
  demographic characteristics of, 198b
  diagnosis of, 205-206
  family and caregiver issues associated with, 208
  interdisciplinary care in, 206-208
  pathophysiology of, 205
  pressure ulcers and, 86
  risk factors for, 205b
Mammography
  in breast cancer diagnosis, 494, 495f
  digital, in breast cancer diagnosis, 495
Manipulative therapies, 30-33
Mannitol (Osmitrol), side effects and nursing considerations
  for, 46t
Marinol (dronabinol), for malnutrition, 206
Mask, for oxygen administration, 116t
Mast cell stabilizers, for chronic obstructive pulmonary disease, 114t
Mastectomy
  indications for, 498b
  types of, 498
Matulane (procarbazine)
  for lung cancer, 511t
  side effects of, 445t
Mavik (trandolapril), for hypertension, 188t
Maxair (pirbuterol), for chronic obstructive pulmonary disease, 114t
Maxalt (rizatriptan), for migraines, 320t
Mazanor (mazindol), for weight loss, 210t
Mazindol (Sanorex, Mazanor), for weight loss, 210t
Mechlorethamine (Mustargen, nitrogen mustard)
  for lung cancer, 511t
  side effects of, 445t
Meclizine (Antivert, Bonine, Antrizine)
  side effects and nursing considerations for, 57t
  for traumatic brain injury, 340t
Meclofenamate (Meclomen)
  for headaches, 319t
  for joint and connective tissue disorders, 397t
Meclomen (meclofenamate)
  for headaches, 319t
  for joint and connective tissue disorders, 397t
Mediastinum, radiation side effects on, 442t
Medical management, of spinal cord injury, 373
Medical oncologist
  in cancer care, 443-446
  in sarcoma care, 557-558

Medical social worker
  in anorexia nervosa care, 201-202
  in arterial ulcer care, 103
  in binge eating disorder care, 204
  in blood malignancy care, 158-159
  in brain tumor care, 463
  in breast cancer care, 502-503
  in Buerger's disease care, 191
  in cancer care, 451
  in chronic pancreatitis care, 257
  in colorectal cancer care, 522
  in Cushing's syndrome care, 305
  in dementia care, 359
  in diabetes mellitus care, 294
  in epilepsy care, 328
  in eye disorder care, 39
  in fibromyalgia care, 422
  in head and neck cancer care, 487
  in HIV/AIDS, 582
  in interdisciplinary team, 18
  in liver disease care, 251-252
  in low back pain care, 433
  in lung cancer care, 513
  in malnutrition care, 206
  in osteomyelitis care, 426
  in osteoporosis care, 419
  in Paget's disease care, 430
  in pressure ulcer care, 95
  in Raynaud's phenomenon care, 193
  in rheumatoid arthritis care, 404
  in sarcoma care, 562
  in spinal cord cancer care, 467
  in spinal cord injury care, 373-374
  in stroke care, 334
  in systemic lupus erythematosus care, 406
  in tuberculosis care, 132
  in ulcerative colitis care, 233-234
  in urinary bladder cancer care, 530
  in venous stasis disease care, 101
  in wound care, 95
Medications. *See also* Drug(s).
  ophthalmic, 45-46t
Medrol (methylprednisolone), for cortisol excess/deficiency,
  304t
Medrysone (HMS Liquifilm), side effects and nursing considerations
  for, 45t
Megace (megestrol), side effects of, 445t
Megestrol (Megace), side effects of, 445t
Meglitinides, for diabetes mellitus, 291t
Melanoma, malignant, 80, 80b
Melphalan (Alkeran), side effects of, 445t
Ménière's disease, 53
  pathophysiology of, 57
Meninges, of brain, 460f
Menthol, side effects and nursing considerations for, 72t
Meperidine (Demerol), for migraine rescue, 322t
Mephenytoin (Mesantoin), for seizure disorders, 319t
6-Mercaptopurine (6-MP, Purinethol)
  side effects of, 445t
  for ulcerative colitis, 232
Meridia (sibutramine), for weight loss, 210t
Mesantoin (mephenytoin), for seizure disorders, 319t
Metabolic disorders
  associated with arthritis, 408-409
  skin signs associated with, 64t
Metabolic profile, comprehensive, in coronary artery disease
  diagnosis, 164t
Metahydrin (trichlormethiazide), for hypertension, 185t
Metaproterenol (Alupent), for chronic obstructive pulmonary
  disease, 114t
Metformin (Glucophage), for diabetes mellitus, 291t
Methazolamide (Neptazane), side effects and nursing considerations
  for, 45t

Methimazole (Tapazole), for hyperthyroidism, 298, 299t
Methotrexate (MTX, Amethopterin, Rheumatrex)
    for Crohn's disease, 231
    for joint and connective tissue disorders, 397t
    for lung cancer, 511t
    for neuromuscular disorders, 383t
    for sarcomas, 560t
    side effects of, 445t
Methoxsalen (Oxsoralen), side effects and nursing considerations
        for, 73t
Methyclothiazide (Enduron), for hypertension, 185t
Methyl CCNU (semustine), side effects of, 445t
Methyldopa (Aldomet), for hypertension, 186t
Methylphenidate (Ritalin), for brain disorders, 322t
Methylprednisolone (Medrol, Solu-Medrol)
    for chronic obstructive pulmonary disease, 114t
    for cortisol excess/deficiency, 304t
    for neuromuscular disorders, 383t
Methysergide (Sansert), for migraines, 320t
Metoclopramide (Reglan), for gastroesophageal reflux disease and
        peptic ulcer, 217t
Metolazone (Zaroxolyn), for hypertension, 185t
Metoprolol (Lopressor), for hypertension, 186t
MetroGel (metronidazole 0.75%), side effects and nursing considerations
        for, 73t
Metronidazole 0.75% (MetroGel), side effects and nursing considerations
        for, 73t
Metronidazole (Flagyl), for *Helicobacter pylori* infection, 223t
Miacalcin (calcitonin), for musculoskeletal disorders, 416t
Mibefradil (Posicor), for hypertension, 188t
Micardis (telmisartan), for hypertension, 188t
Microcytic anemia, 136-137
Micronase (glyburide), for diabetes mellitus, 292t
Midamor (amiloride), for hypertension, 185t
Miglitol (Glyset), for diabetes mellitus, 291t
Migraine, 315
    clinical manifestations of, 317
    disability assessment scale for, 317b
Migranal (dihydroergotamine), for migraines, 320t
Miliary tuberculosis, 129
Milk thistle, for hepatitis C, 253t
Mind-body therapy, 28-29
Mineral oil, side effects and nursing considerations for, 73t
Mineralocorticoids, for cortisol excess/deficiency, 304t
Minipress (prazosin), for hypertension, 186t
Minoxidil (Loniten), for hypertension, 187t
Miochol (acetylcholine), side effects and nursing considerations
        for, 46t
Miostat (carbachol), side effects and nursing considerations for, 46t
Miotics, side effects and nursing considerations for, 46t
Mithracin (mithramycin, plicamycin)
    for musculoskeletal disorders, 417t
    side effects of, 445t
Mithramycin (Mithracin, plicamycin)
    for musculoskeletal disorders, 417t
    side effects of, 445t
Mitomycin (Mutamycin)
    for lung cancer, 511t
    side effects of, 445t
Mitotane (Lysodren)
    for cortisol excess/deficiency, 304t
    side effects of, 445t
Mitoxantrone (Novantrone), side effects of, 445t
Mitral valve disorders, 175-176, 176f
MM. *See* Multiple myeloma (MM).
Moexipril (Univasc), for hypertension, 188t
Moisture, pressure ulcers and, 85
Moles, assessment format for, 63, 69f
Monoamine oxidase (MAO) inhibitors, for neuromuscular disorders,
        383t
Monoclonal antibodies
    for cancer, indications and side effects of, 447t
    for neuromuscular disorders, 383t, 384t

Monoclonal factors, recombinant, for hemophilia, 145t
Monopril (fosinopril), for hypertension, 188t
Montelukast (Singular), for chronic obstructive pulmonary disease,
        115t
Motor paralytic bladder, 274
Motrin (ibuprofen)
    for headaches, 319t
    for joint and connective tissue disorders, 397t
Mouth, dry, complicating head and neck cancers, 478-479, 479b
6-MP (6-mercaptopurine). *See* 6-Mercaptopurine (6-MP, Purinethol).
MS (multiple sclerosis), 384-385
MTX (methotrexate)
    for Crohn's disease, 231
    for lung cancer, 511t
    for sarcomas, 560t
    side effects of, 445t
Muci-fradin (neomycin), 72t
Mucositis, complicating cancer treatment, nursing interventions for,
        450b
Multiple hereditary exostosis, musculoskeletal tumors with, 555b
Multiple myeloma, overview of, 149
Multiple myeloma (MM), 156-157, 157b
Multiple sclerosis (MS), 384-385
Mupirocin (Bactroban), 72t
Muscle relaxants
    for musculoskeletal disorders, 417t
    for neuromuscular disorders, 383t
Muscle trismus, complicating head and neck cancers, 481-482
Musculoskeletal system
    cancers of, 553-564
        assessment of, 553, 554b
        diagnosis of, 553-554
        hereditary conditions with, 555b
        sarcomas as, 554-563. *See also* Sarcomas.
    disorders of, 412-435
        ethnic variations in, 412
        fibromyalgia as, 420-422
        low back pain as, 430-433. *See also* Low back pain (LBP).
        osteomyelitis as, 423-427. *See also* Osteomyelitis.
        osteoporosis as, 412-419. *See also* Osteoporosis.
        Paget's disease as, 427-430. *See also* Paget's disease.
        skin signs associated with, 64t
Mustargen (mechlorethamine), for lung cancer, 511t
Mutamycin (mitomycin)
    for lung cancer, 511t
    side effects of, 445t
Myambutol (ethambutol), for tuberculosis, 130t
Mycobacterium avium-intracellulare complex infection, in HIV/AIDS,
        568, 569t
    nursing interventions for, 575t
Mydriatics, side effects and nursing considerations for, 46t
Myelogenous leukemia, chronic, 150-153
Myeloma, multiple, 156-157
Mylanta (aluminum hydroxide with magnesium hydroxide), for
        gastroesophageal reflux disease and peptic ulcer, 216t
Myleran (busulfan), side effects of, 444t
Myochrysine (gold sodium thiomalate), for joint and connective tissue
        disorders, 397t
Myxedema, 296

N

Nadolol (Corgard)
    for hypertension, 186t
    for thyroid disorders, 299t
Nalfon (fenoprofen)
    for headaches, 319t
    for joint and connective tissue disorders, 397t
Naprosyn (naproxen)
    for headaches, 319t
    for joint and connective tissue disorders, 397t
Naproxen (Aleve, Naprosyn)
    for headaches, 319t
    for joint and connective tissue disorders, 397t

Naqua (trichlormethiazide), for hypertension, 185t
Naratriptan (Amerge), for migraines, 320t
Narcotics, in lung cancer care, 511
Nasal cannula, for oxygen administration, 116t
Nasal cavity, 473f
    function, anatomic relationships, and cancer features of, 474t
Nasopharynx, 473f
    function, anatomic relationships, and cancer features of, 474t
Natacyn (natamycin), side effects of, 45t
Natamycin (Natacyn), side effects of, 45t
National Center for Complementary and Alternative Medicine (NCCAM), 21
    research priorities of, 22b
Native Americans, end-of-life care and, 454t
Naturetin (bendroflumethiazide), for hypertension, 185t
Naturopathic medicine, 26
Nausea, complicating cancer treatment, nursing interventions for, 450b
Navelbine (vinblastine, vinorelbine)
    for lung cancer, 511t
    side effects of, 445t
Neck, cancers of, 470-491. *See also* Head and neck, cancers of.
Nedocromil (Tilade), for chronic obstructive pulmonary disease, 114t
Nelfinavir (Viracept), for HIV/AIDS, 578t
Nembutal (pentobarbital sodium), for brain disorders, 319t
Neptazane (methazolamide), side effects and nursing considerations for, 45t
Neomycin (Muci-fradin), 72t
Neosporin (bacitracin), 72t
Nerves, spinal, 368, 368b, 369f
Neumega (oprelvekin)
    for cancer, indications and side effects of, 447t
    for lung cancer, 511t
Neupogen (filgrastim)
    for cancer, indications and side effects of, 447t
    for lung cancer, 511t
Neurofibromatosis, musculoskeletal tumors with, 555b
Neurofibrosarcoma, general treatments for, 556t
Neurogenic bladder, 273
Neuroleptics
    for cancer symptom management, 448t
    for traumatic brain injury, 340t
Neurologic disorders, skin signs associated with, 65t
Neurologist
    in dementia care, 351
    in epilepsy care, 326
    in stroke care, 332
    in traumatic brain injury care, 339
Neuroma, acoustic, 53
Neuromuscular disorders, 378-392
    amyotrophic lateral sclerosis as, 390
    assessment of, 378-380, 379b
    case study on, 391-392
    complementary and alternative therapies for, 384
    diagnosis of, 380, 381t
    end-of-life issues in, 391
    ethical considerations on, 391, 391b
    family and caregiver issues in, 391
    Guillain-Barré syndrome as, 386
    Huntington's disease as, 388-389
    interdisciplinary care for, 380-382, 383-384t
    multiple sclerosis as, 384-385
    Parkinson's disease as, 387-388
    rehabilitation focus in, 390-391
Neuromusculoskeletal disorders, secondary to spinal cord injury, 371-372
Neuronitis, vestibular, pathophysiology of, 57
Neurontin (gabapentin), for brain disorders, 320t
Neuropsychiatrist, in traumatic brain injury care, 339
Neuropsychologist, in traumatic brain injury care, 339
Neurosurgeon, in epilepsy care, 326
Nevi, assessment format for, 63, 69f

Nevirapine (Viramune), for HIV/AIDS, 577t
Nexium (esomeprazole)
    for gastroesophageal reflux disease and peptic ulcer, 217t
    for *Helicobacter pylori* infection, 223t
Niacin deficiency, skin signs associated with, 64t
Nicardipine (Cardene), for hypertension, 188t
Nicotine. *See also* Smoking.
Nicotine products, in chronic obstructive pulmonary disease management, 115t
Nicotinic acid deficiency, skin signs associated with, 64t
Nifedipine (Procardia), for hypertension, 188t
Nimodipine (Nimotop), for brain disorders, 321t
Nimotop (nimodipine), for brain disorders, 321t
Nipent (pentostatin), side effects of, 445t
Nipride (sodium nitroprusside), for hypertension, 187t
Nisoldipine (Sular), for hypertension, 188t
Nissen fundoplication, for gastroesophageal reflux disease, 219, 219f
Nitrates, for coronary artery disease, 166
Nitrogen mustard (mechlorethamine), side effects of, 445t
Nitroglycerin (Tridil), for hypertension, 187t
Nivea lotion, 73t
Nizatidine (Axid), for gastroesophageal reflux disease and peptic ulcer, 217t
Nocturnal dialysis, 267-268
Nodule, 67t
Noise-induced hearing loss, 54
Nolvadex (tamoxifen), side effects of, 445t
Non-Hodgkin's lymphoma, 154, 155t
    AIDS-related, 569t, 571-572
        nursing interventions for, 576t
    international prognostic index for, 155b
    treatment of, 155-156
Nonnucleoside reverse transcriptase inhibitors, for HIV/AIDS, 577t
Nonsteroidal antiinflammatory drugs (NSAIDs)
    for headaches, 319t
    peptic ulcer disease and, 220, 222b
    for rheumatoid arthritis, 403
Norfloxacin (Noroxin), nursing considerations for, 45t
Normodyne (labetalol), for hypertension, 187t
Noroxin (norfloxacin), nursing considerations for, 45t
Norton scale risk assessment tool, for pressure ulcers, 86, 89t
Nortriptyline (Pamelor), for urinary incontinence, 277t
Norvasc (amlodipine), for hypertension, 188t
Norvir (ritonavir), for HIV/AIDS, 578t
Novantrone (mitoxantrone), side effects of, 445t
Novocolchine (colchicine), for joint and connective tissue disorders, 398t
NSAIDs. *See* Nonsteroidal antiinflammatory drugs (NSAIDs).
Nuclear cardiology, in coronary artery disease diagnosis, 164t
Nucleoside reverse transcriptase inhibitors, for HIV/AIDS, 577t
Nucleotide reverse transcriptase inhibitor, for HIV/AIDS, 577t
Nurse(s)
    in acromegaly care, 311
    in Addison's disease care, 306-307
    in age-related macular degeneration care, 40
    in anorexia nervosa care, 200-201
    in arterial ulcer care, 102-103
    in asthma care, 120
    in binge eating disorder care, 204
    in bladder disorder care, 280-281, 281t
    in blood disorder care, 146
    in blood malignancy care, 158
    in brain tumor care, 462-463
    in breast cancer care, 501-502
    in cancer care, 446-447, 450-451, 450b
    in cataract care, 41
    in cervical cancer care, 540
    in cholelithiasis care, 254
    in chronic kidney disease care, 266
    in chronic liver disease care, 249-250
    in chronic obstructive pulmonary disease care, 112-113

Nurse(s) *(Continued)*
   in chronic pancreatitis care, 256-257
   in colorectal cancer care, 522
   in Crohn's disease care, 231
   in Cushing's syndrome care, 303
   in dementia care, 354
   in diabetes mellitus care, 293-294
   in diabetic foot ulcer care, 104
   in diabetic retinopathy care, 43
   in diverticular disease care, 235
   in endometrial cancer care, 542
   in epilepsy care, 327
   in eye disorder care, 37-38
   in fibromyalgia care, 421-422
   in gastroesophageal reflux disease care, 218
   in glaucoma care, 44
   in gout care, 409
   in head and neck cancer care, 486
   in headache care, 318, 323
   in hearing loss care, 55
   in HIV/AIDS care, 574, 575-576t
   in irritable bowel syndrome care, 237
   in liver cancer care, 524
   in low back pain care, 432
   in lung cancer care, 512
   in malabsorption syndrome care, 239
   in malnutrition care, 206
   in neuromuscular disorder care, 381-382
   in obesity care, 209
   in osteoarthritis care, 396
   in osteomyelitis care, 425
   in osteoporosis care, 418
   in ovarian cancer care, 537
   in Paget's disease care, 429
   in pancreatic cancer care, 525-526
   in peptic ulcer disease care, 224
   in prostate cancer care, 550
   in renal cell carcinoma care, 528
   in rheumatoid arthritis care, 403
   in sarcoma care, 559-561
   in skin disorder care, 66, 69
   in spinal cord cancer care, 466
   in spinal cord injury care, 373
   in stroke care, 333-334
   in systemic lupus erythematosus care, 406
   in systemic sclerosis care, 407-408
   in testicular cancer care, 547
   in thyroid disorder care, 300
   in traumatic brain injury care, 340
   in tuberculosis care, 131-132
   in ulcerative colitis care, 232-233, 234b
   in urinary bladder cancer care, 529
   in vaginal cancer care, 546
   in vestibular disorder care, 60
   in vulvar cancer care, 544
   wound, ostomy, and continence
     in pressure ulcer care, 93, 95
     in venous stasis disease care, 101
Nurse practitioner. *See also* Primary provider.
   in eye disorder care, 37
   in interdisciplinary team, 16
Nursing centers, 13
Nursing practice model, 4, 4f
Nutrition
   deficits in, pressure ulcers and, 86
   in HIV/AIDS management, 580-581, 581b, 582b
   in skin disorder management, 66
Nutritional anemia, 204-205
   demographic characteristics of, 198b
Nutritional care, for chronic kidney disease, 266
Nutritional disorders, 197-198, 205-211. *See also* Eating disorders.
   assessment of, 197-198, 199b
   demographic differences in, 198b

Nutritional disorders *(Continued)*
   malnutrition as, 205-208. *See also* Malnutrition.
   nutritional anemia as, 204-205
   overweight/obesity as, 208-210. *See also* Overweight/obesity.
   undernourishment as, 205-208. *See also* Malnutrition.
Nydrazid (isoniazid), for tuberculosis, 130t
Nystagmus, in vertigo, 58

O

OA. *See* Osteoarthritis (OA).
Obesity, 208-210. *See also* Overweight/obesity.
Obstructive airway disease, 107-125
   assessment of, 107-109
   asthma as, 118-123. *See also* Asthma.
   case study on, 124
   chronic obstructive pulmonary disease as, 109-117. *See also* Chronic obstructive pulmonary disease (COPD).
   end-of-life issues in, 123-124
   ethnic variations in, 108-109
   family and caregiver issues in, 123
   functional health pattern assessment for, 108b
   overview of, 107
   palliative care for, 123-124
Obstructive sleep apnea (OSA), complicating head and neck cancers, 483, 483b
Oby-trim (phentermine), for weight loss, 210t
Occupational therapist
   in arterial ulcer care, 103
   in bladder disorder care, 281-282
   in blood malignancy care, 158
   in brain tumor care, 463
   in breast cancer care, 502
   in cancer care, 451
   in cardiac rehabilitation, 178
   in chronic obstructive pulmonary disease care, 113
   in Cushing's syndrome care, 305
   in dementia care, 359
   in diabetes mellitus care, 294
   in diabetic foot ulcer care, 105
   in diabetic retinopathy care, 43
   in eye disorder care, 38-39
   in fibromyalgia care, 422
   in HIV/AIDS care, 581
   in interdisciplinary team, 17-18
   in liver disease care, 252
   in neuromuscular disorder care, 382, 382f
   in osteoarthritis care, 399
   in osteoporosis care, 419
   in Raynaud's phenomenon care, 193
   in rheumatoid arthritis care, 404
   in sarcoma care, 561-562
   in spinal cord injury care, 373
   in stroke care, 334-335
   in systemic sclerosis care, 408
   in tuberculosis care, 132-133
   in venous stasis disease care, 101
Octreotide (Sandostatin), for acromegaly, 310, 310t
Ocufen (flurbiprofen), side effects and nursing considerations for, 45t
Ocular prosthesis, care of, 48b
Ofloxacin (Floxin), for tuberculosis, 131t
Okuda staging system, for liver cancer, 523t
Oligodendromas, 460
Ollier's disease, musculoskeletal tumors with, 555b
Olmesartan (Benicar), for hypertension, 188t
Omeprazole (Prilosec), for gastroesophageal reflux disease and peptic ulcer, 217t
Oncologist
   in breast cancer care, 499-500
   in cervical cancer care, 539-540
   in colorectal cancer care, 521
   in endometrial cancer care, 542
   in liver cancer care, 523

Oncologist *(Continued)*
  medical
    in cancer care, 443-446
    in sarcoma care, 557-558
  in ovarian cancer care, 536-537
  in pancreatic cancer care, 525
  radiation
    in breast cancer care, 500-501
    in cancer care, 439-442
    in colorectal cancer care, 522
    in sarcoma care, 558-559
  in renal cell carcinoma care, 528
  surgical, in sarcoma care, 556-557
  in testicular cancer care, 547
  in urinary bladder cancer care, 529
  in vaginal cancer care, 545
  in vulvar cancer care, 543-544
Oncovin (vincristine)
  for sarcomas, 560t
  side effects of, 445t
Ondansetron (Zofran), for brain disorders, 322t
Ophthaine (proparacaine), nursing considerations for, 45t
Ophthalmologist
  in age-related macular degeneration care, 40
  in cataract care, 41
  in eye disorder care, 38
  in glaucoma care, 44
Ophthetic (proparacaine), nursing considerations for, 45t
Opiate analgesics, for migraine rescue, 322t
Opioids
  for cancer symptom management, 448t
  in head and neck cancer care, 485-486
  in lung cancer care, 511
Opportunistic infections, in HIV/AIDS, 568-571, 569t
Oprelvekin (Neumega)
  for cancer, indications and side effects of, 447t
  for lung cancer, 511t
Oral cavity, 473f
  function, anatomic relationships, and cancer features of,
    474t
Oretic (hydrochlorothiazide), for hypertension, 185t
Organs, radiosensitivity of, 441t
Orinase (tolbutamide), for diabetes mellitus, 292t
Orlistat (Xenical), for weight loss, 210t
Oropharynx, 473f
  function, anatomic relationships, and cancer features of,
    474t
Orthopedic surgeon, in low back pain care, 432
Orthotist
  in arterial ulcer care, 103
  in diabetic foot ulcer care, 105
Osmitrol (mannitol), side effects and nursing considerations
    for, 46t
Osmotics
  for cancer symptom management, 449t
  side effects and nursing considerations for, 46t
Ossification, heterotopic, secondary to spinal cord injury, 372
Osteitis deformans, 427-430. *See also* Paget's disease.
Osteoarthritis (OA), 393-400
  clinical manifestations of, 395
  complementary and alternative therapies for, 399-400,
    401b
  diagnosis of, 395
  functional assessment instruments for, 395b
  interdisciplinary care for, 395-399
  pain of, managing, recommendations for, 399b
  pathophysiology of, 394-395
  rheumatoid arthritis compared with, 401t
Osteomyelitis
  clinical manifestations of, 424
  complementary and alternative therapies for, 426
  diagnosis of, 424
  ethical considerations on, 427

Osteomyelitis *(Continued)*
  interdisciplinary care for, 424-426
  pathophysiology of, 423
  staging system for, 423b
Osteopenia, definition of, 413b
Osteoporosis, 412-419
  case study on, 433-434
  clinical manifestations of, 413-414, 414f
  complementary and alternative therapies for, 419
  definitions of, 413b
  diagnosis of, 414-415
  interdisciplinary care for, 415-419
  pathophysiology of, 412-413
  preventing and managing, 415b
  risk factors for, 413b
  secondary to spinal cord injury, 372
Osteoradionecrosis, complicating head and neck cancers,
    481
Osteosarcoma, general treatments for, 556t
Ostomy, for ulcerative colitis, nursing care for, 232-233,
    234b
Otoscope, in hearing loss assessment, 50-51, 51b, 51f
Ototoxic agents, exposure to, 53
Outpatient clinics, 14
Ovarian cancer, 533-537
  advanced, nursing interventions for, 538b
  assessment of, 535
  case study on, 550-551
  clinical manifestations of, 535, 536b
  diagnosis of, 535-536
  ethnic differences in, 535b
  interdisciplinary care for, 536-537
  pathophysiology of, 533-535
  signs and symptoms of, 536b
  skin signs associated with, 64t
Overflow incontinence, 273
Overweight/obesity, 208-210
  clinical manifestations of, 208
  diagnosis of, 208
  interdisciplinary care of, 208-210
  pathophysiology of, 208
Oxaliplatin (Eloxatin)
  for colorectal cancer, 521
  side effects of, 445t
Oxcarbazepine (Trileptal), for brain disorders, 320t
Oxitropium (Oxivent), for chronic obstructive pulmonary
    disease, 114t
Oxivent (oxitropium), for chronic obstructive pulmonary
    disease, 114t
Oxsoralen (methoxsalen), side effects and nursing considerations
    for, 73t
Oxybutynin (Ditropan), for urinary incontinence, 277t
Oxycodone, with acetaminophen or aspirin (Percodan, Percocet, Tylox),
    for joint and connective tissue disorders, 398t
Oxygen therapy
  for chronic obstructive pulmonary disease, equipment for, guidelines
    for care of, 117b
  in chronic obstructive pulmonary disease
    delivery methods for, 116t
    devices for administration of, 116t
    safety tips for, 117b
  in chronic obstructive pulmonary disease management, 113
Oxymetholone (Anadrol-50), side effects of, 445t

P

Paclitaxel (Taxol), side effects of, 445t
Paget's disease
  bones affected by, 427t
  clinical manifestations of, 427-428, 428f
  diagnosis of, 428-429
  interdisciplinary care for, 429-430
  pathophysiology of, 427
  skin signs associated with, 65t

Pain
  central poststroke, 331
  chronic, 6
  cultural responses to, 6
  in head and neck cancers, management of, 485-486
  low back, 430-433. *See also* Low back pain (LBP).
  in lung cancer, management of, 512
  management of, 6b
  secondary to spinal cord injury, 372
  shoulder, after stroke, 331-332
Palliative care
  for breast cancer, 503
  end-of-life, 456
  for head and neck cancers, 487-488
  for HIV/AIDS, 583
  for lung cancer, 514
  for obstructive airway disease, 123
Pamelor (nortriptyline), for urinary incontinence, 277t
Pamidronate (Aredia), for musculoskeletal disorders, 416t
Pancreas
  cancer of, 524-526
    incidence of, 517t
    risk factors for, 517t
  hormones of, effects of, 285t
Pancreatic enzymes
  for cirrhosis, 248b
  teaching points related to, 526b
Pancreatitis
  chronic, 255-258
  demographic differences in, 244t
Panlobular emphysema, 111
Pantoprazole (Protonix)
  for gastroesophageal reflux disease and peptic ulcer, 217t
  for *Helicobacter pylori* infection, 232t
Papanicolaou (Pap) smear testing, in cervical cancer
    diagnosis, 537
Papule, 67t
Paralytic bladder, 273-274
Paranasal sinuses, function, anatomic relationships, and cancer
    features of, 474t
Paraneoplastic syndromes, 437b
Paraplatin (carboplatin), side effects of, 444t
Paraplegia, 362
Parkinson's disease (PD), 349, 387-388
Parlodel (bromocriptine), for acromegaly, 310, 310t
Paroxetine (Paxil), for musculoskeletal disorders, 417t
Parse's theory on human becoming, 2-3
Pastor, in interdisciplinary team, 18-19
Patient
  with chronic pancreatitis, education for, 256t
  education for, on peginterferon and ribavirin therapy, 251t
  with gastroesophageal reflux disease, education of, 218t
  in interdisciplinary team, 15-16
  with liver disease, education for, 250t
Patient Self-Determination Act (1990), 452b
Paxil (paroxetine), for musculoskeletal disorders, 417t
PD (Parkinson's disease), 387-388
Peganone (ethotoin), for seizure disorders, 319t
Peginterferon
  for hepatitis C, 249
  therapy with, patient and family education on, 251t
Pelvic exenteration, for cervical cancer, 539, 541f
Pelvic muscle exercises, for urinary incontinence, 276-277
Pelvic tumor, general treatments for, 556t
Penbutolol (Levatol), for hypertension, 186t
Penciclovir (Denavir), side effects and nursing considerations
    for, 73t
Penicillamine (Cuprimine, Depen), for joint and connective tissue
    disorders, 397t
Pentobarbital sodium (Nembutal), for brain disorders, 319t
Pentostatin (Nipent), side effects of, 445t
Pepcid (famotidine), for gastroesophageal reflux disease and
    peptic ulcer, 217t

Peptic ulcer disease, 220-225
  clinical manifestations of, 221-222
  complementary and alternative therapies for, 225
  complications of, 221
  demographic differences in, 214t
  diagnosis of, 222
  epidemiology of, 221b
  Helicobacter pylori infection and, 220, 221b
  interdisciplinary care for, 222-225
  nonsteroidal antiinflammatory drugs and, 220, 222b
  pathophysiology of, 220-221
Pepto-Bismol (bismuth subsalicylate)
  for gastroesophageal reflux disease and peptic ulcer, 216t
  for *Helicobacter pylori* infection, 224t
Percocet (oxycodone with acetaminophen), for joint and connective
    tissue disorders, 398t
Percodan (oxycodone with acetaminophen), for joint and connective
    tissue disorders, 398t
Performance, Alzheimer's disease and, by stage, 353t
Periarteritis nodosa, skin signs associated with, 65t
Perindopril (Aceon), for hypertension, 188t
Perioral dermatitis, 76-77
Peripheral blood cell transplantation, for breast cancer, 501
Peripheral nervous system, disorders of, vertigo in, 56-57
Persantine (dipyridamole), for brain disorders, 321t
Persistent vegetative state, 341-343
Person, impact of chronic illness and disability on, 6-7
PET. *See* Positron emission tomography (PET).
Petrolatum, side effects and nursing considerations for, 73t
Pharmaceuticals, in wound care, 92t
Pharmacist
  in chronic pancreatitis care, 257
  in coronary artery disease care, 165
  in diabetic foot ulcer care, 105
Phendimetrazine (Bontril, Plegine, Prelu-2, X-Trozine), for weight
    loss, 210t
Phenobarbital (Luminal), for brain disorders, 319t
Phenol, side effects and nursing considerations for, 72t
Phenothiazines, for cancer symptom management, 449t
Phenotypic testing, in HIV/AIDS, 579
Phentermine (Adipex-P, Fastin, Ionamin, Oby-trim), for weight
    loss, 210t
Phentolamine (Regitine), for hypertension, 186t
Phenylephrine (AK-Dilate), side effects and nursing considerations
    for, 46t
Phenytoin (Dilantin)
  for brain tumors, 462t
  for seizure disorders, 319t
Phlebotomy
  for hemochromatosis, 146
  for polycythemia, 142
Phospholine Iodide (echothiophate), side effects and nursing
    considerations for, 46t
Photosensitivity, drugs causing, 71t
Physiatrist
  in stroke care, 332
  in traumatic brain injury care, 339
Physical functions, Alzheimer's disease and, by stage, 353t
Physical therapist
  in arterial ulcer care, 103
  in bladder disorder care, 281-282
  in blood malignancy care, 158
  in brain tumor care, 463
  in breast cancer care, 502
  in Buerger's disease care, 191
  in cancer care, 451
  in cardiac rehabilitation, 177-178
  in chronic arterial occlusive disease care, 190
  in chronic obstructive pulmonary disease care, 113
  in Cushing's syndrome care, 303-305
  in dementia care, 354, 359
  in diabetes mellitus care, 294
  in diabetic foot ulcer care, 105

Physical therapist *(Continued)*
in fibromyalgia care, 422
in HIV/AIDS care, 581
in interdisciplinary team, 16-17
in liver disease care, 252
in low back pain care, 432-433
in lung cancer care, 513
in neuromuscular disorder care, 382
in osteoarthritis care, 399
in osteomyelitis care, 425-426
in osteoporosis care, 418-419
in Paget's disease care, 430
in pressure ulcer care, 95
in Raynaud's phenomenon care, 193
in rheumatoid arthritis care, 403-404
in sarcoma care, 561-562
in spinal cord injury care, 373
in stroke care, 334
in systemic sclerosis care, 408
in thyroid disorder care, 300
in tuberculosis care, 132-133
in venous stasis disease care, 101
in vestibular disorder care, 60
in wound care, 95
Physician(s). *See also* Primary provider.
in eye disorder care, 37
in interdisciplinary team, 16
in neuromuscular disorder care, 381
Physostigmine (Isopto Eserine), side effects and nursing considerations
for, 46t
Phytotherapeutic agents, for urinary incontinence, 279t
Pick's disease
clinical manifestations of, 351
pathophysiology of, 348-349
Pigmentation disorders, 78
Pilocarpine (Isopto Carpine), side effects and nursing considerations
for, 46t
Pindolol (Visken), for hypertension, 187t
Pioglitazone (Actos), for diabetes mellitus, 292t
Pirbuterol (Maxair), for chronic obstructive pulmonary
disease, 114t
Piroxicam (Feldene)
for headaches, 319t
for joint and connective tissue disorders, 397t
Pituitary gland, hormones of, effects of, 285t
Plant alkaloids
for lung cancer, 511t
for sarcomas, 560t
Plaque, 67t
Plaquenil (hydroxychloroquine), for joint and connective tissue
disorders, 397t
Platinol (cisplatin)
for lung cancer, 511t
for sarcomas, 560t
side effects of, 444t
Plavix (clopidogrel), for brain disorders, 321t
Plegine (phendimetrazine), for weight loss, 210t
Plendil (felodipine), for hypertension, 188t
Plicamycin (Mithracin, Mithramycin), for musculoskeletal disorders, 417t
PLISSIT model for sexual counseling, 533b
PML (progressive multifocal leukoencephalopathy), AIDS-related,
569t, 572
nursing interventions for, 576t
Pneumocystis carinii pneumonia, in HIV/AIDS, 569t, 570
nursing interventions for, 575t
Pneumonia
pneumocystic carinii, in HIV/AIDS, 569t, 570
Pneumocystis carinii, in HIV/AIDS, nursing interventions for, 575t
secondary to spinal cord injury, 369
Podiatrist
in arterial ulcer care, 103
in diabetes mellitus care, 294
in diabetic foot ulcer care, 105

Polycythemia, 135, 141-142
Polyneuropathies, chronic sensory, skin signs associated
with, 65t
Pontocaine (tetracaine), nursing considerations for, 45t
Posicor (mibefradil), for hypertension, 188t
Positron emission tomography (PET), in breast cancer
diagnosis, 495
Potassium-sparing diuretics, for hypertension, 185t
Prandin (repaglinide), for diabetes mellitus, 291t
Pravachol (pravastatin), for brain disorders, 321t
Pravastatin (Pravachol), for brain disorders, 321t
Prazosin (Minipress), for hypertension, 186t
Precose (acarbose), for diabetes mellitus, 291t
Prednisolone acetate (Econopred), side effects and nursing
considerations for, 45t
Prednisolone (Delta-Cortef), side effects of, 445t
Prednisolone NA phosphate (Inflamase), side effects and nursing
considerations for, 45t
Prednisone (Deltasone)
for chronic obstructive pulmonary disease, 114t
for Crohn's disease, 231
for joint and connective tissue disorders, 398t
for neuromuscular disorders, 383t
side effects of, 445t
Prelu-2 (phendimetrazine), for weight loss, 210t
Premarin (conjugated estrogen)
for musculoskeletal disorders, 416t
for urinary incontinence, 278t
Premphase (estrogen), for musculoskeletal disorders, 416t
Prempro (estrogen), for musculoskeletal disorders, 416t
Presbycusis, 54
Pressure ulcers
assessment of, measurement in, 90-91
classification of, 87, 90
clinical manifestations of, 85-87, 90-91
diagnosis of, 85-87, 90-91
overview of, 84
pathophysiology of, 85
prevention of, 86-87, 87b
risk assessment for, 86, 88-89t
secondary to spinal cord injury, 370-371
sites of, 85f
treatment of, 91-93
Pressure urticaria, clinical features of, 75t
Prevacid (lansoprazole)
for gastroesophageal reflux disease and peptic ulcer, 217t
for *Helicobacter pylori* infection, 223t
Prilosec (omeprazole), for gastroesophageal reflux disease and
peptic ulcer, 217t
Primary provider
in acromegaly care, 310
in anorexia nervosa care, 200
in arterial ulcer care, 102
in asthma care, 120
in binge eating disorder care, 204
in bladder disorder care, 281
in blood disorder care, 146
in blood malignancy care, 158
in brain tumor care, 463
in breast cancer care, 498
in bulimia nervosa and purging care, 202-203
in cancer care, 439
in cervical cancer care, 539
in cholelithiasis care, 254
in chronic kidney disease care, 266
in chronic obstructive pulmonary disease care, 112
in chronic pancreatitis care, 257
in colorectal cancer care, 520-521
in coronary artery disease care, 165
in Crohn's disease care, 231
in dementia care, 351
in diabetes mellitus care, 289-209
in diabetic foot ulcer care, 104

Primary provider *(Continued)*
in diabetic retinopathy care, 43
in diverticular disease care, 235
in epilepsy care, 326
in eye disorder care, 37
in fibromyalgia care, 421
in gastric cancer care, 518
in gastroesophageal reflux disease care, 220
in gout care, 409
in head and neck cancer care, 484
in headache care, 318
in hearing loss care, 54-55
in HIV/AIDS care, 573-574
in irritable bowel syndrome care, 237
in liver cancer care, 523
in liver disease care, 251
in low back pain care, 432
in malabsorption syndrome care, 239
in malnutrition care, 206
in obesity care, 208-209
in osteoarthritis care, 395-396
in osteomyelitis care, 425
in osteoporosis care, 415
in ovarian cancer care, 536
in Paget's disease care, 429
in pancreatic cancer care, 524
in peptic ulcer disease care, 224
in pressure ulcer care, 93
in prostate cancer care, 549
in renal cell carcinoma care, 527
in rheumatoid arthritis care, 402-403
in sarcoma care, 556
in skin disorder care, 65-66
in spinal cord cancer care, 466
in stroke care, 332
in systemic lupus erythematosus care, 405
in systemic sclerosis care, 407
in testicular cancer care, 547
in thyroid disorder care, 297-298
in traumatic brain injury care, 339
in tuberculosis care, 131
in ulcerative colitis care, 232
in urinary bladder cancer care, 529
in vaginal cancer care, 545
in venous stasis disease care, 101
in vestibular disorder care, 59-60
in vulvar cancer care, 543
Prinivil (lisinopril)
for brain disorders, 321t
for hypertension, 188t
Prinzmetal's angina, 162-163
Private duty care, high-technology, 15
Probenecid (Benemid), for joint and connective tissue disorders, 398t
Procarbazine (Matulane)
for lung cancer, 511t
side effects of, 445t
Procardia (nifedipine), for hypertension, 188t
Procrit (epoetin alfa), for lung cancer, 511t
Progressive multifocal leukoencephalopathy (PML), AIDS-related, 569t, 572
nursing interventions for, 576t
Prokine (sargramostim), for lung cancer, 511t
Prokinetic agent, for gastroesophageal reflux disease and peptic ulcer, 217t
Proleukin (interleukin 2), for cancer, indications and side effects of, 447t
Proparacaine (Ophthaine, Ophthetic), nursing considerations for, 45t
Propine (dipivefrin), side effects and nursing considerations for, 46t
Propoxyphene, with acetaminophen or aspirin (Darvocet, Darvon), for joint and connective tissue disorders, 398t

Propranolol (Inderal)
for brain disorders, 320t
for hypertension, 187t
for thyroid disorders, 299t
Propylthiouracil (PTU), for hyperthyroidism, 298, 299t
Proscar (finasteride), for urinary incontinence, 279t
Prostate cancer, 547-550
clinical manifestations of, 549
complementary and alternative therapies for, 550
diagnosis of, 549
ethnic variations in, 548
interdisciplinary care for, 549-550
pathophysiology of, 549
Prosthesis, ocular, care of, 48b
Protease inhibitors
for chronic obstructive pulmonary disease, 115t
for HIV/AIDS, 578t
Proton pump inhibitors
for gastroesophageal reflux disease and peptic ulcer, 217t
for *Helicobacter pylori* infection, 223t
Protonix (pantoprazole)
for gastroesophageal reflux disease and peptic ulcer, 217t
for *Helicobacter pylori* infection, 223t
Proventil (albuterol), for chronic obstructive pulmonary disease, 114t
Prozac (fluoxetine)
for brain disorders, 322t
for musculoskeletal disorders, 417t
Pruritus, 71, 74
in pancreatic cancer, management strategies for, 525b
Pseudoephedrine (Sudafed), for urinary incontinence, 278t
Psoriasis, 77-78, 77f
PsoriGel (coal tar), side effects and nursing considerations for, 73t
Psychological functions, Alzheimer's disease and, by stage, 353t
Psychologist, in blood malignancy care, 158-159
Psychoneuroimmunology, 28
Psychosocial disorders, secondary to spinal cord injury, 370
Psychostimulants
for brain disorders, 322t
for traumatic brain injury, 340t
Psychotherapist, in brain tumor care, 463
PTU (propylthiouracil), for hyperthyroidism, 298, 299t
Public health care, 14
Pulmonary embolus, secondary to spinal cord injury, 368
Pulmonary rehabilitation, in chronic obstructive pulmonary disease management, 113
Purging, in bulimia nervosa, 202-203
Purinethol (6-mercaptopurine)
side effects of, 445t
for ulcerative colitis, 232
Pustule, 68t
Pyrazinamide (PZA), for tuberculosis, 130t
Pyridostigmine, for neuromuscular disorders, 384t
PZA (pyrazinamide), for tuberculosis, 130t

Q

Quadriplegia, 362
Quality-of-life issues, in breast cancer survivors, 497
Quality-of-life scales, for head and neck cancer patients, 485b
Quinapril (Accupril), for hypertension, 188t

R

Rabeprazole (Aciphex)
for gastroesophageal reflux disease and peptic ulcer, 217t
for *Helicobacter pylori* infection, 223t
Radiation oncologist
in breast cancer care, 500-501
in cancer care, 439-442
in colorectal cancer care, 522
in sarcoma care, 558-559

Radiation therapy
  for brain tumors, 461-462
  for breast cancer, 500-501
  for cervical cancer, 540
  for endometrial cancer, 542
  external, for cancer, 440-441
  internal, for cancer, 441-442
  for lung cancer, 510
  for ovarian cancer, 536-537
  personal care related to, 441b
  for prostate cancer, 549
  for sarcomas, 558-559
    side effects of, 560t
  site-specific side effects of, 442t
  for testicular cancer, 547
  for vaginal cancer, 545
  for vulvar cancer, 544
Radiograph, chest, in coronary artery disease diagnosis,
    163t
Radiosensitivity, of body organs and tissues, 441t
Raloxifene (Evista), for musculoskeletal disorders, 416t
Ramipril (Altace), for hypertension, 188t
Ranitidine bismuth citrate (Tritec)
  for gastroesophageal reflux disease and peptic ulcer,
    217t
  for *Helicobacter pylori* infection, 223t
Ranitidine (Zantac), for gastroesophageal reflux disease and
    peptic ulcer, 217t
Raynaud's phenomenon, 192-193
Recombinant interferon alpha, for chronic myelogenous leukemia,
    152
Recombinant monoclonal factors, for hemophilia, 145t
Reflex neurogenic bladder, 273
Reflex sympathetic dystrophy, secondary to spinal cord injury,
    368
Reflexology, 31
  maps for, 32f
Refusal of treatment, 453b
Regional enteritis, 228, 230-231
Regitine (phentolamine), for hypertension, 186t
Reglan (metoclopramide), for gastroesophageal reflux disease and
    peptic ulcer, 217t
Rehabilitation
  for breast cancer survivor, 497-498, 503
  cardiac, 177-178
  for HIV/AIDS, 582-583
  in neuromuscular disorders, focus of, 390-391
Rehabilitation facility, 12-13, 12t
Rehabilitation specialist
  in stroke care, 335
  in traumatic brain injury care, 340-341
Reiki, 31-33
Remicade (infliximab), for Crohn's disease, 231
Reminyl (galantamine), for Alzheimer's disease, 351
Renal cell carcinoma, 526-528
Repaglinide (Prandin), for diabetes mellitus, 291t
Reproductive system
  cancers of, 532-552
    assessment of, 533, 534b
    cervical cancer as, 537-540. *See also* Cervix, cancer of.
    endometrial cancer as, 540-542
    ovarian cancer as, 533-537. *See also* Ovary(ies), cancer of.
    prostate cancer as, 547-550. *See also* Prostate, cancer of.
    risk factors associated with, 535t
    testicular cancer as, 546-547, 548b
    vaginal cancer as, 544-546
    vulvar cancer as, 542-544
  disorders of, skin signs associated with, 65t
Rescriptor (delavirdine), for HIV/AIDS, 577t
Reserpine (Serpasil), for hypertension, 186t
Resistance testing, in HIV/AIDS, 579
Resorcinol (Bicozene), 72t
Respiratory disorders, skin signs associated with, 65t

Respiratory therapist
  in asthma care, 121
  in coronary artery disease care, 165
Respiratory therapy, for chronic obstructive pulmonary disease,
    115-116
Retention, urinary, 274
  differential diagnosis of, 276t
  medications contributing to, 281b
Retin-A (tretinoin 0.025-0.1%), side effects and nursing considerations
    for, 73t
Retinitis pigmentosa, nursing considerations for, 47t
Retinopathy, diabetic, 41-43, 43f
Retrovir (zidovudine), for HIV/AIDS, 576, 577t
Rhabdomyosarcoma, general treatments for, 556t
Rheumatic diseases, American Rheumatism Association classification
    of, 394b
Rheumatic heart disease, skin signs associated with, 65t
Rheumatoid arthritis (RA), 401-404
  case study on, 410-411
  classification of, 402b
  clinical manifestations of, 402
  diagnosis of, 402
  interdisciplinary care for, 402-404
  osteoarthritis compared with, 401t
  pathophysiology of, 402
  progression in, stages of, 402b
Rheumatrex (methotrexate), for joint and connective tissue disorders,
    397t
Rhinocort (budesonide), for chronic obstructive pulmonary disease,
    114t
Ribavirin
  for hepatitis C, 249
  therapy with, patient and family education on, 251t
Riboflavin, skin signs associated with, 64t
Ridaura (auranofin), for joint and connective tissue disorders,
    397t
RIF (rifampin), for tuberculosis, 130t
Rifampin (RIF), for tuberculosis, 130t
Rilutek (riluzole), for neuromuscular disorders, 383t
Riluzole (Rilutek), for neuromuscular disorders, 383t
Rinne test, in hearing loss assessment, 52
Risedronate (Actonel), for osteoporosis, 415, 416t, 417
Ritalin (methylphenidate), for brain disorders, 322t
Ritonavir + lopinavir (ABT-378r, Kaletra), for HIV/AIDS, 578t
Ritonavir (Norvir), for HIV/AIDS, 578t
Rivastigmine (Exelon), for Alzheimer's disease, 351
Rizatriptan (Maxalt), for migraines, 320t
Rofecoxib (Vioxx)
  for headaches, 319t
  for joint and connective tissue disorders, 397t
Rolaids (calcium carbonate)
  for gastroesophageal reflux disease and peptic ulcer, 216t
  for osteoporosis, 417-418
Romycin (erythromycin), nursing considerations for, 45t
Rosacea, 76
Rosiglitazone (Avandia), for diabetes mellitus, 292t
Roux-en-Y esophagojejunostomy, 517
Rural outreach programs, 13

S

Sacral cord syndrome, 363f, 365
St. John's wort, for hepatitis C, 253t
Salicylic acid
  1-2%, side effects and nursing considerations for, 72t
  4% (Sebulex), side effects and nursing considerations for, 72t
Salivary glands, function, anatomic relationships, and cancer
    features of, 475t
Salmeterol (Serevent), for chronic obstructive pulmonary disease,
    114t
Sandimmune (cyclosporin), for joint and connective tissue disorders,
    397t
Sandostatin (octreotide), for acromegaly, 310, 310t
Sanorex (mazindol), for weight loss, 210t

Sansert (methysergide), for migraines, 320t
Sarcomas, 554-563
    caregiver issues on, 563
    case study on, 563-564
    clinical manifestations of, 555
    complementary and alternative therapies for, 562-563
    ethical considerations on, 563
    family issues on, 563
    general treatments for, 556t
    interdisciplinary care for, 555-562
    Kaposi's, AIDS-related, 569t, 571
        nursing interventions for, 576t
    pathophysiology of, 554-555
    primary bone, 555
    primary soft tissue, 555
Sargramostim (Leukine, Prokine)
    for cancer, indications and side effects of, 447t
    for lung cancer, 511t
Saw palmetto, for urinary incontinence, 279t
Scale, 68t
Schisandra, for hepatitis C, 253t
SCI. See Spinal cord injury (SCI).
Scleroderma, skin signs associated with, 64t
Sclerosis, systemic, 406-408
Scoliosis, acquired, secondary to spinal cord injury,
        372
Sebulex (salicylic acid 4%), side effects and nursing
        considerations for, 72t
Sectral (acebutolol), for hypertension, 186t
Sedation, terminal, 453b
Seizures, 323-328. See also Epilepsy.
    classification of, 325t
    triggering events for, 324b
Selective estrogen receptor modulators, for musculoskeletal
        disorders, 416t
Selective serotonin reuptake inhibitors (SSRIs)
    for brain disorders, 322t
    for musculoskeletal disorders, 417t
    for neuromuscular disorders, 384t
Self-identity, 7
Semustine (Methyl CCNU), side effects of, 445t
Senior citizen centers, 14
Sensory paralytic bladder, 273-274
Serevent (salmeterol), for chronic obstructive pulmonary disease,
        114t
Serotonin agonists, for migraines, 320t
Serotonin antagonists, for cancer symptom management,
        449t
Serpasil (reserpine), for hypertension, 186t
Sertraline (Zoloft)
    for brain disorders, 322t
    for musculoskeletal disorders, 417t
Serum sickness, skin signs associated with, 64t
Sexual counseling, PLISSIT model for, 533b
Shark cartilage therapy, 29
Shear, pressure ulcers and, 85
Shifting perspectives model, 4-5, 5f
Shingles, HIV/AIDS, 569t, 571
Shoulder pain, after stroke, 331-332
Sibutramine (Meridia), for weight loss, 210t
Sick syndrome, euthyroid, 296
Sickle cell anemia, 135, 142-143
Silver dressings, in wound care, 92t
Simvastin (Zocor), for brain disorders, 321t
Sinequan (doxepin)
    for musculoskeletal disorders, 417t
    for urinary incontinence, 277t
Singular (montelukast), for chronic obstructive pulmonary disease,
        115t
Sinuses, paranasal, function, anatomic relationships, and cancer features
        of, 474t
Skelid (tiludronate), for musculoskeletal disorders, 416t
Skilled nursing facility, 13

Skin
    alterations in, complicating head and neck cancers, 476
    disorders of, 63-82
        assessment of, 63, 65, 66b, 67-69f
        benign, 71-
        chronic, functional health pattern assessment for, 70b
        complementary and alternative therapies for, 71b, 74b
        drug therapy for, 70-71, 72-73t
        end-of-life care for, 81
        family and caregiver issues on, 81
        interdisciplinary care for, 65-66, 69-70
        premalignant and malignant, 78-81
        secondary to spinal cord injury, 370-371
        treatment modalities for, 71b
    lesions of, common, 67-69t
    problems of, stoma-related, treatment of, 530t
    protection of, 66, 69
    wounds of, 83-106. See also Wounds.
SLE. See Systemic lupus erythematosus (SLE).
Sleep apnea, obstructive, complicating head and neck cancers,
        483, 483b
Sleep disorders, complicating head and neck cancers, 483
Smoking
    arterial ulcers and, 102
    cessation of, strategies for, 508b
    chronic arterial occlusive disease and, 189
    coronary artery disease and, 166
Social functions, Alzheimer's disease and, by stage, 353t
Social isolation, 7
Social worker, medical. See Medical social worker.
Society, impact of chronic illness and disability on, 8-9
Sodium, foods high in, 172t
Sodium nitroprusside (Nipride), for hypertension, 187t
Soft tissues, sarcomas of, primary, 555
Solar urticaria, clinical features of, 75t
Solganal (aurothioglucose), for joint and connective tissue disorders,
        397t
Solu-Cortef (hydrocortisone), for joint and connective tissue disorders,
        398t
Solu-Medrol (methylprednisolone), for chronic obstructive pulmonary
        disease, 114t
Somatostatin analogs, for acromegaly, 310, 310t
Somatostatins, for cancer symptom management, 449t
Sorrow, chronic, 8
Spastic colon, 236-238
Spasticity, secondary to spinal cord injury, 371
Specialists, in HIV/AIDS care, 574
Speech pathologist, in brain tumor care, 463
Speech therapist
    in dementia care, 360
    in head and neck cancer care, 486-487
    in neuromuscular disorder care, 382
    in stroke care, 335
    in traumatic brain injury care, 340
Spinal cord
    ascending tracts of, 367, 367f
    cancers of, 464-467
        clinical manifestations of, 464-465, 465b
        complementary and alternative therapies for, 467
        diagnosis of, 465
        interdisciplinary care for, 465-467
        pathophysiology of, 464
    descending tracts of, 367-368, 367f
    injury to (SCI), 362-377
        anterior, 363f, 365
        assessment of, 364-365, 365f, 366f, 367b
        case study on, 375-376
        common syndromes of, 363f
        complementary and alternative therapies for, 374
        demographic data on, 363
        diagnosis of, 367b, 372
        disabilities secondary to
            cardiopulmonary, 368-370

Spinal cord *(Continued)*
    cardiovascular, 368
    clinical manifestations of, 368-372
    gastrointestinal, 370
    genitourinary, 370
    neuromusculoskeletal, 371-372
    psychosocial, 370
    skin, 370-371
  ethical considerations on, 375
  family and caregiver issues on, 374-375
  functional outcomes in, 367t
  interdisciplinary care of, 372-374
  life expectancies in, 362, 364t
  neurologic classification of, 366f
  pathophysiology of, 367-368
  skin signs associated with, 65t
  spinal nerves of, 368, 368b, 369f
Spiriva (tiotropium), for chronic obstructive pulmonary disease, 114t
Spironolactone (Aldactone), for hypertension, 185t
Splenectomy, in sickle cell anemia, 142
Spondylolisthesis, low back pain in, 431
Spondylolysis, low back pain in, 431
Squamous cell carcinoma, 79-80
Statins, for brain disorders, 321t
Status epilepticus, 325
Stavudine (D4T, Zerit), for HIV/AIDS, 577t
Steroids, for cancer symptom management, 449t
Stimulants, for cancer symptom management, 449t
Stoma, urinary
  care of, in ulcerative colitis, 232-233, 243b
  nursing interventions for, 529b
  skin problems related to, treatment of, 530t
Stomach
  cancer of, 517-518, 520
    skin signs associated with, 64t
  disorders of, peptic ulcer disease as, 220-225. *See also* Peptic ulcer disease.
  nervous, 236-238
Stool softeners
  for cancer symptom management, 448t
  for cirrhosis, 248b
  for neuromuscular disorders, 383t, 384t
Streptomycin, for tuberculosis, 130t
Streptozocin (Zanosar), side effects of, 445t
Stress incontinence, 272-273
  case study on, 282-283
Stretta procedure, for gastroesophageal reflux disease, 219
Stroke
  aspiration after, interventions to prevent, 335b
  assessment of, 332, 332b
  case study on, 343-344
  clinical manifestations of, 330-332
  communication after, strategies to enhance, 334b
  deficits related to, by site of blockage, 331t
  diagnosis of, 332
  end-of-life issues on, 336
  ethnic variations in, 328-329
  family and caregiver issues on, 336
  interdisciplinary care for, 332-335
  mortality from, 329t
  pathophysiology of, 329-330
  risk factors associated with, 330t
Subacute care settings, 11, 12t
Succinimides, for seizure disorders, 319t
Sudafed (pseudoephedrine), for urinary incontinence, 278t
Suicide, secondary to spinal cord injury, 370
Sular (nisoldipine), for hypertension, 188t
Sulfasalazine (Azulfidine)
  for Crohn's disease, 231
  for joint and connective tissue disorders, 397t
  for ulcerative colitis, 232

Sulfinpyrazone (Anturane), for joint and connective tissue disorders, 398t
Sulfonylureas, for diabetes mellitus, 292t
Sulfur 4-10%, 72t
Sulindac (Clinoril)
  for headaches, 319t
  for joint and connective tissue disorders, 397t
Sumatriptan (Imitrex), for migraines, 320t
Surgeon
  in bladder disorder care, 280
  in breast cancer care, 498-499
  in cancer care, 439
  in cervical cancer care, 539
  in colorectal cancer care, 521
  in Crohn's disease care, 231
  in endometrial cancer care, 542
  in gastric cancer care, 518
  in liver cancer care, 523
  in lung cancer care, 510
  in obesity care, 209-210
  orthopedic, in low back pain care, 432
  in osteomyelitis care, 425
  in osteoporosis care, 415
  in ovarian cancer care, 536
  in Paget's disease care, 429
  in pancreatic cancer care, 525
  in prostate cancer care, 549
  in renal cell carcinoma care, 527-528
  in skin disorder care, 69-70
  in testicular cancer care, 547
  in thyroid disorder care, 298
  in ulcerative colitis care, 232
  in urinary bladder cancer care, 529
  in vaginal cancer care, 545
  in vulvar cancer care, 543
Surgery
  for brain tumors, 461
Surgical oncologist, in sarcoma care, 556-557
Sustiva (efavirenz), for HIV/AIDS, 577t
Swallowing, difficulty, complicating head and neck cancers, 480, 480b
Synovial sarcoma, general treatments for, 556t
Synthroid (levothyroxine), for hypothyroidism, 298-300, 299t
Syphilis, skin signs associated with, 65t
Syringomyelia
  secondary to spinal cord injury, 372
  skin signs associated with, 65t
Systemic lupus erythematosus (SLE), 404-406, 405f
  skin signs associated with, 64t
Systemic sclerosis, 406-408

T

T-cell lymphoma, 80-81
T-cell receptor peptides, for neuromuscular disorders, 383t, 384t
Tagamet (cimetidine), for gastroesophageal reflux disease and peptic ulcer, 217t
Tamoxifen (Nolvadex), side effects of, 445t
Tamsulosin (Flomax), for urinary incontinence, 279t
Tapazole (methimazole), for hyperthyroidism, 298, 299t
Tasosartan (Veridia), for hypertension, 188t
Taste alterations, complicating head and neck cancers, 479-480
Tavist (clemastine), nursing considerations for, 72t
Taxol (paclitaxel), side effects of, 445t
Taxotere (Docetaxel), side effects of, 445t
TB. *See* Tuberculosis (TB).
TBI. *See* Traumatic brain injury (TBI).
3TC (lamivudine), for HIV/AIDS, 577t
TCAs. *See* Tricyclic antidepressants (TCAs).
Tearisol, side effects and nursing considerations for, 46t
Tears Naturale, side effects and nursing considerations for, 46t

Tears Plus, side effects and nursing considerations for, 46t
Tegison (etretinate), side effects and nursing considerations for, 73t
Tegretol (carbamazepine)
    for brain disorders, 320t
    for brain tumors, 462t
Telehealth care, 15
Telmisartan (Micardis), for hypertension, 188t
Tenex (guanfacine), for hypertension, 186t
Teniposide (Vumon), side effects of, 445t
Tenofovir (Viread), for HIV/AIDS, 577t
Tenormin (atenolol), for hypertension, 186t
Tension-type headache (TTH), 314-315
    clinical manifestations of, 315, 317
Tenuate (diethylpropion), for weight loss, 210t
Tenuate Dospan (diethylpropion), for weight loss, 210t
Terazosin (Hytrin)
    for hypertension, 186t
    for urinary incontinence, 278t
Terbutaline (Brethine), for chronic obstructive pulmonary disease, 114t
Terminal sedation, 453b
Testicular cancer, 546-547, 548b
Tetracaine (Pontocaine), nursing considerations for, 45t
Tetracycline (Achromycin)
    for *Helicobacter pylori* infection, 223t
    side effects and nursing considerations for, 72t
Tetraplegia, 362
6-TG (6-thioguanine), side effects of, 445t
Thalassemias
    clinical manifestations of, 138-139
    pathophysiology of, 136-137
    treatment of, 139
Theo-Dur (theophylline), for chronic obstructive pulmonary disease, 114t
Theophylline (Theo-Dur, Aerolate), for chronic obstructive pulmonary disease, 114t
Therapists, in neuromuscular disorder care, 382
Thiamine deficiency, skin signs associated with, 64t
Thiazide diuretics, for hypertension, 185t
Thiazolidinediones, for diabetes mellitus, 292t
6-Thioguanine (6-TG), side effects of, 445t
Thiotepa, side effects of, 445t
Thoracic tumors, manifestations of, 465t
Thromboangiitis obliterans, 191
    skin signs associated with, 65t
Thrombosis, deep vein, secondary to spinal cord injury, 368
Thyroid gland
    disorders of, 295-300
        clinical manifestations of, 296, 296f
        diagnosis of, 296-297, 298t
        interdisciplinary care of, 297-300
        pathophysiology of, 295-296
        skin signs associated with, 64t
    function, anatomic relationships, and cancer features of, 475t
    hormones of, effects of, 285t
Thyroid-stimulating hormone level, in coronary artery disease diagnosis, 165t
Thyroiditis
    Hashimoto's, 296
    types of, characteristics of, 297t
Thyroxine (T$_4$), 295
TIA (transient ischemic attack), 330
Tigan (trimethobenzamide), for brain disorders, 322t
Tilade (nedocromil), for chronic obstructive pulmonary disease, 114t
Tiludronate (Skelid), for musculoskeletal disorders, 416t
Time management, 7
Timolol (Blocadren, Timoptic)
    for brain disorders, 320t
    for hypertension, 187t
    side effects and nursing considerations for, 46f

Timoptic (timolol), side effects and nursing considerations for, 46t
Tinnitus, 54
Tiotropium (Spiriva), for chronic obstructive pulmonary disease, 114t
Tissues
    radiosensitivity of, 441t
    soft, sarcomas of, primary, 555
Titralac (calcium carbonate)
    for gastroesophageal reflux disease and peptic ulcer, 216t
    for osteoporosis, 417-418
Tizanidine (Zanaflex), for brain disorders, 321t
Tobacco. *See* Smoking.
Tobramycin (Tobrex), nursing considerations for, 45t
Tobrex (tobramycin), nursing considerations for, 45t
Tofranil (imipramine), for urinary incontinence, 277t
Toileting, Alzheimer's disease and, by stage, 352t
Tolazamide (Tolinase), for diabetes mellitus, 292t
Tolbutamide (Orinase), for diabetes mellitus, 292t
Tolectin (tolmetin)
    for headaches, 319t
    for joint and connective tissue disorders, 397t
Tolinase (tolazamide), for diabetes mellitus, 292t
Tolmetin (Tolectin)
    for headaches, 319t
    for joint and connective tissue disorders, 397t
Tolterodine (Detrol), for urinary incontinence, 277t
Tomography, positron emission, in breast cancer diagnosis, 495
Topamax (topiramate), for brain disorders, 320t
Topiramate (Topamax), for brain disorders, 320t
Torsemide (Demadex), for hypertension, 185t
Torvastatin (Lipitor), for brain disorders, 321t
Toxoplasmosis, in HIV/AIDS, 569t, 570-571
    nursing interventions for, 575t
Trandate (labetalol), for hypertension, 187t
Trandolapril (Mavik), for hypertension, 188t
Transient ischemic attack (TIA), 330
Transparent dressings, in wound care, 92t
Transplantation
    bone marrow
        allogenic, for chronic myelogenous leukemia, 152
        for breast cancer, 501
    kidney, 268-269
    peripheral blood cell, for breast cancer, 501
Transtracheal tube, for oxygen administration, 116t
Tranxene (clorazepate), for seizure disorders, 320t
Trastuzumab (Herceptin), for cancer, indications and side effects of, 447t
Trauma, spinal cord. *See* Spinal cord, injury to (SCI).
Traumatic brain injury (TBI), 336-341
    assessment of, 338-339, 339b
    behavioral consequences of, 338, 338b
    clinical manifestations of, 337-338, 337f
    diagnosis of, 338
    family and caregiver issues on, 341
    Functional Independence Measure in, 339
    interdisciplinary care for, 339-341
    pain from, 338
    pathophysiology of, 336-337
    psychological consequences of, 338, 338b
Treadmill test, in coronary artery disease diagnosis, 163t
Treatment, withdrawal of, 453b
Tretinoin 0.025-0.1% (Retin-A), side effects and nursing considerations for, 73t
Triamcinolone (Aristocort)
    for chronic obstructive pulmonary disease, 114t
    for joint and connective tissue disorders, 398t
Triamterene (Dyrenium), for hypertension, 185t
Trichlormethiazide (Metahydrin, Naqua), for hypertension, 185t

Tricyclic antidepressants (TCAs)
    for brain disorders, 321t
    for musculoskeletal disorders, 417t
    for urinary incontinence, 277t
Tridil (nitroglycerin), for hypertension, 187t
Trifluridine (Viroptic), nursing considerations for, 45t
Triiodothyronine (T₃), 295
Trileptal (oxcarbazepine), for brain disorders, 320t
Trimethaphan (Arfonad), for hypertension, 188t
Trimethobenzamide (Tigan), for brain disorders, 322t
Triptans, for migraines, 320t
Trismus, muscle, complicating head and neck cancers,
        481-482
Tritec (ranitidine bismuth citrate)
    for gastroesophageal reflux disease and peptic ulcer,
        217t
    for *Helicobacter pylori* infection, 223t
Trusopt (dorzolamide), side effects and nursing considerations
        for, 45t
TTH. *See* Tension-type headache (TTH).
Tuberculosis (TB), 126-134
    assessment of, 126, 127b
    caregiver issues on, 133
    case study on, 133-134
    classification of, 127b
    clinical manifestations of, 129
    diagnosis of, 129
    dissemination of, 128f
    drug therapy for, 130-131, 130t, 131t
    ethical considerations on, 133
    ethnic variations in, 126
    family issues on, 133
    in HIV/AIDS, 568, 569t
        nursing interventions for, 575t
    human immunodeficiency virus coinfection with, 129
        drug therapy for, 131
    interdisciplinary care of, 129-133
    latent, 129
    miliary, 129
    overview of, 126
    pathophysiology of, 128-129
    risk factors for, 127b
Tumor(s)
    bone, general treatments for, 556t
    brain, 458-464. *See also* Brain, tumors of.
    fungating, complicating head and neck cancers, 477-478,
        478t
    grading systems for, 438b
    spinal cord, 464-467. *See also* Spinal cord, cancers of.
Tums (calcium carbonate)
    for gastroesophageal reflux disease and peptic ulcer, 216t
    for osteoporosis, 417-418
Tuning fork, in hearing loss assessment, 51-52
Two-dimensional echocardiogram, in coronary artery disease
        diagnosis, 164t
Tylenol (acetaminophen), for joint and connective tissue disorders,
        398t
Tylenol No. 3, No. 4 (codeine with acetaminophen), for joint and
        connective tissue disorders, 398t
Tylox (oxycodone with aspirin), for joint and connective tissue
        disorders, 398t

U
Ulcer(s), 69
    arterial, 101-103, 102f, 189-190
    diabetic foot, 102f, 103-105
    lower extremity, 95-105
        arterial ulcers as, 101-103, 102f, 189-190
        diabetic foot ulcer as, 103-105
        overview of, 95-96
        venous stasis disease as, 96-101. *See also* Venous stasis
            disease.
    pressure, 84-95. *See also* Pressure ulcers.

Ulcerative colitis, 231-234
    case study on, 239-240
    clinical manifestations of, 231-232
    demographic differences in, 229t
    diagnosis of, 232
    interdisciplinary care for, 232-234
    pathophysiology of, 231
    skin signs associated with, 64t
Ultra Tears, side effects and nursing considerations for, 46t
Undernourishment, 205-208. *See also* Malnutrition.
Uniform Health Decisions Act (1993), 452b
Univasc (moexipril), for hypertension, 188t
Uracil mustard, side effects of, 445t
Urea
    5-10%, 73t
    20-40%, 72t
Urea (Ureaphil), side effects and nursing considerations for, 46t
Ureaphil (urea), side effects and nursing considerations for, 46t
Urecholine (bethanechol), for urinary incontinence, 279t
Urge incontinence, 272
Uricosurics, for joint and connective tissue disorders, 398t
Urinary bladder, disorders of, 271-283. *See also* Bladder,
        urinary, disorders of.
Urinary incontinence, 272-273
    causes/contributing factors to, identification and management
        of, 275t
    medications associated with, 276b
    medications for, 277-279t, 277-280
Urinary stoma
    nursing interventions for, 529b
    skin problems related to, treatment of, 530t
Urinary tract infection, secondary to spinal cord injury,
        370
Urticaria, 74-75
    chronic, common types of, 75t
Uterus, cancer of, skin signs associated with, 64t

V

Vagina, cancer of, 544-546
Vaginal cones, for urinary incontinence, 277
Valium (diazepam)
    for brain disorders, 322t
    for seizure disorders, 320t
    side effects and nursing considerations for, 57t
Valproate (Depakote, Depakene), for brain disorders,
        320t
Valproic acid (Depakene), for brain tumors, 462t
Valsalva's maneuver, for bladder emptying, 280
Valsartan (Diovan), for hypertension, 188t
Valvular heart disease, 175-176
Varicose veins, 193-194
Vascular dementia, clinical manifestations of, 351
Vascular disorders, 181-196
    assessment of, 181, 182b
    Buerger's disease as, 191-192
    case study on, 195-196
    chronic arterial occlusive disease as, 189-190
    complementary and alternative therapies for, 194-195
    hypertension as, 181-189. *See also* Hypertension (HTN).
    Raynaud's phenomenon as, 192-193
    varicose veins as, 193-194
Vasodilators, for hypertension, 187t
Vasotec (enalapril)
    for brain disorders, 321t
    for hypertension, 188t
Vasotec Injection (enalaprilat), for hypertension, 188t
Vegetative state
    criteria for, 341b
    persistent, 341-343
Veins, varicose, 193-194
Velban (vinblastine, vinorelbine)
    for lung cancer, 511t
    side effects of, 445t

Venous stasis disease, 96-101
  clinical manifestations of, 96-97, 96f, 97f
  diagnosis of, 96-97, 97t
  interdisciplinary care of, 101
  pathophysiology of, 96
  treatment of, 98-99t, 100-101
Ventilator failure, secondary to spinal cord injury, 370
Ventolin (albuterol), for chronic obstructive pulmonary disease, 114t
VePesid (etoposide)
  for lung cancer, 511t
  side effects of, 444t
Verapamil (Calan, Isoptin)
  for brain disorders, 321t
  in hypertension, 188t
Veridia (tasosartan), for hypertension, 188t
Vertebrae
  injuries to, 365
  spinal nerves associated with, 368b
Vertigo, 54
  benign paroxysmal positional, 56-57
    Dix-Hallpike test for, 58, 58b
  differentiating characteristics of, 58t
  dizziness differentiated from, 56
  in vestibular disorders, 56
Vesicle, 68t
Vestibular disorders, 56-61
  assessment of, 58-59
  case study on, 61-62
  clinical manifestations of, 59, 59b
  complementary and alternative therapy for, 60-61
  drug therapy for, 57t, 60
  interdisciplinary care for, 59-60
  pathophysiology of, 56-57
Vestibular neuronitis, pathophysiology of, 57
Vicodin (hydrocodone with aspirin), for joint and connective tissue
    disorders, 398t
Vidarabine (Vira-A), nursing considerations for, 45t
Videx (didanosine), for HIV/AIDS, 577t
Vinblastine (Navelbine, Velban)
  for lung cancer, 511t
  side effects of, 445t
Vincristine (Oncovin)
  for sarcomas, 560t
  side effects of, 445t
Vindesine (Eldisine), side effects of, 445t
Vinorelbine (Navelbine, Velban)
  for lung cancer, 511t
  side effects of, 445t
Vioxx (rofecoxib)
  for headaches, 319t
  for joint and connective tissue disorders, 397t
Vira-A (vidarabine), nursing considerations for, 45t
Viracept (nelfinavir), for HIV/AIDS, 578t
Viramune (nevirapine), for HIV/AIDS, 577t
Viread (tenofovir), for HIV/AIDS, 577t
Viroptic (trifluridine), nursing considerations for, 45t
Virus, human immunodeficiency. *See* Human immunodeficiency
    virus (HIV).
Vision
  altered, functional health pattern assessment for, 38b
  impaired, complicating head and neck cancers, 482
  low
    definition of, 35
    strategies for daily living with, 39b
    symptoms of, 39b
Vision therapist
  in age-related macular degeneration care, 40
  in diabetic retinopathy care, 43
  in eye disorder care, 39
Visken (pindolol), for hypertension, 187t
Vistaril (hydroxyzine), 72t
Visual impairment, definition of, 35
Vitamin A deficiency, skin signs associated with, 64t

Vitamin B$_1$ deficiency, skin signs associated with, 64t
Vitamin B$_2$ deficiency, skin signs associated with, 64t
Vitamin B$_{12}$ deficiency, anemia in, 137-138
  clinical manifestations of, 139
  treatment of, 140-141
Vitamin K, foods high in, 174t
Vitamins, for cirrhosis, 248b
Vitiligo, 78
Vivelle (estrogen), for musculoskeletal disorders, 416t
Voice test, in hearing loss assessment, 51
Voiding, scheduled, for neurogenic bladder, 276
Voltaren (diclofenac)
  for headaches, 319t
  for joint and connective tissue disorders, 397t
  side effects and nursing considerations for, 45t
Vomiting, complicating cancer treatment, nursing interventions
    for, 450b
VP-16, for sarcomas, 560t
Vulva, cancer of, 542-544
Vumon (teniposide), side effects of, 445t

W

Warfarin (Coumadin)
  for atrial fibrillation, 174
  for brain disorders, 321t
Wasting syndrome, AIDS-related, 569t, 572
  nursing interventions for, 576t
Weber's test, in hearing loss assessment, 51
Weight loss
  in lung cancer, 512
  medications for, 210t
Wellbutrin (bupropion), for chronic obstructive pulmonary disease,
    115t
Wellness, in foreground of shifting perspectives model, 5
Wheal, 67t
Whisper test, in hearing loss assessment, 51
Will, Living, 452b
Withdrawal of treatment, 453b
Wounds, 83-106
  care of
    interdisciplinary, 93, 95
    products for, 91-92t
    seven steps in, with product examples, 94t
  complications of, prevention of, nursing interventions for,
    561b
  healing of, nutrients and, 86t
  lower extremity ulcers as, 95-105
  management of, functional health pattern assessment for,
    84b
  pressure ulcers as, 84-95. *See also* Pressure ulcers.
Wytensin (guanabenz), for hypertension, 186t

X

X-Trozine (phendimetrazine), for weight loss, 210t
Xanthine derivatives, for chronic obstructive pulmonary disease,
    114t
Xenical (orlistat), for weight loss, 210t
Xerostomia
  complicating cancer treatment, nursing interventions for, 450b
  complicating head and neck cancers, 478-479, 479b

Z

Zafirlukast (Accolate), for chronic obstructive pulmonary disease,
    115t
Zalcitabine (DDC, Hivid), for HIV/AIDS, 577t
Zanaflex (tizanidine), for brain disorders, 321t
Zanosar (streptozocin), side effects of, 445t
Zantac (ranitidine), for gastroesophageal reflux disease and peptic ulcer,
    217t
Zarontin (ethosuximide), for seizure disorders, 319t
Zaroxolyn (metolazone), for hypertension, 185t
Zebeta (bisoprolol), for hypertension, 186t
Zerit (stavudine), for HIV/AIDS, 577t

Zestril (lisinopril)
    for brain disorders, 321t
    for hypertension, 188t
Ziagen (abacavir), for HIV/AIDS, 577t
Zidovudine (AZT, Retrovir), for HIV/AIDS, 576,
    577t
Zileuton (Zyflo), for chronic obstructive pulmonary
    disease, 115t
Zocor (simvastin), for brain disorders, 321t
Zofran (ondansetron), for brain disorders, 322t
Zolmitriptan (Zomig), for migraines, 320t

Zoloft (sertraline)
    for brain disorders, 322t
    for musculoskeletal disorders, 417t
Zomig (zolmitriptan), for migraines, 320t
Zovirax (acyclovir), side effects and nursing considerations
    for, 73t
Zyflo (Zileuton), for chronic obstructive pulmonary disease,
    115t
Zyloprim (allopurinol), for joint and connective tissue disorders,
    398t
Zyrtec (cetirizine), nursing considerations for, 72t